Basic Health Profession Skills

Customized Updated 8th Edition

Simmers/Fanger/Asuncion

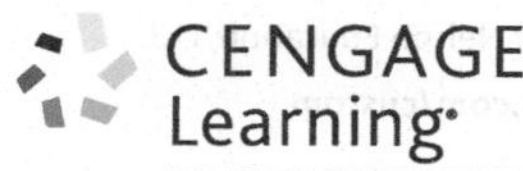

Australia • Brazil • Japan • Korea • Mexico • Singapore • Spain • United Kingdom • United States

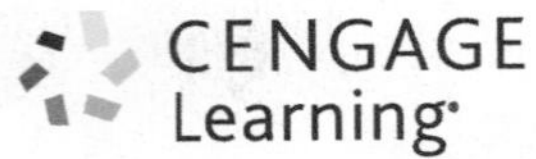

Basic Health Profession Skills: Customized Updated 8th Edition

DHO Health Science Updated, 8th Edition
Simmers/Asuncion

DHO Health Science Updated Student Workbook, 8th Edition
Simmers/Asuncion

Dimensional Analysis (OWM), 1st Edition
Fanger

For product information and technology assistance, contact us at
Cengage Learning Customer & Sales Support, 1-800-354-9706
For permission to use material from this text or product,
submit all requests online at **cengage.com/permissions**
Further permissions questions can be emailed to
permissionrequest@cengage.com

This book contains select works from existing Cengage Learning resources and was produced by Cengage Learning Custom Solutions for collegiate use. As such, those adopting and/or contributing to this work are responsible for editorial content accuracy, continuity and completeness.

ISBN: 978-1-337-31913-3

Cengage Learning
20 Channel Center Street
Boston, MA 02210
USA

Cengage Learning is a leading provider of customized learning solutions with office locations around the globe, including Singapore, the United Kingdom, Australia, Mexico, Brazil, and Japan. Locate your local office at:
www.international.cengage.com/region.

Cengage Learning products are represented in Canada by Nelson Education, Ltd.

For your lifelong learning solutions, visit **www.cengage.com/custom.**

Visit our corporate website at **www.cengage.com.**

Brief Contents

From:
DHO Health Science Updated, 8th Edition
Simmers | Asuncion

From:
Dimensional Analysis (OWM), 1st Edition
Fanger

From:
DHO Health Science Updated, 8th Edition
Simmers | Asuncion

From:
Dimensional Analysis (OWM), 1st Edition
Fanger

From:
DHO Health Science Updated, 8th Edition
Simmers | Asuncion

From:
DHO Health Science Updated Student Workbook, 8th Edition
Simmers | Asuncion

2 Health Care Systems

CHAPTER OBJECTIVES

After completing this chapter, you should be able to:

- Describe at least eight types of private health care facilities.
- Analyze at least three government health services agencies and the services offered by each.
- Describe at least three services offered by voluntary or nonprofit agencies.
- Explain the purpose of organizational structures in health care facilities.
- Compare the basic principles of at least four different health insurance plans.
- Define, pronounce, and spell all key terms.

KEY TERMS

Agency for Healthcare Research and Quality (AHRQ)
assisted living facilities
Centers for Disease Control and Prevention (CDC)
clinics
concierge medicine
dental offices
emergency care services
fee-for-service compensation
Food and Drug Administration (FDA)
genetic counseling centers
health departments
health insurance plans
Health Insurance Portability and Accountability Act (HIPAA)
health maintenance organizations (HMOs)
home health care
hospice
hospitals
independent living facilities
industrial health care centers
laboratories
long-term care facilities (LTCs or LTCFs)
managed care
Medicaid
medical offices
Medicare
Medigap policy
mental health facilities
National Institutes of Health (NIH)
nonprofit agencies
Occupational Safety and Health Administration (OSHA)
Office of the National Coordinator for Health Information Technology (ONC)
optical centers
organizational structure
Patient Protection and Affordable Care Act (PPACA)
pharmaceutical services
preferred provider organization (PPO)
rehabilitation facilities
school health services
The Joint Commission (TJC)
TRICARE
U.S. Department of Health and Human Services (USDHHS)
value-based compensation
voluntary agencies
Workers' compensation
World Health Organization (WHO)

2:1 Private Health Care Facilities

Today, health care systems include the many agencies, facilities, and personnel involved in the delivery of health care. According to U.S. government statistics, health care is one of the largest and fastest-growing industries in the United States. This industry employs more than 17 million workers in more than 200 different health care careers. It attracts people with a wide range of educational backgrounds because it offers multiple career options. By the year 2020, health care employment is expected to increase by 5.6 million jobs to more than 22.1 million workers. Health care spending in the United States is projected to increase from more than $2.9 trillion in 2013 to $4.6 trillion in 2020.

Many different health care facilities provide services that are a part of the industry called *health care* (Figure 2–1). Most private health care facilities require a fee for services. In some cases, grants and contributions provide some financial support for these facilities. A basic description of the various facilities will help provide an understanding of the many different types of services included under the umbrella of the health care industry.

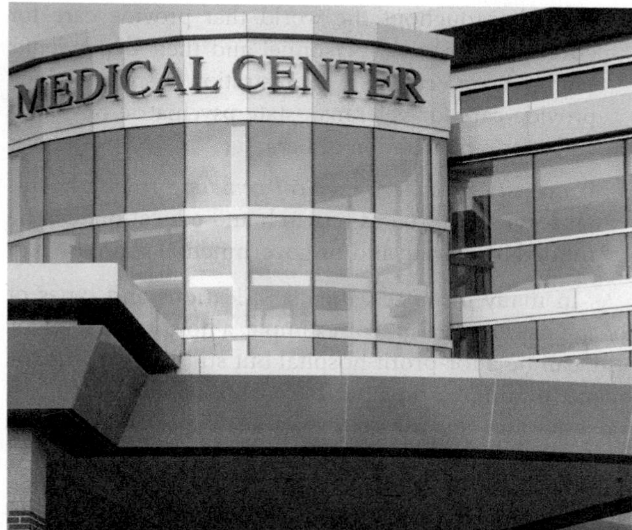

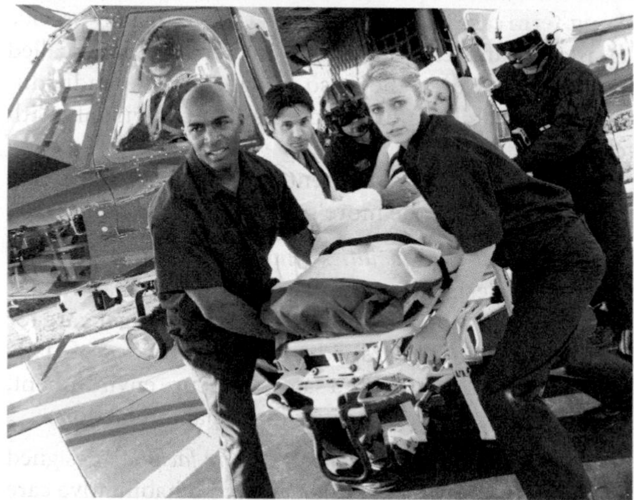

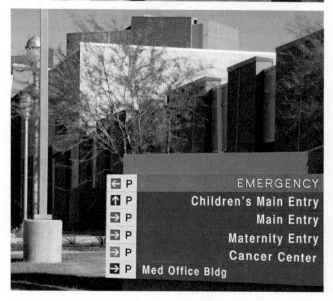

FIGURE 2–1 Different health care facilities. Top image, © iStock.com/Steve Shepard; middle Image, © iStock.com/Catherine Yeulet; and bottom image, © iStock.com/Paul Hill

Hospitals

Hospitals are one of the major types of health care facilities. They vary in size and types of services provided. Some hospitals are small and serve the basic needs of a community; others are large, complex centers offering a wide range of services including diagnosis, treatment, education, and research. Hospitals are also classified as private or proprietary (operated for profit), religious, nonprofit or voluntary, and government, depending on the sources of income received by the hospital.

There are many different types of hospitals. Some of the more common ones include:

- *General hospitals:* treat a wide range of conditions and age groups; usually provide diagnostic, medical, surgical, and emergency care services
- *Specialty hospitals:* provide care for special conditions or age groups; examples include burn hospitals, oncology (cancer) hospitals, pediatric (children's) hospitals, psychiatric hospitals (dealing with mental diseases and disorders), orthopedic hospitals (dealing with bone, joint, or muscle diseases), and rehabilitative hospitals (offering services such as physical and occupational therapy)
- *Government hospitals:* operated by federal, state, and local government agencies; include the many facilities

located throughout the world that provide care for government service personnel and their dependents; examples are Veterans Administration hospitals (which provide care for veterans), state psychiatric hospitals, and state rehabilitation centers

- *University or college medical centers:* provide hospital services as well as research and education; can be funded by private and/or governmental sources

In many instances, the classifications and types of hospitals can overlap. For example, a hospital in a major city can be a for-profit hospital but still receive government funding. A hospital can also be a general hospital but offer specialty services such as oncology and pediatrics.

Long-Term Care Facilities

Long-term care facilities (LTCs or LTCFs) mainly provide assistance and care for elderly patients, usually called *residents*. However, they also provide care for individuals with disabilities or handicaps and individuals with chronic or long-term illnesses.

There are many different types of long-term care facilities. Some of the more common ones include:

- *Residential care facilities (nursing homes or geriatric homes):* designed to provide basic physical and emotional care for individuals who can no longer care for themselves; help individuals with activities of daily living (ADLs), provide a safe and secure environment, and promote opportunities for social interactions
- *Extended care facilities or skilled care facilities:* designed to provide skilled nursing care and rehabilitative care to prepare patients* or residents for return to home environments or other long-term care facilities; some have *subacute units* designed to provide services to patients who need rehabilitation to recover from a major illness or surgery, treatment for cancer, or treatments such as kidney dialysis or heart monitoring
- **Independent living facilities** and **assisted living facilities**: allow individuals who can care for themselves to rent or purchase an apartment in the facility; provide services such as meals, housekeeping, laundry, transportation, social events, and basic medical care (such as assisting with medications)

Most assisted or independent living facilities are associated with nursing homes, extended care facilities, and/or skilled care facilities. This arrangement allows an individual to move readily from one level of care to the next when health needs change. Many long-term care facilities also offer special services such as the delivery of meals to the homes of older adults, the chronically ill, or people with disabilities. Some facilities offer senior citizen or adult day care centers, which provide social activities and other services for older people. The need for long-term care facilities has increased dramatically because of the large increase in the number of older people. Many health care career opportunities are available in these facilities, and there is a shortage of nurses and other trained personnel.

Medical Offices

Medical offices vary from offices that are privately owned by one physician to large complexes that operate as corporations and employ many physicians and other health care professionals. Medical services obtained in these facilities can include diagnosis (determining the nature of an illness), treatment, examination, basic laboratory testing, minor surgery, and other similar care. Some physicians treat a wide variety of illnesses and age groups, but others specialize in and handle only certain age groups or conditions. Examples of specialties include pediatrics (infants and children), cardiology (diseases and disorders of the heart), and obstetrics (care of pregnant women).

Concierge Medicine

Concierge medicine, or *retainer medicine*, is a type of personalized health care. In exchange for an annual or monthly fee, an enhanced level of care is provided by a primary care physician. The physician is able to care for fewer patients while having more availability. The rates and services vary among providers.

Dental Offices

Dental offices vary in size from offices that are privately owned by one or more dentists to dental clinics that employ a group of dentists. In some areas, major retail or department stores operate dental clinics. Dental services can include general care provided to all age groups or specialized care offered to certain age groups or for certain dental conditions.

Clinics or Satellite Centers

Clinics, also called *satellite clinics* or *satellite centers*, are health care facilities found in many types of health care. Some clinics are composed of a group of medical or dental doctors who share a facility and other personnel. Other clinics are operated by private groups who provide special care. Examples include:

*In some health care facilities, patients are referred to as *clients*. For the purposes of this text, *patient* will be used.

- *Surgical clinics or surgicenters:* perform minor surgical procedures; frequently called "one-day" surgical centers because patients are sent home immediately after they recover from their operations
- *Urgent, walk-in, or emergency care clinics:* provide first aid or emergency care to ill or injured patients
- *Rehabilitation clinics:* offer physical, occupational, speech, and other similar therapies
- *Substance abuse clinics:* provide rehabilitation for drug and alcohol abuse
- *Specialty clinics:* provide care for specific diseases; examples include diabetic clinics, kidney dialysis centers, and oncology (cancer) clinics
- *Outpatient clinics:* usually operated by hospitals or large medical groups; provide care for outpatients (patients who are not admitted to the hospital)
- *Health department clinics:* may offer clinics for pediatric health care, treatment of sexually transmitted diseases, treatment of respiratory disease, immunizations, and other special services
- *Medical center clinics:* usually located in colleges or universities; offer clinics for various health conditions; offer care and treatment and provide learning experiences for medical students

Optical Centers

Optical centers can be individually owned by an ophthalmologist or optometrist, or they can be part of a large chain of stores. They provide vision examinations, prescribe eyeglasses or contact lenses, and check for the presence of eye diseases.

Emergency Care Services

Emergency care services provide special care for victims of accidents or sudden illness. Facilities providing these services include ambulance services, both private and governmental; rescue squads, frequently operated by fire departments; emergency care clinics and centers; emergency departments operated by hospitals; and helicopter or airplane emergency services that rapidly transport patients to medical facilities for special care.

Laboratories

Laboratories are often a part of other facilities but can operate as separate health care services. Medical laboratories can perform special diagnostic tests such as blood or urine tests. Dental laboratories can prepare dentures (false teeth) and many other devices used to repair or replace teeth. Medical and dental offices, small hospitals, clinics, and many other health care facilities frequently use the services provided by laboratories.

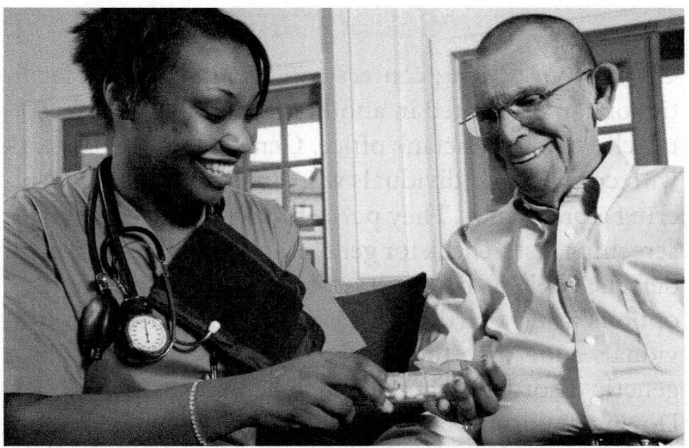

FIGURE 2–2 Many types of health care can be provided in a patient's home. © iStock.com/Steve Debenport

Home Health Care

Home health care agencies are designed to provide care in a patient's home (Figure 2–2). Older adults and people with disabilities frequently use the services of these agencies. Examples of such services include nursing care, personal care, therapy (physical, occupational, speech, respiratory), and homemaking (food preparation, cleaning, and other household tasks). Health departments, hospitals, private agencies, government agencies, and nonprofit or volunteer groups can offer home care services.

Hospice

Hospice agencies provide care for people who are terminally ill and who usually have life expectancies of 6 months or less. Care can be provided in a person's home or in a hospice facility. Hospice offers palliative care, or care that provides support and comfort and is directed toward allowing the person to die with dignity. Psychological, social, spiritual, and financial counseling are provided for both the patient and the family. Hospice also provides support to the family following a patient's death.

Mental Health Facilities

Mental health facilities treat patients who have mental disorders and diseases. Examples of these facilities include guidance and counseling centers, psychiatric clinics and hospitals, chemical abuse treatment centers (dealing with alcohol and drug abuse), and physical abuse treatment centers (dealing with child abuse, spousal abuse, and geriatric [elder] abuse).

Genetic Counseling Centers

Genetic counseling centers can be independent facilities or can be located in another facility such as a hospital, clinic, or physician's office. Genetic counselors work with couples or individuals who are pregnant or considering a pregnancy. They perform prenatal (before birth) screening tests, check for genetic abnormalities and birth defects, explain the results of the tests, identify medical options when a birth defect is present, and help the individuals cope with the psychological issues caused by a genetic disorder. Examples of genetic disorders include Down's syndrome and cystic fibrosis. Counselors frequently consult with couples before a pregnancy if the woman is in her late childbearing years, has a family history of genetic disease, or is of a specific race or nationality with a high risk for genetic disease.

Rehabilitation Facilities

Rehabilitation facilities are located in hospitals, clinics, and/or private centers. They provide care to help patients who have physical or mental disabilities obtain the maximum self-care and function. Services may include physical, occupational, recreational, speech, and hearing therapy.

Health Maintenance Organizations

Health maintenance organizations (HMOs) are both health care delivery systems and a type of health insurance. They provide total health care services that are primarily directed toward preventive health care for a fee that is usually fixed and prepaid. Services include examinations, basic medical services, health education, and hospitalization or rehabilitation services as needed. Some HMOs are operated by large industries or corporations; others are operated by private agencies. They often use the services of other health care facilities including medical and dental offices, hospitals, rehabilitative centers, home health care agencies, clinics, and laboratories.

Industrial Health Care Centers

Industrial health care centers or *occupational health clinics* are found in large companies or industries. Such centers provide health care for employees of the industry or business by performing basic examinations, teaching accident prevention and safety, and providing emergency care. Major resort industries, such as Disney, may also provide emergency health care to visitors.

School Health Services

School health services are found in schools and colleges. These services provide emergency care for victims of accidents and sudden illness; perform tests to check for health conditions such as speech, vision, and hearing problems; promote health education; and maintain a safe and sanitary school environment. Many school health services also provide counseling.

Pharmaceutical Services

Pharmaceutical services, also called pharmacies, chemists, or drug stores, link health science with chemical science. A pharmacist prepares and dispenses medications and provides expertise on drug therapy. They also ensure patient safety through education. Pharmaceutical services can be found in many settings, including hospitals, community stores, clinics, nursing homes, and even online. In addition to prescription drugs, many pharmaceutical services also offer over-the-counter drugs (for conditions such as pain, colds, and allergies), vitamins, and herbal remedies.

2:2 Government Agencies

In addition to the government health care facilities mentioned previously, other health services are offered at the international, national, state, and local levels. Government services are tax supported. Examples of government agencies include:

- **World Health Organization** (WHO): an international agency sponsored by the United Nations; compiles statistics and information on disease, publishes health information, and investigates and addresses serious health problems throughout the world; the main objective of the WHO, per its constitution, "is the attainment by all people of the highest possible level of health care"; Internet address: *www.who.int*
- **U.S. Department of Health and Human Services** (USDHHS): a national agency that deals with the health problems in the United States; its goal is to protect the health of all Americans, especially those people who are in need; provides more grant money than any other federal agency; Internet address: *www.hhs.gov*
- **National Institutes of Health** (NIH): a division of the USDHHS; involved in researching disease and conducting scientific studies; Internet address: *www.nih.gov*
- **Centers for Disease Control and Prevention** (CDC): another division of the USDHHS; concerned with the causes, spread, and control of diseases in populations (Figure 2–3); Internet address: *www.cdc.gov*

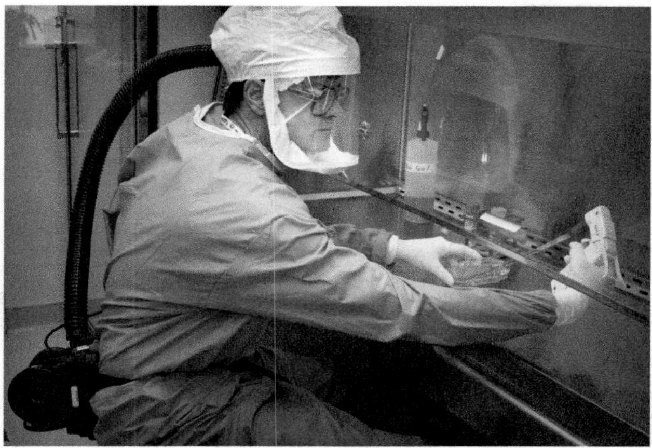

FIGURE 2–3 The Centers for Disease Control and Prevention (CDC) deals with the causes, spread, and control of diseases in populations. CDC/James Gathany

- **Food and Drug Administration (FDA)**: a federal agency responsible for regulating food and drug products sold to the public; also protects the public by regulating things such as medical devices, cosmetics, and cell phones; Internet address: *www.fda.gov*
- **Agency for Healthcare Research and Quality (AHRQ)**: a federal agency established to improve the quality, safety, efficiency, and effectiveness of health care for Americans; Internet address: *www.ahrq.gov*
- **Occupational Safety and Health Administration (OSHA)**: establishes and enforces standards that protect workers from job-related injuries and illnesses; issues standards on things such as limits on chemical and radiation exposure and use of personal protective equipment; Internet address: *www.osha.gov*
- **Office of the National Coordinator for Health Information Technology (ONC)**: leads national efforts to build a private and secure nationwide health information exchange; its goal is to improve health care by allowing health information to be exchanged quickly among providers. Internet address: *www.healthit.gov*
- **Health departments**: provide health services as directed by the U.S. Department of Health and Human Services (USDHHS); also provide specific services needed by the state or local community; examples of services include immunization for disease control, inspections for environmental health and sanitation, communicable disease control, collection of statistics and records related to health, health education, clinics for health care and prevention, and other services needed in a community; Internet address: *www.hhs.gov*; use the search box to locate the web address of a specific state or local health department

2:3 Voluntary or Nonprofit Agencies

Voluntary agencies, frequently called **nonprofit agencies**, are supported by donations, membership fees, fundraisers, and federal or state grants. They provide health services at the national, state, and local levels.

The Joint Commission is a nonprofit, U.S.-based organization that was created to ensure that patients receive the safest, highest quality care in any health care setting. Meeting the standards of the Joint Commission is recognized as a symbol of quality. In many states, a Joint Commission accreditation is required to receive Medicaid reimbursement. Its Internet address is *www.jointcommission.org*.

Other examples of nonprofit agencies include the American Cancer Society, American Heart Association, American Respiratory Disease Association, American Diabetes Association, National Mental Health Association, Alzheimer's Association, National Kidney Foundation, Leukemia and Lymphoma Society, March of Dimes Foundation, American Red Cross, and Autism Speaks. Many of these organizations have national offices as well as branch offices in states and/or local communities.

As indicated by their names, many such organizations focus on one specific disease or group of diseases. Each organization typically studies the disease, provides funding to encourage research directed at curing or treating the disease, and promotes public education regarding the information obtained through research. These organizations also provide special services to victims of disease, such as purchasing medical equipment and supplies, providing treatment centers, and supplying information regarding other community agencies that offer assistance.

Nonprofit agencies employ many health care workers in addition to using volunteers to provide services.

2:4 Organizational Structure

All health care facilities must have some type of **organizational structure**. The structure may be complex, as in larger facilities, or simple, as in smaller facilities. Organizational structure always, however, encompasses a line of authority or chain of command. The organizational structure should indicate areas of responsibility and lead to the most efficient operation of the facility.

A sample organizational chart for a large general hospital is shown in Figure 2–4. This chart shows organization by department. Each department, in turn, can have an organizational chart similar to the one shown for the

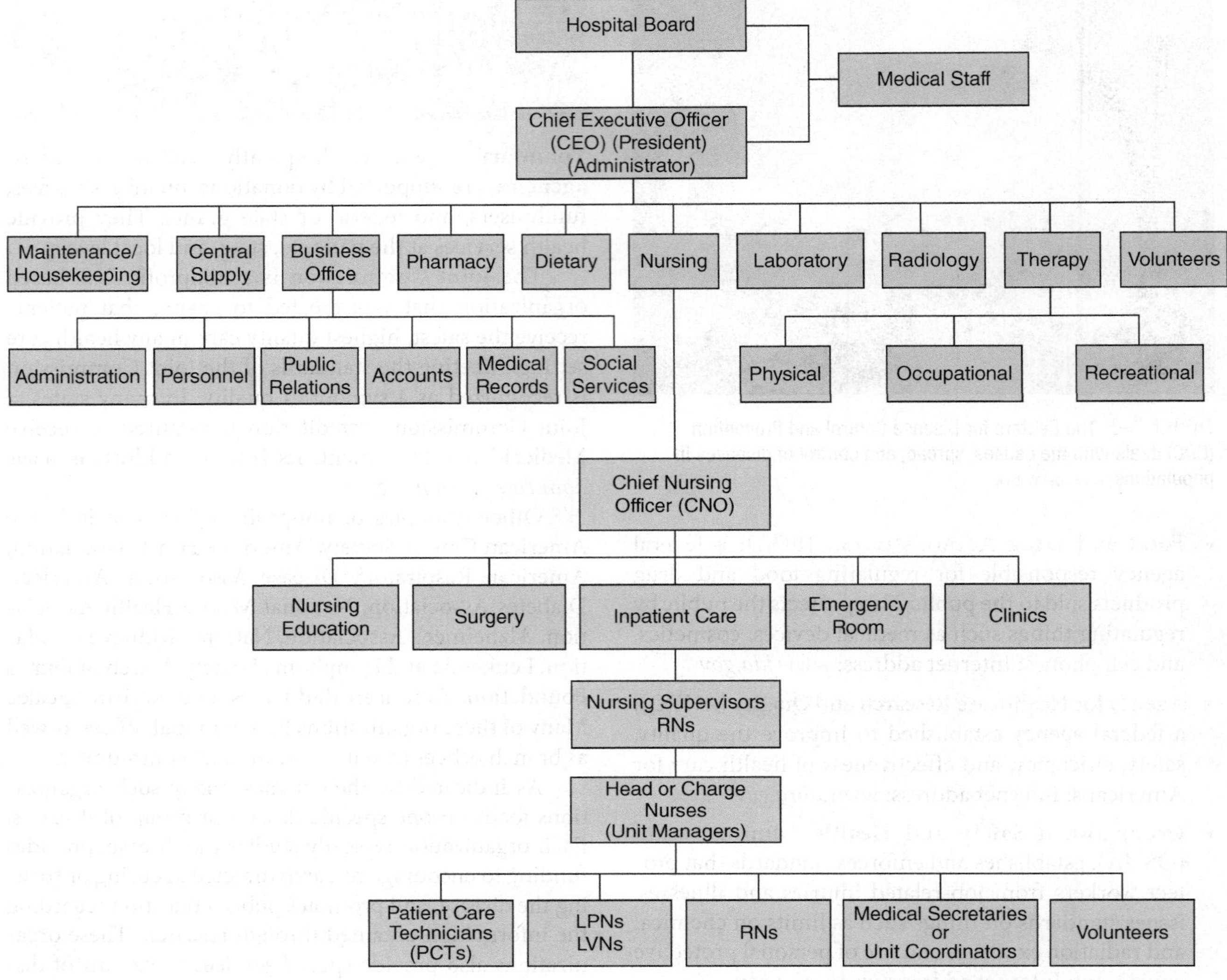

FIGURE 2–4 **A sample hospital organizational chart.**

nursing department in Figure 2–4. A sample organizational chart for a small medical office is shown in Figure 2–5. The organizational structure will vary with the size of the office and the number of people employed.

In both organizational charts illustrated, the lines of authority are clearly indicated. It is important for health care workers to identify and understand their respective positions in a given facility's organizational structure so they will know their lines of authority and understand who the immediate supervisors in charge of their work are. Health care workers must always take questions, reports, and problems to their immediate supervisors, who are responsible for providing the necessary assistance. If immediate supervisors cannot answer the question or solve the problem, it is their responsibility to take the situation to the next level in the organizational chart. It is also important for health care workers to understand the functions and goals of the organization.

2:5 Health Insurance Plans

The cost of health care is a major concern of everyone who needs health services. Statistics show that the cost of health care is more than 17 percent of the gross national product (the total amount of money the country's population spent on all goods and services). Also, health care costs are increasing much faster than other costs of living. To pay for the costs of health care, most people rely on **health insurance plans**. Without insurance, the cost of an illness can mean financial disaster for an individual or family.

Health insurance plans are offered by several thousand insurance agencies. A common example is Blue Cross/Blue Shield (Figure 2–6). In this type of plan, a *premium*, or a fee the individual pays for insurance coverage, is paid to the insurance company. When the

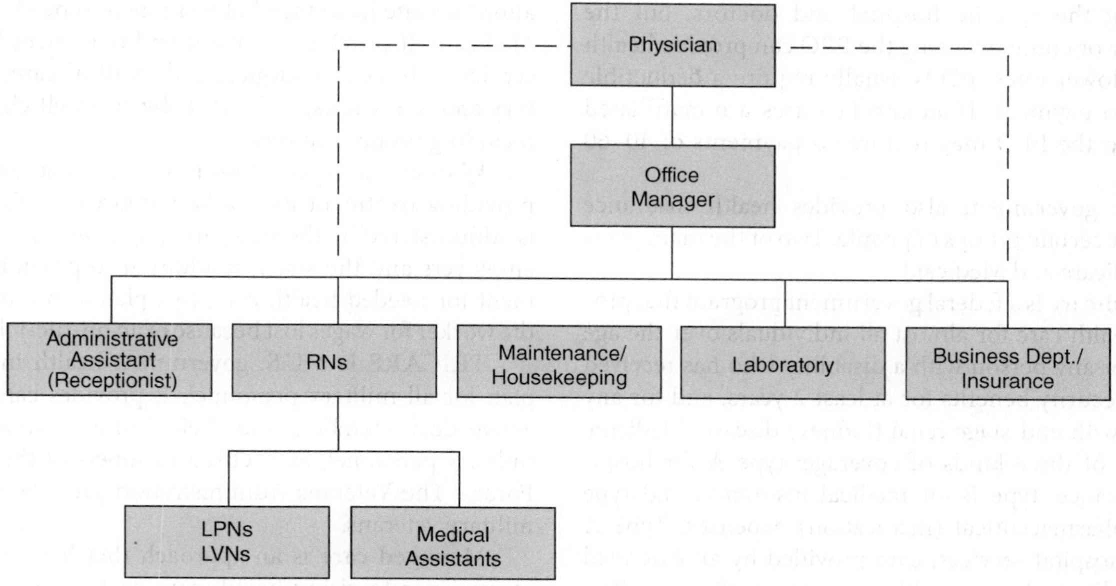

FIGURE 2–5 A sample medical office organizational chart.

insured individual incurs health care expenses covered by the insurance plan, the insurance company pays for the services. The amount of the premium payment and the type of services covered vary from plan to plan. Common insurance terms include:

- *Deductibles:* amounts that must be paid by the patient for medical services before the policy begins to pay
- *Co-insurance:* requires that specific percentages of expenses are shared by the patient and insurance company; for example, in an 80–20 percent co-insurance plan, the company pays 80 percent of covered expenses, and the patient pays the remaining 20 percent
- *Co-payment:* a specific amount of money a patient pays for a particular service, for example, $20 for each physician visit regardless of the total cost of the visit

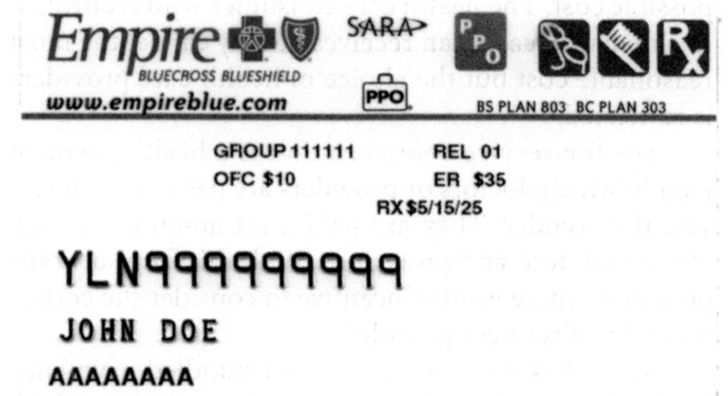

FIGURE 2–6 Health insurance plans help pay for the costs of health care. Courtesy of Empire Blue Cross and Blue Shield

Many individuals have insurance coverage through their places of employment (called employer-sponsored health insurance or group insurance), where the premiums are paid by the employer. In most cases, the individual also pays a percentage of the premium. Private policies are also available for purchase by individuals.

A health maintenance organization (HMO) is another type of health insurance plan that provides a managed care plan for the delivery of health care services. A monthly fee or premium is paid for membership, and the fee stays the same regardless of the amount of health care used. The premium can be paid by an employer and/or an individual. The care provided is directed toward preventive-type health care. Therefore, an individual insured under this type of plan has ready access to health examinations and early treatment and detection of disease. Because most other types of insurance plans do not cover routine examinations and preventive care, an individual insured by an HMO can therefore theoretically maintain a better state of health. The disadvantage of an HMO is that the insured is required to use only HMO-affiliated health care providers (doctors, laboratories, hospitals) for health care. If a nonaffiliated health care provider is used instead, the insured usually must pay for the care.

A **preferred provider organization (PPO)** is another type of managed care health insurance plan usually provided by large industries or companies to their employees. The PPO forms a contract with certain health care agencies, such as a large hospital and specific doctors and dentists, to provide certain types of health care at reduced rates. Employees are restricted to using the specific hospital and doctors, but the industry or company using the PPO can provide health care at lower rates. PPOs usually require a deductible and a co-payment. If an enrollee uses a nonaffiliated provider, the PPO may require co-payments of 40–60 percent.

The government also provides health insurance plans for certain groups of people. Two of the main plans are Medicare and Medicaid.

Medicare is a federal government program that provides health care for almost all individuals over the age of 65, for any person with a disability who has received Social Security benefits for at least 2 years, and for any person with end-stage renal (kidney) disease. Medicare consists of three kinds of coverage: type A for hospital insurance, type B for medical insurance, and type D for pharmaceutical (medication) expenses. Type A covers hospital services, care provided by an extended care facility or home health care agency after hospitalization, and hospice care for people who have terminal illnesses. Type B offers additional coverage for doctors' services, outpatient treatments, therapy, clinical laboratory services, and other health care. The individual does pay a premium for type B coverage and also must pay an initial deductible for services. In addition, Medicare pays for only 80 percent of these medical services; the individual must either pay the balance or have another insurance policy to cover the expenses.

A **Medigap policy** is a health insurance plan that helps pay medical expenses not covered by Medicare. These policies are offered by private insurance companies and require the enrollee to pay a premium. Medigap policies must meet specific federal guidelines. They provide options that allow enrollees to choose how much coverage they want to purchase.

Medicaid is a medical assistance program that is jointly funded by the federal government and state governments but operated by individual states. Benefits and individuals covered under this program vary slightly from state to state because each state has the right to establish its own eligibility standards, determine the type and scope of services, set the rate of payment for services, and administer its own program. In most states, Medicaid pays for the health care of individuals with low incomes, children who qualify for public assistance, and individuals who are physically disabled or blind. Generally, all state Medicaid programs provide hospital services, physician's care, long-term care services, and some therapies. In some states, Medicaid offers dental care, eye care, and other specialized services.

The Children's Health Insurance Program (CHIP) was established in 1997 to provide health care to uninsured children of working families who earn too little to afford private insurance but too much to be eligible for Medicaid. It provides inpatient and outpatient hospital services, physician's surgical and medical care, laboratory and X-ray tests, and well-baby and well-child care, including immunizations.

Workers' compensation is a health insurance plan providing treatment for workers injured on the job. It is administered by the state, and payments are made by employers and the state. In addition to providing payment for needed health care, this plan also reimburses the worker for wages lost because of an on-the-job injury.

TRICARE is a U.S. government health insurance plan for all military personnel. It provides care for all active duty members and their families, survivors of military personnel, and retired members of the Armed Forces. The Veterans Administration provides care for military veterans.

Managed care is an approach that has developed in response to rising health care costs. Employers, as well as insurance companies who pay large medical bills, want to ensure that such money is spent efficiently rather than wastefully. The principle behind managed care is that all health care provided to a patient must have a purpose. A second opinion or verification of need is frequently required before care can be provided. Every effort is made to provide preventive care and early diagnosis of disease to avoid the high cost of treating disease. For example, routine physical examinations, well-baby care, immunizations, and wellness education to promote good nutrition, exercise, weight control, and healthy living practices are usually provided under managed care. Employers and insurance companies create a network of doctors, specialists, therapists, and health care facilities that provide care at the most reasonable cost. HMOs and PPOs are the main providers of managed care, but many private insurance companies are establishing health care networks to provide care to their subscribers. As these health care networks compete for the consumer dollar, they are required to provide quality care at the lowest possible cost. The health care consumer who is enrolled in a managed care plan receives quality care at the most reasonable cost but the choice of health care providers is restricted.

Fee-for-service compensation is a health payment plan in which doctors or providers are paid for each service they render. They are paid a set amount for each office visit, test, and procedure. With this form of compensation, there is little incentive to consider the cost or necessity of services provided.

Value-based compensation, or bundled payments, is a health payment plan in which doctors are paid for their performance. This form of compensation takes into account quality, cost, patient satisfaction, and patient outcomes. Doctors and providers are paid a certain amount for each diagnosis or disease. This type of plan has been met with resistance because the uniqueness of each patient and each disease complicates the idea of placing a measurable value on each case.

Health insurance plans do not solve all the problems of health care costs, but they do help many people by paying for all or part of the cost of health services. However, as the cost of insurance increases, many employers are less willing to offer health care insurance. Individuals with chronic illnesses often find they cannot obtain insurance coverage if their place of employment changes. This is one reason the federal government passed the **Health Insurance Portability and Accountability Act (HIPAA)** in 1996. This act has five main components:

- *Health Care Access, Portability, and Renewability:* limits exclusions on preexisting conditions to allow for the continuance of insurance even with job changes, prohibits discrimination against an enrollee or beneficiary based on health status, guarantees renewability in multiemployer plans, and provides special enrollment rights for individuals who lose insurance coverage in certain situations such as divorce or termination of employment
- *Preventing Health Care Fraud and Abuse; Administrative Simplification and Medical Liability Reform:* establishes methods for preventing fraud and abuse and imposes sanctions or penalties if fraud or abuse does occur, reduces the costs and administration of health care by adopting a single set of electronic standards to replace the wide variety of formats used in health care, provides strict guidelines for maintaining the confidentiality of health care information and the security of health care records, and recommends limits for medical liability. The confidentiality requirement is discussed in more detail in Section 5:1 under Privacy Act.
- *Tax-Related Health Provisions:* promotes the use of medical savings accounts (MSAs) by allowing tax deductions for monies placed in the accounts, establishes standards for long-term care insurance, allows for the creation of state insurance pools, and provides tax benefits for some health care expenses
- *Application and Enforcement of Group Health Plan Requirements:* establishes standards that require group health care plans to offer portability, access, and renewability to all members of the group
- *Revenue Offsets:* provides changes to the Internal Revenue Code for HIPAA expenses

Compliance with all HIPAA regulations was required by April 2004 for all health care agencies. These regulations have not solved all of the problems of health care insurance, but they have provided consumers with more access to insurance and greater confidentiality in regard to medical records. In addition, standardization of electronic health care records, reductions in administrative costs, increased tax benefits, and decreased fraud and abuse in health care have reduced health care costs for everyone.

Major changes to health care insurance have been provided by the **Patient Protection and Affordable Care Act (PPACA)**, also called the *Affordable Care Act (ACA)*. This act was signed into law in March 2010, and by 2014 most of the provisions of the act were in place. The primary provisions of this law are:

- Guaranteed issue that requires all insurers to charge the same premium to all applicants of the same gender, age, and geographic location, regardless of preexisting conditions
- Prohibits insurance companies from rescinding coverage to any individual as long as premiums are paid
- Expands Medicaid eligibility to include families and individuals with incomes up to 133 percent of the poverty level unless a particular state opts out of this requirement
- Creates affordable insurance exchanges in every state that provide a more organized and competitive market for insurance, offers a choice of plans to individuals or small businesses, and establishes common rules regarding the offering and pricing of insurance
- Mandates that all individuals secure minimum health insurance and imposes a fine on those who do not obtain insurance under the shared responsibility rules; special exemptions do exist such as financial hardship, religious beliefs, individuals who are American Indians, individuals for whom the lowest cost health care plan exceeds 8 percent of income, and individuals who have income below the lowest tax filing threshold
- Provides subsidies for low-income families, individuals, or very small businesses, on a sliding income scale of between 100 percent and 400 percent of the poverty level, to purchase insurance through a health insurance exchange
- Allows a young adult to be covered under a parent's policy up to age 26
- Provides increased enrollment for Medicaid and CHIP
- Enforces a "shared responsibility payment" or fine per full-time employee that must be made by any firm that employs more than 50 people and does not offer health insurance

- Improves benefits for Medicare and prescription drug coverage
- Allows a restructuring of Medicare reimbursement from fee-for-service to bundled payments; for example, a specific amount is paid to a group of physicians for treating a patient with a specific diagnosis instead of individual payments for each treatment provided
- Gives a small business tax credit to qualified small businesses and nonprofit organizations that provide health insurance for employees
- Establishes a national voluntary insurance program that allows individuals to purchase community living assistance services and support for long-term care

TODAY'S RESEARCH TOMORROW'S HEALTH CARE

Nature as a Pharmacy?

Throughout history, many medicines have been derived from natural resources. Examples include aspirin, which comes from willow bark; penicillin, which comes from fungus; and the cancer drug Taxol, which comes from the Pacific yew tree. Recognizing this, many scientists believe that nature is a pharmaceutical gold mine and are exploring the vast supply of materials present in the oceans and on the earth.

The National Cancer Institute (NCI) has more than 50,000 samples of plants and 10,000 samples of marine organisms stored in Frederick, Maryland. Every sample is crushed into a powder and made into extracts that can be tested against human cancer cells. Over 110,000 extracts of these samples are available to other scientists who evaluate their effectiveness against conditions such as viral diseases and infections. To date, more than 4,000 extracts have shown promise and are being used in more advanced studies. One compound, Halichondrin B, labeled "yellow slimy" by researchers, is an extract taken from a deep-sea sponge found in New Zealand. Scientists created a synthetic version of the active component in Halichondrin B, called E7389. After extensive testing, the drug Eribulin, which was created from this compound, was approved by the FDA in 2010 as a treatment for metastatic breast cancer. Bristol-Myers received FDA approval for another drug, Ixabepilone, that is extracted from garden soil bacteria and is also used to treat metastatic breast cancer. Wyeth's drug Rapamune was isolated from soil on Easter Island and approved for preventing kidney rejection after transplants. Another novel drug involves photodynamic activity. A substance called psoralen is obtained from a Nile-dwelling weed called ammi. Psoralen is inactive until it is exposed to light. When it is activated, it attaches to the DNA of cancer cells and kills them. Research led to the approval of a psoralen-like drug that is exposed to certain wavelengths of light and used to treat some forms of lymphoma, a cancer of white blood cells. By creating synthetic versions of the compounds, scientists are preserving natural resources while also benefiting from them.

Other natural products are now being tested and modified. Clinical trials are being conducted on ecteinascidin, which is a substance obtained from a sea creature called a tunicate (a marine organism that spends most of its life attached to docks or rocks). Lab tests show it is safe for humans and that it may be an effective treatment for soft-tissue sarcomas (tumors of the muscles, tendons, and supportive tissues).

Other unique studies involve cone snails found in the reefs surrounding Australia, Indonesia, and the Philippines. These animals produce a unique venom containing nerve toxins. Some of these venoms are being studied as pain relievers because they block pain signals from reaching the brain. Researchers in Oslo, Norway, are studying and testing plant extracts from the sweet wormwood plant and the bark of the cinchona tree to determine if an effective drug can be created to destroy both the malaria parasite and the mosquitoes that carry the parasite. An intriguing bioluminescent bacterium named *Vibrio fischeri* has researchers trying to develop antibiotics that prevent bacterial resistance. This special bacterium emits light when it senses that there are enough bacteria to draw prey that can be used as sources of nourishment, a phenomenon called "quorum sensing," similar to the "safety in numbers" concept. When there are enough of these bacteria, they signal each other and produce an enzyme that creates light. Disease-producing bacteria also use quorum sensing, and when a quorum is reached, they form slimy, sticky biofilms and produce toxins that make people sick. If researchers can develop a class of antibiotics that disrupt the signals bacteria use to sense a quorum or destroy the biofilms that are formed, they can destroy the action of the bacteria and render them harmless. Because the drugs do not kill the bacteria, the bacteria would be less likely to develop resistance. As scientists continue to explore all that nature has to offer, it is possible they will find cures for many cancers, diseases, and infections.

- Establishes a Prevention and Public Health Fund to create programs that promote good health and prevent disease
- Provides additional support for medical research and the National Institutes of Health
- Requires minimum health insurance standards and removes annual and lifetime coverage caps
- Eliminates co-payments for insurance benefits that have been mandated as essential coverage benefits such as those for specified preventive care services
- Requires insurance companies to spend at least 80 percent to 85 percent of premiums collected on medical costs or to refund excess money to the insured individuals
- Mandates that insurance companies provide coverage for individuals participating in clinical trials

STUDENT: **Go to the workbook and complete the assignment sheet for Chapter 2, Health Care Systems.**

CHAPTER 2 SUMMARY

Health care, one of the largest and fastest growing industries in the United States, encompasses many different types of facilities that provide health-related services. These include hospitals, long-term care facilities, medical and dental offices, clinics, laboratories, industrial and school health services, and many others. Government and nonprofit or voluntary agencies also provide health care services. All health care facilities require different health care workers at all levels of training.

Organizational structure is important in all health care facilities. The structure can be complex or simple, but it should show a line of authority or chain of command within the facility and indicate areas of responsibility.

Many types of health insurance plans are available to help pay the costs of health care. Insurance does not usually cover the entire cost of care, however. It is important for consumers to be aware of the types of coverage provided by their respective insurance plans.

INTERNET SEARCHES

Use the search engines suggested in Chapter 12:9 in this text to search the Internet for additional information about the following topics:

1. **Private health care facilities:** Search for information on each of the specific types of facilities; for example, hospitals, hospice care, or emergency care services.
2. **Government agencies:** Search for more detailed information about the activities of the World Health Organization, U.S. Department of Health and Human Services, National Institutes of Health, Centers for Disease Control and Prevention, Food and Drug Administration, Agency for Healthcare Research and Quality, Occupational Safety and Health Administration, and Office of the National Coordinator for Health Information Technology.
3. **Voluntary or nonprofit agencies:** Search for information about the purposes and activities of organizations such as the Joint Commission, American Cancer Society, American Heart Association, American Respiratory Disease Association, American Diabetes Association, National Mental Health Association, March of Dimes Foundation, and the American Red Cross.
4. **Health insurance:** Search the Internet to find specific names of companies that are health maintenance organizations or preferred provider organizations. Check to see how their coverage for individuals is the same or how it is different.
5. **Government health care insurance:** Search the Internet to learn about benefits provided under Medicare, Medicaid, and the Children's Health Insurance Program.
6. **Patient Protection and Affordable Care Act (PPACA):** Search for information about how this act helps individuals obtain insurance. Evaluate what benefits consumers receive from this act and how it has changed health insurance for individuals in the United States.

REVIEW QUESTIONS

1. Differentiate between private or proprietary, religious, nonprofit or voluntary, and government types of hospital.
2. Identify at least six (6) different types of private health care facilities by stating the functions of the facility. Provide specific examples of the care received at each facility.
3. Name each of the following government agencies and briefly describe its function:
   a. CDC
   b. FDA
   c. NIH
   d. OSHA
   e. USDHHS
   f. WHO
   g. ONC
4. Why is it important for every health care worker to know the organizational structure for his/her place of employment?
5. Create an organizational chart for a health care facility.
6. What does the term *deductible* mean in regard to health insurance policies? *Co-insurance? Co-payment? Premium?*
7. An insurance policy has a co-payment of 70–30 percent. If an emergency department bill is $660.00, what amount will the patient have to pay?
8. Review the five (5) components of HIPAA. Create three (3) examples of how a health care facility or a health care worker could be in violation of HIPAA regulations.
9. Does the Patient Protection and Affordable Care Act provide health care insurance to every individual living in the United States? Why or why not?

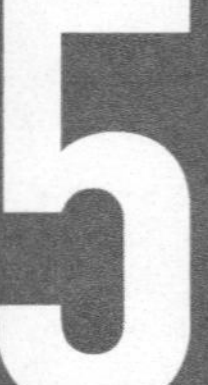

5 Legal and Ethical Responsibilities

CHAPTER OBJECTIVES

After completing this chapter, you should be able to:

- Provide one example of a situation that might result in legal action for each of the following: malpractice; negligence; assault and battery; invasion of privacy; false imprisonment; abuse; and defamation.
- Describe how contract laws affect health care.
- Define *privileged communications* and explain how they apply to health care.
- State the legal regulations that apply to health care records.
- Define HIPAA and explain how it provides confidentiality for health care information.
- List at least six basic rules of ethics for health care personnel.
- List at least six rights of the patient who is receiving health care.
- Justify at least eight professional standards by explaining how they help meet legal/ethical requirements.
- Define, pronounce, and spell all key terms.

KEY TERMS

abuse
advance directives
agent
assault and battery
civil law
confidentiality *(con"-fih-den-chee"-ahl'-ih-tee)*
Consumer Bill of Rights and Responsibilities
contract
criminal law
defamation *(deff'-ah-may'-shun)*
Designation of Health Care Surrogate
Durable Power of Attorney (POA)
ethics *(eth'-iks)*
expressed contracts
false imprisonment
health care records
Health Insurance Portability and Accountability Act (HIPAA)
implied contracts
informed consent
invasion of privacy
legal
legal disability
libel *(ly'-bull)*
living wills
malpractice
negligence *(neg'-lih-gents)*
Omnibus Budget Reconciliation Act (OBRA) of 1987
Patient Protection and Affordable Care Act (PPACA)
Patient Self-Determination Act (PSDA)
patients' rights
privileged communications
Resident's Bill of Rights
scope of practice
slander
tort

5:1 Legal Responsibilities

Introduction

In every aspect of life, there are certain laws and legal responsibilities formulated to protect you and society. An excellent example is the need to obey traffic laws when driving a motor vehicle. A worker in any health care career also has certain responsibilities. Being aware of and following legal regulations is important for your own protection, the protection of your employer, and the safety and well-being of the patient.

Legal responsibilities are those that are authorized or based on law. A law is a rule that must be followed. Laws are created and enforced by the federal, state, or local governments. Health care workers must follow any laws that affect health care. In addition, *health care professionals/workers are also required to know and follow the state laws that regulate their respective licenses or registrations or set standards for their respective professions.* Failure to meet your legal responsibilities can result in legal action against you and your employer.

Two main types of laws affect health care workers: criminal laws and civil laws.

- **Criminal law**: focuses on behavior known as crime; deals with the wrongs against a person, property, or society; examples include practicing in a health profession without having the required license, illegal possession of drugs, misuse of narcotics, theft, sexual assault, and murder
- **Civil law**: focuses on the legal relationships between people and the protection of a person's rights; in health care, civil law usually involves torts and contracts

Torts

A **tort** is a wrongful act that does not involve a contract. It is called a civil wrong instead of a crime. A tort occurs when a person is harmed or injured because a health care provider does not meet the established or expected standards of care. Many different types of torts can lead to legal action. These offenses may be quite complex and may be open to different legal interpretations. Some of the more common torts include the following:

- **Malpractice**: Malpractice can be interpreted as "bad practice" and is commonly called "professional negligence." It can be defined as the failure of a professional to use the degree of skill and learning commonly expected in that individual's profession, resulting in injury, loss, or damage to the person receiving care. Examples might include a physician not administering a tetanus injection when a patient has a puncture wound, or a nurse performing minor surgery without having any training.
- **Negligence**: Negligence can be described as failure to give care that is normally expected of a person in a particular position, resulting in injury to another person (Figure 5–1). Examples include falls and injuries that occur when siderails are left down, using or not reporting defective equipment, infections caused by the use of nonsterile instruments and/or supplies, and burns caused by improper heat or radiation treatments.
- **Assault and battery**: Assault includes a threat or attempt to injure, and battery includes the unlawful touching of another person without consent. They are closely related and often used together. Examples of assault and battery include performing a procedure after a patient has refused to give permission, threatening a patient, and improper handling or rough treatment of a patient while providing care.

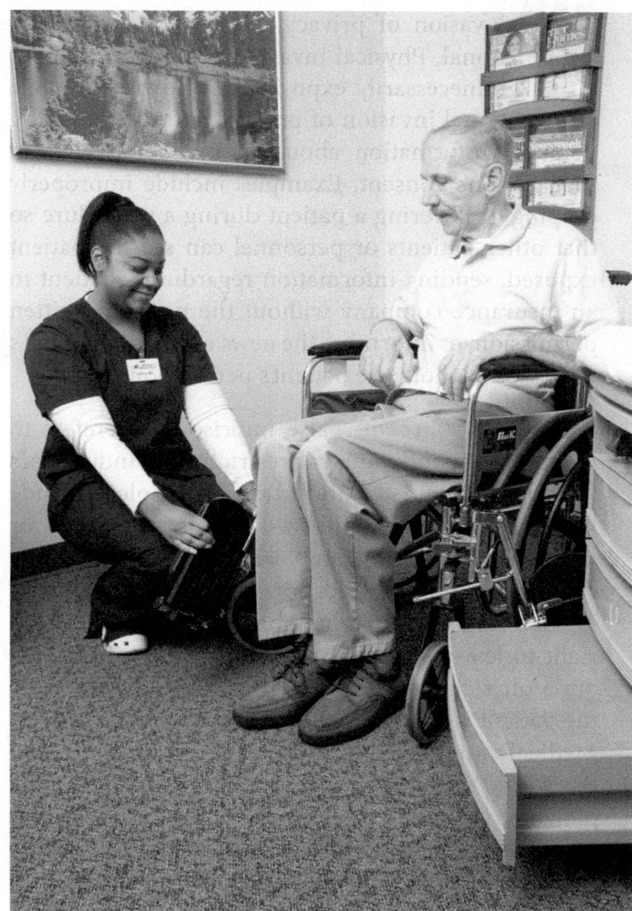

FIGURE 5–1 A medical assistant could be charged with negligence if a patient is injured because the foot rests on a wheelchair are not moved up and out of the way before the patient is transferred out of the chair.

It is important to remember that patients must give consent for any care and that they have the right to refuse care. Some procedures or practices require written consent from the patient. Examples include surgery, certain diagnostic tests, experimental procedures, treatment of minors (individuals younger than legal age, which varies from state to state) without parental consent, and even simple things such as siderail releases for a patient who wants siderails left down when other factors indicate that the siderails should be up to protect the patient. Verbal consent is permitted in other cases, but the law states that this must be "informed consent." **Informed consent** is permission granted voluntarily by a person who is of sound mind and who has been instructed, in terms the person can understand, about all the risks involved. It is important to remember that a person has the right to withdraw consent at any time. Therefore, all procedures must be explained to the patient, and no procedure should be performed if the patient does not give consent.

- HIPAA **Invasion of privacy**: There are two kinds of invasion of privacy, physical and informational. Physical invasion of privacy includes unnecessarily exposing an individual, while informational invasion of privacy refers to revealing personal information about an individual without that person's consent. Examples include improperly draping or covering a patient during a procedure so that other patients or personnel can see the patient exposed, sending information regarding a patient to an insurance company without the patient's written permission, or informing the news media of a patient's condition without the patient's permission.
- **False imprisonment**: False imprisonment refers to restraining an individual or restricting an individual's freedom without authorization. Examples include keeping patients hospitalized against their will or applying physical restraints without proper authorization or with no justification.

  It is important to remember that patients have the right to leave a hospital or health care facility without a physician's permission. If this situation occurs, the patient is usually asked to sign an AMA (Against Medical Advice) form. If the patient refuses to sign the form, this refusal must be documented in the patient's record and the physician must be notified.

  Physical restraints, devices used to limit a patient's movements, are discussed in detail in Chapter 22:12. They should be used *only* to protect patients from harming themselves or others and when all other measures to control the situation have failed. A physician's order must be obtained before they are used, and strict guidelines must be observed while they are in use.
- **Abuse**: Abuse includes any care that results in physical harm, pain, or mental anguish. Examples of types of abuse include:
  - *Physical abuse:* hitting, forcing people against their will, restraining movement, depriving people of food or water, and not providing physical care
  - *Verbal abuse:* speaking harshly, swearing or shouting, using inappropriate words to describe a person's race or nationality, and writing threats or abusive statements
  - *Psychological abuse:* threatening harm; denying rights; belittling, intimidating, or ridiculing the person; and threatening to reveal information about the person
  - *Sexual abuse:* any sexual touching or act, using sexual gestures, and suggesting sexual behavior, even if the patient is willing or tries to initiate it

  Patients may experience abuse before entering a health care facility. *Domestic abuse* occurs when an intimate partner uses threats, manipulation, aggression, or violent behavior to maintain power and control over another person. If abuse is directed toward a child, it is *child abuse*. If it is directed toward an older person, it is *elder abuse*. Health care providers must be alert to the signs and symptoms that may indicate patients in their care are victims of abuse. These may include:
  - unexplained bruises, fractures, burns, or injuries
  - signs of neglect such as poor personal hygiene
  - irrational fears or a change in personality
  - aggressive or withdrawn behavior
  - patient statements that indicate abuse or neglect

  Many of the other torts can lead to charges of abuse, or a charge of abuse can occur alone. Laws in all states require that any form of abuse be reported to the proper authorities. Even though the signs and symptoms do not always mean a person is being abused, their presence indicates a need for further investigation. Health care workers are required to report any signs or symptoms of abuse to their immediate supervisor or to the individual in the health care facility responsible for reporting suspicions to the proper authorities.
- **Defamation**: Defamation occurs when false statements either cause a person to be ridiculed or damage the person's reputation. Incorrect information given out in error can result in defamation. If the information is spoken, it is **slander**; if it is written, it is **libel**. Examples include reporting that a patient has an infectious disease to a government agency when laboratory results are inaccurate, telling others that a person has a drug problem when actually another medical condition exists, or saying that a coworker is incompetent.

Contracts

In addition to tort laws, contract laws also affect health care. A **contract** is an agreement between two or more parties. Most contracts have three parts:

- *Offer:* a health care facility or provider has a treatment or services they can offer to a patient; a competent individual offers to be a patient
- *Acceptance:* a patient makes an appointment with the health care facility or provider and accepts the treatment or services offered; the health care facility or provider accepts the individual as a patient
- *Consideration:* the patient receives treatment or services; the health care facility or provider receives payment from the patient

Contracts in health care are implied or expressed. **Implied contracts** are those obligations that are understood without verbally expressed terms. For example, when a qualified health care worker prepares a medication and a patient takes the medication, it is implied that the patient accepts this treatment. **Expressed contracts** are stated in distinct and clear language, either orally or in writing. An example is a surgery permit. Promises of care must be kept. Therefore, all risks associated with treatment must be explained completely to the patient (Figure 5–2).

All parties entering into a contract must be free of **legal disability**. A person who has a legal disability does not have the legal capacity to form a contract. Examples of people who have legal disabilities are minors (individuals under legal age), mentally incompetent persons, individuals under the influence of drugs that alter the mental state, and semiconscious or unconscious people. In such cases, parents, guardians, or others permitted by law must form the contract for the individual.

A contract requires that certain standards of care be provided by competent, qualified individuals. If the contract is not performed according to the agreement, the contract is breached. Failure to provide care and/or giving improper care on the part of the health provider, or failure on the part of the patient to pay according to the consideration, can be considered a breach of contract and cause for legal action.

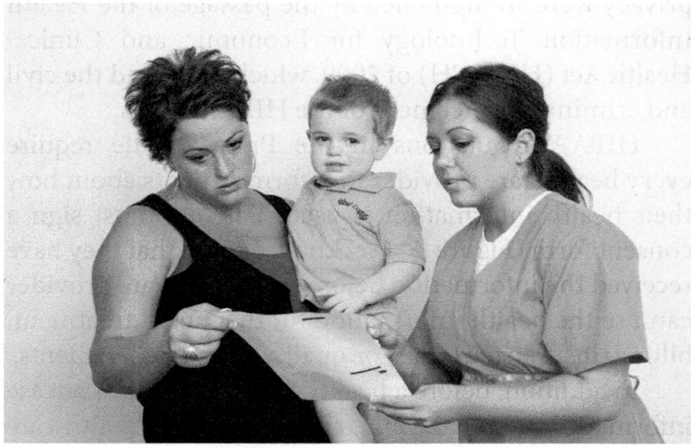

FIGURE 5–2 All risks of treatment must be explained to a patient before asking the patient for permission to administer treatment.

Comm

To comply with legal mandates, an interpreter/translator must be used when a contract is explained to an individual who does not speak English. In addition, many states require the use of interpreter services for individuals who are deaf or hard of hearing. Most health care agencies have a list of interpreters who can be used in these situations. At times, an English-speaking relative or friend of the patient can also serve as an interpreter.

A final important consideration in contract law is the role of the **agent**. When a person works under the direction or control of another person, the employer is called the *principal*, and the person working under the employer is called the *agent*. The principal is responsible for the actions of the agent and can be required to pay or otherwise compensate people who have been injured by the agent. For example, if a dental assistant tells a patient "your dentures will look better than your real teeth," the dentist may have to compensate the patient financially should this statement prove false. Health care workers should therefore be aware of their role as agents of their employers and work to protect the interests of their employers.

Privileged Communications

Comm

Privileged communications are another important aspect of legal responsibility. Privileged communications comprise all information given to health care personnel by a patient. By law, this information must be kept confidential and shared only with other members of the patient's health care team. It cannot be told to anyone else without the written consent of the patient. The consent should state what information is to be released, to whom the information should be given, and any applicable time limits. Certain information is exempt by law and must be reported in accordance with facility policy. Examples of exempt information are births and deaths; injuries caused by violence (such as assault and battery, abuse, or stabbings) that may require police involvement; drug abuse; communicable diseases; and sexually transmitted diseases.

Health care records are also considered privileged communications. Such records contain information about the care provided to the patient. Although the records belong to the health care provider (for example, the physician, dentist, hospital, or long-term care facility), the patient has a right to obtain a copy of any information in the record. Health care records can be used as legal records in a court of law. Erasures are therefore not allowed on such records. Errors should be crossed out with a single line so the material is still readable. Correct information should then be inserted, initialed, and dated. If necessary, an explanation for the correction should also be provided. Health care records must be properly maintained, kept confidential, and retained for the amount of time required by state law. When records are disposed of after the legal time for retention, they should be burned or shredded to maintain confidentiality.

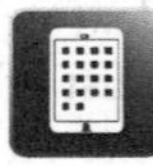

The growing use of electronic health records (EHRs) has created a dilemma in maintaining confidentiality (Figure 5–3). In a large health care facility such as a hospital, many different individuals may have access to a patient's records. For this reason, health care providers are creating safeguards to maintain computer confidentiality. Some examples include limiting the personnel who have access to such records, requiring the use of iris scans or fingerprints to access records, using codes to prevent access to certain information, requiring passwords to access specific information on records, and constantly monitoring and evaluating computer use.

In 2009, under the American Recovery and Reinvestment Act (ARRA), the Health Information Technology for Economic and Clinical Health Act (HITECH) was enacted. Its purpose was to promote the adoption and meaningful use of health information technology. As a result of this act, the Office of the National Coordinator for Health Information (ONC) was authorized to establish programs to improve health care quality, safety, and efficiency through the use and transfer of electronic health records (EHRs) in a secure network exchange. The ONC established a national electronic health record exchange called a *health information exchange (HIE)* that is being developed with the help of government funding. The HIE allows all medical facilities to electronically transfer and receive patient electronic health records. The HIE provides many benefits to patients and facilities, including:

- A greater degree of patient safety with quick access to medical history and lab tests
- Better-coordinated care across different health care facilities and across different levels of specialization within those facilities
- Patient access to the EHR
- Information for research and public health monitoring
- Reduction in health care costs due to eliminating repetition of the same tests in different facilities

One problem of the HIE is coordinating the system so that all facilities use compatible software that can interpret the information. Policies and standards are being developed to solve this communication problem. However, the biggest challenge for the HIE is keeping the transferred information secure. If the networks for all transferring facilities are not completely secure, then the security of the health care records can be compromised. This is a major issue that will need to be monitored continually with use of the HIE.

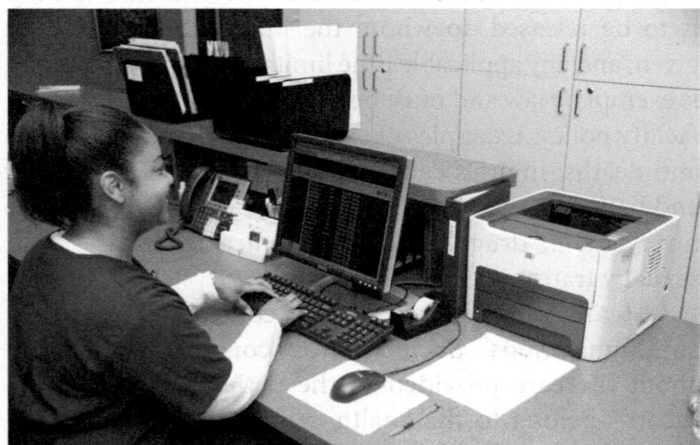

FIGURE 5–3 The growing use of electronic health records (EHRs) has created the need to limit access to computers to maintain confidentiality.

Privacy Act

HIPAA

The federal government is concerned about protecting privileged communications and maintaining confidentiality of health care records. In the **Health Insurance Portability and Accountability Act (HIPAA)** of 1996, Congress required the U.S. Department of Health and Human Services (USDHHS) to establish standards to protect health information. The USDHHS published the *Standards for Privacy of Individually Identifiable Health Information* (commonly called the Privacy Rule), which went into effect in 2003. These standards provide federal protection for privacy of health information in all states. These mandates for privacy were strengthened by the passage of the Health Information Technology for Economic and Clinical Health Act (HITECH) of 2009, which increased the civil and criminal enforcement of the HIPAA codes.

HIPAA regulations in the Privacy Rule require every health care provider to inform patients about how their health information is used. Patients must sign a consent form (Figure 5–4) acknowledging that they have received the information before any health care provider can use the health information for diagnosis, treatment, billing, insurance claims, or quality of care assessments.

In addition, before a health care provider can release information to anyone else, such as another health care provider, attorney, insurance company, federal or state agency, or even other members of the patient's family,

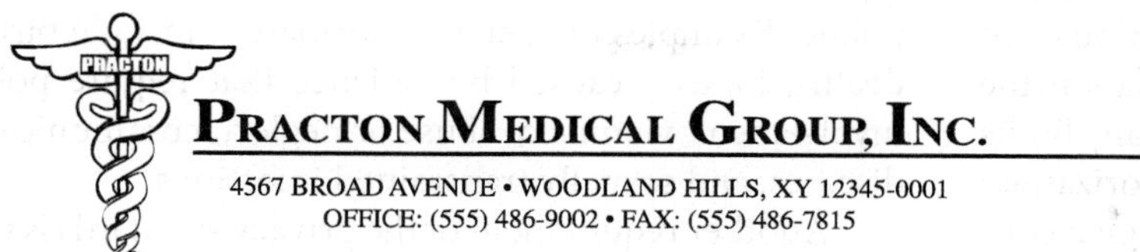

Fran Practon, M.D.
Gerald Practon, M.D.

CONSENT TO THE USE AND DISCLOSURE OF HEALTH INFORMATION

I understand that this organization originates and maintains health records which describe my health history, symptoms, examination, test results, diagnoses, treatment, and any plans for future care or treatment. I understand that this information is used to:

- plan my care and treatment
- communicate among health professionals who contribute to my care
- apply my diagnosis and services, procedures, and surgical information to my bill
- verify services billed by third-party payers
- assess quality of care and review the competence of health care professionals in routine health care operations

I further understand that:

- a complete description of information uses and disclosures is included in a *Notice of Information Practices* which has been provided to me
- I have a right to review the notice prior to signing this consent
- the organization reserves the right to change their notice and practices
- any revised notice will be mailed to the address I have provided prior to implementation
- I have the right to object to the use of my health information for directory purposes
- I have the right to request restrictions as to how my health information may be used or disclosed to carry out treatment, payment, or health care operations
- the organization is not required to agree to the restrictions requested
- I may revoke this consent in writing, except to the extent that the organization has already taken action in reliance thereon.

☐ I request the following restrictions to the use or disclosure of my health information.

____

June 29, 20XX	*June 29, 20XX*
Date	Notice Effective Date
Consuelo Hernandez	
Signature of Patient or Legal Representative	Witness
Signature	Title
Date	_____Accepted_____Rejected

FIGURE 5–4 Example of a Health Insurance Portability and Accountability Act (HIPAA) required form granting consent for the use and disclosure of health information.

a patient must sign an authorization form for the release of this information (Figure 5–5). This authorization form must identify the purpose or need for the information, the extent of the information that may be released, any limits on the release of information, the date of authorization, and the signature of the person authorized to give consent. These requirements are used to ensure the privacy and confidentiality of a patient's health care information. The only exception to these regulations is for the release of information about diseases or injuries that must be reported by law to protect the safety and welfare of the public. Examples of exempt information include births, deaths, injuries caused by violence that require police involvement, victims of abuse or neglect, communicable diseases, and sexually transmitted infections.

Another requirement of the privacy standards is that patients must be able to see and obtain copies of their medical records. Many health care agencies provide a *patient portal* or an Internet site patients can use to access their electronic health records (EHRs). In addition, every

AUTHORIZATION FOR RELEASE OF INFORMATION

Section A: Must be completed for all authorizations.

I hereby authorize the use or disclosure of my individually identifiable health information as described below.
I understand that this authorization is voluntary. I understand that if the organization authorized to receive the information is not a health plan or health care provider, the released information may no longer be protected by federal privacy regulations.

Patient name: Hilda F. Goodman **ID Number:** 4309

Identity of person/organization disclosing protected health information

Persons/organizations providing information:
Practon Medical Group, Inc
4567 Broad Avenue
Woodland Hills, XY 12345-4700

Persons/organizations receiving information:
Jennifer P. Lee, MD
400 North M Street
Anytown, XY 54098-1235

Identity of those authorized to use protected health information

Specific description of information [including from and to date(s)]:
Complete medical records from 4-22-XX to 9-15-XX

Specific description of information to be used or disclosed with dates

Section B: Must be completed only if a health plan or a health care provider has requested the authorization.

Purpose for disclosure

1. The health plan or health care provider must complete the following:
   a. What is the purpose of the use or disclosure? Patient relocating to another city
   b. Will the health plan or health care provider requesting the authorization receive financial or in-kind compensation in exchange for using or disclosing the health information described above? Yes__ No X
2. The patient or the patient's representative must read and initial the following statements:
   a. I understand that my health care and the payment for my health care will not be affected if I do not sign this form.
   Initials: hfg
   b. I understand that I may see and copy the information described on this form if I ask for it, and that I get a copy of this form after I sign it.
   Initials: hfg

Section C: Must be completed for all authorizations.

The patient or the patient's representative must read and initial the following statements:

Expiration date

1. I understand that this authorization will expire on 12 / 31 / 20XX (DD/MM/YR).
   Initials: hfg

Individual's right to revoke this authorization in writing

2. I understand that I may revoke this authorization at any time by notifying the providing organization in writing, but if I do it will not have any effect on any actions they took before they received the revocation.
   Initials: hfg

Redisclosure conditions

3. I understand that any disclosure of information carries with it the potential for an unauthorized redisclosure and the information may not be protected by federal confidentiality rules.
   Initials: hfg

Individual's signature

Hilda F. Goodman
Signature of patient or patient's representative
(Form MUST be completed before signing)

September 15, 20XX
Date

Date of signature

Printed name of patient's representative:________

Relationship to the patient:________

FIGURE 5–5 Example of an authorization form to release health information.

patient must be provided with information on how to file a complaint against a health care provider who violates the privacy act. Health care providers must be aware of these standards and make every effort to protect the privacy and confidentiality of a patient's health care information.

Regulation of Health Care Providers

All states have laws, regulations, and licensing boards that govern health care providers. The regulations usually determine the **scope of practice**, or the procedures, processes, and actions that health care providers are legally permitted to perform in keeping with the terms of their professional license or registration. Failure to abide by the regulations can result in the suspension or loss of a license or registration.

The federal government has established national standards that regulate health care. Some of the regulations are mandated by federal laws. A few examples of these laws include:

- Health Insurance Portability and Accountability Act (HIPAA)
- Health Information Technology for Economic and Clinical Health Act (HITECH)
- Americans with Disabilities Act (ADA)
- Patient Self-Determination Act (PSDA)
- Genetic Information Non-Discrimination Act (GINA)
- Mental Health Parity Act (MHPA)
- Newborns' and Mothers' Health Protection Act (NMHPA)
- Omnibus Budget Reconciliation Act (OBRA) of 1987
- Patient Protection and Affordable Care Act (PPACA)

Health care providers are responsible for knowing and following the provisions of these laws. In addition, federal agencies such as the Centers for Disease Control and Prevention (CDC), the Occupational Safety and Health Administration (OSHA), the Centers for Medicare and Medicaid Services (CMS), the Food and Drug Administration (FDA), the National Highway Traffic Safety Administration (NHTSA), and the U.S. Department of Health and Human Services (USDHHS) issue standards and regulations. For example, OSHA established *Bloodborne Pathogen Standards* that must be followed by all health care facilities and health care workers. The NHTSA Office of EMS established the educational standards for emergency medical services. The CDC developed *Standard Precautions* and *Transmission Based Precautions*.

Professional organizations in all of the health care careers assist in the establishment of educational requirements for the career, professional standards that should be observed, certification and/or registration requirements that must be met, and a code of ethics or conduct that must be followed. The organizations strive to establish standards that are followed by every individual working in the career field. In addition, they monitor legislative and regulatory actions and advocate for laws that affect the health care career. Again, every health care worker in the specific career field must be aware of and follow these professional guidelines and standards.

In addition, most health care agencies have specific rules, regulations, and standards that determine the activities performed by individuals employed in different positions. These standards are usually in the facility's policy or procedure manual. Every health care worker should read and follow the guidelines presented in the manual.

Legal

Standards and regulations can vary from state to state, and even from agency to agency. It is important to remember that you are liable, or legally responsible, for your own actions regardless of what anyone tells you or what position you hold. Therefore, when you undertake a particular position of employment in a health care agency, *it is your responsibility to learn exactly what you are legally permitted to do and to familiarize yourself with your exact responsibilities.*

5:2 Ethics

Legal responsibilities are determined by law. **Ethics** are a set of principles relating to what is morally right or wrong. Ethics provide a standard of conduct or code of behavior. This allows a health care provider to analyze information and make decisions based on what people believe is right and good conduct. Modern health care advances, however, have created many ethical dilemmas for health care providers. Some of these dilemmas include:

- Should a person have the right to euthanasia (assisted death) if he or she is terminally ill and in excruciating pain?
- Should a patient be told that a health care provider has AIDS?
- When should life support be discontinued?
- Do parents have a religious right to refuse a life-saving blood transfusion for their child?
- Can a health care facility refuse to provide expensive treatment such as a bone marrow transplant if a patient cannot pay for the treatment?
- Who decides whether a 75-year-old patient or a 56-year-old patient gets a single kidney available for transplant?

- Should people be allowed to sell organs for use in transplants?
- If a person can benefit from marijuana, should a physician be allowed to prescribe it as a treatment?
- Should animals be used in medical research even if it results in the death of the animal?
- Should genetic researchers be allowed to transplant specific genes to create the "perfect" human being?
- Should human beings be cloned?
- Should aborted embryos be used to obtain stem cells for research, especially as scientists may be able to use the stem cells to cure diseases such as diabetes, osteoporosis, and Parkinson's?

Although there are no easy answers to any of these questions, some guidelines are provided by an ethical code. Most of the national organizations affiliated with the different health care professions have established ethical codes for personnel in their respective occupations. Although such codes differ slightly, most contain the same basic principles:

- Put the saving of life and the promotion of health above all else.
- Make every effort to keep the patient as comfortable as possible and to preserve life whenever possible.
- Respect the patient's choice to die peacefully and with dignity when all options have been discussed with the patient and family and/or predetermined by advance directives.
- Treat all patients equally, regardless of race, religion, social or economic status, gender, age, or nationality. Bias, prejudice, and discrimination have no place in health care.
- Provide care for *all* individuals to the best of your ability.
- Maintain a competent level of skill consistent with your particular health care career.
- Stay informed and up to date, and pursue continuing education as necessary.
- 

Maintain **confidentiality**. Confidentiality means that information about the patient must remain private and can be shared *only* with other members of the patient's health care team. A legal violation can occur if a patient suffers personal or financial damage when confidential information is shared with others, including family members. Information obtained from patients should not be repeated or used for personal gain. Gossiping about patients is ethically wrong.
- Refrain from immoral, unethical, and illegal practices. If you observe others taking part in illegal actions, report such actions to the proper authorities. Failure to report these actions may result in legal actions taken against you.
- Show loyalty to patients, coworkers, and employers. Avoid negative or derogatory statements, and always express a positive attitude.
- Be sincere, honest, and caring. Treat others as you want to be treated. Show respect and concern for the feelings, dignity, and rights of others.

When you enter a health care career, learn the code of ethics for that career. Make every effort to abide by the code and to become a competent and ethical health care worker. In doing so, you will earn the respect and confidence of patients, coworkers, and employers.

5:3 Patients' Rights

Federal and state legislation requires health care agencies to have written policies concerning **patients' rights**, or the factors of care that patients can expect to receive. Agencies expect all personnel to respect and honor these rights.

The Department of Health and Human Services implemented a **Consumer Bill of Rights and Responsibilities** in 1998 that must be recognized and honored by health care providers. This bill of rights states, in part, that patients have the right to:

- Receive accurate, easily understood information and assistance in making informed health care decisions about their health care plans, professionals, and facilities
- A choice of health care providers that is sufficient to ensure access to appropriate high-quality health care
- Access emergency health services when and where the need arises
- Fully participate in all decisions related to their health care (Figure 5–6)
- Be represented by parents, guardians, family members, or other conservators if they are unable to fully participate in treatment decisions
- Considerate and respectful care
- Not be discriminated against in the delivery of health care services based on race, ethnicity, national origin, religion, gender, age, mental or physical disability, sexual orientation, genetic information, or source of payment

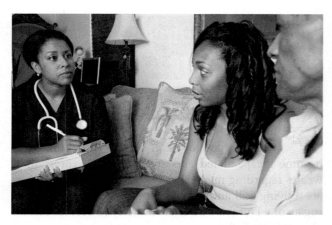

FIGURE 5–6 Patients have the right to fully participate in all decisions related to their health care. © iStock.com/Steve Debenport

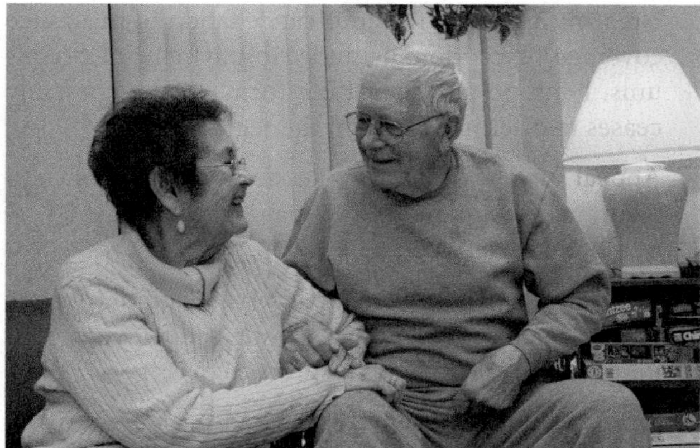

FIGURE 5–7 A married couple in a long-term care facility has the legal right to share a room if both members of the couple are residents in the facility.

- Communicate with health care providers in confidence and have the confidentiality of their individually identifiable health care information protected
- Review and copy their own medical records and request amendments to their records
- A fair and efficient process for resolving differences with their health care plans, health care providers, and the institutions that serve them, including a rigorous system of internal review and an independent system of external review

OBRA

Residents in long-term care facilities are guaranteed certain rights under the **Omnibus Budget Reconciliation Act (OBRA) of 1987**. Every long-term care facility must inform residents or their guardians of these rights and a copy must be posted in each facility. This is often called a **Resident's Bill of Rights**, and it states, in part, that a resident has the right to:

- Free choice regarding physician, treatment, care, and participation in research
- Freedom from abuse and chemical or physical restraints
- Privacy and confidentiality of personal and clinical records
- Accommodation of needs and choice regarding activities, schedules, and health care
- Voice grievances without fear of retaliation or discrimination
- Organize and participate in family/resident groups and in social, religious, and community activities
- Information about medical benefits, medical records, survey results, deficiencies of the facility, and advocacy groups, including the ombudsman program (state representative who checks on resident care and violations of rights)
- Manage personal funds and use personal possessions
- Unlimited access to immediate family or relatives and to share a room with his or her spouse, if both are residents (Figure 5–7)
- Remain in the facility and not be transferred or discharged except for medical reasons, the welfare of the resident or others, failure to pay, or if the facility either cannot meet the resident's needs or ceases to operate

The **Patient Protection and Affordable Care Act (PPACA)**, commonly called the *Affordable Care Act (ACA)*, also guarantees certain rights pertaining to health insurance coverage. Some of the main provisions of this act state, in part, that consumers have the right to:

- An easy-to-understand summary of insurance benefits and coverage
- Coverage for essential health benefits such as emergency care, hospitalization, prescription drugs, maternity care, and newborn care
- Preventive care for specific procedures at no cost to the consumer
- Coverage even if a pre-existing illness or condition exists
- Coverage to age 26 under a parent's health care plan if eligible
- Choose any available participating primary care provider as their doctor
- Receive care for emergency medical conditions at any emergency care facility without pre-authorization and without higher co-payments for out-of-network services
- No annual or lifetime limits on health care benefits

- No arbitrary withdrawal or cancellation of insurance coverage (exceptions include no payment of premiums, lying on an application form, or the company ceases to offer insurance in the region)
- Appeal any health care plan decision if the health insurance company denies payment for a medical treatment or service
- A review by an independent organization (outside review) if a health insurance company denies payment for a claim or terminates insurance coverage
- A refund of a percentage of their premiums if an insurance company does not spend at least 80–85 percent of premiums paid on health care versus administrative costs such as salaries and marketing

All states have adopted these rights, and some have added additional rights. It is important to check state law and obtain a list of the rights established in your state. Health care workers can face job loss, fines, and even imprisonment if they do not follow and grant established patients' or residents' rights. By observing these rights, the health care worker helps ensure the patient's safety, privacy, and well-being, and provides quality care at all times.

5:4 Advance Directives for Health Care

Advance directives for health care, also known as *legal directives*, are legal documents that allow individuals to state what medical treatment they want or do not want in the event that they become incapacitated and are unable to express their wishes regarding medical care. The two main directives are a living will and a Designation of Health Care Surrogate or a Durable Power of Attorney (POA) for Health Care (Figure 5–8).

Living wills are documents that allow individuals to state what measures should or should not be taken to prolong life when their conditions are terminal (death is expected). The document must be signed when the individual is competent and witnessed by two adults who cannot benefit from the death. Most states now have laws that honor living wills and allow life-sustaining procedures to be withheld. A living will frequently results in a Do Not Resuscitate (DNR) order for a terminally ill individual. The DNR order means that cardiopulmonary resuscitation is not performed when

INSTRUCTIONS

FLORIDA ADVANCE DIRECTIVE – PAGE 1 OF 5

Part One. Designation of Health Care Surrogate

PRINT YOUR NAME

Name: ______________________
(Last) (First) (Middle Initial)

In the event that I have been determined to be incapacitated to provide informed consent for medical treatment and surgical and diagnostic procedures, I wish to designate as my surrogate for health care decisions:

PRINT THE NAME, HOME ADDRESS AND TELEPHONE NUMBER OF YOUR SURROGATE

Name: ______________________

Address: ______________________

______________________ Zip Code: __________

Phone: ______________________

If my surrogate is unwilling or unable to perform his or her duties, I wish to designate as my alternate surrogate:

PRINT THE NAME, HOME ADDRESS AND TELEPHONE NUMBER OF YOUR ALTERNATE SURROGATE

Name: ______________________

Address: ______________________

______________________ Zip Code: __________

Phone: ______________________

I fully understand that this designation will permit my designee to make health care decisions and to provide, withhold, or withdraw consent on my behalf; to apply for public benefits to defray the cost of health care; and to authorize my admission to or transfer from a health care facility.

When making health care decisions for me, my health care surrogate should think about what action would be consistent with past conversations we have had, my treatment preferences as expressed in Part Two (if I have filled out Part Two), my religious and other beliefs and values, and how I have handled medical and other important issues in the past. If what I would decide is still unclear, then my health care surrogate should make decisions for me that my health care surrogate believes are in my best interest, considering the benefits, burdens, and risks of my current circumstances and treatment options.

FLORIDA ADVANCE DIRECTIVE - PAGE 2 OF 5

ADD OTHER INSTRUCTIONS, IF ANY, REGARDING YOUR ADVANCE CARE PLANS

THESE INSTRUCTIONS CAN FURTHER ADDRESS YOUR HEALTH CARE PLANS, SUCH AS YOUR WISHES REGARDING HOSPICE TREATMENT, BUT CAN ALSO ADDRESS OTHER ADVANCE PLANNING ISSUES, SUCH AS YOUR BURIAL WISHES

ATTACH ADDITIONAL PAGES IF NEEDED

Additional instructions (optional): ______________________

FIGURE 5–8 **Advance directives include a living will that allows an individual to state what measures should or should not be taken to prolong life, and a designation of a health care surrogate that allows an individual to appoint another person to make health care decisions if the individual is unable to make his or her own decisions.** Visit caringinfo.org for more information.

INSTRUCTIONS	**FLORIDA ADVANCE DIRECTIVE – PAGE 3 OF 5**
	Part Two. Declaration
PRINT THE DATE	Declaration made this ________ day of ____________, ________, (day) (month) (year)
PRINT YOUR NAME	I, ______________________________, willfully and voluntarily make known my desire that my dying not be artificially prolonged under the circumstances set forth below, and I do hereby declare that:
	If at any time I am incapacitated and (initial all that apply)
INITIAL EACH THAT APPLIES	______ I have a terminal condition, or ______ I have an end-stage condition, or ______ I am in a persistent vegetative state
	and if my attending or treating physician and another consulting physician have determined that there is no reasonable medical probability of my recovery from such condition, I direct that life-prolonging procedures be withheld or withdrawn when the application of such procedures would serve only to prolong artificially the process of dying, and that I be permitted to die naturally with only the administration of medication or the performance of any medical procedure deemed necessary to provide me with comfort care or to alleviate pain.
	It is my intention that this declaration be honored by my family and physician as the final expression of my legal right to refuse medical or surgical treatment and to accept the consequences for such refusal.
© 2005 National Hospice and Palliative Care Organization. 2011 Revised.	

	FLORIDA ADVANCE DIRECTIVE - PAGE 4 OF 5
ORGAN DONATION (OPTIONAL)	ORGAN DONATION (OPTIONAL) I hereby make this anatomical gift, if medically acceptable, to take effect on death. The words and marks below indicate my desires: I give (initial one choice below):
	_____ any needed organs, tissues, or eyes for the purpose of transplantation, therapy, medical research, or education;
INITIAL ONLY ONE OF THE FOUR OPTIONS	_____ only the following organs, tissues, or eyes for the purpose of transplantation, therapy, medical research, or education: ______________________________ ______________________________
	_____ my body for anatomical study if needed. Limitations or special wishes, if any: ______________________________ ______________________________
IF YOU HAVE ALREADY ARRANGED TO DONATE YOUR ORGANS TO A SPECIFIC DONEE, INITIAL THIS OPTION, AND INDICATE THE DETAILS OF YOUR ARRANGEMENT HERE	_____ I have already arranged to donate _____ Any needed organs, tissues, or eyes, _____ The following organs, tissues, or eyes: ______________________________ ______________________________ to the following donee:____________________ Phone:____________________ Address:____________________ ______________ Zip Code:__________
© 2005 National Hospice and Palliative Care Organization. 2011 Revised.	

	FLORIDA ADVANCE DIRECTIVE - PAGE 5 OF 5
	Part Three. Execution
PRINT YOUR NAME	I, ______________________________, understand the full impact of this declaration, and I am emotionally and mentally competent to make this declaration. I further affirm that this designation is not being made as a condition of treatment or admission to a health care facility.
SIGN AND DATE THE DOCUMENT	Signed: ____________________ Date: ____________________
TWO WITNESSES MUST SIGN AND PRINT THEIR ADDRESSES	Witness 1: Signed: ____________________ Address: ____________________ Witness 2: Signed: ____________________ Address: ____________________
OPTIONAL PRINT THE NAMES AND ADDRESSES OF THOSE WHO YOU WANT TO KEEP COPIES OF THIS DOCUMENT	(Optional) I will notify and send a copy of this document to the following persons other than my surrogate, so they may know who my surrogate is: Name: ____________________ Address: ____________________ Name: ____________________ Address: ____________________
© 2005 National Hospice and Palliative Care Organization. 2011 Revised.	*Courtesy of Caring Connections* *1731 King St., Suite 100, Alexandria, VA 22314* *www.caringinfo.org, 800/658-8898*

FIGURE 5–8 ***(Continued)*** Visit caringinfo.org for more information.

the patient stops breathing. The patient is allowed to die with peace and dignity. At times, this is extremely difficult for health care workers to honor. It is important to remember that many individuals believe that the quality of life is important and a life on support systems has no meaning or purpose for them.

A **Designation of Health Care Surrogate**, also called a **Durable Power of Attorney (POA)** for Health Care, is a document that permits an individual (known as a principal) to appoint another person (known as an agent) to make any decisions regarding health care if the principal should become unable to make decisions. This includes providing or withholding specific medical or surgical procedures, hiring or dismissing health care providers, spending or withholding funds for health care, and having access to medical records. Although they are most frequently given to spouses or adult children, POAs can be given to any qualified adult. To meet legal requirements, the POA must be signed by the principal, agent, and one or two adult witnesses.

A federal law, called the **Patient Self-Determination Act (PSDA)** of 1990, mandates that all health care facilities receiving any type of federal aid comply with the following requirements:

- Inform every adult, both orally and in writing, of their right under state law to make decisions concerning medical care, including the right to refuse treatment and right-to-die options
- Provide information and assistance in preparing advance directives
- Document any advance directives on the patient's record
- Provide written statements to implement the patient's rights in the decision-making process
- Affirm that there will be no discrimination or effect on care because of advance directives
- Educate the staff on the medical and legal issues of advance directives

The PSDA ensures that patients are informed of their rights and have the opportunity to determine the care they will receive.

All health care workers must be aware of and honor advance or legal directives. In addition, health care workers should give serious consideration to preparing their own advance directives.

5:5 Professional Standards

Legal responsibilities, ethics, patients' rights, and advance directives all help determine the type of care provided by health care workers. By following certain standards at all times, you can protect yourself, your employer, and the patient. Some of the basic standards are:

- *Perform only those procedures for which you have been trained and you are legally permitted to do.* Never perform any procedure unless you are qualified. The necessary training may be obtained from an educational facility, from your employer, or in special classes provided by an agency. If you are asked to perform any procedure for which you are not qualified, it is your responsibility to state that you have not been trained and to refuse to do it until you receive the required instruction. If you are not legally permitted to either perform a procedure or to sign documents, it is your responsibility to refuse to do so because of legal limitations.
- *Use approved, correct methods while performing any procedure.* Follow specific methods taught by qualified instructors in educational facilities, or observe and learn procedures from your employer or authorized personnel. Most health care facilities have an approved procedure manual that explains the step-by-step methods for performing tasks. Use this manual or read the manufacturer's instructions for specific equipment or supplies.
- *Obtain proper authorization before performing any procedure.* In some health care careers, you will obtain authorization directly from the doctor, therapist, or individual in charge of a patient's care (Figure 5–9). In other careers, you will obtain authorization by checking written orders. In careers where you have neither access to patients' records nor direct contact with the individuals in charge of care, an immediate supervisor will interpret orders and then direct you to perform procedures.
- *Identify the patient.* In some health care facilities, patients wear identification bands. If this is the case, check this name band (Figure 5–10). In addition, state the patient's name clearly, repeating it if necessary. For example, say "Miss Jones?" followed by "Miss Sandra Jones?" to be sure you have the correct patient. Some health care facilities now use bar codes on patient identification bands. A scanner is used to check the bar code and verify the identity of the patient. Some long-term care facilities use photo IDs for patients because sometimes the patients are disoriented and are not able to state their name.
- *Obtain the patient's consent before performing any procedure.* Always explain a procedure briefly or state what you are going to do, and obtain the patient's consent. It is best to avoid statements such as "May I take your blood pressure?" because the patient can say "No." By stating, "The doctor would like me to

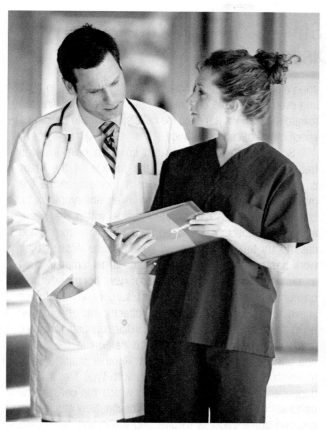

FIGURE 5–9 Obtain proper authorization before performing any procedure on a patient. © iStock.com/Eric Hood

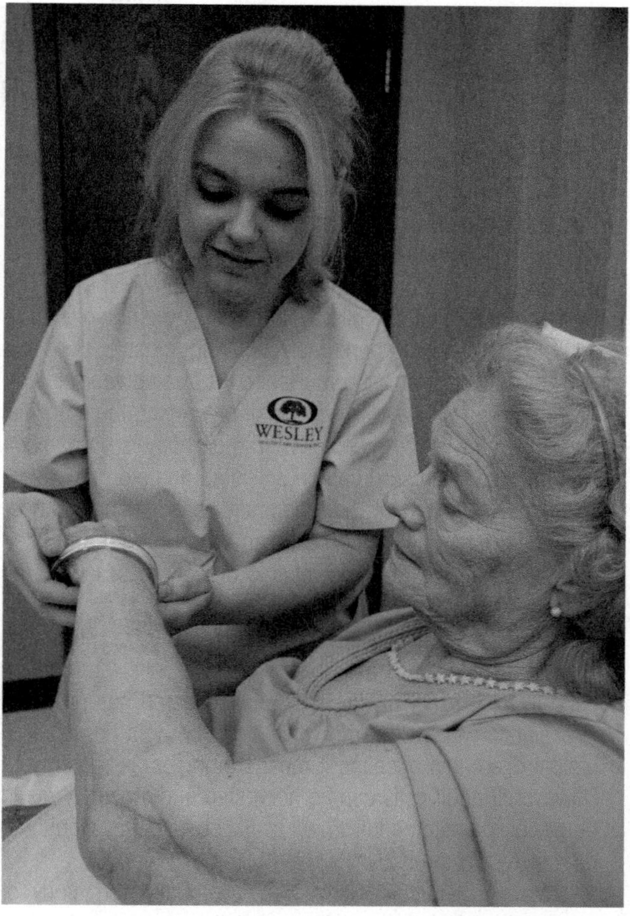

FIGURE 5–10 If a name band is present, use it to identify the patient.

check your blood pressure," you are identifying the procedure and obtaining consent by the patient's acceptance or lack of objection. If a patient refuses to allow you to perform a procedure, check with your immediate supervisor. Some procedures require written consent from the patient. Follow the agency policy with regard to such procedures. Never sign your name as a witness to any written consent or document unless you are authorized to do so.

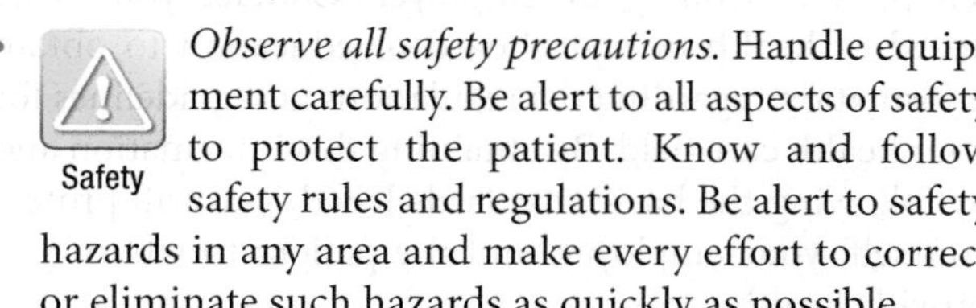

- Safety *Observe all safety precautions.* Handle equipment carefully. Be alert to all aspects of safety to protect the patient. Know and follow safety rules and regulations. Be alert to safety hazards in any area and make every effort to correct or eliminate such hazards as quickly as possible.
- HIPAA *Keep all information confidential.* This includes oral and written information. Ensure that you do not place patient records in any area where they can be seen by unauthorized individuals. Do not reveal any information contained in the records without proper authorization and patient consent. If you are reporting specific information about a patient to your immediate supervisor, ensure that your conversation cannot be heard by others. Avoid discussing patients with others at home, in social situations, in public places, or anywhere outside the agency.

- Comm *Think before you speak and carefully consider everything you say.* Do not reveal information to the patient unless you are specifically permitted to do so.
- *Treat all patients equally regardless of race, religion, social or economic status, gender, age, or nationality.* Provide care for *all* individuals to the best of your ability.
- *Accept no tips or bribes for the care you provide.* You receive a salary for your services, and the care you provide should not be influenced by the amount of money a patient can afford to pay. A polite refusal, such as "I'm sorry, I am not allowed to accept tips," is usually the best way to handle this situation. An exception to this rule is if a patient or family member brings the entire floor/unit a thank-you gift such as cookies or candy.

TODAY'S RESEARCH TOMORROW'S HEALTH CARE

Frozen Stem Cells That Cure Major Diseases?

Stem cells are a major area of research today. Stem cells are important because they can become any of the specialized cell types needed in the human body. They can turn into muscle cells in the heart, nerve cells in the brain, or cells that secrete the insulin needed by a patient with diabetes. The major sources of stem cells are a developing embryo (infant); adult tissues such as bone marrow, brain, muscle, skin, and liver; and blood from the umbilical cord of a newborn infant. Currently, parents have the option of preserving the umbilical cord blood for its stem cells. When their baby is born, blood from the umbilical cord can be collected and stored in liquid nitrogen. If the child later develops a disease such as cancer and needs stem cells, the cells can be recovered and used for the transplant. The cost of this procedure still limits its widespread use.

Scientists the world over are finding ways to grow stem cells and force them to generate special cells that can be used to treat injury or disease. Early research has proved it is easier to work with embryonic cells, but this has created ethical dilemmas because it means embryos are destroyed. However, if adult cells can be harvested and grown, it would be easier to use an adult's own cells because they would not be rejected by the body.

Many scientists believe that, eventually, the study of stem cells will help explain how cells grow and develop. Conditions such as cancer and birth defects are caused by abnormal cell division. If scientists can learn how the abnormal development occurs, they could find ways to treat and even prevent the conditions. Major research is directed toward learning what makes the cells specialize to become a specific type of cell in the body.

Some of the latest research on stem cells involves treatment for heart disease. If the muscle of the heart is deprived of oxygen because of a blocked artery, the muscle cells die. Researchers are using embryonic cells, cardiac stem cells that naturally reside within the heart, myoblasts (muscle stem cells), and umbilical cord blood cells to try to repair damaged heart tissue. Most of their work has been performed on rats or larger animals such as pigs. However, some experiments have been performed on humans undergoing open-heart surgery. Initial studies showed that stem cells injected directly into the injured heart tissue appeared to improve cardiac function. However, much more research is needed to determine the safety and effectiveness of this treatment. Another major area of research is directed toward patients with Type 1 or insulin-dependent diabetes, a condition in which the cells of the pancreas do not produce sufficient insulin. New studies are showing some success in directing embryonic stem cells in a cell culture to form insulin-producing cells that could eventually be transplanted into a person with diabetes. Again, years of intensive research will be required before this is an effective treatment for diabetes, but stem cells do offer exciting promise for future therapies.

- *If any error occurs or you make a mistake, report it immediately to your supervisor.* Never try to hide or ignore an error. Make every effort to correct the situation as soon as possible, and take responsibility for your actions.
- *Behave professionally in dress, language, manners, and actions.* Take pride in your profession and in the work you do. Promote a positive attitude at all times.

Even when standards are followed, errors leading to legal action sometimes still occur. Liability insurance constitutes an additional form of protection in such cases. Many insurance companies offer policies at reasonable cost for health care workers and students. Some companies will even issue liability protection under a homeowner's policy or through a liability policy that protects the person against all liabilities, not just those related to their profession.

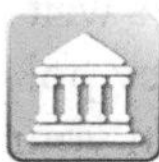
Legal

Again, remember that it is your responsibility to understand the legal and ethical implications of your particular health care career. Never hesitate to ask specific questions or to request written policies from your employer. Contact your state board of health or state board of education to obtain information regarding the regulations and guidelines for your health care field. By obtaining this information and by following the basic standards listed, you will protect yourself, your employer, and the patient to whom you provide health care.

STUDENT: **Go to the workbook and complete the assignment sheet for Chapter 5, Legal and Ethical Responsibilities.**

CHAPTER 5 SUMMARY

All health care professionals and workers have legal and ethical responsibilities that exist to protect the health care worker and employer and to provide for the safety and well-being of the patient.

Legal responsibilities in health care usually involve torts and contracts. Torts are wrongful acts that do not involve contracts. Examples of torts that can lead to legal action include malpractice, negligence, assault and battery, invasion of privacy, false imprisonment, abuse, and defamation. A contract is an agreement between two or more parties. Contracts create obligations that must be met by all involved individuals. If a contract is not performed according to the agreement, the contract is breached, and legal action can occur.

Understanding privileged communications is another important aspect of legal responsibilities. A health care worker must be aware that all information given by a patient is confidential and should not be told to anyone other than members of the patient's health care team without the written consent of the patient. Health care records are also privileged communications and can be used as legal records in a court of law.

All health care providers must know and follow all of the regulations that determine which procedures, processes, and actions they can legally perform. These regulations are determined by many sources including scope of practice, state laws, state licensing/registration boards, federal laws, federal agencies, professional organizations, and health care agencies. Because standards and regulations vary from state to state, and even from agency to agency, health care providers are responsible for determining what they are legally permitted to do.

Ethical responsibilities are based not on law, but rather, on what is morally right or wrong. Most health care careers have established codes of ethics that provide standards of conduct or codes of behavior. Health care workers should make every effort to abide by the codes of ethics established for their given professions.

Health care workers must respect patients' rights. Health care facilities have written policies concerning the factors of care that patients can expect to receive. All personnel must respect and honor these rights.

Advance directives for health care are legal documents that allow individuals to state what medical treatment they want or do not want in the event that they become incapacitated. The two main examples are a living will and a Designation of Health Care Surrogate or Durable Power of Attorney for Health Care. As a result of a federal law called the Patient Self-Determination Act (PSDA), any health care facility receiving federal funds must provide patients with information regarding and assistance in preparing advance or legal directives.

Professional standards of care provide guidelines for meeting legal responsibilities, ethics, and patients' rights. Every health care worker should follow these standards at all times. In addition, all health care workers should know and follow the state laws that regulate their respective careers.

INTERNET SEARCHES

Use the search engines suggested in Chapter 12:9 in this text to search the Internet for additional information about the following topics:

1. **Torts:** Search for additional information or actual legal cases involving malpractice, negligence, assault and battery, invasion of privacy, false imprisonment, and defamation.
2. **Abuse:** Research domestic violence or abuse, child abuse, and elder abuse to determine how victims might react, signs and symptoms indicative of abuse, and information about how to help these victims.
3. **Contracts:** Search for information about the components of a contract and legal cases in health care caused by a breach of contract.
4. **Federal laws:** Search for additional information about federal laws that regulate health care providers or health care facilities.
5. **Ethics:** Use Internet addresses for professional organizations (see Chapter 3) to find two or three different codes of ethics; compare and contrast these codes of ethics.
6. **Patient's rights:** Search for complete copies of a patient's or resident's bill of rights; compare and contrast the different bills of rights.
7. **Advance directives:** Search for different examples of a living will and a designation of health care surrogate or durable power of attorney for health care; compare the different forms.
8. **Patient Self-Determination Act of 1990:** Locate a copy of this act or information about the purposes of this act (*Hint:* check federal legislation websites).
9. **Insurance:** Search for different types of liability insurance for health care providers; determine what different policies cover and their cost.

REVIEW QUESTIONS

1. Choose a specific health care profession (e.g., dental hygienist, physical therapist) and create a situation where this individual might be subject to legal action for each of the following torts: malpractice, negligence, assault, battery, invasion of privacy, false imprisonment, abuse, and defamation.
2. Differentiate between slander and libel.
3. What is the difference between an implied contract and an expressed contract?
4. You are employed as a geriatric assistant. A resident tells you that he is saving sleeping pills so he can commit suicide. He has terminal cancer and is in a great deal of pain. What should you do? Why?
5. What is HIPAA? Identify three (3) specific ways that HIPAA protects the privacy and confidentiality of health care information.
6. What is the PPACA? How does it influence health care insurance plans?
7. Obtain at least two (2) different codes of ethics for health professions by contacting professional organizations or searching the Internet. Compare these codes of ethics.
8. Mr. Gonzales is a healthy 55-year-old man with a living will that contains a DNR (Do Not Resuscitate) order for terminal conditions. He goes into cardiac arrest as a result of an allergic reaction to an injection of dye for a laboratory test. Should cardiopulmonary resuscitation (CPR) be started? Why or why not?
9. How does a living will differ from a Designation of Health Care Surrogate?
10. List five (5) different patient or resident rights.
11. Identify six (6) professional standards by explaining why they are important to meet legal responsibilities, ethics, or patient's rights.
12. There is a major shortage of kidneys available for transplant. Should an individual be allowed to sell a kidney to another individual in renal failure who needs the kidney in order to live and is willing to pay for the kidney? Why or why not?

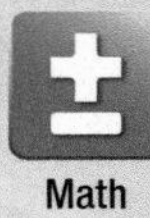

13 Medical Math*

CHAPTER OBJECTIVES

After completing this chapter, you should be able to:

- Perform basic math calculations on whole numbers, decimals, fractions, percentages, and ratios.
- Convert between the following numerical forms: decimals, fractions, percentages, and ratios.
- Round off numbers correctly.
- Solve mathematical problems with proportions.
- Express numbers using Roman numerals.
- Estimate angles from a reference plane.
- Use household, metric, and apothecary units to express length, volume, and weight.
- Convert between the Fahrenheit and Celsius temperature scales.
- Express time using the 24-hour clock (military time).
- Define, pronounce, and spell all key terms.

KEY TERMS

angles
apothecary system *(ah-pa' -the-ker-E)*
Celsius
centigrade
decimals
degrees
estimating
Fahrenheit
fractions
household system
improper fractions
metric system
military time
nomenclature *(no' -men-kla-shure)*
percentages
proportion
ratios
reciprocal *(ree-si' -pre-kal)*
reference plane
Roman numerals
rounding numbers
whole numbers

* This chapter has been adapted from Dakota Mitchell's and Lee Haroun's textbook entitled *Introduction to Health Care*, 2/E, Cengage Learning, 2007. Our sincere thanks to these authors for allowing the use of their material in this textbook.

Introduction

Working in health care requires the use of math skills to measure and perform various types of calculations. There are applications in all types of occupations:

- Calculating medication dosages
- Taking height and weight readings
- Measuring the amount of intake (fluids consumed or infused) and output (fluids expelled, e.g., urine, vomit)
- Billing and bookkeeping tasks
- Performing lab tests
- Mixing cleaning solutions

Safety

Errors in math can have negative effects on patients. For example, administering the wrong dosage of medication is a serious mistake and can harm the patient. Health care workers must strive for 100 percent accuracy. *If there is any doubt, it is essential to ask your supervisor or a qualified coworker to double-check calculations.*

13:1 Basic Calculations

To work safely in health care, it is essential to be able to add, subtract, multiply, and divide whole numbers, decimals, fractions, and percentages. Health care workers also need to understand equivalents when using decimals, fractions, and percentages (Figure 13–1).

Many health care workers use small calculators to assist them with calculations. During your health science studies, some instructors will allow the use of calculators, and others will not. It is always best to know how to do the basic functions by "long hand" (without a calculator). Calculators can quit working at any time during a test or at the workplace. In addition, some professional examinations required for licensure or certification do not allow the use of calculators.

Whole Numbers

Whole numbers are what we traditionally use to count (1, 2, 3, . . .). They do not contain fractions or decimals. For example, 30 is a whole number, while 30½ and 30.5 are not. Health care workers must be able to accurately add, subtract, multiply, and divide whole numbers.

ADDITION OF WHOLE NUMBERS

Addition is adding two or more numbers together to find the *sum*, or total. A few examples of how addition is used in health care include:

- Counting and totaling supplies for an inventory
- Adding oral (by mouth) intake
- Adding intravenous or IV (into a vein) intake
- Measuring and totaling output from the body such as amounts of urine
- Completing statistical information such as the total number of patients diagnosed with lung cancer or the total number of surgeries performed in a hospital in a 1-year period

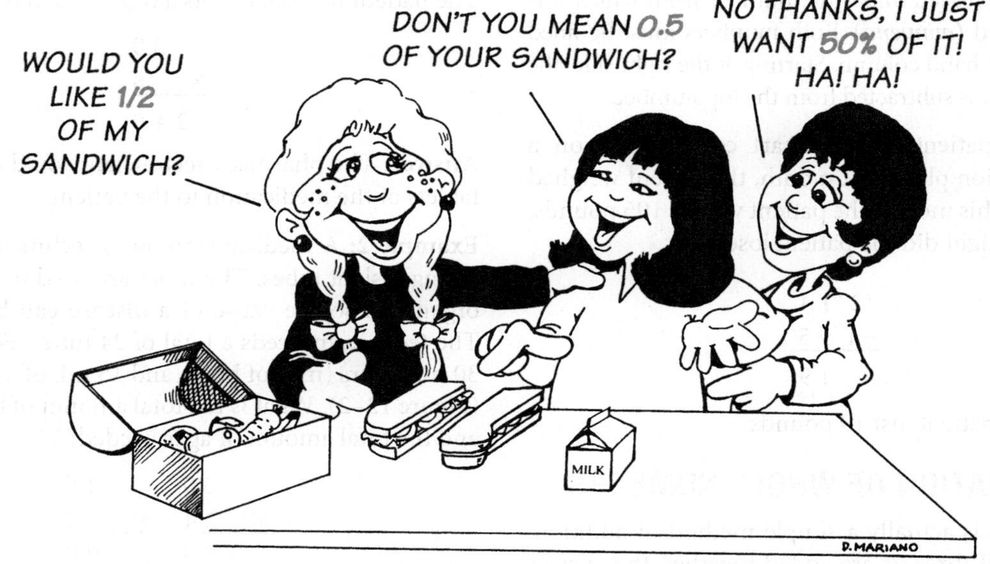
WOULD YOU LIKE 1/2 OF MY SANDWICH?
DON'T YOU MEAN 0.5 OF YOUR SANDWICH?
NO THANKS, I JUST WANT 50% OF IT! HA! HA!
MILK
D. MARIANO

FIGURE 13–1 An easy way to remember how to convert decimals, percentages, and fractions is to think of this humorous cartoon.

To add whole numbers together, the numbers are placed in a column and lined up on the right side of the column. The columns are then added together starting with the column on the right.

Example: A nurse assistant must encourage a patient to drink large amounts of fluid. For lunch, the patient drank 240 milliliters (mL) of milk, 120 mL of coffee, 45 mL of water, and 60 mL of juice. What is the total amount of fluids the patient drank?

$$\begin{array}{r} {}^{+1}240 \\ 120 \\ 45 \\ +\ 60 \\ \hline 465 \end{array}$$

Answer: The patient drank 465 mL of fluid.

SUBTRACTION OF WHOLE NUMBERS

Subtraction is the process of taking a number away from another number to find the *difference*, or *remainder*, between the numbers. A few examples of how subtraction is used in health care include:

- Determining weight loss or gain
- Maintaining an inventory of supplies
- Calculating a pulse deficit (difference between the number of times a heart beats and the actual pulse it creates)
- Performing laboratory tests
- Reporting statistical information such as number of deaths from a particular disease

To subtract whole numbers, the number to be subtracted *(subtrahend)* is placed under the number from which it is to be subtracted *(minuend)*. Both numbers must be lined up on the right-hand column. Starting at the right side, the bottom number is subtracted from the top number.

Example: A patient with a heart condition is on a weight-reduction plan. Last month, the patient weighed 214 pounds. This month, the patient weighs 195 pounds. How much weight did the patient lose?

$$\begin{array}{r} {}^{1}2\,{}^{0}1\,4 \\ -1\,9\,5 \\ \hline 1\,9 \end{array}$$

Answer: The patient lost 19 pounds.

MULTIPLICATION OF WHOLE NUMBERS

Multiplication is actually a simple method of addition. For example, if three *7s* are added together, the answer or sum is *21* (7 + 7 + 7 = 21). If the number *7* is multiplied by *3*, the answer or product is *21* (7 × 3 = 21). A few examples of how multiplication is used in health care include:

- Maintaining payroll records including hours worked and salary earned
- Performing laboratory tests
- Determining the magnification power of a microscope
- Calculating prescription amounts such as the number of pills a patient should receive for a 30-day supply of medication
- Calculating caloric requirement based on body weight

To multiply whole numbers, write the number to be multiplied *(multiplicand)* first. If possible, use the largest number as the multiplicand. Under the multiplicand, write the number of times it is to be multiplied *(multiplier)*, making sure the numbers are lined up on the right side. Then multiply every number in the multiplicand by every number in the multiplier. After all of the multipliers are used, the products obtained are added together to get the answer.

Example 1: A pharmacy technician is preparing a prescription for a patient. The physician ordered a dosage of 2 tablets after meals and at bedtime every day. How many tablets should the technician dispense for a 30-day supply of the medication?

First it is necessary to determine how many tablets the patient would require each day. The patient would take 2 tablets of the medication 4 times daily, once after 3 meals and once at bedtime.

$$\begin{array}{r} 2 \\ \times 4 \\ \hline 8 \end{array}$$

The patient needs 8 tablets a day for 30 days.

$$\begin{array}{r} 30 \\ \times\ \ 8 \\ \hline 240 \end{array}$$

Answer: The pharmacy technician would dispense 240 tablets of the medication to the patient.

Example 2: A medical laboratory technician is preparing agar slant tubes. The tubes are used to grow microorganisms so the cause of a disease can be identified. The technician needs a total of 24 tubes. For each tube, 30 milliliters (mL) of broth and 15 mL of agar is needed (Figure 13–2). What is the total amount of broth needed and the total amount of agar needed?

$$\begin{array}{r} 30 \\ \times\ 24 \\ \hline 120 \\ +\ 60\ \ \\ \hline 720 \end{array} \qquad \begin{array}{r} 15 \\ \times\ 24 \\ \hline 60 \\ +\ 30\ \ \\ \hline 360 \end{array}$$

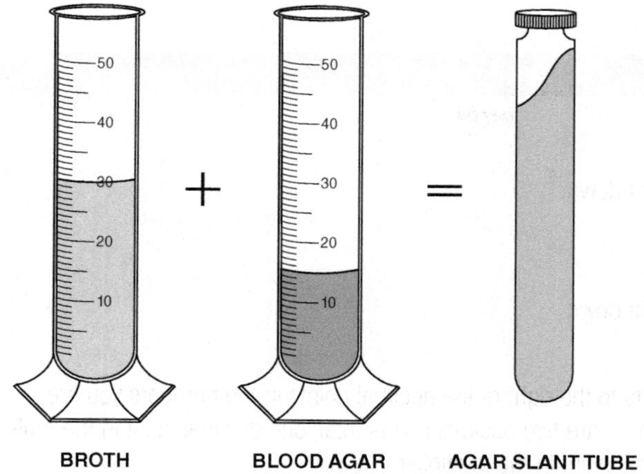

FIGURE 13–2 How much broth and agar is needed to fill 24 agar slant tubes?

Answer: The laboratory technician needs 720 mL of broth and 360 mL of agar to prepare 24 agar slant tubes.

DIVISION OF WHOLE NUMBERS

Division is a simple method used to determine how many times one number is present in another number. A few examples of how division is used in health care include:

- Calculating diets and amounts of nutrients allowed
- Determining cost per item while ordering bulk supplies or equipment
- Performing laboratory tests
- Compiling statistics on diseases and death rates
- Calculating budgets and salaries

Division involves the use of two numbers: a dividend and a divisor. The number to be divided is the *dividend.* The *divisor* is the number of times the dividend is to be divided. It is important to position these numbers correctly to obtain an answer, or *quotient.*

Example: A student doing research learns that statistics show 569,484 people die of cancer each year. On average, how many people die of cancer each month? (*Hint:* Remember that there are 12 months in a year.)

```
       4 7 4 5 7
 1 2 √ 5 6 9 4 8 4
     - 4 8
       8 9
     - 8 4
         5 4
       - 4 8
           6 8
         - 6 0
             8 4
           - 8 4
               0
```

Answer: On average, 47,457 people die of cancer each month.

Decimals

Decimals are one way of expressing parts of numbers or anything else that has been divided into parts. The parts are expressed in units of 10. That is, decimals represent the number of tenths, hundredths, thousandths, and so on that are available. For example, 0.7 represents 7 of the 10 parts into which something has been divided. When reading decimals verbally, it is necessary to know the place values for the decimals (digits to the right of the decimal point) and that the decimal point is read as "and" (Figure 13–3). For example:

- 0.5 is read "five tenths"
- 1.5 is read "one and five tenths"
- 1.50 is read "one and fifty hundredths"
- 1.500 is read "one and five hundred thousandths"
- 1.5000 is read "one and five thousand ten thousandths"

Note that a zero is placed to the left of the decimal point if the number begins to the right of the point. This is necessary to prevent errors from occurring if the decimal point is not seen.

Decimals are added, subtracted, multiplied, and divided in the same way as whole numbers. The most common mistake is incorrect placement of the decimal point (Table 13–1).

A few examples of how decimals are used in health care include:

- Determining medication dosages
- Performing laboratory tests
- Calculating dietary requirements or restrictions
- Measuring respiratory function
- Maintaining payroll records

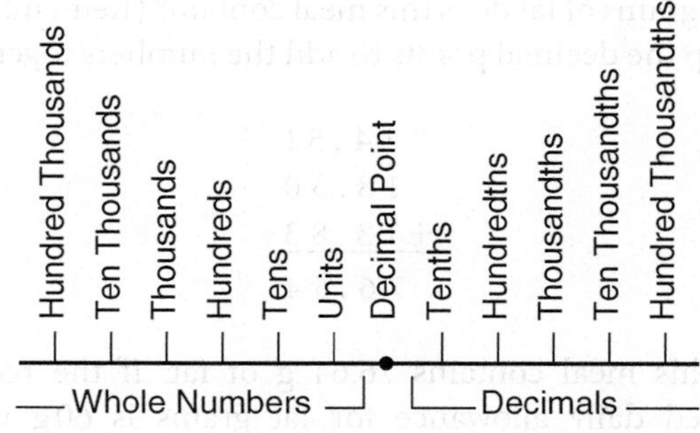

FIGURE 13–3 The position of the number to the left or the right of the decimal point is its place value. The value of each place left of the decimal point is 10 times that of the place to its right. The value of each place right of the decimal point is one-tenth the value of the place to its left.

TABLE 13–1 Working with Decimals

Function	Example	Key Points
Add: (+)	1.5 + 2.25 3.75	1. Line up the decimal points. 2. Add the numbers. 3. Bring the decimal point straight down.
Subtract: (−)	3.75 − 1.25 2.50	1. Line up the decimal points. 2. Subtract the numbers. 3. Bring the decimal point straight down.
Multiply: (×)	2.5 × 2.5 125 + 50 6.25	1. Multiply the numbers. 2. Count the total number of digits to the right of the decimal points in the numbers you are multiplying. In this example, there are two decimal points total, one decimal point in the multiplicand of 2.5 and one decimal point in the multiplier of 2.5. 3. Count the same number of places in your answers. Start to the right of the last digit in your answer and move that number of places to the left. This is where the decimal point is placed. In this example, the decimal point was moved two places to the left.
Divide: (÷)	2.5)50.5 25.)505.0 20.2 25)505.0 50 5 −0 50 50 0	1. Move the decimal point to the right in the number you are dividing by (divisor) to make it a whole number. In this example, the decimal point is moved one place to the right to change 2.5 to 25. 2. Move the decimal point the same number of places to the right in the number being divided (dividend). Add zeros if necessary. In this example, the decimal point in the dividend is moved one place to the right (50.5 to 505.0) because the decimal point was moved one place to the right in the divisor. 3. Divide the numbers. 4. Place the decimal point in the answer by moving it straight up from the dividend, or number that was divided.

- Billing charges on patient accounts
- Determining exposure to radiation
- Totaling the cost of supplies and equipment orders

Example: A dietitian is teaching teenagers about the high levels of fat in fast food. She notes that there are 44.51 grams (g) of fat in a bacon cheese-burger, 18.3 g in a large serving of fries, and 13.83 g in a milkshake. How many grams of fat does this meal contain? (Remember to line up the decimal points to add the numbers together.)

```
  44.51
  18.30
+13.83
  76.64
```

This meal contains 76.64 g of fat. If the recommended daily allowance for fat grams is 60 g in an 1,800-calorie diet, how many extra grams of fat are present in just this one meal? To solve this, subtract the recommended daily allowance from the total number of fat grams in the meal. Add zeros to the right of the decimal point to make it easier to subtract the numbers.

```
  76.64
− 60.00
  16.64
```

Answer: This fast-food meal contains 76.64 g of fat, which is 16.64 g more than is recommended for an entire day of meals.

Fractions

Fractions are another way of expressing numbers that represent parts of a whole. A few examples of how fractions are used in health care include:

- Measuring solutions for laboratory tests
- Calculating height and weight
- Measuring head circumference on an infant
- Mixing solutions such as disinfectants for infection control

- Preparing dental materials and trimming dental models
- Mixing infant formulas or tube feedings
- Calculating dosages for certain medications

A fraction has a *numerator* (top number) and a *denominator* (bottom number). An example of a fraction is $\frac{3}{10}$, where 3 is the numerator and 10 is the denominator.

The 3 tells how many parts are present. The 10 tells how many parts make up the whole (Figure 13–4). The fraction $\frac{3}{10}$ has been *reduced* to its lowest terms because no number can be divided evenly into both the numerator and denominator.

Some fractions must be *reduced* to their lowest terms. An example is $\frac{4}{8}$. Both the numerator and denominator can be divided evenly by $4: 4 \div 4 = 1$ and $8 \div 4 = 2$. As a result, $\frac{4}{8} = \frac{1}{2}$.

Improper fractions have numerators that are larger than the denominators. To reduce these fractions, divide the denominator into the numerator. The result will be a whole number or a mixed number (whole number and a fraction). For example:

- The fraction $\frac{12}{4}$ would be reduced to the whole number 3 ($12 \div 4 = 3$)
- The fraction $\frac{11}{4}$ would be reduced to the mixed number $2\frac{3}{4}$ ($11 \div 4 = 2\frac{3}{4}$)

Performing calculations with fractions is not difficult, but it does require following a series of steps. These are described in Table 13–2. When adding and subtracting fractions, it is necessary to change all the denominators to the same number to perform the calculations. This is known as *converting the fractions*. To do this, find a number that each denominator can divide into evenly. Then adjust the numerators to maintain an equivalent fraction. For example, to add $\frac{1}{2} + \frac{1}{3}$, convert both fractions to sixths $= \frac{3}{6} + \frac{2}{6} = \frac{5}{6}$. The denominators 2 and 3 both divide into 6 evenly, so 6 is the new denominator. Then multiply the numerator by the number of times the old denominator divides into the new denominator (2 divides into 6 three times, so 1×3 then creates the new fraction of $\frac{3}{6}$; 3 divides into 6 two times, so 1×2 then creates the new fraction of $\frac{2}{6}$).

Multiplying fractions is straightforward. First multiply the two numerators and then the two denominators. For example, $\frac{2}{3} \times \frac{2}{5}$ is $\frac{4}{15}$ ($2 \times 2 = 4$ and $3 \times 5 = 15$).

Dividing fractions requires the dividing fraction to be *inverted* (turned upside down). The new, upside-down fraction is called the **reciprocal**. The numerators and denominators are then multiplied to get the answer. For example, $\frac{1}{2} \div \frac{2}{3} = \frac{1}{2} \times \frac{3}{2} = \frac{3}{4}$.

Study the examples in Table 13–2 to see how to add, subtract, multiply, and divide fractions. Then review these examples:

Example 1: A dental assistant has $\frac{1}{2}$ ounce of disinfectant solution in one bottle and $\frac{2}{3}$ ounce in a second bottle. Can the two bottles be combined in a $1\frac{1}{2}$-ounce bottle? To solve this, add $\frac{1}{2}$ and $\frac{2}{3}$ together using the following steps:

First think of a number that both *2* and *3* divide into evenly. The answer is 6.

$$6 \div 2 = 3 \qquad 6 \div 3 = 2$$

Then multiply the numerator by the number of times the old denominator goes into 6.

$$1 \times 3 = 3 \quad \frac{1}{2} = \frac{3}{6}$$
$$2 \times 2 = 4 \quad \frac{2}{3} = \frac{4}{6}$$

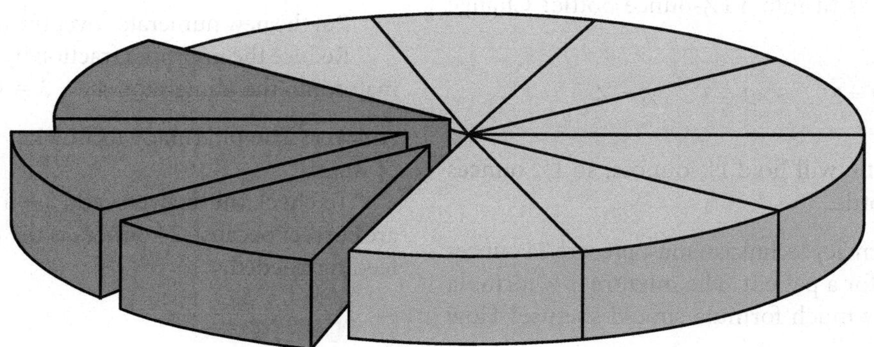

$$\frac{\text{Part or Numerator}}{\text{Whole or Denominator}} = \frac{3}{10}$$

FIGURE 13–4 A fraction is a comparison of parts (numerator) to a whole (denominator).

TABLE 13–2 Working with Fractions

Function	Example	Key Points
Add: (+)	$\frac{1}{5}=\frac{6}{30}$ $+\frac{1}{6}=\frac{5}{30}$ $=\frac{11}{30}$	1. If the denominators are not the same, find a number both denominators divide into evenly. 2. Multiply the numerators by the number of times the old denominators divide into the new denominator. 3. Add the numerators. 4. Place the new numerator over the denominator. 5. Reduce the fraction, if necessary.
Subtract: (−)	$\frac{1}{5}=\frac{6}{30}$ $-\frac{1}{6}=\frac{5}{30}$ $=\frac{1}{30}$	1. If the denominators are not the same, find a number both denominators divide into evenly. 2. Multiply the numerators by the number of times the old denominators divide into the new denominator. 3. Subtract the numerators. 4. Place the new numerator over the denominator. 5. Reduce the fraction, if necessary.
Multiply: (×)	$\frac{1}{5}\times\frac{1}{6}=\frac{1}{30}$	1. Multiply numerators. 2. Multiply denominators. 3. Reduce the fraction, if necessary.
Divide: (÷)	$\frac{1}{5}\div\frac{1}{6}=\frac{1}{5}\times\frac{6}{1}=\frac{6}{5}=1\frac{1}{5}$	1. Invert the dividing fraction. 2. Multiply numerators. 3. Multiply denominators. 4. Reduce the fraction, if necessary.

Now add the two numerators together and place the answer over the common denominator.

$$3/6 + 4/6 = 7/6$$

The fraction $7/6$ is an improper fraction because the numerator is larger than the denominator. Divide the denominator into the numerator.

$$7 \div 6 = 1\,1/6 \text{ ounces}$$

Will $1\,1/6$ ounces fit into a $1\,1/2$-ounce bottle? Change the $1/2$ to sixths.

$$6 \div 2 = 3 \qquad 3 \times 1 = 3 \qquad 1/2 = 3/6$$

Answer: The bottle will hold $1\,3/6$ ounces, so $1\,1/6$ ounces will fit into the bottle.

Example 2: A pharmacy technician must prepare 24 ounces of a tube feeding for a patient. The mixture is $1/3$ formula and $2/3$ water. How much formula should she use? How much water?

To determine the amount of formula, multiply 24 (write as the fraction $24/1$) by $1/3$:

$$24/1 \times 1/3 = ?$$

Multiply the numerators: $24 \times 1 = 24$.
Multiply the denominators: $1 \times 3 = 3$

Put the new numerator over the new denominator: $24/3$.
Reduce the improper fraction by dividing the denominator into the numerator: $24 \div 3 = 8$.

Answer: The pharmacy technician will need 8 ounces of formula. To determine the amount of water, multiply 24 by $2/3$:

$$24/1 \times 2/3 = ?$$

Multiply the numerators: $24 \times 2 = 48$.
Multiply the denominators: $3 \times 1 = 3$.
Put the new numerator over the new denominator: $48/3$.
Reduce the improper fraction by dividing the denominator into the numerator: $48 \div 3 = 16$.

Answer: The pharmacy technician will need 16 ounces of water.

To check the answers, add $8 + 16 = 24$. The answers are correct because 24 ounces is the total amount of tube feeding needed.

Percentages

Percentages are used to express either a whole or part of a whole. The whole is expressed as 100 percent (100%). Refer to Figure 13–4 and imagine this as a hot apple pie sliced into 10 equal pieces. The 10 slices together equal the whole, or 100%, of the pie. 100 divided by 10 equals 10. Therefore, each slice represents 10% of the pie. If each slice is 10%, then three slices represent 30% of the pie.

A few examples of how percentages are used in health care include:

- Recording statistics such as the percentage of people who die of lung cancer
- Preparing solutions for laboratory tests
- Mixing solutions for infection control such as a 10 percent bleach solution
- Calculating the amount of tax that must be subtracted from a salary check
- Determining dietary requirements or calculating special (therapeutic) diets

When working with percentages, it is easier to convert the percentage to a decimal and then perform the addition, subtraction, multiplication, and division. Converting percentages to decimals is explained in Table 13–3.

Look at the pie chart in Figure 13–5 that shows emergency department admissions for a one-month period. Then use this information to find the answers to the following questions on percentages.

Example 1: What is the total percentage of people admitted due to heart attacks or respiratory problems?

The percentage admitted for heart attacks was 11.8%.

The percentage admitted for respiratory problems was 8.8%.

These two percentages can be added together by lining up the decimal points:

$$\begin{array}{r} 11.8\% \\ +\ 8.8\% \\ \hline 20.6\% \end{array}$$

Answer: 20.6 percent of the people were admitted with heart attacks or respiratory problems.

Example 2: If a total of 364 patients were admitted to the emergency department during the one-month period, how many people were admitted because of an auto accident?

Check the pie chart: 26.1 percent of the admissions were for auto accidents.

TABLE 13–3 Converting Decimals, Fractions, and Percentages

Converting	Example	Key Points
Decimals to fractions	0.75 = 75/100 $\frac{75}{100} = \frac{75}{100} \div \frac{25}{25} = \frac{3}{4}$	1. Drop the decimal point. 2. Position the number over its placement value (Figure 13–3). 3. If necessary, reduce the fraction.
Decimals to percentages	5.275 = 5.275 × 100 = 527.5 527.5%	1. Move the decimal point two places to the right because percentages are based on 100. This is the same as multiplying by 100. 2. Add the percentage sign.
Fractions to decimals	3/5 = 3 ÷ 5 = 0.6	1. Divide the numerator by the denominator.
Fractions to percentages	7/8 = 7 ÷ 8 = 0.875 0.875 × 100 = 87.5 87.5%	1. Divide the numerator by the denominator. 2. Move the decimal point two places to the right because percentages are based on 100. This is the same as multiplying by 100. 3. Add the percentage sign.
Percentages to decimals	125.5% = 125.5 125.5 ÷ 100 = 1.255	1. Remove the percentage sign. 2. Move the decimal point two places to the left because percentages are based on 100. This is the same as dividing by 100.
Percentages to fractions	5% = 5 $\frac{5}{100} = \frac{5 \div 5}{100 \div 5} = \frac{1}{20}$	1. Remove the percentage sign. 2. Place the number over 100. 3. If appropriate, reduce the fraction to its lowest terms.
Percentages to ratios	75% = 75 75:100	1. Remove the percentage sign. 2. Create a ratio using the former percentage and the number 100. 3. Insert a colon (:) between the numbers.
Ratios to percentages	1:2 = 1 ÷ 2 = 0.5 0.5 × 100 = 50 50 = 50%	1. Divide the number on the left of the colon or ratio sign by the number on the right of the ratio sign. 2. Move the decimal point two places to the right. Add zero(s) if necessary. This is the same as multiplying by 100. 3. Add the percentage sign.

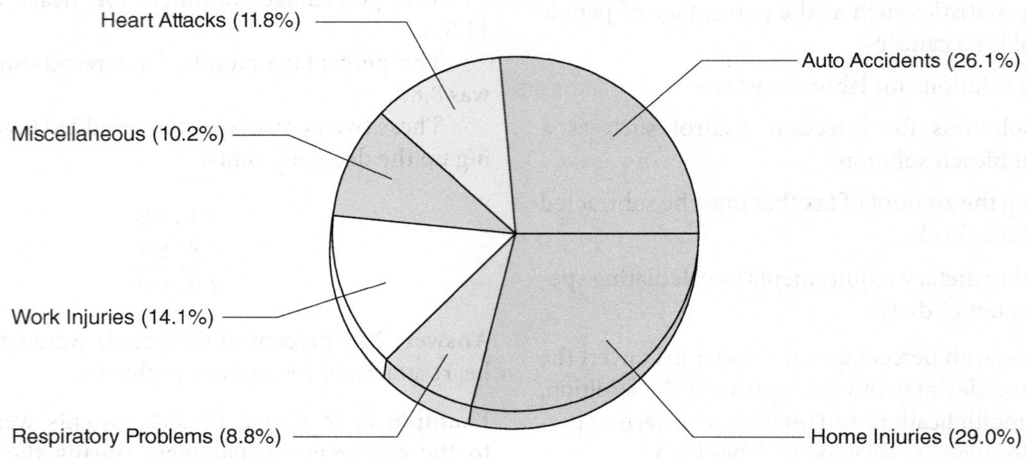

FIGURE 13–5 Causes for emergency department admissions in a one-month period.

First convert the 26.1 percent to decimals:

26.1% = 26.1 (Remove percent sign)

26.1 ÷ 100 = 0.261 (Divide by 100 to convert to a decimal)

Now multiply the total number of patients, or 364, by 0.261:

```
      3 6 4
  × 0 . 2 6 1
      3 6 4
    2 1 8 4
    7 2 8
    9 5 0 0 4. = 95.004 = 95
```

Starting at the right side, move the decimal point the same number of places to the left as it is in the multiplier. Because 0.261 has three decimal places, 95.004 is the correct answer.

Answer: A total of 95 people were admitted to the emergency department because of auto accidents. Note that the *4* at the end of the answer was ignored. When percentages are calculated, answers are often rounded to whole numbers.

Ratios

Ratios show relationships between numbers or like values: how many of one number or value is present as compared with the other. For example, a bleach and water solution with a 1:2 ratio means that one part of bleach is added for every two parts of water. This relationship applies regardless of the units used:

- 1 cup of bleach and 2 cups of water
- 1 quart of bleach and 2 quarts of water
- ½ cup of bleach and 1 cup of water
- ¼ cup of bleach and ½ cup of water

The use of ratios to express the strength of a solution is commonly seen in health care. Solution strengths are also frequently expressed as percentages. A 50-percent bleach solution is the same as the 1:2 ratio. Conversions between ratios and percentages are explained in the next section.

Converting Decimals, Fractions, Percentages, and Ratios

Decimals, fractions, and percentages all express parts of a whole. The cartoon in Figure 13–1 humorously portrayed how they are related: the fraction ½, the decimal 0.5, and the percentage 50% all represent the same amount of the sandwich. The steps used to convert between these numerical forms are shown in Table 13–3.

Rounding Numbers

Rounding numbers means changing them to the nearest ten, hundred, thousand, and so on. Deciding which to use depends on the size of the original number and the degree of accuracy required. Deciding whether to round up or round down depends on the digits (numbers) located to the right of the value chosen for rounding. The following examples illustrate how these rules are applied:

Example 1: When rounding to the nearest 10: look at the digit to the right of the tens place (the ones place). If the number is 5 or greater, round up. If it is less than 5, round down.

8<u>8</u> rounds up to 90
8<u>3</u> rounds down to 80

TABLE 13–4 **Rounding Numbers**

Round the Number 1,234.5678 to the Nearest:	Result	Comments
Whole number	1,234.5678 = 1,235	The digit to the right of the whole number (1,234) is 5, so you round up one number.
Tens	1,234.5678 = 1,230	The digit to the right of the tens place is 4, so you round down.
Hundreds	1,234.5678 = 1,200	The digit to the right of the hundreds place is 3, so you round down.
Thousands	1,234.5678 = 1,000	The digit to the right of the thousands place is 2, so you round down.
Tenths	1,234.5678 = 1,234.6	The digit to the right of the tenths place is 6, so you round up.
Hundredths	1,234.5678 = 1,234.57	The digit to the right of the hundredths place is 7, so you round up.
Thousandths	1,234.5678 = 1,234.568	The digit to the right of the thousandths place is 8, so you round up.
Ten thousandths	1,234.56780 = 1,234.5678	No change.

Example 2: When rounding to the nearest 100, look at the digit to the right of the hundreds place (the tens place). If the number is 5 or greater, round up. If it is less than 5, round down.

67 rounds up to 100
133 rounds down to 100
668 rounds up to 700
621 rounds down to 600

Example 3: When rounding to the nearest 1,000, look at the digit to the right of the thousands place (the hundreds place). If the number is 5 or greater, round up. If it is less than 5, round down.

7777 rounds up to 8,000
7355 rounds down to 7,000

All numbers can be rounded. Review Figure 13–3 and study the examples in Table 13–4.

Solving Problems with Proportions

A **proportion** is a statement of equality between two ratios. For example, the proportion 2:6 = 3:9 means that 2 is related to 6 in the same way that 3 is related to 9. It is verbalized as "two is to six as three is to nine."

Proportions are used to solve many math problems in health care. Some common examples include:

- Calculating height to feet and inches
- Calculating weight to pounds and ounces
- Determining the proper dosage of a medicine
- Calculating a flow rate for IV (intravenous, or into a vein) solutions
- Determining measurements to mix solutions
- Interpreting laboratory test results

Proportions are useful for determining an amount needed when three of the terms in the proportion are known.

Example 1: A pharmacy technician has to prepare 500 milliliters (mL) of a 5% boric acid solution. How many grams (g) of boric acid crystals will he use?

First calculate that a 5% boric acid solution equals 0.05 or 5/100 or 5:100 or 5 g of boric acid in every 100 mL of solution. Three of the terms in the proportion are known:

- 5 g of boric acid crystal
- 100 mL of solution
- 500 mL of solution required

The proportion is set up as follows:

$$\frac{5\text{ g}}{x\text{ g}} = \frac{100\text{ mL}}{500\text{ mL}}$$

Note that the unit measurements on each side of the equation are the same (grams per milliliters).

To solve this problem, follow these steps:

Cross multiply:

$$\frac{5\text{ g}}{x\text{ g}} = \frac{100\text{ mL}}{500\text{ mL}}$$

$$5 \times 500 = 100 \times x \qquad 2{,}500 = 100\,x$$

Divide each side by the number in front of x:

$$100x \div 100 = x \text{ and } 2{,}500 \div 100 = 25$$

$$x = 25\text{g}$$

The complete proportion is:

$$\frac{5\text{ g}}{25\text{ g}} = \frac{100\text{ mL}}{500\text{ mL}}$$

Answer: The pharmacy technician must use 25 g of boric acid crystals to prepare 500 mL of a 5% boric acid solution.

Converting units of measurement is another common application of proportions. When a patient's height is measured, the height bar on most medical scales provides the measurement in inches. This must be converted to feet and inches.

Example 2: A medical assistant measures the height of a small child at 36 inches. How many feet are in 36 inches? Three of the terms in the proportion are known:

- 36 inches
- 12 (the number of inches in 1 foot)
- 1 foot

The proportion is set up as follows:

$$\frac{1 \text{ foot}}{x \text{ feet}} = \frac{12 \text{ inches}}{36 \text{ inches}}$$

To solve this problem, follow these steps:
Cross multiply:

$$\frac{1 \text{ foot}}{x \text{ feet}} \gtrless \frac{12 \text{ inches}}{36 \text{ inches}}$$

$$12 \times x = 1 \times 36 \qquad 12x = 36$$

Divide each side by the number in front of x:

$$12x \div 12 = x \text{ and } 36 \div 12 = 3$$

$$x = 3 \text{ feet}$$

The completed proportion is:

$$\frac{1 \text{ foot}}{3 \text{ feet}} = \frac{12 \text{ inches}}{36 \text{ inches}}$$

Answer: The small child is 3 feet tall.

Note: *If a child is 38 inches tall, 12 would divide into 38 three times with a remainder of 2. The child's height would be recorded as 3 feet, 2 inches tall.*

Another common application of proportions in health care is to find the value of an unknown when calculating the dosage of medications.

Example 3: A physician orders a patient to have 50 milligrams (mg) of a medication. When the nurse checks, he notes that the medication is only available in 12.5-mg tablets. How many tablets should he give the patient?

Set up the proportion with the three known facts:

$$\frac{1 \text{ tablet}}{x \text{ tablets}} = \frac{12.5 \text{ mg}}{50 \text{ mg}}$$

Cross multiply:

$$\frac{1 \text{ tablet}}{x \text{ tablets}} \gtrless \frac{12.5 \text{ mg}}{50 \text{ mg}}$$

$$12.5 \times x = 1 \times 50 \qquad 12.5x = 50$$

Divide each side by the number in front of x:

$$12.5x \div 12.5 = x \text{ and } 50 \div 12.5 = 4$$

$$x = 4 \text{ tablets}$$

The completed proportion is:

$$\frac{1 \text{ tablet}}{4 \text{ tablets}} = \frac{12.5 \text{ mg}}{50 \text{ mg}}$$

Answer: 4 tablets are needed to equal 50 mg.

Example 4: A pharmacy technician reviews a prescription that orders amoxicillin suspension 300 milligrams (mg) by mouth three times a day. The amoxicillin suspension that is available is labeled 400 mg/2 mL. How many mL must be dispensed for a 10-day supply?

First calculate the amount of amoxicillin that is required for a single dose. Three of the terms in the proportion are known:

- 300 mg of amoxicillin
- 400 mg of amoxicillin
- 2 mL of suspension

The proportion is set up as follows:

$$\frac{400 \text{ mg}}{300 \text{ mg}} = \frac{2 \text{ mL}}{x \text{ mL}}$$

To solve this problem, follow these steps:

Cross multiply:

$$\frac{400 \text{ mg}}{300 \text{ mg}} \gtrless \frac{2 \text{ mL}}{x \text{ mL}}$$

$$2 \times 300 = 400 \times x \qquad 600 = 400x$$

Divide each side by the number in front of x:

$$400x \div 400 = x \text{ and } 600 \div 400 = 1.5$$

$$x = 1.5 \text{ mL}$$

The complete proportion is:

$$\frac{400 \text{ mg}}{300 \text{ mg}} = \frac{2 \text{ mL}}{1.5 \text{ mL}}$$

Answer: The amount of amoxicillin required for a single dose of 300 mg is 1.5 mL.

Now calculate the number of mL needed per day. Since the patient is taking the medication 3 times a day, multiply by 3:

$$3 \times 1.5 \text{ mL} = 4.5 \text{ mL}$$

Finally calculate how many mL will be needed for a 10-day supply. Multiply the 4.5 mL daily dose by 10:

$$10 \times 4.5 \text{ mL} = 45 \text{ mL}$$

Answer: The pharmacy technician must dispense 45 mL of the amoxicillin suspension for a 10-day supply.

13:2 Estimating

Health care workers must work carefully and thoughtfully when performing calculations. An important skill to help check work is anticipating the results. This involves **estimating**—calculating the approximate answer—and judging if the calculated results seem reasonable. If calculations are performed without thought and answers simply accepted, errors can go unnoticed. It is easy for mistakes to occur when you're working in a hurry. Numbers can be placed in the wrong order, decimal points misplaced, or operations carried out incorrectly. Knowing when an answer "just doesn't look right" serves as an alert to double-check the results. Working on "automatic pilot" is not acceptable when using math in the workplace.

Learning to estimate and detect incorrect answers takes practice and thought. There are a few guidelines to make estimating useful. First, use rounding to get numbers that are easier to mentally compute.

- For example, when multiplying 47 times 83, round 47 up to 50 and 83 down to 80. Multiplying 50 times 80 is much easier to multiply mentally than the original numbers.
- Second, watch place values carefully. In the 50 times 80 example, if 5 is multiplied times 8, two zeros must be added to the quick result of 40. This means the result must be approximately 4,000, *not* 40 or 400.
- Third, look at the size of the answer. Does it make sense? For example, when multiplying whole numbers, the answer should be larger than either of the numbers in the problem. When dividing numbers, it should be smaller.
- Fourth, be careful about placing decimal points. Remember that everything to the right of the point is a fraction. Even 0.99999 does not equal 1.0.

Estimates can also be useful in planning at health care agencies. For example, an estimate can be made for the approximate number of slides a cytologist (an individual who studies cells on slides) could examine in an 8-hour day. If a cytologist examines 12 slides the first hour, 16 slides the second hour, 11 slides the third hour, and 14 slides the fourth hour, an average number of slides per hour can be calculated. By adding the four numbers together and dividing by 4, an average of 13.25 slides per hour is the result. In an 8-hour period, the cytologist could examine 106 (8×13.25) slides. This estimate could be used to plan the daily workload of the cytologist. This does not mean that the cytologist will examine 106 slides in one day. She may examine more or fewer slides. However, the estimate is a good approximation of what could occur and allows the health care agency to determine employees needed and workloads that can be completed.

13:3 Roman Numerals

The traditional numbering system we use every day is referred to as Arabic numerals (1, 2, 3, . . .). In health care, it is necessary to know Roman numerals because they are used for some medications, solutions, and ordering systems. You may also see some files or materials organized using Roman numerals. When using **Roman numerals**, remember the following key points:

- All numbers can be expressed by using seven key numerals:

  I = 1

  V = 5

  X = 10

  L = 50

  C = 100

  D = 500

  M = 1000

- If a smaller numeral is placed in front of a larger numeral, the smaller numeral is *subtracted* from the larger numeral. For example:

  IV = 1 is placed before the 5, so it is subtracted ($5 - 1 = 4$)

- If a smaller numeral is placed after a larger numeral, the smaller numeral is *added* to the larger numeral. For example:

  VI = 1 is placed after the 5, so it is added ($5 + 1 = 6$)

- When the same numeral is placed next to itself it is added. For example:

  III = $1 + 1 + 1 = 3$

  XX = $10 + 10 = 20$

  XIX = this has two of the same numerals with a smaller numeral in the middle, but the rules still apply ($10 + 10 - 1 = 19$ OR $10 + (10 - 1) = 10 + 9 = 19$)

- The same numeral is *not* placed next to itself more than three times. For example:

  XXX = 30

  XL = 40 (XXXX is not correct)

  To express 40, subtract 10 from the 50 symbol to get XL

- When Roman numerals are used with medication dosages, the lowercase (i, v, x, l, c, d, m) may be used rather than uppercase (capital letters). For example, ii = 2, iv = 4, xix = 19.

Study Table 13–5 to practice converting between Arabic and Roman numerals.

TABLE 13–5 Arabic and Roman Numeral Conversion Chart

Arabic	Roman	Arabic	Roman
1	I	23	XXIII
2	II	24	XXIV
3	III	25	XXV
4	IV	26	XXVI
5	V	27	XXVII
6	VI	28	XXVIII
7	VII	29	XXIX
8	VIII	30	XXX
9	IX	40	XL
10	X	50	L
20	XX	100	C
21	XXI	500	D
22	XXII	1000	M

13:4 Angles

Angles are used in health care when injecting medications, describing joint movement, and indicating bed positions. **Angles** are always defined by comparison to a **reference plane**, a real or imaginary flat surface from which the angle is measured. The distance between the plane and the line of the angle is measured in units called **degrees**. For example, if a flat stick is placed on a table (the reference plane), the angle is at 0 degrees. If the stick is moved to a straight up position (perpendicular to the table), there is a 90-degree angle to the table. Moving the stick halfway between these two positions creates a 45-degree angle. Rotating the stick all the way around the arc and returning to the reference point creates a complete circle and represents 360 degrees (Figure 13–6). The following examples illustrate how angles are used in health care:

Example 1: Angles for injecting needles vary, depending on the type of medication or procedure being performed (Figure 13–7). Note that in this case the reference plane is the surface of the skin.

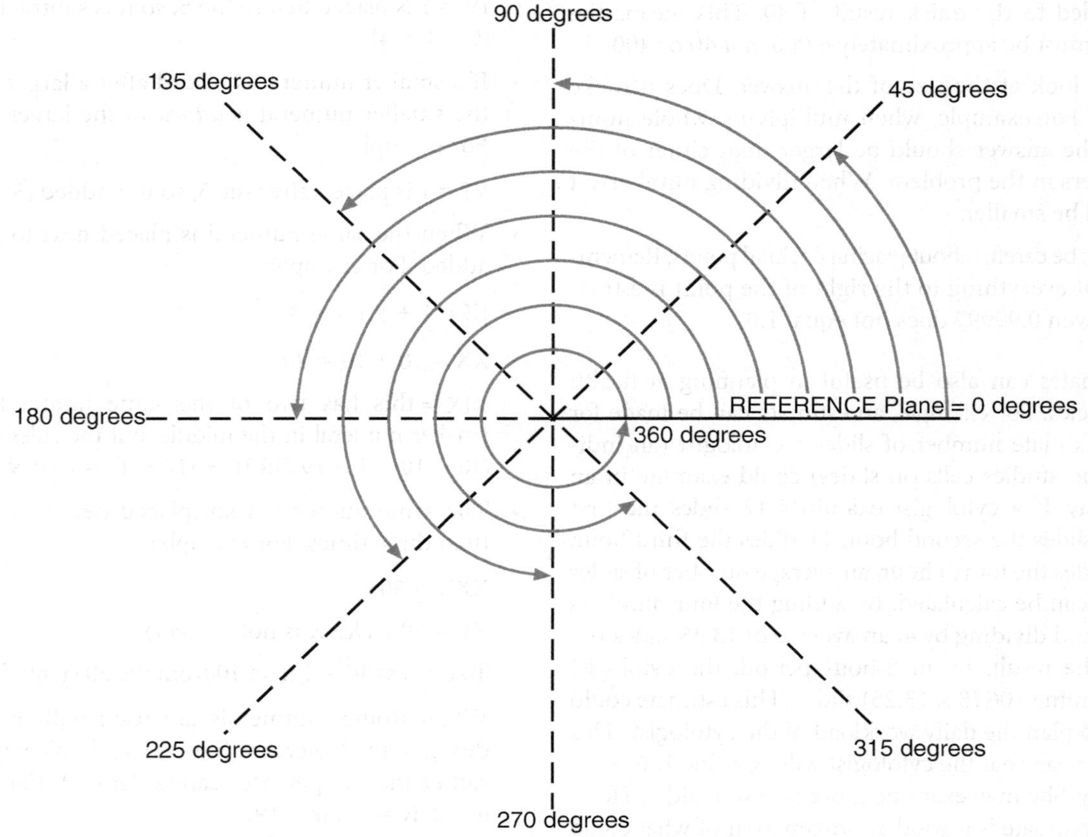

FIGURE 13–6 All angles are expressed in relation to a real or imaginary reference plane.

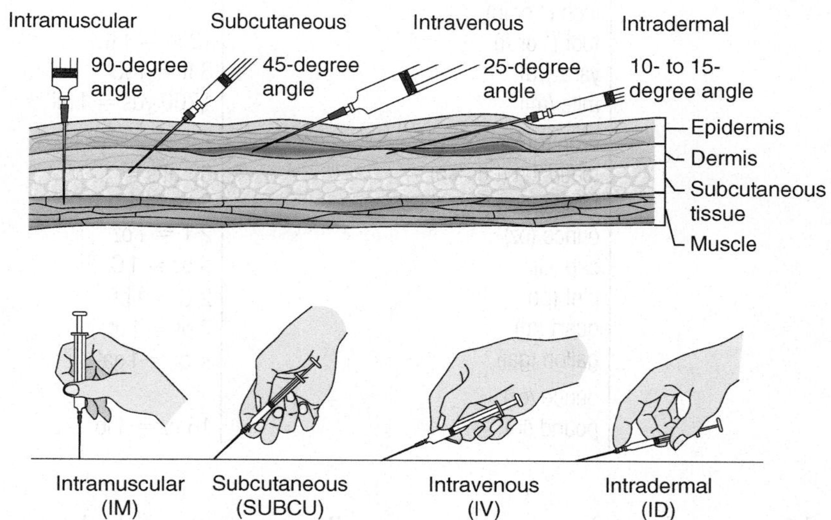

FIGURE 13–7 **The correct angle must be used when inserting needles for administration of injections.**

Example 2: When describing the angle of extremities (arms and legs), the body in a full upright position is the reference plane (Figure 13–8). Each joint (e.g., elbow, knee, hip) in the body has a normal range it is intended to move within. Physicians, physical therapists, physician's assistants, certified nurse practitioners, and other qualified professionals may assess the range of a patient's joint compared with this normal range to chart loss of function or progress of recovery.

Example 3: After surgery on a joint (e.g., hip or knee replacement), the physician or other authorized individual will order that the joint not be moved more than a certain number of degrees to prevent the new joint from "popping" out of place.

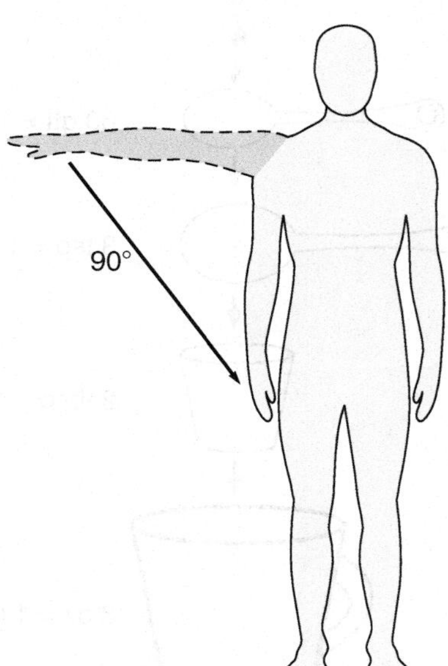

FIGURE 13–8 **Body in full upright position with right arm lifted to 90-degree angle.**

Example 4: Sometimes the physician will order that the head of the bed must be elevated by 30 to 45 degrees at all times. This is usually ordered to aid in respiration or to prevent aspiration (stomach contents entering the lungs). In this situation, the bed in the flat position is the reference plane.

13:5 Systems of Measurement

Basic skills in calculation are applied when learning and using the various systems of measurement used in health care. Each system has its own terminology for designating distance (length), capacity (volume), and mass (weight). Converting between these systems requires the use of the skills presented in this chapter. The three systems used in health care are household, metric, and apothecary. Each system has its own **nomenclature** (method of naming).

Household System

The **household system**, or U.S. customary or English system, is probably the method of measurement most familiar to students who are educated in the United States (Table 13–6). Note that "ounce" is used as both a measurement of capacity/volume and mass/weight. Health care workers use both. Liquids, such as an 8-ounce glass

TABLE 13–6 **Household Measurement System**

Type of Measurement	Nomenclature	Common Equivalents
Distance/Length	inch (″ or in) foot (′ or ft) yard (yd) mile (mi)	12 in = 1 ft 3 ft = 1 yd 1,760 yds = 1 mi
Capacity/Volume	drop (gtt) teaspoon (t or tsp) tablespoon (T or tbsp) ounce (oz) cup (C) pint (pt) quart (qt) gallon (gal)	60 gtts = 1 t 3 t = 1 T 2 T = 1 oz 8 oz = 1 C 2 C = 1 pt 2 pt = 1 qt 4 qt = 1 gal
Mass/Weight	ounce (oz) pound (lb)	16 oz = 1 lb

of water, are measured in terms of capacity or volume. Determining mass or weight, such as with a 6-pound 12-ounce infant, is done by weighing with a scale. The various units of measurements in the household system relate to each other and can be converted among themselves. For example, volume/capacity is measured in drops, teaspoons, tablespoons, ounces, cups, pints, quarts, and gallons. Knowing the equivalencies of these units enables you to calculate each one in terms of the others (Figure 13–9).

When the basic equivalents are known, unknown measurements can be determined using proportions. Suppose that 3 tablespoons of a liquid are needed, but the only measuring device available is a cup marked in ounces (oz). How many ounces are in 3 tablespoons (3 T)? Knowing that 2 T = 1 oz, the proportion would be set up as follows:

$$\frac{2\text{ T}}{3\text{ T}} = \frac{1\text{ oz}}{x\text{ oz}}$$

$$2x = 3$$

$$2x \div 2 = 3 \div 2$$

$$x = 1.5\text{ oz}$$

Answer: There are 1.5 ounces in 3 tablespoons.

The next example involves measurement of height. If a patient is 63 inches tall and asks how many feet that is, the calculation would use the following proportion:

$$\frac{12\text{ inches}}{63\text{ inches}} = \frac{1\text{ foot}}{x\text{ feet}}$$

$$12x = 63$$

$$12x \div 12 = 63 \div 12$$

$$x = 5.25\text{ feet}$$

Because most people do not say they are 5.25 feet tall, the decimal of 0.25 feet can be converted to inches. The following proportion can be used:

$$\frac{1\text{ foot}}{0.25\text{ ft}} = \frac{12\text{ inches}}{x\text{ inches}}$$

Cross multiply:

$$1 \times x = 1x \qquad 12 \times 0.25 = 3$$

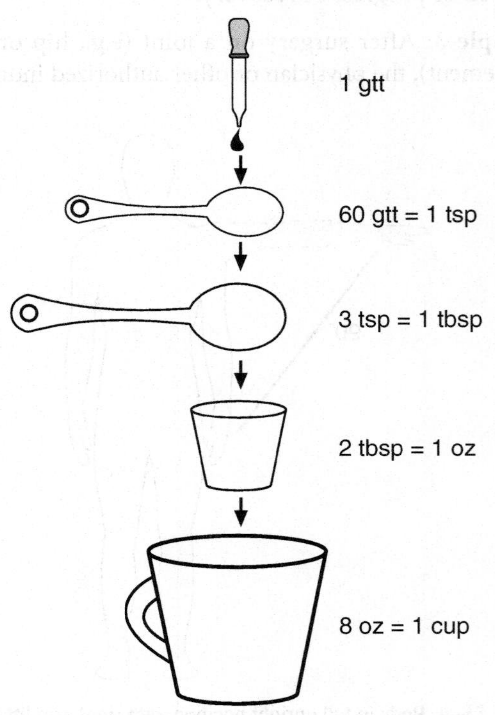

FIGURE 13–9 **Common household measurements used in health care.**

Divide both by 1 to find the value of x:

$$1x \div 1 = x \quad 3 \div 1 = 3$$

The value of x is 3 inches. The patient is 5 feet 3 inches tall.

Metric System

The **metric system**, frequently called the International System of Units or simply SI, is more accurate than the household system. Converting between numbers is easier because everything is based on a unit of 10. The nomenclature for the metric units is as follows:

- Distance/length: meter (m)
- Capacity/volume: liter (L)
- Mass/weight: gram (g)

The meter, liter, and gram are modified by adding the appropriate prefix to express larger or smaller units (Table 13–7).

Because metric units are based on multiples of 10, conversions within the metric system are calculated by multiplying or dividing by 10, 100, 1,000, and so on:

- 1 *kilo*liter = 1,000 × 1 liter = 1,000 liters
- 1 *hecto*liter = 100×1 liter = 100 liters
- 1 *deca*liter = 10 × 1 liter = 10 liters
- 1 *deci*liter = 0.1 × 1 liter = 0.1 liter
- 1 *centi*liter = 0.01 × 1 liter = 0.01 liter
- 1 *milli*liter = 0.001 × 1 liter = 0.001 liter

A shortcut for performing these operations is to move the decimal point the number of places indicated by the prefix. Here are three examples:

Example 1: Multiplying by 10 means moving the decimal point one place to the right. This may require adding one or more zeros. Multiplying 4.2 by 10 = 42. Dividing by 10 means moving the decimal point one place to the left. Dividing 4.2 by 10 = 0.42.

Example 2: Multiplying by 100 means moving the decimal point two places to the right. This may require adding one or more zeros. Multiplying 4.2 by 100 = 420. Dividing by 100 means moving the decimal point two places to the left. Dividing 4.2 by 100 = 0.042.

Example 3: Multiplying by 1,000 means moving the decimal point three places to the right. This may require adding one or more zeros. Multiplying 4.2 by 1,000 = 4,200. Dividing by 1,000 means moving the decimal point three places to the left. Dividing 4.2 by 1,000 = 0.0042.

Converting units within the metric system is accomplished by moving the decimal point. See Figure 13–10 for a visual representation of decimal placement. Examples of how this is used in health care include:

Example 1: A physician orders 2 grams (g) of a medication. The medication is available in 1,000-milligram (mg) tablets. The 2 g must be changed to milligrams. The conversion is made as follows:

- *Milli* is in the third place to the right of *gram.* Move the decimal point three places to the right toward milligrams: 2 = 2,000.
- Change unit name to milligrams: 2,000 milligrams.
- The proper dose would be 2,000 mg, or two 1,000-mg tablets.

Example 2: A physical therapist measures a distance at 1,000 centimeters, but must know the distance in kilometers to check a patient's progress. The conversion is made as follows:

- *Centi* is five decimal places to the right of *kilo,* so move the decimal point five places to the left *toward* kilo. Add zeros as needed: 1,000 = 0.01.

TABLE 13–7 **Common Prefixes of the Metric System**

Prefix	Meaning	Examples	Meaning of Examples
kilo	1,000 times	kilogram kilometer kiloliter	1,000 grams 1,000 meters 1,000 liters
hecto	100 times	hectogram	100 grams
deca (also "deka")	10 times	decaliter	10 liters
meter, liter, gram	Whole units of measurement		
deci	1/10	decigram	1/10 of a gram
centi	1/100	centimeter	1/100 of a meter
milli	1/1,000	milliliter	1/1,000 of a liter
micro	1/1,000,000	microgram	1/1,000,000 of a gram

PREFIX	KILO-	HECTO-	DEKA-	BASE	DECI-	CENTI-	MILLI-	DECIMILLI-	CENTIMILLI-	MICROMILLI-
Common Units	kilogram			gram liter meter		centimeter	milligram milliliter millimeter			microgram
Value to Base	1,000	100	10	1.0	0.1	0.01	0.001	0.0001	0.00001	0.000001

FIGURE 13–10 Comparison of common metric units used in health care.

- Change unit name to kilometers: 0.01 kilometer.
- 1,000 centimeters equals 0.01 kilometer.

In addition to moving the decimal point the correct number of places, it is critical that it be moved in the correct direction. This can be confusing. The easiest way is to determine whether the answer should be a larger or smaller number and then just move the decimal point accordingly:

- If converting from a larger to a smaller prefix (e.g., *kilo* to *milli*), the answer will be larger. It takes more smaller units to make up the larger unit.
- If converting from a smaller to a larger prefix (e.g., *milli* to *kilo*), the answer will be smaller. Many small units can be contained in a smaller number of large units.

A common health care application of the metric system is in the measurement of medications. Two units that represent the same amount are milliliters (mL) and cubic centimeters (cc). Both units measure volume and they are often interchanged when dispensing liquids. For example, 1 mL = 1 cc, 2 mL = 2 cc, and so forth. It is also worth noting that 1 mL or cc has a weight of 1 g (Figure 13–11). In most health care careers, milliliters (mL) are the unit of choice.

Apothecary System

The **apothecary system** is the oldest and least used of the three systems of measurement presented. Even though it is used very infrequently, it is still necessary to be familiar with these units of measurements (Table 13–8). Health care workers must be able to convert within the system as well as to convert to the metric system.

Roman numerals can be used in conjunction with the apothecary system, and may be seen in uppercase or lowercase. If lowercase is used, the Roman numeral for 1 is written with a line and a dot or as $\bar{\text{i}}$. The Roman numeral for 2 is written as $\overline{\text{ii}}$. A commonly used abbreviation that originated with the apothecary system is $\overline{\text{ss}}$, which means "half." For example, 2½ would be written as $\overline{\text{iiss}}$.

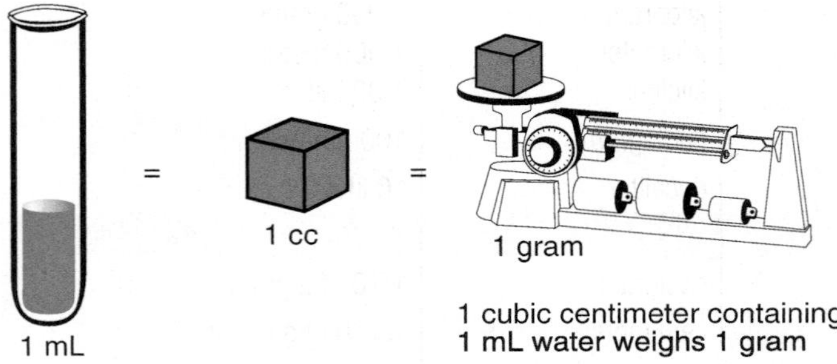

FIGURE 13–11 The metric units that measure weight and volume are related.

DIMENSIONAL ANALYSIS

Dimensional analysis is a systematic problem-solving method. It is often referred to as the problem-solving method of choice because it provides a straightforward way to set up problems, gives a clear understanding of the principles of the problem, helps the learner to organize, visualize and evaluate data, assists in determining whether the setup of the problem is correct, and even confirms that you have arrived at the answer to the problem. It is less prone to errors than solving problems by ratio and proportion method. It is most often used when two quantities are directly proportional to each other in the system of measurements, as in Chemistry. This approach to solving conversion problems works on a **Fraction Method**.

Problem Solving By Dimensional Analysis

There are four elements required in order to use this problem solving method.

1. **Given quantity:** the beginning point of the problem (what is given in the problem)
2. **Required:** what is required as the answer to the problem
3. **Unit path:** What path (road) to take from what is given to what is required. It is the series of conversions necessary to achieve the answer to the problem. There could be more than one pathway.
4. **Conversion factors:** For each of the unit path, there must be a corresponding conversion factor (equivalents necessary to convert between systems of measurement and to allow unwanted units to be cancelled from the problem).

Below is an example of the problem-solving method, showing the placement of basic terms used in dimensional analysis

UNIT PATH

Given Quantity	***Conversion Factor For Given Quantity***	***Conversion Factor For Wanted Quantity***	***Conversion Computation***		***Wanted Quantity***
1 liter (L)	1000 mL	1 oz	1 X 1000 X 1 oz	1000	= 33.3 ounces
	1 liter (L)	30 mL	1 X 30	30	

Once the given quantity is identified, the unit path leading to the wanted quantity is established. The problem-solving method of dimensional analysis can be explained using the following five steps.

1. Identify the *given quantity* in the problem.
2. Identify the *wanted quantity* in the problem.
3. Establish the *unit path* from the given quantity to the wanted quantity using equivalents as *conversions factors.*
4. Set up the problem to permit cancellation of unwanted units.
5. Multiply the numerators, multiply the denominators then divide the product of the numerators by the product of the denominators to provide the numerical value of the wanted quantity.

The following example uses the five steps to solve a problem using dimensional analysis.

EXAMPLE #1: 1 liter (L) equals how many ounces (oz): **OR**
How many ounces are in 1 L?

Step #1: Identify the *given quantity* in the problem.

Need to know: What is the given quantity?

Answer: ***The given quantity is 1 L.***

U N I T P A T H

Given Quantity	*Conversion Factor For Given Quantity*	*Conversion Factor For Wanted Quantity*	*Conversion Computation*			*Wanted Quantity*
1 liter (L)					=	

Step #2: Identify the *wanted quantity* in the problem.

Need to know: What is the wanted quantity?

Answer: ***The wanted quantity is the number of ounces (oz) in 1 L.***

U N I T P A T H

Given Quantity	*Conversion Factor For Given Quantity*	*Conversion Factor For Wanted Quantity*	*Conversion Computation*			*Wanted Quantity*
1 liter (L)					= oz	

THINKING THROUGH THE PROBLEM

Dimensional analysis is a problem-solving method that uses the same terms as fractions, specifically numerators and denominators.

The ***numerator*** = the top portion of the problem

The ***denominator*** = the bottom portion of the problem

Some problems will have a given quantity and a wanted quantity that contain only numerators. Other problems will have a given quantity and a wanted quantity that contain both a numerator and a denominator.

Step #3: Establish the *unit path* from the given quantity to the wanted quantity by selecting the equivalents that will be used as conversion factors.

Need to know: What conversion factors are needed in the unit path that will convert the given quantity to the wanted quantity?

Answer: ***given quantity of 1 L = 1000 mL***
wanted quantity of 1 oz = 30 mL

UNIT PATH

Given Quantity	Conversion Factor For Given Quantity	Conversion Factor For Wanted Quantity	Conversion Computation			Wanted Quantity
1 liter (L)	1000 mL / 1 liter (L)	1 oz / 30 mL				= oz

Step #4: Write the units path for the problem so that each unit cancels out the preceding unit until all unwanted units are canceled from the problem except the wanted quantity.

Need to know: What is the wanted quantity that remains in the unit path after canceling unwanted units?

Answer:

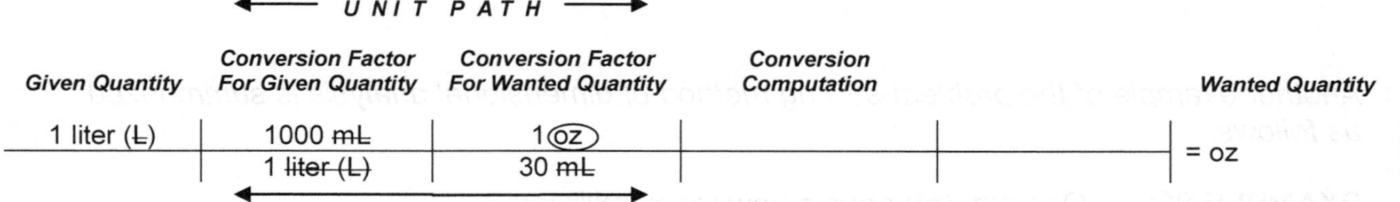

THINKING THROUGH THE PROBLEM

Each conversion factor is a ratio of unit that equals 1. The conversion factors are set up to cancel out the preceding unit. The wanted quantity must be within the numerator portion of the problem to identify that the problem is set up correctly. Carefully choose each conversion factor and ensure that it is correctly placed in the numerator or denominator portion of the problem to allow the unwanted units to be canceled from the problem. If you are unable to cancel unwanted units because both units are numerators or denominators, then the problem is not set up correctly. The units need to be opposite each other to be canceled from the problem.

Step #5: After the unwanted units are canceled from the problem, only the numerical values remain. Multiply the numerators, multiply the denominators and divide the product of the numerators by the product of the denominators to provide the numerical value for the wanted quantity.

Need to know:

- What is the product of the numerators?
- What is the product of the denominators?
- After multiplying the numerators and the denominators and dividing the product of the numerators by the product of the denominators, what is the numerical value for the wanted quantity?

Answer: The wanted quantity is 33.3 oz and the answer to the problem.

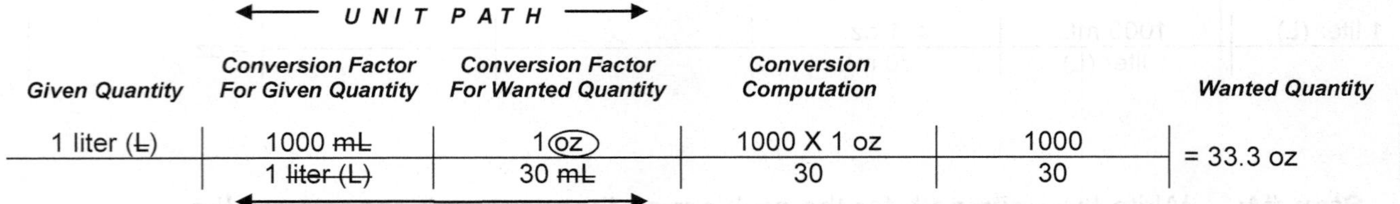

← UNIT PATH →

Given Quantity	*Conversion Factor For Given Quantity*	*Conversion Factor For Wanted Quantity*	*Conversion Computation*		*Wanted Quantity*
1 liter (~~L~~)	1000 ~~mL~~ / 1 ~~liter (L)~~	1 (oz) / 30 ~~mL~~	1000 X 1 oz / 30	1000 / 30	= 33.3 oz

THINKING THROUGH THE PROBLEM

Ounce is the wanted quantity in the problem and is the remaining unit left in the problem after the unwanted units are canceled from the problem. Ounce is correctly placed in the numerator portion of the problem to correspond with the wanted quantity in the numerator portion of the problem.

Another example of the problem-solving method of dimensional analysis is summarized as follows:

EXAMPLE #2: One pint (pt) equals how many milliliters?
Or: How many milliliters are in 1 pint?

Step #1: Identify the given quantity in the problem.

Need to know: What is the given quantity?

Answer: The given quantity is 1 pint.

1 pt		=

Step #2: Identify the wanted quantity in the problem.

Need to know: What is the wanted quantity?

Answer: The wanted quantity is the number of milliliters (ml) in 1 pint.

1 pt		= mL

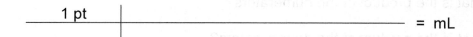

Step #3: Establish the unit path from the given quantity to the wanted quantity by selecting the equivalents that will be used as conversion factors.

Need to know: What conversion factors are needed in the unit path that will convert the given quantity to the wanted quantity?

Answer: Given quantity of 1 pint = 16 ounces

1 ounce (oz) = 30 mL the wanted quantity unit

Step #4: Write the unit path for the problem so that each unit cancels out the preceding unit until all unwanted units are canceled from the problem except the wanted quantity.

Need to know: What is the wanted quantity that remains in the unit path after canceling all unwanted units?

Answer:

1 ~~pt~~	16 ~~oz~~	30 mL	1X16X30 (mL)	= 480 mL
	1 ~~pt~~	1 ~~oz~~	1X1X1	

Step #5: After the unwanted units are canceled from the problem only the numerical value remain. Multiply the numerators, multiply the denominators, and divide the product of the numerators by the product of the denominators to provide the numerical value for the wanted quantity.

Need to know:

- What is the product of the numerators?
- What is the product of the denominators?
- After multiplying the numerators and the denominators and dividing the product of the numerators by the product of the denominators, what is the numerical value for the wanted quantity?

Answer:

1 ~~pt~~	16~~oz~~	30 ~~mL~~			=	$\frac{480\text{ mL}}{1}$	= 480 mL
	1 ~~pt~~	1 ~~oz~~					

Practice Exercises

1. Problem: 10 mL = How many L?

   Given quantity =

   Wanted quantity =

10 mL		= L

2. Problem: 120 lb = How many kg?

   Given quantity =

   Wanted quantity =

120 lb		= kg

3. Problem: 5 grains (gr) = How many mg? (1 gr = 60 mg)

   Given quantity =

   Wanted quantity =

5 gr		= mg

4. Problem: 2 g = How many (grains) gr?

   Given quantity =

   Wanted quantity =

2 g		= gr

5. Problem: 5 dram (dr) = How many mL? (1 dr = 5 ml)

   Given quantity =

   Wanted quantity =

5 dr		= mL

6. Problem: 8 dram = How many oz?

Given quantity =

Wanted quantity =

8 dr | = oz

7. Problem: 10 (minims) m = How many drams? (1 dr = 5 ml), (1 ml = 15 m)

Given quantity =

Wanted quantity =

10 m | = dr

8. Problem: 35 kg = How many lb?

Given quantity =

Wanted quantity =

35 kg | = lb

9. Problem: 10 mL = How many tsp? (1 tsp = 5 ml)

Given quantity =

Wanted quantity =

10 mL | = tsp

10. Problem: 30 mL = How many tbs? (1 tbs = 15 ml)

Given quantity =

Wanted quantity =

30 mL | = tbs

11. Problem: 0.25 g = How many mg?

Given quantity =

Wanted quantity =

0.25 g		= mg

12. Problem: 350 mcg = How many mg?

Given quantity =

Wanted quantity =

350 mcg		= mg

13. Problem: 0.75 L = How many mL?

Given quantity =

Wanted quantity =

0.75 L		= mL

14. Problem: 3.5 mL = How many minims (m)?

Given quantity =

Wanted quantity =

3.5 mL		= m

15. Problem: 225 (minims) m = How many tsp?

Given quantity =

Wanted quantity =

225 m		= tsp

This chapter has introduced the learner to the problem-solving method of dimensional analysis with a step-by-step explanation and an opportunity to practice solving problems involving common equivalents. To demonstrate your understanding of dimensional analysis and conversions between systems of measurement, complete the following practice problems.

Practice Problems

1. Problem: ¾ mL = How many m?

2. Problem: gtt XV = How many m?

3. Problem: 5/6 gr = How many mg?

4. Problem: How many mL in 3 oz?

5. Problem: 0.5 mg = How many mcg?

6. Problem: gtt XLV = How many mL?

7. Problem: How many mL in 3 qt?

8. Problem: 4 gal = How many qt? (1 gal = 4 qt)

9. Problem: 1.5 cup = How many mL? (1 cup = 120 mL)

10. Problem: oz XIIss = How many glasses? (1 glass = 180 mL)

ANSWERS TO DIMENSIONAL ANALYSIS PRACTICE EXERCISES

1. 0.01L
2. 54.55 Kg
3. 300 mg
4. 33.33 grains
5. 25 mL
6. 1.33 oz
7. 0.13 dram
8. 77 lbs
9. 2 tsp
10. 2 tbs
11. 250 mg
12. 0.35 mg
13. 750 mL
14. 17.5 m
15. 3 tsp

ANSWERS TO DIMENSIONAL ANALYSIS PROBLEMS

1. 11.25 m
2. 15 m
3. 50 mg
4. 90 mL
5. 500 mcg
6. 3 mL
7. 3000 cc
8. 16 qt
9. 180 cc
10. 0.2 glass or 1/5 glass

Table of Equivalence: Metric, Apothecary, and Household Systems

There are some equivalents in one system have equivalents in another system; however, equivalents are not exact measures, and you will see discrepancies. Several tables have been developed illustrating conversions/equivalents. Sometimes drug companies use equivalents that may be different for a measure. A common discrepancy is with grains, which is an apothecary measure.

Roman Numerals: ss = ½, I or i = 1, V = 5, X = 10, L = 50, C = 100, D = 500, M = 1000

Know these common equivalents:

Metric	Apothecary	Household
1 ml	**(minims) m 15**	**15 gtts (drops)**
5 ml	**(dram) 1**	**1 t, 1 tsp**
15 ml		**1 T, tbs**
1 Kg = 1000 gm		**2.2 lbs**
1 g = 1000 mg		
1 mg = 1000 mcg		
60 mg	**grain 1**	
90 mg	**grain 1 ½**	
30 ml	**(ounce) 1**	**1 oz**
		1 pt = 16 oz.
		1 qt = 32 oz.
1 L = 1000 ml		
2.54 cm		**1 inch**
°C = (°F – 32) * 5/9		**°F = (°C * 9/5) + 32**

gr = grain
dr = dram
oz = (fluid) ounces
m = minim
g = gm = gram
kg = kilogram

mg = milligram
ml = milliliter
L = liter
lb = pound
mcg = microgram

cm = centimeter
gtt(s) = drop(s)
T, tbs = tablespoon
t, tsp = teaspoon

1 lb = 0.454 kgs

13:6 Temperature Conversion

Thermometers using **Fahrenheit** (F) as the measuring unit are more familiar to people living in the United States. The **Celsius** (C) or **centigrade** (C) system of measurement, however, is frequently seen in medical practice and in other countries. One way to start understanding the difference between the two systems is to compare how each one expresses the boiling and freezing points of water:

Boiling points: 212°F = 100°C

Freezing points: 32°F = 0°C

See Figure 13–12 for a comparison of Fahrenheit (F) and Celsius (C) thermometers and Table 13–10 for a conversion chart. Health care workers may have to convert between the Fahrenheit and Celsius systems when a conversion chart is not available. Table 13–11 contains the formulas for conversion. There is a fraction and a decimal approach that give the same results. Deciding which to use depends on whether you have stronger skills working with fractions or decimals. All the formulas include parentheses. These are used to indicate that the enclosed calculation must be performed first. For example, the steps to solve the formula (°F − 32) × 5/9 = °C are to first subtract 32 from the value for °F and *then* multiply that value by 5/9.

TABLE 13–10 Fahrenheit–Celsius Conversion Chart

Fahrenheit	Celsius
32 (freezing point)	0 (freezing point)
95	35
96	35.6
97	36.1
97.4	36.3
98	36.7
98.6	37
99	37.2
99.4	37.4
100	37.8
101	38.3
102	38.9
103	39.4
104	40
212 (boiling point)	100 (boiling point)

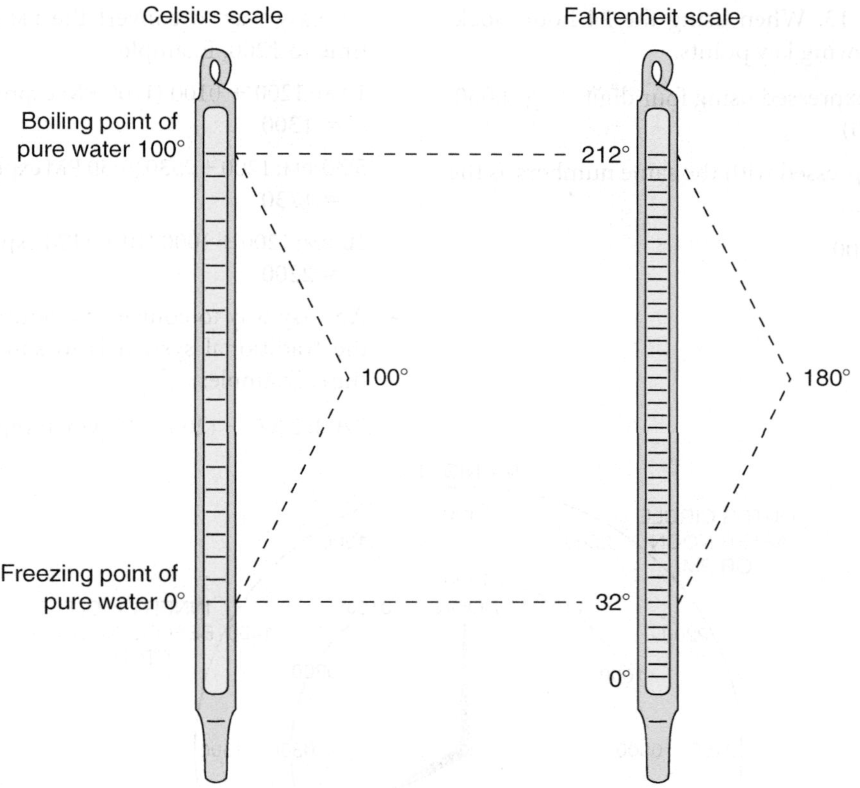

FIGURE 13–12 **Comparison of Fahrenheit and Celsius (Centigrade) temperature scales.**

TABLE 13–11 Temperature Scale Conversion Formulas

Convert From	Fraction Formula	Decimal Formula
Celsius to Fahrenheit	(°C × 9/5) + 32 = °F Example: 37°C (37 × 9/5) + 32 = °F 333/5 + 32 = °F 66.6 + 32 = 98.6°F	(°C × 1.8) + 32 = °F Example: 37°C (37 × 1.8) + 32 = °F 66.6 + 32 = 98.6°F
Fahrenheit to Celsius	(°F − 32) × 5/9 = °C Example: 101°F (101 − 32) × 5/9 = °C 69 × 5/9 = °C 345/9 = 38.3°C (rounded to nearest tenth)	(°F − 32) × 0.5556 = °C OR (°F − 32) ÷ 1.8 = °C Example: 101°F (101 − 32) × 0.5556 = °C 69 × 0.5556 = 38.3°C (rounded to nearest tenth) OR (101 − 32) ÷ 1.8 = °C 69 ÷ 1.8 = 38.3°C (rounded to nearest tenth)

13:7 Military Time

Military time is frequently used in health care to avoid the confusion created by the AM and PM used in the traditional system to designate the correct time. The problem with the traditional system is that if the AM or PM is omitted or misread, an error of 12 hours is made. Errors in recording times are unacceptable in health care. For example, accuracy is critical when entering data on a patient chart, reporting when medications are given, or signing off on physician orders.

When **military time** is the standard used, all time designations are made with the 24-hour clock. The 12th hour is at 12 noon, or 12 PM, and the 24th hour is at 12 midnight, or 12 AM. At 12 midnight, the clock starts again at zero since there are 24 hours in a day.

See Figure 13–13. When using the 24-hour clock, remember the following key points:

- Time is always expressed using four digits (e.g., 0030, 0200, 1200, 1700)
- AM hours are expressed with the same numbers as the traditional clock:

  12 Midnight: 0000

  1 AM: 0100

  5:30 AM: 0530

  10 AM: 1000

  12 Noon: 1200

- An easy way to convert the PM hours is to add the time to 1200. Example:

  1 PM: 1200 + 0100 (1:00 PM expressed in four digits) = 1300

  5:30 PM: 1200 + 0530 (5:30 PM expressed in four digits) = 1730

  10 PM: 1200 + 1000 (10:00 PM expressed in four digits) = 2200

- An easy way to convert PM hours in military time to the traditional system is to subtract 1200 from the time. Example:

  2200: 2200 − 1200 = 10 which represents 10 PM

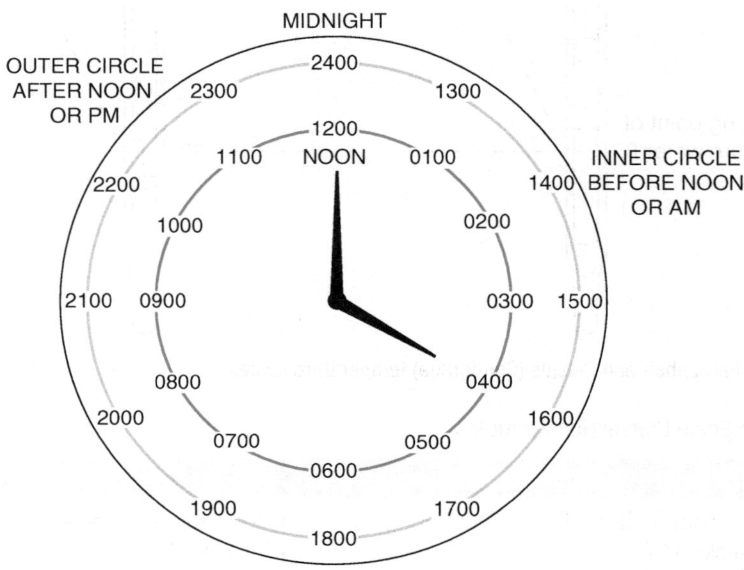

FIGURE 13–13 The military clock is based on a 24-hour day.

TABLE 13–12 **Military (24-Hour Clock) and Traditional Time Conversion Chart**

Traditional	24-Hour Time	Traditional	24-Hour Time
12:01 AM	0001	12:01 PM	1201
12:30 AM	0030	12:30 PM	1230
1:00 AM	0100	1:00 PM	1300
2:00 AM	0200	2:00 PM	1400
3:00 AM	0300	3:00 PM	1500
4:00 AM	0400	4:00 PM	1600
5:00 AM	0500	5:00 PM	1700
6:00 AM	0600	6:00 PM	1800
7:00 AM	0700	7:00 PM	1900
8:00 AM	0800	8:00 PM	2000
9:00 AM	0900	9:00 PM	2100
10:00 AM	1000	10:00 PM	2200
11:00 AM	1100	11:00 PM	2300
12:00 noon	1200	12:00 midnight	2400

1845: 1845 − 1200 = 645 which represents 6:45 PM

1330: 1330 − 1200 = 130 which represents 1:30 PM

- When times are verbalized, there is a specific way in which it is expressed:

  0200 = oh two hundred hours

  0938 = oh nine thirty eight hours

  1300 = thirteen hundred hours

  1301 = thirteen oh one hours

  1730 = seventeen thirty hours

  2200 = twenty-two hundred hours

Study Table 13–12 to practice converting between traditional and military times.

STUDENT: Go to the workbook and complete the assignment sheet for Chapter 13, Medical Math.

TODAY'S RESEARCH TOMORROW'S HEALTH CARE

Scorpions and Snakes to Cure Cancer?

Eighty percent of cancerous brain tumors are gliomas and they affect more than 18,000 people every year in the United States. Gliomas grow at a rapid rate and can kill a person in a matter of weeks. In most cases, surgical removal of the tumors will destroy too much brain tissue or the tumors grow back quickly if they are surgically removed, so treatment is extremely limited. Few patients live more than 6 to 12 months after the tumor is diagnosed.

Now there is hope for people with gliomas. Dr. Harald Sontheimer, working with a research team at the University of Alabama at Birmingham, discovered that a giant Israeli golden scorpion secretes a venom that is safe to humans but paralyzes muscles of a cockroach. The toxic molecules of the venom target a specific protein on the muscles of the cockroach, killing the cockroach. Through research, Sonteheimer found that the same protein is present on the cancerous glioma cells. Researchers were then able to develop TM-601, a synthetic version of the venom. In the first clinical trials conducted at Cedars-Sinai Medical Center in California, 18 patients with advanced reoccurring gliomas had the tumors removed. Then a single low dose of radioactive iodine attached to TM-601 was injected into a small tube inserted in the surgical area where the tumor was removed. The TM-601 attached to the glioma cells and the radioactive iodine was able to target the specific cancer cells. Very few side effects were noted. While most patients survived approximately 6–10 months, two women were still alive almost 3 years after treatment. More advanced clinical trials are now underway. Other researchers are using chlorotoxin from the scorpion venom to determine if it will be an effective carrier for gene therapy to treat brain, prostate, colorectal, and skin cancers. In Israel, Dr. Michael Gurevitz is leading a team of scientists at Tel Aviv University who are investigating ways the scorpion venom can be used for analgesic (pain relief) applications. The researchers believe that the venom interacts with sodium channels in the muscular and nervous system to block the sensation of pain without causing additional or other dangerous side effects. Other medical researchers are evaluating if the scorpion venom is effective for treating neurological conditions such as epilepsy or seizure disorders.

Snake venom is also a major area of research. Some scientists are trying to use snake venom to destroy the blood vessels that supply cancerous tumors with nourishment and fluid. If access to nourishment is restricted, tumors will not be able to grow. A research team at the University of South California is using mice to determine if a protein in copperhead snake venom can inhibit the growth of breast cancer. Initial studies showed a 60 to 70 percent reduction in the growth rate of breast tumors in the mice treated with the protein. However, it will be several years before the venom protein will be available for human tests. Finally, researchers at the University of Northern Colorado are studying snake venom from the prairie rattler and rear-fanged snakes to determine if it is effective against melanoma (skin), colon, or breast cancer. One of the leading causes of death will be eliminated if research finds that readily available venom from scorpions and snakes can cure a cancerous tumor.

CHAPTER 13 SUMMARY

Work in health care requires the use of math skills to measure and perform various types of calculations. To work safely in health care, it is essential to be able to add, subtract, multiply, and divide whole numbers, decimals, fractions, and percentages. An understanding of equivalents when using decimals, fractions, and percentages is also needed.

An important skill to help check work is anticipating the results. Learning to estimate and detect incorrect answers takes practice and thought.

Roman numerals are used in health care for some medications, solutions, and ordering systems. Angles are used when injecting medications, describing joint movement, and indicating bed positions.

The three systems of measurement used in health care are household, metric, and apothecary. Health care work sometimes requires that units from one system of measurement be converted to those of another. This requires knowledge of the equivalencies between the units of the systems. Health care workers may have to convert between the Fahrenheit and Celsius systems of temperature measurement, because the Celsius or centigrade system of measurement is frequently seen in medical practice.

Military time is frequently used in health care to avoid the confusion created by the AM and PM used in the traditional system. Errors in recording times are unacceptable in health care. Accuracy is critical, such as when entering data on a patient chart, reporting when medications are given, or signing off on physicians orders.

Health care workers must work carefully and thoughtfully when performing calculations. Errors in math can have serious effects on the patient; therefore, health care workers must strive for 100 percent accuracy.

INTERNET SEARCHES

Use the search engines suggested in Chapter 12:9 in this text to search the Internet for additional information about the following topics:

1. **Math:** Search words such as math, basic math, basic calculations, fractions, and percentages.
2. **Roman numerals:** Search for additional information about using Roman numerals.
3. **Measurement:** Search words such as measurement, mass/weight, volume, converting measures, metric system, and equivalents.
4. **Temperature:** Search for information on Fahrenheit, centigrade, Celsius, and converting temperatures.
5. **Military time:** Search words such as time, military time, and 24-hour clock.

REVIEW QUESTIONS

1. A patient's oral intake is being measured. For breakfast, he drinks 240 milliliters (mL) of coffee, 120 mL of juice, and 60mL of water. What is the total fluid intake?
2. A patient is on a diet to lose weight. Last month, she weighed 172 pounds. This month, she weighs 159 pounds. How much weight did she lose?
3. A physical therapist is buying elastic bandages. Each roll costs $3.25. How much would 30 rolls cost?
4. A central supply worker orders 12 new stethoscopes for a total cost of $108.48. How much does each stethoscope cost?
5. A pharmacy technician reviews a prescription for an antibiotic. The patient must take 2 1/2 tablets every 4 hours for 6 days. How many tablets should the technician dispense?
6. A surgical nurse works $1\frac{1}{4}$ hours in preoperative (before surgery) care, $2\frac{1}{2}$ hours in the operating room, and $3\frac{3}{4}$ hours in the recovery room. What is the total number of hours worked?
7. An electrocardiograph technician knows that one small block on electrocardiographic paper represents $\frac{1}{25}$ of a second. How many seconds are represented by 150 small blocks?
8. A laboratory technician counts 7,742 leukocytes (white blood cells). If 36% of the leukocytes are lymphocytes, how many lymphocytes are present?
9. A pharmacy technician must prepare 250 mL of a 2.5% dextrose solution. How many grams of dextrose are needed?
10. A doctor orders 500 mg of Sumycin for a patient. Sumycin, an antibiotic, is available in 250-mg capsules. How many capsules should be given to the patient?
11. A cough medicine is ordered for a child. The child must take 1 teaspoon every 4 hours. How many ounces should be dispensed for an 8-day supply of cough medicine?
12. A medical assistant orders MM pairs of gloves. How many gloves were ordered?
13. How many liters are in 2.5 kiloliters?
14. A patient drinks 90 mL of water. How many ounces did the patient drink?
15. A doctor orders a saline irrigation with 2,000 mL. How many quarts of solution must be used?
16. An emergency medical technician must report to work at 1830. What does this mean in traditional time?
17. Convert 70 degrees Fahrenheit to Celsius.
18. Convert 28 degrees Celsius to Fahrenheit.

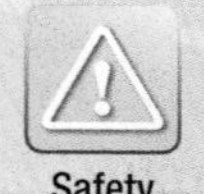

14 Promotion of Safety

CHAPTER OBJECTIVES

After completing this chapter, you should be able to:

- Define *body mechanics*.
- Use correct body mechanics while performing procedures in the laboratory or clinical area.
- Observe all safety standards established by OSHA, especially the Occupational Exposure to Hazardous Chemicals Standard and the Bloodborne Pathogen Standard.
- Follow safety regulations stated while performing in the laboratory area.
- Observe all regulations for patient safety while performing procedures on a student partner in the laboratory or clinical area, or on a patient in any area.
- List the four main classes of fire extinguishers.
- Relate each class of fire extinguisher to the specific fire(s) for which it is used.
- Simulate the operation of a fire extinguisher by following the directions on the extinguisher and specific measures for observing fire safety.
- Locate and describe the operation of the nearest fire alarm.
- Describe in detail the evacuation plan for the laboratory area according to established school policy.
- Define, pronounce, and spell all key terms.

KEY TERMS

base of support
Bloodborne Pathogen Standard
body mechanics
ergonomics
fire extinguishers
Occupational Exposure to Hazardous Chemicals Standard
Occupational Safety and Health Administration (OSHA)
Safety Data Sheet (SDS)
safety standards

LEGAL ALERT

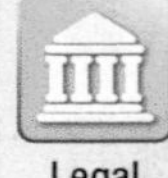

Before performing any procedures in this chapter, know and follow the standards and regulations established by the scope of practice; federal laws and agencies; state laws; state or national licensing, registration, or certification boards; professional organizations; professional standards; and agency policies.

It is your responsibility to learn exactly what you are legally permitted to do and to perform only procedures for which you have been trained.

14:1 Using Body Mechanics

To prevent injury to yourself and others while working in the health care field, it is important that you observe good body mechanics and maintain correct posture.

Body mechanics refers to the way in which the body moves and maintains balance while making the most efficient use of all its parts. Basic rules for body mechanics are provided as guidelines to prevent strain and help maintain muscle strength.

There are four main reasons for using good body mechanics:

- Muscles work best when used correctly.
- The correct use of muscles makes lifting, pulling, and pushing easier.
- The correct application of body mechanics prevents unnecessary fatigue and strain and saves energy.
- The correct application of body mechanics prevents injury to self and others.

Eight basic rules of good body mechanics include:

- Maintain a broad **base of support** by keeping the feet 8–10 inches apart, placing one foot slightly forward, balancing weight on both feet, and pointing the toes in the direction of movement.
- Bend from the hips and knees to get close to an object, and keep your back straight (Figure 14–1A). Do not bend at the waist.
- Use the strongest muscles to do the job. The larger and stronger muscles are located in the shoulders, upper arms, hips, and thighs. Back muscles are weak.
- Use the weight of your body to help push or pull an object. Whenever possible, push, slide, or pull rather than lift.
- Carry heavy objects close to the body (Figure 14–1B). Also, stand close to any object or person being moved.
- Avoid twisting your body as you work. Turn with your feet and entire body when you change direction of movement.

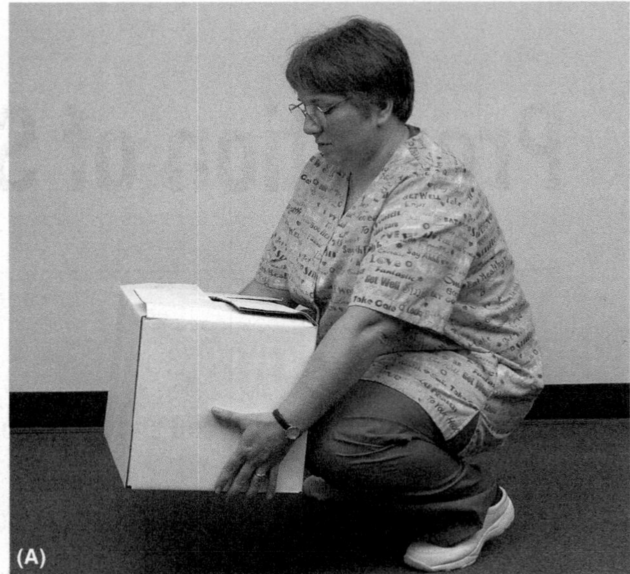

FIGURE 14–1A Bend from the hips and knees to get close to an object.

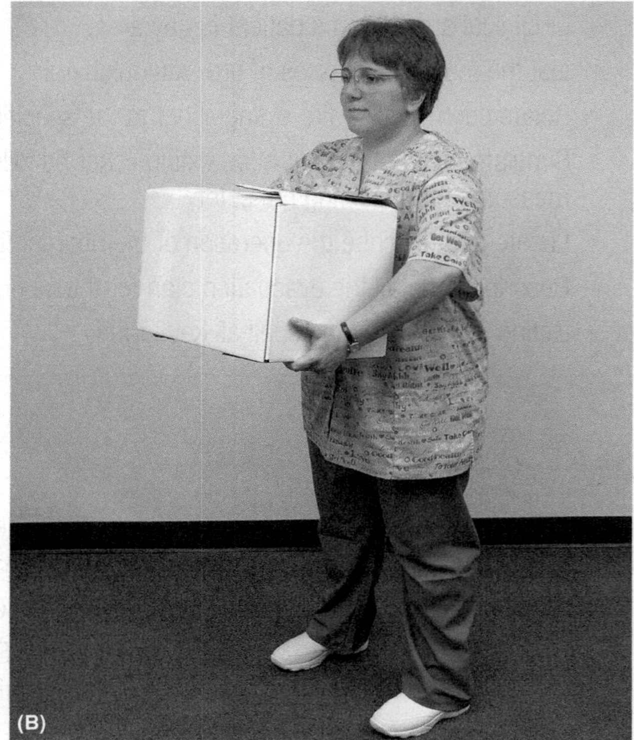

FIGURE 14–1B Maintain a broad base of support while carrying objects close to the body.

- Avoid bending for long periods.
- If a patient or object is too heavy for you to lift alone, always get help. Mechanical lifts, transfer (gait) belts, wheelchairs, and other similar types of equipment are also available to help lift and move patients.

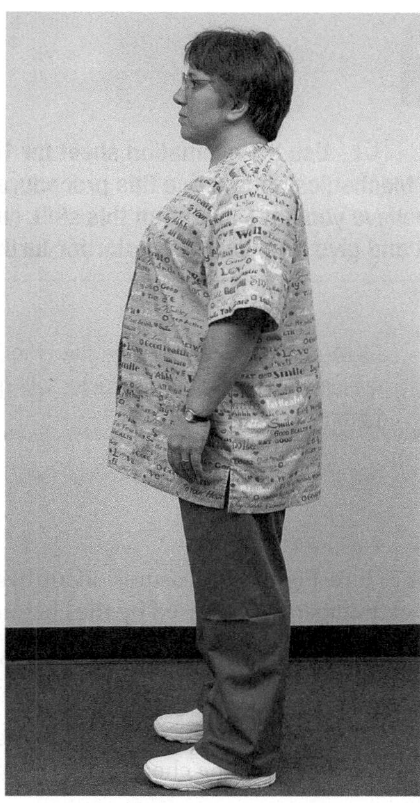

FIGURE 14–2 Correct posture puts less stress on muscles and prevents fatigue.

Good posture is also an essential part of correct body mechanics. Aligning the body correctly puts less stress on muscles and prevents fatigue (Figure 14–2). Basic principles include standing straight with stomach muscles pulled in, shoulders relaxed and pulled back, weight balanced equally on each foot and aligned with the shoulders, and chest and chin held up.

Some health care facilities may require health care workers to wear back supports while lifting or moving patients. These supports are supposed to help prevent back injuries, but their use is controversial. Back supports may provide a false sense of security as an individual tries to lift heavier loads. It is important to remember that a back brace does not increase strength. Back supports may also cause sweating, skin irritation, and increased abdominal pressure. They do remind the wearer to use good body mechanics. If a back support is used, it should be the correct size to provide the maximum benefit. When the worker is performing strenuous tasks, the support should fit snugly. At other times, it should be loosened to decrease abdominal pressure.

STUDENT: Go to the workbook and complete the assignment sheet for 14:1, Using Body Mechanics. Then return and continue with the procedure.

PROCEDURE 14:1

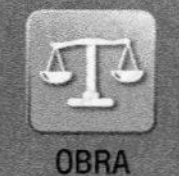

Using Body Mechanics

Equipment and Supplies

Heavy book, bedside stand, bed with wheel locks

Procedure

1. Assemble equipment.
2. Practice correct posture. Stand straight with your feet aligned with your shoulders and your weight supported equally on each foot. Pull in your stomach muscles. Relax your shoulders and pull them back. Hold your chin and chest up. Notice how this helps maintain your spine in a straight line while it also balances all parts of your body.
3. Compare using a narrow base of support to using a broad base of support. Stand on your toes, with your feet close together. Next, stand on your toes with your feet farther apart. Then, stand with your feet flat on the floor but close together. Finally, stand with your feet flat on the floor but approximately 8–10 inches apart and with one foot slightly forward. Balance your weight on both feet. You should feel the best support in the final position because the broad base supports your body weight.
4. Place the book on the floor. Bend from the hips and knees (not the waist) and keep your back straight to pick up the book. Return to the standing position.
5. Place the book between your thumb and fingers, but not touching the palm of your hand, and hold your hand straight out in front of your body. Slowly move your hand toward your body, stopping several times to feel the weight of the book in different positions. Finally, hold the book with your entire hand and bring your hand close to your body. The final position should be the most comfortable.

   NOTE: This illustrates the need to carry heavy objects close to your body and to use the strongest muscles to do the job.
6. Stand at either end of the bed. Release the wheel locks on the bed. Position your feet to provide a broad base of support. Get close to the bed. Use the weight of your body to push the bed forward.

(continues)

PROCEDURE 14:1 (CONT.)

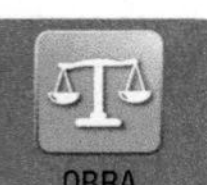

7. Place the book on the bed. Pick up the book and place it on the bedside stand. Avoid twisting your body. Turn with your feet to place the book on the stand.

   NOTE: Remember that holding the book close to your body allows you to use the strongest muscles.
8. Practice the rules of body mechanics by setting up situations similar to those listed in the previous steps. Continue until the movements feel natural to you.
9. Replace all equipment used.

PRACTICE: **Use the evaluation sheet for 14:1, Using Body Mechanics, to practice this procedure. When you believe you have mastered this skill, sign the sheet and give it to your instructor for further action.**

FINAL CHECKPOINT: Using the criteria listed on the evaluation sheet, your instructor will grade your performance.

14:2 Preventing Accidents and Injuries

The **Occupational Safety and Health Administration (OSHA)**, a division of the Department of Labor, establishes and enforces **safety standards** for the workplace. Two main standards affect health care workers:

- The Occupational Exposure to Hazardous Chemicals Standard
- The Bloodborne Pathogen Standard

Chemical Hazards

The **Occupational Exposure to Hazardous Chemicals Standard** requires that employers inform employees of all chemicals and hazards in the workplace. In addition, all manufacturers must provide **Safety Data Sheets (SDSs)**, formerly known as Material Safety Data Sheets (MSDSs), with any hazardous products they sell (Figure 14–3). The SDSs contain 16 standard sections that make it easy to locate and understand information about how to properly and safely handle hazardous chemicals. The SDSs must always be readily accessible and provide the following information:

- Section 1: Identification: identifies the chemical and its recommended use
- Section 2: Hazard(s) Identification: identifies the hazards of the chemical and other warning information
- Section 3: Composition/Information on Ingredients: identifies the ingredients of the chemical
- Section 4: First-Aid Measures: describes the initial care required for people exposed to the chemical
- Section 5: Fire-Fighting Measures: identifies the best way to extinguish a fire caused by the chemical
- Section 6: Accidental Release Measures: recommends how to clean up and contain a spill
- Section 7: Handling and Storage: recommends how to safely handle and store the chemical
- Section 8: Exposure Controls/Personal Protection: indicates the maximum exposure limit and what personal protective equipment is required
- Section 9: Physical and Chemical Properties: identifies physical properties such as look and smell
- Section 10: Stability and Reactivity: describes stability and reactivity hazards of the chemical
- Section 11: Toxicology Information: identifies the health effects of exposure
- Section 12: Ecological Information: identifies the environmental impact of an exposure
- Section 13: Disposal Considerations: identifies how to safely dispose of the chemical
- Section 14: Transport Information: provides guidance on how the chemical can be safely transported
- Section 15: Regulatory Information: identifies other regulations on the chemical that are not indicated elsewhere in SDS
- Section 16: Other Information: states when this SDS was prepared or revised

Chemicals must also be labeled with a hazardous category classification according to the National Fire Protection Association's (NFPA) color code (Figure 14–4). This code alerts the user to health, fire, reactivity, or other specific hazards of the chemical.

MERCURY

Safety Data Sheet

according to the federal final rule of hazard communication revised on 2012 (HazCom 2012)

Date of issue: 11/19/2013

SECTION 1: Identification of the substance/mixture and of the company/undertaking

1.1. Product identifier

Trade name : MERCURY

CAS No : 7439-97-6

Other means of identification : Colloidal Mercury, Quick Silver, Liquid Silver, NCI-C60399, Hydrargyrum

1.2. Relevant identified uses of the substance or mixture and uses advised against

Use of the substance/mixture : Variety of industrial, analytical and research applications.

1.3. Details of the supplier of the safety data sheet

ABC Pharmaceuticals

1234 Chemcial Way
Amalgam Center, AL 31313

1.4. Emergency telephone number

Emergency number : 1-800-555-5656

SECTION 2: Hazards identification

2.1. Classification of the substance or mixture

GHS-US classification

Acute Tox. 1 (Inhalation:dust,mist)	H330
Repr. 1B	H360
STOT RE 1	H372
Aquatic Acute 1	H400
Aquatic Chronic 1	H410

2.2. Label elements

GHS-US labelling

Hazard pictograms (GHS-US) :

GHS06 GHS08 GHS09

Signal word (GHS-US) : Danger

Hazard statements (GHS-US) : H330 - Fatal if inhaled
H360 - May damage fertility or the unborn child
H372 - Causes damage to organs through prolonged or repeated exposure
H400 - Very toxic to aquatic life
H410 - Very toxic to aquatic life with long lasting effects

Precautionary statements (GHS-US) : P201 - Obtain special instructions before use
P202 - Do not handle until all safety precautions have been read and understood
P260 - Do not breathe vapors, gas
P264 - Wash skin, hands thoroughly after handling
P270 - Do not eat, drink or smoke when using this product
P271 - Use only outdoors or in a well-ventilated area
P273 - Avoid release to the environment
P280 - Wear eye protection, protective clothing, protective gloves, Face mask
P284 - [In case of inadequate ventilation] wear respiratory protection
P304+P340 - IF INHALED: Remove person to fresh air and keep comfortable for breathing
P308+P313 - IF exposed or concerned: Get medical advice/attention
P310 - Immediately call a POISON CENTER/doctor/...
P314 - Get medical advice and attention if you feel unwell
P320 - Specific treatment is urgent (see First aid measures on this label)
P391 - Collect spillage
P403+P233 - Store in a well-ventilated place. Keep container tightly closed
P405 - Store locked up
P501 - Dispose of contents/container to comply with applicable local, national and international regulation.

2.3. Other hazards

other hazards which do not result in classification : When inhaled, Mercury will be rapidly distributed throughout the body. During this time, Mercury will cross the blood-brain barrier, and become oxidized to the Hg (II) oxidation state. The oxidized species of Mercury cannot cross the blood-brain barrier and thus accumulates in the

FIGURE 14–3 Read the Safety Data Sheet (SDS) before using any chemical product. LabChem

(continues)

(continued)

MERCURY

Safety Data Sheet

according to the federal final rule of hazard communication revised on 2012 (HazCom 2012)

brain. Mercury in other organs is removed slowly from the body via the kidneys. The average half-time for clearance of Mercury for different parts of the human body is as follows: lung: 1.7 days; head: 21 days; kidney region: 64 days; chest: 43 days; whole body: 58 days. Mercury can be irritating to contaminated skin and eye. Prolonged contact may lead to ulceration of the skin. Allergic reactions (i.e. rashes, welts) may occur in sensitive individuals. Mercury can be irritating to contaminated skin and eyes. Short-term over-exposures to high concentrations of mercury vapors can lead to breathing difficulty, coughing, acute, and potentially fatal lung disorders. Depending on the concentration of inhalation over-exposure, heart problems, damage to the kidney, liver or nerves and effects on the brain may occur.

2.4. Unknown acute toxicity (GHS-US)

No data available

SECTION 3: Composition/information on ingredients

3.1. Substance

Not applicable

Full text of H-phrases: see section 16

3.2. Mixture

Name	Product identifier	%	GHS-US classification
Mercury	(CAS No) 7439-97-6	100	Acute Tox. 2 (Inhalation), H330 Repr. 1B, H360 STOT RE 1, H372 Aquatic Acute 1, H400 Aquatic Chronic 1, H410

SECTION 4: First aid measures

4.1. Description of first aid measures

First-aid measures general : Never give anything by mouth to an unconscious person. If exposed or concerned: Get medical advice/attention.

First-aid measures after inhalation : Remove to fresh air and keep at rest in a position comfortable for breathing. Assure fresh air breathing. Allow the victim to rest. Immediately call a POISON CENTER or doctor/physician. In case of irregular breathing or respiratory arrest provide artificial respiration.

First-aid measures after skin contact : Wash immediately with lots of water (15 minutes)/shower. Remove affected clothing and wash all exposed skin area with mild soap and water, followed by warm water rinse. Seek immediate medical advice.

First-aid measures after eye contact : Rinse immediately and thoroughly, pulling the eyelids well away from the eye (15 minutes minimum). Keep eye wide open while rinsing. Seek medical attention immediately.

First-aid measures after ingestion : Immediately call a POISON CENTER or doctor/physician. Rinse mouth. If conscious, give large amounts of water and induce vomiting. Give water or milk if the person is fully conscious. Obtain emergency medical attention.

4.2. Most important symptoms and effects, both acute and delayed

Symptoms/injuries after inhalation : Short-term over-exposures to high concentrations of mercury vapors can lead to breathing difficulty, coughing, acute, chemical pneumonia, and pulmonary edema (a potentially fatal accumulation of fluid in the lungs) . Depending on the concentration of over-exposure, cardiac abnormalities, damage to the kidney, liver or nerves and effects on the brain may occur. Long-term inhalation over-exposures can lead to the development of a wide variety of symptoms, including the following: excessive salivation, gingivitis, anorexia, chills, fever, cardiac abnormalities, anemia, digestive problems, abdominal pains, frequent urination, an inability to urinate, diarrhea, peripheral neuropathy (numbness, weakness, or burning sensations in the hands or feet), tremors (especially in the hands, fingers, eyelids, lips, cheeks, tongue, or legs), alteration of tendon reflexes, slurred speech, visual disturbances, and deafness. Allergic reactions (i.e. breathing difficulty) may also occur in sensitive individuals.

Symptoms/injuries after skin contact : Symptoms of skin exposure can include redness, dry skin, and pain. Prolonged contact may lead to ulceration of the skin. Allergic reactions (i.e. rashes, welts) may occur in sensitive individuals. Dermatitis (redness and inflammation of the skin) may occur after repeated skin exposures.

Symptoms/injuries after eye contact : Symptoms of eye exposure can include redness, pain, and watery eyes. A symptom of Mercury exposure is discoloration of the lens of the eyes.

Symptoms/injuries after ingestion : If Mercury is swallowed, symptoms of such over-exposure can include metallic taste in mouth, nausea, vomiting, central nervous system effects, and damage to the kidneys. Metallic mercury is not usually absorbed sufficiently from the gastrointestinal tract to induce an acute, toxic response. Damage to the tissues of the mouth, throat, esophagus, and other tissues of the digestive system may occur. Ingestion may be fatal, due to effects on gastrointestinal system and kidneys.

Chronic symptoms : Long-term over-exposure can lead to a wide range of adverse health effects. Anyone using Mercury must pay attention to personality changes, weight loss, skin or gum discolorations, stomach pains, and other signs of Mercury over-exposure. Gradually developing syndromes ("Erethism" and "Acrodynia") are indicative of potentially severe health problems. Mercury can cause the development of allergic reactions (i.e. dermatitis, rashes, breathing difficulty) upon prolonged or repeated exposures. Refer to Section 11 (Toxicology Information) for additional data.

MERCURY

Safety Data Sheet

according to the federal final rule of hazard communication revised on 2012 (HazCom 2012)

4.3. Indication of any immediate medical attention and special treatment needed

Treatment for Mercury over-exposure must be given. The following treatment protocol for ingestion of Mercury is from Clinical Toxicology of Commercial Products (5th Edition, 1984).

SECTION 5: Firefighting measures

5.1. Extinguishing media

Suitable extinguishing media : Foam. Dry powder. Carbon dioxide. Water spray. Sand.

Unsuitable extinguishing media : Do not use a heavy water stream.

5.2. Special hazards arising from the substance or mixture

Fire hazard : Not flammable. Mercury vapors and oxides generated during fires involving this product are toxic.

Reactivity : Stable. Reacts with (some) metals. Mercury can react with metals to form amalgams.

5.3. Advice for firefighters

Firefighting instructions : Use water spray or fog for cooling exposed containers. Exercise caution when fighting any chemical fire. Prevent fire-fighting water from entering environment. Do not allow run-off from fire fighting to enter drains or water courses.

Protective equipment for firefighters : Do not enter fire area without proper protective equipment, including respiratory protection.

Other information : Decontaminate all equipment thoroughly after the conclusion of fire-fighting activities.

SECTION 6: Accidental release measures

6.1. Personal precautions, protective equipment and emergency procedures

General measures : Uncontrolled release should be responded to by trained personnel using pre-planned procedures. Evacuate area. Evacuate personnel to a safe area.

6.1.1. For non-emergency personnel

Emergency procedures : Evacuate unnecessary personnel.

6.1.2. For emergency responders

Protective equipment : Equip cleanup crew with proper protection. In the event of a release under 1 pound: the minimum level "C" Personal Protective Equipment is needed. Triple-gloves (rubber gloves and nitril gloves over latex gloves), chemical resistant suit and boots, hard-hat, and Air-Purifying Respirator with Cartridge appropriate for Mercury.
In the event of a release over 1 pound or when concentration of oxygen in atmosphere is less than 19.5% or unknown, the level "B" Personal Protective Equipments which includes Self-Contained Breathing Apparatus must be worn.

Emergency procedures : Ventilate area.

6.2. Environmental precautions

Prevent entry to sewers and public waters. Notify authorities if liquid enters sewers or public waters. Avoid release to the environment.

6.3. Methods and material for containment and cleaning up

For containment : For larger spills, dike area and pump into waste containers. Put into a labelled container and provide safe disposal.

Methods for cleaning up : There are a variety of methods which can be used to clean-up Mercury spills. Use a commercially available Mercury Spill Kit for small spills. A suction pump with aspirator can also be used during clean-up operations. For larger release, a Mercury vacuum can be used. Calcium polysulfide or excess sulfur can be also used for clean-up. Mercury can migrate into cracks and other difficult-to-clean areas; calcium polysulfide and sulfur can be sprinkled effectively into these areas. Decontaminate the area thoroughly. The area should be inspected visually and with colorimetric tubes for Mercury to ensure all traces have been removed prior to re-occupation by non-emergency personnel. Decontaminate all equipment used in response thoroughly. If such equipments cannot de adequately decontaminated, it must be discarded with other spill residue. Place all spill residues in an appropriate container, seal immediately, and label appropriately. Dispose of in accordance with federal, state, and local hazardous waste disposal requirements. (Refer to Section 13 of this SDS).

6.4. Reference to other sections

See Heading 8. Exposure controls and personal protection.

SECTION 7: Handling and storage

7.1. Precautions for safe handling

Additional hazards when processed : Supervisors and responsible personnel must be aware of personality changes, weight loss, or other sign of Mercury over-exposure in employees using this product; These symptoms can develop gradually and are indicative of potentially severe health effects related to Mercury contamination.

(continues)

(continued)

MERCURY

Safety Data Sheet

according to the federal final rule of hazard communication revised on 2012 (HazCom 2012)

Precautions for safe handling	: As with all chemicals, avoid getting Mercury ON YOU or IN YOU. Do not handle until all safety precautions have been read and understood. Obtain special instructions before use. Wash hands and other exposed areas with mild soap and water before eating, drinking or smoking and when leaving work. Provide good ventilation in process area to prevent formation of vapor. Report all Mercury releases promptly. Open container slowly on a stable surface. Drums, flasks and bottles of this product must be properly labeled. Empty containers may contain residual amounts of Mercury and should be handled with care.
Hygiene measures	: Do not eat, drink or smoke when using this product. Always wash hands and face immediately after handling this product, and once again before leaving the workplace. Remove contaminated clothing immediately.

7.2. Conditions for safe storage, including any incompatibilities

Technical measures	: Follow practice indicated in Section 6. Make certain that application equipment is locked and tagged-out safely. Always use this product in areas where adequate ventilation is provided. Decontaminate equipment thoroughly before maintenance begins.
Storage conditions	: Keep container tightly closed. Store drums, flasks and bottles in a cool, dry location, away from direct sunlight, source of intense heat, or where freezing is possible. Store away from incompatible materials. Material should be stored in secondary container or in a diked area, as appropriate.
Incompatible materials	: Acetylene and acetylene derivatives, amines, ammonia, 3-bromopropyne, boron diiodophosphide, methyl azide, sodium carbide, heated sulfuric acid, methylsilane/oxygen mixtures, nitric acid/alcohol mixtures, tetracarbonylnickel/oxygen mixtures, alkyne/silver perchlorate mixtures, halogens and strong oxidizers. Mercury can attack copper alloys. Mercury can react with many metals (i.e. calcium, lithium, potassium, sodium, rubidium, aluminum) to form amalgams.
Prohibitions on mixed storage	: Mercury can attack copper alloys. Mercury can react with many metals (i.e. calcium, lithium, potassium, sodium, rubidium, aluminum) to form amalgams.
Storage area	: Storage area should be made of fire-resistant materials.
Special rules on packaging	: Inspect all incoming containers before storage to ensure containers are properly labeled and not damaged.

7.3. Specific end use(s)

No additional information available

SECTION 8: Exposure controls/personal protection

8.1. Control parameters

Mercury (7439-97-6)		
USA ACGIH	ACGIH TWA (mg/m³)	0,025 mg/m³
USA OSHA	OSHA PEL (Ceiling) (mg/m³)	0,1 mg/m³

8.2. Exposure controls

Appropriate engineering controls	: Ensure adequate ventilation. Ensure exposure is below occupational exposure limits (where available). Emergency eye wash fountains and safety showers should be available in the immediate vicinity of any potential exposure.
Personal protective equipment	: Avoid all unnecessary exposure. Gloves. Protective clothing. Safety glasses. Mist formation: aerosol mask.

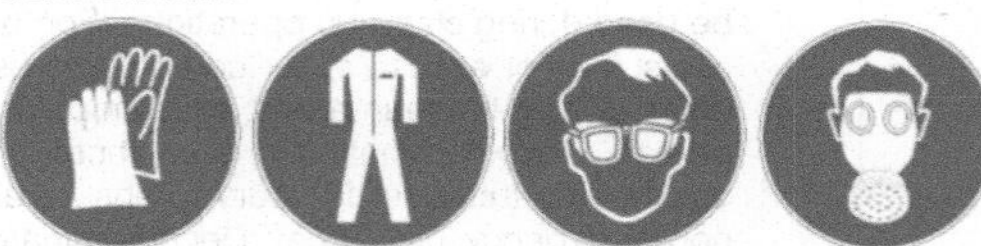

Hand protection	: Wear neoprene gloves for routine industrial use. Use triple gloves for spill response, as stated in Section 6 of this SDS.
Eye protection	: Splash goggles or safety glasses. For operation involving the use of more than 1 pound of Mercury, or if the operation may generate a spray of Mercury, the use of a faceshield is recommended.
Skin and body protection	: Wear suitable protective clothing.
Respiratory protection	: Maintain airborne contaminants concentration below provided exposure limits. If respiratory protection is needed, use only protection authorized in 29 CFR 1910.134 or applicable state regulations. Use supplied air respiration protection if oxygen levels are below 19.5% or are unknown.
Other information	: Do not eat, drink or smoke during use.

SECTION 9: Physical and chemical properties

9.1. Information on basic physical and chemical properties

Physical state	: Liquid
Colour	: Silver white.

MERCURY

Safety Data Sheet

according to the federal final rule of hazard communication revised on 2012 (HazCom 2012)

Odor	:	Odorless.
Odor threshold	:	Not applicable
pH	:	Not applicable
Relative evaporation rate (butylacetate=1)	:	No data available
Melting point	:	No data available
Freezing point	:	-38,87 °C (-37.97 F)
Boiling point	:	No data available
Flash point	:	Not applicable
Self ignition temperature	:	Not applicable
Decomposition temperature	:	No data available
Flammability (solid, gas)	:	No data available
Vapour pressure	:	0,002 mm Hg at 25°C
Relative vapor density at 20 °C	:	6,9 (Air = 1)
Relative density	:	No data available
Relative density of saturated gas/air mixture	:	13,6
Solubility	:	No data available
Log Pow	:	No data available
Log Kow	:	No data available
Viscosity, kinematic	:	No data available
Viscosity, dynamic	:	No data available
Explosive properties	:	No data available
Oxidizing properties	:	No data available
Explosive limits	:	Not applicable

9.2. Other information

No additional information available

SECTION 10: Stability and reactivity

10.1. Reactivity

Stable. Reacts with (some) metals. Mercury can react with metals to form amalgams.

10.2. Chemical stability

Not established.

10.3. Possibility of hazardous reactions

Not established. Hazardous polymerization will not occur.

10.4. Conditions to avoid

Direct sunlight. Extremely high or low temperatures.

10.5. Incompatible materials

Acetylene and acetylene derivatives, amines, ammonia, 3-bromopropyne, boron diiodophosphide, methyl azide, sodium carbide, heated sulfuric acid, methylsilane/oxygen mixtures, nitric acid/alcohol mixtures, tetracarbonylnickel/oxygen mixtures, alkyne/silver perchlorate mixtures, halogens and strong oxidizers. Mercury can attack copper alloys. Mercury can react with many metals (i.e. calcium, lithium, potassium, sodium, rubidium, aluminum) to form amalgams.

10.6. Hazardous decomposition products

If this product is exposed to extremely high temperature in the presence of oxygen or air, toxic vapor of mercury and mercury oxides will be generated.

SECTION 11: Toxicological information

11.1. Information on toxicological effects

Acute toxicity	:	Fatal if inhaled.
Skin corrosion/irritation	:	Not classified pH: Not applicable
Serious eye damage/irritation	:	Not classified pH: Not applicable
Respiratory or skin sensitisation	:	Not classified
Germ cell mutagenicity	:	Not classified Based on available data, the classification criteria are not met
Carcinogenicity	:	Not classified

(continues)

(continued)

MERCURY

Safety Data Sheet

according to the federal final rule of hazard communication revised on 2012 (HazCom 2012)

Mercury (7439-97-6)	
IARC group	3

Reproductive toxicity : May damage fertility or the unborn child.
Based on available data, the classification criteria are not met

Specific target organ toxicity (single exposure) : Not classified

Specific target organ toxicity (repeated exposure) : Causes damage to organs through prolonged or repeated exposure.
Based on available data, the classification criteria are not met
Causes damage to organs through prolonged or repeated exposure

Aspiration hazard : Not classified
Based on available data, the classification criteria are not met

Potential adverse human health effects and symptoms : Based on available data, the classification criteria are not met. Fatal if inhaled.

Symptoms/injuries after inhalation : Short-term over-exposures to high concentrations of mercury vapors can lead to breathing difficulty, coughing, acute,chemical pneumonia, and pulmonary edema (a potentially fatal accumulation of fluid in the lungs) . Depending on the concentration of over-exposure, cardiac abnormalities, damage to the kidney, liver or nerves and effects on the brain may occur. Long-term inhalation over-exposures can lead to the development of a wide variety of symptoms, including the following: excessive salivation, gingivitis, anorexia, chills, fever, cardiac abnormalities, anemia, digestive problems, abdominal pains, frequent urination, an inability to urinate, diarrhea, peripheral neuropathy (numbness, weakness, or burning sensations in the hands or feet), tremors (especially in the hands, fingers, eyelids, lips, cheeks, tongue, or legs), alteration of tendon reflexes, slurred speech, visual disturbances, and deafness. Allergic reactions (i.e. breathing difficulty) may also occur in sensitive individuals.

Symptoms/injuries after skin contact : Symptoms of skin exposure can include redness, dry skin, and pain. Prolonged contact may lead to ulceration of the skin. Allergic reactions (i.e. rashes, welts) may occur in sensitive individuals. Dermatitis (redness and inflammation of the skin) may occur after repeated skin exposures.

Symptoms/injuries after eye contact : Symptoms of eye exposure can include redness, pain, and watery eyes. A symptom of Mercury exposure is discoloration of the lens of the eyes.

Symptoms/injuries after ingestion : If Mercury is swallowed, symptoms of such over-exposure can include metallic taste in mouth, nausea, vomiting, central nervous system effects, and damage to the kidneys. Metallic mercury is not usually absorbed sufficiently from the gastrointestinal tract to induce an acute, toxic response. Damage to the tissues of the mouth, throat, esophagus, and other tissues of the digestive system may occur. Ingestion may be fatal, due to effects on gastrointestinal system and kidneys.

Chronic symptoms : Long-term over-exposure can lead to a wide range of adverse health effects. Anyone using Mercury must pay attention to personality changes, weight loss, skin or gum discolorations, stomach pains, and other signs of Mercury over-exposure. Gradually developing syndromes ("Erethism" and "Acrodynia") are indicative of potentially severe health problems. Mercury can cause the development of allergic reactions (i.e. dermatitis, rashes, breathing difficulty) upon prolonged or repeated exposures. Refer to Section 11 (Toxicology Information) for additional data.

SECTION 12: Ecological information

12.1. Toxicity

Ecology - water : Very toxic to aquatic life. Toxic to aquatic life with long lasting effects.

Mercury (7439-97-6)	
LC50 fishes 1	0,5 mg/l (Exposure time: 96 h - Species: Cyprinus carpio)
EC50 Daphnia 1	5,0 µg/l (Exposure time: 96 h - Species: water flea)
LC50 fish 2	0,16 mg/l (Exposure time: 96 h - Species: Cyprinus carpio [semi-static])

12.2. Persistence and degradability

MERCURY (7439-97-6)	
Persistence and degradability	May cause long-term adverse effects in the environment.

12.3. Bioaccumulative potential

MERCURY (7439-97-6)	
Bioaccumulative potential	Not established.

12.4. Mobility in soil

No additional information available

12.5. Other adverse effects

Other information : Avoid release to the environment.

MERCURY

Safety Data Sheet

according to the federal final rule of hazard communication revised on 2012 (HazCom 2012)

SECTION 13: Disposal considerations

13.1. Waste treatment methods

Waste disposal recommendations	: Dispose in a safe manner in accordance with local/national regulations. Waste disposal must be in accordance with appropriate federal, state, and local regulations. This product, if unaltered by use, should be recycled. If altered by use, recycling may be possible. Consult Bethlehem Apparatus Company for information. If Mercury must be disposed of as hazardous waste, it must be handled at a permitted facility or as advised by your local hazardous waste regulatory authority.
Ecology - waste materials	: Hazardous waste due to toxicity. Avoid release to the environment.

SECTION 14: Transport information

In accordance with DOT

14.1. UN number

UN-No.(DOT)	: 2809
DOT NA no.	UN2809

14.2. UN proper shipping name

DOT Proper Shipping Name	: Mercury
Department of Transportation (DOT) Hazard Classes	: 8 - Class 8 - Corrosive material 49 CFR 173.136
Hazard labels (DOT)	: 8 - Corrosive substances 6.1 - Toxic substances

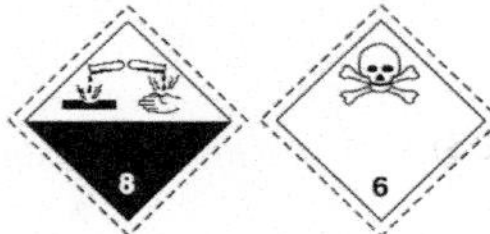

DOT Symbols	: A - Material is regulated as a hazardous material only when be transported by air, W - Material is regulated as a hazardous material only when be transported by water
Packing group (DOT)	: III - Minor Danger
DOT Packaging Exceptions (49 CFR 173.xxx)	: 164
DOT Packaging Non Bulk (49 CFR 173.xxx)	: 164
DOT Packaging Bulk (49 CFR 173.xxx)	: 240

14.3. Additional information

Other information	: No supplementary information available.

Overland transport

No additional information available

Transport by sea

DOT Vessel Stowage Location	: B - (i) The material may be stowed "on deck" or "under deck" on a cargo vessel and on a passenger vessel carrying a number of passengers limited to not more than the larger of 25 passengers, or one passenger per each 3 m of overall vessel length; and (ii) "On deck only" on passenger vessels in which the number of passengers specified in paragraph (k)(2)(i) of this section is exceeded.
DOT Vessel Stowage Other	: 40 - Stow "clear of living quarters",97 - Stow "away from" azides

Air transport

DOT Quantity Limitations Passenger aircraft/rail (49 CFR 173.27)	: 35 kg
DOT Quantity Limitations Cargo aircraft only (49 CFR 175.75)	: 35 kg

SECTION 15: Regulatory information

15.1. US Federal regulations

Mercury (7439-97-6)	
Listed on the United States TSCA (Toxic Substances Control Act) inventory Listed on SARA Section 313 (Specific toxic chemical listings)	
EPA TSCA Regulatory Flag	S - S - indicates a substance that is identified in a proposed or final Significant New Uses Rule.
SARA Section 313 - Emission Reporting	1,0 %

15.2. International regulations

CANADA

(continues)

(continued)

MERCURY

Safety Data Sheet

according to the federal final rule of hazard communication revised on 2012 (HazCom 2012)

Mercury (7439-97-6)	
Listed on the Canadian DSL (Domestic Sustances List) inventory.	
WHMIS Classification	Class D Division 1 Subdivision A - Very toxic material causing immediate and serious toxic effects Class D Division 2 Subdivision A - Very toxic material causing other toxic effects Class E - Corrosive Material

EU-Regulations

Mercury (7439-97-6)
Listed on the EEC inventory EINECS (European Inventory of Existing Commercial Chemical Substances) substances.

Classification according to Regulation (EC) No. 1272/2008 [CLP]

Classification according to Directive 67/548/EEC or 1999/45/EC

Not classified

15.2.2. National regulations

Mercury (7439-97-6)
Listed on the AICS (the Australian Inventory of Chemical Substances) Listed on Inventory of Existing Chemical Substances (IECSC) Listed on the Korean ECL (Existing Chemical List) inventory. Listed on New Zealand - Inventory of Chemicals (NZIoC) Listed on Inventory of Chemicals and Chemical Substances (PICCS) Poisonous and Deleterious Substances Control Law Pollutant Release and Transfer Register Law (PRTR Law) Listed on the Canadian Ingredient Disclosure List

15.3. US State regulations

Mercury (7439-97-6)				
U.S. - California - Proposition 65 - Carcinogens List	U.S. - California - Proposition 65 - Developmental Toxicity	U.S. - California - Proposition 65 - Reproductive Toxicity - Female	U.S. - California - Proposition 65 - Reproductive Toxicity - Male	No significance risk level (NSRL)
	Yes			

SECTION 16: Other information

Other information : None.

Full text of H-phrases: see section 16:

Acute Tox. 1 (Inhalation:dust,mist)	Acute toxicity (inhalation:dust,mist) Category 1
Acute Tox. 2 (Inhalation)	Acute toxicity (inhalation) Category 2
Aquatic Acute 1	Hazardous to the aquatic environment — AcuteHazard, Category 1
Aquatic Chronic 1	Hazardous to the aquatic environment — Chronic Hazard, Category 1
Repr. 1B	Reproductive toxicity Category 1B
STOT RE 1	Specific target organ toxicity (repeated exposure) Category 1
H330	Fatal if inhaled
H360	May damage fertility or the unborn child
H372	Causes damage to organs through prolonged or repeated exposure
H400	Very toxic to aquatic life
H410	Very toxic to aquatic life with long lasting effects

NFPA health hazard : 3 - Short exposure could cause serious temporary or residual injury even though prompt medical attention was given.

NFPA fire hazard : 0 - Materials that will not burn.

NFPA reactivity : 0 - Normally stable, even under fire exposure conditions, and are not reactive with water.

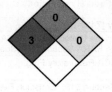

SDS US (GHS HazCom 2012)

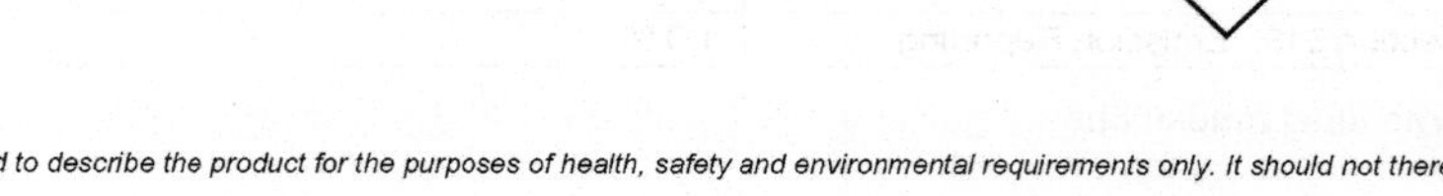

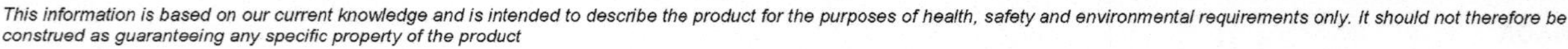

This information is based on our current knowledge and is intended to describe the product for the purposes of health, safety and environmental requirements only. It should not therefore be construed as guaranteeing any specific property of the product

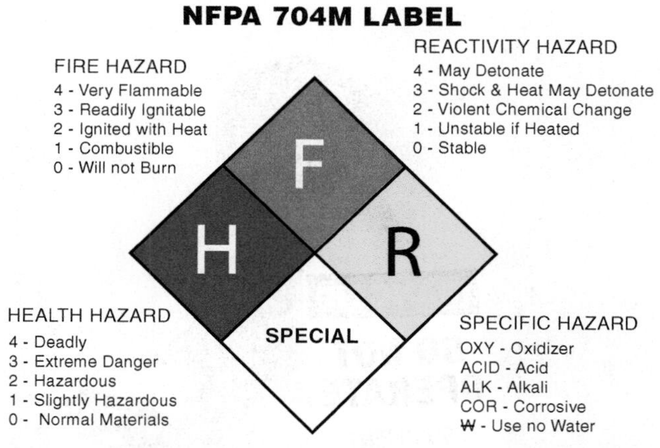

NFPA 704M LABEL

FIRE HAZARD
4 - Very Flammable
3 - Readily Ignitable
2 - Ignited with Heat
1 - Combustible
0 - Will not Burn

REACTIVITY HAZARD
4 - May Detonate
3 - Shock & Heat May Detonate
2 - Violent Chemical Change
1 - Unstable if Heated
0 - Stable

F
H
R
SPECIAL

HEALTH HAZARD
4 - Deadly
3 - Extreme Danger
2 - Hazardous
1 - Slightly Hazardous
0 - Normal Materials

SPECIFIC HAZARD
OXY - Oxidizer
ACID - Acid
ALK - Alkali
COR - Corrosive
W̶ - Use no Water

FIGURE 14–4 The NFPA label identifies specific hazards of chemicals.

The Occupational Exposure to Hazardous Chemicals Standard also mandates that all employers train employees to follow the proper procedures or policies with regard to:

- Identifying the types and locations of all chemicals or hazards
- Locating and using the SDS manual containing all of the safety data sheets; SDSs must be readily accessible for all hazardous chemicals used
- Reading and interpreting chemical labels and hazard signs
- Using personal protective equipment (PPE) such as masks, gowns, gloves, and goggles
- Locating cleaning equipment and following the correct methods for managing spills and disposal of chemicals
- Reporting accidents or exposures and documenting any incidents that occur

Bloodborne Pathogen Standard

The **Bloodborne Pathogen Standard** has mandates to protect health care providers from diseases caused by exposure to body fluids. Examples of body fluids include blood and blood components, urine, stool, semen, vaginal secretions, cerebrospinal fluid, saliva, mucus, and other similar fluids. Three diseases that can be contracted by exposure to body fluids include hepatitis B, caused by the hepatitis B virus; hepatitis C, caused by the hepatitis C virus; and acquired immune deficiency syndrome (AIDS), caused by the human immunodeficiency virus (HIV). The mandates of this standard are discussed in detail in Chapter 15:4. Isolation precautions required while caring for patients who have communicable disease are found under *transmission-based precautions* in Chapter 15:9 of this text.

Environmental Safety

Ergonomics is an applied science used to promote the safety and well-being of a person by adapting the environment and using techniques to prevent injuries. Ergonomics includes correctly placing furniture and equipment, training in required muscle movements, avoiding repetitive motions, and being aware of the environment to prevent injuries. The prevention of accidents and injury centers around people and the immediate environment. The health care worker must be conscious of personal and patient/resident safety at all times. In addition, every health care worker must be alert to unsafe situations and report them immediately. Examples include burned-out lightbulbs, frayed electrical cords, scalding water in a sink or bath area, missing floor tiles or torn carpet, and other similar hazards.

Environmental hazards in health care facilities can also endanger patients, health care personnel, other individuals, and the environment. Radiation exposure is a major concern in radiology departments and dental offices. In dental offices, a lead apron should be used to cover the patient before dental radiographs are taken. In addition, the dental worker taking the radiographs usually stands outside the room to activate the machine and obtain the radiograph. In radiology departments, all machines that emit radiation waves must be checked frequently to make sure they are operating correctly and not leaking radiation. Radiographers should stand behind a protective shield when activating the machines. To ensure that the level of exposure is safe, personnel in these departments wear badges that measure exposure to radiation. Another substance that can cause radiation exposure is radioactive iodine. This substance is used to diagnose thyroid problems and treat thyroid diseases. After it has been given to a patient, small amounts of radiation are present in the neck area for several days. This is a beneficial treatment for the patient, but precautions must be taken to protect the patient's family and friends. Contact must be limited, especially with children and pregnant women. No eating utensils or food should be shared. Other radioactive substances used to treat cancer present the same problems. An example is radioactive seeds that are used to treat prostate cancer in men. At times, patients are even kept in isolation for several days to prevent radiation exposure to others.

Medications and gases can be an environmental hazard. Antineoplastic drugs used to treat different cancers can be hazardous to health care personnel and pregnant individuals and must be handled with care. In operating rooms and dental offices, nitrous oxide, a gas used as an anesthetic, may cause spontaneous abortions in pregnant women. Mercury used in dental offices and thermometers can present a danger to people and the environment if it is not disposed of correctly.

In the same way, individuals and the environment can be harmed by improper disposal of biohazard wastes such as needles and syringes. Contaminated wastes containing body fluids, such as blood, can spread disease if they are not destroyed properly. All health care workers are responsible for identifying the specific hazards that present a danger to themselves, others in society, and the environment, and for taking proper precautions to deal with those hazards.

Legal

In addition, every health care worker must accept the responsibility to use good judgment in all situations, ask questions when in doubt, and follow approved policies and procedures to create a safe environment. Always remember that a health care worker has a legal responsibility to protect the patient from harm and injury.

EQUIPMENT AND SOLUTIONS SAFETY

Basic rules that must be followed when working with equipment and solutions include:

- Do *not* operate or use any equipment until you have been instructed on how to use it.
- Read and follow the operating instructions for all major pieces of equipment. If you do not understand the instructions, ask for assistance.
- Do *not* operate any equipment if your instructor/immediate supervisor is not in the room.
- Report any damaged or malfunctioning equipment immediately. Make no attempt to use it. Some facilities use a lockout tag system for damaged electrical or mechanical equipment. A locking device is placed on the equipment to prevent the equipment from being used (Figure 14–5).
- Do not use frayed or damaged electrical cords. Do not use a plug if the third prong for grounding has been broken off. Never use excessive force to insert a plug into an outlet.
- Never handle any electrical equipment with wet hands or around water.
- Store all equipment in its proper place. Unused equipment should not be left in a patient's room, a hallway, or a doorway.
- When handling any equipment, observe all safety precautions that have been taught.
- Read SDSs before using any hazardous chemical solutions.
- Check the NFPA code on a chemical to determine the specific hazards associated with the chemical.
- Never use solutions from bottles that are not labeled.

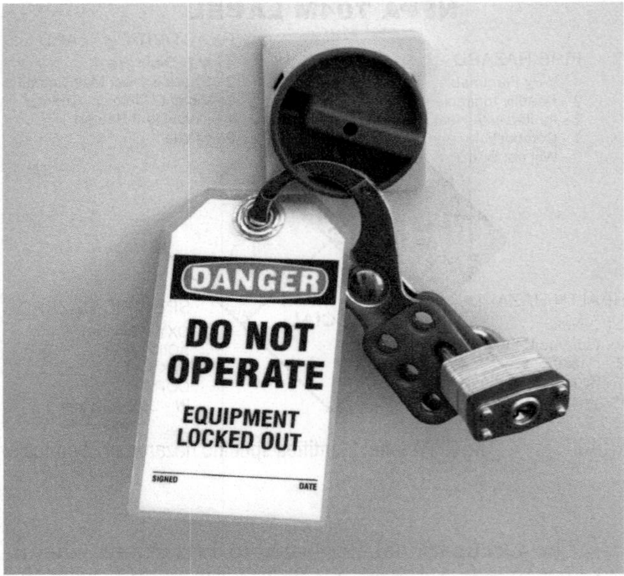

FIGURE 14–5 Some facilities use a lockout tag system for damaged equipment to prevent anyone from using the equipment.
©iStock.com/Brandon Clark

- Read the labels of solution bottles at least three times during use to be sure you have the correct solution (Figure 14–6).
- Do *not* mix any solutions together unless instructed to do so by your instructor/immediate supervisor or you can verify that they are compatible.
- Some solutions can be injurious or poisonous. Avoid contact with your eyes and skin. Avoid inhaling any fumes emitted by a solution. Use only as directed.
- Store all chemical solutions in a locked cabinet or closet following the manufacturer's recommendations. For example, some solutions must be kept at room temperature, while others must be stored in a cool area.

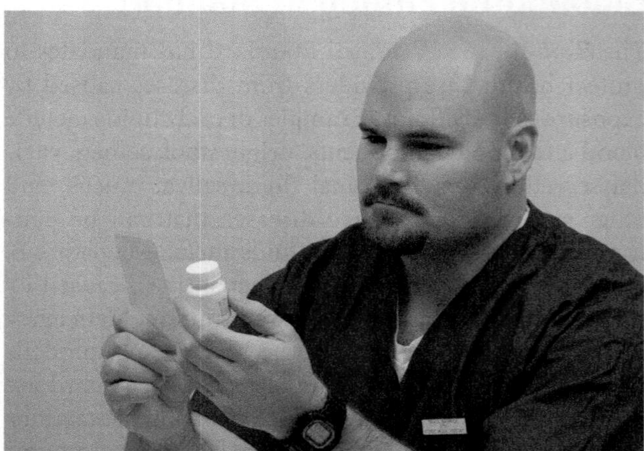

FIGURE 14–6 Read the label on a solution bottle at least three times to be sure you have the correct solution.

- Dispose of chemical solutions according to the instructions provided on the SDS for the solution.
- If you break any equipment or spill any solutions, immediately report the incident to your instructor/immediate supervisor. You will be told how to dispose of the equipment or how to remove the spilled solution (Figure 14–7).

PATIENT/RESIDENT SAFETY

Basic rules that must be followed to protect a patient or resident include:

- Do *not* perform any procedure on patients unless you have been instructed to do so. Make sure you have the proper authorization. Follow instructions carefully. Ask questions if you do not understand. Use correct or approved methods while performing any procedure. Avoid shortcuts or incorrect techniques.
- Provide privacy for all patients. Knock on the door before entering any room (Figure 14–8A). Speak to the patient and identify yourself. Ask for permission to enter before going behind closed privacy curtains. Close the door and draw curtains for privacy before beginning a procedure on a patient (Figure 14–8B).
- Always identify your patient. Be absolutely positive that you have the correct patient. Check the identification wristband, if present. Ask the patient to state his or her name. Repeat the patient's name at least twice. Check the name on the patient's bed and on the patient's record.
- Always explain the procedure so the patient knows what you are going to do (Figure 14–8C). Answer any questions and make sure you have the patient's consent before performing any procedure. Never perform a procedure if a patient refuses to allow you to do so.
- Observe the patient closely during any procedure. If you notice any change, immediately report this. Be alert to the patient's condition at all times.
- Frequently check the patient area, waiting room, office rooms, bed areas, or home environment for safety hazards. Report all unsafe situations immediately to the proper person or correct the safety hazard.
- Before leaving a patient/resident in a bed, observe all safety checkpoints. Make sure the patient is in a comfortable position. Check the bed to be sure that the

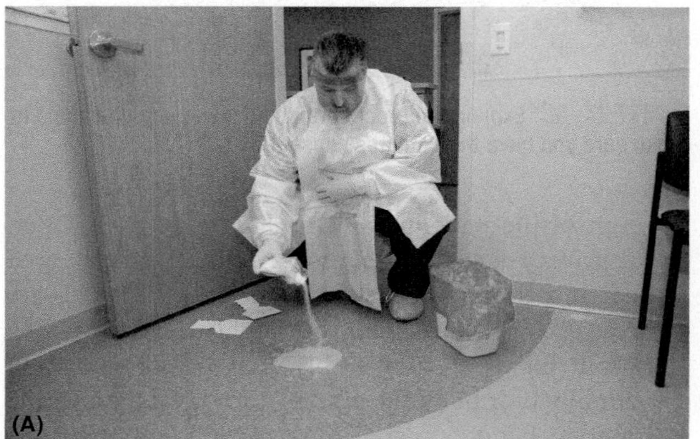

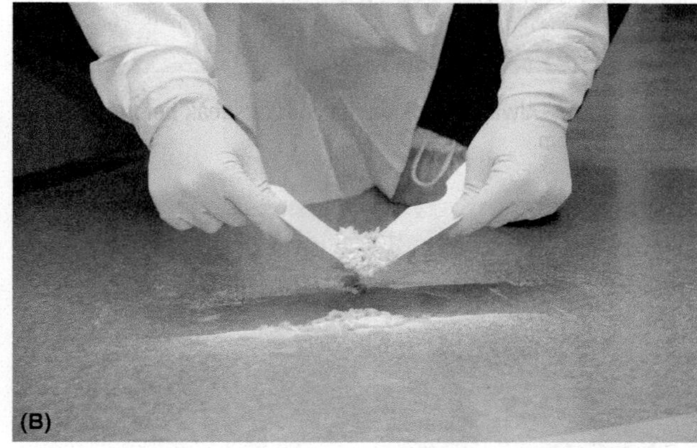

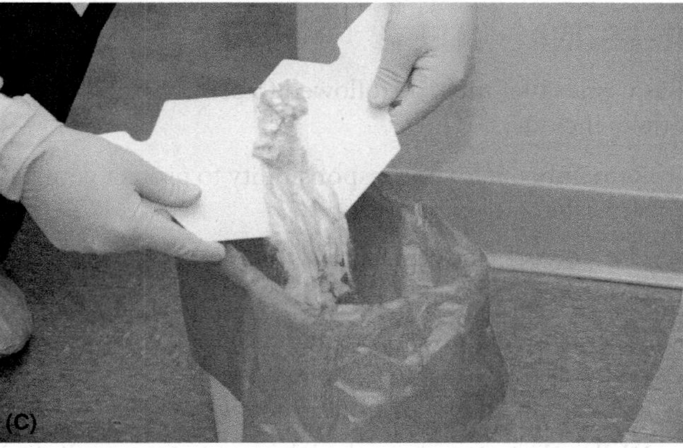

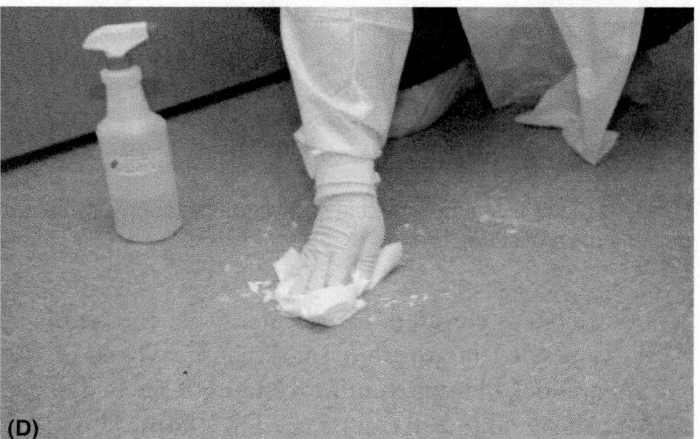

FIGURE 14–7 To clean a spill: (A) pour coagulating powder on the spill. (B) When the material has been absorbed, pick up the residue and (C) place it in a biohazard container. (D) Clean the area thoroughly with a disinfecting solution.

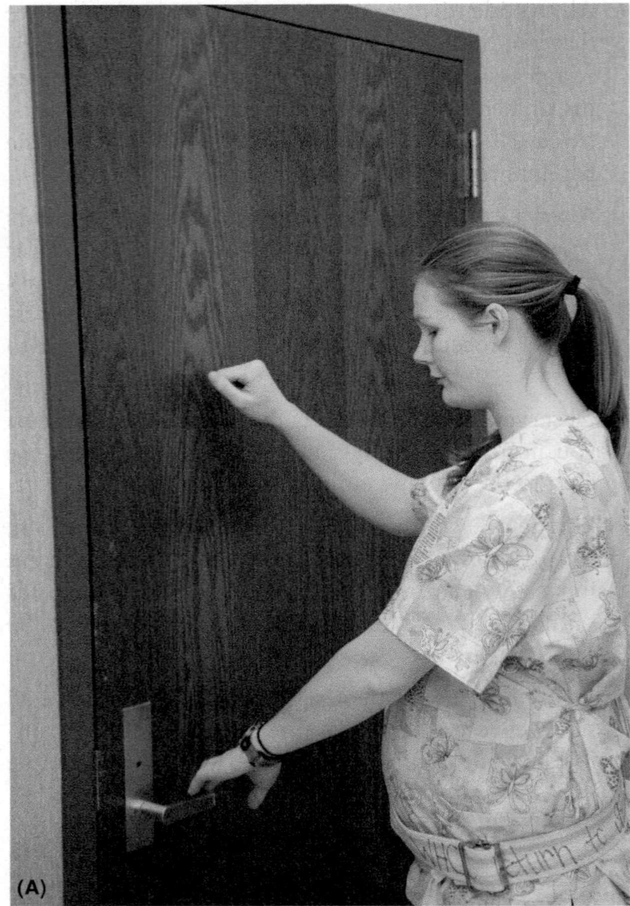

FIGURE 14–8A Always knock on the door or speak before entering a patient's room.

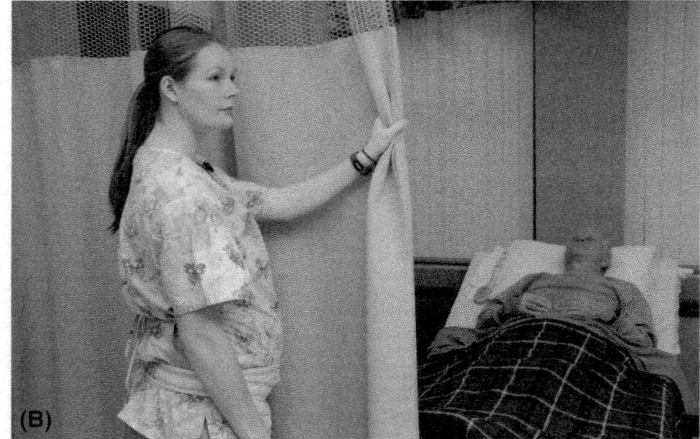

FIGURE 14–8B Close the door and draw curtains for privacy before beginning a procedure.

side rails are elevated, if indicated; that the bed is at the lowest level to the floor; and that the wheels on the bed are locked to prevent movement of the bed. Place the call signal (a bell can be used in a home situation) and other supplies such as the telephone, television remote control, fresh water, and tissues within easy

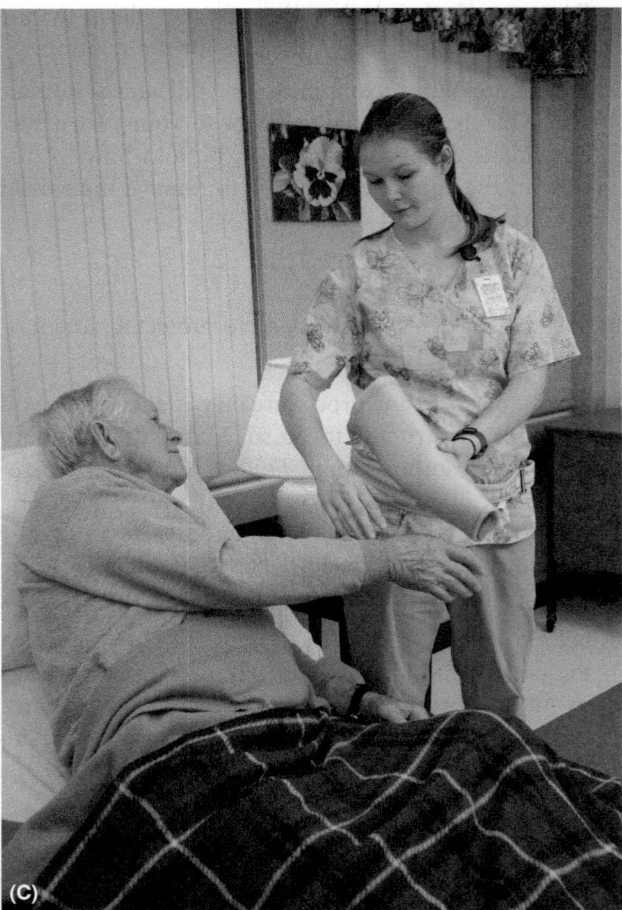

FIGURE 14–8C Explain the procedure and answer any questions to make sure you have the patient's consent.

reach of the patient/resident (Figure 14–9A). Open the privacy curtains if they were closed. Leave the area neat and clean, and make sure no safety hazards are present. Wash your hands thoroughly (Figure 14–9B). If your hands are not visibly dirty or contaminated with blood or body fluids, they can be cleaned with a waterless hand cleaner (Figure 14–9C).

PERSONAL SAFETY

Basic rules that must be followed to protect yourself and others include:

- Remember, it is your responsibility to protect yourself and others from injury.
- Use correct body mechanics while performing any procedure.
- Wear the required personal protective equipment (PPE) as discussed in Chapter 15:4. This may include a gown, mask, gloves, and protective eyewear.
- Walk—do *not* run—in the laboratory area or clinical area, in hallways, and especially on stairs. Keep to the

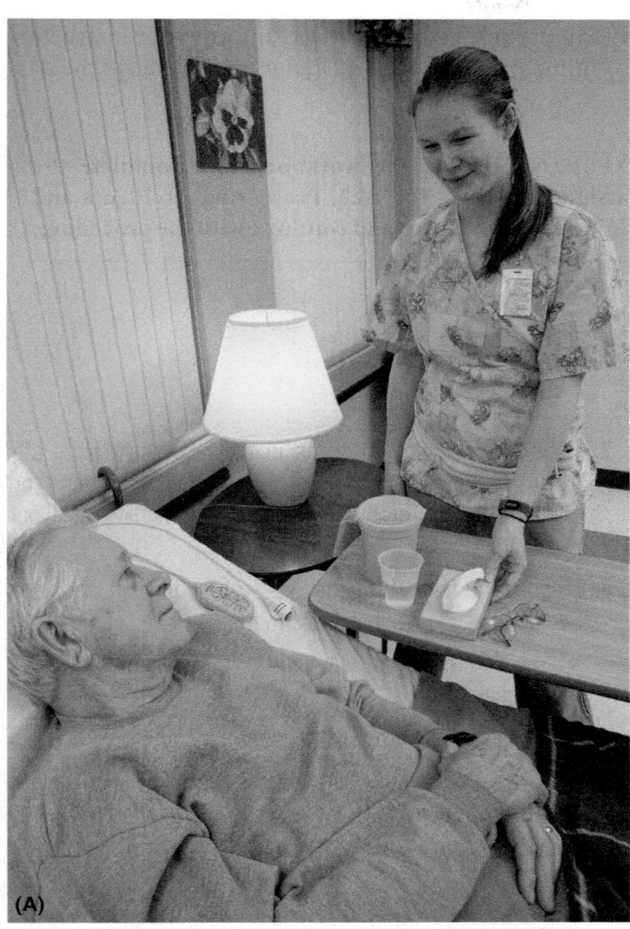

FIGURE 14–9A Lower the bed and place the call signal and other supplies within easy reach of the patient before leaving a patient.

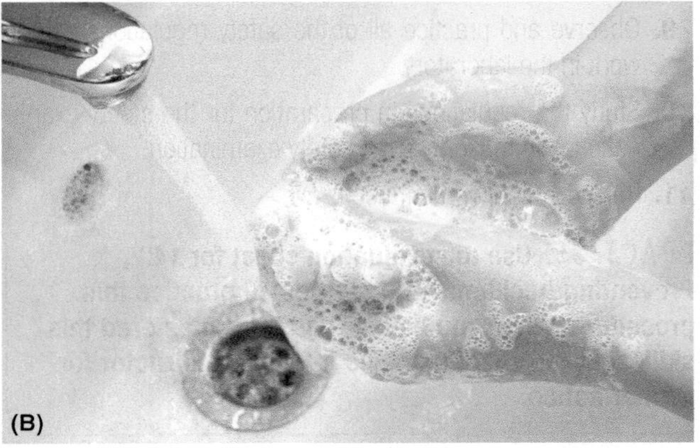

FIGURE 14–9B Wash your hands before and after any procedure, and any time they become contaminated during a procedure.

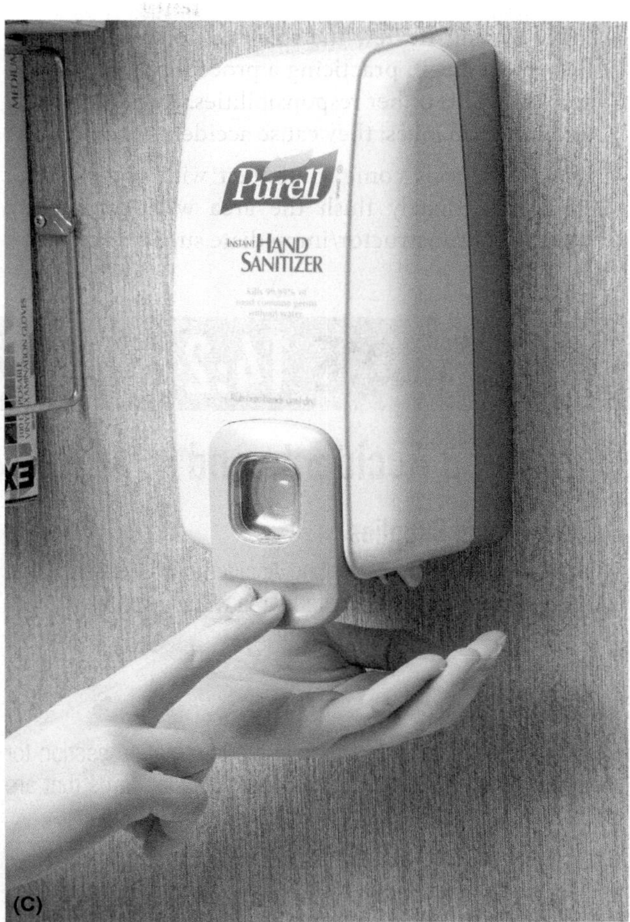

FIGURE 14–9C If your hands are not visibly dirty or contaminated with blood or body fluids, they can be cleaned with a waterless hand cleaner.

right and watch carefully at intersections to avoid collisions. Use handrails on stairways.

- Promptly report any personal injury or accident, no matter how minor, to your instructor/immediate supervisor.
- If you see an unsafe situation or a violation of a safety practice, report it to your instructor/immediate supervisor promptly.
- Keep all areas clean and neat with all equipment and supplies in their proper locations at all times.
- Wash your hands frequently. Hands should always be washed before and after any procedure, and any time they become contaminated during a procedure (refer to Figure 14–9B).
- Keep your hands away from your face, eyes, mouth, and hair.
- Dry your hands thoroughly before handling any electrical equipment.
- Wear safety glasses when instructed to do so and in any situations that might result in possible eye injury.
- While working with your partner in patient simulations, observe all safety precautions taught in caring

for a patient. Review the role each of you will have before you begin practicing a procedure so each person knows his or her responsibilities. Avoid horseplay and practical jokes; they cause accidents.

- If any solutions come in contact with your skin or eyes, immediately flush the area with cool water. Inform your instructor/immediate supervisor.
- If a particle gets in your eye, inform your instructor/immediate supervisor. Do *not* try to remove the particle or rub your eye.

STUDENT: **Go to the workbook and complete the assignment sheet for 14:2, Preventing Accidents and Injuries. Then return and continue with the procedure.**

PROCEDURE 14:2

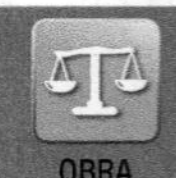

Preventing Accidents and Injuries

Equipment and Supplies

Information section on Preventing Accidents and Injuries, several bottles of solutions, laboratory area with equipment

Procedure

1. Assemble equipment.
2. Review the safety standards in the information section for Preventing Accidents and Injuries. Note standards that are not clear and ask your instructor for an explanation.
3. Examine several bottles of solutions. Read the labels carefully. Read the safety or danger warnings on the bottles. Read SDSs provided with hazardous chemicals. Check the NFPA label and note specific hazards.
4. Practice reading the label three times to be sure you have the correct solution. Read the label before taking the bottle off the shelf, before pouring from the bottle, and after you have poured from the bottle.
5. Look at major pieces of equipment in the laboratory. Read the operating instructions for the equipment. Do *not* operate the equipment until you are taught how to do it correctly.
6. Role-play the following situations by using another student as a patient.
   - Show ways to provide privacy for the patient.
   - Identify the patient.
   - Explain a procedure to the patient.
   - Observe the patient during a procedure. List points you should observe to note a change in the patient's condition.
7. Check various patient areas in the laboratory. Note any safety hazards that may be present. Discuss how you can correct the problems. Report your findings to your instructor.
8. Discuss the following situations with another student and decide how you would handle them:
   - You see an unsafe situation or a violation of a safety practice
   - You see a wet area on the laboratory counter
   - You get a small cut on your hand while using a glass slide
   - A solution splashes on your arm
   - A particle gets in your eye
   - A piece of equipment is not working correctly
   - A bottle of solution does not have a label
   - You break a glass beaker
9. Observe and practice all of the safety regulations as you work in the laboratory.
10. Study the regulations in preparation for the safety examination. You must pass the safety examination.
11. Replace all equipment used.

PRACTICE: **Use the evaluation sheet for 14:2, Preventing Accidents and Injuries, to practice this procedure. When you believe you have mastered this skill, sign the sheet and give it to your instructor for further action.**

FINAL CHECKPOINT: Using the criteria listed on the evaluation sheet, your instructor will grade your performance.

14:3 Observing Fire Safety

Health care providers must know three basic facts about fires: how they start, how to prevent them, and how to respond when they occur.

Fires need three things in order to start (Figure 14–10):

- *Oxygen:* present in the air
- *Fuel:* any material that will burn
- *Heat:* sparks, matches, flames

The major cause of fires is carelessness with smoking and with matches. Other causes include misuse of electricity (overloaded circuits, frayed electrical wires, improperly grounded plugs), defects in heating systems, spontaneous ignition, improper rubbish disposal, and arson.

Fire Extinguishers

Fire extinguishers are classified and labeled according to the kind of fire they extinguish. The main classes are:

- *Class A:* used on fires involving combustibles such as paper, cloth, plastic, and wood
- *Class B:* used on fires involving flammable or combustible liquids such as gasoline, oil, paint, grease, and cooking fat
- *Class C:* used on electrical fires such as fuse boxes, appliances, wiring, and electrical outlets; the C stands for nonconductive; if possible, the electricity should be turned off before using an extinguisher on an electrical fire

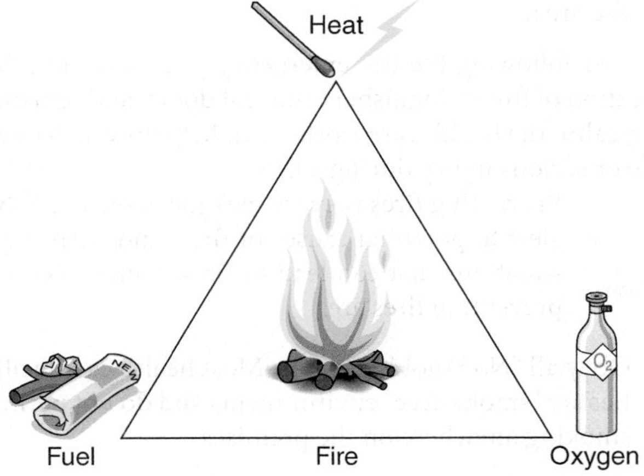

FIGURE 14–10 The fire triangle shows the three things needed to start a fire.

- *Class D:* used on burning or combustible metals; often specific for the type of metal being used and not used on any other types of fires

Many different types of fire extinguishers are available. The main types include:

- *Water:* contains pressurized water and should only be used on Class A fires
- *Carbon dioxide:* contains carbon dioxide gas that provides a smothering action on the fire by forming a cloud of cool ice or snow that displaces the air and oxygen; leaves a powdery, snow-like residue that irritates the skin and eyes and can be dangerous if inhaled; most effective on Class B or C fires
- *Dry chemical:* contains a chemical that acts to smother a fire; type BC extinguishers contain potassium bicarbonate or sodium bicarbonate, which leaves a mildly corrosive residue that must be cleaned up as soon as possible; type ABC extinguishers contain monoammonium phosphate, a yellow powder that leaves a sticky residue that can damage electrical appliances such as computers; both residues can irritate the skin and eyes; used on Class A, B, or C fires
- *Halon:* contains a gas that interferes with the chemical reaction that occurs when fuels burn; used on electrical equipment because it does not leave a residue and will not damage appliances such as computers; most effective on Class C fires

Most fire extinguishers are labeled with a diagram and/or a letter showing the type of fire for which they are effective (Figure 14–11). Many extinguishers are used on different types of fires and will be labeled with more than one diagram or letter. In addition, some extinguishers put all of the diagrams on the label; however, a diagonal red line is drawn through any diagram that depicts a fire for which the extinguisher should not be used. For example, if a diagonal red line is drawn through the diagram for electrical fires, it means the extinguisher should not be used on any electrical fire. Health care workers must become familiar with the types and locations of fire extinguishers in their place of employment so they are prepared to act when a fire occurs.

In case of fire, the main rule is to remain calm. If your personal safety is endangered, evacuate the area according to the stated method and sound the alarm. If the fire is small, confined to one area, and your safety is not endangered, determine what type of fire it is and use the proper extinguisher.

CLASSES OF FIRE EXTINGUISHERS

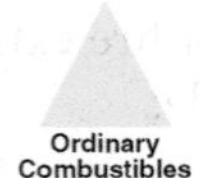

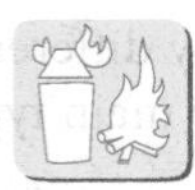

CLASS A

Used for fires of ordinary combustibles such as wood, paper, cloth, and plastics

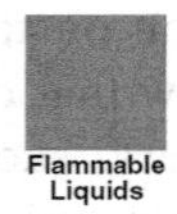

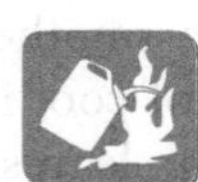

CLASS B

Used for fires of flammable liquids and gases such as paint, gasoline, oil, grease, and cooking fats

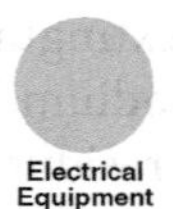

CLASS C

Used for electrical fires such as fuse boxes, wiring, electrical outlets, and appliances; if possible, turn off the electricity before using an extinguisher on this type of fire

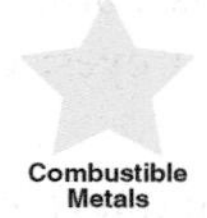

CLASS D

Used on burning or combustible metals such as magnesium, titanium, and sodium; specific for the type of metal; not used on other types of fires

FIGURE 14–11 Fire extinguishers contain diagrams and/or letters to show the type of fire on which they should be used.

Fire Emergency Plan

While working in a health care facility, know and follow the fire emergency plan established by the facility. The plan usually states that all patients and personnel in immediate danger should be moved from the area. The alarm should be activated as quickly as possible (Figure 14–12). All doors and windows should be closed, if possible, to prevent drafts, which cause fire to spread more rapidly. Electrical equipment and oxygen should be shut off. Elevators should never be used during a fire. The acronym *RACE* is frequently used to remember the important steps. *RACE* stands for:

- *R* = Rescue anyone in immediate danger. Move patients to a safe area. If the patient can walk, escort him or her to a safe area. At times it may be necessary to move a patient in a bed or use the bed sheets as lift sheets to carry a patient to a safe area.
- *A* = Activate the alarm. Sound the alarm and give the location and type of fire.
- *C* = Contain the fire. Close windows and doors to prevent drafts. Shut off electrical equipment and oxygen if your safety is not endangered.
- *E* = Extinguish the fire or evacuate the area. If the fire is small and contained, and you are not in danger, locate the correct fire extinguisher to extinguish the fire. If the fire is large or spreading rapidly, or if you or a patient/resident are in danger, evacuate the area.

By following the fire emergency plan, knowing the location of fire extinguishers and exit doors, and remaining calm, the health care worker can help prevent loss of life or serious injury during a fire.

Preventing fires is everyone's job. Constantly be alert to potential causes of fires, and correct all situations that can lead to fires. Some rules for preventing fires are:

- Obey all "No Smoking" signs. Most health care facilities are "smoke-free" environments and do not permit smoking anywhere on the premises.
- Extinguish matches, cigarettes, and any other flammable items completely. Do not empty ashtrays into trash cans or plastic bags that can burn. Always empty ashtrays into separate metal cans or containers partially filled with sand or water.

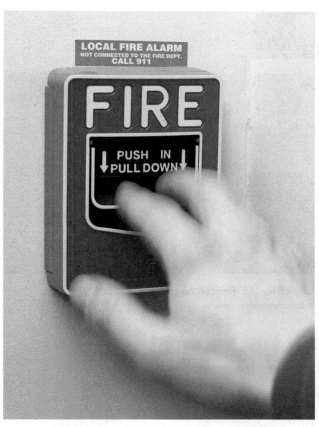

FIGURE 14–12 When a fire occurs, the fire alarm should be activated as quickly as possible. © Andre Blais/Shutterstock.com

- Dispose of all waste materials in proper containers.
- Before using electrical equipment, check for damaged cords or improper grounding. Avoid overloading electrical outlets.
- Store flammable materials such as kerosene or gasoline in proper containers and in a safe area. If you spill a flammable liquid, wipe it up immediately.
- Do not allow clutter to accumulate in rooms, closets, doorways, or traffic areas. Make sure no equipment or supplies block any fire exits.
- When oxygen is in use, observe special precautions. Post a "No Smoking—Oxygen in Use" sign. Remove all smoking materials, candles, lighters, and matches from the room. Avoid the use of electrically operated equipment whenever possible. Do not use flammable liquids such as alcohol, nail polish, and oils. Avoid static electricity by using cotton blankets, sheets, and gowns.

Disaster Plans

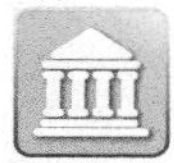
Legal

In addition to fires, other types of disasters may occur. Examples include tornadoes, hurricanes, earthquakes, floods, and bomb threats. In any type of disaster, stay calm, follow the policy of the health care facility, and provide for the safety of yourself and the patient. It is important to note that health care workers are legally responsible for familiarizing themselves with disaster policies so appropriate action can be taken when a disaster strikes.

STUDENT: **Go to the workbook and complete the assignment sheet for 14:3, Observing Fire Safety. Then return and continue with the procedure.**

PROCEDURE 14:3

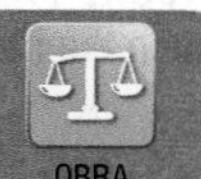
OBRA

Observing Fire Safety

Equipment and Supplies

Fire alarm box, fire extinguishers

Procedure

1. Read the information section on Observing Fire Safety.
2. Learn the four classes of fire extinguishers and know for which kind of fire each type is used.
3. Locate the nearest fire alarm box. Read the instructions on how to operate the alarm. Be sure you could set off the alarm in case of a fire.
4. Locate any fire extinguishers in the laboratory or clinical area. Look for extinguishers in both the room and surrounding building. Identify each extinguisher and the kind of fire for which it is meant to be used.
5. Learn how to operate a fire extinguisher. Read the manufacturer's operating instructions carefully. Work with a practice extinguisher or do a mock demonstration.

Safety

CAUTION: Do *not* discharge a real extinguisher in the laboratory or clinical area.

a. Check the extinguisher type to be sure it is the proper one to use for the mock fire (Figure 14–13A).

(continues)

PROCEDURE 14:3 (CONT.)

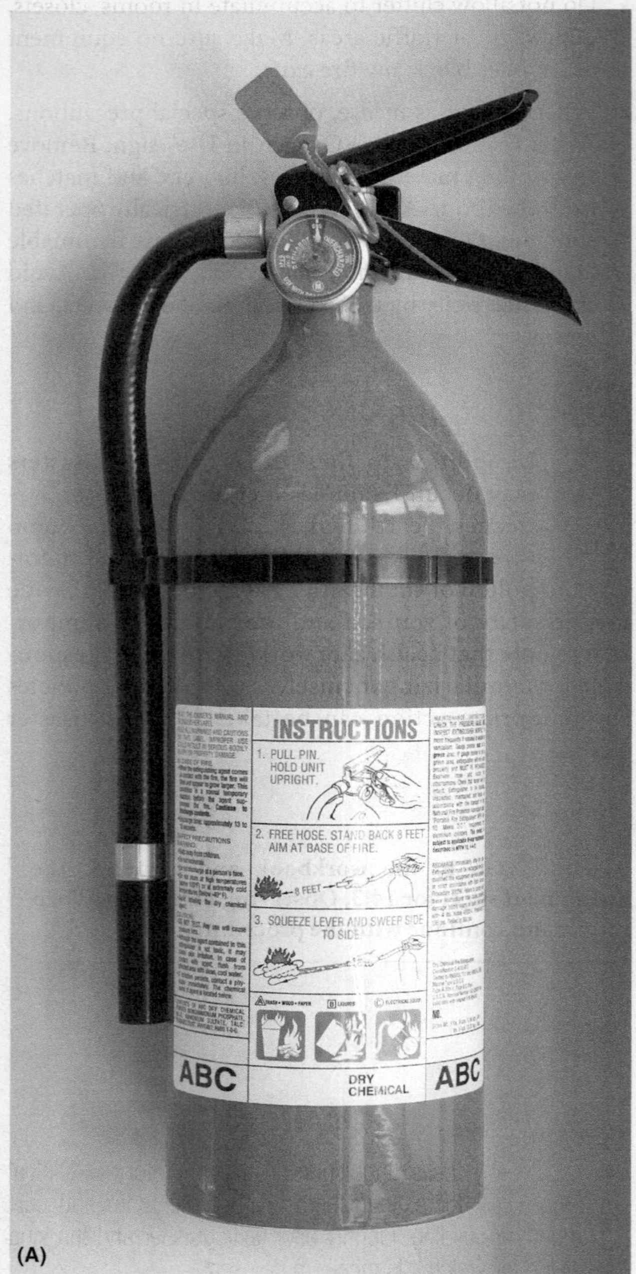

FIGURE 14–13A Check the extinguisher type to make sure it is the correct one to use. © Rob Byron/Shutterstock.com

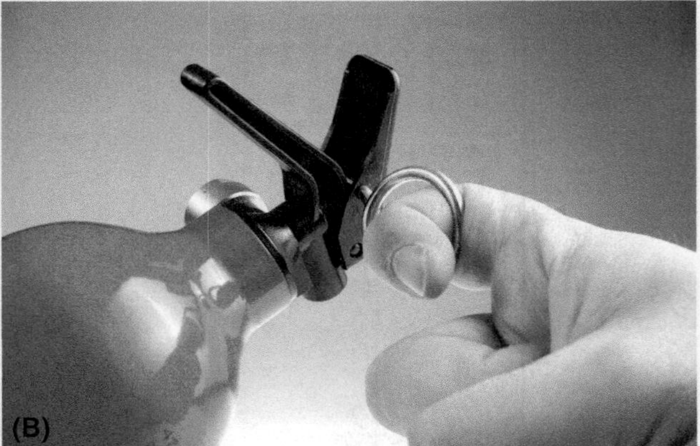

FIGURE 14–13B Release the pin on the fire extinguisher.
© iStock.com/Alessandro D'Alessandro

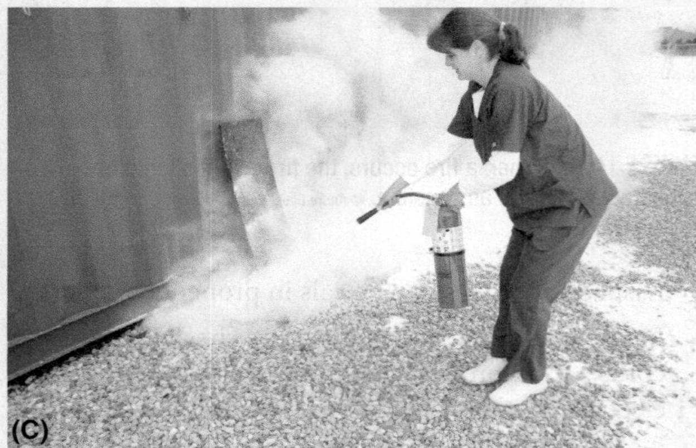

FIGURE 14–13C Aim the nozzle at the near edge of the fire, and push the handle to discharge the extinguisher.

b. Locate the lock or pin at the top handle. Release the lock following the manufacturer's instructions (Figure 14–13B).

NOTE: During a mock demonstration, only pretend to release the lock.

c. Grasp the handle to hold the extinguisher firmly in an upright position.

d. Stand approximately 6–10 feet from the near edge of the fire.

e. Aim the nozzle at the fire (Figure 14–13C).

f. Discharge the extinguisher. Use a side-to-side motion. Spray toward the near edge of the fire at the bottom of the fire.

CAUTION: Do not spray into the center or top of the fire, because this will cause the fire to spread in an outward direction.

PROCEDURE 14:3 (CONT.)

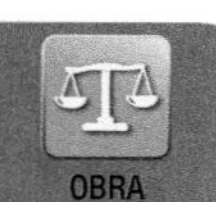

g. Continue with the same side-to-side motion until the fire is extinguished.

NOTE: The word *PASS* can help you remember the correct steps:

P = Pull the pin.

A = Aim the extinguisher at the near edge and bottom of the fire.

S = Squeeze the handle to discharge the extinguisher.

S = Sweep the extinguisher from side to side at the base of the fire.

h. At all times, stay a safe distance from the fire to avoid personal injury.

Safety

CAUTION: Avoid contact with residues from chemical extinguishers.

i. After an extinguisher has been used, it must be recharged or replaced. Another usable extinguisher must be put in position when the extinguisher is removed.

6. Check the policy in your area for evacuating the laboratory or clinical area during a fire. Practice the method and know the locations of all exits.

NOTE: Remember to remain calm and avoid panic.

7. Replace all equipment used.

PRACTICE: **Use the evaluation sheet for 14:3, Observing Fire Safety, to practice this procedure. When you believe you have mastered this skill, sign the sheet and give it to your instructor for further action.**

Check

FINAL CHECKPOINT: Using the criteria listed on the evaluation sheet, your instructor will grade your performance.

PRACTICE: **Study the safety regulations throughout Chapter 14 in preparation for the safety examination.**

Check

FINAL CHECKPOINT: Take the safety examination and obtain a passing grade to demonstrate your knowledge of safety.

TODAY'S RESEARCH TOMORROW'S HEALTH CARE

Draino for Blood Vessels?

Cardiovascular (heart and blood vessel) disease is the leading cause of death in the United States. Fatty plaques, caused mainly by an accumulation of LDL (low-density lipoprotein, or "bad" cholesterol), block the flow of blood in arterial walls, triggering a heart attack or stroke. HDL (high-density lipoprotein, or "good" cholesterol) helps protect the body from cardiovascular disease. HDL carries fats to the liver for disposal, helps prevent clots, and decreases inflammation in the blood vessels. For years, researchers have tried to find ways to increase the level of HDL while decreasing the level of LDL in the blood.

Scientists may have found the key to solve this problem in a small village in Italy. They discovered that residents of this village seemed to be immune to heart disease. Research showed that these individuals have a mutant gene that produces a powerful version of HDL. Scientists have produced a synthetic version of this HDL called *apo A-1 Milano*. When it was injected into a small group of volunteer heart patients, plaque in blood vessels was reduced by 4 percent and no new plaque buildup occurred. Scientists called it a miracle "blood vessel Draino." However, *apo A-1 Milano* is expensive to produce because it is a protein. It also must be injected into the body by an intravenous infusion, making it even more costly and inconvenient. Recently the rights to *apo A-1 Milano* were acquired by The Medicines Company, which named the compound *MDCO-215*. The company is conducting extensive research to create a medicine from this compound and begin clinical studies.

Scientists are also evaluating other methods to increase levels of HDL. They have discovered an enzyme called the *cholesteryl ester transfer protein* that appears to reduce HDL levels and increase the levels of harmful LDL. Research is being conducted on new drugs that will block this enzyme. Who knows which approach will be most successful, but scientists will find the answer.

CHAPTER 14 SUMMARY

Safety is the responsibility of every health care provider. It is essential that established safety standards be observed by everyone. This protects the worker, the employer, and the patient.

One important aspect of safety is the correct use of body mechanics. Body mechanics refer to the way the body moves and maintains balance while making the most efficient use of all of its parts. Practicing basic principles of good body mechanics prevents strain and maintains muscle strength. In addition, correct body mechanics make lifting, pulling, and pushing easier.

Knowing and following basic safety standards is also important. In this chapter, basic standards are listed in regard to the use of equipment and solutions, patient safety, and personal safety. It is important for everyone to learn and follow the established standards at all times.

An awareness of the causes and prevention of fires is essential. Every health care worker should be familiar with the types and use of fire extinguishers. In addition, every facility has a fire emergency plan. By following the fire emergency plan or other disaster plan, knowing the location of fire extinguishers and exit doors, and remaining calm, the health care provider can help prevent loss of life or serious injury during a fire or a disaster.

INTERNET SEARCHES

Use the search engines suggested in Chapter 12:9 in this text to search the Internet for additional information about the following topics:

1. **Federal regulations:** Obtain more information about federal safety regulations by searching the sites of the Occupational Safety and Health Administration (OSHA), Occupational Exposure to Hazardous Chemicals Standard, National Fire Protection Association's (NFPA) chemical code, Bloodborne Pathogen Standard, and Safety Data Sheets (SDSs).
2. **Ergonomics:** Search for additional information about ergonomics and environmental safety.
3. **Diseases:** Obtain information about the causative agents and methods of transmission for hepatitis B and C and acquired immune deficiency syndrome (AIDS).
4. **Fire safety:** Search for information about fire prevention and fire safety.
5. **Fire extinguishers:** Search for various manufacturers of fire extinguishers and obtain information about the types of extinguishers, their main uses, precautions for handling, and safety rules that must be observed while using these extinguishers.
6. **Disasters:** Obtain information about safety procedures that must be followed for tornadoes, floods, hurricanes, earthquakes, bomb threats, and explosions.

REVIEW QUESTIONS

1. Define *body mechanics* and list four (4) reasons why it is important to use good body mechanics.
2. You are using an electrical microhematocrit centrifuge to spin blood. You see smoke coming from the back of the machine. What should you do?
3. List four (4) safety precautions that must be followed while using solutions.
4. Identify three (3) things that must be done before performing any procedure on a patient.
5. State five (5) checkpoints that must be observed before leaving a patient/resident in bed.
6. What is a SDS? Why is it used?
7. What is the NFPA? Why is it important for health care providers?
8. Identify the three (3) things fires need in order to start.
9. List five (5) rules that must be followed while oxygen is in use.
10. What does the acronym *RACE* stand for?
11. Create a chart showing the four (4) main types of fire extinguishers and the type of fire for which each is effective.
12. What does the acronym *PASS* stand for?

15 Infection Control

CHAPTER OBJECTIVES

After completing this chapter, you should be able to:

- Identify five classes of microorganisms by describing the characteristics of each class.
- List the six components of the chain of infection.
- Differentiate between antisepsis, disinfection, and sterilization.
- Define bioterrorism and identify at least four ways to prepare for a bioterrorism attack.
- Wash hands following aseptic technique.
- Observe standard precautions while working in the laboratory or clinical area.
- Wash, wrap, and autoclave instruments, linen, and equipment.
- Operate an autoclave with accuracy and safety.
- Follow basic principles of chemical disinfection.
- Clean instruments with an ultrasonic unit.
- Open sterile packages with no contamination.
- Don sterile gloves with no contamination.
- Prepare a sterile dressing tray with no contamination.
- Change a sterile dressing with no contamination.
- Don and remove a transmission-based isolation mask, gloves, and gown.
- Relate specific basic tasks to the care of a patient in a transmission-based isolation unit.
- Define, pronounce, and spell all key terms.

KEY TERMS

acquired immune deficiency syndrome (AIDS)
aerobic
airborne precautions
anaerobic
antisepsis *(ant"-ih-sep'-sis)*
asepsis *(a-sep'-sis)*
autoclave
bacteria
bioterrorism
cavitation *(kav"-ih-tay'-shun)*
chain of infection
chemical disinfection
clean
communicable disease
contact precautions
contaminated
disinfection

KEY TERMS (CONT.)

droplet precautions
Ebola
endogenous
epidemic
exogenous
fomites
fungi *(fun' -guy)*
helminths
hepatitis B
hepatitis C
infectious agent
microorganism *(my-crow-or' -gan-izm)*
mode of transmission
nonpathogens
opportunistic
pandemic
pathogens *(path' -oh-jenz')*
personal protective equipment (PPE)
portal of entry
portal of exit
protective (reverse) isolation
protozoa *(pro-toe-zo' -ah)*
reservoir
rickettsiae *(rik-et' -z-ah)*
standard precautions
sterile
sterile field
sterilization
susceptible host
transmission-based precautions
ultrasonic units
viruses

Related Health Careers

- Central/Sterile Supply Worker
- Epidemiologists
- Housekeepers/Sanitary Managers
- Infection Preventionists
- Infectious Disease Physician
- Microbiologists
- Surgical Technologists

LEGAL ALERT

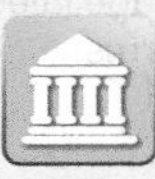
Legal

Before performing any procedures in this chapter, know and follow the standards and regulations established by the scope of practice; federal laws and agencies; state laws; state or national licensing, registration, or certification boards; professional organizations; professional standards; and agency policies.

It is your responsibility to learn exactly what you are legally permitted to do and to perform only procedures for which you have been trained.

15:1 Understanding the Principles of Infection Control

Science

OBRA

Understanding the basic principles of infection control is essential for any health care worker in any field of health care. The principles described in this unit provide a basic knowledge of how disease is transmitted and the main ways to prevent disease transmission.

A **microorganism**, or microbe, is a small, living organism that is not visible to the naked eye. It must be viewed under a microscope. Microorganisms are found everywhere in the environment, including on and in the human body. Many microorganisms are part of the normal flora (plant life adapted for living in a specific environment) of the body and are beneficial in maintaining certain body processes. These are called **nonpathogens**. Other microorganisms cause infection and disease and are called **pathogens**, or germs. At times, a microorganism that is beneficial in one body system can become pathogenic when it is present in another body system. For example, a bacterium called *Escherichia coli* (*E. coli*) is part of the natural flora of the large intestine. If *E. coli* enters the urinary system, however, it causes an infection.

To grow and reproduce, microorganisms need certain things. Most microorganisms prefer a warm environment, and body temperature is ideal. Darkness is also preferred by most microorganisms, and many are killed quickly by sunlight. In addition, a source of food and moisture is needed. Some microorganisms, called

aerobic organisms, require oxygen to live. Others, called **anaerobic** organisms, live and reproduce in the absence of oxygen. The human body is the ideal supplier of all the requirements of microorganisms.

Classes of Microorganisms

There are many different classes of microorganisms. In each class, some microorganisms are pathogenic to humans. The main classes include bacteria, protozoa, fungi, rickettsia, viruses, and helminths.

BACTERIA

Bacteria are simple, one-celled organisms that multiply rapidly. They are classified by shape and arrangement. *Cocci* are round or spherical in shape (Figure 15-1). If cocci occur in pairs, they are diplococci. Diplococci bacteria cause diseases such as gonorrhea, meningitis, and pneumonia. If cocci occur in chains, they are streptococci. A common streptococcus causes a severe sore throat (strep throat) and rheumatic fever. *Streptococcus pyogenes*, also called *Strep A* or flesh-eating strep, causes necrotizing fasciitis that destroys tissues and can result in amputation or death (Figure 15-2). If cocci occur in clusters or groups, they are staphylococci. These are the most common pyogenic (pus-producing) microorganisms. Staphylococci cause infections such as boils, urinary tract infections, wound infections, and toxic shock. Rod-shaped bacteria are called *bacilli* (Figure 15-3). They can occur singly, in pairs, or in chains. Many bacilli contain flagella, which are thread-like projections that are similar to tails and allow the organisms to move. Bacilli also have the ability to form spores, or thick-walled capsules, when conditions for growth are poor. In the spore form, bacilli are extremely difficult to kill. Diseases caused by different types of bacilli include tuberculosis, tetanus, pertussis (whooping cough), botulism, diphtheria, and typhoid. Bacteria that are spiral or corkscrew in shape are called *spirilla* (Figure 15-4). These include the comma-shaped vibrio and the corkscrew-shaped spirochete. Diseases caused by spirilla include syphilis and cholera.

Antibiotics are used to kill bacteria. However, due to the overuse and misuse of antibiotics, some strains of bacteria have become antibiotic-resistant, which means that the antibiotic is no longer effective against the bacteria. If a bacterium becomes resistant to several

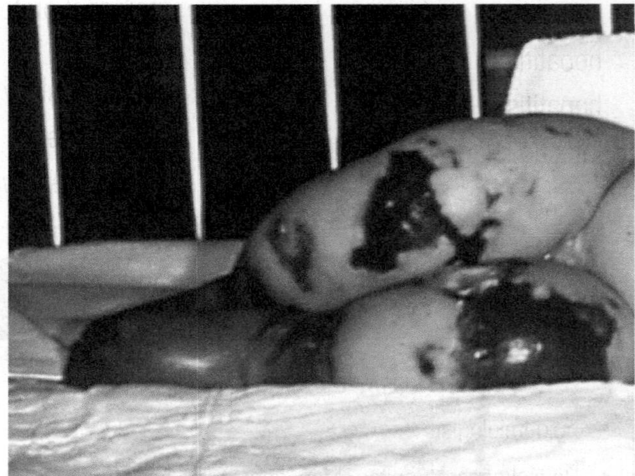

FIGURE 15–2 ***Streptococcus pyogenes*, also called *Strep A* or flesh-eating strep, causes necrotizing fasciitis that destroys tissues and can result in amputation or death if not treated immediately.**
Courtesy of the CDC.

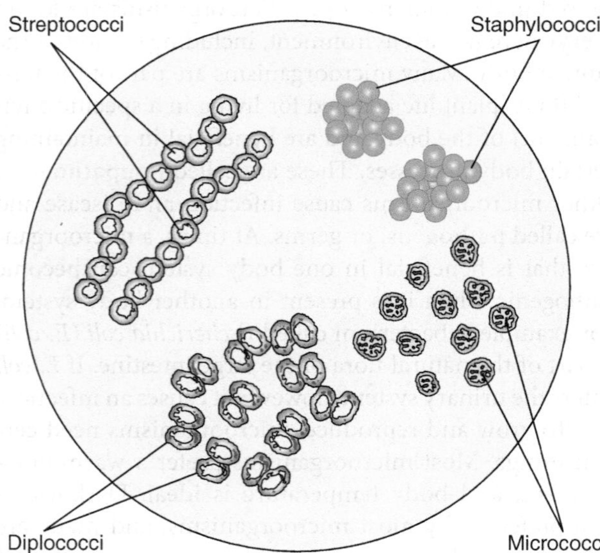

FIGURE 15–1 Kinds of cocci bacteria.

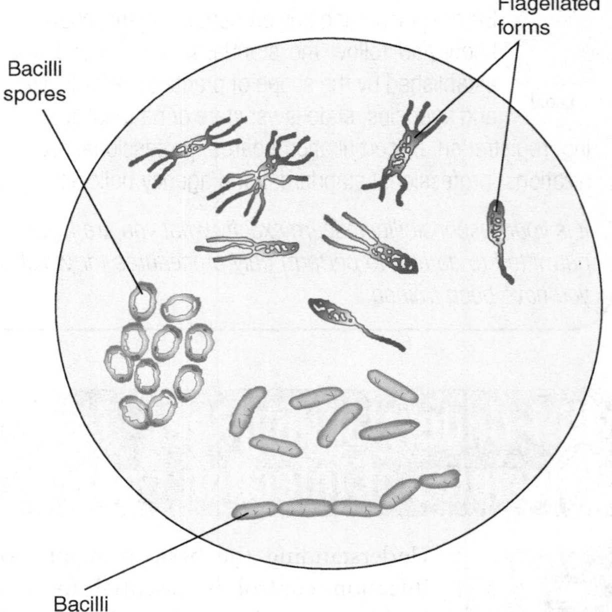

FIGURE 15–3 Bacilli bacteria.

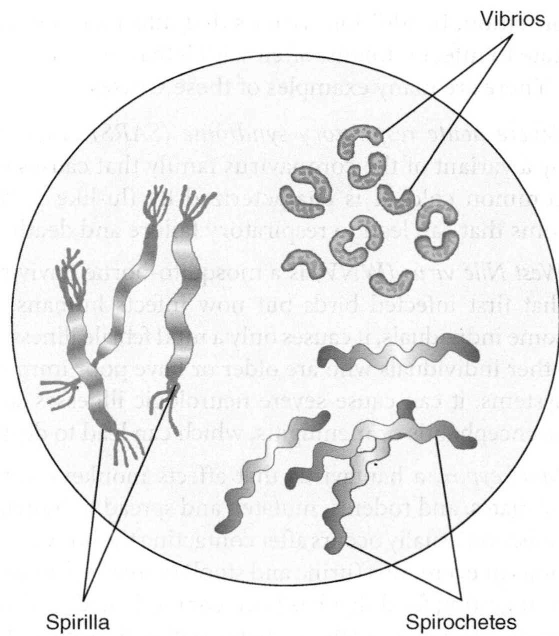

FIGURE 15–4 Spirilla bacteria.

drugs, it is called multidrug resistant, or a "superbug." Methicillin-resistant staphylococcus aureas (MRSA) is an example. It causes a severe staph infection that is difficult to treat because it is resistant to many different antibiotics. Vancomycin-resistant enterococcus (VRE) is a bacterium that is resistant to vancomycin and several other drugs. Because no single antibiotic can eliminate VRE, drug combinations are often used to treat it. *Extended spectrum beta lactamase* (ESBL)-producing bacterium developed from an increased use of beta lactam antibiotics such as penicillin and ampicillin. ESBL is resistant to many antibiotics. Multidrug-resistant *acinetobacter baumannii* (MRAB) is an example of a bloodstream infection that is difficult to treat due to drug resistance. In some cases, *A. baumannii* has been resistant to all drugs tested. *Carbapenem-resistant enterobacteriaceae* (CRE) are resistant to most antibiotics and can cause pneumonia, kidney and bladder disease, and septicemia (pathogenic organisms in the bloodstream). All antibiotic-resistant bacterium are a major concern because they are difficult to treat, they cause increased hospital stays, and they increase the cost of health care. A major campaign has been launched to push for less antibiotic use, unless specifically indicated, to help prevent drug resistance.

PROTOZOA

Protozoa are one-celled animal-like organisms often found in decayed materials, animal or bird feces, insect bites, and contaminated water (Figure 15-5). Many contain flagella, which allow them to move freely. Some protozoa are pathogenic and cause diseases such as malaria, amebic dysentery (intestinal infection), trichomonas, and African sleeping sickness.

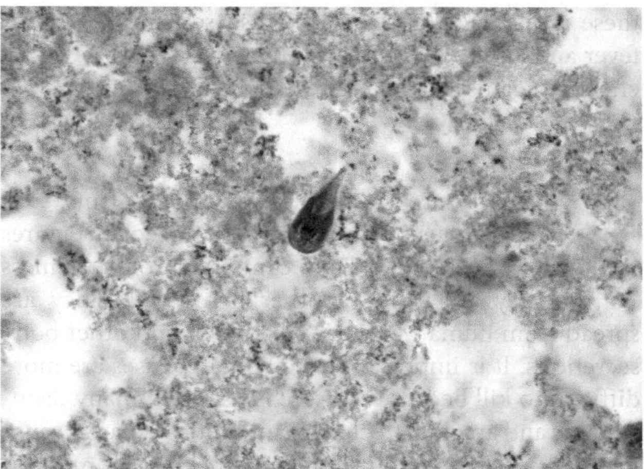

FIGURE 15–5 An intestinal protozoan, *Giardia intestinalis*, is the blue stained mass in the center of the photo. Courtesy CDC/DPDx-Melanie Moser.

FUNGI

Fungi are simple, plant-like organisms that live on dead organic matter. Yeasts and molds are two common forms that can be pathogenic. They cause diseases such as ringworm, athlete's foot, histoplasmosis, yeast vaginitis, and thrush (Figure 15-6). Antibiotics do not kill fungi. Antifungal medications are available for many of the pathogenic fungi, but they are expensive, must be taken internally for a long period, and may cause liver damage.

RICKETTSIAE

Rickettsiae are parasitic microorganisms, which means they cannot live outside the cells of another living organism. They are commonly found in fleas, lice, ticks, and mites, and are transmitted to humans by the bites of

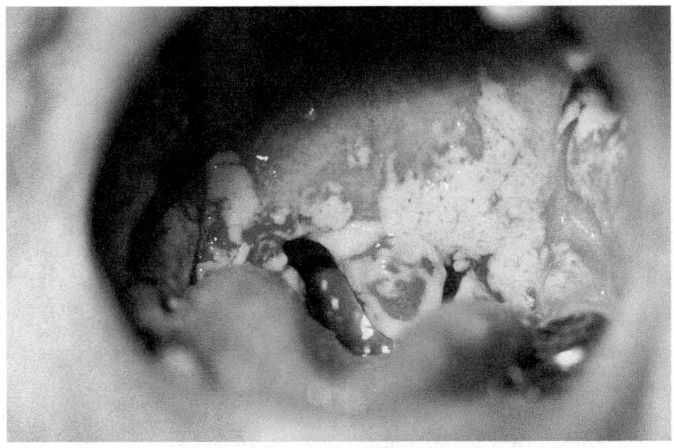

FIGURE 15–6 The yeast (fungus) called *thrush* causes these characteristic white patches on the tongue and in the mouth. Courtesy CDC.

these insects. Rickettsiae cause diseases such as typhus fever and Rocky Mountain spotted fever. Antibiotics are effective against many different rickettsiae.

VIRUSES

OBRA

Viruses are the smallest microorganisms, visible only using an electron microscope (Figures 15-7A and B). They cannot reproduce unless they are inside another living cell. They are spread from human to human by blood and other body secretions. It is important to note that viruses are more difficult to kill because they are resistant to many disinfectants and are not affected by antibiotics. Viruses cause many diseases including the common cold, measles, mumps, chicken pox, herpes, warts, influenza, and polio. New and different viruses emerge constantly because viruses are prone to mutating and changing genetic information. In addition, viruses that infect animals can mutate to infect humans, often with lethal results.

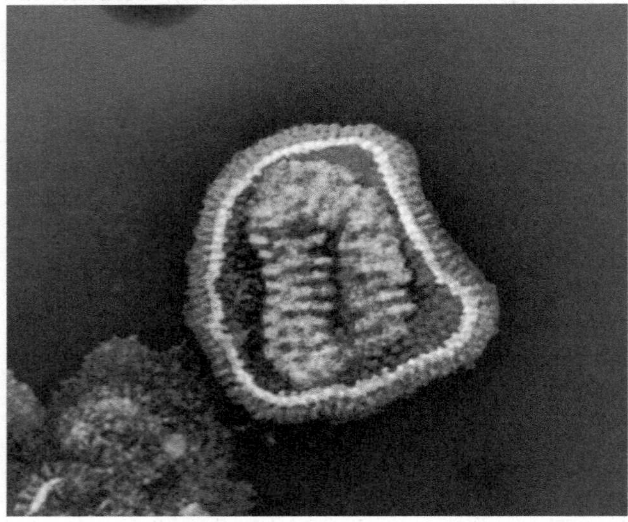

FIGURE 15–7A **Electron micrograph of the influenza virus.** Courtesy CDC/Erskine L. Palmer, Ph.D.; M.L. Martin. Photo credit: Frederick Murphy.

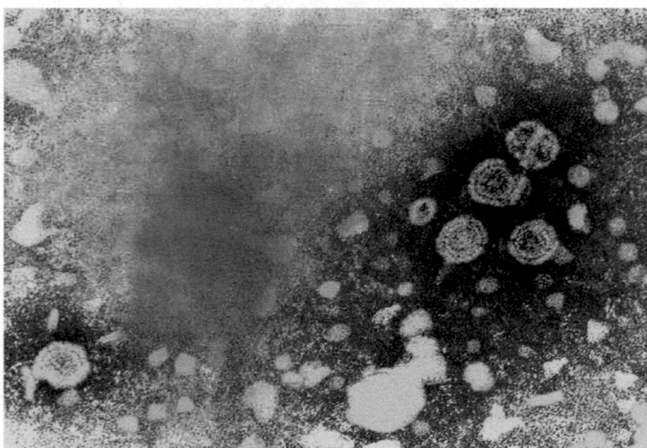

FIGURE 15–7B **Electron micrograph of the hepatitis B virus.** Courtesy CDC/Dr. Erskine Palmer.

There are many examples of these viruses:

- *Severe acute respiratory syndrome (SARS)* is caused by a variant of the coronavirus family that causes the common cold. It is characterized by flu-like symptoms that can lead to respiratory failure and death.
- *West Nile virus (WNV)* is a mosquito-borne flavivirus that first infected birds but now infects humans. In some individuals, it causes only a mild febrile illness. In other individuals who are older or have poor immune systems, it can cause severe neurologic illnesses such as encephalitis or meningitis, which can lead to death.
- *Monkeypox*, a hantavirus that affects monkeys, other primates, and rodents, mutated and spread to humans. Infection usually occurs after contacting the body secretions or excretions (urine and stool) of infected animals or ingesting food that has been contaminated by fluids from infected animals. A major outbreak occurred in the American Southwest when infected prairie dogs contaminated food with fecal material. Monkeypox is similar to smallpox. It causes severe flu-like symptoms, lymphadenopathy (disease of the lymph nodes), and pustules that cause severe scarring of the skin. If the eyes are infected, blindness can occur. It can be prevented and treated with a smallpox vaccination.
- Filoviruses such as **Ebola** and *Marburg* first affected primates and then spread to humans. These viruses cause hemorrhagic fever, a disease that begins with flu-like symptoms, fever, chills, headache, myalgia (muscle pain), and a skin rash. It quickly progresses to jaundice, pancreatitis, liver failure, massive hemorrhaging throughout the body, delirium, shock, and death. Most outbreaks of hemorrhagic fever have occurred in Africa, but isolated cases have appeared in other parts of the world when individuals were in contact with infected primates. A major epidemic of Ebola occurred in West Africa in 2014. It is discussed in detail in Chapter 2:1 of this text under *Pandemics*.
- The *H5N1* virus that causes avian or bird flu has devastated bird flocks in many countries. The infection has appeared in humans, but most cases have resulted from contact with infected poultry or contaminated surfaces. The spread from one person to another has been reported only rarely. However, because the death rate for bird flu is between 50 and 60 percent, a major concern is that the *H5N1* virus will mutate and spread more readily.
- *H1N1*, or swine flu, was declared a global pandemic in 2009. The virus spreads quickly and causes flu-like symptoms. In severe cases, it results in pneumonia, respiratory distress or failure, and, in some cases,

death. As with the bird flu, it rarely spreads from one person to another. Most cases result from contact with infected hogs.

In addition to these viruses, there are three other viral diseases of major concern to the health care worker: hepatitis B, hepatitis C, and acquired immune deficiency syndrome (AIDS).

Hepatitis B, or serum hepatitis, is caused by the HBV virus and is transmitted by blood, serum, and other body secretions. It affects the liver and can lead to the destruction and scarring of liver cells. A vaccine has been developed to protect individuals from this disease, but this vaccine is expensive and involves a series of three injections. Under federal law, employers must provide the vaccination at no cost to any health care worker with occupational exposure to blood or other body secretions that may carry the HBV virus. An individual does have the right to refuse the vaccination, but a written record must be kept proving that the vaccine was offered.

Hepatitis C is caused by the hepatitis C virus, or HCV, and is transmitted by blood and blood-containing body fluids. Many individuals who contract the disease are asymptomatic (display no symptoms); others have mild symptoms that are often diagnosed as influenza or flu. In either case, HCV can cause serious liver damage. At present, there is no preventive immunization, but a vaccine is being developed. Both HBV and HCV are extremely difficult to destroy. These viruses can even remain active for several days in dried blood. Health care workers must take every precaution to protect themselves from hepatitis viruses.

Acquired immune deficiency syndrome (AIDS) is caused by the human immunodeficiency virus (HIV) and suppresses the immune system. An individual with AIDS cannot fight off many cancers and infections that would not affect a healthy person. Presently, there is no cure, and no vaccine is available, so it is important for the health care worker to take precautions to prevent the spread of this disease.

HELMINTHS

Helminths are multicellular parasitic organisms commonly called *worms* or *flukes*. They are transmitted to humans when humans ingest the eggs or larvae in contaminated food, ingest meat contaminated with the worms, or get bitten by infected insects. Some worms can also penetrate the skin to enter the body. Examples of helminths include hookworms, which attach to the small intestine and can infect the heart and lungs (Figure 15-8); ascariasis, which live in the small intestine and can cause an obstruction of the intestine; trichinella spiralis, which causes trichinosis and is contracted by eating raw or inadequately cooked pork products; enterobiasis, which is commonly called *pinworm* and mainly affects young children; and taenia solium or the pork tapeworm, which is contracted by eating inadequately cooked pork.

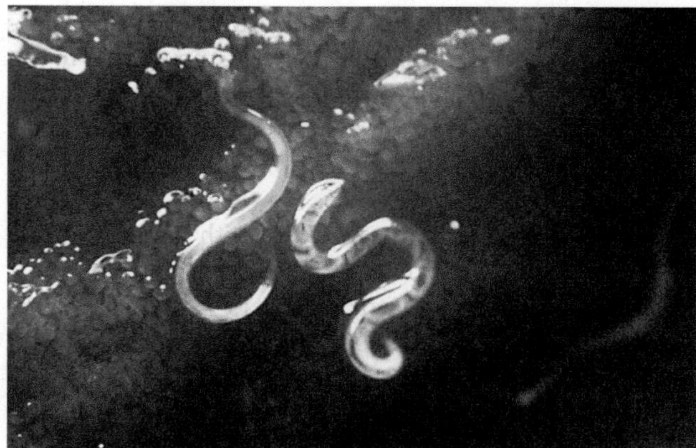

FIGURE 15–8 Hookworms attached to the mucosal lining of the intestine are one type of helminth. Courtesy CDC.

Types of Infection

Pathogenic microorganisms cause infection and disease in different ways. Some pathogens produce poisons, called *toxins*, which harm the body. An example is the bacillus that causes tetanus, which produces toxins that damage the central nervous system. Some pathogens cause an allergic reaction in the body, resulting in a runny nose, watery eyes, and sneezing. Other pathogens attack and destroy the living cells they invade. An example is the protozoan that causes malaria; it invades red blood cells and causes them to rupture.

Infections and diseases are also classified as endogenous, exogenous, hospital-acquired, or opportunistic. **Endogenous** means the infection or disease originates within the body. These include metabolic disorders, congenital abnormalities, tumors, and infections caused by microorganisms within the body. **Exogenous** means the infection or disease originates outside the body. Examples include pathogenic organisms that invade the body, radiation, chemical agents, trauma, electric shock, and temperature extremes. A *hospital-acquired* or *healthcare-associated infection* (HAI) (formerly referred to as *nosocomial*) is an infection acquired by an individual in a health care facility such as a hospital or long-term care facility. Hospital-acquired infections are usually present in the facility and transmitted by health care workers to the patient. Many of the pathogens transmitted in this manner are antibiotic-resistant and can cause serious and even life-threatening infections in patients. Common examples are staphylococcus, pseudomonas, and enterococci. Infection-control programs are used in health care facilities to prevent and deal with HIAs.

The infection control professionals that run these programs are called *infection preventionists*, according to the Association for Professionals in Infection Control and Epidemiology (APIC). Their job is to reduce the incidence of HAIs. **Opportunistic** infections are those that occur when the body's defenses are weak. These diseases do not usually occur in individuals with intact immune systems. Examples include the development of a yeast infection called *candidiasis*, Kaposi's sarcoma (a rare type of cancer), or *Pneumocystis jiroveci* pneumonia in individuals who have AIDS.

Chain of Infection

For disease to occur and spread from one individual to another, certain conditions must be met. These conditions are commonly called the **chain of infection** (Figure 15-9). The parts of the chain include:

- **Infectious agent**: a pathogen, such as a bacterium or virus that can cause a disease
- **Reservoir**: an area where the infectious agent can live; some common reservoirs include the human body, animals, the environment, and **fomites**, or objects contaminated with infectious material that contains the pathogens. Common fomites include doorknobs, bedpans, urinals, linens, instruments, and specimen containers.
- **Portal of exit**: a way for the infectious agent to escape from the reservoir in which it has been growing. In the human body, pathogens can leave the body through urine, feces, saliva, blood, tears, mucous discharge, sexual secretions, and draining wounds.
- **Mode of transmission**: a way that the infectious agent can be transmitted to another reservoir or host where it can live. The pathogen can be transmitted in different ways. One way is by *direct contact*, which includes person-to-person contact (physical or sexual contact) or contact with a body secretion containing the pathogen. Contaminated hands are one of the most common sources of direct contact transmission. Another way is by *indirect contact*, when the pathogen is transmitted from contaminated substances such as food, air, soil, insects, feces, clothing, instruments, and equipment. Examples include touching contaminated equipment and spreading the pathogen on the hands, breathing

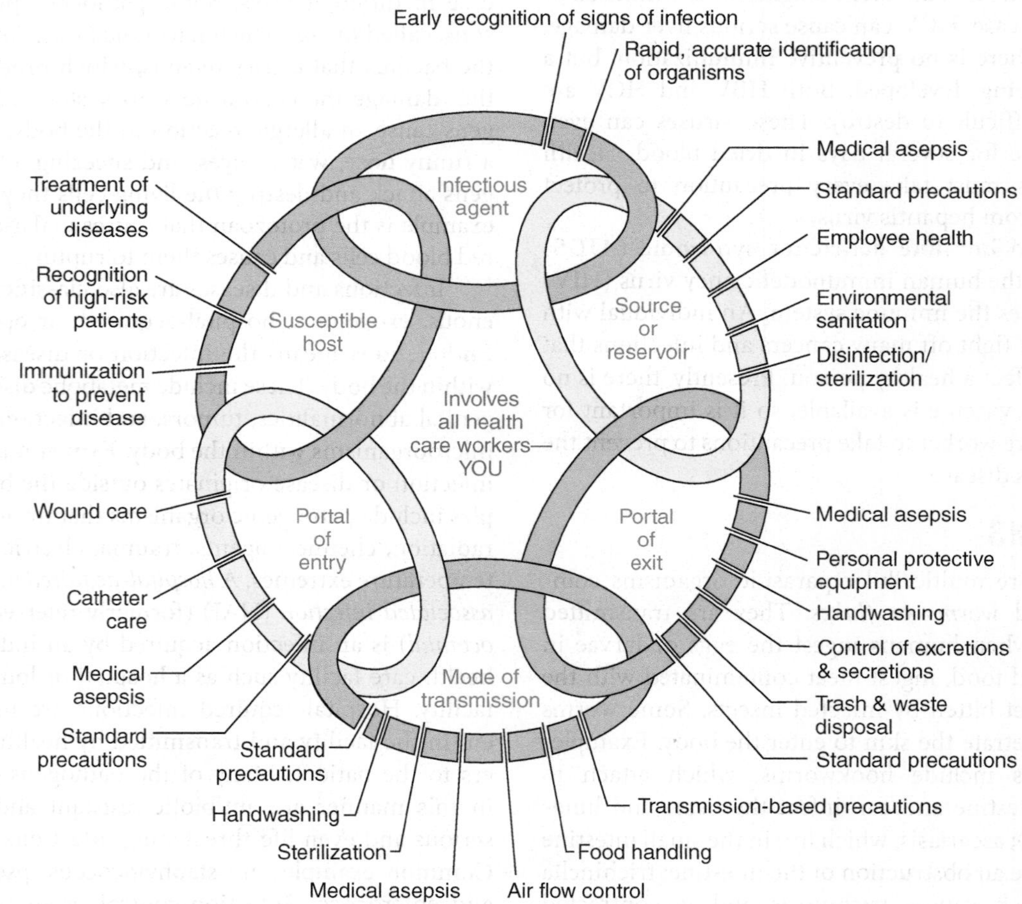

FIGURE 15–9 Note the components in the chain of infection and the ways in which the chain can be broken.

in droplets carrying airborne infections, and contacting *vectors* (insects, rodents, or small animals), such as being bitten by an insect carrying a pathogen.

- **Portal of entry**: a way for the infectious agent to enter a new reservoir or host. Some ways pathogens can enter the body are through breaks in the skin, breaks in the mucous membrane, the respiratory tract, the digestive tract, the genitourinary tract, and the circulatory system. If the defense mechanisms of the body are intact and the immune system is functioning, a human can frequently fight off the infectious agent and not contract the disease. Body defenses include:

  Mucous membrane: lines the respiratory, digestive, and reproductive tracts and traps pathogens

  Cilia: tiny, hair-like structures that line the respiratory tract and propel pathogens out of the body

  Coughing and sneezing: expels pathogens out of the body

  Hydrochloric acid: destroys pathogens in the stomach

  Tears in the eye: contain bacteriocidal (bacteria-killing) chemicals

  Fever: high temperatures destroy some pathogens

  Inflammation: leukocytes, or white blood cells, destroy pathogens

  Immune response: body produces antibodies, which are protective proteins that combat pathogens, and protective chemicals secreted by cells, such as interferon and complement

- **Susceptible host**: a person likely to get an infection or disease, usually because body defenses are weak

Health care workers must constantly be aware of the parts in the chain of infection. If any part of the chain is eliminated, the spread of disease or infection will be stopped. A health care worker who is aware of this can follow practices to interrupt or break this chain and prevent the transmission of disease. It is important to remember that pathogens are everywhere and that preventing their transmission is a continuous process.

Aseptic Techniques

A major way to break the chain of infection is to use aseptic techniques while providing health care. **Asepsis** is defined as the absence of disease-producing microorganisms, or pathogens.

Sterile means free from all organisms, both pathogenic and nonpathogenic, including spores and viruses. **Contaminated** means that organisms and pathogens are present. Any object or area that may contain pathogens is considered to be contaminated. Aseptic techniques are directed toward maintaining cleanliness and eliminating or preventing contamination. Common aseptic techniques include handwashing, good personal hygiene, use of disposable gloves when contacting body secretions or contaminated objects, proper cleaning of instruments and equipment, and thorough cleaning of the environment.

Various levels of aseptic control are possible. These include:

- **Antisepsis**: Antiseptics prevent or inhibit growth of pathogenic organisms but are not effective against spores and viruses. They can usually be used on the skin. Common examples include alcohol and betadine.
- **Disinfection**: This is a process that uses chemical disinfectants to destroy or kill pathogenic organisms. It is not always effective against spores and viruses. Disinfectants can irritate or damage the skin and are used mainly on objects, not people. Some common disinfectants are bleach solutions and zephirin.
- **Sterilization**: This is a process that destroys all microorganisms, both pathogenic and nonpathogenic, including spores and viruses. Steam under pressure, gas, radiation, and chemicals can be used to sterilize objects. An autoclave is the most common piece of equipment used for sterilization.

In the sections that follow, correct methods of aseptic techniques are described. It is important for the health care worker to know and use these methods in every aspect of providing health care to prevent the spread and transmission of disease.

STUDENT: **Go to the workbook and complete the assignment sheet for 15:1, Understanding the Principles of Infection Control.**

15:2 Bioterrorism

Introduction

Bioterrorism is the use of microorganisms, or biologic agents, as weapons to infect humans, animals, or plants. Throughout history, microorganisms have been used in biologic warfare. Some examples include:

- The Tartar army throwing bodies of dead plague victims over the walls of a city called Caffa in 1346, causing an epidemic of plague in the city
- The British army providing Delaware Indians with blankets and handkerchiefs contaminated with smallpox in 1763, resulting in a major outbreak of smallpox among the Indian population

- The Germans using a variety of animal and human pathogens in World War I
- The Japanese military using prisoners of war to experiment with many different pathogens in World War II
- The United States, Canada, the Soviet Union, and the United Kingdom developing biologic weapons programs until the late 1960s
- The release of sarin gas in Tokyo in 1995
- An unknown individual or individuals sending anthrax through the mail in the United States in 2001

Today, there is a major concern that these biologic agents will be used not only in wars but also against unsuspecting civilians.

Biologic Agents

Many different microorganisms can cause diseases in humans, animals, and plants. However, only a limited number are considered to be ideal for bioterrorism. Six characteristics of the "ideal" microorganism include:

- Inexpensive and readily available or easy to produce
- Spread through the air by winds or ventilation systems and inhaled into the lungs of potential victims, or spread by ingesting contaminated food or water
- Survives sunlight, drying, and heat
- Causes death or severe disability and public panic
- Easily transmitted from person to person
- Difficult to prevent or has no effective treatment

The Centers for Disease Control and Prevention (CDC) has identified and classified major bioterrorism agents. High-priority agents that have been identified include:

- *Smallpox:* Smallpox is a highly contagious infectious disease that is caused by a variola virus (Figure 15-10). A smallpox vaccination can provide protection against some types of smallpox, but one type, hemorrhagic smallpox, is usually fatal. Until the 1970s, people were vaccinated against smallpox. However, after many years with no reported cases, the vaccinations were no longer required. Now, with the threat of a smallpox bioterrorism attack, the U.S. government has started a new vaccination program. The program encourages first responders, police, fire department, and health care personnel to be vaccinated.
- *Anthrax:* Anthrax is an infectious disease caused by the spores of bacteria called *Bacillus anthracis*. The spores are highly resistant to destruction and can live in soil for years. Grazing animals such as cattle, sheep, and goats eat the contaminated soil and become infected.

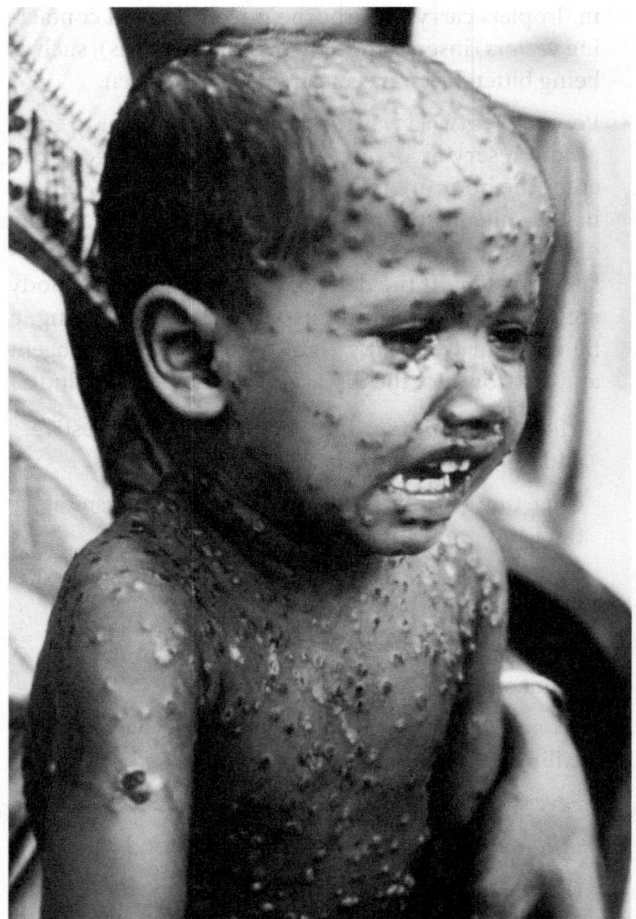

FIGURE 15–10 Smallpox is a highly contagious infectious disease caused by a variola virus. Courtesy CDC/Dr. Michael Schwartz.

Humans develop anthrax by exposure through the skin (cutaneous) (Figure 15-11), by eating undercooked or raw infected meat (gastrointestinal), or by inhaling the spores (pulmonary). Cutaneous and gastrointestinal anthrax are usually treated successfully with antibiotics, but some victims die. Inhalation anthrax causes death in more than 80 percent of its victims. An anthrax vaccine is available for prevention, and the military has an active vaccination program.

- *Plague:* This is an infectious disease that is caused by bacteria called *Yersinia pestis*. Usually plague is transmitted by the bites of infected fleas. In some cases, the organism enters the body through a break in the skin or by contact with the tissue of an infected animal (bubonic plague). Rats, rock squirrels, prairie dogs, and chipmunks are the most common sources of plague in the United States. If the disease is not treated immediately with antibiotics, the infection spreads to the blood (septicemic plague) and lungs (pneumonic plague), and causes death. No vaccine for plague is available in the United States.

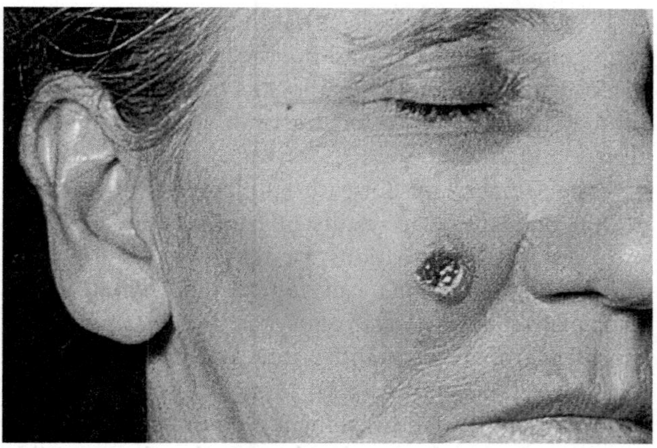
FIGURE 15–11 Cutaneous (skin) anthrax is usually treated successfully with antibiotics. Courtesy CDC.

- *Botulism:* Botulism is a paralytic illness caused by a nerve toxin produced by bacteria called *Clostridium botulinum*. Three main types of botulism exist. One type is caused by eating foods that contain the toxin. A second type is caused by the presence of the toxin in a wound or injury to the skin. A third type occurs in infants who eat the spores that then grow in the intestine and release the toxin. The toxin rapidly causes muscle paralysis. If it is not treated with an antitoxin, the paralysis spreads to the respiratory muscles and causes death.
- *Tularemia:* This is an infectious disease caused by bacteria called *Francisella tularensis*. This bacteria is commonly found in animals such as rats, rabbits, and insects (ticks and deerflies). Humans get the disease through the bite of an infected animal or insect, by eating contaminated food, by drinking contaminated water, or by breathing in the bacteria. The disease causes death if it is not treated with appropriate antibiotics. Currently, the Food and Drug Administration (FDA) is reviewing a vaccine, but it is not available in the United States.
- *Hemorrhagic fever:* This is an infectious disease caused by a filovirus. Two filoviruses have been identified: the Ebola virus and the Marburg virus. The source of these viruses is still being researched, but the common belief is that the viruses are transmitted from animals such as bats, monkeys, and chimpanzees. Once the viruses affect a human, the disease is spread rapidly from person to person by contact with body fluids. Treatment is supportive care with fluid and electrolyte replacement, respiratory support, and management of symptoms. Several experimental antiviral therapies were used during the 2014 outbreak of Ebola in West Africa, but none have proven to be effective in humans. In the 2014 outbreak, it is estimated that more than 70 percent of the infected people died.

Many other pathogenic microorganisms can be used in a bioterrorism attack. In fact, any pathogenic organism could be used in a bioterrorism attack. For this reason, health care workers must be constantly alert to the threat of infection with a biologic agent.

Preparing for Bioterrorism

A bioterrorism attack could cause an epidemic and public health emergency. Large numbers of infected people would place a major stress on health care facilities. Fear and panic could lead to riots, social disorder, and disregard for authority. For these reasons, the Bioterrorism Act of 2002 was passed by Congress and signed into law in June 2002. This act requires the development of a comprehensive plan against bioterrorism to increase the security of the United States.

Preparing for bioterrorism will involve government at all levels—local, regional, state, and national (Figure 15-12). Some of the major aspects of preparation include:

- Community-based surveillance to detect early indications of a bioterrorism attack
- Notification of the public when a high-risk situation is detected
- Strict infection-control measures and public education about the measures
- Funding for studying pathogenic organisms, developing vaccines, researching treatments, and determining preventive actions
- Strict guidelines and restrictions for purchasing and transporting pathologic microorganisms
- Mass immunization, especially for military, first responders, police, fire department, and health care personnel

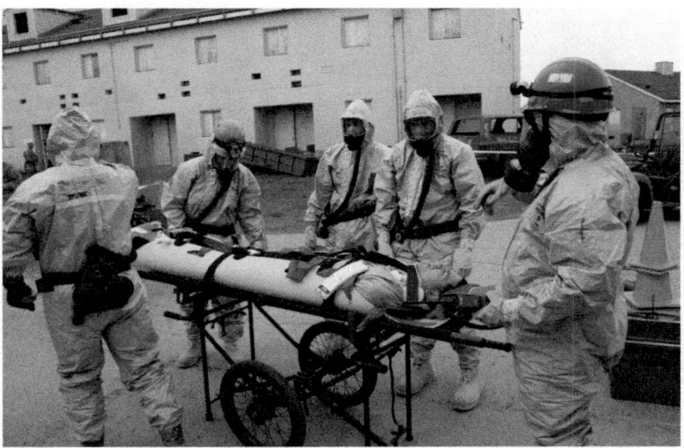
FIGURE 15–12 Response to a bioterrorism attack involves preparing and training emergency personnel at all government levels—local, regional, state, and federal. Courtesy U.S. Army/Photo by Lt. Col. Richard Goldenberg.

- Increased protection of food and water supplies
- Training personnel to properly diagnose and treat infectious diseases
- Establishing emergency management policies
- Criminal investigation of possible threats
- Improving the ability of health care facilities to deal with an attack by increasing emergency department space, preparing decontamination areas, and establishing isolation facilities
- Improving communications so information about bioterrorism is transmitted quickly and efficiently

Every health care worker must constantly be alert to the threat of bioterrorism. In today's world, it is likely that an attack will occur. Careful preparation and thorough training can limit the effect of the attack and save the lives of many people.

STUDENT: Go to the workbook and complete the assignment sheet for 15:2, Bioterrorism.

15:3 Washing Hands

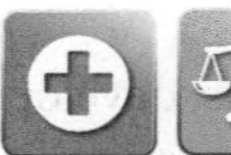

Handwashing is a basic task required in any health care occupation. The method described in this unit has been developed to ensure that a thorough cleansing occurs. An aseptic technique is a method followed to prevent the spread of germs or pathogens. *Handwashing is the single most important method used to practice aseptic technique* (Figure 15–13). Handwashing is also the most effective way to prevent the spread of infection.

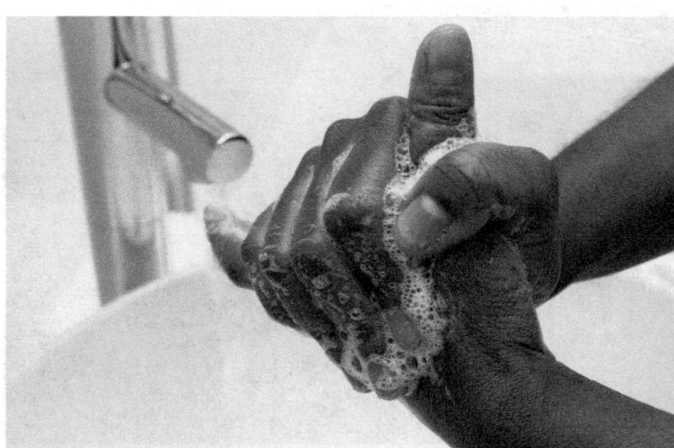

FIGURE 15–13 Handwashing is the most important method used to practice aseptic technique. © iStock.com/Jo Unruh.

The hands are a perfect medium for the spread of pathogens. Thoroughly washing the hands helps prevent and control the spread of pathogens from one person to another. It also helps protect the health care worker from disease and illness.

The Centers for Disease Control and Prevention (CDC) published the results of handwashing research and new recommendations for hand hygiene in 2002. The recommendations call for regular handwashing using plain soap and water, antiseptic handwashing using an antimicrobial soap and water, and antiseptic hand rubs (waterless handwashing) using alcohol-based hand cleaners. Regular handwashing is recommended for routine cleansing of the hands when the hands are visibly dirty or soiled with blood or other body fluids. Antiseptic handwashing is recommended before invasive procedures, in critical care units, while caring for patients on specific organism transmission-based precautions, and in specific circumstances defined by the infection-control program of the health care facility. Antiseptic hand rubs are recommended if the hands are not visibly dirty or are not soiled with blood or body fluids.

Handwashing should be performed frequently. The World Health Organization (WHO) has developed guidelines for handwashing called *My 5 Moments for Hand Hygiene*. The five essential times for handwashing include:

- Before touching a patient
- Before a clean or aseptic procedure
- After body fluid exposure or risk of exposure
- After touching a patient
- After touching the patient's surroundings

In addition, handwashing should be done:

- When you arrive at the facility and immediately before leaving the facility
- After contact with a patient's intact skin (for example, after taking a blood pressure)
- Before moving from a contaminated body site to a clean body site during patient care (for example, before washing the patient's hands after removing a bedpan)
- Any time the hands become contaminated during a procedure
- Before applying and immediately after removing gloves
- Any time gloves are torn or punctured
- Before and after handling any specimen
- After contact with any soiled or contaminated item

- After picking up any item off the floor
- After personal use of the bathroom
- After you cough, sneeze, or use a tissue
- Before and after any contact with your mouth or mucous membranes, such as eating, drinking, smoking, applying lip balm, or inserting or removing contact lenses

The recommended method for handwashing is based on the following principles; they should be observed whenever hands are washed:

- Soap is used as a cleansing agent because it aids in the removal of germs through its sudsy action and alkali content. Pathogens are trapped in the soapsuds and rinsed away. Liquid soap from a dispenser should be used whenever possible because bar soap can contain microorganisms.
- Warm water should be used. This is less damaging to the skin than hot water. It also creates a better lather with soap than does cold water.
- Friction must be used in addition to soap and water. This action helps rub off pathogens from the surface of the skin.
- All surfaces on the hands must be cleaned. This includes the palms, the backs/tops of the hands, and the areas between the fingers.
- Fingertips must be pointed downward. The downward direction prevents water from getting on the forearms and then running down to contaminate the clean hands.
- Dry paper towels must be used to turn the faucet on and off. This action prevents contamination of the hands from pathogens on the faucet. A dry towel must be used because pathogens can travel more readily through a wet towel.

Nails also harbor dirt and pathogens, and must be cleaned during the handwashing process. An orange/cuticle stick can be used. Care must be taken to use the blunt end of the stick because the pointed end can injure the nailbeds. A brush can also be used to clean the nails. If a brush or orange stick is not available or the nails are not visibly dirty, the nails can be rubbed against the palm of the opposite hand to get soap under the nails. Most health care facilities prohibit the use of artificial nails or extenders and require that nails be kept short, usually less than ¼-inch long. Artificial or long nails can harbor organisms and increase the risk for infection for both the patient and health care worker. In addition, long nails can puncture or tear gloves.

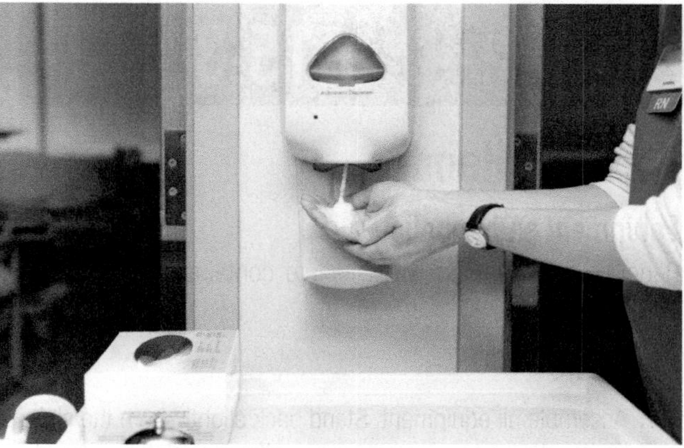

FIGURE 15–14 Waterless handwashing using an alcohol-based hand cleaner is an effective way to clean hands that are not visibly soiled. © iStock.com/Nancy Louie.

Waterless hand cleaning with an alcohol-based gel, lotion, or foam has been proved safe for use during routine patient care. Its use is recommended when the hands are not visibly dirty and are not contaminated with blood or body fluids (Figure 15-14). Most waterless hand cleaning products contain alcohol to provide antisepsis and a moisturizer to prevent drying of the skin. It is important to read the manufacturer's instructions before using any product. Usually a small amount of the alcohol-based cleaner is applied to the palm of the hands. The hands are then rubbed vigorously so the solution is applied to all surfaces of the hands, fingers, nails, and wrists. The hands should be rubbed until they are dry, usually at least 20 seconds. Most manufacturers recommend that the hands be washed with soap and water after 6–10 cleanings with the alcohol-based product. In addition, if the hands are visibly soiled, or if there has been contact with blood or body fluid, the hands must be washed with soap and water.

Many facilities conduct handwashing audits. Staff are evaluated by trained observers during the WHO's five moments for hand hygiene to ensure that handwashing is done correctly and at the appropriate times. In addition, an ultraviolet black light and special lotion can be used to test how clean hands are. Any germs that remain will glow under the light.

Every health care facility has written policies for hand hygiene as a part of their standard precautions manual. Health care workers must become familiar with and follow these policies to prevent the spread of infection.

STUDENT: **Go to the workbook and complete the assignment sheet for 15:3, Washing Hands. Then return and continue with the procedure.**

PROCEDURE 15:3

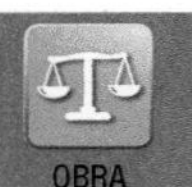

Washing Hands

Equipment and Supplies

Paper towels, running water, waste container, hand brush or orange/cuticle stick, soap

Procedure

1. Assemble all equipment. Stand back slightly from the sink so you do not contaminate your uniform or clothing. Avoid touching the inside of the sink with your hands as it is considered contaminated. Remove any rings and push your wristwatch up above your wrist.
2. Turn the faucet on by holding a paper towel between your hand and the faucet (Figure 15–15A). Regulate the temperature of the water and let water flow over your hands. Discard the towel in the waste container.

   NOTE: Water should be warm.

   CAUTION: Hot water will burn your hands.
3. With your fingertips pointing downward, wet your hands.

   NOTE: Washing in a downward direction prevents water from getting on your forearms and then running back down to contaminate your hands.
4. Use soap to create a lather on your hands.
5. Put the palms of your hands together and rub them using friction and a circular motion for at least 15 seconds.
6. Put the palm of one hand on the back of the other hand. Rub together several times. Repeat this after reversing the position of your hands (Figure 15–15B).
7. Interlace the fingers on both hands and rub them back and forth (Figure 15–15C).
8. Encircle your wrist with the palm and fingers of the opposite hand. Use a circular motion to clean the front, back, and sides of the wrist. Repeat for the opposite wrist.
9. Clean the nails with an orange/cuticle stick or hand brush if they are visibly dirty or if this is the first hand cleaning of the day (Figures 15-15D and E). If the nails are not visibly dirty, they can be cleaned by rubbing them against the palm of the opposite hand.

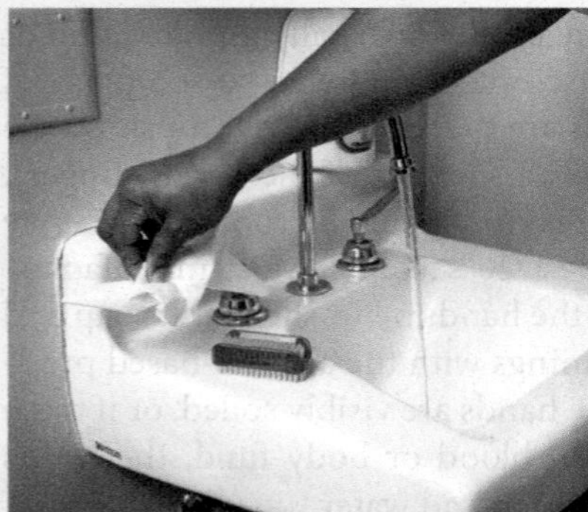

FIGURE 15–15A Use a dry towel to turn the faucet on.

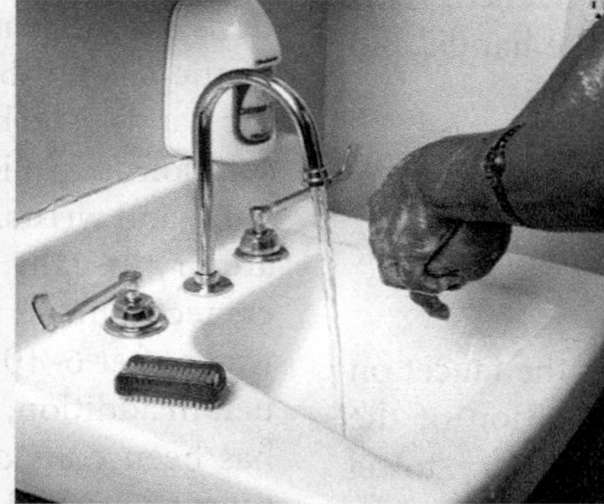

FIGURE 15–15B Point the fingertips downward and use the palm of one hand to clean the back of the other hand.

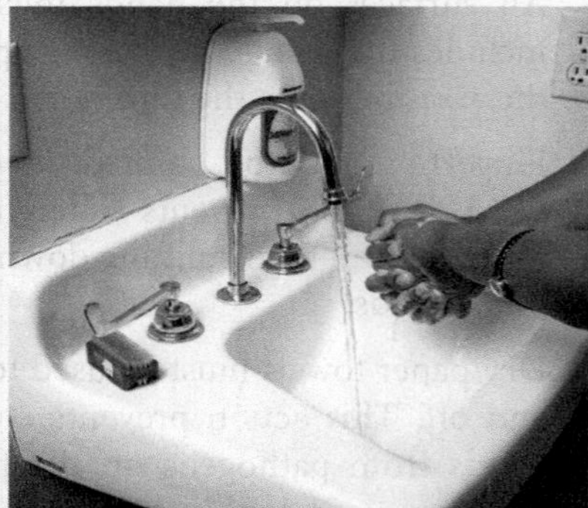

FIGURE 15–15C Interlace the fingers to clean between the fingers.

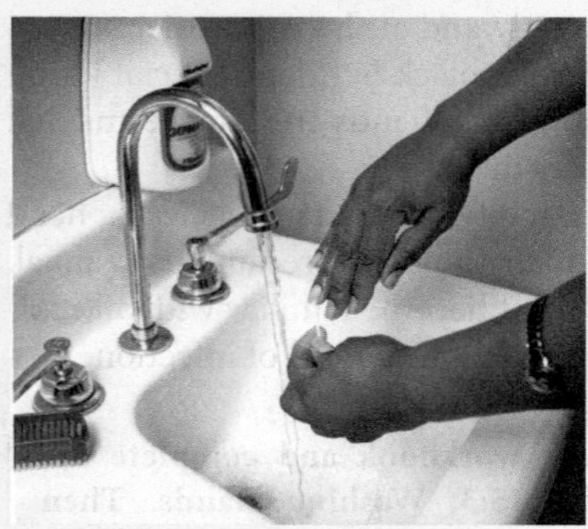

FIGURE 15–15D The blunt end of an orange stick can be used to clean the nails.

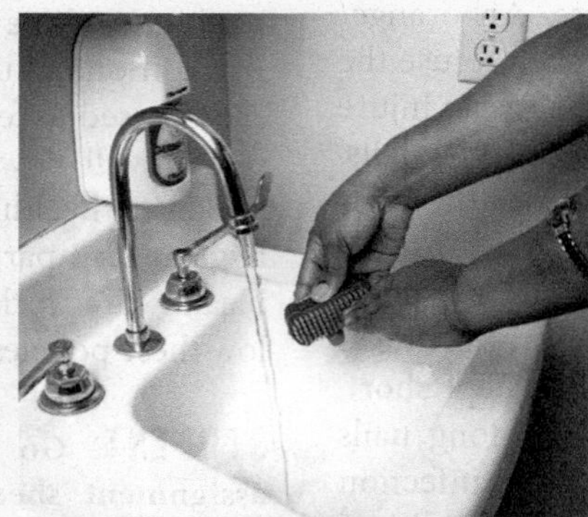

FIGURE 15–15E A hand brush can also be used to clean the nails.

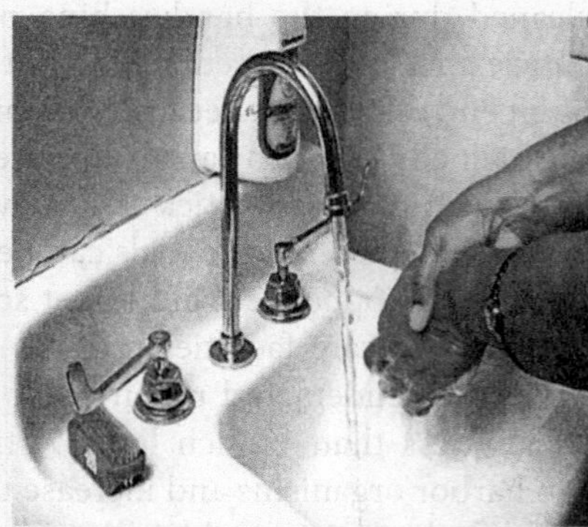

FIGURE 15–15F With the fingertips pointing downward, rinse the hands thoroughly.

(continues)

PROCEDURE 15:3 (CONT.)

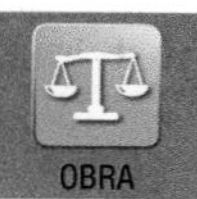

CAUTION: Use the blunt end of orange/cuticle stick to avoid injury.

NOTE: Steps 3 through 9 ensure that all parts of both hands are clean.

NOTE: Many health care facilities require washing the hands for 40–60 seconds (2014 WHO recommendation is 40–60 seconds). This is equivalent to singing the "Happy Birthday" song twice.

10. Rinse your hands from the forearms down to the fingertips, keeping fingertips pointed downward (Figure 15–15F).
11. Use a clean paper towel to dry hands thoroughly, from tips of fingers to wrist. Discard the towel in the waste container.
12. Use another dry paper towel to turn off the faucet.

CAUTION: Wet towels allow passage of pathogens.

13. Discard all used towels in the waste container. Leave the area neat and clean.
14. Apply a water-based hand lotion if desired.

PRACTICE: **Go to the workbook and use the evaluation sheet for 15:3, Washing Hands, to practice this procedure. When you believe you have mastered this skill, sign the sheet and give it to your instructor for further action.**

FINAL CHECKPOINT: Using the criteria listed on the evaluation sheet, your instructor will grade your performance.

15:4 Observing Standard Precautions

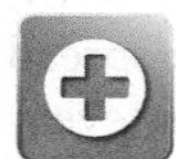

To prevent the spread of pathogens and disease, the chain of infection must be broken. The standard precautions discussed in this unit are an important way health care workers can break this chain.

Bloodborne Pathogens Standard

One of the main ways that pathogens are spread is by blood and body fluids. Three pathogens of major concern are the hepatitis B virus (HBV), the hepatitis C virus (HCV), and the human immunodeficiency virus (HIV), which causes AIDS. Consequently, extreme care must be taken at all times when an area, object, or person is contaminated with blood or body fluids. In 1991, the Occupational Safety and Health Administration (OSHA) established *Bloodborne Pathogen Standards* that must be followed by all health care facilities. The employer faces civil penalties if the regulations are not implemented by the employer and followed by the employees. These regulations require all health care facility employers to:

- Develop a written exposure control plan, and update it annually, to minimize or eliminate employee exposure to bloodborne pathogens.
- Identify all employees who have occupational exposure to blood or potentially infectious materials such as semen, vaginal secretions, and other body fluids.
- Provide hepatitis B vaccine free of charge to all employees who have occupational exposure, and obtain a written release form signed by any employee who does not want the vaccine.
- Provide **personal protective equipment (PPE)** such as gloves, gowns, lab coats, masks, and face shields in appropriate sizes and in accessible locations.
- Provide adequate handwashing facilities and supplies.
- Ensure that the worksite is maintained in a clean and sanitary condition, follow measures for immediate decontamination of any surface that comes in contact with blood or infectious materials, and dispose of infectious waste correctly.
- Enforce rules of no eating, drinking, smoking, applying cosmetics or lip balm, handling contact lenses, and mouth pipetting or suctioning in any area that can be potentially contaminated by blood or other body fluids.
- Provide appropriate containers that are color coded (fluorescent orange or orange-red) and labeled for contaminated sharps (needles, scalpels) and other infectious or biohazard wastes.
- Post signs at the entrance to work areas where there is occupational exposure to biohazardous materials. Label any item that is biohazardous with the red

biohazard symbol (Figure 15-16). The label must show both the symbol and the word "biohazard."

- Provide a confidential medical evaluation and follow-up for any employee who has an exposure incident. Examples might include an accidental needlestick or the splashing of blood or body fluids on the skin, eyes, or mucous membranes.
- Provide training about the regulations and all potential biohazards to all employees at no cost during working hours, and provide additional education as needed when procedures or working conditions are changed or modified.

In 2014 the CDC established more stringent precautions because of an outbreak of Ebola in West Africa. These requirements are discussed in detail in Chapter 15:9 of this text.

Needlestick Safety Act

In 2001, OSHA revised its Bloodborne Pathogen Standards in response to Congress passing the *Needlestick Safety and Prevention Act* in November 2000. This act was passed after the Centers for Disease Control and Prevention (CDC) estimated that 600,000 to 800,000 needlesticks occur each year, exposing health care workers to bloodborne pathogens. Employers are required to:

- *Identify and use effective and safer medical devices.* OSHA defines safer devices as sharps with engineered injury protections, and includes, but is not limited to, devices such as syringes with a sliding sheath that shields the needle after use, needles that retract into a syringe after use, shielded or retracting catheters that can be used to administer intravenous medications or fluids, and intravenous systems that administer medication or fluids through a catheter port or connector site using a needle housed in a protective covering (Figure 15-17). OSHA also encourages the use of needleless systems, which include, but are not limited to, intravenous medication delivery systems that administer medication or fluids through a catheter port or connector site using a blunt cannula or other non-needle connection, and jet injection systems that deliver subcutaneous or intramuscular injections through the skin without using a needle.
- *Incorporate changes in annual updates of the exposure control plan.* Employers must include changes in technology that eliminate or reduce exposure to bloodborne pathogens in the annual update and document the implementation of any safer medical devices.
- *Solicit input from nonmanagerial employees who are responsible for direct patient care.* Employees who provide patient care and are exposed to injuries from contaminated sharps must be included in a multidisciplinary team that identifies, evaluates, and selects safer medical devices, and determines safer work practice controls.
- *Maintain a sharps injury log.* Employers with more than 11 employees must maintain a sharps injury log to help identify high-risk areas and evaluate ways to decrease injuries. Each injury recorded must protect the confidentiality of the injured employee but must state the type and brand of device involved in the incident, the work area or department where the exposure injury occurred, and a description of how the incident occurred.

Standard Precautions

Employers are also required to make sure that every employee uses standard precautions at all times to prevent contact with blood or other potentially infectious materials. **Standard precautions** (Figure 15-18) are rules developed by the CDC to prevent the spread of infection. According to standard precautions, every body fluid must be considered a potentially infectious

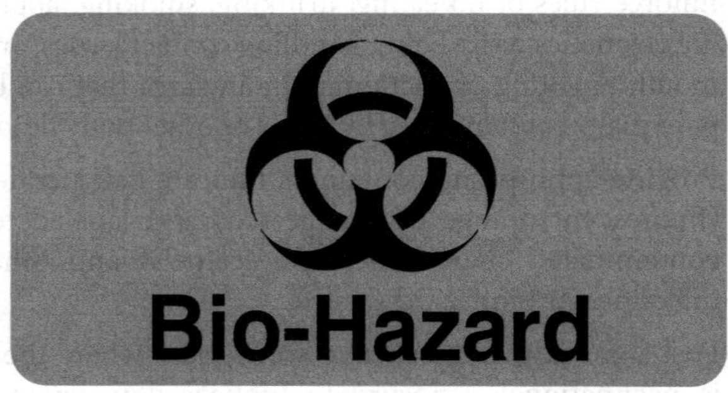

FIGURE 15–16 The universal biohazard symbol indicates a potential source of infection.

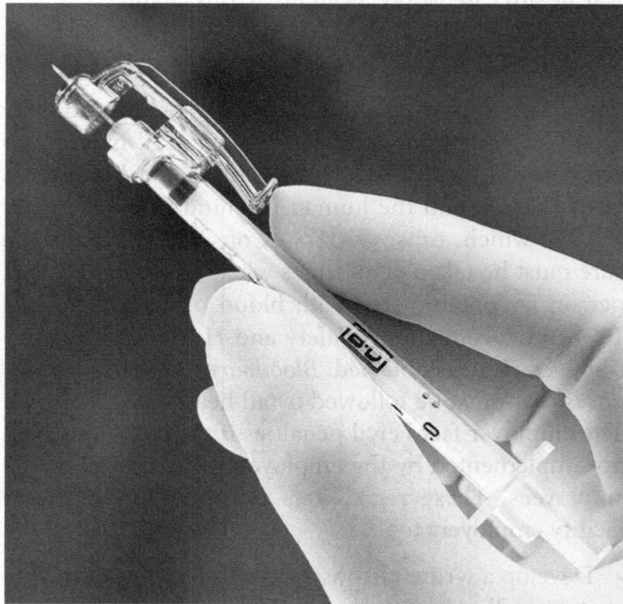

FIGURE 15–17 The Safety-Glide syringe is one example of a safer device to prevent needlesticks. Photo reprinted courtesy of BD [Becton, Dickinson and Company].

STANDARD PRECAUTIONS

Assume that every person is potentially infected or colonized with an organism that could be transmitted in the healthcare setting.

Hand Hygiene

Avoid unnecessary touching of surfaces in close proximity to the patient.

When hands are visibly dirty, contaminated with proteinaceous material, or visibly soiled with blood or body fluids, wash hands with soap and water.

If hands are not visibly soiled, or after removing visible material with soap and water, decontaminate hands with an alcohol-based hand rub. Alternatively, hands may be washed with an antimicrobial soap and water.

Perform hand hygiene:

- Before having direct contact with patients.
- After contact with blood, body fluids or excretions, mucous membranes, nonintact skin, or wound dressings.
- After contact with a patient's intact skin (e.g., when taking a pulse or blood pressure or lifting a patient).
- If hands will be moving from a contaminated-body site to a clean-body site during patient care.
- After contact with inanimate objects (including medical equipment) in the immediate vicinity of the patient.
- After removing gloves.

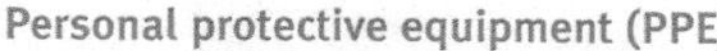

Personal protective equipment (PPE)

Wear PPE when the nature of the anticipated patient interaction indicates that contact with blood or body fluids may occur.

Before leaving the patient's room or cubicle, remove and discard PPE.

Gloves

Wear gloves when contact with blood or other potentially infectious materials, mucous membranes, nonintact skin, or potentially contaminated intact skin (e.g., of a patient incontinent of stool or urine) could occur.

Remove gloves after contact with a patient and/or the surrounding environment using proper technique to prevent hand contamination. Do not wear the same pair of gloves for the care of more than one patient.

Change gloves during patient care if the hands will move from a contaminated body-site (e.g., perineal area) to a clean body-site (e.g., face).

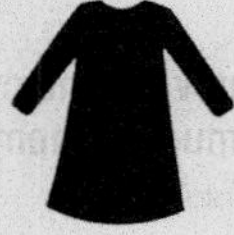

Gowns

Wear a gown to protect skin and prevent soiling or contamination of clothing during procedures and patient-care activities when contact with blood, body fluids, secretions, or excretions is anticipated.

Wear a gown for direct patient contact if the patient has uncontained secretions or excretions.

Remove gown and perform hand hygiene before leaving the patient's environment.

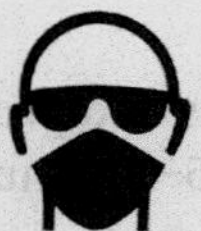

Mouth, nose, eye protection

Use PPE to protect the mucous membranes of the eyes, nose and mouth during procedures and patient-care activities that are likely to generate splashes or sprays of blood, body fluids, secretions and excretions.

During aerosol-generating procedures wear one of the following: a face shield that fully covers the front and sides of the face, a mask with attached shield, or a mask and goggles.

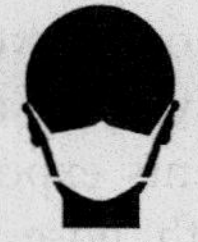

Respiratory Hygiene/Cough Etiquette

Educate healthcare personnel to contain respiratory secretions to prevent droplet and fomite transmission of respiratory pathogens, especially during seasonal outbreaks of viral respiratory tract infections.

Offer masks to coughing patients and other symptomatic persons (e.g., persons who accompany ill patients) upon entry into the facility.

Patient-care equipment and instruments/devices

Wear PPE (e.g., gloves, gown), according to the level of anticipated contamination, when handling patient-care equipment and instruments/devices that are visibly soiled or may have been in contact with blood or body fluids.

Care of the environment

Include multi-use electronic equipment in policies and procedures for preventing contamination and for cleaning and disinfection, especially those items that are used by patients, those used during delivery of patient care, and mobile devices that are moved in and out of patient rooms frequently (e.g., daily).

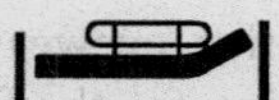

Textiles and laundry

Handle used textiles and fabrics with minimum agitation to avoid contamination of air, surfaces and persons.

SPR

FIGURE 15–18 Standard precautions must be observed while working with all patients. Reprinted with Permission from Brevis Corporation [www.brevis.com].

material, and all patients must be considered potential sources of infection, regardless of their disease or diagnosis. Standard precautions must be used in any situation where health care providers may contact:

- Blood or any fluid that may contain blood
- Body fluids, secretions, and excretions, such as mucus, sputum, saliva, cerebrospinal fluid, urine, feces, vomitus, amniotic fluid (surrounding a fetus), synovial (joint) fluid, pleural (lung) fluid, pericardial (heart) fluid, peritoneal (abdominal cavity) fluid, semen, and vaginal secretions
- Mucous membranes
- Nonintact skin
- Tissue or cell specimens

The basic rules of standard precautions include:

- *Handwashing:* Hands must be washed before and after contact with any patient. If hands or other skin surfaces are contaminated with blood, body fluids, secretions, or excretions, they must be washed immediately and thoroughly with soap and water. If hands are not visibly soiled, an alcohol-based hand cleaner can be used. Hands must always be washed immediately before donning and immediately after removing gloves.
- *Gloves:* Gloves (Figure 15-19) must be worn whenever contact with blood, body fluids, secretions, excretions, mucous membranes, tissue specimens, or nonintact skin is possible; when handling or cleaning any contaminated items or surfaces; when performing any invasive (entering the body) procedure; and when performing venipuncture or blood tests. Rings must be removed before putting on gloves to avoid puncturing the gloves. Gloves must be changed after contact with each patient and even between tasks or procedures on the same patient if there is any chance the gloves are contaminated. Gloves should not be worn out of patient rooms or care areas. Hands must be washed immediately after gloves are removed. Care must be taken while removing gloves to avoid contamination of the skin. Gloves must *not* be washed or disinfected for reuse because washing may allow penetration of liquids through undetected holes and disinfecting agents may cause deterioration of the gloves.
- *Gowns:* Gowns must be worn during any procedure that may cause splashing or spraying of blood, body fluids, secretions, or excretions. This helps prevent contamination of clothing or uniforms. Contaminated gowns must be handled according to agency policy and local and state laws. Gowns should only be worn once and then discarded. Gowns should not be worn out of patient rooms or care areas. Wash hands immediately after removing a gown.

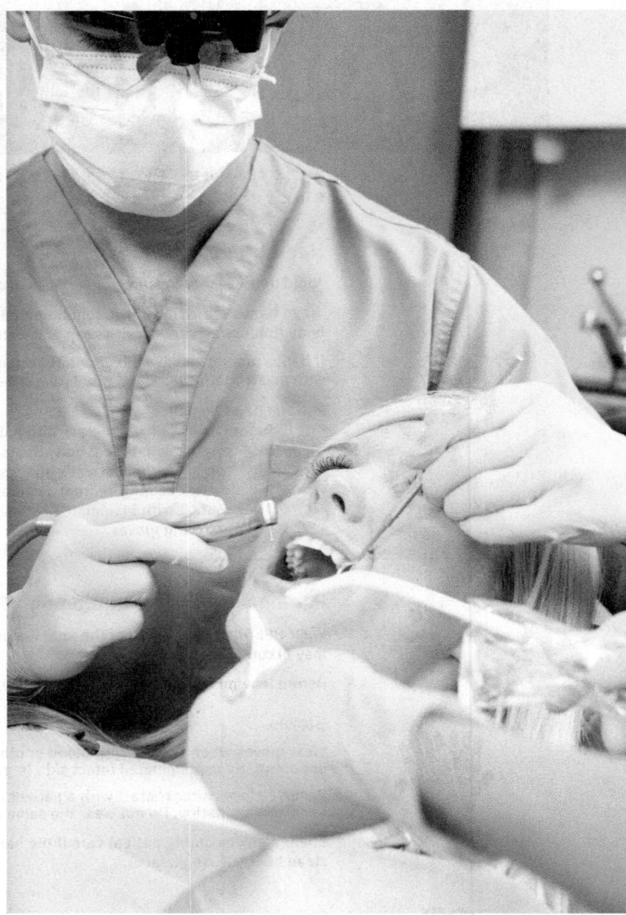

FIGURE 15–19 Gloves must be worn whenever contact with blood, body fluids, secretions, excretions, mucous membranes, or nonintact skin is possible. © Tyler Olson/Shutterstock.com.

- *Masks and Eye Protection:* Masks and protective eyewear or face shields (Figure 15-20) must be worn during procedures that may produce splashes or sprays of blood, body fluids, secretions, or excretions. Examples include irrigation of wounds, suctioning, dental procedures, delivery of a baby, and surgical procedures. This prevents exposure of the mucous membranes of the mouth, nose, and eyes to any pathogens.

  Masks must be used once and then discarded. In addition, masks should be changed every 30 minutes or anytime they become moist or wet. They should be removed by grasping the ties or elastic strap. Mask should not be worn out of patient rooms or care areas and should not be left dangling around the neck. Hands must be washed immediately after the mask is removed. Protective eyewear or face shields should provide protection for the front, top, bottom, and sides of the eyes. If eyewear is not disposable, it must be cleaned and disinfected before it is reused.

- *Sharps:* To avoid accidental cuts or punctures, extreme care must be taken while handling sharp objects. Whenever possible, safe needles or needleless devices must be used. Disposable needles must never be bent or broken after use. They must be left uncapped and attached to the syringe and placed in a leakproof, puncture-resistant sharps container (Figure 15-21). The sharps container must be labeled with a red biohazard symbol. Surgical blades, razors, and other sharp objects must also be discarded in the sharps container.

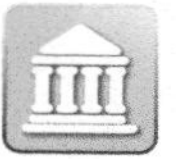
Legal

The sharps containers must *not* be emptied or reused. Federal, state, and local laws establish regulations for the disposal of sharps containers.

- *Spills or Splashes:* Spills or splashes of blood, body fluids, secretions, or excretions must be wiped up immediately. Gloves must be worn while wiping up the area with disposable cleaning cloths. The area must then be cleaned with a disinfectant solution such as a 10 percent bleach solution. Furniture or equipment contaminated by the spill or splash must be cleaned and disinfected immediately. For large spills, an absorbent powder may be used to soak up the fluid. After the fluid is absorbed, the powder is swept up and placed in an infectious waste container (Figure 15-22).
- *Resuscitation Devices:* Mouthpieces or resuscitation devices should be used to avoid mouth-to-mouth resuscitation. These devices should be placed in

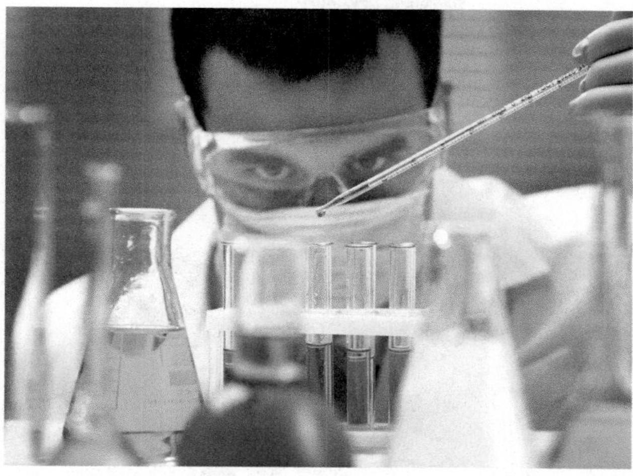

FIGURE 15–20 **Gloves, a gown, a mask, and protective eyewear must be worn during any procedure that may produce droplets or cause splashing of blood, body fluids, secretions, or excretions.**

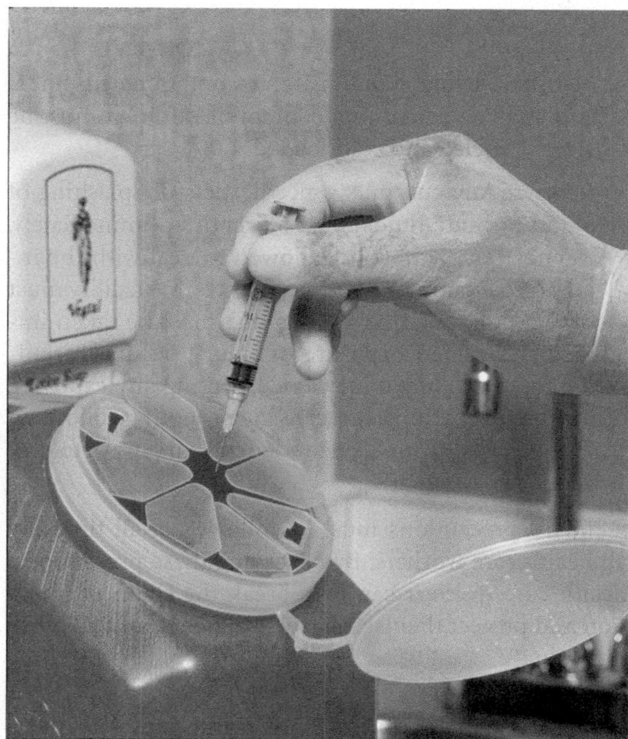

FIGURE 15–21 **All needles and sharp objects must be discarded immediately in a leakproof, puncture-resistant sharps container.**

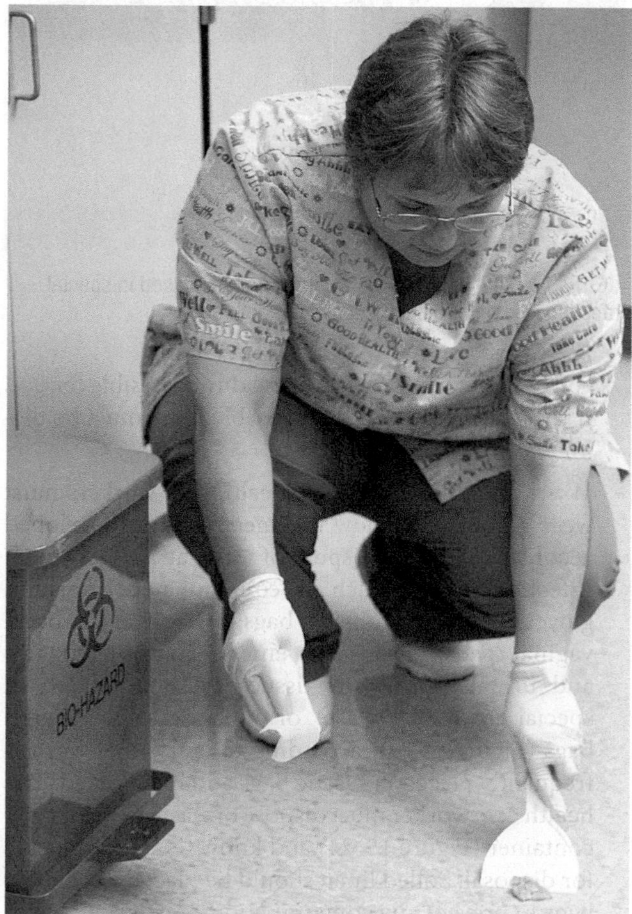

FIGURE 15–22 **An absorbent powder may be used to soak up a spill of blood, body fluids, secretions, or excretions. Gloves must be worn while picking up the solidified spill.**

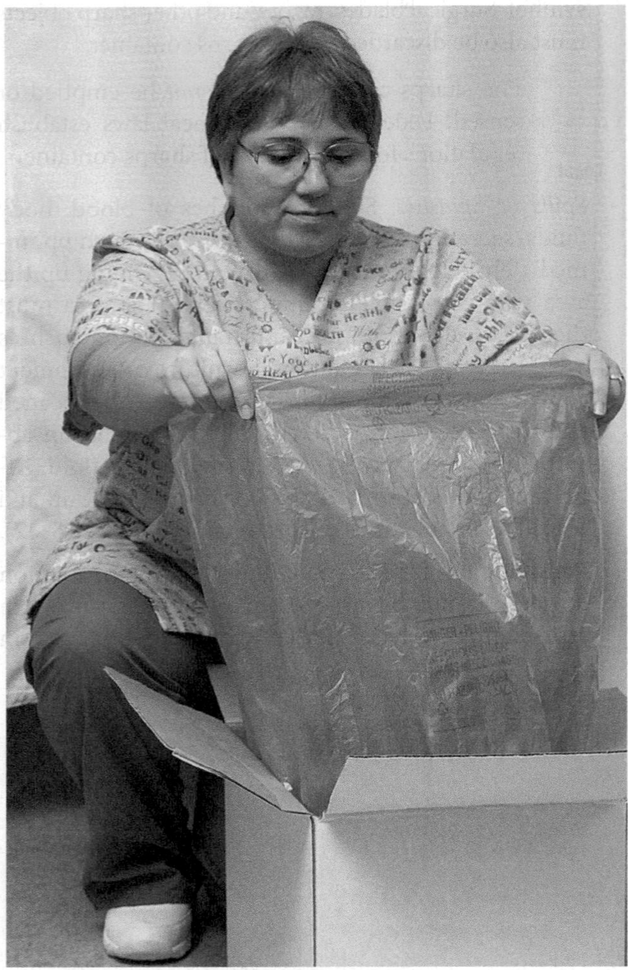

FIGURE 15–23 All infectious wastes must be placed in special infectious waste or biohazardous material bags.

convenient locations and be readily accessible for use. If these devices are not disposable, they must be disinfected between patient use.

- *Waste and Linen Disposal:* Health care workers must wear gloves and follow the agency policy developed according to law to dispose of waste and soiled linen. Infectious wastes such as contaminated dressings; gloves; urinary drainage bags; incontinence pads; vaginal pads; disposable emesis basins, bedpans, and urinals; and body tissues must be placed in special infectious waste or biohazardous material bags (Figure 15-23) according to law. Other trash is frequently placed in plastic bags and incinerated. The health care worker must dispose of waste in the proper container (Figure 15-24) and know the requirements for disposal. Soiled linen should be placed in laundry bags to prevent any contamination. Linen soiled with blood, body fluids, or excretions is placed in a special bag for contaminated linen and is usually soaked in a disinfectant before being laundered. Gloves must

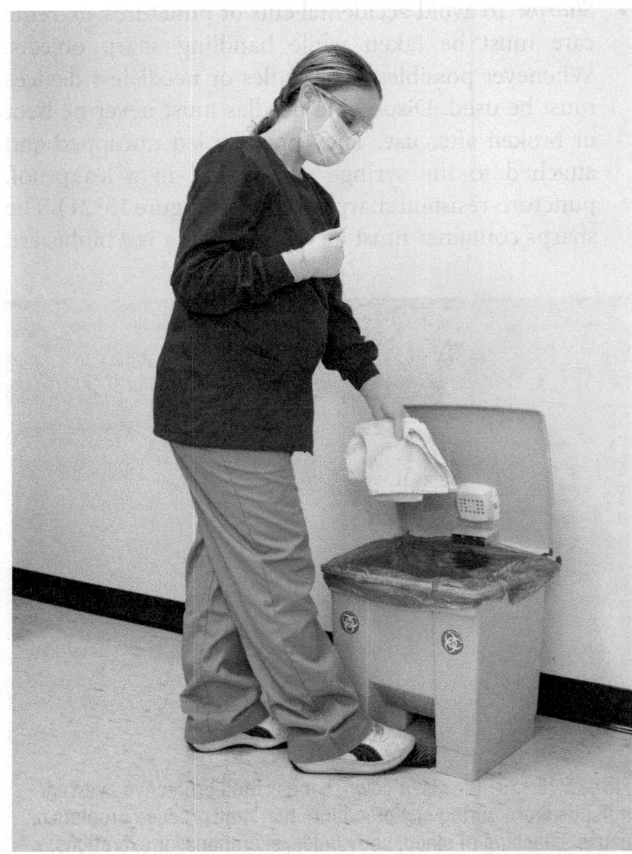

FIGURE 15–24 The health care worker must know the requirements for disposal of waste materials and dispose of wastes in the proper containers.

be worn while handling any contaminated linen, and any bag containing contaminated linen must be clearly labeled and color coded.

- *Injuries:* Any cut, injury, needlestick, or splashing of blood or body fluids must be reported immediately. Agency policy must be followed to deal with the injury or contamination. Every health care facility must have a policy stating actions that must be taken immediately when exposure or injury occurs, including reporting any injury, documenting any exposure incident, recording the care given, noting follow-up to the exposure incident, and identifying ways to prevent a similar incident.

Standard precautions must be followed at all times by all health care workers. By observing these precautions, health care workers can help break the chain of infection and protect themselves, their patients, and all other individuals.

STUDENT: **Go to the workbook and complete the assignment sheet for 15:4, Observing Standard Precautions. Then return and continue with the procedure.**

PROCEDURE 15:4

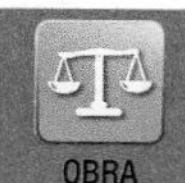

OBRA

Observing Standard Precautions

Equipment and Supplies

Disposable gloves, infectious waste bags, needle and syringe, sharps container, gown, masks, protective eyewear, resuscitation devices

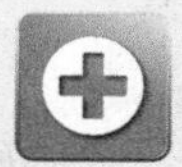

Precaution

NOTE: This procedure will help you learn standard precautions. It is important for you to observe these precautions at all times while working in the laboratory or clinical area.

Procedure

1. Assemble equipment.
2. Review the precautions in the information section for Observing Standard Precautions. Note points that are not clear, and ask your instructor for an explanation.
3. Practice handwashing according to Procedure 15:3. Identify at least six times that hands must be washed according to standard precautions.
4. Name four instances when gloves must be worn to observe standard precautions. Put on a pair of disposable gloves. Practice removing the gloves without contaminating the skin. With a gloved hand, grasp the cuff of the glove on the opposite hand, handling only the outside of the glove (Figure 15–25A). Pull the glove down and turn it inside out while removing it (Figure 15–25B). Take care not to touch the skin with the gloved hand. Grasp the contaminated glove in the palm of the gloved hand (Figure 15–25C). Using the ungloved hand, slip the fingers under the cuff of the glove on the opposite hand (Figure 15–25D). Touching only the inside of the glove and taking care not to touch the skin, pull the glove down and turn it inside out while removing it (Figure 15–25E). Place the gloves in an infectious waste container (Figure 15–25F). Wash your hands immediately.
5. Practice putting on a gown. State when a gown is to be worn. To remove the gown, touch only the inside. Fold the contaminated gown so the outside is folded inward. Roll it into a bundle and place it in an infectious waste container if it is disposable, or in a bag for contaminated linen if it is not disposable.

Safety

CAUTION: If a gown is contaminated, gloves should be worn while removing the gown.

NOTE: Folding the gown and rolling it prevents transmission of pathogens.

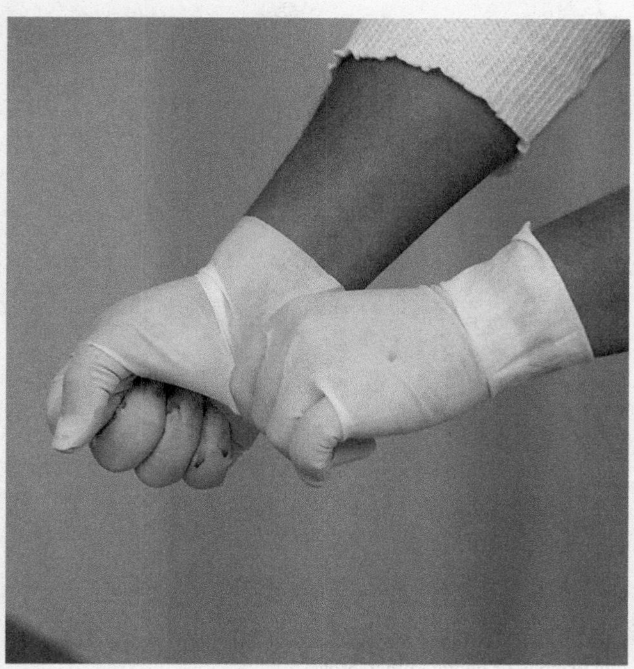

FIGURE 15–25A To remove the first glove, use a gloved hand to grasp the outside of the glove on the opposite hand.

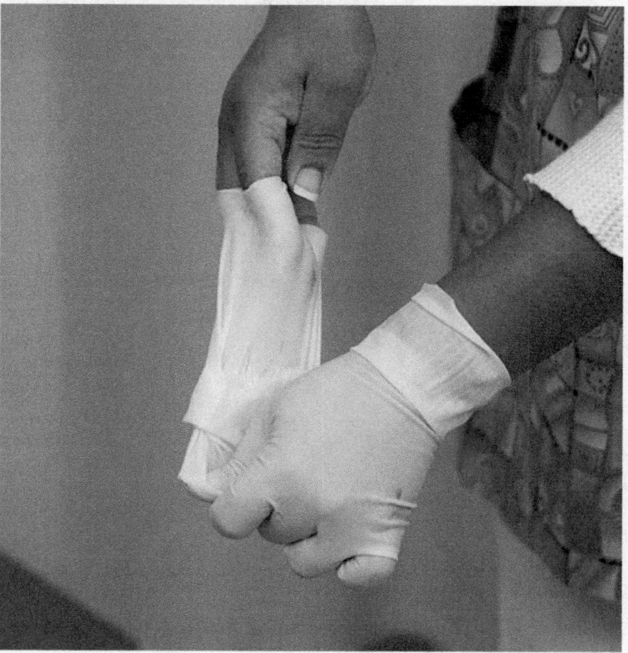

FIGURE 15–25B Pull the glove down and turn it inside out while removing it.

(continues)

PROCEDURE 15:4 (CONT.)

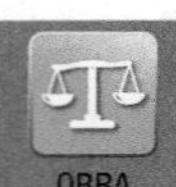

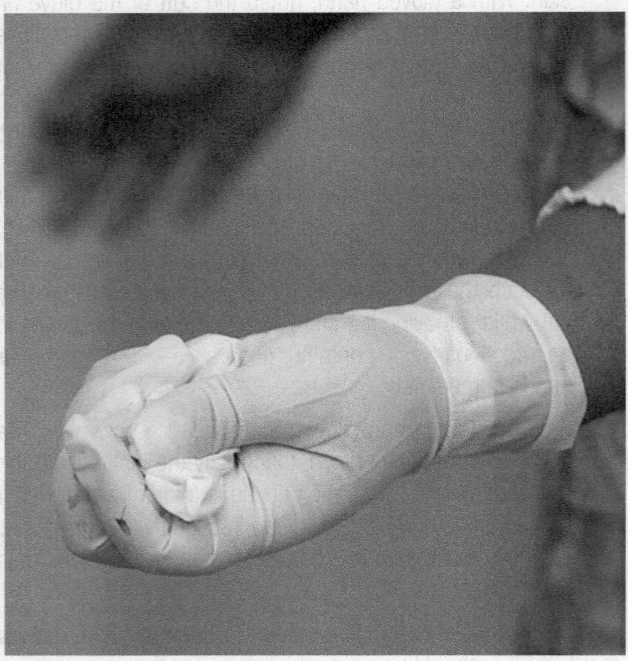

FIGURE 15–25C Grasp the contaminated glove in the palm of the gloved hand.

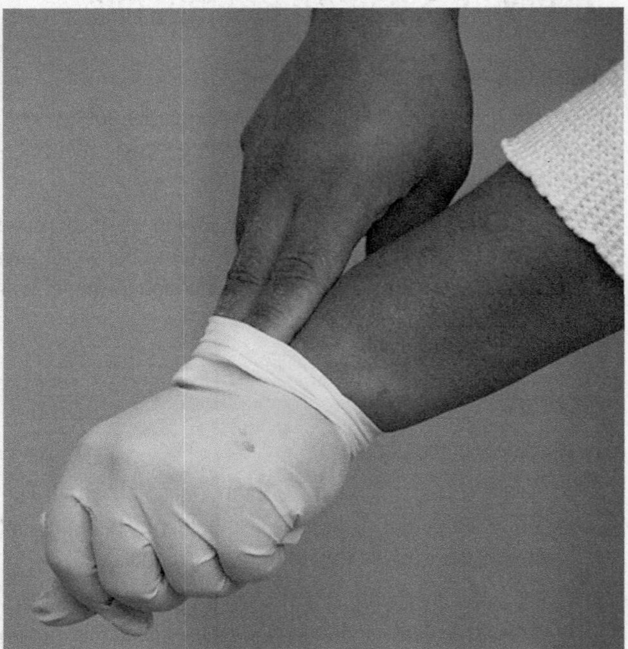

FIGURE 15–25D To remove the second glove, slip the fingers of the ungloved hand inside the cuff of the glove.

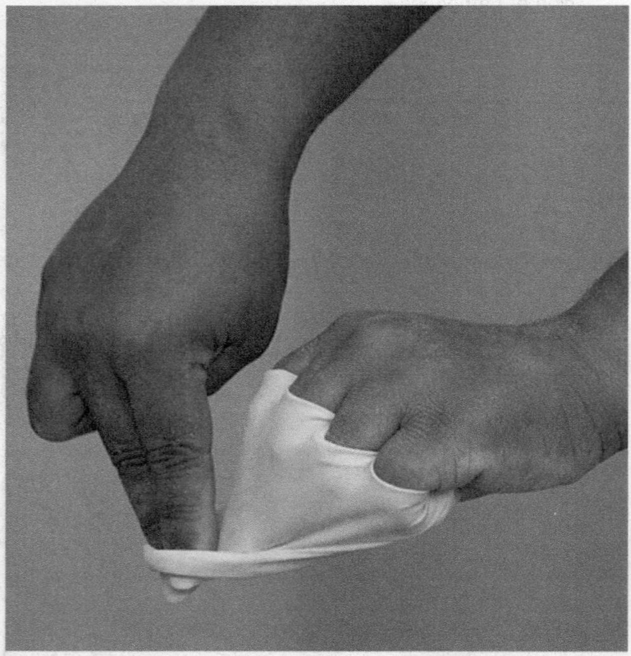

FIGURE 15–25E Touch only the inside of the glove while pulling it down and turning it inside out.

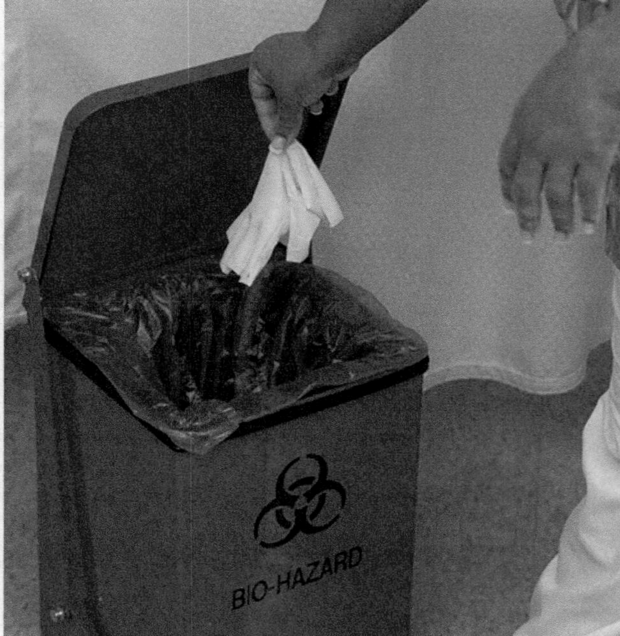

FIGURE 15–25F Place the gloves in an infectious-waste container and wash your hands immediately.

PROCEDURE 15:4 (CONT.)

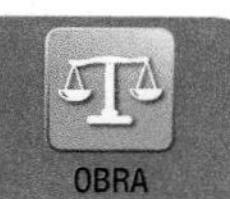

6. Practice putting on a mask and protective eyewear. To remove the mask, handle it by the ties only. Clean and disinfect protective eyewear after use.
7. Practice proper disposal of sharps. Uncap a needle attached to a syringe, taking care not to stick yourself with the needle. Place the entire needle and syringe in a sharps container. Never recap a needle. State the rules regarding disposal of the sharps container.
8. Spill a small amount of water on a counter. Pretend that it is blood. Put on gloves and use disposable cloths or gauze to wipe up the spill. Put the contaminated cloths or gauze in an infectious waste bag. Use clean disposable cloths or gauze to wipe the area thoroughly with a disinfectant agent (Figure 15–26). Put the cloths or gauze in the infectious waste bag, remove your gloves, and wash your hands.
9. Practice handling an infectious waste bag. Fold down the top edge of the bag to form a cuff at the top of the bag. Wear gloves to close the bag after contaminated wastes have been placed in it. Put your hands under the folded cuff and gently expel excess air from the bag. Twist the top of the bag shut and fold down the top edges to seal the bag. Secure the fold with tape or a tie according to agency policy (Figure 15–27).
10. Examine mouthpieces and resuscitation devices that are used for resuscitation. You will be taught to use these devices when you learn cardiopulmonary resuscitation (CPR).

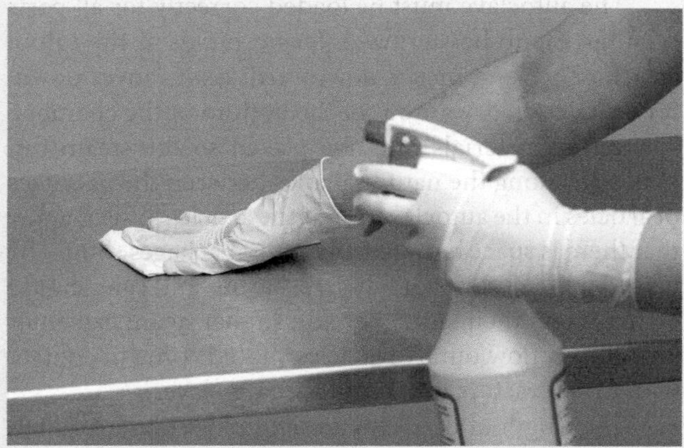

FIGURE 15–26 Wear gloves to spray the contaminated counter with a disinfectant. Then wipe the counter clean with a disposable cloth or gauze.

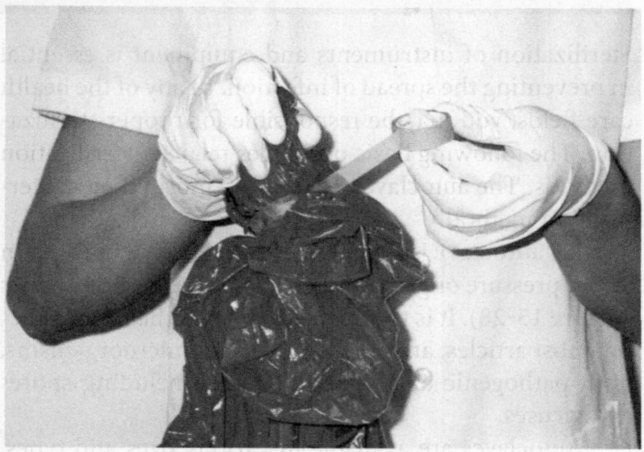

FIGURE 15–27 After folding down the top edge of the infectious waste bag, tie or tape it securely.

11. Discuss the following situations with another student and determine which standard precautions should be observed:
    - A patient has an open sore on the skin and pus is seeping from the area. You are going to bathe the patient.
    - You are cleaning a tray of instruments that contains a disposable surgical blade and a needle with syringe.
    - A tube of blood drops to the floor and breaks, spilling the blood on the floor.
    - Drainage from dressings on an infected wound has soiled the linen on the bed you are changing.
    - You work in a dental office and are assisting a dentist while a tooth is being extracted (removed).
12. Replace all equipment used.

PRACTICE: Go to the workbook and use the evaluation sheet for 15:4, Observing Standard Precautions. When you believe you have mastered this skill, sign the sheet and give it to your instructor for further action.

FINAL CHECKPOINT: Using the criteria listed on the evaluation sheet, your instructor will grade your performance.

15:5 Sterilizing with an Autoclave

Sterilization of instruments and equipment is essential in preventing the spread of infection. In any of the health care fields, you may be responsible for proper sterilization. The following basic principles relate to sterilization methods. The autoclave is the safest, most efficient sterilization method.

An **autoclave** is a piece of equipment that uses steam under pressure or gas to sterilize equipment and supplies (Figure 15-28). It is the most efficient method of sterilizing most articles, and it will destroy all microorganisms, both pathogenic and nonpathogenic, including spores and viruses.

Autoclaves are available in various sizes and types. Offices and health clinics usually have smaller units, and hospitals or surgical areas have large floor models. A pressure cooker can be used in home situations.

Before any equipment or supplies are sterilized in an autoclave, they must be prepared properly. All items must be washed thoroughly and then rinsed. Oily substances can often be removed with alcohol or ether. Any residue left on articles will tend to bake and stick to the article during the autoclaving process.

Items that are to remain sterile must be wrapped before they are autoclaved. A wide variety of wraps are available. The wrap must be a material that will allow for the penetration of steam during the autoclaving process. Samples of wraps include muslin, autoclave paper, special plastic or paper bags, and autoclave containers (Figure 15-29).

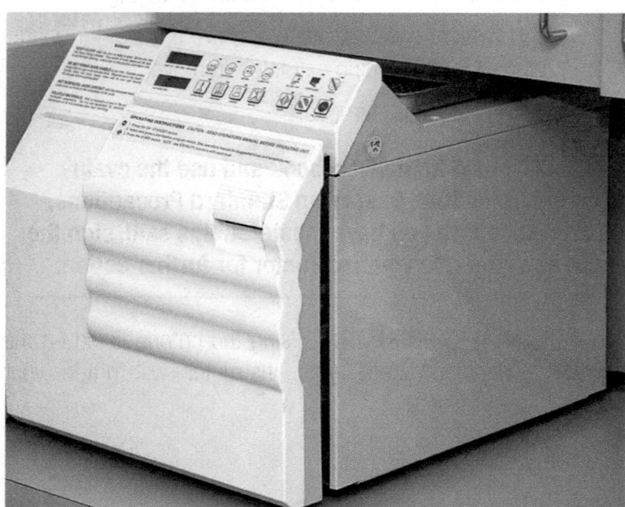

FIGURE 15–28 An autoclave uses steam under pressure to sterilize items.

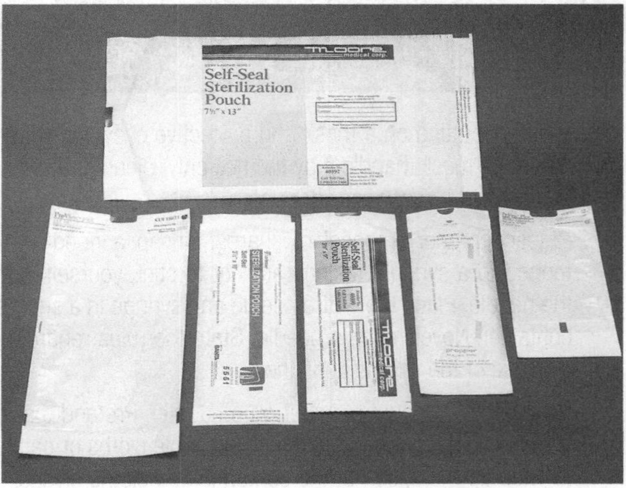

FIGURE 15–29 Special plastic or paper autoclave bags can be used to sterilize instruments.

Autoclave indicators are used to ensure that articles have been sterilized (Figure 15-30). Examples of indicators include autoclave tape, sensitivity marks on bags or wraps, and indicator capsules. The indicator is usually placed on or near the article when the article is put into the autoclave. Indicators can also be placed in the center of a package, such as a tray of instruments, to show that sterilization of the entire package has occurred. The indicator will change appearance during the autoclaving process because of the length of time and the temperature, which lead to sterilization. Learn how to recognize that an article is sterile by reading the directions provided with indicators.

The autoclave must be loaded correctly for all parts of an article to be sterilized. Steam builds at the top of the chamber and moves downward. As it moves down, it pushes cool, dry air out of the bottom of the chamber. Therefore, materials must be placed so the steam can penetrate along the natural planes between the packages of articles in the autoclave. Place the articles in such a way that there is space between all pieces. Packages should be placed on the sides, not flat. Jars, basins, and cans should be placed on their sides, not flat, so that steam can enter and air can flow out. No articles should come in contact with the sides, top, or door of the autoclave.

The length of time and amount of pressure required to sterilize different items varies (Figure 15-31). *It is important to check the directions that come with the autoclave.* Because different types of articles require different times and pressures, it is important to separate loads so that all articles sterilized at one time require the same time and pressure. For example, rubber tubings usually require a relatively short time and can be damaged by long exposure. Certain instruments and needles require a longer

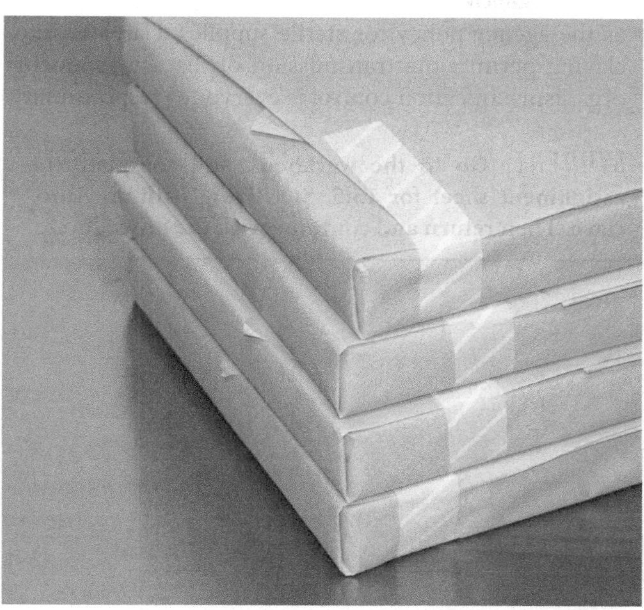

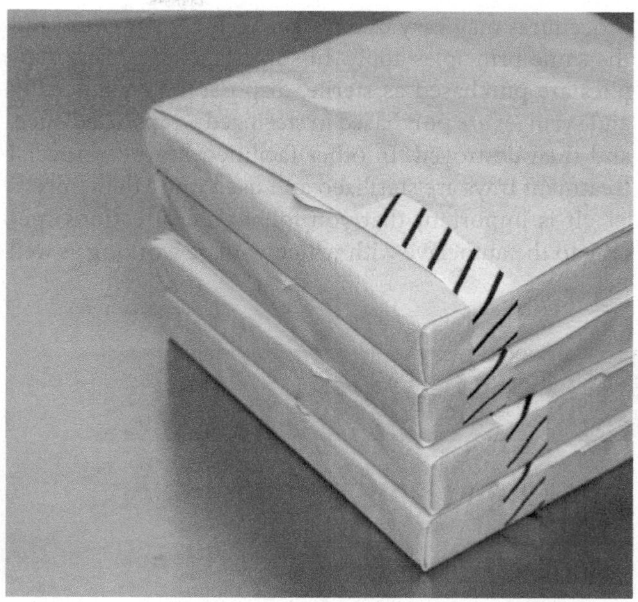

FIGURE 15–30 Autoclave indicators change color to show that sterilization has occurred: (A) before sterilization and (B) after sterilization.
Courtesy, SPSmedical Supply Corp.

Articles	Time at 250° to 254°F (121° to 123°C)
Glassware: empty, inverted Instruments: metal in covered or open, padded or unpadded tray Needles, unwrapped Syringes: unassembled, unwrapped Instruments, metal combined with other materials in covered and/or padded tray	15 minutes
Instruments wrapped in double-thickness muslin Flasked solutions, 75–250 mL Rubber products: gloves, catheters, and tubings	20 minutes
Syringes: unassembled, individually packed in muslin or paper Needles, individually packaged in glass tubes or paper Dressings wrapped in paper or muslin (small packs only) Flasked solutions, 500–1,000 mL Sutures: silk, cotton, or nylon; wrapped in paper or muslin Treatment trays wrapped in muslin or paper	30 minutes

FIGURE 15–31 The length of time required to sterilize different items varies.

time to ensure sterilization; therefore, items of this type should not be sterilized in the same load as rubber tubings.

Wet surfaces permit rapid infiltration of organisms, so it is important that all items are thoroughly dry before being removed from the autoclave. The length of drying time varies. Follow the manufacturer's instructions.

Sterilized items must be stored in clean, dustproof areas. Items usually remain sterile for 30 days after autoclaving. However, if the wraps loosen or tear, if they become wet, or if any chance of contamination occurs, the items should be rewrapped and autoclaved again.

NOTE: *At the end of the 30-day sterile period—providing that the wrap has not loosened, been torn, or gotten wet—remove the old autoclave tape from the package, replace with a new, dated tape, and resterilize according to correct procedure.*

Some autoclaves are equipped with a special door that allows the autoclave to be used as a dry-heat sterilizer. Dry heat involves the use of a high temperature for a long period. The temperature is usually a minimum of 320°F–350°F (160°C–177°C). The minimum time is usually 60 minutes. Dry-heat sterilization is a good method for sterilizing instruments that may corrode, such as knife blades, or items that would be destroyed by the moisture in steam sterilization, such as powders. Dry heat should never be used on soft rubber goods because the heat will destroy the rubber. Some types of plastic will also melt in dry heat. An oven can be used for dry-heat sterilization in home situations.

Procedures 15:5A and 15:5B describe wrapping articles for autoclaving and autoclaving techniques. These procedures may vary in different agencies and areas, but the same principles apply. In some facilities, many supplies are purchased as sterile, disposable items; needles and syringes are purchased in sterilized wraps, used once, and then destroyed. In other facilities, however, special treatment trays are sterilized and used more than once.

It is important that you follow the directions specific to the autoclave with which you are working as well as the agency policy for sterile supplies. Careless autoclaving permits the transmission of disease-producing organisms. Infection control is everyone's responsibility.

STUDENT: Go to the workbook and complete the assignment sheet for 15:5, Sterilizing with an Autoclave. Then return and continue with the procedures.

PROCEDURE 15:5A

Wrapping Items for Autoclaving

Equipment and Supplies

Items to wrap: instrument, towel, bowl; autoclave wrap: paper, muslin, plastic or paper bag; autoclave tape or indicator; disposable or utility gloves; pen or autoclave marker; masking tape (if autoclave tape is not used)

Procedure

1. Assemble equipment.
2. Wash hands. Put on gloves.

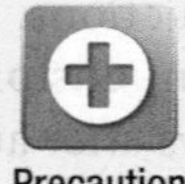
Precaution

CAUTION: If the items to be autoclaved may be contaminated with blood, body fluids, or tissues, gloves must be worn while cleaning the items.

3. Sanitize the items to be sterilized. Instruments, bowls, and similar items should be cleaned thoroughly in soapy water (Figure 15–32). Rinse the items well in cool water to remove any soapy residue. Then rinse well with hot water. Dry the items with a towel. After the items are sanitized and dry, remove the gloves and wash hands.

   NOTE: If stubborn stains are present, it may be necessary to soak the items.

   NOTE: Check the teeth on serrated (notched like a saw) instruments. Scrub with a brush as necessary.

4. To prepare linen for wrapping, check first to make sure it is clean and dry. Fold the linen in half lengthwise. If it is very wide, fold lengthwise again. Fanfold or accordion pleat the linen from end to end until a compact package is formed (Figure 15–33A). All folds should be the same size. Fold back one corner on the top fold (Figure 15–33B). This provides a piece to grab when opening the linen.

   NOTE: Fanfolding linens allows for easy handling after sterilization.

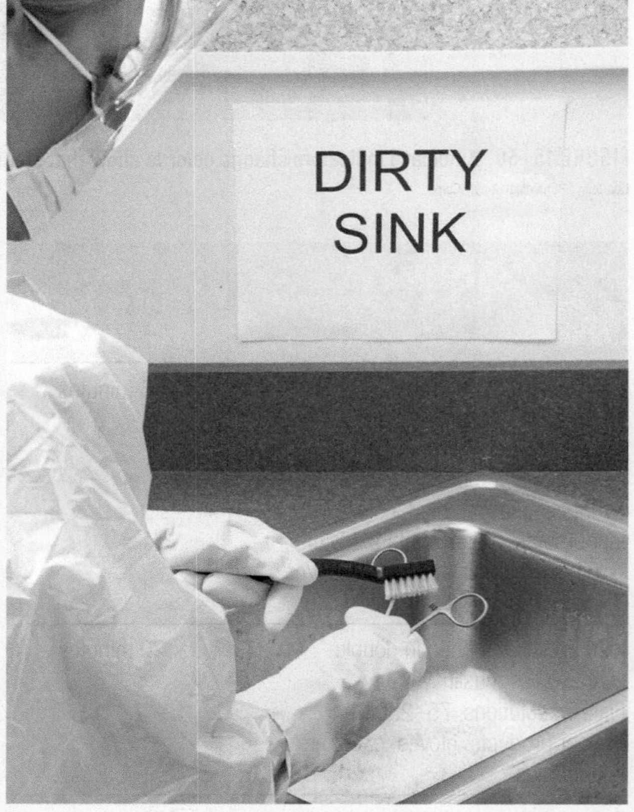

FIGURE 15–32 **Wear gloves to scrub instruments thoroughly with soapy water.**

5. Select the correct wrap for the item. Make sure the wrap is large enough to enclose the item to be wrapped.

   NOTE: Double-thickness muslin, disposable paper wraps, and plastic or paper bags are the most common wraps.

6. With the wrap positioned at a diagonal angle and one corner pointing toward you, place the item to be sterilized in the center of the wrap (Figure 15–34A)

   NOTE: Make sure that hinged instruments are open so the steam can sterilize all edges.

PROCEDURE 15:5A (CONT.)

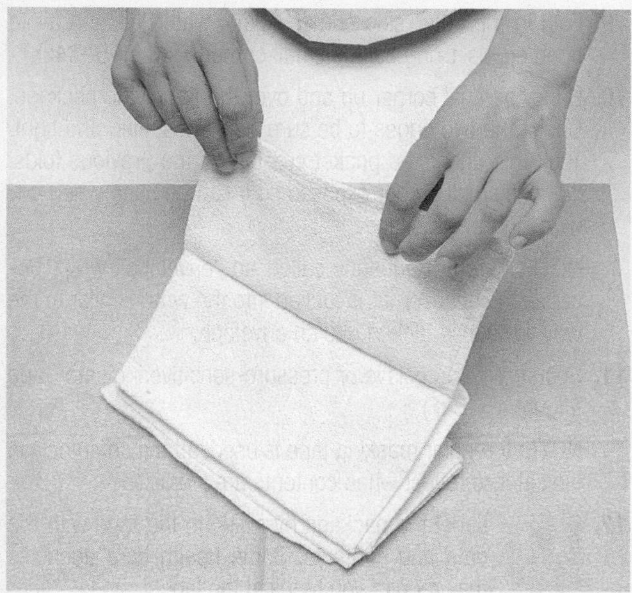

FIGURE 15–33A Fanfold clean, dry linen so all the folds are the same size.

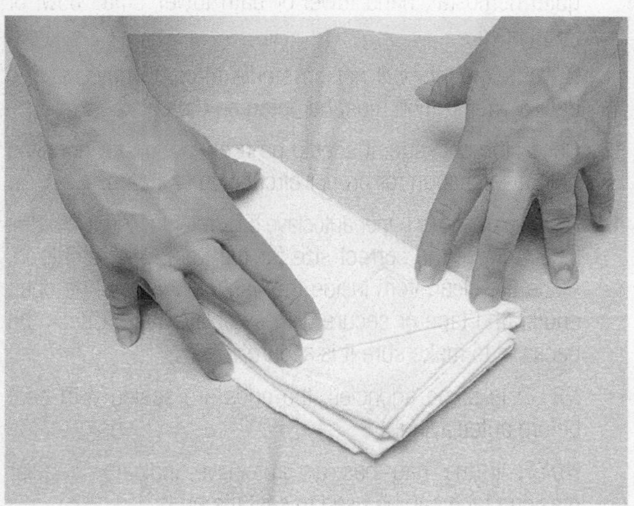

FIGURE 15–33B Fold back one corner on the top fold of the linen.

7. Fold up the bottom corner to the center (Figure 15–34B). Double back a small corner (Figure 15–34C).
8. Fold a side corner over to the center. Make sure the edges are sealed and that there are no air pockets. Bring back a small corner (Figure 15–34D).

Safety

CAUTION: Any open areas at corners will allow pathogens to enter.

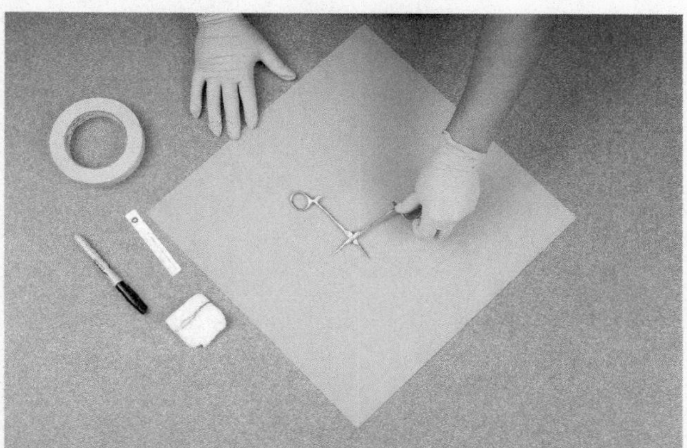

FIGURE 15–34A Place the instrument in the center of the wrap.

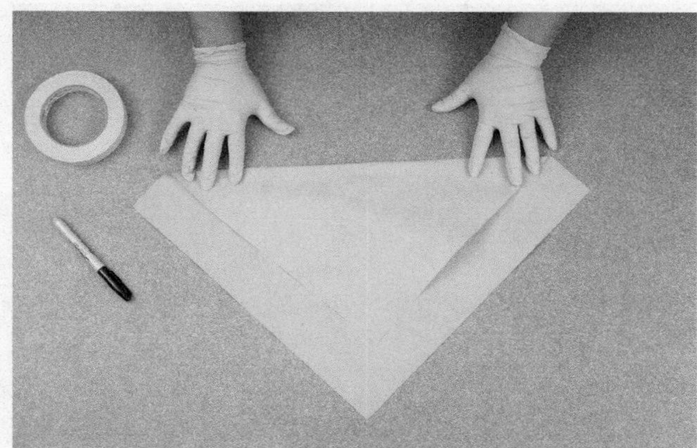

FIGURE 15–34B Fold up the bottom corner to the center.

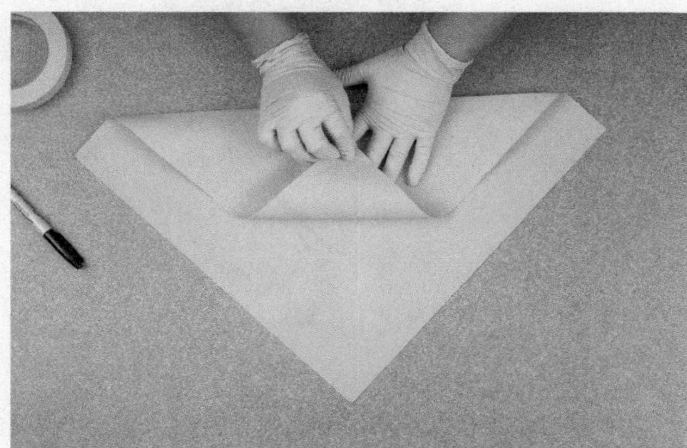

FIGURE 15–34C Turn a small corner back to form a tab.

(continues)

PROCEDURE 15:5A (CONT.)

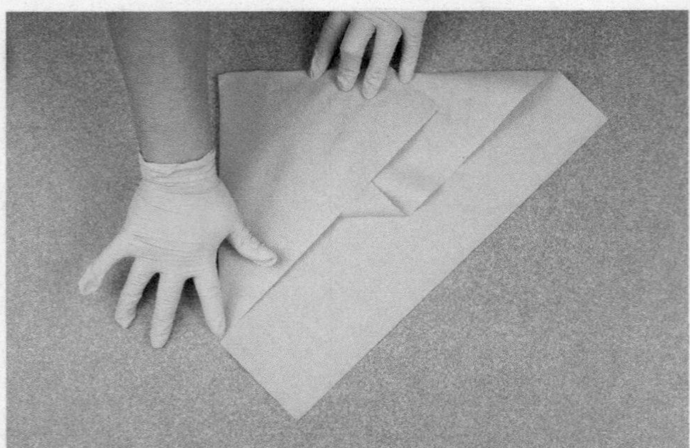

FIGURE 15–34D **Fold in one side to the center.**

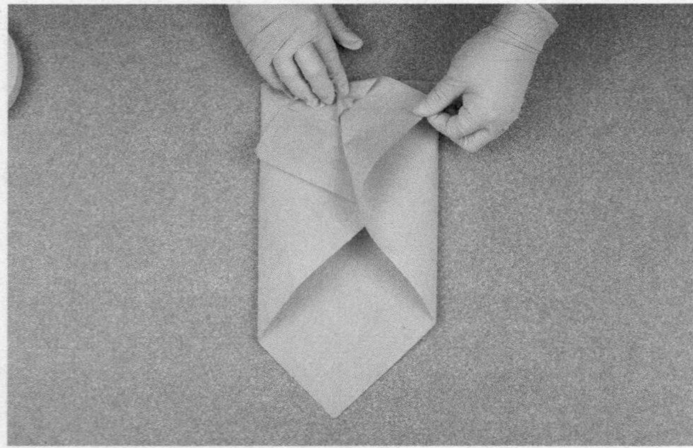

FIGURE 15–34E **Fold in the opposite side and fold back a tab.**

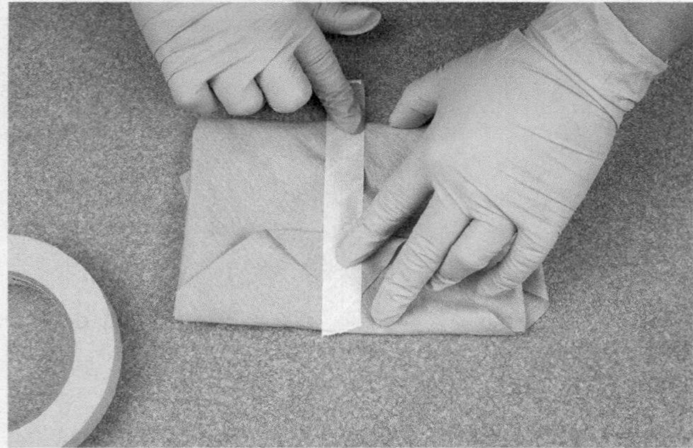

FIGURE 15–34F **Secure the package with pressure-sensitive autoclave tape.**

9. Fold in the other side corner. Again, watch for and avoid open edges. Bring back a small corner (Figure 15–34E).
10. Bring the final corner up and over the top of the package. Check the two edges to be sure they are sealed and tight. Tuck this under the pocket created by the previous folds. Leave a small corner exposed so it can be used when unwrapping the package.

    NOTE: This is frequently called an "envelope" wrap, because the final corner is tucked into the wrap similar to the way the flap is tucked into an envelope.
11. Secure with autoclave or pressure-sensitive indicator tape (Figure 15–34F).

    NOTE: If regular masking tape is used, attach an autoclave indicator to reflect when contents are sterilized.
12. Comm Label the package by marking the tape with the date and contents. Some health care agencies may require you to initial the label.

    NOTE: For certain items, the type or size of item should be noted, for example, curved hemostat or mosquito hemostat, hand towel or bath towel, small bowl or large bowl.

    NOTE: Contents will not be sterile after 30 days, so the date of sterilization must be noted on the package.
13. Check the package. It should be firm enough for handling but loose enough for proper circulation of steam.
14. To use a plastic or paper autoclave bag (refer to Figure 15–29), select or cut the correct size for the item to be sterilized. Place the clean item inside the bag. Double fold the open end(s) and tape or secure with autoclave tape. Check the package to make sure it is secure.

    NOTE: In some agencies, the ends are sealed with heat before autoclaving.

    NOTE: If the bag has an autoclave indicator, regular masking tape can be used to seal the ends.
15. Replace all equipment used.
16. Wash hands.

PRACTICE: **Go to the workbook and use the evaluation sheet for 15:5A, Wrapping Items for Autoclaving, to practice this procedure. When you believe you have mastered this skill, sign the sheet and give it to your instructor for further action.**

Check

FINAL CHECKPOINT: Using the criteria listed on the evaluation sheet, your instructor will grade your performance.

PROCEDURE 15:5B

Loading and Operating an Autoclave

NOTE: Follow the operating instructions for your autoclave. The basic principles of loading apply to all autoclaves.

Equipment and Supplies

Autoclave, distilled water, small pitcher or measuring cup, items wrapped or prepared for autoclaving, time chart for autoclave, 15:5 information section.

Procedure

Review the information section for 15:5, Sterilizing with an Autoclave. Then proceed with the following activities. You should read through the procedure first, checking against the diagram. Then practice with an autoclave.

1. Assemble equipment.
2. Wash and dry hands thoroughly.
3. Check the three-prong plug and the electrical cord. If either is damaged or prongs are missing, do not use the autoclave. If no problems are present, plug the cord into a wall outlet.
4. Use distilled water to fill the reservoir to within 2½ inches below the opening or to the level indicated on the autoclave.
   NOTE: Distilled water prevents the collection of mineral deposits and prolongs the life and effectiveness of the autoclave.
5. Check the pressure gauge to make sure it is at zero.

Safety

CAUTION: Never open the door unless the pressure is zero.

6. Open the safety door by following the manufacturer's instructions. Some door handles require an upward and inward pressure; others require a side-pressure technique.
7. Load the autoclave. Make sure all articles have been prepared correctly. Check for autoclave indicators, secure wraps, and correct labels. Separate loads so all items require the same time, temperature, and pressure. Place packages on their sides. Place bowls or basins on their sides so air and steam can flow in and out of the containers (Figure 15–35). Make sure there is space between the packages so the steam can circulate.
   NOTE: Check to make sure no large packages block the steam flow to smaller packages. Place large packages on the bottom.

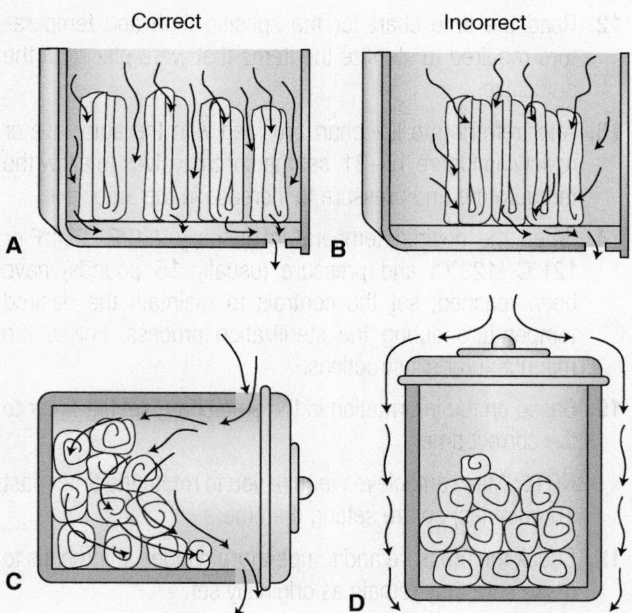

FIGURE 15–35 Packages should be placed on their sides and separated to allow steam to penetrate all sides of the packages: (A) correct placement; (B) incorrect placement. Bowls or basins should be placed on their sides so steam can flow in and out of the containers: (C) correct placement; (D) incorrect placement. Courtesy of STERIS Corporation.

Safety

CAUTION: Make sure no item comes in contact with the sides, top, or door of the autoclave chamber.

8. Follow the instructions for filling the chamber with the correct amount of water. Most autoclaves have a "Fill" setting on the control. Allow water to enter the chamber until the water covers the fill plate inside the chamber.
9. When the correct amount of water is in the chamber, follow the instructions for stopping the flow of water. In many autoclaves, turning the control valve to "Sterilize" stops the flow of water from the reservoir.
10. Check the load in the chamber to be sure it is properly spaced. The chamber can also be loaded at this point, if this has not been done previously.
11. Close and lock the door.

Safety

CAUTION: Be sure the door is securely locked; check by pulling slightly.

(continues)

PROCEDURE 15:5B (CONT.)

12. Read the time chart for the specific time and temperature required to sterilize the items that were placed in the autoclave.
13. After referring to the chart provided with the autoclave or reviewing Figure 15–31, set the control valves to allow the temperature and pressure to increase in the autoclave.
14. When the desired temperature (usually 250°F–254°F or 121°C–123°C) and pressure (usually 15 pounds) have been reached, set the controls to maintain the desired temperature during the sterilization process. Follow the manufacturer's instructions.
15. Based on the information in the time chart, set the timer to the correct time.

    NOTE: Many autoclaves require you to rotate the timer past 10 (minutes) before setting the time.
16. Check the pressure and temperature gauges at intervals to make sure they remain as originally set.

    NOTE: Most autoclaves automatically shut off when pressure reaches 35 pounds.
17. When the required time has passed, set the controls so the autoclave will vent the steam from the chamber.
18. Put on safety glasses.

Safety

CAUTION: Never open the door without glasses. The escaping steam can burn the eyes.

19. Check the pressure and temperature gauges. When the pressure gauge is at zero, and the temperature gauge is at or below 212°F, open the door about ½ to 1 inch to permit thorough drying of the contents.

Safety

CAUTION: Do not open the door until pressure is zero.

NOTE: Most autoclaves have a safety lock on the door that does not release until the pressure is at zero.

20. After the autoclaved items are completely dry, remove and store them in a dry, dust-free area.

Safety

CAUTION: Handle supplies and equipment carefully. They may be hot.

21. If there are additional loads to run, leave the main valve in the vent position. This will keep the autoclave ready for immediate use.
22. If this is the final load, turn the autoclave off. Unplug the cord from the wall outlet; do not pull on the cord.

    NOTE: The autoclave must be cleaned on a regular basis. Follow manufacturer's instructions.
23. Replace all equipment used.
24. Wash hands.

PRACTICE: **Go to the workbook and use the evaluation sheet for 15:5B, Loading and Operating an Autoclave, to practice this procedure. When you believe you have mastered this skill, sign the sheet and give it to your instructor for further action.**

Check

FINAL CHECKPOINT: Using the criteria listed on the evaluation sheet, your instructor will grade your performance.

15:6 Using Chemicals for Disinfection

Many health care fields require the use of chemicals for aseptic control. Certain points that must be observed while using the chemicals are discussed in the following section.

Chemicals are frequently used for aseptic control. Many chemicals do not kill spores and viruses; therefore, chemicals are not a method of sterilization. Because sterilization does not occur, **chemical disinfection** is the appropriate term (rather than *cold sterilization*, a term sometimes used). A few chemicals will kill spores and viruses, but these chemicals frequently require that instruments be submerged in the chemical for 10 or more hours. It is essential to read the entire label to determine the effectiveness of a product before using any chemical.

Chemicals are used to disinfect instruments that do not penetrate body tissue. Many dental instruments, percussion hammers, scissors, and similar items are examples. In addition, chemicals are used to disinfect thermometers and other items that would be destroyed by the high heat used in the autoclave.

Proper cleaning of all instruments or articles is essential. Particles or debris on items may contaminate the chemicals and reduce their effectiveness. In addition, all items must be rinsed thoroughly because the presence of soap can also reduce the effectiveness of chemicals. The articles must be dry before being placed in the disinfectant to keep the chemical at its most effective strength.

Some chemical solutions used as disinfectants are 90 percent isopropyl alcohol, formaldehyde–alcohol, 2 percent phenolic germicide, 10 percent bleach (sodium hypochlorite) solution, glutaraldehyde, iodophor, Lysol, Cidex, and benzalkonium (Zephiran). The manufacturer's directions should be read completely before using any solution. Some solutions must be diluted or mixed before use. The directions will also specify the recommended time for the most thorough disinfection.

Chemical solutions can cause rust to form on certain instruments, so antirust tablets or solutions are frequently added to the chemicals. Again, it is important to read the directions provided with the tablets or solution. If improperly used, antirust substances may cause a chemical reaction with a solution and reduce the effectiveness of the chemical disinfectant.

The container used for chemical disinfection must be large enough to accommodate the items. In addition, the items should be separate so each one will come in contact with the chemical. A tight-fitting lid must be placed on the container while the articles are in the solution to prevent evaporation, which could affect the strength of the solution. The lid also decreases the chance of dust or airborne particles falling into the solution.

The chemical disinfectant must completely cover the article. This is the only way to be sure that all parts of the article will be disinfected.

Before removing items from solutions, health care workers must wash their hands. Sterile gloves or sterile pick-ups or transfer forceps may be used to remove the instruments from the solution. The items should be rinsed with sterile water to remove any remaining chemical solution. After rinsing, the instruments are placed on a sterile or clean towel to dry, and then stored in a drawer or dust-free closet.

Solutions must be changed frequently. Some solutions can be used more than once, but others must be discarded after one use. Follow the manufacturer's instructions. However, any time contamination occurs or dirt is present in the solution, discard it. A fresh solution must be used.

STUDENT: **Go to the Workbook and complete the assignment sheet for 15:6, Using Chemicals for Disinfection. Then return and continue with the procedure.**

PROCEDURE 15:6

Using Chemicals for Disinfection

Equipment and Supplies

Chemicals, container with tight-fitting lid, basin, soap, water, instruments, brush, sterile pick-ups or transfer forceps, sterile towel, sterile gloves, eye protection, disposable gloves

Procedure

1. Assemble equipment.
2. Wash hands. Put on disposable or heavy-duty utility gloves and eye protection.

   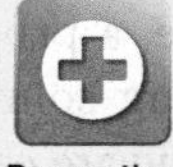
   Precaution

   NOTE: Wear gloves if any of the instruments or equipment may be contaminated with blood or body fluids. Wear eye protection if there is any chance splashing will occur.
3. Wash all instruments or equipment thoroughly. Use warm soapy water. Use the brush on serrated edges of instruments.

   NOTE: All tissue and debris must be removed from the item or it will not be disinfected.
4. Rinse the item in cool water to remove soapy residue. Then rinse well with hot water. Dry all instruments or equipment thoroughly.

   NOTE: Water on the instruments or equipment will dilute the chemical disinfectant.
5. Check the container. Make sure the lid fits securely.

   NOTE: A loose cover will permit entrance of pathogens and/or evaporation of the chemical solution.
6. Place instruments in the container. Make sure there is a space between instruments. Leave hinged edges open so the solution can flow between the surfaces.
7. Carefully read label instructions about the chemical solution. Some solutions must be diluted. Check the manufacturer's recommended soaking time.

   Safety

   CAUTION: Reread instructions to be sure the solution is safe to use on instruments.

   NOTE: An antirust substance must be added to some solutions.

(continues)

PROCEDURE 15:6 (CONT.)

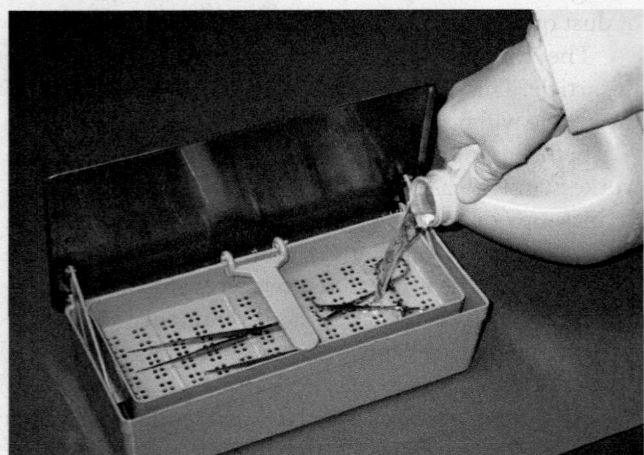

FIGURE 15–36 **Pour the chemical disinfectant into the container until all instruments are covered with the solution.**

8. Pour the solution into the container slowly to avoid splashing. Make sure that all instruments are covered (Figure 15–36). Close the lid of the container.

   NOTE: Read label three times: before pouring, while pouring, and after pouring.

   Safety

   CAUTION: Avoid splashing the chemical on your skin. Improper handling of chemicals may cause burns or injuries.

9. Remove gloves. Wash hands.
10. Leave the instruments in the solution for the length of time recommended by the manufacturer.

    NOTE: The usual soaking time is 20–30 minutes.

    NOTE: If the solution requires a long period (for example, 10–12 hours) for disinfecting, label the container with the date and time the process began, ending date and time, and your initials.

11. When instruments have soaked the correct amount of time, use sterile gloves or sterile pick-ups or transfer forceps to remove the instruments from the solution. Hold the instruments over a sink or basin and pour sterile water over them to rinse them thoroughly. Place them on a sterile towel to dry. A second sterile towel is sometimes used to dry the instruments or to cover the instruments while they are drying. Store the instruments in special drawers, containers, or dust-free closets.

    NOTE: Some contamination occurs when instruments are exposed to the air. In some cases, such as with external instruments, this minimal contamination will not affect usage.

12. Replace all equipment used.

    Safety

    CAUTION: If the disinfectant solution can be used again, label the container with the name of the disinfectant, date, and number of days it can be used according to manufacturer's instructions. When solutions cannot be reused, dispose of the solution according to the manufacturer's instructions.

13. Remove gloves. Wash hands.

PRACTICE: Go to the workbook and use the evaluation sheet for 15:6, Using Chemicals for Disinfection, to practice this procedure. When you believe you have mastered this skill, sign the sheet and give it to your instructor for further action.

Check

FINAL CHECKPOINT: Using the criteria listed on the evaluation sheet, your instructor will grade your performance.

15:7 Cleaning with an Ultrasonic Unit

Ultrasonic units are used in many dental and medical offices and in other health agencies to remove dirt, debris, blood, saliva, and tissue from a large variety of instruments before sterilizing them. Ultrasonic cleaning uses sound waves to clean. When the ultrasonic unit is turned on, the sound waves produce millions of microscopic bubbles in a cleaning solution. When the bubbles strike the items being cleaned, they explode, a process known as **cavitation**, and drive the cleaning solution onto the article. Accumulated dirt and residue are easily and gently removed from the article.

Ultrasonic cleaning is not sterilization because spores and viruses remain on the articles. If sterilization is desired, other methods must be used after the ultrasonic cleaning.

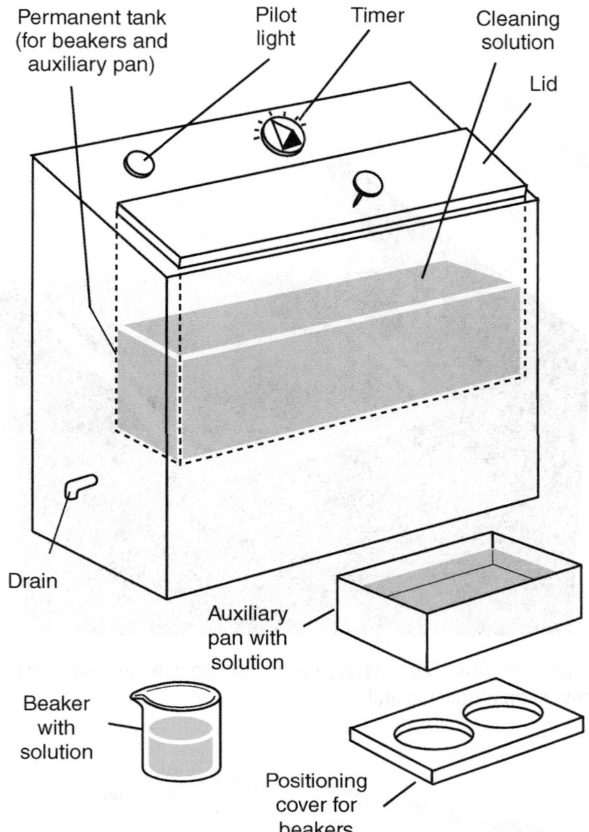

FIGURE 15–37 Parts of an ultrasonic cleaning unit.

Only ultrasonic solutions should be used in the unit. Different solutions are available for different materials. A general, all-purpose cleaning solution is usually used in the permanent tank and to clean many items. There are other specific solutions for alginate, plaster and stone removal, and tartar removal. The solution chart provided with the ultrasonic unit will state which solution should be used. It is important to read labels carefully before using any solutions. Some solutions must be diluted before use, and some can be used only on specific materials. All solutions are toxic. They can also cause skin irritation, so contact with the skin and eyes should be avoided. Solutions should be discarded when they become cloudy or contaminated, or if cleaning results are poor.

The permanent tank of the ultrasonic unit (Figure 15-37) must contain a solution at all times. A general, all-purpose cleaning solution is used most of the time. Glass beakers or auxiliary pans or baskets can then be placed in the permanent tank. The items to be cleaned and the proper cleaning solution are then put in the beakers or pans. The bottoms of the beakers or pans must always be positioned below the level of the solution present in the permanent tank. In this way, cavitation can be transmitted from the main tank and through the solution to the items being cleaned in the beakers or pans. The ultrasonic unit should never be operated without solutions in both containers. In addition, the items being cleaned must be submerged in the cleaning solution.

Many different items can be cleaned in an ultrasonic unit. Examples include instruments, dental impression trays, glass products, and most jewelry. The ultrasonic unit should not be used on jewelry with pearls or pasted stones. The sound waves can destroy the pearls or the paste holding the stones. Before cleaning, most of the dirt or particles should be brushed off the items being cleaned. It is better to clean a few articles at a time and avoid overloading the unit. If items are close together, the cavitation is poor because the bubbles cannot strike all parts of the items being cleaned.

The glass beakers used in the ultrasonic unit are made of a type of glass that allows the passage of sound waves. After continual use, the sound waves etch the bottom of the beakers. A white, opaque coating forms. The beakers must be discarded and replaced when this occurs. After each use, the beakers should be washed with soap and water and rinsed thoroughly to remove any soapy residue. They must be dry before being filled with solution because water in the beaker can dilute the solution.

The permanent tank of the unit must be drained and cleaned at intervals based on tank use or the appearance of the solution in the tank. A drain valve on the side of the tank is opened to allow the solution to drain. The tank is then wiped with a damp cloth or disinfectant. Another damp cloth or disinfectant is used to wipe off the outside of the unit. The unit should never be submerged in water to clean it. After cleaning, a fresh solution should be placed in the permanent tank.

The manufacturer's instructions must be read carefully before using any ultrasonic unit. Most manufacturers provide cleaning charts that state the type of solution and time required for a variety of cleaning problems. Each time an item is cleaned in an ultrasonic unit, the chart should be used to determine the correct cleaning solution and time required.

STUDENT: **Go to the workbook and complete the assignment sheet for 15:7, Cleaning with an Ultrasonic Unit. Then return and continue with the procedure.**

PROCEDURE 15:7

Cleaning with an Ultrasonic Unit

Equipment and Supplies

Ultrasonic unit, permanent tank with solution, beakers, auxiliary pan or basket with covers, beaker bands, cleaning solutions, transfer forceps or pick-ups, paper towels, gloves, brush, soap, water for rinsing, articles for cleaning, solution chart

Procedure

1. Assemble all equipment.
2. 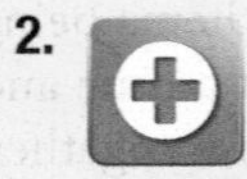
Precaution
Wash hands. Put on gloves if any items may be contaminated with blood, body fluids, secretions, or excretions.

   NOTE: Use heavy-duty utility gloves if instruments are sharp.
3. Use a brush and soap and water to remove any large particles of dirt from articles to be cleaned. Rinse articles thoroughly. Dry items.

   NOTE: Rinsing is important because soap may interact with the cleaning solution.
4. Check the permanent tank to be sure it has enough cleaning solution. An all-purpose cleaning solution is usually used in this tank.

   Safety
   CAUTION: Never run the unit without solution in the permanent tank.

   NOTE: Many solutions must be diluted before use; if new solution is needed, read the instructions on the bottle.
5. Pour the proper cleaning solution into the auxiliary pan or beakers.

   NOTE: Use the cleaning chart to determine which solution to use.

   Safety
   CAUTION: Read label before using.

   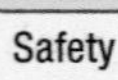

   Safety
   CAUTION: Handle solutions carefully. Avoid contact with skin and eyes.
6. Place the beakers, basket, or auxiliary pan into the permanent tank (Figures 15–38A and B). Use beaker positioning covers and beaker bands. Beaker bands are large bands that circle the beakers to hold them in position and keep them from hitting the bottom of the permanent tank.

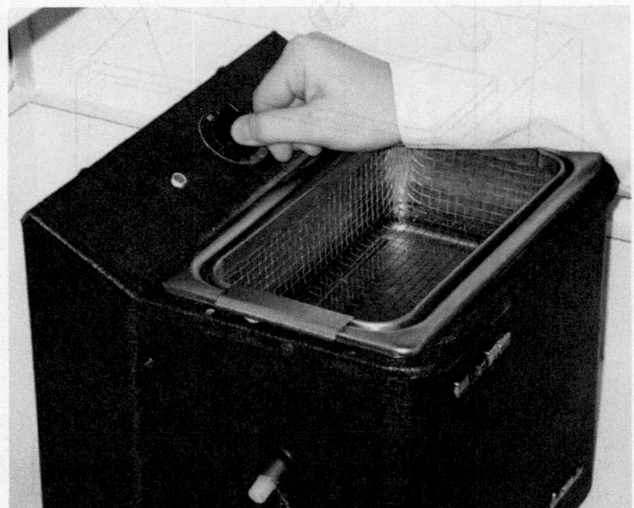

FIGURE 15–38A The auxiliary basket can be used to clean larger items in an ultrasonic unit.

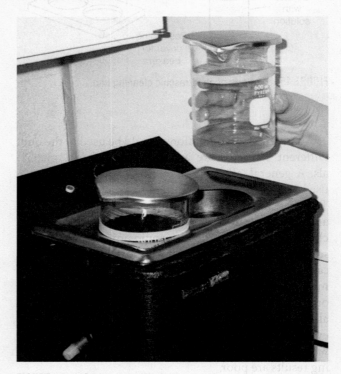

FIGURE 15–38B Glass beakers can be used to clean smaller items in an ultrasonic unit.

7. Check to be sure that the bottoms of the beakers, basket, or pan are below the level of solution in the permanent tank.

   NOTE: For sonic waves to flow through solutions in the beakers, basket, or pan, the two solution levels must overlap.

PROCEDURE 15:7 (CONT.)

8. Place articles to be cleaned in the beakers, basket, or pan. Be sure the solution completely covers the articles. Do not get solution on your hands.

   NOTE: Remember that pearls or pasted stones cannot be cleaned in an ultrasonic unit.

9. Turn the timer past 5 (minutes) and then set the proper cleaning time. Use the cleaning chart to determine the correct amount of time required for the items. Most articles are cleaned in 2–5 minutes.

10. Check that the unit is working. You should see a series of bubbles in both solutions. This is called *cavitation*.

Safety

CAUTION: Do not get too close. Solution can spray into your face and eyes. Use beaker lids to prevent spray.

11. When the timer stops, cleaning is complete. Use transfer forceps or pick-ups to lift articles from the basket, pan, or beakers. Place the articles on paper towels. Then rinse the articles thoroughly under running water.

Safety

CAUTION: Avoid contact with skin. Solutions are toxic.

12. Allow articles to air-dry or dry them with paper towels. Inspect the articles for cleanliness. If they are not clean, repeat the process.

13. Periodically change solutions in the permanent tank and auxiliary containers. Do this when solutions become cloudy or cleaning has not been effective. To clean the permanent tank, place a container under the side drain to collect the solution. Then open the valve and drain the solution from the tank. Wash the inside with a damp cloth or disinfectant. To clean the auxiliary pans or beakers, discard the solution. (It can be poured down the sink, but allow water to run for a time after disposing of the solution.) Then wash the containers and rinse thoroughly.

    NOTE: If the bottoms of beakers are etched and white, the beakers must be discarded and replaced.

14. Clean and replace all equipment used. Make sure all beakers are covered with lids.

15. Wash hands.

PRACTICE: Go to the workbook and use the evaluation sheet for 15:7, Cleaning with an Ultrasonic Unit, to practice this procedure. When you believe you have mastered this skill, sign the sheet and give it to your instructor for further action.

Check

FINAL CHECKPOINT: Using the criteria listed on the evaluation sheet, your instructor will grade your performance.

15:8 Using Sterile Techniques

Many procedures require the use of sterile techniques to protect the patient from further infection. *Surgical asepsis* refers to procedures that keep an object or area free from living organisms. The main facts are presented here.

Sterile means "free from all organisms," including spores and viruses. **Contaminated** means that organisms and pathogens are present. While working with sterile supplies, it is important that correct techniques be followed to maintain sterility and avoid contamination. It is also important that you are able to recognize sterile surfaces and contaminated surfaces.

A clean, uncluttered working area is required when working with sterile supplies. A sterile object must never touch a nonsterile object. If other objects are in the way, it is easy to contaminate sterile articles. If sterile articles touch the skin or any part of your clothing, they are no longer sterile. Because any area below the waist is considered contaminated, sterile articles must be held away from and in front of the body and above the waist.

Once a **sterile field** has been set up (for example, a sterile towel has been placed on a tray), never reach across the top of the field. Microorganisms can drop from your arm or clothing and contaminate the field. Always reach in from either side to place additional articles on the field. Keep the sterile field in constant view. Never turn your back to a sterile field. Avoid coughing, sneezing, or talking over the sterile field because airborne particles can fall on the field and contaminate it. A person must remain alert and honest to properly maintain a sterile field.

The 2-inch border around the sterile field (towel-covered tray) is considered contaminated. Therefore, 2 inches around the outside of the field must not be used when sterile articles are placed on the sterile field.

All sterile items must be checked carefully before they are used. If the item was autoclaved and dated, most health care facilities believe the date should not be more

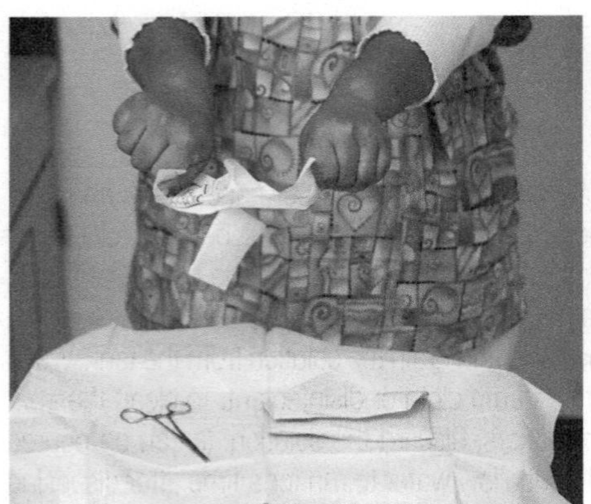
FIGURE 15–39A Sterile items can be dropped from the wrapper onto the sterile field.

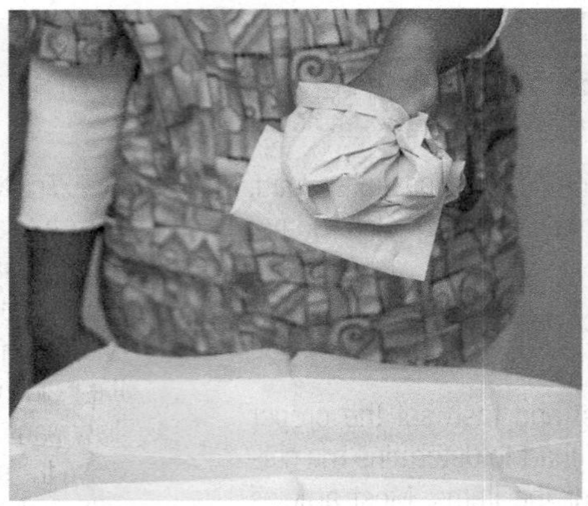
FIGURE 15–39B By using the wrap as a mitten, sterile supplies can be placed on a sterile field.

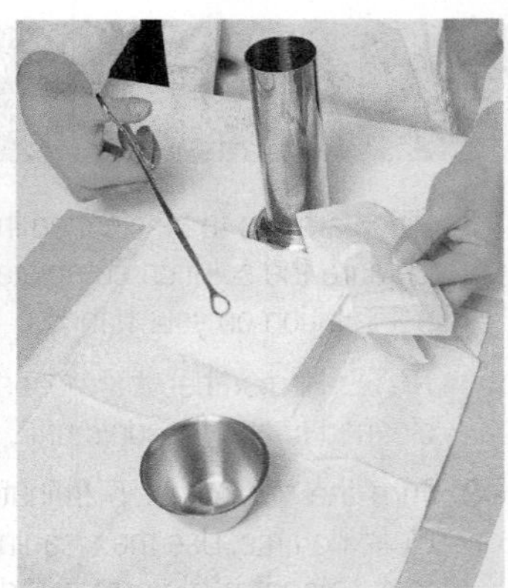
FIGURE 15–39C Sterile transfer forceps or pick-ups can be used to grasp sterile items and place them on a sterile field.

than 30 days from autoclaving. Follow agency guidelines for time limits. If tears or stains are present on the package, the item should *not* be used because it could be contaminated. If there are any signs of moisture on the package, it has been contaminated and should *not* be used.

Organisms and pathogens travel quickly through a wet surface, so the sterile field must be kept dry. If a sterile towel or article gets wet, contamination has occurred. It is very important to use care when pouring solutions into sterile bowls or using solutions around a sterile field.

Various techniques can be used to remove articles from sterile wraps, depending on the article being unwrapped. Some common techniques are the drop, mitten, and transfer-forceps techniques:

- *Drop technique:* This technique is used for gauze pads, dressings, and small items. The wrapper is partially opened and then held upside down over the sterile field. The item drops out of the wrapper and onto the sterile field (Figure 15-39A). It is important to keep fingers back so the article does not touch the skin as it falls out of the wrapper. It is also important to avoid touching the inside of the wrapper.
- *Mitten technique:* This technique is used for bowls, drapes, linen, and other similar items. The wrapper is opened and its loose ends are grasped around the wrist with the opposite hand (Figure 15-39B). In this way, a mitten is formed around the hand that is still holding the item (for example, a bowl). With the mitten hand, the item can be placed on the sterile tray.
- *Transfer forceps:* These are used for cotton balls, small items, or articles that cannot be removed by the drop or mitten techniques. Either sterile gloves or sterile transfer forceps (pick-ups) are used. Sterile transfer forceps or pick-ups are removed from their container of disinfectant solution and used to grasp the article from the opened package. The item is removed from the opened, sterile wrap and placed on the sterile field (Figure 15-39C). The transfer forceps must be pointed in a downward direction. If they are pointed upward, the solution will flow back to the handle, become contaminated, and return to contaminate the sterile tips when they are being used to pick up items. In addition, care must be taken not to touch the sides or rim of the forceps container while removing or inserting the transfer forceps. Also, the transfer forceps must be shaken gently to get rid of excess disinfectant solution before they are used.

Make sure the sterile tray is open and you are ready to do the sterile procedure *before* putting the sterile gloves on your hands. Sterile gloves are considered sterile on the outside and contaminated on the inside (side against the skin). Once they have been placed on the hands, it is important to hold the hands away from the body and above the waist to avoid contamination. Handle only sterile objects while wearing sterile gloves.

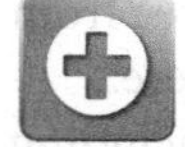
Precaution

If at any time during a procedure there is any suspicion that you have contaminated any article, start over. Never take a chance on using contaminated equipment or supplies.

A wide variety of commercially prepared sterile supplies is available. Packaged units are often set up for special procedures, such as changing dressings. Many agencies use these units instead of setting up special trays. Observe all sterile principles while using these units and read any directions provided with the units.

STUDENT: **Go to the workbook and complete the assignment sheet for 15:8, Using Sterile Techniques. Then return and continue with the procedures.**

PROCEDURE 15:8A

Opening Sterile Packages

Equipment and Supplies

Sterile package of equipment or supplies, a table or other flat surface, sterile field (tray with sterile towel)

Procedure

1. Assemble equipment.
2. Wash hands.
3. Take equipment to the area where it will be used. Check the autoclave indicator and date on the package. Check the package for stains, tears, moisture, or evidence of contamination. Do *not* use the package if there is any evidence of contamination.

   NOTE: Contents are not considered sterile if 30 days have elapsed since autoclaving.
4. Pick up the package with the tab or sealed edge pointing toward you. If the item is small, it can be held in the hand while being unwrapped. If it is large, place it on a table or other flat surface.
5. Loosen the wrapper fastener (usually tape).
6. Check to be sure the package is away from your body. If it is on a table, make sure it is not close to other objects.

   NOTE: Avoid possible contamination by keeping sterile supplies away from other objects.
7. Open the distal (furthest) flap of the wrapper by grasping the outside of the wrapper and pulling it away from you (Figure 15–40A).

   Safety

   CAUTION: Do not reach across the top of the package. Reach around the package to open it.
8. With one hand, raise a side flap and pull laterally (sideways) away from the package (Figure 15–40B).

   Safety

   CAUTION: Do not touch the inside of the wrapper at any time.
9. With the opposite hand, open the other side flap by pulling the tab to the side (Figure 15–40C).

   NOTE: Always reach in from the side. Never reach across the top of the sterile field or across any opened edges.

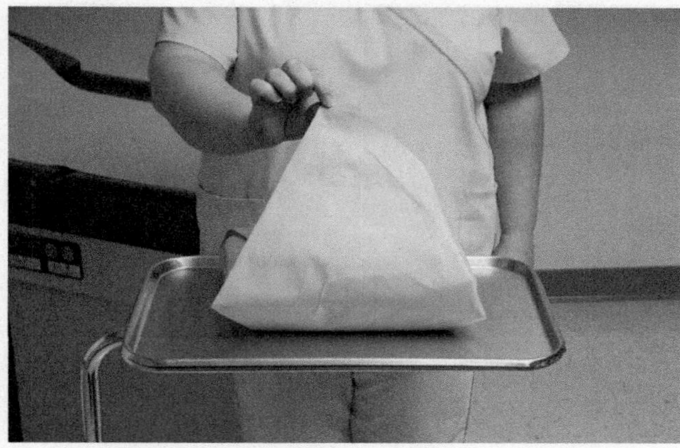

FIGURE 15–40A To open a sterile package, open the top flap away from you, handling only the outside of the wrap.

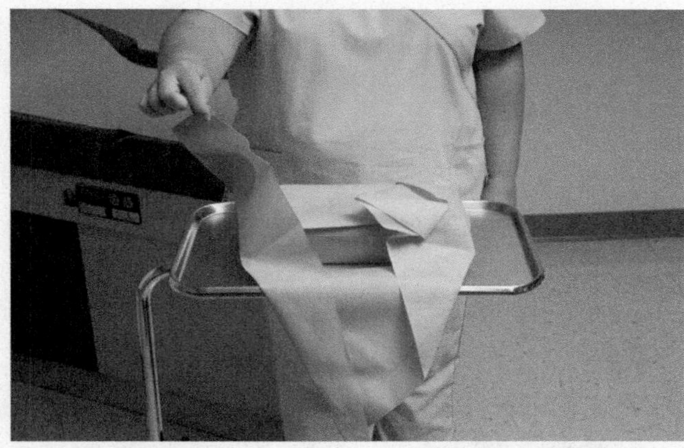

FIGURE 15–40B Open one side by pulling the wrap out to the side.

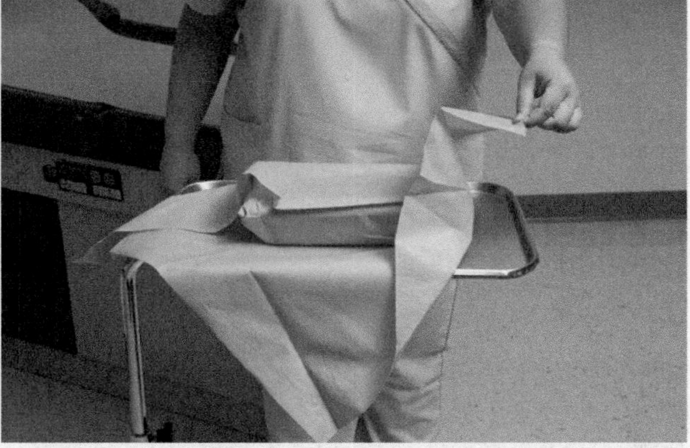

FIGURE 15–40C Open the opposite side by pulling the wrap out to the opposite side.

(continues)

PROCEDURE 15:8A (CONT.)

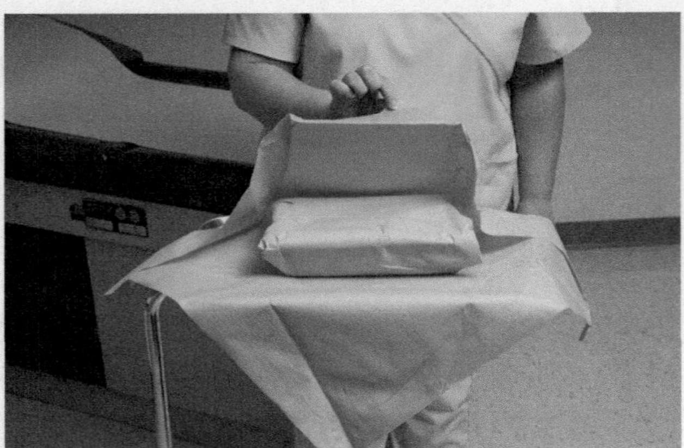

FIGURE 15–40D **Open the side nearest to you by pulling back on the wrap.**

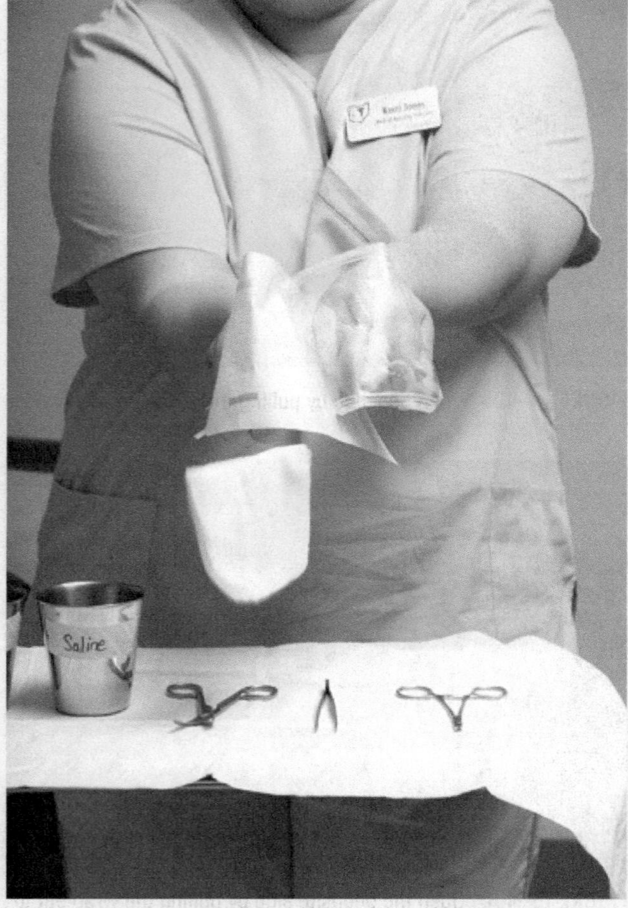

FIGURE 15–40E **Separate the ends of the wrap and hold the package upside down to allow the contents to drop onto the sterile tray.**

10. Open the proximal (closest) flap by lifting the flap up and toward you. Then drop it over the front of your hand (or the table) (Figure 15–40D).

Safety

CAUTION: Be careful not to touch the inside of the package or the contents of the package.

11. Transfer the contents of the sterile package using one of the following techniques:

a. *Drop:* Separate the ends of the wrap and pull apart gently. Avoid touching the inside of the wrap. Secure the loose ends of the wrap and hold the package upside down over the sterile field. Allow the contents to drop onto the sterile tray (Figure 15–40E).

b. *Mitten:* Grasp the contents securely by holding on to the outside of the wrapper as you unwrap it. With your free hand, gather the loose edges of the wrapper together and hold them securely around your wrist. This can be compared to making a mitten of the wrapper (with the sterile equipment on the outside of the mitten). Place the item on the sterile tray or hand it to someone who is wearing sterile gloves (refer to Figure 15–39B).

c. *Transfer forceps:* Remove forceps from their sterile container, taking care not to touch the side or rim of the container with the forceps. Hold the forceps pointed downward. Shake them gently to remove excess disinfectant solution. Take care not to touch anything with the forceps. Use the forceps to grasp the item in the package and then place the item on the sterile tray (Figures 15–40F and G).

NOTE: The method of transfer depends on the sterile item being transferred.

Safety

CAUTION: If at any time during the procedure there is any suspicion that you have contaminated any article, start over. Never take a chance on using equipment for a sterile procedure if there is any possibility that the equipment is contaminated.

12. Replace all equipment used.

13. Wash hands.

PRACTICE: **Go to the workbook and use the evaluation sheet for 15:8A, Opening Sterile Packages, to practice this procedure. When you believe you have mastered this skill, sign the sheet and give it to your instructor for further action.**

PROCEDURE 15:8A (CONT.)

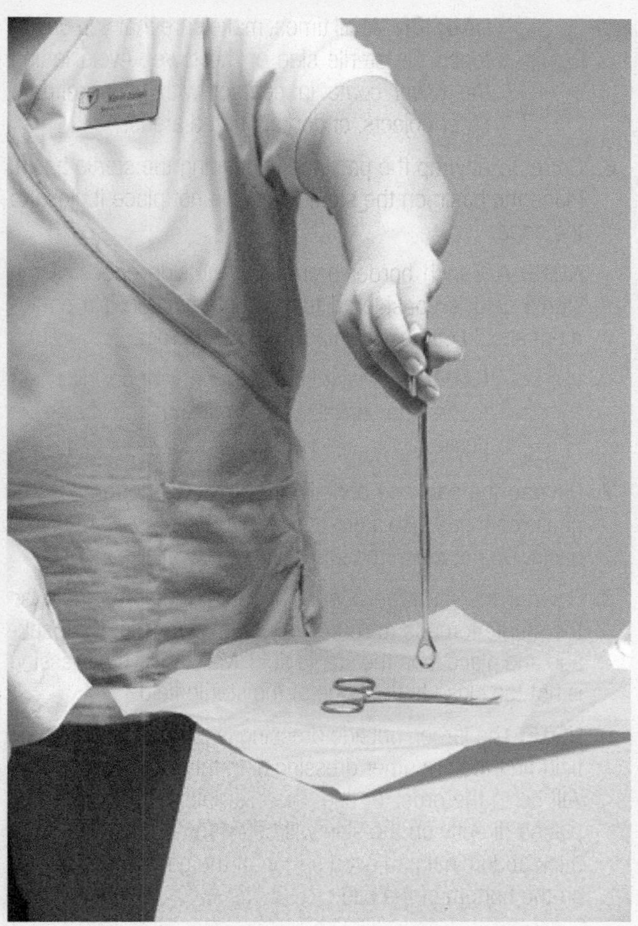

FIGURE 15–40F **Hold the forceps pointed downward while picking up the sterile instrument that needs to be transferred.**

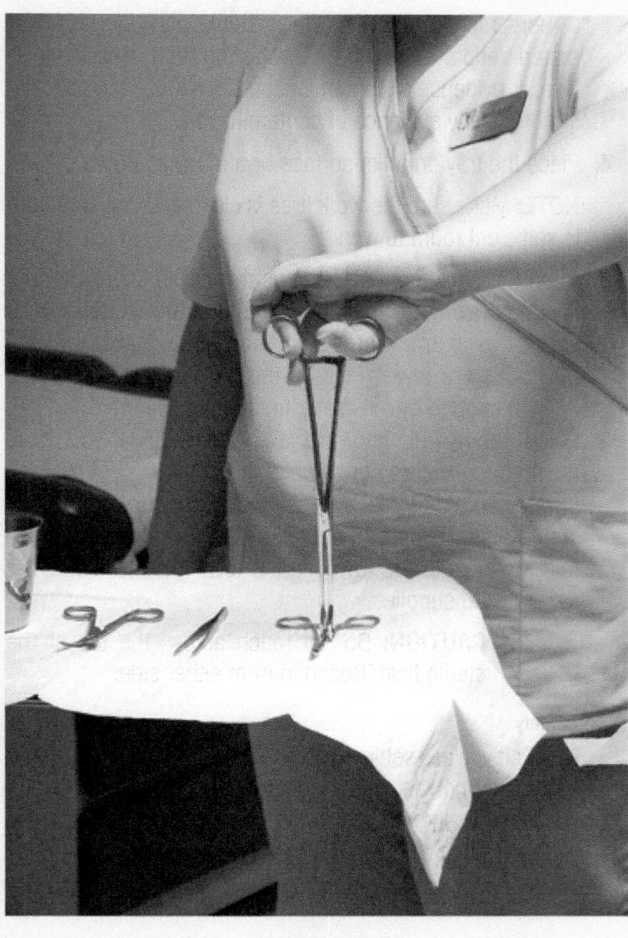

FIGURE 15–40G **Place the instrument on the sterile tray.**

Check

FINAL CHECKPOINT: Using the criteria listed on the evaluation sheet, your instructor will grade your performance.

PROCEDURE 15:8B

Preparing a Sterile Dressing Tray

Equipment and Supplies

Tray or Mayo stand, sterile towels, sterile basin, sterile cotton balls or gauze sponges, sterile dressings (different sizes), antiseptic solution, forceps in disinfectant solution

Procedure

1. Assemble all equipment.
2. Wash hands.
3. Check the date and autoclave indicator for sterility. If more than 30 days have elapsed, use another package with

(continues)

PROCEDURE 15:8B (CONT.)

a more recent date. Put the unsterile package aside for resterilization. Check the package for stains, tears, moisture, or evidence of contamination. Do not use the package if there is any evidence of contamination.

4. Place the tray on a flat surface or a Mayo stand.

   NOTE: Make sure the work area is clean and dry, and there is sufficient room to work.

5. Open the package that contains the sterile towel. Be sure it is held away from your body. Place the wrapper on a surface away from the tray or work area. Touch only the outside of the towel. Pick up the towel at its outer edge. Allow it to open by releasing the fanfolds (Figure 15–41A). Place the towel with the outer side (side you have touched) on the tray or Mayo stand (Figure 15–41B). The untouched, or sterile, side will be facing up to create a sterile field. Holding the outside edges of the towel, fanfold the back of the towel so the towel can be used later to cover the supplies.

   Safety

   CAUTION: Do not reach across the top of the sterile field. Reach in from either side.

   NOTE: If you are setting up a relatively large work area, one towel may not be large enough when fanfolded to cover the supplies. In such a case, you will need a second sterile towel (later) to cover your sterile field.

   Safety

   CAUTION: At all times, make sure that you do not touch the sterile side of the towel. Avoid letting the towel come in contact with your uniform, other objects, or contaminated areas.

6. Correctly unwrap the package containing the sterile basin. Place the basin on the sterile field. Do not place it close to the edge.

   NOTE: A 2-inch border around the outside edges of the sterile field is considered to be contaminated. No equipment should come in contact with this border.

   Safety

   CAUTION: Make sure that the wrapper does not touch the towel while placing the basin in position.

7. Unwrap the package containing the sterile cotton balls or gauze sponges. Use a dropping motion to place them in the basin. Do not touch the basin with the wrapper.

8. Unwrap the package containing the larger dressing. Use the sterile forceps to remove the dressing from the package and place it on the sterile field. Make sure the dressing is not too close to the edge of the sterile field.

   NOTE: The larger, outside dressing is placed on the sterile field first (before other dressings). In this way, the supplies will be in the order of use. For example, gauze dressings placed directly on the skin will be on top of the pile, and a thick abdominal pad used on top of the gauze pads will be on the bottom of the pile.

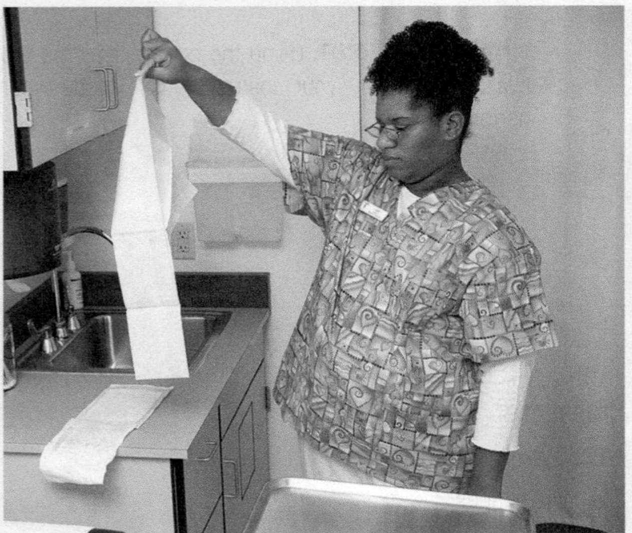

FIGURE 15–41A Pick up the sterile towel at its outer edge and allow it to open by releasing the fanfolds.

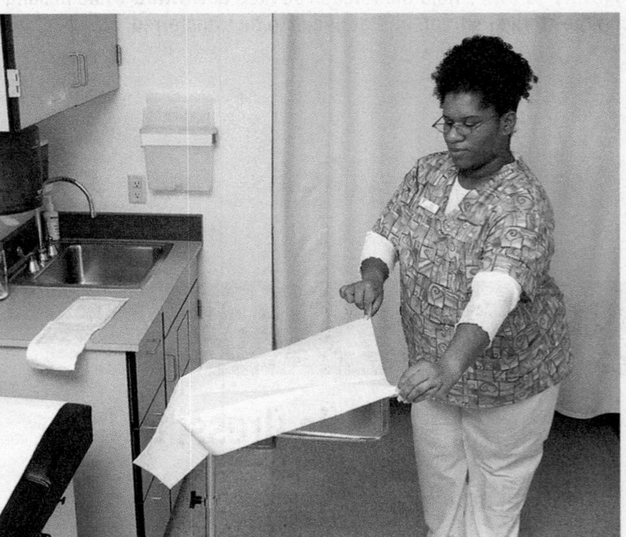

FIGURE 15–41B Place the towel on the Mayo stand without reaching across the top of the towel.

PROCEDURE 15:8B (CONT.)

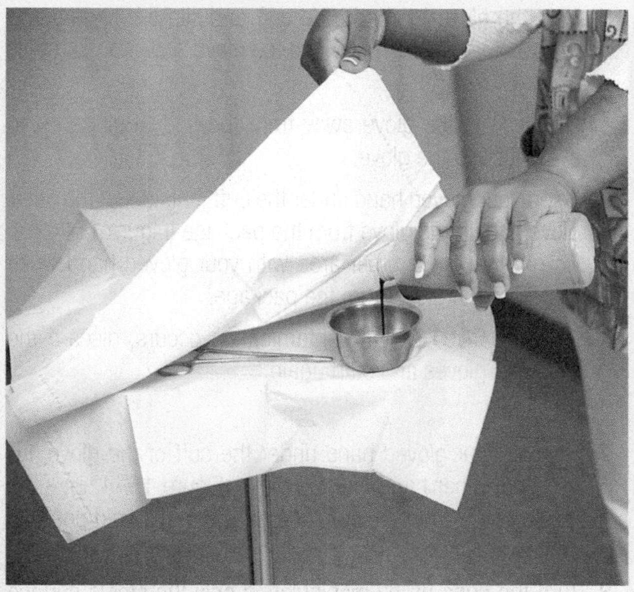

FIGURE 15–41C **Avoid splashing the solution onto the sterile field while pouring it into the basin.**

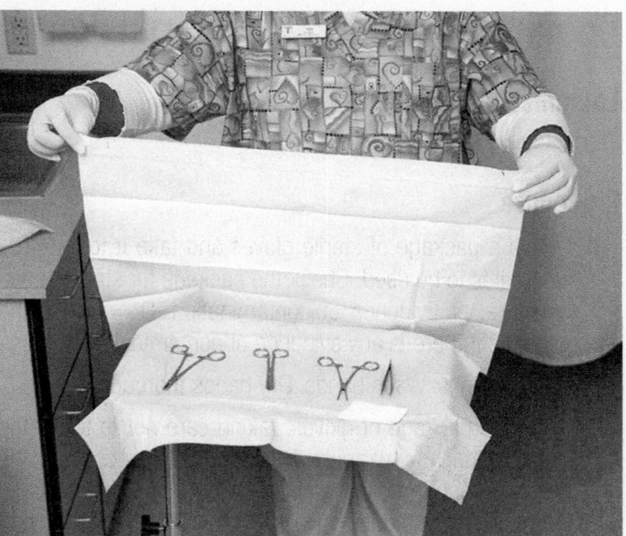

FIGURE 15–41D **Use a second sterile towel to cover the first sterile towel and protect the sterile field, taking care not to reach across the field.**

NOTE: The forceps must be lifted straight up out of the container and must *not* touch the side or rim of the container. Keep the tips pointed down and above the waist at all times. Shake off excess disinfectant solution.

9. Unwrap the inner dressings correctly. Use the sterile forceps to place them on top of the other dressings on the sterile field, or use a drop technique.

   NOTE: Dressings are now in a pile; the dressing that will be used first is on the top of the pile.

   NOTE: The number and type of dressings needed is determined by checking the patient being treated.

10. Open the bottle containing the correct antiseptic solution. Place the cap on the table, with the inside of the cap facing up. Pour a small amount of the solution into the sink to clean the lip of the bottle. Then hold the bottle over the basin and pour a sufficient amount of the solution into the basin (Figure 15–41C).

Safety

CAUTION: Make sure that no part of the bottle touches the basin or the sterile field. Pour carefully to avoid splashing. If the sterile field gets wet, the entire tray will be contaminated, and you must begin again.

11. Check the tray to make sure all needed equipment is on it.
12. Pick up the fanfolded edge of the towel by placing one hand on each side edge of the towel on the underside, or contaminated side. Do not touch the sterile side. Keep your hands and arms to the side of the tray, and bring the towel forward to cover the supplies.

    NOTE: A second sterile towel may be used to cover the supplies if the sterile field is too large to be covered by the one fanfolded towel (Figure 15–41D).

Safety

CAUTION: Never reach across the top of the sterile tray.

13. Once the sterile tray is ready, never allow it out of your sight. Take it to the patient area and use it immediately. If you need more equipment, you must take the tray with you. This is the only way to be completely positive that the tray does not become contaminated.
14. Replace equipment.
15. Wash hands.

PRACTICE: **Go to the workbook and use the evaluation sheet for 15:8B, Preparing a Sterile Dressing Tray, to practice this procedure. When you believe you have mastered this skill, sign the sheet and give it to your instructor for further action.**

Check

FINAL CHECKPOINT: Using the criteria listed on the evaluation sheet, your instructor will grade your performance.

PROCEDURE 15:8C

Donning and Removing Sterile Gloves

Equipment and Supplies

Sterile gloves

Procedure

1. Obtain a package of sterile gloves and take it to the area where it is to be used. Check the package for stains, tears, moisture, or evidence of contamination. Do *not* use the package if there is any evidence of contamination.
2. Remove rings. Wash hands. Dry hands thoroughly.
3. Open the package of gloves, taking care not to touch the inside of the inner wrapper. The inner wrapper contains the gloves. Reach in from the sides to open the inner package and expose the sterile gloves (Figure 15–42A). The folded cuffs will be nearest to you.

Safety

CAUTION: If you touch the *inside* of the package (where the gloves are), get a new package and start again.

4. The glove for the right hand will be on the right side and the glove for the left hand will be on the left side of the package. With the thumb and forefinger of the nondominant hand, pick up the top edge of the folded-down cuff (inside of glove) of the glove for the dominant hand. Remove the glove carefully (Figure 15–42B).

Safety

CAUTION: Do *not* touch the outside of the glove. This is sterile. Only the part that will be next to the skin can be touched. Remember, unsterile touches unsterile and sterile touches sterile.

5. Hold the glove by the inside cuff and slip the fingers and thumb of your other hand into the glove. Pull it on carefully (Figure 15–42C).

   NOTE: Hold the glove away from the body. Pull gently to avoid tearing the glove.

6. Insert your gloved hand under the cuff (outside) of the other glove and lift the glove from the package (Figure 15–42D). Do not touch any other area with your gloved hand while removing the glove from the package.

Safety

CAUTION: If contamination occurs, discard the gloves and start again.

7. Holding your gloved hand under the cuff of the glove, insert your other hand into the glove (Figure 15–42E). Keep the thumb of your gloved hand tucked in to avoid possible contamination.
8. Turn the cuffs up by manipulating only the sterile surface of the gloves (sterile touches sterile). Go up under the folded cuffs, pull out slightly, and turn cuffs over and up (Figure 15–42F). Do not touch the inside of the gloves or the skin with your gloved hand.
9. Interlace the fingers to position the gloves correctly, taking care not to touch the skin with the gloved hands (Figure 15–42G).

Safety

CAUTION: If contamination occurs, start again with a new pair of gloves.

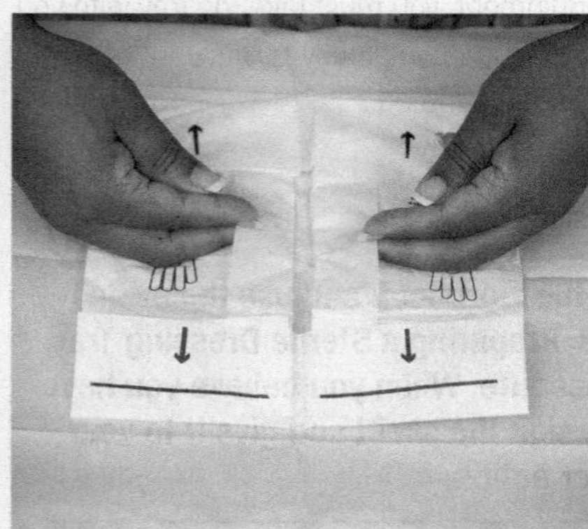

FIGURE 15–42A **Reach in from the sides to open the inner package and expose the sterile gloves.**

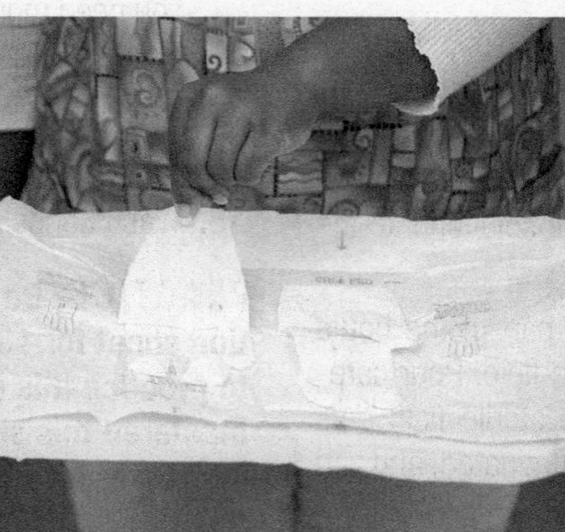

FIGURE 15–42B **Pick up the first glove by grasping the glove on the top edge of the folded-down cuff.**

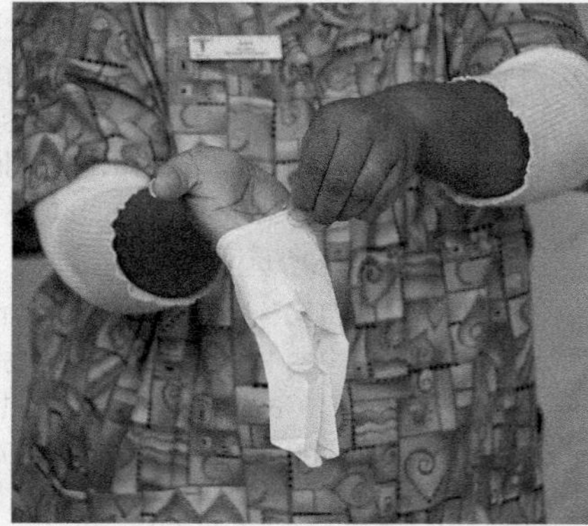

FIGURE 15–42C **Hold the glove securely by the cuff and slip the opposite hand into the glove.**

PROCEDURE 15:8C (CONT.)

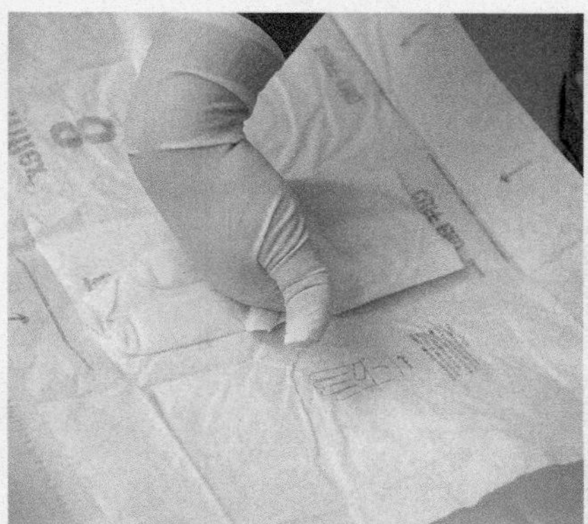
FIGURE 15–42D Slip the gloved fingers under the cuff of the second glove to lift it from the package.

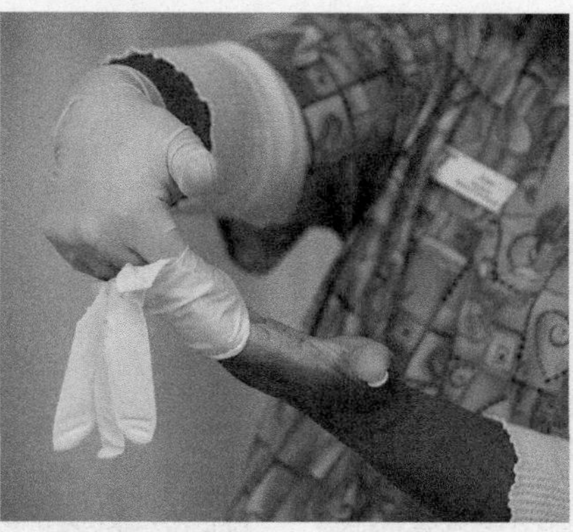
FIGURE 15–42E Hold the gloved hand under the cuff while inserting the other hand into the glove.

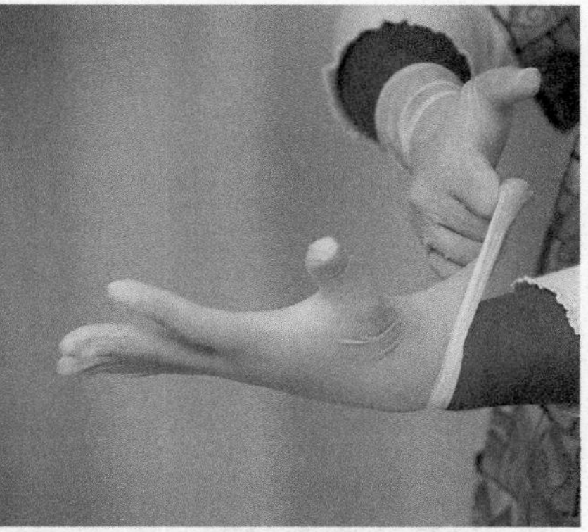
FIGURE 15–42F Insert the gloved fingers under the cuff, pull out slightly, and turn the cuffs over and up without touching the inside of the gloves or the skin.

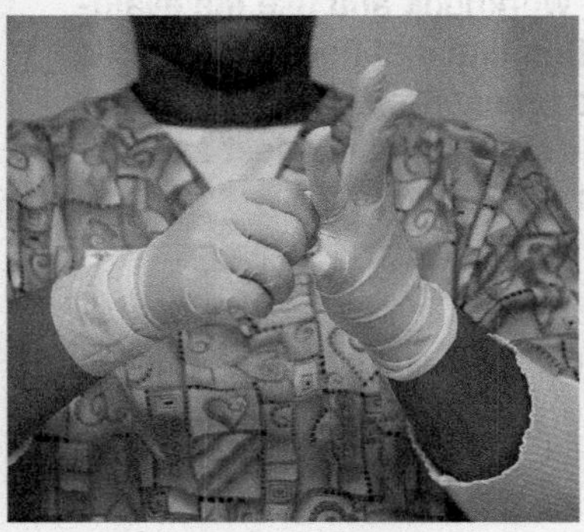
FIGURE 15–42G Interlace the fingers to position the gloves correctly, taking care not to touch the skin with the gloved hands.

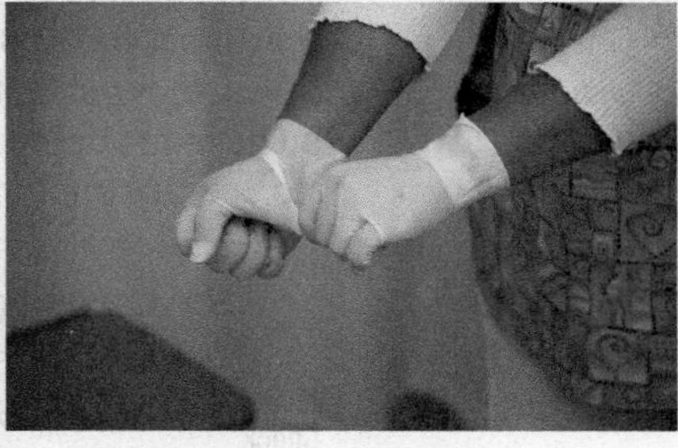
FIGURE 15–42H Use a gloved hand to grasp the other glove by the outside of the cuff.

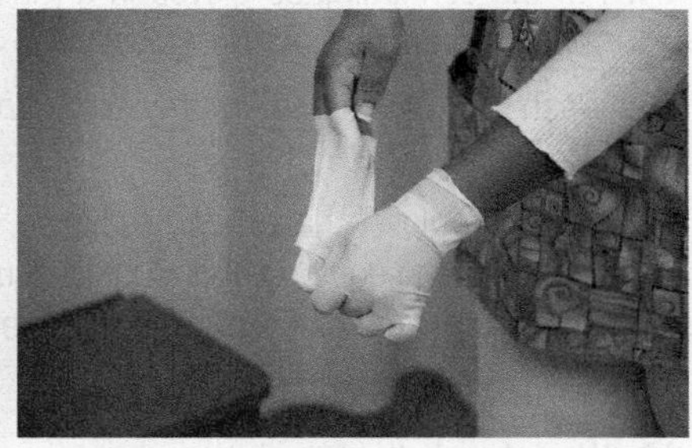
FIGURE 15–42I Remove the glove by pulling it down over the hand and turning it inside out.

10. Do not touch anything that is not sterile once the gloves are in place. Gloves are applied for the purpose of performing procedures requiring sterile technique. During the procedure, they will become contaminated with organisms related to the patient's condition, for example, wound drainage, blood, or other body discharges. Even a clean, dry wound may contaminate gloves.

NOTE: Gloved hands should remain in position above the waist. Do *not* allow them to fall below waist.

11. After the procedure requiring sterile gloves is completed, dispose of all contaminated supplies before removing the gloves.

NOTE: This reduces the danger of cross-infection caused by handling contaminated supplies without glove protection.

12. To remove the gloves, use one gloved hand to grasp the other glove by the outside of the cuff (Figure 15–42H). Taking care not to touch the skin, remove the glove by pulling it down over the hand (Figure 15–42I). It will be wrong side out when removed.

NOTE: This prevents contamination of your hands by organisms picked up during performance of the procedure. Now you must consider the outside of the gloves contaminated, and the area inside, next to your skin, clean.

13. Insert your bare fingers inside the second glove (Figure 15–42J). Remove the glove by pulling it down gently, taking care not to touch the outside of the glove with your bare fingers (Figure 15–42K). It will be wrong side out when removed.

Safety

CAUTION: Avoid touching your uniform or any other object with the contaminated gloves.

(continues)

PROCEDURE 15:8C (CONT.)

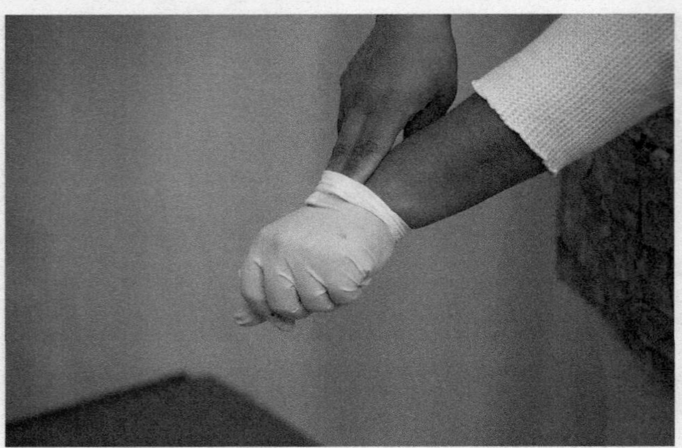

FIGURE 15–42J Insert your bare fingers inside the top of the second glove.

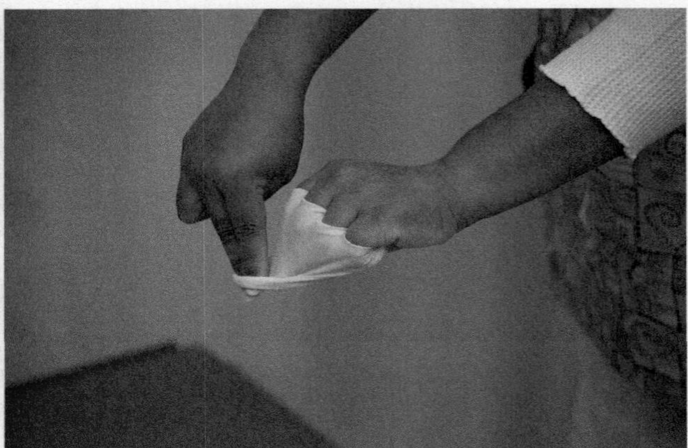

FIGURE 15–42K Pull the glove down gently, taking care to not touch the outside of the glove with your fingers.

14. Put the contaminated gloves in an infectious waste container immediately after removal.
15. Wash your hands immediately and thoroughly after removing gloves.
16. Once the gloves have been removed, do not handle any contaminated equipment or supplies such as soiled dressings or drainage basins. Protect yourself.
17. Replace equipment if necessary.
18. Wash hands thoroughly.

PRACTICE: **Go to the workbook and use the evaluation sheet for 15:8C, Donning and Removing Sterile Gloves, to practice this procedure. When you believe you have mastered this skill, sign the sheet and give it to your instructor for further action.**

Check

FINAL CHECKPOINT: Using the criteria listed on the evaluation sheet, your instructor will grade your performance.

PROCEDURE 15.8D

Changing a Sterile Dressing

Equipment and Supplies

Sterile tray with basin, solution, gauze sponges and pads (or a prepared sterile dressing package); sterile gloves; adhesive or nonallergic tape; disposable gloves; infectious waste bag; pen or computer

Procedure

1. Check doctor's written orders or obtain orders from immediate supervisor.

   NOTE: Dressings should *not* be changed without orders.

   NOTE: The policy of your agency will determine how you obtain orders for procedures.

2. Assemble equipment. Check autoclave indicator and date on all equipment. If more than 30 days have elapsed, use another package with a more recent date. Put the unsterile package aside for resterilization.
3. Wash hands thoroughly.
4. Prepare a sterile tray as previously taught in Procedure 15:8B or obtain a commercially prepared sterile dressing package.

   NOTE: Prepared packages are used by some agencies.

   Safety

   CAUTION: Never let the tray out of your sight after it has been prepared.

5. Take all necessary equipment to the patient area. Place it where it will be convenient for use yet free from possible contamination by other equipment.

PROCEDURE 15:8D (CONT.)

6. Comm Introduce yourself. Identify the patient. Explain the procedure. Close the door and/or windows to avoid drafts and flow of organisms into the room.
7. Close the door or draw curtains to provide privacy for the patient. If the patient is in a bed, elevate the bed to a comfortable working height and lower the siderail. Expose the body area needing the dressing change. Use sheets or drapes as necessary to prevent unnecessary exposure of the patient.
8. Fold down a 2- to 3-inch cuff on the top of the infectious waste bag. Position it in a convenient location. Tear off the tape you will need later to secure the clean dressing. Place it in an area where it will be available for easy access.
9. Precaution Put on disposable, nonsterile gloves. Gently but firmly remove the tape from the soiled dressing. Discard it in the infectious waste bag. Hold the skin taut and then lift the dressing carefully, taking care not to pull on any surgical drains. Note the type, color, and amount of drainage on the dressing. Discard dressing in the infectious waste bag.

   NOTE: Surgical drains are placed in some surgical incisions to aid in the removal of secretions. Care must be taken to avoid moving the drains when the dressing is removed.
10. Check the incision site. Observe the type and amount of remaining drainage, color of drainage, and degree of healing.

   Comm
   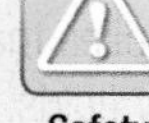
   Safety

   CAUTION: Report any unusual observations immediately to your supervisor. Examples are bright red blood, pus, swelling, abnormal discharges at the wound site, or patient complaints of pain or dizziness.
11. Remove disposable gloves and place in infectious waste bag. Immediately wash your hands.

   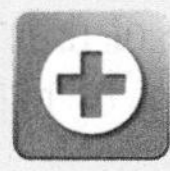
   Precaution

   CAUTION: Nonsterile disposable gloves should be worn while removing dressings to avoid contamination of the hands or skin by blood or body discharge.
12. Fanfold the top cover back to uncover the sterile field.

   Safety

   CAUTION: Handle only the contaminated side (outside) of the towel. The side in contact with the tray's contents is the sterile side.

   NOTE: If a prepared package is used, open it at this time.
13. Don sterile gloves as previously taught in Procedure 15:8C.
14. Using thumb and forefinger or dressing forceps, pick up a gauze sponge from the basin. Squeeze it slightly to remove any excess solution. Warn the patient that the solution may be cool.
15. Cleanse the wound using a circular motion (Figure 15–43A).

   NOTE: Begin near the center of the wound and move outward or away from the wound. Make an ever-widening circle. Discard the wet gauze sponge after use. Never go back over the same area with the same gauze sponge. Repeat this procedure until the area is clean, using a new gauze sponge each time.
16. Do not cleanse directly over the wound unless there is a great deal of drainage or it is specifically ordered by the physician. If this is to be done, use sterile gauze and wipe with a single stroke from the top to the bottom. Discard the soiled gauze. Repeat as necessary, using a new sterile gauze sponge each time.
17. The wound is now ready for clean dressings. Lift the sterile dressings from the tray and place them lightly on the wound (Figure 15–43B). Make sure they are centered over the wound.

   NOTE: The inner dressing is usually made up of 4-by-4-inch gauze sponges.
18. Apply outer dressings until the wound is sufficiently protected (Figure 15–43C).

   NOTE: Heavier dressings such as abdominal pads are usually used.

   NOTE: The number and size of dressings needed will depend on the amount of drainage and the size of the wound.
19. Place the precut tape over the dressing at the proper angle. Check to make sure that the dressing is secure and the ends are closed.

   NOTE: Tape should be applied so it runs opposite from body action or movement (Figure 15–43D). It should be the correct width for the dressing. It should be long enough to support the dressing, but it should not be too long because it may irritate the patient's skin.

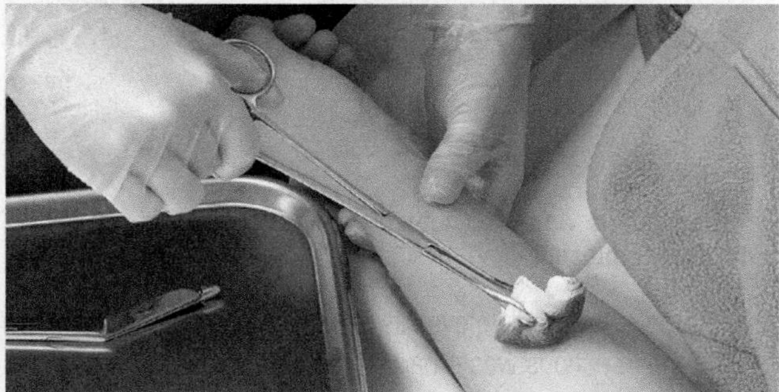

FIGURE 15–43A Use a circular motion to clean the wound, starting at the center of the wound and moving in an outward direction.

(continues)

PROCEDURE 15:8D (CONT.)

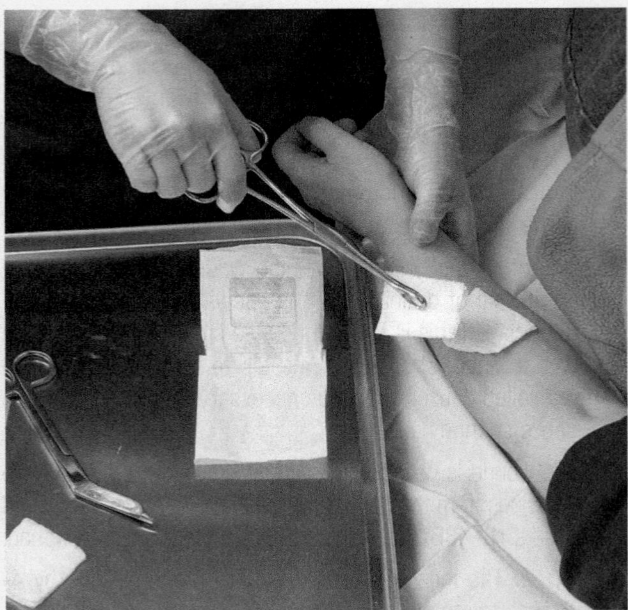

FIGURE 15–43B **Position the inner sterile dressings so they are centered over the wound.**

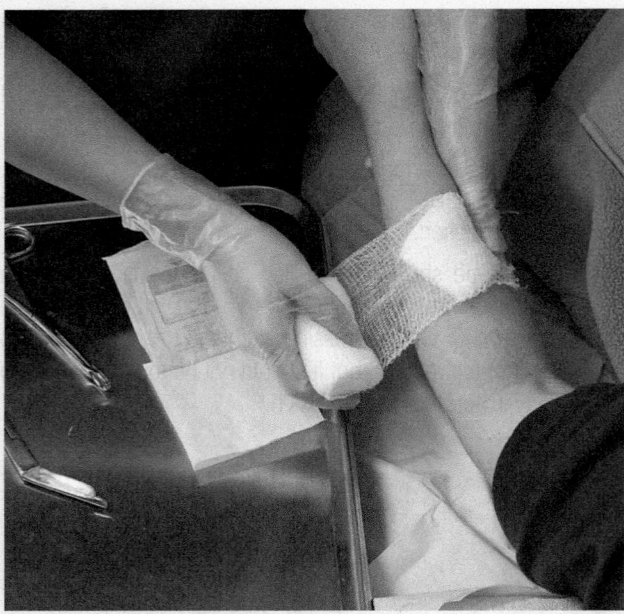

FIGURE 15–43C **Apply the outer dressings until the wound is sufficiently protected.**

20. Remove the sterile gloves as previously taught. Discard them in the infectious waste bag. Immediately wash your hands.
21. Check to be sure the patient is comfortable and that safety precautions have been observed before leaving the area.

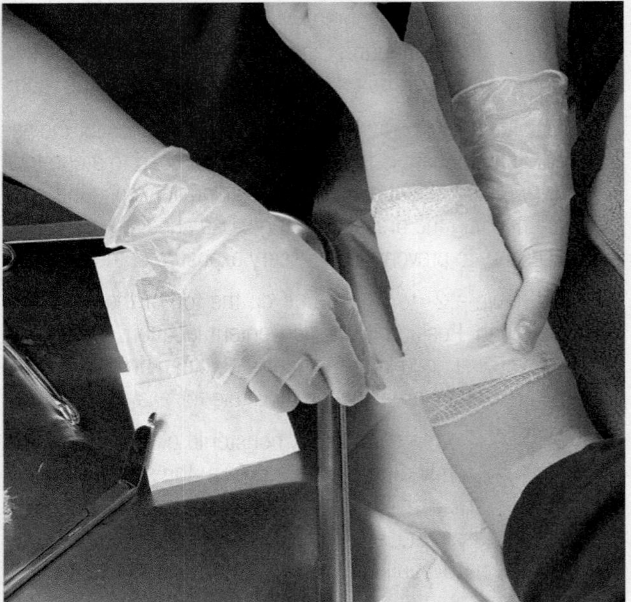

FIGURE 15–43D **Tape should be applied so that it runs opposite to body action or movement.**

22. Put on disposable, nonsterile gloves. Clean and replace all equipment used. Tie or tape the infectious waste bag securely. Dispose of it according to agency policy.

Safety

CAUTION: Disposable, nonsterile gloves should be worn to provide a protective barrier while cleaning equipment or supplies that may be contaminated by blood or body fluids.

23. Remove disposable gloves. Wash hands thoroughly. Protect yourself from possible contamination.
24. Comm — Record the following information on the patient's chart or enter it into the computer: date, time, dressing change, amount and type of drainage, and any other pertinent information, or tell this information to your immediate supervisor.

EXAMPLE: 1/8/—, 9:00 A.M. Dressing changed on right abdominal area. Small amount of thick, light yellow discharge noted on dressings. No swelling or inflammation apparent at incision site. Sterile dressing applied. Your signature and title.

NOTE: Report any unusual observations immediately.

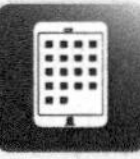

EHR

NOTE: In health care agencies using electronic health records (EHRs), also known as electronic medical records (EMRs), the information is entered directly into the patient's record on a computer.

PROCEDURE 15:8D (CONT.)

PRACTICE: Go to the workbook and use the evaluation sheet for 15:8D, Changing a Sterile Dressing, to practice this procedure. When you believe you have mastered this skill, sign the sheet and give it to your instructor for further action.

Check

FINAL CHECKPOINT: Using the criteria listed on the evaluation sheet, your instructor will grade your performance.

15:9 Maintaining Transmission-Based Precautions

Introduction

OBRA

In health occupations, you will deal with many different diseases/disorders. Some diseases are communicable and require isolation. A **communicable disease** is caused by a pathogenic organism that can be easily transmitted to others. An **epidemic** occurs when the communicable disease spreads rapidly from person to person and affects a large number of people at the same time. A **pandemic** exists when the outbreak of disease occurs over a wide geographic area and affects a high proportion of the population. Because individuals can travel readily throughout the world, a major concern is that worldwide pandemics will become more and more frequent.

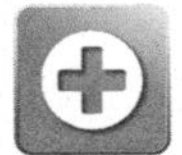
Precaution

Transmission-based precautions are a method or technique of caring for patients who have communicable diseases. Examples of communicable diseases are tuberculosis, wound infections, and pertussis (whooping cough). Standard precautions, discussed in information section 15:4, Observing Standard Precautions, do not eliminate the need for specific transmission-based precautions. Standard precautions are used on all patients. Transmission-based precautions are used to provide extra protection against specific diseases or pathogens to prevent their spread.

Communicable diseases are spread in many ways. Some examples include direct contact with the patient; contact with dirty linen, equipment, and/or supplies; and contact with blood, body fluids, secretions, and excretions such as urine, feces, droplets (from sneezing, coughing, or spitting), and discharges from wounds. Transmission-based precautions are used to limit contact with pathogenic organisms. These techniques help prevent the spread of the disease to other people and protect patients, their families, and health care providers.

The type of transmission-based precautions used depends on the causative organism of the disease, the way the organism is transmitted, and whether the pathogen is antibiotic resistant (not affected by antibiotics). Personal protective equipment (PPE) is used to provide protection from the pathogen. Some transmission-based precautions require the use of gowns, gloves, face shields, and masks (Figure 15–44), while others require the use of only a mask.

Two terms are extensively used in transmission-based precautions: *contaminated* and *clean*. These words refer to the presence of organisms on objects.

- **Contaminated**, or dirty, means that objects contain disease-producing organisms. These objects must not be touched unless the health care worker is protected by gloves, gown, and other required items.

  NOTE: The outside and waist ties of the gown, protective gloves, and mask are considered contaminated.

- **Clean** means that objects or parts of objects do *not* contain disease-producing organisms and therefore have minimal chance of spreading the disease. Every effort must be made to prevent contamination of these objects or parts of objects.

  NOTE: The insides of the gloves and gown are clean, as are the neckband, its ties, and the mask ties.

The Centers for Disease Control and Prevention (CDC) in conjunction with the National Center for Infectious Diseases (NCID) and the Hospital Infection Control Practices Advisory Committee (HICPAC) has recommended four main classifications of precautions that

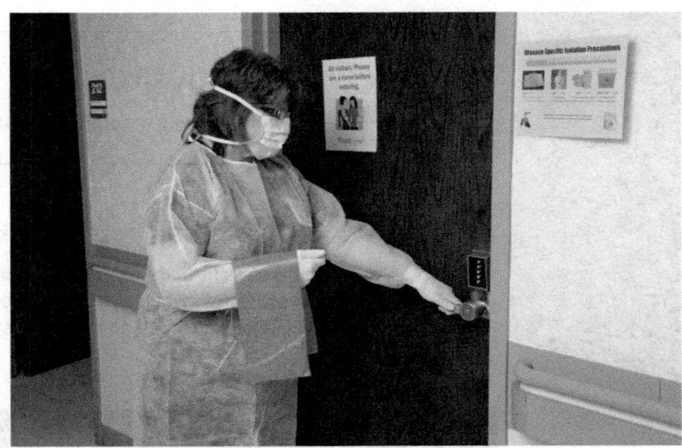

FIGURE 15–44 Some transmission-based precautions require the use of gowns, gloves, and a mask, while others require the use of only a mask.

must be followed: standard, airborne, droplet, and contact. Health care facilities are provided with a list of infections/conditions that shows the type and duration of precautions needed for each specific disease. In this way, facilities can follow the guidelines to determine the type of transmission-based isolation that should be used along with the specific precautions that must be followed.

Standard Precautions

Standard precautions (discussed in information section 15:4, Observing Standard Precautions) are used on all patients. In addition, a patient must be placed in a private room if the patient contaminates the environment or does not (or cannot be expected to) assist in maintaining appropriate hygiene. Every health care worker must be well informed about standard precautions and must follow the recommendations for the use of gloves, gowns, and face masks when conditions indicate their use.

Airborne Precautions

Airborne precautions (Figure 15-45) are used for patients known or suspected to be infected with pathogens transmitted by airborne droplet nuclei. These are small particles of evaporated droplets that contain

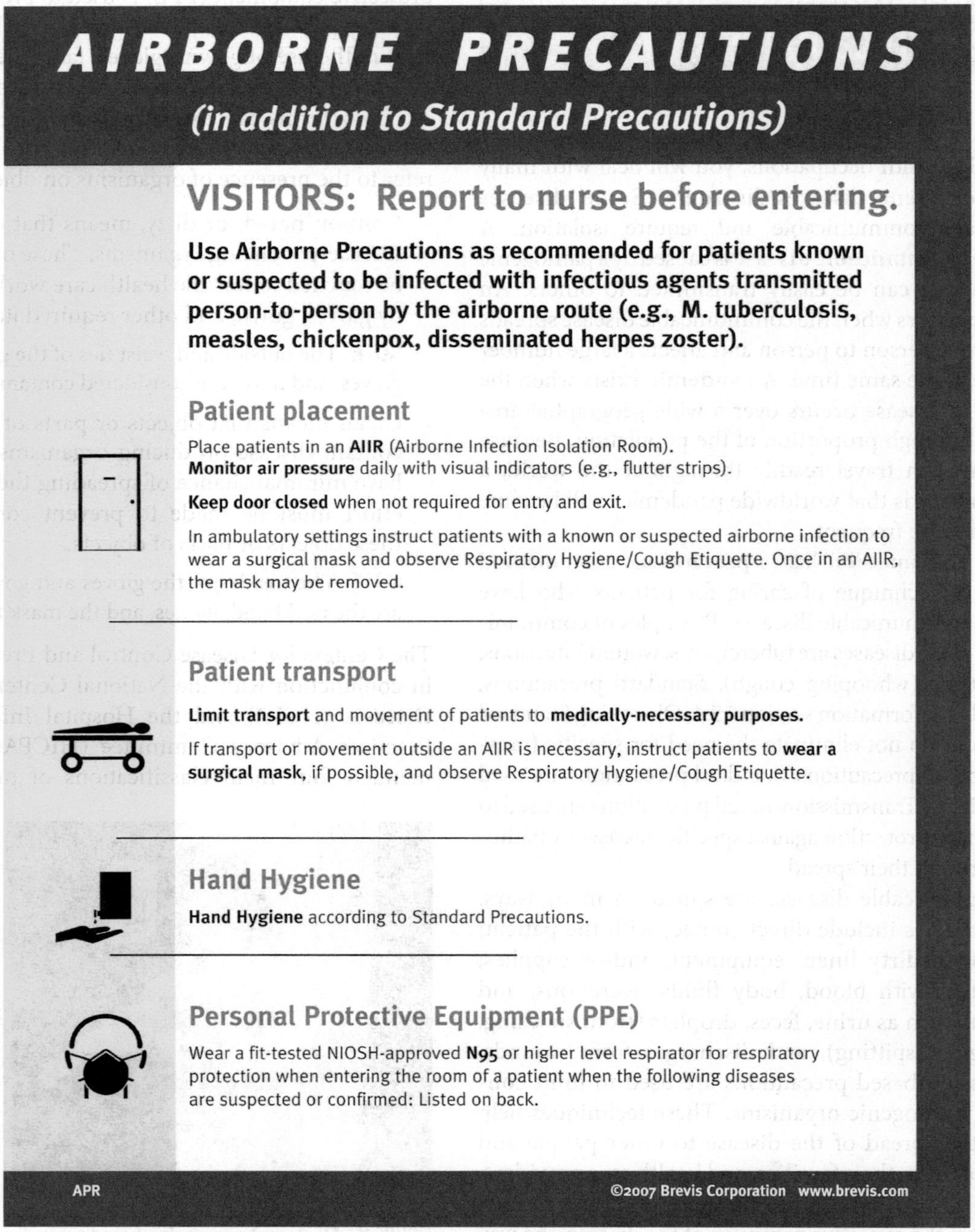

AIRBORNE PRECAUTIONS

(in addition to Standard Precautions)

VISITORS: Report to nurse before entering.

Use Airborne Precautions as recommended for patients known or suspected to be infected with infectious agents transmitted person-to-person by the airborne route (e.g., M. tuberculosis, measles, chickenpox, disseminated herpes zoster).

Patient placement

Place patients in an **AIIR** (Airborne Infection Isolation Room).
Monitor air pressure daily with visual indicators (e.g., flutter strips).

Keep door closed when not required for entry and exit.

In ambulatory settings instruct patients with a known or suspected airborne infection to wear a surgical mask and observe Respiratory Hygiene/Cough Etiquette. Once in an AIIR, the mask may be removed.

Patient transport

Limit transport and movement of patients to **medically-necessary purposes.**

If transport or movement outside an AIIR is necessary, instruct patients to **wear a surgical mask**, if possible, and observe Respiratory Hygiene/Cough Etiquette.

Hand Hygiene

Hand Hygiene according to Standard Precautions.

Personal Protective Equipment (PPE)

Wear a fit-tested NIOSH-approved **N95** or higher level respirator for respiratory protection when entering the room of a patient when the following diseases are suspected or confirmed: Listed on back.

APR

FIGURE 15–45 Airborne precautions. Reprinted with Permission from Brevis Corporation [www.brevis.com].

microorganisms and remain suspended in the air or on dust particles. Examples of diseases requiring these isolation precautions are rubella (measles), varicella (chicken pox), tuberculosis, and severe acute respiratory syndrome (SARS). Standard precautions are used at all times. In addition, the following precautions must be taken:

- The patient must be placed in an airborne infection isolation room (AIRR), and the door should be kept closed.
- Air in the room must be discharged to outdoor air or filtered before being circulated to other areas.
- Each person who enters the room must wear respiratory protection in the form of an N95, P100, or more powerful filtering mask such as a high-efficiency particulate air (HEPA) mask (Figures 15–46A and B). These masks contain special filters to prevent the entrance of the small airborne pathogens. The masks must be fit tested to make sure they create a tight seal each time they are worn by a health care provider. Men with facial hair cannot wear a standard filtering mask because a beard prevents an airtight seal. Men with facial hair can use a special HEPA-filtered hood.
- People susceptible to measles or chicken pox should not enter the room.
- If at all possible, the patient should not be moved from the room. If transport is essential, however, the patient must wear a surgical mask during transport to minimize the release of droplets into the air.

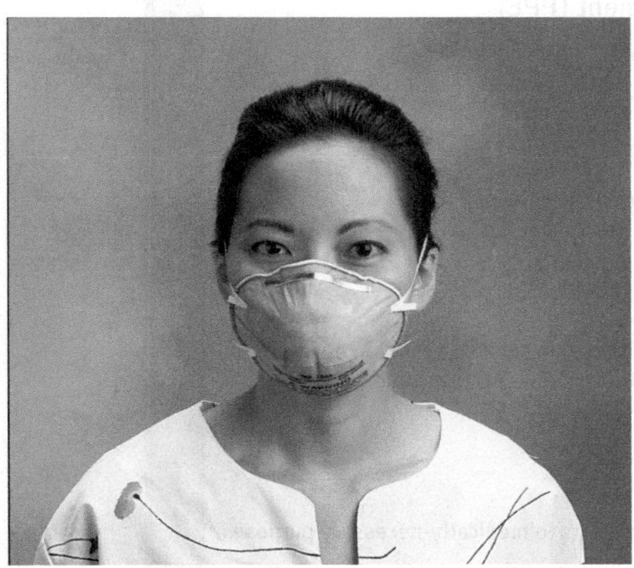

FIGURE 15–46A The N95 respirator mask. Courtesy of 3M Company, St. Paul, MN.

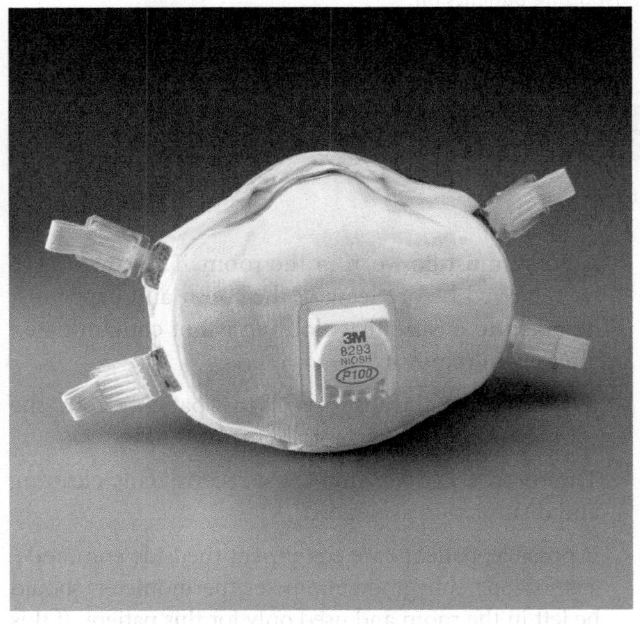

FIGURE 15–46B The P100 respirator mask. Courtesy of 3M Company, St. Paul, MN.

Droplet Precautions

Droplet precautions (Figure 15-47) must be followed for a patient known or suspected to be infected with pathogens transmitted by large-particle droplets expelled during coughing, sneezing, talking, or laughing. Examples of diseases requiring these isolation precautions include *Haemophilus influenzae* meningitis and pneumonia; *Neisseria* meningitis and pneumonia; multidrug-resistant *Streptococcus* meningitis, pneumonia, sinusitis, and otitis media; diphtheria; *Mycoplasma* pneumonia; pertussis; adenovirus; mumps; and severe viral influenza. Standard precautions are used at all times. In addition, the following precautions must be taken:

- The patient should be placed in a private room. If a private room is not available and the patient cannot be placed in a room with a patient who has the same infection, a distance of at least 3 feet should separate the infected patient and other patients or visitors.
- Masks must be worn when entering the room.
- If transport or movement of the patient is essential, the patient must wear a surgical mask.

Contact Precautions

Contact precautions (Figure 15-48) must be followed for any patients known or suspected to be infected with *epidemiological* (capable of spreading rapidly from person to person, an epidemic) microorganisms that can be transmitted by either direct or indirect contact. Examples of diseases requiring these precautions include any gastrointestinal, respiratory, skin, or wound infections caused by multidrug-resistant organisms; diapered or incontinent patients with enterohemorrhagic *E. coli, Shigella,* hepatitis A, or rotavirus; viral or hemorrhagic conjunctivitis or fevers; and any skin infections that are highly contagious or that may occur on dry skin, such as diphtheria, herpes simplex virus, impetigo, pediculosis (head or body lice), scabies, and staphylococcal

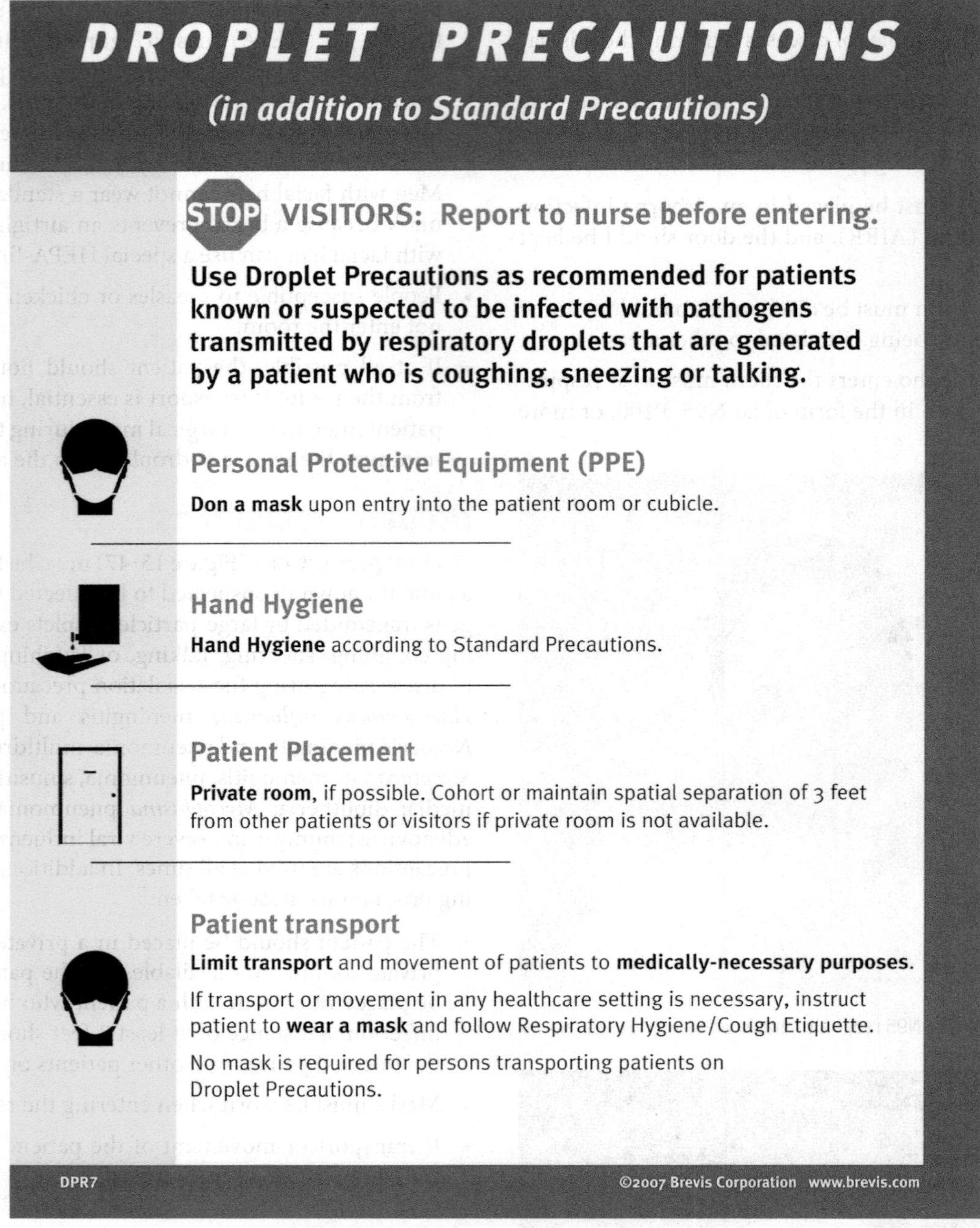

DROPLET PRECAUTIONS
(in addition to Standard Precautions)
STOP
VISITORS: Report to nurse before entering.
Use Droplet Precautions as recommended for patients known or suspected to be infected with pathogens transmitted by respiratory droplets that are generated by a patient who is coughing, sneezing or talking.
Personal Protective Equipment (PPE)
Don a mask upon entry into the patient room or cubicle.
Hand Hygiene
Hand Hygiene according to Standard Precautions.
Patient Placement
Private room, if possible. Cohort or maintain spatial separation of 3 feet from other patients or visitors if private room is not available.
Patient transport
Limit transport and movement of patients to medically-necessary purposes.
If transport or movement in any healthcare setting is necessary, instruct patient to wear a mask and follow Respiratory Hygiene/Cough Etiquette.
No mask is required for persons transporting patients on Droplet Precautions.
DPR7
©2007 Brevis Corporation www.brevis.com

FIGURE 15–47 Droplet precautions. Reprinted with Permission from Brevis Corporation [www.brevis.com].

infections. Standard precautions are used at all times. In addition, the following precautions must be taken:

- The patient should be placed in a private room or, if a private room is not available, in a room with a patient who has an active infection caused by the same organism.
- Gloves must be worn when entering the room.
- Gloves must be changed after having contact with any material that may contain high concentrations of the microorganism, such as wound drainage or fecal material.
- Gloves must be removed before leaving the room, and the hands must be washed with an antimicrobial agent.
- A gown must be worn in the room. The gown must be removed before leaving the room and care must be taken to ensure that clothing is not contaminated after gown removal.
- Movement and transport of the patient from the room should be for essential purposes only.
- The room and items in it must receive daily cleaning and disinfection as needed.
- If possible, patient-care equipment (bedside commode, stethoscope, sphygmomanometer, thermometer) should be left in the room and used only for this patient. If this

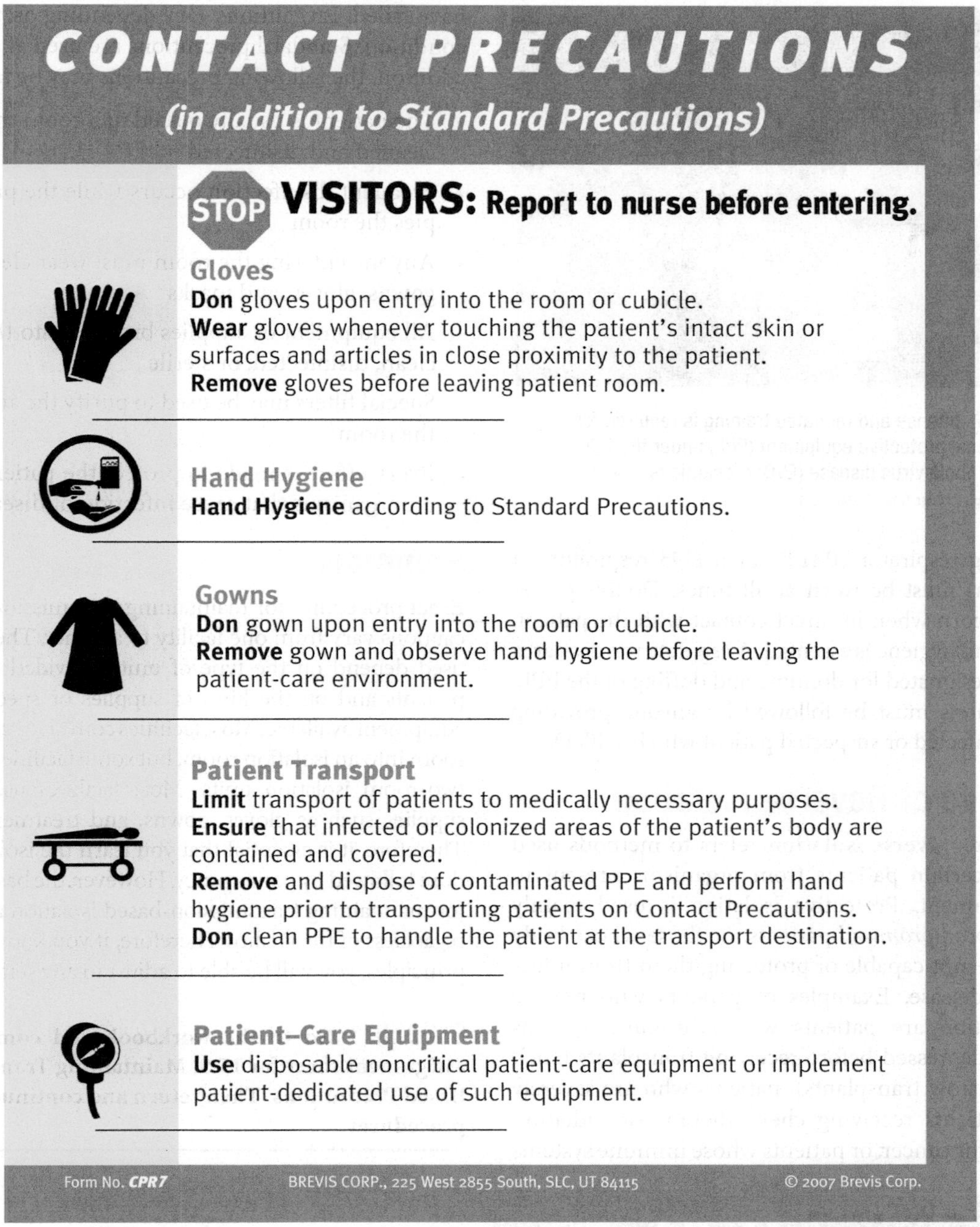

CONTACT PRECAUTIONS

(in addition to Standard Precautions)

STOP **VISITORS: Report to nurse before entering.**

Gloves

Don gloves upon entry into the room or cubicle.
Wear gloves whenever touching the patient's intact skin or surfaces and articles in close proximity to the patient.
Remove gloves before leaving patient room.

Hand Hygiene

Hand Hygiene according to Standard Precautions.

Gowns

Don gown upon entry into the room or cubicle.
Remove gown and observe hand hygiene before leaving the patient-care environment.

Patient Transport

Limit transport of patients to medically necessary purposes.
Ensure that infected or colonized areas of the patient's body are contained and covered.
Remove and dispose of contaminated PPE and perform hand hygiene prior to transporting patients on Contact Precautions.
Don clean PPE to handle the patient at the transport destination.

Patient–Care Equipment

Use disposable noncritical patient-care equipment or implement patient-dedicated use of such equipment.

Form No. ***CPR7*** BREVIS CORP., 225 West 2855 South, SLC, UT 84115 © 2007 Brevis Corp.

FIGURE 15–48 Contact precautions. Reprinted with Permission from Brevis Corporation [www.brevis.com].

is not possible, all equipment must be cleaned and disinfected before being used on another patient.

Ebola Virus Disease (EVD) Precautions

The first Ebola outbreak to reach epidemic proportions occurred in West Africa in 2014. In October of 2014, the CDC formulated more stringent infection control guidelines to be used when caring for patients with confirmed or suspected Ebola virus disease (EVD). These guidelines call for strict enforcement of standard, contact, and droplet precautions. The patient is to be placed in an airborne infection isolation room (AIIR) with restricted visitation. Medical equipment is dedicated to the patient whenever possible. The use of needles and blood draws are limited to necessity only. In addition, personal protective equipment (PPE) is a high priority. Intense and repeated training must be done to ensure that the correct PPE is used and that it is put on (donned) and taken off (doffed) properly (Figure 15-49). The proper order and procedure for donning and doffing is essential. The guidelines require a second trained staff member to supervise the donning and doffing of the PPE at all times. The PPE must cover all of the skin, head, neck, body, and feet. A powered

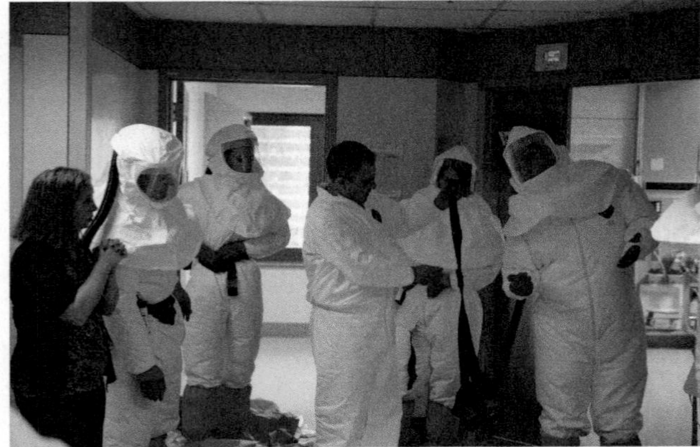

FIGURE 15–49 **Intense and repeated training is required for donning personal protective equipment (PPE) under the CDC guidelines for Ebola virus disease (EVD) precautions.** Courtesy of the CDC/U.S. DoD, Army Sgt. 1st Class Tyrone C. Marshall, Jr.

air-purifying respirator (PAPR) or a N95 respirator (at a minimum) must be worn at all times. Double gloves should be worn when in direct contact with the patient. Diligent hand hygiene is essential. A separate room or area should be designated for donning and doffing of the PPE. All precautions must be followed by anyone providing care to an infected or suspected patient who has EVD.

Protective or Reverse Isolation

Protective or reverse isolation refers to methods used to protect certain patients from organisms present in the environment. Protective isolation is used mainly for *immunocompromised* patients, or those whose body defenses are not capable of protecting them from infections and disease. Examples of patients who require this protection are patients whose immune systems have been depressed before receiving transplants (such as bone marrow transplants), patients who are severely burned, patients receiving chemotherapy or radiation treatments for cancer, or patients whose immune systems have failed. Precautions vary depending on the patient's condition. Standard precautions are used at all times. In addition, the following precautions may be taken:

- The patient is usually placed in a room that has been cleaned and disinfected
- Frequent disinfection occurs while the patient occupies the room
- Anyone entering the room must wear clean or sterile gowns, gloves, and masks
- All equipment or supplies brought into the room are clean, disinfected, or sterile
- Special filters may be used to purify the air that enters the room
- Every effort is made to protect the patient from microorganisms that cause infection or disease

Summary

Exact procedures for maintaining transmission-based precautions vary from one facility to another. The procedures used depend on the type of units provided for isolation patients and on the kind of supplies or special isolation equipment available. Most facilities convert a regular patient room into an isolation room, but some facilities use special, two-room isolation units. Most facilities use disposable supplies such as gloves, gowns, and treatment packages. Therefore, it is essential that you learn the isolation procedure followed by your agency. However, the basic principles for maintaining transmission-based isolation are the same regardless of the facility. Therefore, if you know these basic principles, you will be able to adjust to any setting.

STUDENT: **Go to the workbook and complete the assignment sheet for 15:9, Maintaining Transmission-Based Precautions. Then return and continue with the procedures.**

PROCEDURE 15:9A

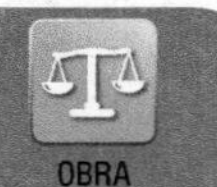

OBRA

Donning and Removing Transmission-Based Isolation Garments

OBRA

NOTE: The following procedure deals with contact transmission-based precautions. For other types of transmission-based precautions, follow only the steps that apply.

Equipment and Supplies

Isolation gown, surgical mask, gloves, small plastic bag, linen cart or container, infectious waste container, paper towels, sink with running water

Procedure

1. Assemble equipment.

   NOTE: In many agencies, clean isolation garments and supplies are kept available on a cart outside the isolation unit or in the outer room of a two-room unit. A waste container should be positioned just inside the door.

PROCEDURE 15:9A (CONT.)

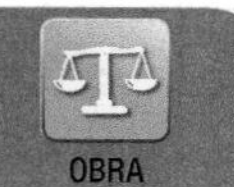

2. Wash hands.
3. Remove rings and place them in your pocket or pin them to your uniform.
4. Remove your watch and place it in a small plastic bag or centered on a clean paper towel. If placed on a towel, handle only the bottom part of the towel; do not touch the top.

   NOTE: The watch will be taken into the room and placed on the bedside stand for taking vital signs. Because it cannot be sterilized, it must be kept clean.

   NOTE: In some agencies, a plastic-covered watch is left in the isolation room or the room has a clock with a second hand.
5. Put on the mask. Secure it under your chin. Make sure to cover your mouth and nose. Handle the mask as little as possible. Tie the mask securely behind your head and neck. Tie the top ties first and the bottom ties second (Figure 15–50A).

   NOTE: The tie bands on the mask are considered clean. The mask is considered contaminated.

   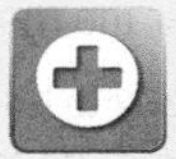

   CAUTION: The mask is considered to be contaminated after 30 minutes in isolation or anytime it gets wet. If you remain in isolation longer than 30 minutes, or if the mask gets wet, you must wash your hands, and remove and discard the old mask. Then wash your hands again, and put on a clean mask.
6. If uniform sleeves are long, roll them up above the elbows before putting on the gown.
7. Lift the gown by placing your hands inside the shoulders.

   NOTE: The inside of the gown and the ties at the neck are considered clean.

   NOTE: Most agencies use disposable gowns that are discarded after use.

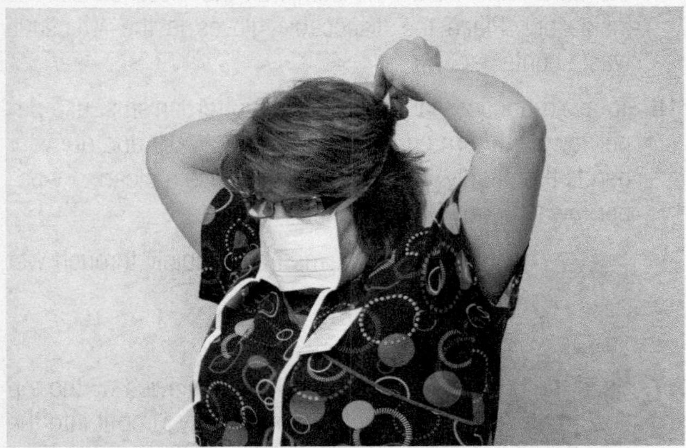

FIGURE 15–50A Put on the mask, tying the top ties before the bottom ties.

8. Work your arms into the sleeves of the gown by gently twisting (Figure 15–50B). Take care not to touch your face with the sleeves of the gown.
9. Place your hands *inside* the neckband, adjust until it is in position, and then tie the bands at the back of your neck (Figure 15–50C).
10. Reach behind and fold the edges of the gown over so that the uniform is completely covered. Tie the waistbands (Figure 15–50D). Some waistbands are long enough to wrap around your body before tying.
11. If gloves are to be worn, put them on. Make sure that the cuff of each glove comes over the top of the cuff of the gown (Figure 15–50E). In this way, there are no open areas for organisms to enter.

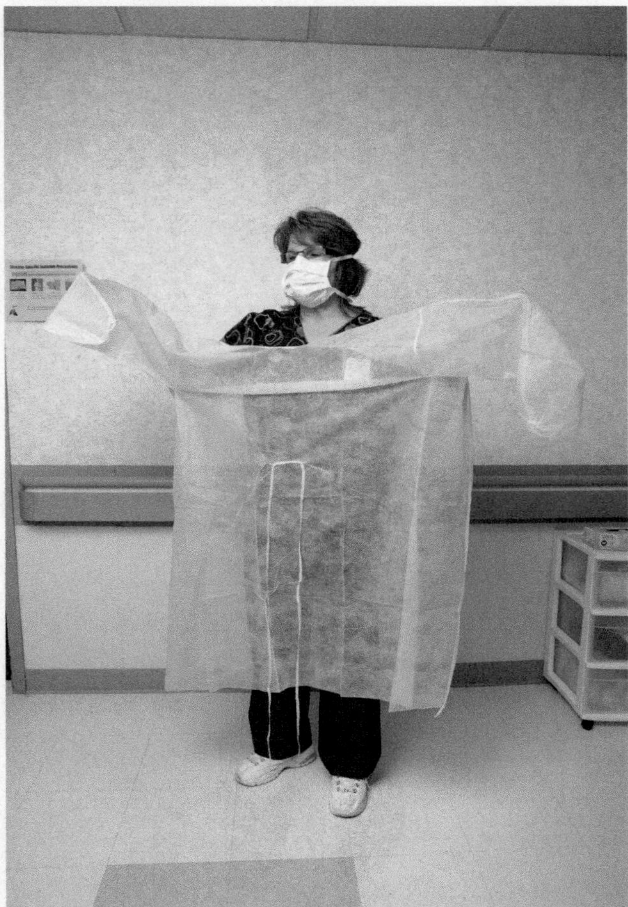

FIGURE 15–50B After tying the mask in place, put on the gown by placing your hands inside the shoulders to ease your arms into the sleeves.

(continues)

PROCEDURE 15:9A (CONT.)

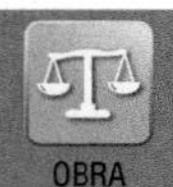

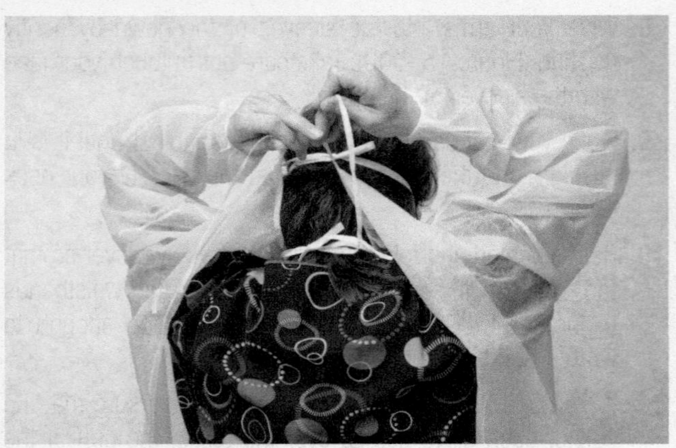

FIGURE 15–50C Slip your fingers inside the neckband to tie the gown at the neck.

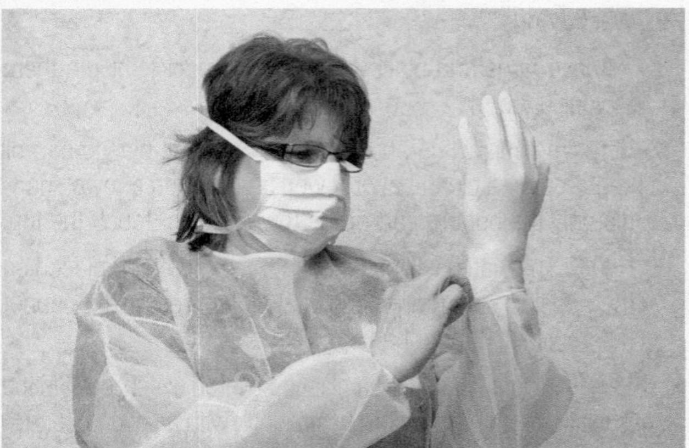

FIGURE 15–50E Put on gloves, making sure that the cuff of each glove is over the top of the cuff on the gown.

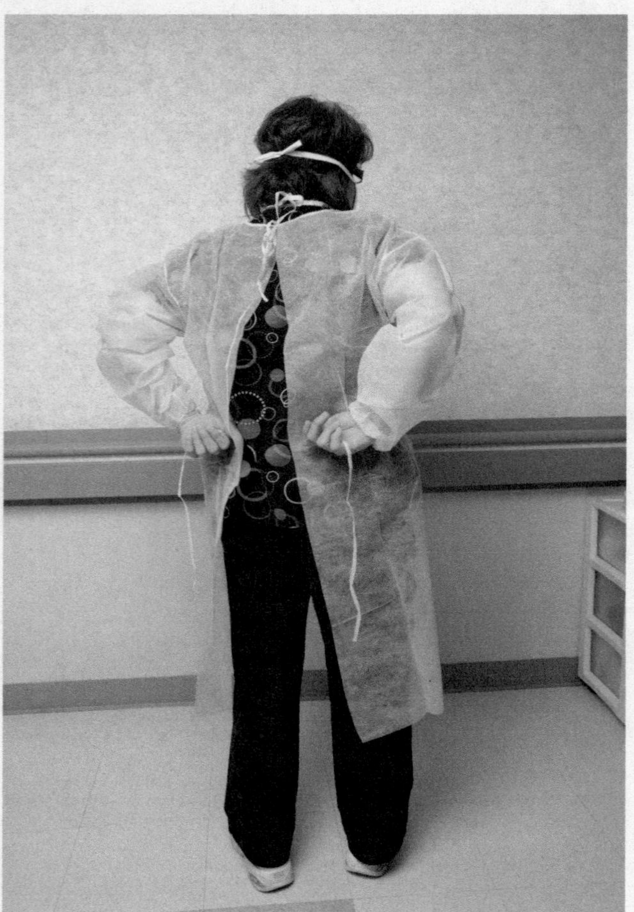

FIGURE 15–50D Tie the waist ties and make sure the back edges of the gown overlap to cover your uniform.

12. You are now ready to enter the isolation room. Double-check to be sure you have all equipment and supplies that you will need for patient care before you enter the room.
13. When patient care is complete, you will be ready to remove isolation garments. In a two-room isolation unit, go to the outer room. In a one-room unit, remove garments while you are standing close to the inside of the door. Take care to avoid touching the room's contaminated articles.
14. Untie the waist ties (Figure 15–51A), and loosen the gown at the waist.

    NOTE: The waist ties are considered contaminated.
15. If gloves are worn, remove the first glove by grasping the outside of the cuff with the opposite gloved hand. Pull the glove over the hand so that the glove is inside out (Figure 15–51B). Remove the second glove by placing the bare hand inside the cuff. Pull the glove off so it is inside out. Place the disposable gloves in the infectious waste container.
16. To avoid unnecessary transmission of organisms, use paper towels to turn on the water faucet. Wash and dry your hands thoroughly. When they are dry, use a clean, dry paper towel to turn off the faucet.

    CAUTION: Organisms travel rapidly through wet paper towels.
17. Untie the bottom ties of the mask first followed by the top ties. Holding the mask by the top ties only, drop it into the infectious waste container (Figure 15–51C).

PROCEDURE 15:9A (CONT.)

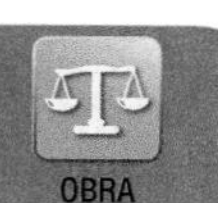
OBRA

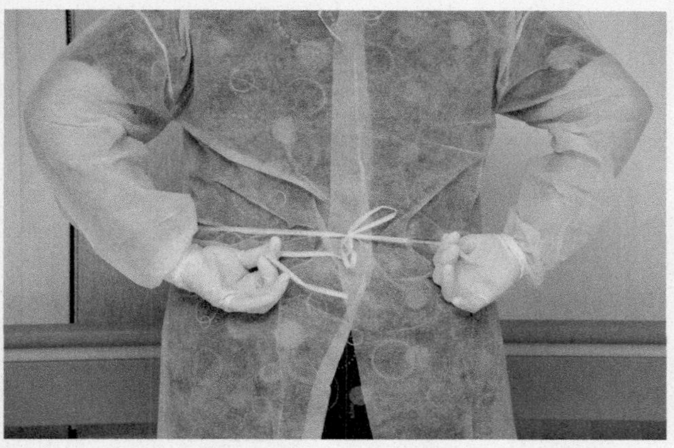

FIGURE 15–51A **Untie the waist ties of the gown before removing the gloves.**

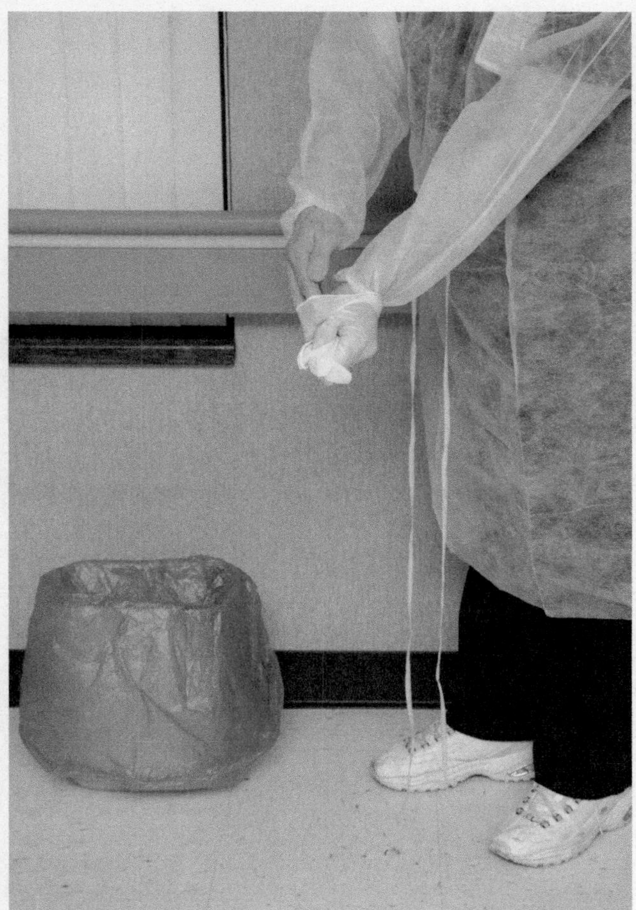

FIGURE 15–51B **To remove the gloves, pull them over the hand so the glove is inside out.**

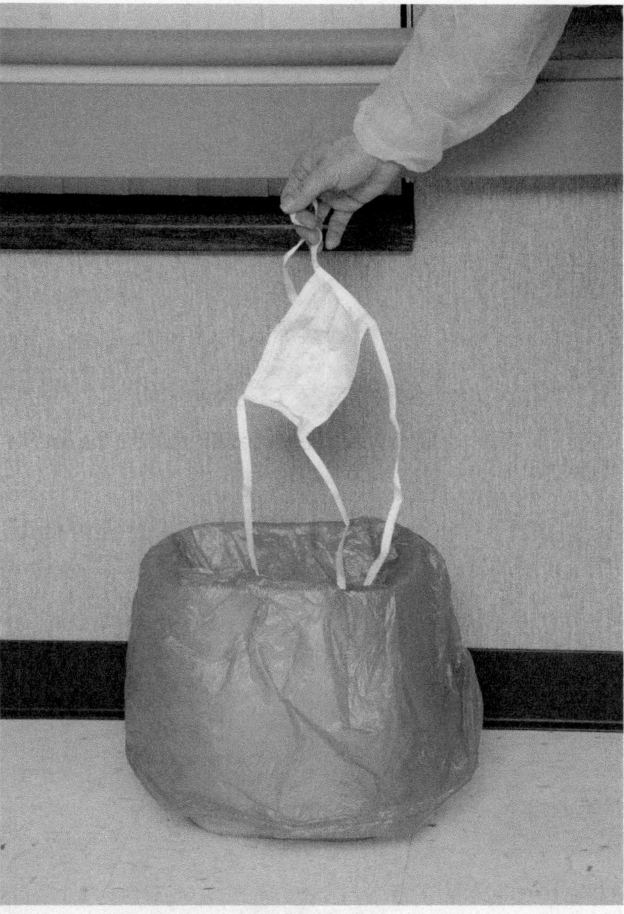

FIGURE 15–51C **Remove the mask and hold only the top ties to drop it in an infectious-waste container.**

NOTE: The ties of the mask are considered clean. Do not touch any other part of the mask, because it is considered contaminated.

18. Untie the neck ties (Figure 15–51D). Loosen the gown at the shoulders, handling only the inside of the gown.

NOTE: The neck ties are considered clean.

19. Slip the fingers of one hand inside the opposite cuff. Do *not* touch the outside. Pull the sleeve down over the hand (Figure 15–51E).

Safety

CAUTION: The outside of the gown is considered contaminated and should not be touched.

20. Using the gown-covered hand, pull the sleeve down over the opposite hand (Figure 15–51F).

(continues)

PROCEDURE 15:9A (CONT.)

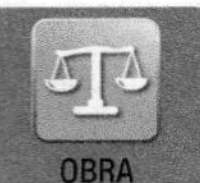

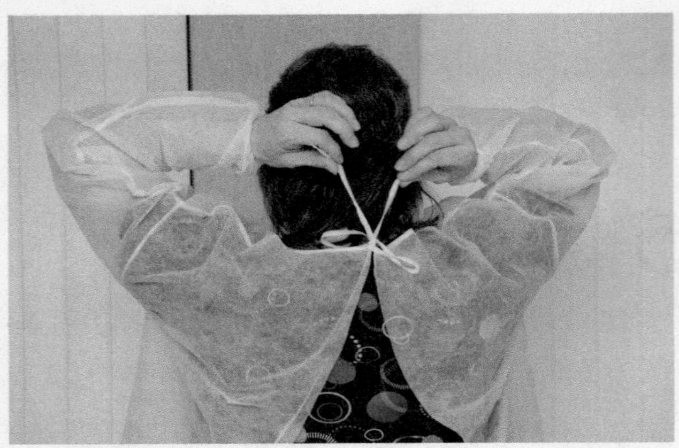

FIGURE 15–51D **Untie the neck ties but avoid touching the outside of the gown.**

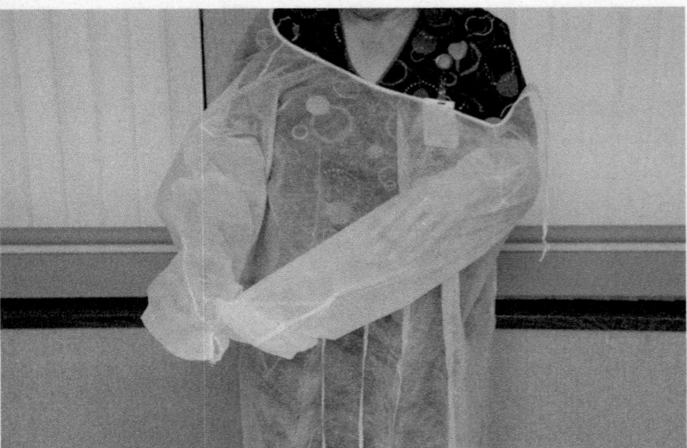

FIGURE 15–51F **Using the gown-covered hand, grasp the outside of the gown on the opposite arm and pull the gown down over the hand.**

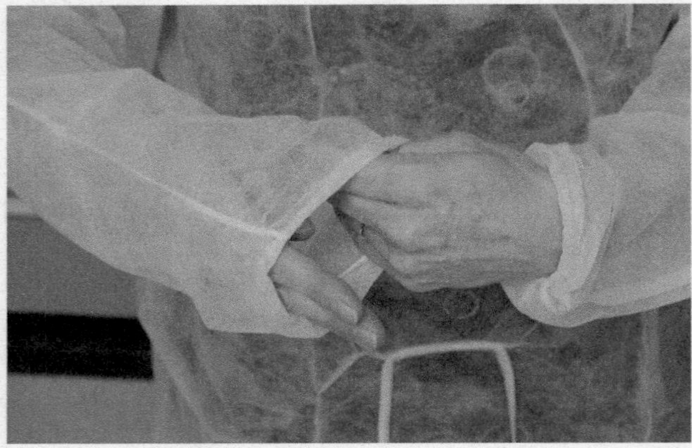

FIGURE 15–51E **To remove the gown, slip the fingers of one hand under the cuff of the opposite arm to pull the gown down over the opposite hand.**

21. Ease your arms and hands out of the gown. Keep the gown in front of your body and keep your hands away from the outside of the gown. Use as gentle a motion as possible.

NOTE: Excessive flapping of the gown will spread organisms.

22. With your hands inside the gown at the shoulders, bring the shoulders together and turn the gown so that it is inside out (Figure 15–51G). In this manner, the outside of the contaminated gown is on the inside. Fold the gown in half and then roll it together. Place it in the infectious waste container (Figure 15–51H).

NOTE: Avoid excess motion during this procedure because motion causes the spread of organisms.

23. Wash hands thoroughly. Use dry, clean paper towels to operate the faucets.

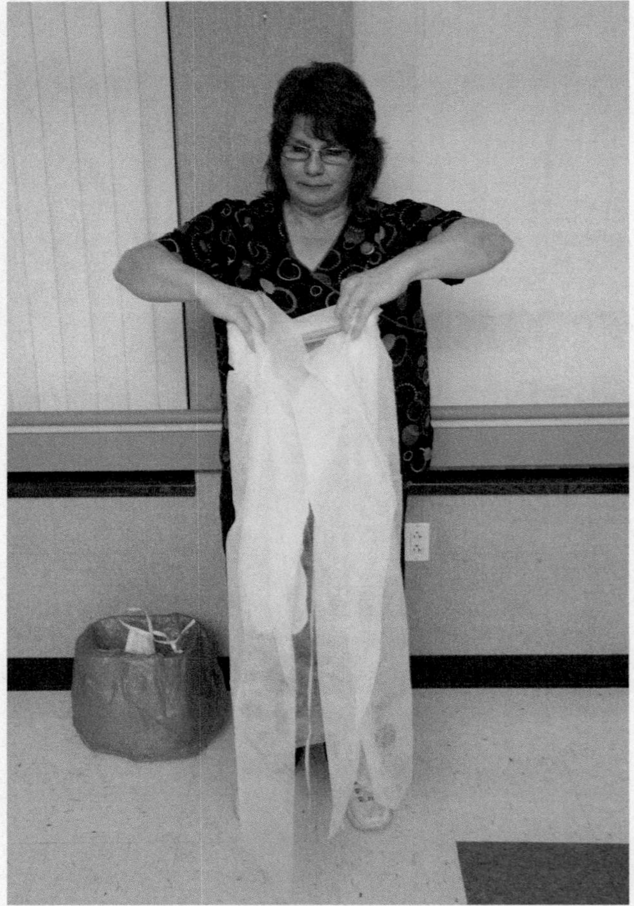

FIGURE 15–51G **With your hands inside the gown at the shoulders, bring the shoulders together and turn the gown so it is inside out, with the contaminated side on the inside.**

PROCEDURE 15:9A (CONT.)

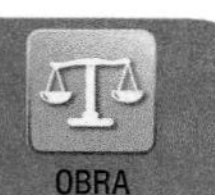

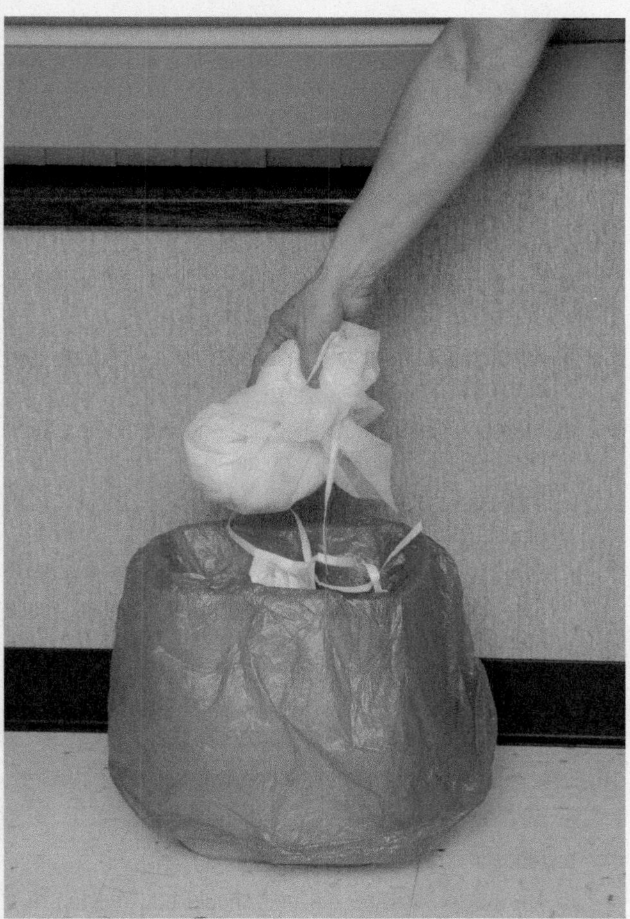

FIGURE 15–51H After folding the gown, discard it in an infectious-waste container.

24. Touch only the inside of the plastic bag to remove your watch. Discard the bag in the waste container. If the watch is on a paper towel, handle only the "clean," top portion (if necessary). Discard the towel in the infectious waste container.

25. Use a clean paper towel to open the door. Discard the towel in the waste container before leaving the room.

CAUTION: The inside of the door is considered contaminated.

NOTE: The waste container should be positioned just inside the door of the room.

26. After leaving the isolation room, wash hands thoroughly. This will help prevent the spread of the disease. It also protects you from the illness.

PRACTICE: **Go to the workbook and use the evaluation sheet for 15:9A, Donning and Removing Transmission-Based Isolation Garments, to practice this procedure. When you believe you have mastered this skill, sign the sheet and give it to your instructor for further action.**

FINAL CHECKPOINT: Using the criteria listed on the evaluation sheet, your instructor will grade your performance.

PROCEDURE 15:9B

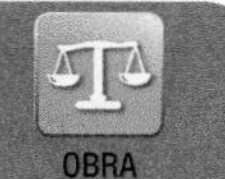

Working in a Hospital Transmission-Based Isolation Unit

Equipment and Supplies

Clothes hamper, two laundry bags, two trays, dishes, cups, bowls, waste container lined with a plastic bag, infectious waste bags, bags, tape, pencil, pen, paper

Procedure

1. Assemble all equipment.

   NOTE: Any equipment or supplies to be used in the isolation room must be assembled before entering the room.

2. Wash hands.

3. Put on appropriate isolation garments as previously instructed.

4. Tape paper to the outside of the isolation door. This will be used to record vital signs.

(continues)

PROCEDURE 15:9B (CONT.)

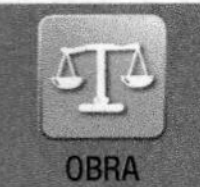
OBRA

5. Enter the isolation room. Take all needed equipment into the room.

6. Introduce yourself. Greet and identify patient. Provide patient care as needed.

Comm

NOTE: All care is provided in a routine manner. However, transmission-based isolation garments must be worn as ordered.

7. To record vital signs:
   a. Take vital signs using the watch in the plastic bag. (If the watch is not in a plastic bag, hold it with the bottom part of a paper towel.) Use other equipment in the room as needed.
   b. Open the door touching only the inside, or contaminated side.
   c. Using a pencil, record the vital signs on the paper taped to the door. Do *not* touch the outside of the door at any time.

NOTE: The pencil remains in the room because it is contaminated.

8. To transfer food into the isolation unit:
   a. The transfer of food requires two people; one person must stay outside the unit and one inside.
   b. The person inside the isolation unit picks up the empty tray in the room and opens the door, touching only the inside of the door.
   c. The person outside holds the tray while the dishes are being transferred (Figure 15–52).

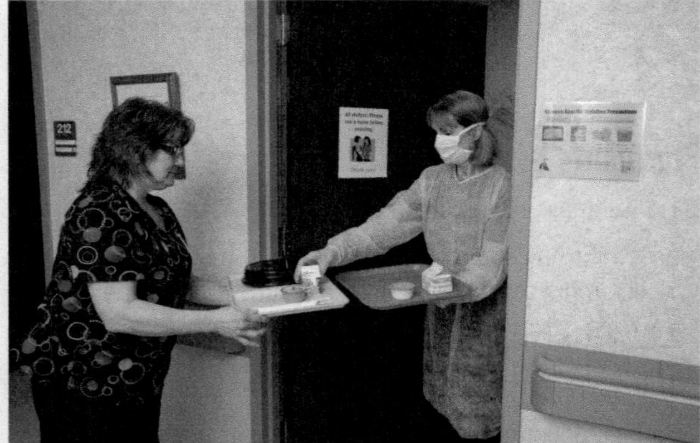

FIGURE 15–52 To transfer food into an isolation unit, a health worker holds the tray so the worker in isolation can transfer the food onto the tray kept inside the unit.

   d. When transferring food, the two people should handle the opposite sides of the dishes. In this manner, one person will not touch the other person.
   e. Glasses should be held near the top by the transfer person on the outside. The transfer person on the inside should receive the glasses by holding them on the bottom.

9. To dispose of leftover food or waste:
   a. Liquids can be poured down the sink or flushed down the toilet.
   b. Soft foods such as mashed potatoes or cooked vegetables can be flushed down the toilet.
   c. Hard particles of food, such as bone, should be placed in the plastic-lined trash container.
   d. Disposable utensils or dishes should be placed in the plastic-lined trash container.
   e. Metal utensils should be washed and kept in the isolation room to be used as needed for other meals. These utensils, however, are contaminated. When they are removed from the isolation room, they must be disinfected or double bagged and labeled before being sent for decontamination and reprocessing.

10. To transfer soiled linen from the unit, two people are required:
   a. All dirty linen should be folded and rolled.
   b. Place linen in the isolation linen bag.
   c. The person outside the unit should cuff the top of a clean infectious waste laundry bag and hold it. Hands should be kept on the inside of the bag's cuff to avoid contamination.
   d. The person in isolation should seal the isolation linen bag. The bag is then placed inside the outer bag, which is being held by the person outside (Figure 15–53).
   e. The outer bag should be folded over at the top and taped by the person outside. The bag should be labeled as "BIOHAZARDOUS LINEN."
   f. At all times, no direct contact should occur between the two people transferring linen.

NOTE: Many agencies use special isolation linen bags. Hot water dissolves the bags during the washing process. Therefore, no other personnel handle the contaminated linen after it leaves the isolation unit.

11. To transfer trash from the isolation unit, two people are required:
   a. Any trash in the isolation room should be in plastic bags. Any trash or disposable items contaminated with blood, body fluids, secretions, or excretions should be placed in infectious waste bags.

PROCEDURE 15:9B (CONT.)

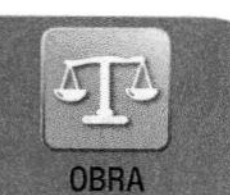

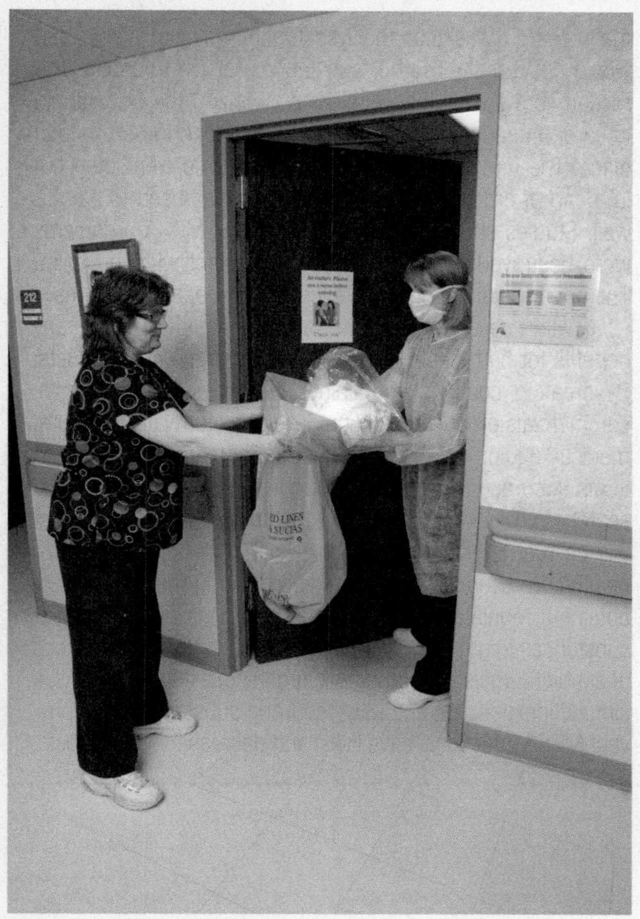

FIGURE 15–53 **To transfer linen from an isolation unit, the worker in the unit places the sealed bag containing the infectious linen inside a second bag held by a "clean" worker outside the unit.**

b. When the bag is full, expel excess air by pushing gently on the bag.

c. Tie a knot at the top of the bag to seal it or fold the top edge twice and tape it securely.

d. Place this bag inside a cuffed biohazardous waste bag held by a "clean" person outside the unit.

e. The outside person then ties the outer bag securely or tapes the outer bag shut.

f. The double-bagged trash should then be burned. Double-bagged infectious waste is autoclaved before incineration or disposal as infectious waste according to legal requirements.

g. At all times, direct contact between the two people transferring trash must be avoided.

12. To transfer equipment from the isolation unit, two people are required:

a. Thoroughly clean and disinfect all equipment in the unit.

b. After cleaning, place equipment in a plastic bag or special isolation bag. Label the bag with the contents and the word "ISOLATION."

c. After folding the bag down twice at the top, tape the bag shut.

d. A second person outside the isolation room should hold a second, cuffed infectious waste bag.

e. The person in isolation places the sealed, contaminated bag inside the bag being held outside the unit. The person in isolation should have no direct contact with the clean bag.

f. The person outside the unit turns down the top of the infectious waste bag twice and securely tapes the bag. The outside person then labels the bag with the contents, for example, "ISOLATION DISHES."

g. The double-bagged material is then sent to Central Supply or another designated area for sterilization and/or decontamination.

13. The transmission-based isolation unit must be kept clean and neat at all times. Equipment no longer needed should be transferred out of the unit using the appropriate isolation technique.

14. Comm Before leaving an isolation room, ask the patient whether a urinal or bedpan is needed. This will save time and energy by reducing the need to return to provide additional patient care shortly after leaving. Also, before leaving, check all safety and comfort points to make sure patient care is complete.

15. Remove isolation garments as previously instructed in Procedure 15:9A.

16. Wash hands thoroughly.

PRACTICE: **Go to the workbook and use the evaluation sheet for 15:9B, Working in a Hospital Transmission-Based Isolation Unit, to practice this procedure. When you believe you have mastered this skill, sign the sheet and give it to your instructor for further action.**

FINAL CHECKPOINT: Using the criteria listed on the evaluation sheet, your instructor will grade your performance.

TODAY'S RESEARCH TOMORROW'S HEALTH CARE

Paint Away Those Germs?

Healthcare-associated infections (HAIs) are a major problem for health care providers. The Centers for Disease Control and Prevention (CDC) estimates that one out of every 20 patients receiving health care may acquire an HAI. In addition, the CDC estimates that HAIs in hospitals alone result in 10 billion dollars of excess medical costs every year. Methicillin-resistant *Staphylococcus aureus*, commonly called MRSA, is one of the most common HAIs. MRSA is a bacterium that causes severe infections in humans. It is difficult to treat because it is resistant to many antibiotics, which means the antibiotics will not eliminate the organism.

Now, thanks to biotechnology researchers at the Rensselaer Polytechnic Institute and Albany Medical College in New York, it may be possible to use paint to kill MRSA germs. The researchers studied a naturally occurring enzyme, lysostaphin, that is used by non-pathogenic (non-disease producing) strains of staphylococcus bacteria to defend themselves against *Staphylococcus aureus*. Lysostaphin is harmless to humans and toxic only to MRSA. It is not an antibiotic to which bacteria could become resistant, and it does not leach chemicals into the environment. Lysostaphin kills MRSA bacteria by slicing open the cell wall, causing the MRSA cell to literally explode and die. One problem encountered during the research was that the lysostaphin was not stable and would not remain in other substances for long periods. The researchers solved this problem by packing the lysostaphin in carbon nanotubes, tiny structures that lock the enzyme in place. The nanotubes containing the enzyme were then put in a can of ordinary house paint, which was used to paint a wall. Studies showed that 100 percent of MRSA organisms were destroyed when they came in contact with the paint. The paint remained effective even after repeated washings.

Within several years, this research could provide many benefits for both health care and other commercial products. By creating coatings containing nanotubes of lysostaphin, commercials products could be developed for walls, furniture, medical equipment, food-processing equipment, and even items such as shoes or hospital gowns. One of the lead researchers, Dr. Jonathan Dordick, estimates that the product will be ready for commercial use within 1–2 years and for health care use after 3 or more years due to the necessity of obtaining regulatory approval. It is also possible that similar substances might be discovered that will eliminate other types of antibiotic-resistant pathogenic organisms. If this happens, a simple, inexpensive, naturally occurring substance could prevent MRSA infections, save lives, and decrease medical costs.

CHAPTER 15 SUMMARY

Understanding the basic principles of infection control is essential for any health care worker in any health care field. Disease is caused by a wide variety of pathogens, or germs. An understanding of the types of pathogens, methods of transmission, and the chain of infection allows health care workers to take precautions to prevent the spread of disease.

Bioterrorism is the use of microorganisms as weapons to infect humans, animals, or plants. The CDC has identified and classified agents that could be used for bioterrorism. In today's world, it is likely that an attack will occur. Every health care worker must constantly be alert to the threat of bioterrorism. Careful preparation of a comprehensive plan against bioterrorism and thorough training of all individuals can limit the effect of the attack and save the lives of many people.

Asepsis is defined as "the absence of disease-producing microorganisms, or pathogens." Various levels of aseptic control are possible. Antisepsis refers to methods that prevent or inhibit the growth of pathogenic organisms. Proper handwashing and using an ultrasonic unit to clean instruments and supplies are examples of antisepsis methods. Disinfection is a process that uses chemical disinfectants to destroy or kill pathogenic organisms, but it is not always effective against spores and viruses. Sterilization is a process that destroys all microorganisms, including spores and viruses. The use of an autoclave is an example of a sterilization method. Instruments and equipment are properly prepared, and then processed in the autoclave to achieve sterilization.

Following the standard precautions established by the CDC helps prevent the spread of pathogens by way of blood, body fluids, secretions, and excretions. The standard precautions provide guidelines for handwashing; wearing gloves; using gowns, masks, and protective eyewear when splashing is likely; proper handling and disposal of contaminated sharp objects; proper disposal of contaminated waste; and proper methods to wipe up spills of blood, body fluids, secretions, and excretions. Every health care worker must be familiar with and follow the recommended standard precautions while working with all patients.

Sterile techniques are used in specific procedures, such as changing dressings. Health care workers must learn and follow sterile techniques when they are required to perform these procedures.

Transmission-based precautions are used for patients who have communicable diseases, or diseases that are easily transmitted from one person to another. An awareness of the major types of transmission-based precautions presented in this unit will help the health care worker prevent the transmission of communicable diseases.

Infection control must be followed when performing any and every health care procedure. By learning and following the principles discussed in this unit, health care workers will protect themselves, patients, and others from disease.

INTERNET SEARCHES

Use the search engines suggested in Chapter 12:9 in this text to search the Internet for additional information about the following topics:

1. **Organizations regulating infection control:** Find the organization sites for the Occupational Safety and Health Administration (OSHA), Centers for Disease Control and Prevention (CDC), National Center for Infectious Diseases (NCID), and the Hospital Infection Control Practices Advisory Committee (HICPAC) to obtain information about regulations governing infection control.
2. **Microbiology:** Search for specific information about bacteria (you can also search for specific types such as *Escherichia coli*), protozoa, fungi, rickettsiae, and viruses.
3. **Diseases:** Obtain information about the method of transmission, signs and symptoms, treatment, and complications for diseases such as hepatitis B, hepatitis C, acquired immune deficiency syndrome (AIDS), Ebola, and specific diseases listed by the discussion of microorganisms in this unit.
4. **Infections:** Research endogenous infections, exogenous infections, hospital-acquired infections, and opportunistic infections.
5. **Bioterrorism:** Find information about pathogens that can be used as weapons, how they are spread, methods for prevention or treatment of diseases caused by these pathogens, and bioterrorism preparedness plans developed as a result of the Bioterrorism Act of 2002.
6. **Foreign trip:** Plan a trip to an exotic foreign country; research the Internet to determine specific health precautions that must be taken during your stay, and determine which immunizations you will need before the trip.
7. **Infection control:** Locate and read the Bloodborne Pathogen Standards, Needlestick Safety and Prevention Act, Standard Precautions, and Transmission-Based Precautions (airborne precautions, droplet precautions, contact precautions, and Ebola virus disease (EVD) precautions).
8. **Medical supply companies:** Search for names of specific medical supply companies to research products available such as autoclaves, chemical disinfectants, and spill clean-up kits.

REVIEW QUESTIONS

1. List the classifications of bacteria by shape and give two (2) examples of diseases caused by each class.
2. Draw the chain of infection and identify three (3) ways to break each section of the chain.
3. Differentiate between antisepsis, disinfection, and sterilization.
4. Develop a plan showing at least five (5) ways you can protect yourself and your family from a bioterrorism attack.
5. List eight (8) times the hands must be washed.
6. Name the different types of personal protective equipment (PPE) and state when each type must be worn to meet the requirements of standard precautions.
7. What level of infection control is achieved by an ultrasonic cleaner? Chemicals? An autoclave?
8. Name three (3) methods that can be used to place sterile items on a sterile field. Identify the types of items that can be transferred by each method.
9. List the three (3) main types of transmission-based precautions and the basic principles that must be followed for each type.
10. What special precautions for personal protective equipment (PPE) must be followed under the CDC guidelines for Ebola virus disease (EVD)?

16 Vital Signs

CHAPTER OBJECTIVES

After completing this chapter, you should be able to:

- List the five main vital signs.
- Convert Fahrenheit to Celsius, or vice versa.
- Read a clinical thermometer to the nearest two-tenths of a degree.
- Measure and record oral temperature accurately.
- Measure and record rectal temperature accurately.
- Measure and record axillary temperature accurately.
- Measure and record tympanic (aural) temperature accurately.
- Measure and record temporal temperature accurately.
- Measure and record radial pulse to an accuracy within ±2 beats per minute.
- Count and record respirations to an accuracy within ±1 respiration per minute.
- Measure and record apical pulse to an accuracy within ±2 beats per minute.
- Measure and record blood pressure to an accuracy within ±2 mm of actual reading.
- State the normal range for oral, axillary, and rectal temperature; pulse; respirations; and systolic and diastolic pressure.
- Define, pronounce, and spell all key terms.

KEY TERMS

apical pulse *(ape' -ih-kal)*
apnea *(ap' -nee" -ah)*
arrhythmia *(ah-rith' -me-ah)*
aural temperature
axillary temperature
blood pressure
bradycardia *(bray' -dee-car' -dee-ah)*
bradypnea *(brad" -ip-nee' -ah)*
character
Cheyne-Stokes *(chain' -stokes")*
clinical thermometers
cyanosis
diastolic *(die" -ah-stall' -ik)*
dyspnea *(dis(p)' -nee" -ah)*
electronic thermometers
fever
homeostasis *(home" -ee-oh-stay' -sis)*
hypertension
hyperthermia *(high-pur-therm' -ee-ah)*
hypotension
hypothermia *(high-po-therm' -ee-ah)*
oral temperature

KEY TERMS (CONT.)

orthopnea *(of″-thop-nee′-ah)*
pain
pulse
pulse deficit
pulse pressure
pyrexia
rales (rawls)
rate
rectal temperature
respirations
rhythm
sphygmomanometer *(sfig″-moh-ma-nam′-eh-ter)*
stethoscope *(steth′-uh-scope)*
systolic *(sis″-tall′-ik)*
tachycardia *(tack″-eh-car′-dee-ah)*
tachypnea *(tack″-ip-nee′-ah)*
temperature
temporal scanning thermometers
temporal temperature
tympanic thermometers
vital signs
volume
wheezing

LEGAL ALERT

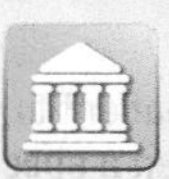

Before performing any procedures in this chapter, know and follow the standards and regulations established by the scope of practice; federal laws and agencies; state laws; state or national licensing, registration, or certification boards; professional organizations; professional standards; and agency policies.

It is your responsibility to learn exactly what you are legally permitted to do and to perform only procedures for which you have been trained.

16:1 Measuring and Recording Vital Signs

Vital signs are defined as various determinations that provide information about the basic body conditions of the patient. The five main vital signs are temperature, pulse, respirations, blood pressure, and pain. Other important vital signs that provide information about the patient's condition include the color of the skin, the size of the pupils in the eyes and their reaction to light, the level of consciousness, and the patient's response to stimuli. As a health care worker, it will be your responsibility to measure and record the vital signs of patients. It is essential that vital signs be accurate. They are often the first indication of a disease or abnormality in the patient.

Temperature is a measurement of the balance between heat lost and heat produced by the body. Temperature can be measured in the mouth (oral), rectum (rectal), armpit (axillary), ear (aural), or by the temporal artery in the forehead (temporal). A low or high reading can indicate disease. Most temperatures are measured in degrees on a thermometer that has a Fahrenheit scale. However, some health care facilities are now measuring temperature in degrees on a Celsius (centigrade) scale. A comparison of the two scales is shown in Figure 16–1 and in Appendix C. At times, it may be necessary to convert Fahrenheit temperatures to Celsius, or Celsius to Fahrenheit. The formulas for the conversion are as follows:

- 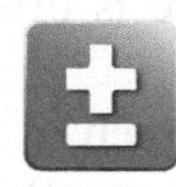

To convert Fahrenheit (F) temperatures to Celsius (C) temperatures, use one of the following formulas:

$$C = (F - 32) \times 5/9 \text{ or } C = (F - 32) \times 0.5556$$

For example, to convert a Fahrenheit temperature of 212 to Celsius, subtract 32 from 212 to get 180. Then multiply 180 by 5/9, or 0.5556, to get the Celsius temperature of 100.0.

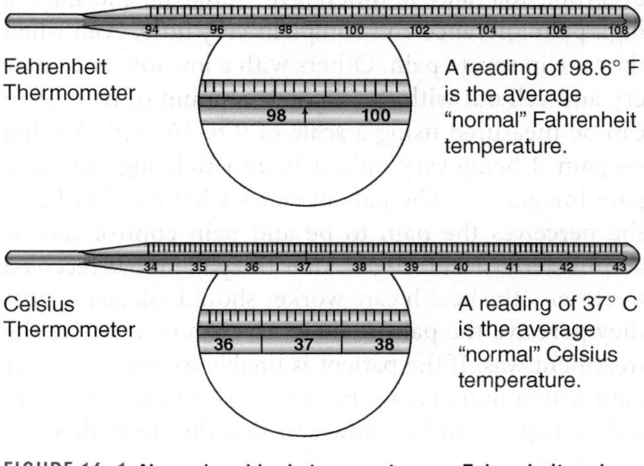

Fahrenheit Thermometer
A reading of 98.6° F is the average "normal" Fahrenheit temperature.

Celsius Thermometer
A reading of 37° C is the average "normal" Celsius temperature.

FIGURE 16–1 Normal oral body temperature on Fahrenheit and Celsius thermometers.

- 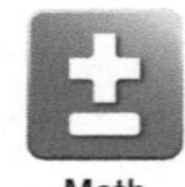

  To convert Celsius (C) temperatures to Fahrenheit (F) temperatures, use one of the following formulas:

$$F = (\tfrac{9}{5} \times C) + 32 \text{ or } F = (1.8 \times C) + 32$$

For example, to convert a Celsius temperature of 37 to Fahrenheit, multiply 37 by $\tfrac{9}{5}$, or 1.8, to get 66.6. Then add 32 to 66.6 to get the Fahrenheit temperature of 98.6.

Pulse is the pressure of the blood felt against the wall of an artery as the heart contracts and relaxes, or beats. The rate, rhythm, and volume are recorded. **Rate** refers to the number of beats per minute, **rhythm** refers to regularity, and **volume** refers to strength, force, or quality. The pulse is usually taken over the radial artery, although it may be felt over any superficial artery that has a bone behind it. Any abnormality can indicate disease.

Respirations reflect the breathing rate of the patient. In addition to the respiration count, the rhythm (regularity) and character (type) of respirations are noted. Abnormal respirations usually indicate that a health problem or disease is present.

Blood pressure is the force exerted by the blood against the arterial walls when the heart contracts or relaxes. Two readings (systolic and diastolic) are noted to show the greatest pressure and the least pressure. Both are very important. Abnormal blood pressure is often the first indication of disease.

Pain is an unpleasant sensation that is perceived in the nervous system when illness or injury occurs. Pain can be acute or chronic. Acute pain lasts for a short amount of time, as with post-operative pain or pain from a physical injury. Chronic pain is long term, as with cancer pain, arthritis, or other on-going illness. When assessing pain it is important to remember that pain is what the person says it is. Only they can describe what they are feeling. Pain is a very individual experience and everyone tolerates it differently. Some people have a high pain tolerance and complain very little, even when they are in severe pain. Others with a low tolerance may cry and yell out with the slightest amount of pain. Pain can be measured using a scale of 0 to 10, with 0 being no pain, 1 being very mild pain and 10 being the worst pain imaginable. The patient states what number he or she perceives the pain to be and pain control can be administered accordingly. After the patient has received treatment, the health care worker should ask again what they perceive the pain to be to assess how effective the treatment was. If the patient is unable to rate his or her pain with a number, a series of faces ranging from very sad to happy can be shown to describe how they are

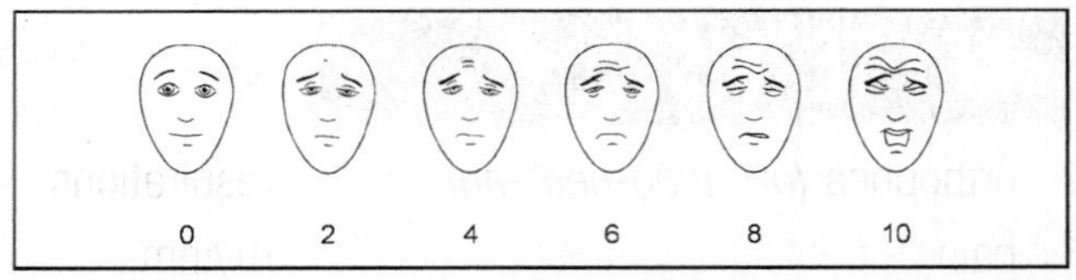

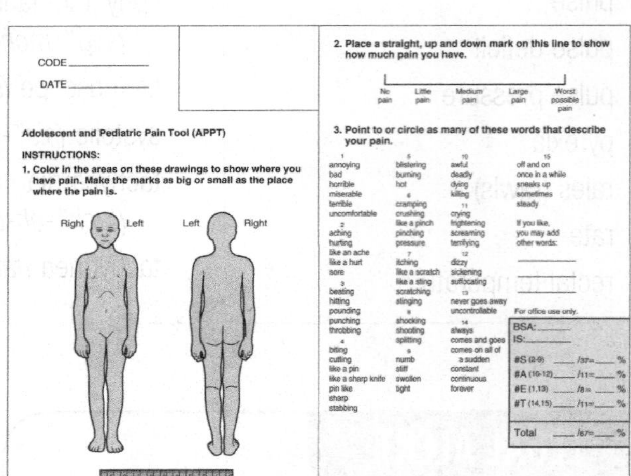

FIGURE 16–2 (A) Pain can be measured by asking the patient to rate the level of pain on a scale of 0 to 10. (B) For children a special scale tool can be used that will allow a child to color an area of the body where they have pain or to circle words that can help describe what they are feeling.

Top image, Hicks CL, von Baeyer CL, Spafford P, van Korlaar I, Goodenough B. Faces Pain-Scale-Revised: Toward a Common Metric in Pediatric Pain Measurement. PAIN 2001; 93: 173-183. With the instructions and translations as found on the website www.iasp-pain.org/FPSR; Bottom image, From Savedra, M., Tesller, M., Holzemer, W., & Ward, J. (1992). University of California, San Francisco, School of Nursing, San Francisco, CA 94143-0606. Copyright © 1989, 1992. Used with permission.

feeling (Figure 16–2). A patient must be assessed for pain frequently because it is often the first sign of a problem.

Another vital sign is the **apical pulse**. This pulse is taken with a stethoscope at the apex of the heart. The actual heartbeat is heard and counted. At times, because of illness, hardening of the arteries, a weak or very rapid radial pulse, or doctor's orders, you will be required to take an apical pulse. Also, because infants and small children have a very rapid radial pulse that is difficult to count, apical pulses are usually taken.

If you note any abnormality or change in any vital sign, it is your responsibility to report this immediately to your supervisor. If you have difficulty obtaining a correct reading, ask another individual to check the patient. Never guess or report an inaccurate reading.

STUDENT: Go to the workbook and complete the assignment sheet for 16:1, Measuring and Recording Vital Signs.

16:2 Measuring and Recording Temperature

OBRA Legal

Body temperature is one of the main vital signs. Guidelines for measuring and recording temperature will vary depending on state laws and policies of health care agencies. It is your legal responsibility to know and follow the guidelines for your state and agency.

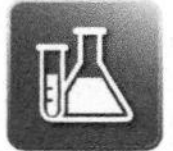
Science

Temperature is defined as "the balance between heat lost and heat produced by the body." Heat is lost through perspiration, respiration, and excretion (urine and feces). Heat is produced by the metabolism of food, and by muscle and gland activity. A constant state of fluid balance, known as **homeostasis**, is the ideal health state in the human body. The rates of chemical reactions in the body are regulated by body temperature. Therefore, if body temperature is too high or too low, the body's fluid balance is affected.

Variations in Body Temperature

The normal range for body temperature is 97°–100° Fahrenheit, or 36.1°–37.8° Celsius (sometimes called centigrade). However, variations in body temperature can occur. Some reasons for variations include:

- *Individual Differences:* some people have accelerated body processes and usually have higher temperatures; others have slower body processes and usually have lower temperatures
- *Time of Day:* body temperature is usually lower in the morning, after the body has rested, and higher in the evening, after muscular activity and daily food intake have taken place
- *Body Sites:* parts of the body where temperatures are taken lead to variations; temperature variations by body site are shown in Table 16–1.

Oral temperatures are taken in the mouth. This is usually the most common, convenient, and comfortable method of obtaining a temperature. Eating, drinking hot or cold liquids, and/or smoking can alter the temperature in the mouth. It is important to make sure the patient has *not* had anything to eat or drink, or has *not* smoked for at least 15 minutes prior to taking the patient's oral temperature. If the patient has done any of these things, explain why you cannot take the temperature and that you will return to do so.

Rectal temperatures are taken in the rectum. This is an internal measurement and is the most accurate of all methods. Rectal temperatures are frequently taken on infants and small children and on patients with hypothermia (below-normal body temperature).

Axillary temperatures are taken in the armpit, under the upper arm. The arm is held close to the body, and the thermometer is inserted between the two folds of skin. A *groin* temperature is taken between the two folds of skin formed by the inner part of the thigh and the lower abdomen. Both axillary and groin are external temperatures and, thus, less accurate.

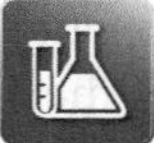
Science

Aural temperatures are taken with a special tympanic thermometer that is placed in the ear or auditory canal. The thermometer detects and measures the thermal, infrared energy radiating from blood vessels in the tympanic membrane, or eardrum. Because this provides a measurement of body core temperature, the range is similar to rectal or internal body temperature. Most tympanic thermometers record temperature in less than 2 seconds; so this is a fast and convenient method for obtaining temperature. However, a drawback to using tympanic thermometers is that inaccurate results will be obtained if the thermometer is not inserted into the ear correctly or if an ear infection or wax buildup is present.

Temporal temperatures are taken with a special temporal scanning thermometer that is passed in a straight line across the forehead, midway between the eyebrows and upper hairline. The thermometer measures the temperature in the temporal artery to provide an accurate measurement of blood temperature. A normal temporal temperature is similar to a rectal temperature, because it measures the temperature inside the body or bloodstream. Because a temporal scanning thermometer is easy to use and usually produces

TABLE 16–1 Temperature Variations by Body Site

	Oral	Rectal and/or Temporal	Axillary and/or Groin
Average Temperature	98.6°F (37°C)	99.6°F (37.6°C)	97.6°F (36.4°C)
Normal Range of Temperature	97.6°F – 99.6°F (36.5°C – 37.5°C)	98.6°F – 100.6°F (37°C – 38.1°C)	96.6°F – 98.6°F (36°C – 37°C)

accurate results, it is a common way to record body temperature. However, if the forehead has a wig or covering on it, is laying on a pillow, or has profuse perspiration on it, an inaccurate result may be obtained.

Body temperatures can be above or below the normal range for a variety of reasons:

- *Causes of increased body temperature:* illness, infection, exercise, excitement, and high temperatures in the environment
- *Causes of decreased body temperature*: starvation or fasting, sleep, decreased muscle activity, mouth breathing, exposure to cold temperatures in the environment, and certain diseases

Very low or very high body temperatures are indicative of abnormal conditions. **Hypothermia** is a low body temperature, below 95°F (35°C) measured rectally. It can be caused by prolonged exposure to cold. Death usually occurs if body temperature drops below 93°F (33.9°C) for a period of time. A **fever** is an elevated body temperature, usually above 101°F (38.3°C) measured rectally. **Pyrexia** is another term for fever. The term *febrile* means a fever is present; *afebrile* means no fever is present or the temperature is within the normal range. Fevers are usually caused by infection or injury. **Hyperthermia** occurs when the body temperature exceeds 104°F (40°C) measured rectally. It can be caused by prolonged exposure to hot temperatures, brain damage, and serious infections. Immediate actions must be taken to lower body temperature, because temperatures above 106°F (41.1°C) can quickly lead to convulsions, brain damage, and death.

Types of Thermometers

Clinical thermometers may be used to record temperatures, but very few health care agencies use them. A clinical thermometer consists of a slender glass tube containing mercury or a heat-reactive mercury-free liquid such as alcohol, which expands when exposed to heat. There are different types of clinical thermometers (Figure 16–3). The glass oral thermometer has a long, slender bulb or a blue tip. A security oral thermometer has a shorter, rounder bulb and is usually marked with a blue tip. A rectal thermometer has a short, stubby, rounded bulb and may be marked with a red tip. In addition, some clinical thermometers have the word "oral" or "rectal" written on their stems. Disposable plastic sheaths may be used to cover the thermometer when it is used on a patient.

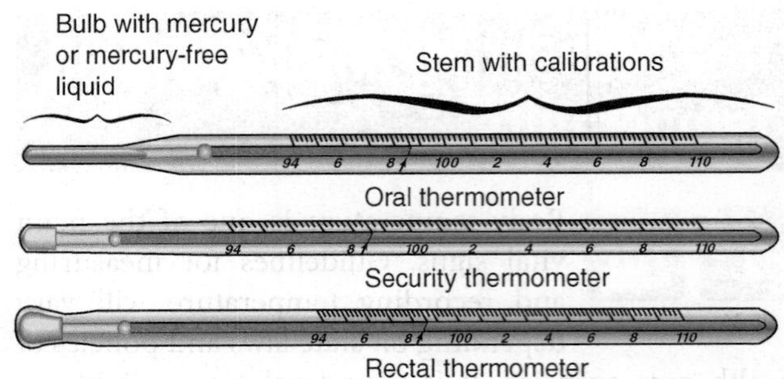

FIGURE 16–3 Types of clinical thermometers.

To avoid the chance of mercury contamination, the Occupational Health and Safety Administration (OSHA), the Environment Protection Agency (EPA), and the American Medical Association (AMA) recommend the use of mercury-free liquid clinical thermometers or digital thermometers. If a clinical thermometer containing mercury breaks, the mercury can evaporate and create a toxic vapor that can harm both humans and the environment. Mercury poisoning attacks the central nervous system in humans. Children, especially those under the age of six, are very susceptible. Mercury can contaminate water supplies and build up in the tissues of fish and animals. Therefore, proper cleanup of a broken clinical thermometer is essential. Only authorized individuals should clean up a mercury spill. *Never* use a vacuum cleaner or broom to clean up mercury because this will break up the beads of mercury and allow them to vaporize more quickly. *Never* pour mercury down a drain or discard it in a toilet because this causes contamination of the water supply. If a mercury-filled thermometer breaks, close doors to other indoor areas and open the windows in the room with the mercury spill to vent any vapors outside. Some facilities have mercury spill kits that provide everything you need to clean up a spill, including an air tight container (refer to Figure 19–72). If this is not available, put on gloves and use two cards or stiff paper to push the droplets of mercury and broken glass into a plastic container with a tight-fitting lid. If necessary, use an eyedropper to pick up the balls of mercury. Shine a flashlight in the area of the spill because the light will reflect off the shiny mercury beads and make them easier to see. Wipe the entire area with a damp sponge. Then place all cleanup material, including the paper, eyedropper, gloves, and sponge, in the plastic container and label it "Mercury for Recycling." Seal the lid tightly and take the container to a mercury recycling center. Most waste disposal companies will accept mercury for recycling. To discard unbroken mercury thermometers, place the intact thermometer in a plastic container with a tight-fitting lid, label it, and take it to a mercury recycling center.

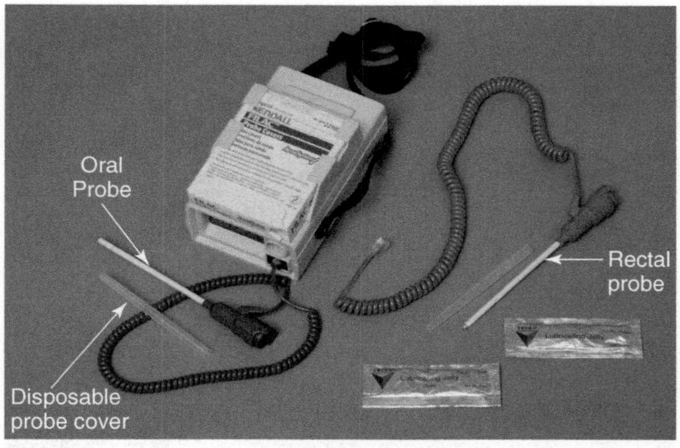

FIGURE 16–4 An electronic thermometer registers the temperature in easy-to-read numbers on a viewer.

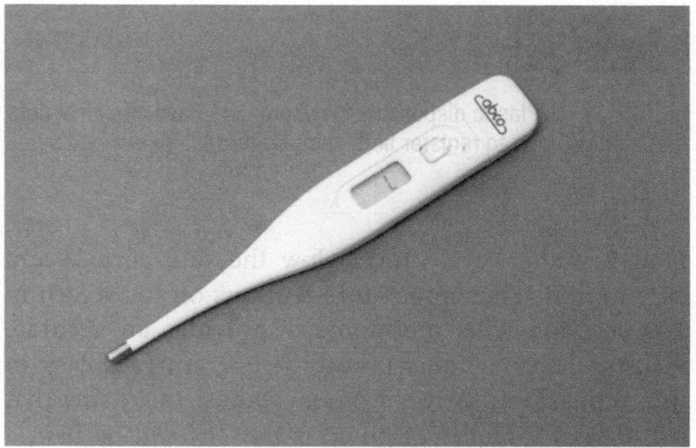
FIGURE 16–5 Electronic digital thermometers are excellent for home use.

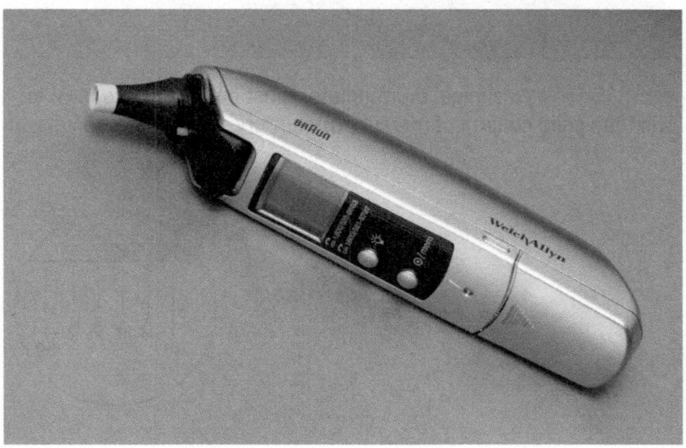
FIGURE 16–6 Tympanic thermometers record the aural temperature in the ear.

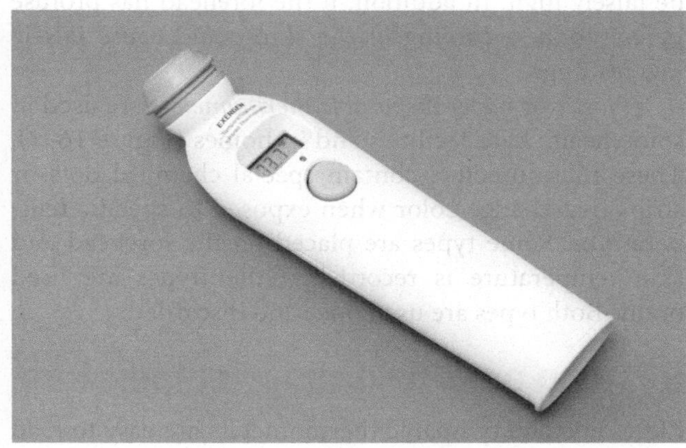
FIGURE 16–7 Temporal scanning thermometers measure the temperature in the temporal artery of the forehead.

Electronic thermometers are used in most health care facilities. This type of thermometer uses a heat sensor to record temperature and displays the temperature on a viewer in a few seconds (Figure 16–4). Electronic thermometers can be used to take oral, rectal, axillary, and/or groin temperatures. Most facilities have electronic thermometers with blue probes for oral or axillary use and red probes for rectal use. To prevent cross-contamination, a disposable cover is placed over the thermometer probe before the temperature is taken. By changing the disposable cover after each use, one unit can be used on many patients. Electronic digital thermometers are excellent for home use because they eliminate the hazard of a mercury spill that occurs when a clinical thermometer is broken (Figure 16–5). The small battery-operated unit usually will register the temperature in about 60 seconds on a digital display screen. Disposable probe covers prevent contamination of the probe.

Tympanic thermometers are specialized electronic thermometers that use an infrared ray to record the aural temperature in the ear (Figure 16–6). A disposable plastic cover is placed on the ear probe. By inserting the probe into the auditory canal and pushing a scan button, the temperature is recorded on the screen within 1–2 seconds. It is important to read and follow instructions while using this thermometer to obtain an accurate reading.

Temporal scanning thermometers are specialized electronic thermometers that use an infrared scanner to measure the temperature in the temporal artery of the forehead (Figure 16–7). The thermometer probe is placed on the forehead and passed in a straight line across the forehead, midway between the eyebrows and upper hairline. In this area, the temporal artery is less

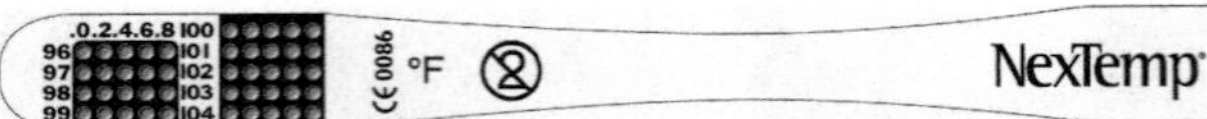

FIGURE 16–8 **Plastic disposable thermometers have chemical dots that change color to register body temperature.** Courtesy Medical Indicators, Inc.

than 2 millimeters (mm) below the skin surface and easy to find. The temperature registers on the screen in 1–2 seconds. This thermometer provides an accurate measurement of internal body temperature, is easy to use, and is noninvasive. It is important to make sure that the area of forehead scanned is not covered by hair, a wig, or a hat. If the person's head is lying on a pillow, the side of the forehead by the pillow should not be used for the measurement. Any type of head covering or a pillow prevents heat from dissipating and causes the reading to be falsely high. In addition, if the forehead has profuse perspiration, a cooling of the skin could cause falsely low readings.

Plastic or *paper disposable thermometers* are used in some health care facilities and in homes (Figure 16–8). These thermometers contain special chemical dots or strips that change color when exposed to specific temperatures. Some types are placed on the forehead and skin temperature is recorded. Other types are used orally. Both types are used once and discarded.

Reading and Recording Temperature

Electronic and tympanic thermometers are easy to read because they have digital displays. Reading a glass clinical thermometer is a procedure that must be practiced. The thermometer should be held at eye level and rotated slowly to find the solid column of mercury or mercury-free liquid (Figure 16–9). The thermometer is read at the point where the liquid line ends. Each long line on a thermometer is read as 1 degree. An exception to this is the long line for 98.6°F (37°C), which is the normal oral body temperature. Each short line represents 0.2 (two-tenths) of a degree. Temperature is always recorded to the next nearest two-tenths of a degree. In Figure 16–10, the line ends at 98.6°F (the inset explains the markings for each line).

To record the temperature, write 98^6 instead of 98.6. This reduces the possibility of making an error in reading. For example, a temperature of 100.2 could easily be read as 102. By writing 100^2, the chance of error decreases. If a temperature is taken orally, it is not necessary to indicate that it is an oral reading. If it is taken rectally, place an (R) beside the recording; if in the axillary area, use an (Ax); if in the eardrum or tympanically (aurally), use an (A) or (T) or

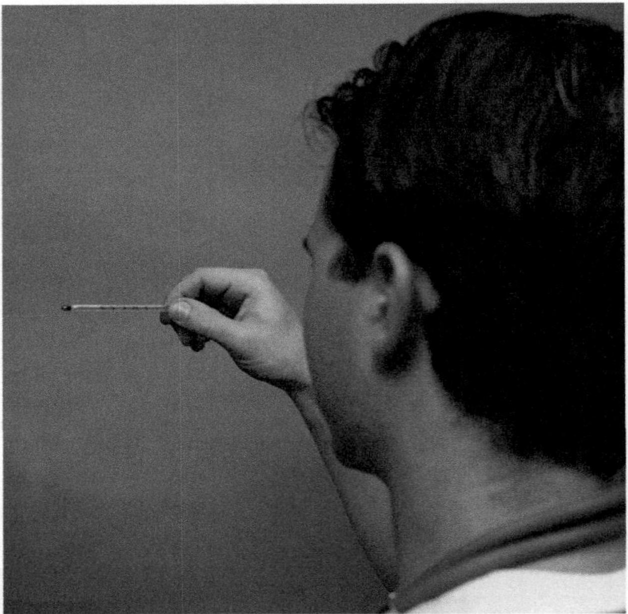

FIGURE 16–9 **A clinical thermometer must be held at eye level to find the solid column of mercury or mercury-free liquid.**

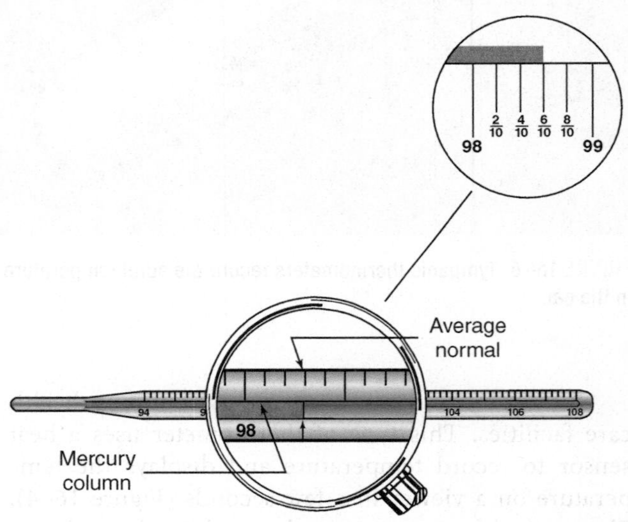

FIGURE 16–10 **Each line on a thermometer equals two-tenths of a degree, so the thermometer shown reads 98.6°F.**

(Tym); and if over the temporal artery, or temporally, use a (TA). For example:

- 98^6 is an oral reading
- 99^6 (R) is a rectal reading
- 97^6 (Ax) is an axillary reading
- 98^6 (A) is an aural reading
- 99^6 (TA) is a temporal artery reading

Cleaning Thermometers

Thermometers must be cleaned thoroughly after use. The procedure used varies with different agencies and types of thermometers. In some agencies, the glass clinical thermometer is washed and rinsed. Cool water is used to prevent breakage and to avoid destroying the column of liquid. The thermometer is then soaked in a disinfectant solution (frequently 70 percent alcohol) for a minimum of 30 minutes before it is used again. Other agencies cover the clinical thermometer with a plastic sheath that is discarded after use (Figure 16–11). The probe on electronic thermometers is covered with a plastic sheath that is discarded after each use. These covers prevent the thermometers from coming into contact with each patient's mouth or skin and prevent transmission of germs. Electronic thermometers all use disposable probes so contamination of the thermometer is limited. Some health care facilities do use disinfectants to wipe the outside of electronic thermometers to prevent the spread of infection between patients. In most cases, it is best to follow the recommendations of the manufacturer for cleaning and proper care of electronic thermometers. Every health care worker should learn and follow the agency's policy for cleaning and care of thermometers.

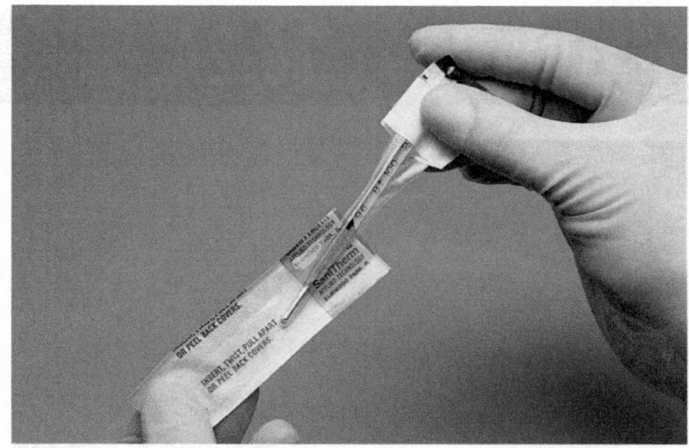

FIGURE 16–11 A clinical thermometer can be covered with a plastic sheath that is discarded after each use.

STUDENT: **Go to the workbook and complete the assignment sheet for 16:2, Measuring and Recording Temperature. Then return and continue with the procedures.**

PROCEDURE 16:2A

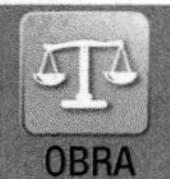

OBRA

Measuring and Recording Oral Temperature with a Clinical Thermometer

Equipment and Supplies

Oral thermometer, plastic sheath (if used), holder with disinfectant solution, tissues or dry cotton balls, container for used tissues, watch with second hand, soapy cotton balls, disposable gloves, notepaper, pen and/or computer

Procedure

1. Assemble equipment.
2. Wash hands and put on gloves.

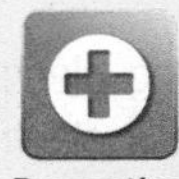

Precaution

CAUTION: Follow standard precautions for contact with saliva or the mucous membrane of the mouth.

3. Introduce yourself. Identify the patient. Explain the procedure.

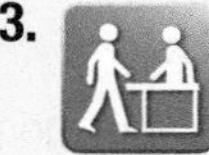

Comm

4. Position the patient comfortably. Ask the patient if he/she has eaten, has had hot or cold fluids, or has smoked in the past 15 minutes.

NOTE: Eating, drinking liquids, or smoking can affect the temperature in the mouth. Wait at least 15 minutes if the patient says "yes" to your question.

5. Remove the clean thermometer by the upper end. Use a clean tissue or dry cotton ball to wipe the thermometer from stem to bulb.

NOTE: If the thermometer was soaking in a disinfectant, rinse first in cool water.

Safety

CAUTION: Hold the thermometer securely to avoid breaking.

(continues)

PROCEDURE 16:2A (CONT.)

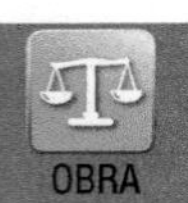

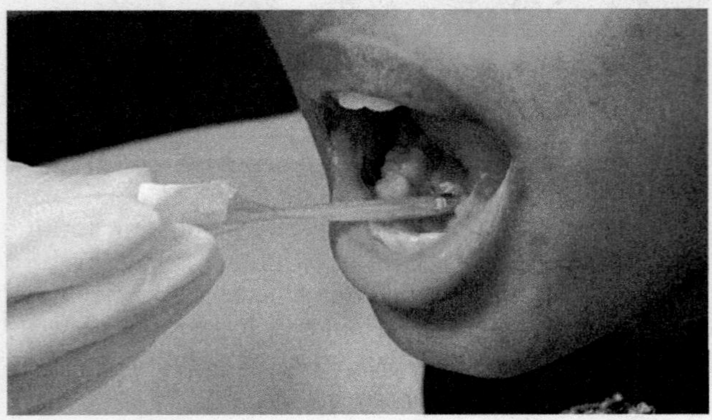

FIGURE 16–12 **Insert the bulb of the thermometer under the patient's tongue (sublingually).**

6. Read the thermometer to be sure it reads 96°F (35.6°C) or lower. Check carefully for chips or breaks.

CAUTION: Never use a cracked thermometer because it may injure the patient.

7. If a plastic sheath is used, place it on the thermometer.
8. Insert the bulb under the patient's tongue, toward the side of the mouth (Figure 16–12). Ask the patient to hold it in place with the lips, and caution against biting it.

   NOTE: Check to be sure patient's mouth is closed.
9. Leave the thermometer in place for 3–5 minutes.

   NOTE: Some agencies require that a clinical thermometer be left in place for 5–8 minutes. Follow your agency's policy.
10. Remove the thermometer. Hold it by the stem and use a tissue or cotton ball to wipe toward the bulb.

    NOTE: If a plastic sheath was used to cover the thermometer, there is no need to wipe the thermometer. Simply remove the sheath, taking care not to touch the part that was in the patient's mouth.

CAUTION: Do ***not*** hold the bulb end. This could alter the reading because of the warmth of your hand.

11. Read the thermometer. Record the reading on notepaper.

    NOTE: Recheck the reading and your notation for accuracy.

    NOTE: If the reading is less than 97°F, reinsert the thermometer in the patient's mouth for 1–2 minutes.
12. Check the patient for comfort and safety before leaving.

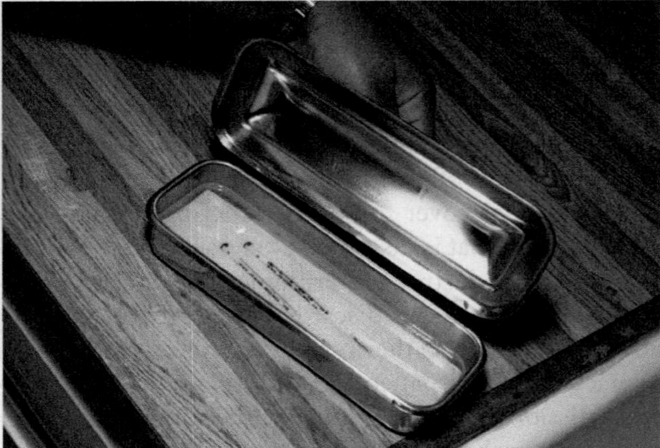

FIGURE 16–13 **Soak the thermometer in a disinfectant solution for a minimum of 30 minutes.**

13. Clean the thermometer following agency policy. General guidelines include:
    a. Wearing gloves, use a soapy cotton ball to wipe the thermometer once from the top to the tip or bulb. Discard the cotton ball.
    b. With the bulb pointed downward, hold the thermometer by the stem and rinse it in cool water.
    c. Hold the thermometer securely between your thumb and index finger. Use a snapping motion of the wrist to shake the thermometer down to 96°F (35.6°C) or lower.
    d. Place the thermometer in a small basin or container filled with a disinfectant solution. Make sure the thermometer is completely covered by the solution (Figure 16–13).
    e. Allow the thermometer to soak for the recommended time, usually 30 minutes.
14. Replace all equipment.
15. Remove gloves and discard in infectious waste container. Wash hands.
16. Record all required information on the patient's chart or enter it into the computer. For example: date and time, T 98^6, your signature and title. Report any abnormal reading to your supervisor immediately.

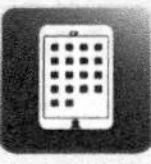

NOTE: In health care agencies using electronic health records (EHRs), also known as electronic medical records (EMRs), the information is entered directly into the patient's record on a computer.

PROCEDURE 16:2A (CONT.)

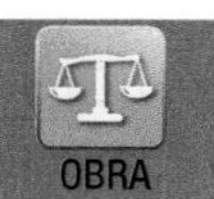

PRACTICE: Go to the workbook and use the evaluation sheet for 16:2A, Measuring and Recording Oral Temperature with a Clinical Thermometer, to practice this procedure. When you believe you have mastered this skill, sign the sheet and give it to your instructor for further action.

Check

FINAL CHECKPOINT: Using the criteria listed on the evaluation sheet, your instructor will grade your performance.

PROCEDURE 16:2B

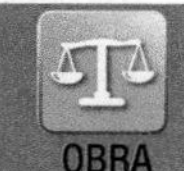

Measuring Oral Temperature with an Electronic Thermometer

Equipment and Supplies

Electronic thermometer with blue probe, sheath (probe cover) gloves, paper, pen and/or computer, container for soiled sheath

Procedure

1. Assemble equipment.

   NOTE: Read the operating instructions for the electronic thermometer so you understand how the particular model operates.

2. Wash hands. Put on gloves if needed.

   Precaution

   CAUTION: Follow standard precautions.

   NOTE: Some health care facilities do not require gloves for an oral temperature taken with an electronic thermometer because there is usually no contact with oral fluids. Follow agency policy.

3. 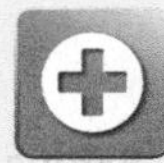 Comm

   Introduce yourself. Identify the patient. Explain the procedure.

4. Position the patient comfortably. Ask the patient if he/she has eaten, has had hot or cold fluids, or has smoked in the past 15 minutes. Wait at least 15 minutes if the patient answers "yes."

5. If the blue probe has to be connected to the thermometer unit, insert the probe into the correct receptacle. If the thermometer has an "on" or "activate" button, push the button to turn on the thermometer.

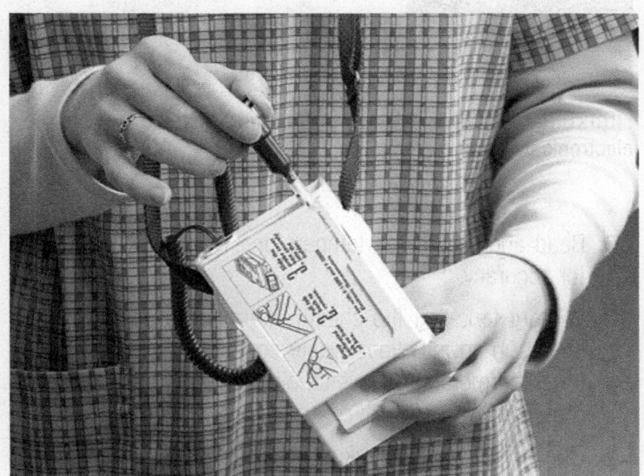

FIGURE 16–14A **Install a probe cover on the thermometer.**

6. Cover the probe with the sheath or probe cover (Figure 16–14A).

7. Insert the covered probe under the patient's tongue toward the side of the mouth. Ask the patient to close his or her mouth but to avoid biting down on the thermometer. Most probes are heavy, so it is usually necessary to hold the probe in position (Figure 16–14B).

8. When the unit signals that the temperature has been recorded, remove the probe.

   NOTE: Many electronic thermometers have an audible "beep." Others indicate that temperature has been recorded when the numbers stop flashing and become stationary.

   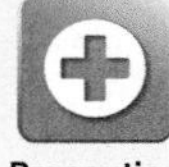

   Precaution

   CAUTION: Do not touch the probe cover. It is contaminated with the patient's saliva.

(continues)

PROCEDURE 16:2B (CONT.)

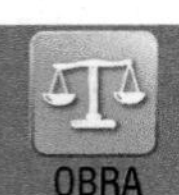

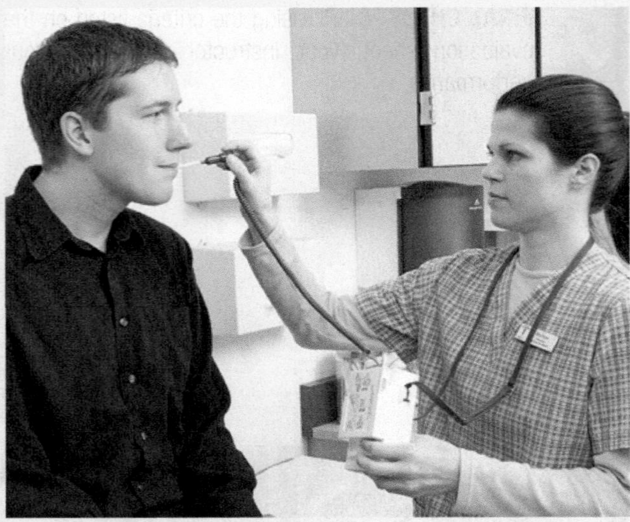

FIGURE 16–14B While taking a temperature, hold the probe of the electronic thermometer in place.

9. Read and record the temperature. Recheck your reading for accuracy.
10. Without touching the sheath or probe cover, discard the sheath in an infectious waste container (Figure 16–14C). Most thermometers have an eject button that is pushed to remove the sheath.
11. Observe all safety checkpoints before leaving the patient.
12. Return the probe to the correct storage position in the thermometer unit. Turn off the unit if this is necessary. Place the unit in the charging stand if the model has a charging unit.
13. Replace all equipment.
14. Remove gloves if worn and discard in an infectious waste container. Wash hands.
15. 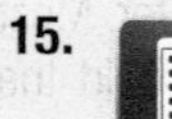  EHR Comm Record all required information on the patient's chart or enter it into the electronic health record (EHR). For example: date and time, T 98^8, your signature and title. Report any abnormal reading immediately to your supervisor.

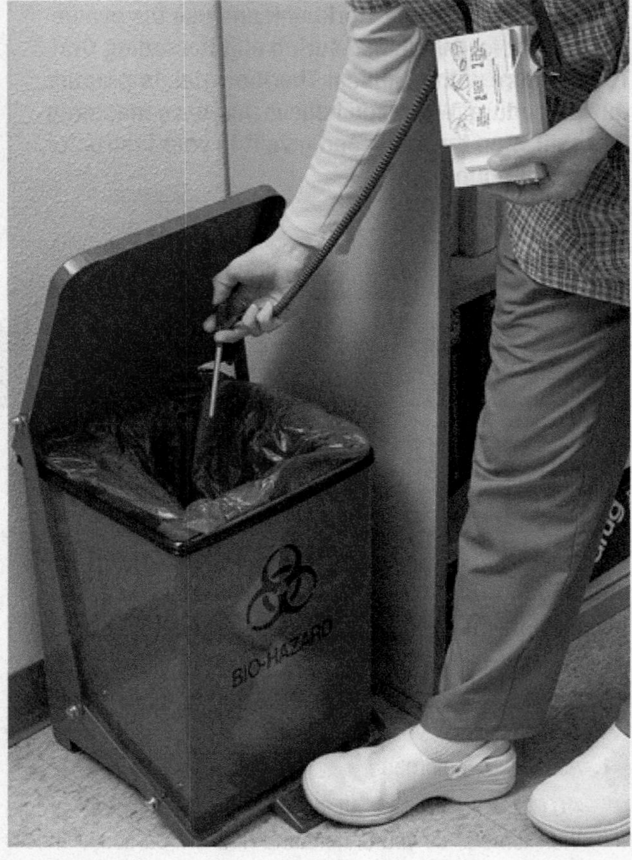

FIGURE 16–14C Discard the probe cover in an infectious-waste container without touching the cover.

PRACTICE: Go to the workbook and use the evaluation sheet for 16:2B, Measuring Oral Temperature with an Electronic Thermometer, to practice this procedure. When you believe you have mastered this skill, sign the sheet and give it to your instructor for further action.

Check

FINAL CHECKPOINT: Using the criteria listed on the evaluation sheet, your instructor will grade your performance.

PROCEDURE 16:2C

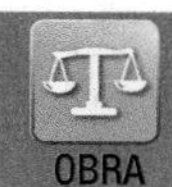

OBRA

Measuring and Recording Rectal Temperature

Equipment and Supplies

Electronic thermometer with red probe or rectal thermometer, plastic sheath or probe cover, lubricant, tissues/cotton balls, waste bag or container, watch with second hand, paper, pen, and/or computer, disposable gloves

NOTE: A manikin is frequently used to practice this procedure.

Procedure

1. Assemble equipment.
2. Wash hands and put on gloves.

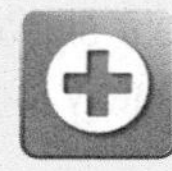

Precaution

CAUTION: Follow standard precautions if contact with rectal discharge is possible.

3.  Comm

Introduce yourself. Identify the patient. Explain the procedure. Screen unit, draw curtains, and/or close door to provide privacy for the patient.

4. Prepare the thermometer.
   a. Insert the red probe on the electronic thermometer. Cover the probe with a disposable sheath or probe cover. Turn the thermometer on.
   b. If a clinical thermometer is being used, remove it from its container. If the thermometer was soaking in a disinfectant, hold it by the stem end and rinse in cool water. Use a dry tissue/cotton ball to wipe from stem to bulb. Check that the thermometer reads 96°F (35.6°C) or lower. Check condition of thermometer. If a plastic sheath is used, position it on the thermometer.

Safety

CAUTION: Breaks in a thermometer can injure the patient. Never use a cracked thermometer.

5. Place a small amount of lubricant on the tissue. Roll the tip of the probe or the bulb end of the thermometer in the lubricant to coat it. Leave the lubricated thermometer on the tissue until the patient is properly positioned.
6. Turn the patient on his or her side. If possible, use Sims' position (lying on left side with right leg bent up near the abdomen). Infants are usually placed on their backs, with legs raised and held securely, or on their abdomens (Figure 16–15).

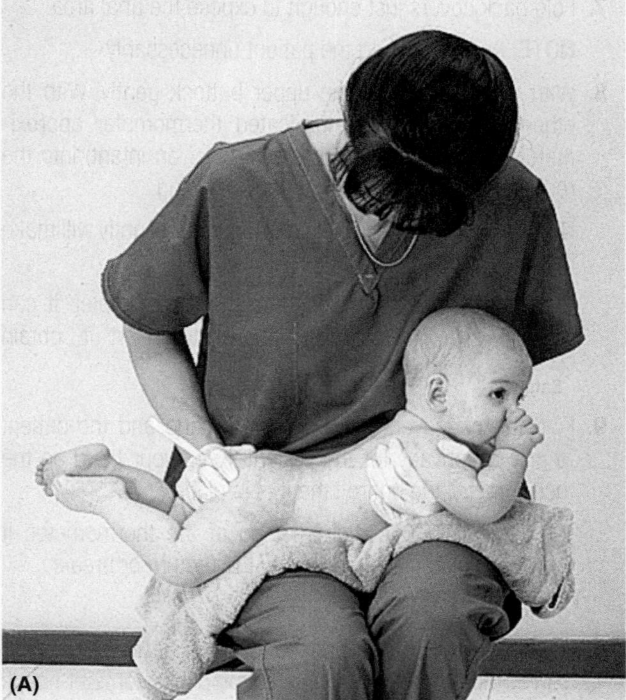
(A)

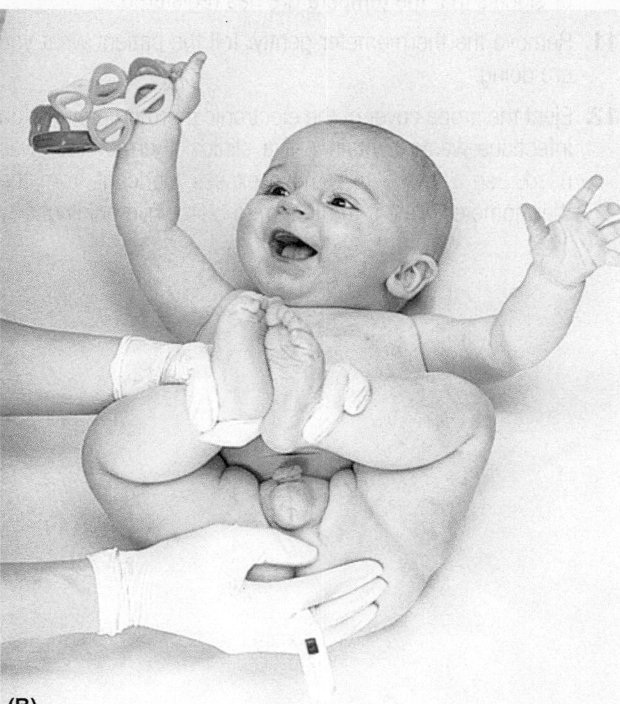
(B)

FIGURE 16–15 **The infant can be positioned on the (A) abdomen or (B) back for a rectal temperature.**

(continues)

PROCEDURE 16:2C (CONT.)

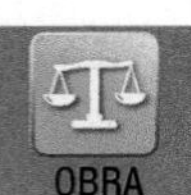

7. Fold back covers just enough to expose the anal area.

   NOTE: Avoid exposing the patient unnecessarily.

8. With one hand, raise the upper buttock gently. With the other hand, insert the lubricated thermometer approximately 1 to 1½ inches (½ to 1 inch for an infant) into the rectum. Tell the patient what you are doing.

   NOTE: At times, rotating the thermometer slightly will make it easier to insert.

   CAUTION: Never force the thermometer. It can break. If you are unable to insert it, obtain assistance.

9. Fold the bedcovers back over your hand and the patient to provide privacy for the patient. Keep your hand on the thermometer the entire time it is in place.

   CAUTION: *Never* let go of the thermometer. It could slide further into the rectum or break.

10. Hold the thermometer in place for 3–5 minutes for a clinical thermometer, or until the electronic thermometer beeps or signals that the temperature has registered.

11. Remove the thermometer gently. Tell the patient what you are doing.

12. Eject the probe cover of the electronic thermometer into an infectious waste container. If a clinical thermometer was used, use a tissue to remove excess lubricant from the thermometer. Wipe it from stem to bulb while holding it by the stem area only. Discard the tissue into an infectious waste container.

13. Read and record. Recheck your reading for accuracy. Remember to place an (R) next to the recording to indicate a rectal temperature was taken.

14. Reposition the patient. Observe all safety checkpoints before leaving the patient.

15. Clean the thermometer following agency policy.

16. Replace all equipment.

17. Remove gloves and discard in infectious waste container. Wash hands.

18. 

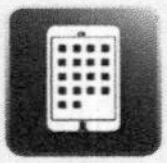

Record all required information on the patient's chart or enter it into the electronic health record (EHR). For example: date and time, T 99^6 (R), your signature and title. Report any abnormal reading immediately to your supervisor.

PRACTICE: Go to the workbook and use the evaluation sheet for 16:2C, Measuring and Recording Rectal Temperature, to practice this procedure. When you believe you have mastered this skill, sign the sheet and give it to your instructor for further action.

FINAL CHECKPOINT: Using the criteria listed on the evaluation sheet, your instructor will grade your performance.

PROCEDURE 16:2D

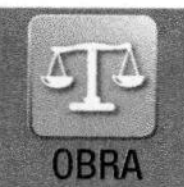
OBRA

Measuring and Recording Axillary Temperature

Equipment and Supplies

Electronic thermometer with blue probe or oral thermometer, probe cover or sheath, disposable gloves (if needed), tissues/towel, waste container, watch with second hand, paper, pen, and/or computer

Procedure

1. Assemble equipment.
2. Wash hands. Put on gloves if necessary.

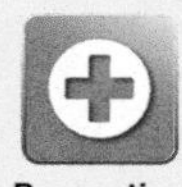
Precaution

CAUTION: Follow standard precautions if contact with open sores or body fluids is possible.

3.  Comm

Introduce yourself. Identify the patient. Explain the procedure.

4. Prepare the thermometer.
   a. Insert the blue probe on the electronic thermometer. Cover the probe with a disposable sheath or probe cover. Turn the thermometer on.
   b. If a clinical thermometer is being used, remove it from its container. Use a tissue to wipe from stem to bulb. Check the thermometer for damaged areas. Read the thermometer to be sure it reads below 96°F (36.5°C). Place a plastic sheath on the thermometer, if used.
5. Expose the axilla and use a towel to pat the armpit dry.
   NOTE: Moisture can alter a temperature reading. Do not rub area hard because this too can alter the reading.
6. Raise the patient's arm and place the tip or bulb end of the thermometer in the hollow of the axilla (Figure 16–16). Bring the arm over the chest or abdomen.
7. Leave the thermometer in place for 10 minutes for a clinical thermometer, or until the electronic thermometer beeps or signals that the temperature has registered.
8. Remove the thermometer. Eject the probe cover of the electronic thermometer into an infectious waste container. If a clinical thermometer was used, use a tissue to wipe from stem to bulb to remove moisture. Hold by the stem end only.

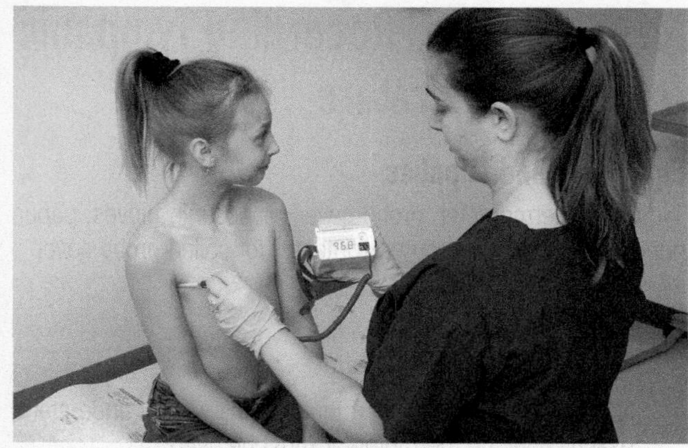

FIGURE 16–16 **To take an axillary temperature, insert the thermometer in the hollow of the axilla or armpit.**

Safety

CAUTION: Holding the bulb end will change the reading.

9. Read and record. Check your reading for accuracy. Remember to mark (Ax) by the recording to indicate axillary temperature.
10. Reposition the patient. Be sure to check for safety and comfort before leaving.
11. Clean the thermometer following agency policy.
12. Replace all equipment used.
13. Remove gloves if worn and discard in an infectious waste container. Wash hands.
14.  Comm 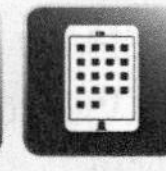 EHR

Record all required information on the patient's chart or enter it into the electronic health record (EHR). For example: date and time, T 97^6 (Ax), your signature and title. Report any abnormal reading immediately to your supervisor.

PRACTICE: Go to the workbook and use the evaluation sheet for 16:2D, Measuring and Recording Axillary Temperature, to practice this procedure. When you believe you have mastered this skill, sign the sheet and give it to your instructor for further action.

Check

FINAL CHECKPOINT: Using the criteria listed on the evaluation sheet, your instructor will grade your performance.

PROCEDURE 16:2E

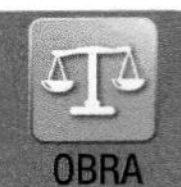

Measuring and Recording Tympanic (Aural) Temperature

Equipment and Supplies

Tympanic thermometer, probe cover, disposable gloves, paper, pencil/pen, and/or computer, container for soiled probe cover

Procedure

1. Assemble equipment.

   NOTE: Read the operating instructions so you understand exactly how the thermometer must be used.

2. Wash hands. Put on gloves if needed.

   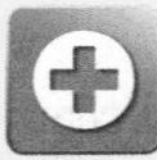
   Precaution

   CAUTION: Follow standard precautions if contact with open sores or body fluids is possible.

3. 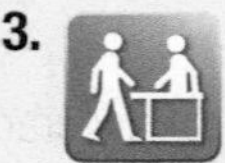
   Comm

   Introduce yourself. Identify the patient. Explain the procedure.

4. Remove the thermometer from its base and turn it on. A *ready* or series of lines will usually appear on the screen.

5. Install a probe cover according to instructions (Figure 16–17A). This will usually activate the thermometer.

6. Position the patient. Infants under 1 year of age should be positioned lying flat with the head turned for easy access to the ear. Small children can be held on the parent's lap, with the head held against the parent's chest for support. Adults who can cooperate and hold the head steady can either sit or lie flat. Patients in bed should have the head turned to the side, and stabilized against the pillow.

7. Hold the thermometer in your right hand to take a temperature in the right ear, and in your left hand to take a temperature in the left ear. With your other hand, pull the ear pinna (external lobe) up and back on any child over 1 year of age and on adults (Figure 16–17B). Pull the ear pinna straight back for infants under 1 year of age.

   NOTE: Pulling the pinna correctly straightens the auditory canal so the probe tip will point directly at the tympanic membrane.

8. Insert the covered probe into the ear canal as far as possible to seal the canal. Do not apply pressure.

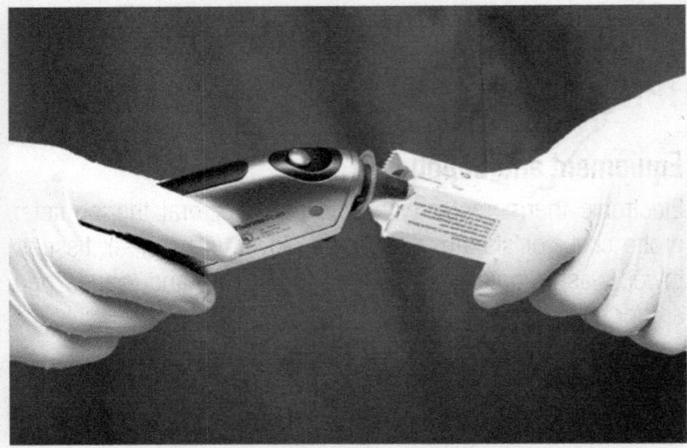

FIGURE 16–17A Install a disposable probe cover on the tympanic thermometer.

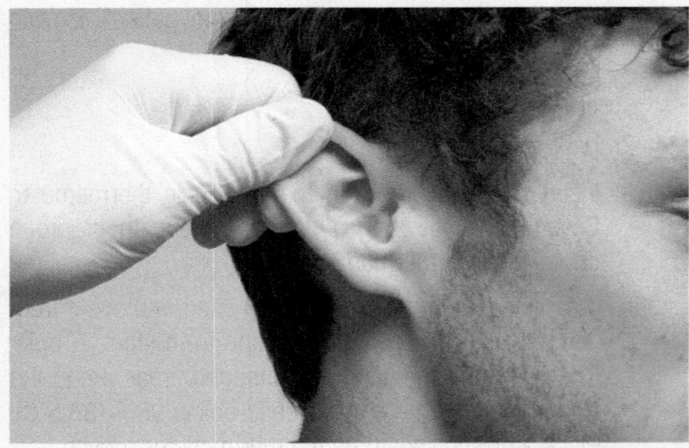

FIGURE 16–17B Before inserting the tympanic thermometer, pull the pinna up and back on adults and children older than 1 year.

9. Rotate the thermometer handle slightly until it is aligned with the patient's jaw. Hold the thermometer steady and press the scan or activation button (Figure 16–17C). Hold it for the required amount of time, usually 1–2 seconds, until the reading is displayed on the screen.

10. Remove the thermometer from the patient's ear. Read and record the temperature. Place an (A), (T), or (Tym) by the recording to indicate tympanic temperature.

    NOTE: The temperature will remain on the screen until the probe cover is removed.

PROCEDURE 16:2E (CONT.)

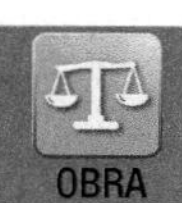

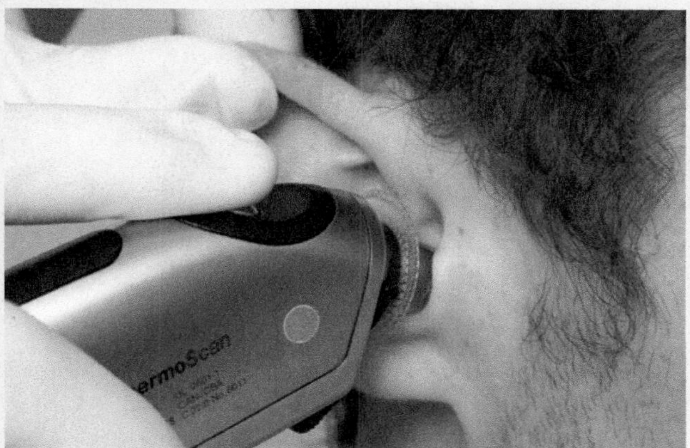

FIGURE 16–17C **After inserting the covered probe of the tympanic thermometer into the ear canal, press the scan or activation button and hold the thermometer steady until the temperature reading is displayed.**

CAUTION: If the temperature reading is low or does not appear to be accurate, change the probe cover and repeat the procedure. The opposite ear can be used for comparison.

11. Press the eject button on the thermometer to discard the probe cover into a waste container.
12. Return the thermometer to its base.
13. Reposition the patient. Observe all safety checkpoints before leaving the patient.
14. Remove gloves if worn and discard in an infectious waste container. Wash hands.
15.  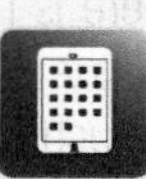 Record all required information on the patient's chart or enter it into the electronic health record (EHR). For example: date and time, T 98° (A), your signature and title. Report any abnormal reading immediately to your supervisor.

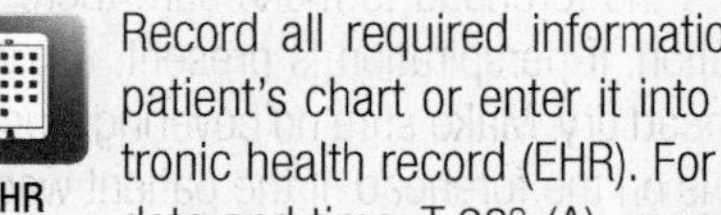

PRACTICE: Go to the workbook and use the evaluation sheet for 16:2E, Measuring and Recording Tympanic (Aural) Temperature, to practice this procedure. When you believe you have mastered this skill, sign the sheet and give it to your instructor for further action.

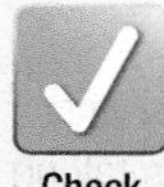

FINAL CHECKPOINT: Using the criteria listed on the evaluation sheet, your instructor will grade your performance.

PROCEDURE 16:2F

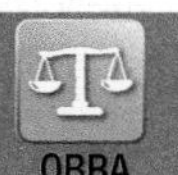

Measuring and Recording Temporal Temperature

Equipment and Supplies

Temporal scanning thermometer, disinfectant wipe or probe cover, paper, pen and/or computer

Procedure

1. Assemble equipment.

   NOTE: Read the operating instructions for the temporal scanning thermometer so you understand how the particular model works.
2. Wash hands.
3.  Introduce yourself. Identify the patient. Explain the procedure.
4. Remove the protective cap on the lens of the thermometer. Hold the thermometer upside down to clean the lens with disinfectant wipe and allow it to dry. Check the lens for cleanliness after it has dried.

   NOTE: Holding the thermometer upside down prevents excess moisture from entering the sensor area. The moisture will not harm the sensor, but a temperature cannot be taken until the sensor lens is dry.

   NOTE: Some temporal thermometers use disposable probe covers. If a probe cover is used, the probe does not have to be cleaned with alcohol.

(continues)

PROCEDURE 16:2F (CONT.)

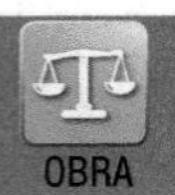
OBRA

5. Position the patient comfortably. Adults who can cooperate and hold the head steady can either sit or lie flat. Infants younger than 1 year should be positioned lying flat on the back. Small children can be held on the parent's lap, with the head held against the parent's chest for support, or lying flat.
6. Check the forehead to make sure there is no sign of perspiration. If perspiration is present, use a towel to pat the forehead dry. Make sure no covering, such as a hat, wig, or hair, is on the forehead. If the patient was lying on a pillow, do not use the side of the forehead that was on the pillow.

Safety

CAUTION: Head coverings or a pillow prevent heat from dissipating from the forehead and cause a falsely high temperature reading.

7. Gently position the probe flat on the center of the forehead, midway between the eyebrow and hairline. Press and hold the scan button.
8. Slide the thermometer across the forehead lightly and slowly (Figure 16–18). Keep the sensor flat and in contact with the skin until you reach the hairline on the side of the face.

   NOTE: The thermometer will emit a beeping sound and a red light will blink to indicate that a measurement is taking place.
9. Release the scan button and remove the thermometer from the head.

   NOTE: If sweating is profuse and you are not able to dry the forehead completely, use a different method to obtain the temperature.
10. Read and record the temperature that is displayed on the thermometer. Double-check your reading.
11. Press and release the activation button quickly to turn off the thermometer. If a probe cover was used, remove and discard the cover. Wipe the lens with a disinfectant wipe and let it air dry. Put the protective cap on the lens to protect the lens.

    NOTE: Most thermometers will turn off automatically after 30 seconds to 1 minute.

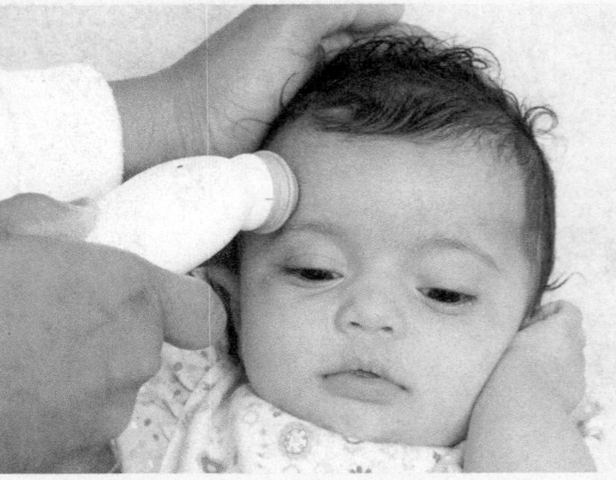

FIGURE 16–18 **To take a temporal temperature, hold the scan button while lightly sliding the thermometer across the forehead midway between the eyebrow and hairline.**

12. Reposition the patient. Observe all safety checkpoints before leaving the patient.
13. Replace all equipment.
14. Wash hands.
15.  Comm 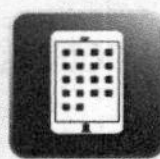 EHR Record all required information on the patient's chart or enter it into the electronic health record (EHR). For example: date and time, T 99^8 (TA), your signature, and your title. Report any abnormal reading immediately to your supervisor.

PRACTICE: **Go to the workbook and use the evaluation sheet for 16:2F, Measuring and Recording Temporal Temperature, to practice this procedure. When you believe you have mastered this skill, sign the sheet and give it to your instructor for further action.**

Check

FINAL CHECKPOINT: Using the criteria listed on the evaluation sheet, your instructor will grade your performance.

16:3 Measuring and Recording Pulse

OBRA

Pulse is a vital sign that you will be required to take. There are certain facts you must know when you take this measurement.

Science

Pulse refers to the pressure of the blood pushing against the wall of an artery as the heart beats and rests. In other words, it is a throbbing of the arteries that is caused by the contractions of the heart. The pulse is more easily felt in arteries that lie fairly close to the skin and can be pressed against a bone by the fingers.

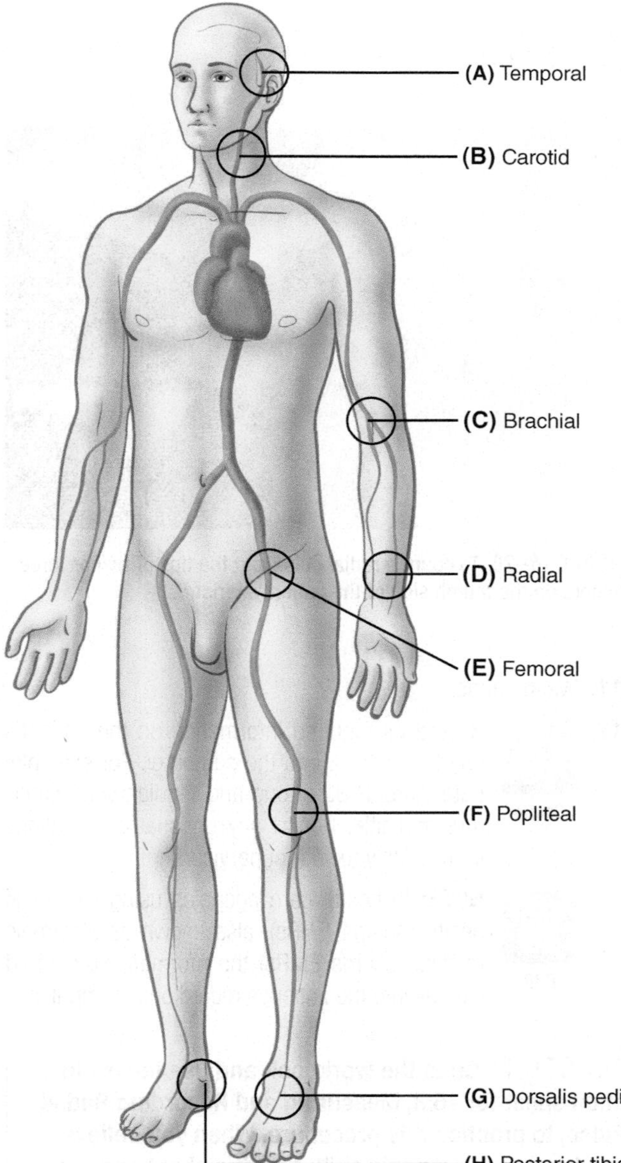

FIGURE 16–19 Major pulse sites.

The pulse can be felt at different arterial sites on the body. Some of the major sites are shown in Figure 16–19 and include:

- *Temporal:* on either side of the forehead
- *Carotid:* at the neck on either side of the trachea
- *Brachial:* inner aspect of forearm at the antecubital space (crease of the elbow)
- *Radial:* at the inner aspect of the wrist, above the thumb
- *Femoral:* at the inner aspect of the upper thigh where the thigh joins with the trunk of the body
- *Popliteal:* behind the knee
- *Dorsalis pedis:* at the top of the foot arch
- *Posterior tibial:* just below and behind the medial malleolus (the bony part of the ankle that sticks out on the inner or big toe side of the leg)

NOTE: *Pulse is usually taken over the radial artery.*

Each time a pulse is measured, three different facts must be noted: the rate, the rhythm, and the volume of the pulse. These facts are important to provide complete information about the pulse. For example, a pulse of 82, strong and regular, is much different than a pulse of 82, weak and very irregular.

The **rate** of the pulse is measured as the number of beats per minute. Pulse rates vary among individuals, depending on age, sex, and body size:

- *Adults:* general range of 60–100 beats per minute
- *Adult men:* 60–70 beats per minute
- *Adult women:* 65–80 beats per minute
- *Children aged over 7:* 70–100 beats per minute
- *Children aged from 1–7:* range of 80–110 beats per minute
- *Infants:* 100–160 beats per minute
- **Bradycardia**: a pulse rate under 60 beats per minute
- **Tachycardia**: a pulse rate over 100 beats per minute (except in children)

NOTE: *Any variations or extremes in pulse rates should be reported immediately.*

Rhythm of the pulse is also noted. Rhythm refers to the regularity of the pulse, or the spacing of the beats. It is described as *regular* or *irregular*. An **arrhythmia** is an irregular or abnormal rhythm, usually caused by a defect in the electrical conduction pattern of the heart.

Volume, or the strength, force, quality, or intensity of the pulse, is also noted. It is described by words such as bounding, *strong, weak,* or *thready*.

Various factors will change pulse rate. Increased, or accelerated, rates can be caused by exercise, stimulant drugs, excitement, fever, dehydration, shock, nervous tension, and other similar factors. Decreased, or slower, rates can be caused by sleep, depressant drugs, heart disease, coma, physical training, and other similar factors.

STUDENT: **Go to the workbook and complete the assignment sheet for 16:3, Measuring and Recording Pulse. Then return and continue with the procedure.**

PROCEDURE 16:3 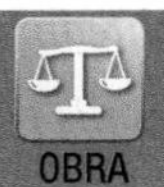

Measuring and Recording Radial Pulse

Equipment and Supplies

Watch with second hand, paper, pen and/or computer

Procedure

1. Assemble equipment.
2. Wash hands.
3.  Introduce yourself. Identify the patient. Explain the procedure.
4. Place the patient in a comfortable position, with the arm supported and the palm of the hand turned downward.

   NOTE: If the forearm rests on the chest, it will be easier to count respirations after taking the pulse.
5. With the tips of your first two or three fingers, locate the pulse on the thumb side of the patient's wrist (Figure 16–20).

   NOTE: Do not use your thumb; use your fingers. The thumb contains a pulse that you may confuse with the patient's pulse.
6. When the pulse is felt, exert slight pressure and start counting. Use the second hand of the watch and count for 1 full minute.

   NOTE: In some agencies, the pulse is counted for 30 seconds and the final number multiplied by 2. To detect irregularities, it is better to count for 1 full minute.
7. While counting the pulse, also note the volume (character or strength) and the rhythm (regularity).
8. Record the following information: date, time, rate, rhythm, and volume. Follow your agency's policy for recording.
9. Check the patient before leaving. Observe all safety precautions to protect the patient.
10. Replace all equipment used.

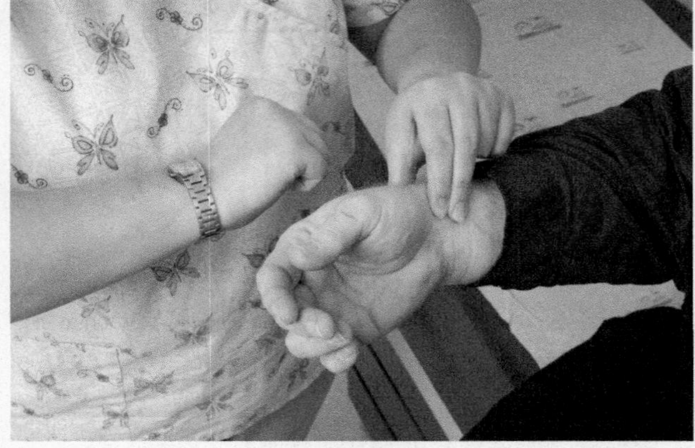

FIGURE 16–20 To count a radial pulse, put the tips of two or three fingers on the thumb side of the patient's wrist.

11. Wash hands.
12.  Record all required information on the patient's chart or enter it into the computer. For example: date, time, P 82 strong and regular, your signature and title. Report any unusual observations immediately to your supervisor.

    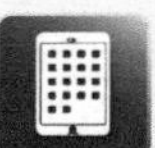 **NOTE:** In health care agencies using electronic health records (EHRs), also known as electronic medical records (EMRs), the information is entered directly into the patient's record on a computer.

PRACTICE: Go to the workbook and use the evaluation sheet for 16:3, Measuring and Recording Radial Pulse, to practice this procedure. When you believe you have mastered this skill, sign the sheet and give it to your instructor for further action.

 **FINAL CHECKPOINT:** Using the criteria listed on the evaluation sheet, your instructor will grade your performance.

16:4 Measuring and Recording Respirations

 Respirations are another vital sign that you must observe, count, and record correctly. This section provides the main points you must note when counting and recording the quality of respirations.

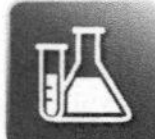 **Respiration** is the process of taking in oxygen (O_2) and expelling carbon dioxide (CO_2) from the lungs and respiratory tract. One respiration consists of one inspiration (breathing in) and one expiration (breathing out).

Each time respiration is measured, three different facts must be noted: the rate, the character, and the rhythm of respirations. These three facts provide complete information about how the patient is breathing.

For example, a respiration measurement of 18, deep and regular, is much different than a measurement of 18, very shallow and irregular.

Rate of respirations counts the numbers of breaths per minute. The normal rate for respirations in adults is a range of 12–20 breaths per minute. In children, respirations are slightly faster than those for adults and average 16–30 per minute. In infants, the rate may be 30–50 per minute.

In addition to rate, the character and rhythm of respirations should be noted. Character refers to the depth and quality of respirations. Words used to describe character include *deep, shallow, labored, difficult, stertorous* (abnormal sounds like snoring), and *moist*. Rhythm refers to the regularity of respirations, or equal spacing between breaths. It is described as *regular* or *irregular*.

The following terminology is used to describe abnormal respirations:

- Dyspnea: difficult or labored breathing
- Apnea: absence of respirations, usually a temporary period of no respirations
- Tachypnea: rapid, shallow respiratory rate above 25 respirations per minute
- Bradypnea: slow respiratory rate, usually below 10 respirations per minute
- Orthopnea: severe dyspnea in which breathing is very difficult in any position other than sitting erect or standing
- Cheyne-Stokes: abnormal breathing pattern characterized by periods of dyspnea followed by periods of apnea; frequently noted in the dying patient
- Rales: bubbling, crackling, or noisy sounds caused by fluids or mucus in the air passages
- Wheezing: difficult breathing with a high-pitched whistling or sighing sound during expiration; caused by a narrowing of bronchioles (as seen in asthma) and/or an obstruction or mucus accumulation in the bronchi
- Cyanosis: a dusky, bluish discoloration of the skin, lips, and/or nail beds as a result of decreased oxygen and increased carbon dioxide in the bloodstream

Respirations must be counted in such a way that the patient is unaware of the procedure. Because respirations are partially under voluntary control, patients may breathe more quickly or more slowly when they become aware of the fact that respirations are being counted. Do not tell the patient you are counting respirations. Also, leave your hand on the pulse site while counting respirations. The patient will think you are still counting pulse and will not be likely to alter the respiratory rate.

STUDENT: **Go to the workbook and complete the assignment sheet for 16:4, Measuring and Recording Respirations. Then return and continue with the procedure.**

PROCEDURE 16:4

OBRA

Measuring and Recording Respirations

Equipment and Supplies

Watch with second hand, paper, pen and/or computer

Procedure

1. Assemble equipment.
2. Wash hands.
3. 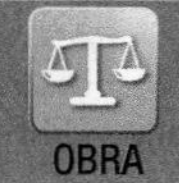 Comm Introduce yourself. Identify the patient.
4. After the pulse rate has been counted, leave your hand in position on the pulse site and count the number of times the chest rises and falls during 1 minute (Figure 16–21).

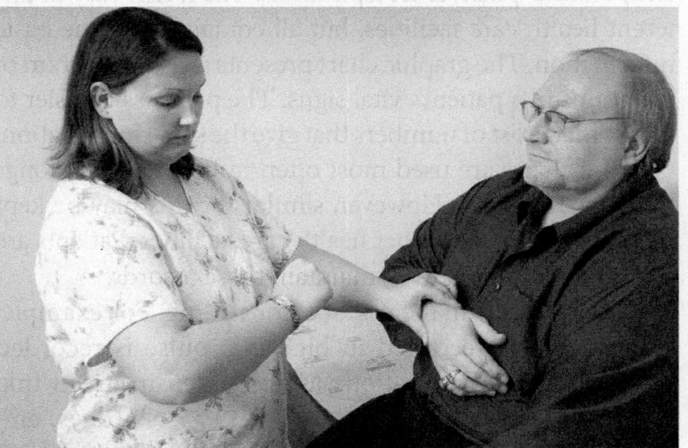

FIGURE 16–21 **Positioning the patient's hand on his chest makes it easier to count pulse and respiration.**

(continues)

PROCEDURE 16:4 (CONT.)

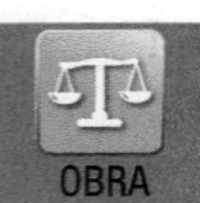

NOTE: This is done so the patient is not aware that respirations are being counted. If patients are aware, they can alter their rate of breathing.

5. Count each expiration and inspiration as one respiration.
6. Note the depth (character) and rhythm (regularity) of the respirations.
7. Record the following information: date, time, rate, character, and rhythm.
8. Check the patient before leaving the area. Observe all safety precautions to protect the patient.
9. Replace all equipment.
10. Wash hands.
11.  Record all required information on the patient's chart or enter it into the computer. For example: date, time, R 16 deep and regular (or even), your signature and title. Report any unusual observations immediately to your supervisor.

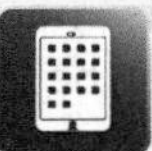

NOTE: In health care agencies using electronic health records (EHRs), also known as electronic medical records (EMRs), the information is entered directly into the patient's record on a computer.

PRACTICE: **Go to the workbook and use the evaluation sheet for 16:4, Measuring and Recording Respirations, to practice this procedure. When you believe you have mastered this skill, sign the sheet and give it to your instructor for further action.**

FINAL CHECKPOINT: Using the criteria listed on the evaluation sheet, your instructor will grade your performance.

16:5 Graphing TPR

In some agencies, you may be required to chart temperature, pulse, and respirations (TPR) on graphic records. This section provides basic information about these records.

Graphic sheets are special records used for recording temperature, pulse, and respirations. The forms vary in different health care facilities, but all contain the same basic information. The graphic chart presents a visual diagram of variations in a patient's vital signs. The progress is easier to follow than a list of numbers that give the same information. Graphic charts are used most often in hospitals and long-term-care facilities. However, similar records may be kept in medical offices or other health care facilities. Patients are sometimes taught how to maintain these records.

Some charts make use of color coding. For example, temperature is recorded in blue ink, pulse is recorded in red ink, and respirations are recorded in green ink. Other agencies use blue ink for 7 AM to 7 PM (days) and red ink for 7 PM to 7 AM (nights). Follow the policy of your institution.

Factors that affect vital signs are often included on the graph. Examples include surgery, medications that lower temperature (such as aspirin), and antibiotics.

 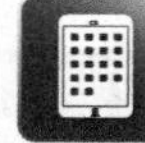

Computer software programs may also be used to create a graphic chart for vital signs. After vital signs have been entered into the computer, the software program records the entries on a graphic chart. The chart can be printed and used as a patient record or kept in a patient's electronic health record (EHR).

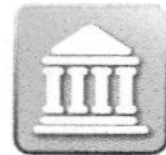

The graph is a medical record, so it must be neat, legible, and accurate. Double-check all information recorded on the graph. If an error occurs, it should be crossed out carefully with red ink and initialed. Correct information should then be inserted on the graph.

STUDENT: **Read the complete procedure for 16:5, Graphing TPR. Then go back and start doing the procedure. Your assignment will follow the procedure.**

PROCEDURE 16:5

Graphing TPR

Equipment and Supplies

Blank TPR graphic sheets in the workbook, TPR sample graph, assignment sheets on graphing in the workbook, pen, ruler, or computer with graphic program

Procedure

1. Assemble equipment.
2. Examine the sample graphic sheet (Figure 16–22). This will vary, depending on the agency. However, most graphic sheets contain time blocks across the top and number blocks for TPRs on the side. Note areas for recording temperature, pulse, and respirations. Refer to the example while completing the procedure steps.
3. Using a blank graphic sheet, fill in patient information in the spaces provided at the top. Write last name first in most cases. Be sure patient identification, hospital, and room number are accurate.

   NOTE: Forms vary. Follow directions as they apply to your form.
4. Fill in the dates in the spaces provided after DATE.

   NOTE: A graphic chart provides a day-to-day visual representation of the variations in a patient's TPRs.
5. If your chart calls for DAY IN HOSPITAL below the dates, enter *Adm* under the first date. This stands for day of

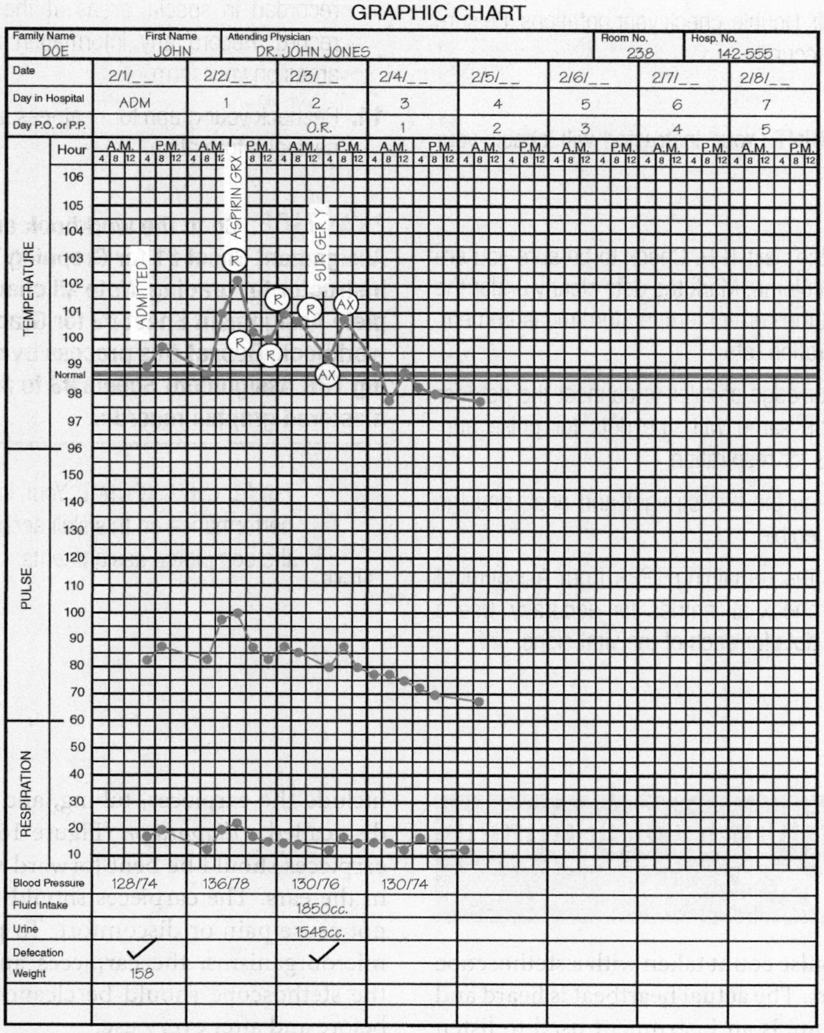

GRAPHIC CHART

Family Name DOE	First Name JOHN	Attending Physician DR. JOHN JONES			Room No. 238	Hosp. No. 142-555		
Date	2/1/__	2/2/__	2/3/__	2/4/__	2/5/__	2/6/__	2/7/__	2/8/__
Day in Hospital	ADM	1	2	3	4	5	6	7
Day P.O. or P.P.			O.R.	1	2	3	4	5
Hour	A.M. 4 8 12 P.M. 4 8 12	A.M. 4 8 12 P.M. 4 8 12	A.M. 4 8 12 P.M. 4 8 12	A.M. 4 8 12 P.M. 4 8 12	A.M. 4 8 12 P.M. 4 8 12	A.M. 4 8 12 P.M. 4 8 12	A.M. 4 8 12 P.M. 4 8 12	A.M. 4 8 12 P.M. 4 8 12
TEMPERATURE (106–96, 98.6 Normal)	ADMITTED	ASPIRIN GR X; R	SURGERY; R; AX					
PULSE (150–60)								
RESPIRATION (50–10)								
Blood Pressure	128/74	136/78	130/76	130/74				
Fluid Intake			1850cc.					
Urine			1545cc.					
Defecation	✓		✓					
Weight	158							

FIGURE 16–22 A sample graphic sheet.

(continues)

PROCEDURE 16:5 (CONT.)

admission. The second date would then be day 1, or first full day in the hospital. The third date would be day 2, and so forth.

6. Some graphs contain a third line, DAYS PO or PP, which means days post-op (after surgery) or postpartum (after delivery of a baby). The day of surgery would be shown as *OR or Surgery*. The next day would be day 1, or first day after surgery. The day of delivery of a baby is shown as *Del*, with the next day as day 1, or first day after delivery. Numbers continue in sequence for each following day.
7. Go to the Assignment Sheet #1. Note the TPRs. On the graphic sheet, find the correct *Date and Time* column. Move down the column until the correct temperature number is found on the side of the chart. Mark this with a dot (•) in the box. Do the same for the pulse and respirations.

Safety

CAUTION: Double-check your notations. Be sure they are accurate.

Check

CHECKPOINT: Your instructor will check your notations.

8. Repeat step 7 for the next TPR. Check to be sure you are in the correct time column. Mark the dots clearly under the time column and at the correct temperature measurement, pulse rate, or respiration rate.
9. Use a straight paper edge or ruler to connect the dots for temperature. Do the same with the dots for pulse and, finally, with the dots for respiration.

   NOTE: A ruler makes the line straight and neat, and the readings are more legible.
10. Continue to graph the remaining TPRs from Assignment Sheet #1. Double-check all entries for accuracy. Use a ruler to connect all dots for each of the vital signs.
11. Any drug that might alter or change temperature or other vital sign is usually noted on the graph in the time column closest to the time when the drug was first given. Turn the paper sideways and write the name of the drug in the correct time column. Aspirin is often recorded in this column because it lowers temperature. A rapid drop in body temperature would be readily explained by the word aspirin in the time column. Antibiotics and medications that alter heart rate are also noted in many cases.
12. Other events in a patient's hospitalization are also recorded in the time column. Examples include surgery and discharge. In some hospitals, if the patient is placed in isolation, this is also noted on the graph.
13. Blood pressure, weight, height, defecation (bowel movements), and other similar kinds of information are often recorded in special areas at the bottom of the graphic record. Record any information required in the correct areas on your form.
14. Recheck your graph for neatness, accuracy, and completeness of information.

PRACTICE: **Go to the workbook and complete Assignment Sheet #1 for Graphing TPR. Give it to your instructor for grading. Note all changes. Then complete Assignment Sheet #2 for Graphing TPR in the workbook. Repeat this process by completing Graphing TPR Assignment Sheets #3 to #5 until you have mastered graphic records.**

Check

FINAL CHECKPOINT: Your instructor will grade your performance on this skill according to the accuracy of the completed assignments.

16:6 Measuring and Recording Apical Pulse

An **apical pulse** is a pulse count taken with a stethoscope at the apex of the heart. The actual heartbeat is heard and counted. A **stethoscope** is an instrument used to listen to internal body sounds. The stethoscope amplifies the sounds so they are easier to hear. Parts of the stethoscope include the earpieces, tubing, and bell or thin, flexible disk called a *diaphragm* (Figure 16–23). The tips of the earpieces should be bent forward when they are placed in the ears. The earpieces should fit snugly but should not cause pain or discomfort. To prevent the spread of microorganisms, the earpieces and bell/diaphragm of the stethoscope should be cleaned with a disinfectant before and after every use.

Usually, a physician orders an apical pulse. It is frequently ordered for patients with irregular heartbeats,

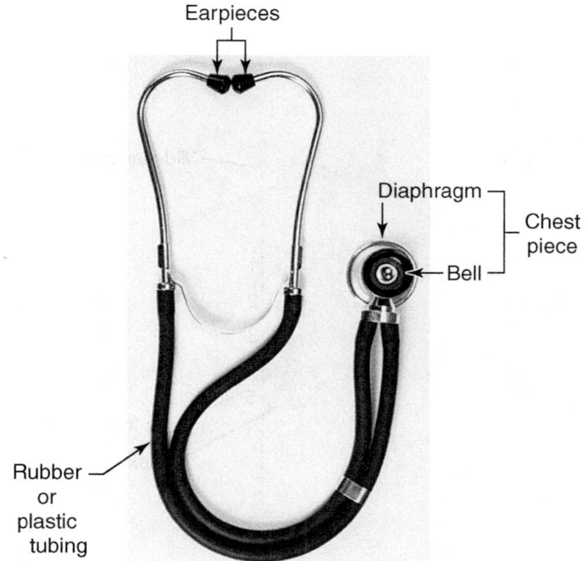

FIGURE 16–23 Parts of a stethoscope.

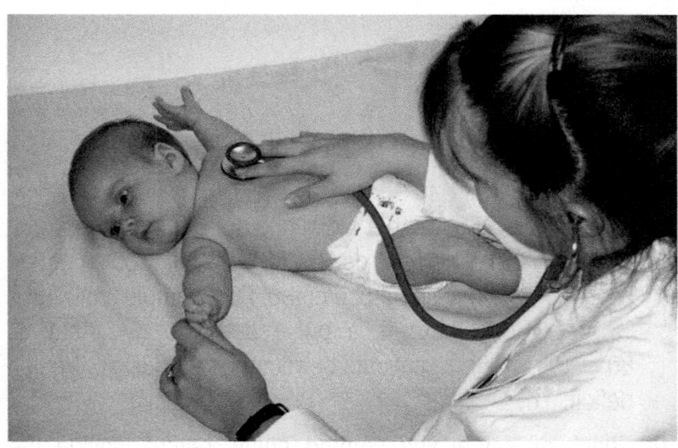

FIGURE 16–24 An apical pulse is frequently taken on infants and small children because their pulses are more rapid.

hardening of the arteries, or weak or rapid radial pulses. Because children and infants have very rapid radial pulse counts, apical pulse counts are usually taken (Figure 16–24). It is generally easier to count a rapid pulse while listening to it through a stethoscope than by feeling it with your fingers.

It is important that you protect the patient's privacy when counting an apical pulse. Avoid exposing the patient during this procedure.

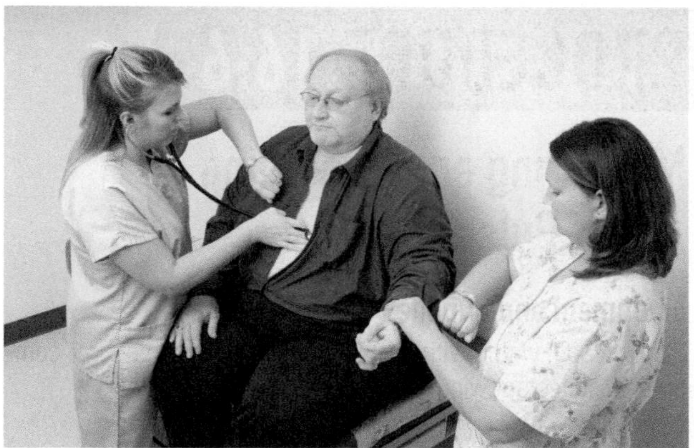

FIGURE 16–25 To determine a pulse deficit, one person should count an apical pulse while another person is counting a radial pulse.

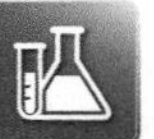

Two separate heart sounds are heard while listening to the heartbeat. The sounds resemble a "lubb-dupp." Each lubb-dupp counts as one heartbeat. The sounds are caused by the closing of the heart valves as blood flows through the chambers of the heart. Any abnormal sounds or beats should be reported immediately to your supervisor.

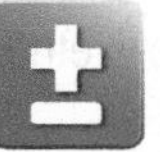

A **pulse deficit** is a condition that occurs with some heart conditions. In some cases, the heart is weak and does not pump enough blood to produce a pulse. In other cases, the heart beats too fast (tachycardia), and there is not enough time for the heart to fill with blood; therefore, the heart does not produce a pulse during each beat. In such cases, the apical pulse rate is higher than the pulse rate at other pulse sites on the body. For the most accurate determination of a pulse deficit, one person should check the apical pulse while a second person checks another pulse site, usually the radial pulse (Figure 16–25). If this is not possible, one person should first check the apical pulse and then immediately check the radial pulse. Then, subtract the rate of the radial pulse from the rate of the apical pulse. The difference is the pulse deficit. For example, if the apical pulse is 130 and the radial pulse is 92, the pulse deficit would be 38 (130 − 92 = 38).

STUDENT: **Go to the workbook and complete the assignment sheet for 16:6, Measuring and Recording Apical Pulse. Then return and continue with the procedure.**

PROCEDURE 16:6

Measuring and Recording Apical Pulse

Equipment and Supplies

Stethoscope, watch with second hand, paper, pen and/or computer, disinfectant wipe

Procedure

1. Assemble equipment. Use a disinfectant to wipe the earpieces and the bell/diaphragm of the stethoscope.
2. Wash hands.
3. 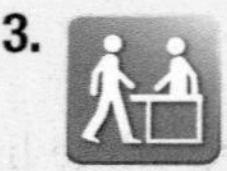
Comm
Introduce yourself. Identify the patient and explain the procedure. If the patient is an infant or child, explain the procedure to the parent(s).

   NOTE: It is usually best to say, "I am going to listen to your heartbeat." Some patients do not know what an apical pulse is.
4. Close the door to the room. Screen the unit or draw curtains around the bed to provide privacy.
5. Uncover the left side of the patient's chest. The stethoscope must be placed directly against the skin.

   NOTE: If the diaphragm of the stethoscope is cold, warm it by placing it in the palm of your hand before placing it on the patient's chest.
6. Place the stethoscope tips in your ears. Locate the apex of the heart, 2–3 inches to the left of the breastbone. Use your index finger to locate the fifth intercostal (between the ribs) space at the midclavicular (collarbone) line (Figure 16–26). Place the bell/diaphragm over the apical region and listen for heart sounds.

   Safety
   CAUTION: Be sure the tips of the stethoscope are facing forward before placing them in your ears.
7. Count the apical pulse for 1 full minute. Note the rate, rhythm, and volume.

   NOTE: Remember to count each lubb-dupp as one beat.
8. If you doubt your count, recheck your count for another minute.
9. Record your reading. Note date, time, rate, rhythm, and volume. Chart according to the agency policy. Some use an A and others use an AP to denote apical pulse.

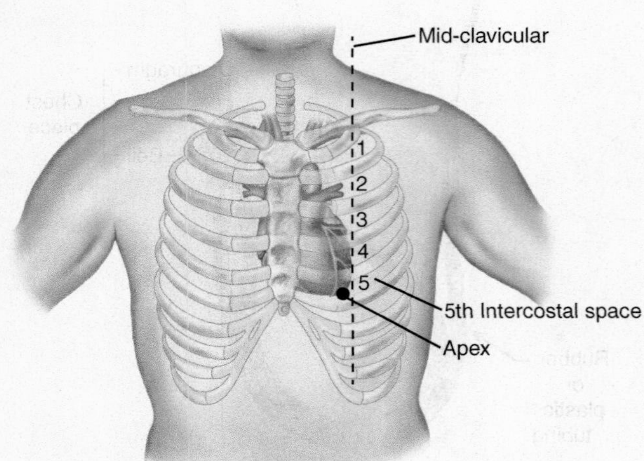

FIGURE 16–26 **Locate the apex of the heart at the fifth intercostal (between the ribs) space by the midclavicular (middle of the collarbone) line.**

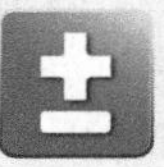
Math
NOTE: If both a radial and apical pulse are taken, it may be recorded as A82/R82. If a pulse deficit exists, it should be noted. For example, with A80/R64, there is a pulse deficit of 16 (that is, $80 - 64 = 16$). This would be recorded as A80/R64 pulse deficit: 16.

10. Check all safety and comfort points before leaving the patient.
11. Use a disinfectant wipe to clean the earpieces and the bell/diaphragm of the stethoscope. If the tubing contacted the patient's skin, wipe the tubing with a disinfectant. Replace all equipment.
12. Wash hands.
13. 
Comm
Record all required information on the patient's chart or enter it into the computer. For example: date, time, AP 86 strong and regular, your signature and title. If any abnormalities or changes were observed, note and report these immediately.

    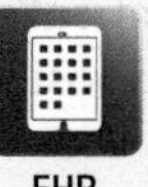
    EHR
    NOTE: In health care agencies using electronic health records (EHRs), also known as electronic medical records (EMRs), the information is entered directly into the patient's record on a computer.

PROCEDURE 16:6A (CONT.)

PRACTICE: Go to the workbook and use the evaluation sheet for 16:6, Measuring and Recording Apical Pulse, to practice this procedure. When you believe you have mastered this skill, sign the sheet and give it to your instructor for further action.

Check

FINAL CHECKPOINT: Using the criteria listed on the evaluation sheet, your instructor will grade your performance.

16:7 Measuring and Recording Blood Pressure

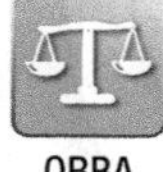
OBRA

Blood pressure (BP) is one of the vital signs you will be required to take. It is important that your recording be accurate and that you understand what the blood pressure reading means.

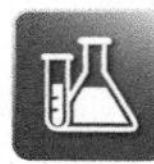
Science

Blood pressure is a measurement of the pressure that the blood exerts on the walls of the arteries during the various stages of heart activity. Blood pressure is read in millimeters (mm) of mercury (Hg) on an instrument known as a *sphygmomanometer.*

There are two types of blood pressure measurements: systolic and diastolic. **Systolic** pressure occurs in the walls of the arteries when the left ventricle of the heart is contracting and pushing blood into the arteries. **Diastolic** pressure is the constant pressure in the walls of the arteries when the left ventricle of the heart is at rest, or between contractions. Blood has moved forward into the capillaries and veins, so the volume of blood in the arteries has decreased.

Normal values and classifications for diastolic and systolic pressure are shown in Table 16–2.

TABLE 16–2 Classifications of Blood Pressure in Adults

	Blood Pressure Level Millimeters of Mercury (mm Hg)		
Category	**Systolic**		**Diastolic**
Normal blood pressure	<120	and	<80
Normal range	100–120	and	60–80
Prehypertension	120–139	or	80–89
Hypertension			
Stage 1 Hypertension	140–159	or	90–99
Stage 2 Hypertension	≥160	or	≥100

Legend: < less than; > greater than or equal to.

Blood pressure is recorded as a fraction. The systolic reading is the top number, or numerator. The diastolic reading is the bottom number, or denominator. For example, a systolic reading of 120 and a diastolic reading of 80 is recorded as 120/80.

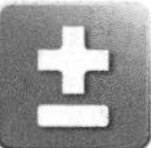
Math

Pulse pressure is the difference between systolic and diastolic pressure. The pulse pressure is an important indicator of the health and tone of arterial walls. A normal range for pulse pressure in adults is 30 to 50 mm Hg. For example, if the systolic pressure is 120 mm Hg and the diastolic pressure is 80 mm Hg, the pulse pressure is 40 mm Hg ($120 - 80 = 40$). The pulse pressure should be approximately one third of the systolic reading. A high pulse pressure can be caused by an increase in blood volume or heart rate, or a decrease in the ability of the arteries to expand.

Prehypertension is indicated when pressures are between 120 and 139 mm Hg systolic or 80 and 89 mm Hg diastolic. Prehypertension is a warning that high blood pressure will develop unless steps are taken to prevent it. Research has proven that prehypertension can harden arteries, dislodge plaque, and block vessels that nourish the heart. Proper nutrition and a regular exercise program are the main treatments for prehypertension.

Hypertension, or high blood pressure, is indicated when pressures are greater than 140 mm Hg systolic and 90 mm Hg diastolic. Common causes include stress, anxiety, obesity, high salt intake, aging, kidney disease, thyroid deficiency, and vascular conditions such as arteriosclerosis. Hypertension is often called a "silent killer" because most individuals do not have any signs or symptoms of the disease. If hypertension is not treated, it can lead to stroke, kidney disease, and/or heart disease.

Hypotension, or low blood pressure, is indicated when pressures are less than 90 mm Hg systolic and 60 mm Hg diastolic. Hypotension may occur with heart failure, dehydration, depression, severe burns, hemorrhage, and shock. *Orthostatic,* or postural, hypotension occurs when there is a sudden drop in both systolic and diastolic pressure when an individual moves from a lying to a sitting or standing position. It is caused by the inability of blood vessels to compensate quickly to the change in position. The individual becomes lightheaded and dizzy, and may experience blurred vision. The symptoms last a few seconds until the blood vessels compensate and more blood is pushed to the brain.

Many factors can influence blood pressure readings. These factors can cause blood pressure to be high or low. Some examples include:

- *Factors causing changes in readings:* force of the heartbeat, resistance of the arterial system, elasticity of the arteries, volume of blood in the arteries, and position of the patient (lying down, sitting, or standing)
- *Factors that may increase blood pressure:* excitement, anxiety, nervous tension, exercise, eating, pain, obesity, smoking, and/or stimulant drugs
- *Factors that may decrease blood pressure:* rest or sleep, depressant drugs, shock, dehydration, hemorrhage (excessive loss of blood), and fasting (not eating)

A **sphygmomanometer** is an instrument used to measure blood pressure in millimeters of mercury (mm Hg). There are three main types of sphygmomanometers: mercury, aneroid, and electronic. The mercury sphygmomanometer has a long column of mercury (Figure 16–27). Each mark on the gauge represents 2 mm Hg. The mercury sphygmomanometer must always be placed on a flat, level surface or mounted on a wall. If it is calibrated correctly, the level of mercury should be at zero when viewed at eye level. Even though the mercury sphygmomanometer has proven to be the most accurate instrument for measuring blood pressure, the Occupational Health and Safety Administration (OSHA) discourages its use because of the possibility of a mercury spill and contamination. The aneroid sphygmomanometer does not have a mercury column (Figure 16–28A). However, it is calibrated in mm Hg. Each line represents 2 mm Hg pressure. When the cuff is deflated, the needle must be on zero (Figure 16–28B).

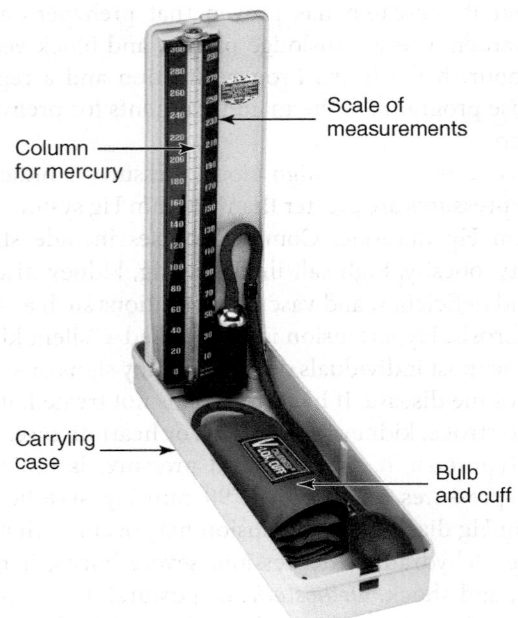

FIGURE 16–27 **The gauge on a mercury sphygmomanometer has a column of mercury.** Courtesy, W.A. Baum Co., Inc.

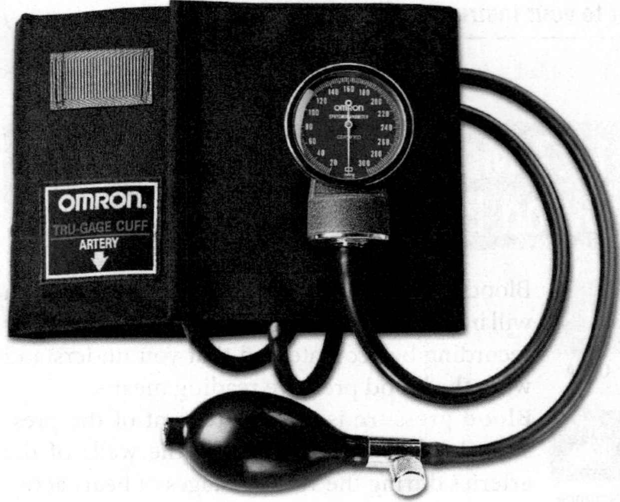

FIGURE 16–28A **The gauge on an aneroid sphygmomanometer does not contain a column of mercury.**
Courtesy, Omron Healthcare, Inc.

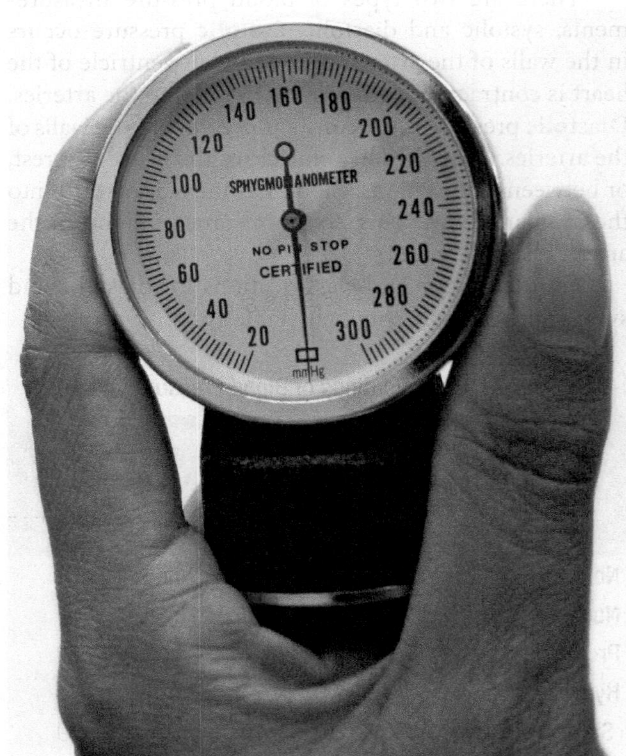

FIGURE 16–28B **If the needle is not on zero when the aneroid cuff is deflated, the sphygmomanometer should not be used until it is recalibrated.** ©iStock.com/Tiburon Studios.

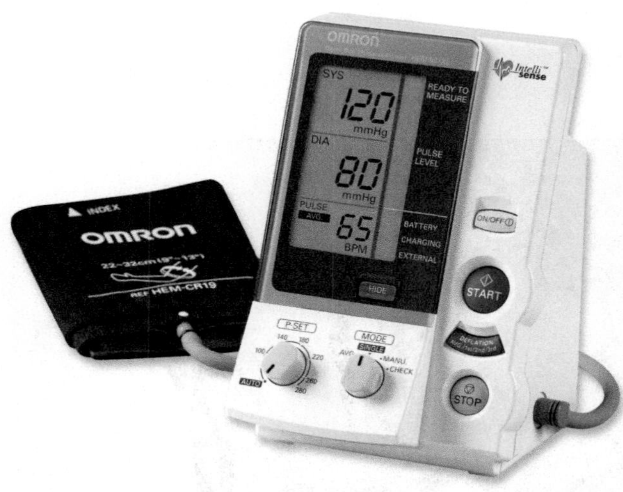

FIGURE 16–29 **Automatic sphygmomanometers provide a digital display of blood pressure and pulse readings.**

Courtesy, Omron Healthcare, Inc.

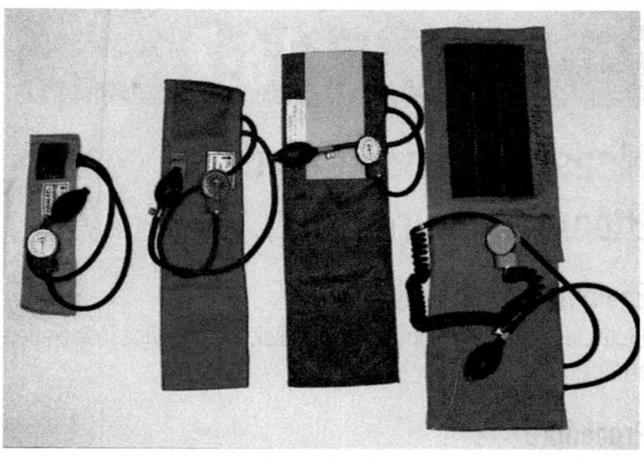

FIGURE 16–30 **It is important to use the correct size cuff because cuffs that are too wide or too narrow will result in inaccurate readings.**

If the needle is not on zero, the sphygmomanometer should not be used until it is recalibrated. Electronic sphygmomanometers are used in many health care facilities. Blood pressure and pulse readings are shown on a digital display after a cuff is placed on the patient. Automatic sphygmomanometers are also available for use. They register the blood pressure after a cuff is positioned on the arm and a start button is activated. They are frequently used by patients who monitor their blood pressure at home. It is important to read and follow the instructions provided with the sphygmomanometer to obtain accurate readings (Figure 16–29).

In order to obtain accurate blood pressure readings, it is important to observe several factors. The American Heart Association (AHA) recommends that the patient sit quietly for at least 5 minutes before blood pressure is taken. The AHA also recommends that two separate readings be taken and averaged, with a minimum wait of 30 seconds between readings.

The size and placement of the sphygmomanometer cuff is also important (Figure 16–30). The cuff contains a rubber bladder that fills with air to apply pressure to the arteries. Cuffs that are too wide or too narrow give inaccurate readings. A cuff that is too small will give an artificially high reading; if it is too large it will give an artificially low reading. To ensure the greatest degree of accuracy, the width of the cuff should be approximately 40 percent of the circumference (distance around) of the patient's upper arm. The length of the bladder should be approximately 80 percent of the circumference of the patient's upper arm. The patient should be seated or lying comfortably and have the forearm supported on a flat surface. The area of the arm covered by the cuff should be at heart level. The arm must be free of any constrictive clothing. The fully deflated cuff should be placed on the arm with the center of the bladder in the cuff directly over the brachial artery, and the lower edge of the cuff 1 to 1½ inches above the antecubital area (bend of the elbow). Disposable cuffs are available for use when strict infection control is needed. They are available in a variety of sizes and help prevent the transmission of disease. If a non-disposable cuff is used, it can be wiped down with a disinfectant wipe between patients.

A final point relating to accuracy is placement of the stethoscope bell/diaphragm. The bell/diaphragm should be placed directly over the brachial artery at the antecubital area and held securely but with as little pressure as possible.

Comm

For a health care worker, a major responsibility is accuracy in taking and recording blood pressure. If you have difficulty obtaining an accurate reading, ask another individual to check the reading. If you note any abnormalities, report these to your supervisor immediately. A physician, physician's assistant, certified nurse practitioner, or other authorized individual will determine whether an abnormal blood pressure is an indication for treatment.

STUDENT: **Go to the workbook and complete the assignment sheets for 16:7, Measuring and Recording Blood Pressure, Reading a Mercury Sphygmomanometer, and Reading an Aneroid Sphygmomanometer. Then return and continue with the procedure.**

PROCEDURE 16:7

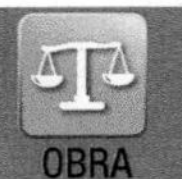

OBRA

Measuring and Recording Blood Pressure

Equipment and Supplies

Stethoscope, sphygmomanometer, disinfectant wipe, paper, pen and/or computer

Procedure

1. Assemble equipment. Use disinfectant wipe to clean the earpieces and bell/diaphragm of the stethoscope.
2. Wash hands.
3. Introduce yourself. Identify the patient. Explain the procedure.

   Comm

   NOTE: If possible, allow the patient to sit quietly for 5 minutes before taking the blood pressure.

   NOTE: Reassure the patient as needed. Nervous tension and excitement can alter or elevate blood pressure.
4. Roll up the patient's sleeve to approximately 5 inches above the elbow. Position the arm so that it is supported, comfortable, and close to the level of the heart. The palm should be up.

   NOTE: If the sleeve constricts the arm, remove the garment. The arm must be bare and unconstricted for an accurate reading.
5. Wrap the deflated cuff around the upper arm 1 to 2 inches above the elbow and over the brachial artery. The center of the bladder inside the cuff should be over the brachial artery.

   CAUTION: Do not pull the cuff too tight. The cuff should be smooth and even.

   Safety
6. Determine the palpatory systolic pressure (Figure 16–31A). To do this, find the radial pulse and keep your fingers on it. Inflate the cuff until the radial pulse disappears. Inflate the cuff 30 mm Hg above this point. Slowly release the pressure on the cuff while watching the gauge. When the pulse is felt again, note the reading on the gauge. This is the palpatory systolic pressure.
7. Deflate the cuff completely. Ask the patient to raise the arm and flex the fingers to promote blood flow. Wait 30–60 seconds to allow blood flow to resume completely.

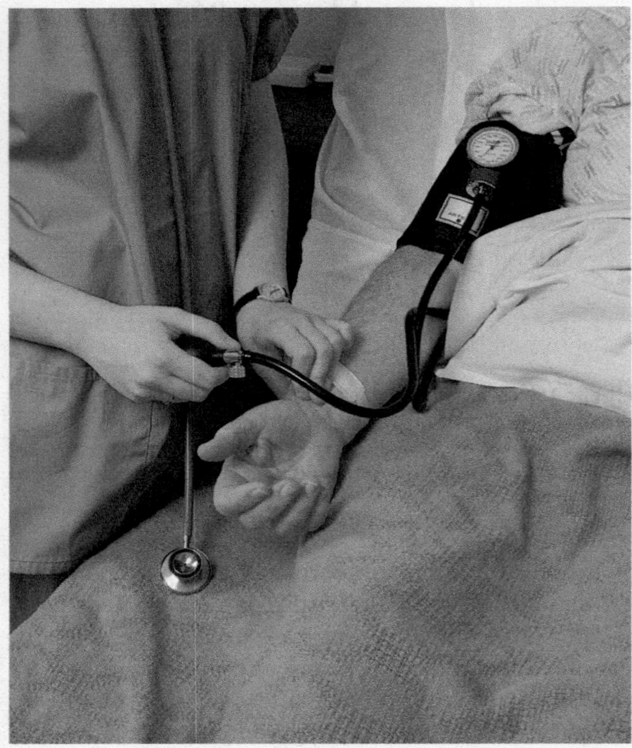

FIGURE 16–31A Determine the palpatory systolic pressure by checking the radial pulse as you inflate the cuff.

8. Use your fingertips to locate the brachial artery (Figure 16–31B). The brachial artery is located on the inner part of the arm at the antecubital space (area where the elbow bends). Place the stethoscope over the artery (Figure 16–31C). Put the earpieces in your ears.

   NOTE: Earpieces should be pointed forward.
9. Check to make sure the tubings are separate and not tangled together.
10. Gently close the valve on the rubber bulb by turning it in a clockwise direction. Inflate the cuff to 30 mm Hg above the palpatory systolic pressure.

    NOTE: Make sure the sphygmomanometer gauge is at eye level.
11. Open the bulb valve slowly and let the air escape gradually at a rate of 2–3 mm Hg per second (or per heartbeat if the heart rate is very slow).

    NOTE: Deflating the cuff too rapidly will cause an inaccurate reading.

PROCEDURE 16:7 (CONT.)

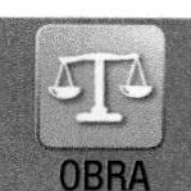

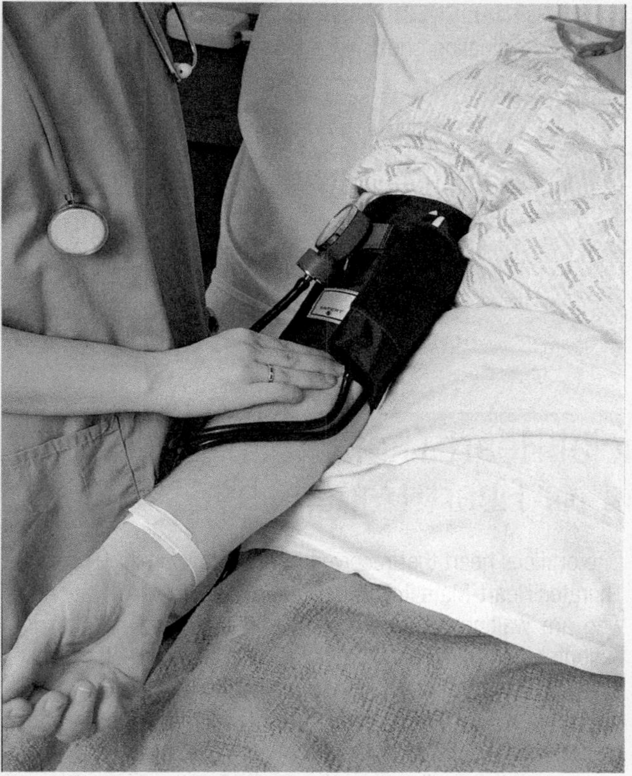

FIGURE 16–31B **Locate the brachial artery on the inner part of the arm at the antecubital space.**

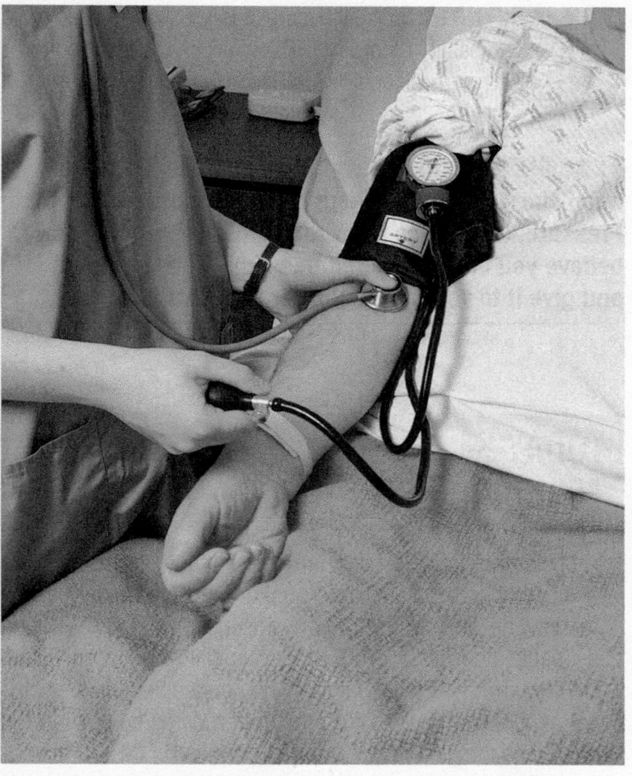

FIGURE 16–31C **Place the stethoscope over the brachial artery as you listen for the blood pressure sounds.**

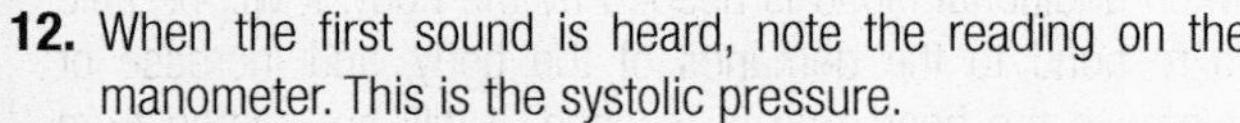

12. When the first sound is heard, note the reading on the manometer. This is the systolic pressure.
13. Continue to release the air until there is an abrupt change of the sound, usually soft or muffled. Note the reading on the manometer. Continue to release the air until the sound changes again, becoming first faint and then no longer heard. Note the reading on the manometer. The point at which the first change in sound occurs is the diastolic pressure in children. The diastolic pressure in adults is the point at which the sound becomes very faint or stops.

    NOTE: If you still hear sound, continue to the zero mark. Record both readings (the change of sound and the zero reading). For a systolic of 122 and a continued diastolic of 78, this can be written as 122/78/0.
14. Continue to listen for sounds for 10–20 mm Hg below the last sound. If no further sounds are heard, rapidly deflate the cuff.
15. If you need to repeat the procedure to recheck your reading, completely deflate the cuff, wait 1 minute, and repeat the procedure. Ask the patient to raise the arm and flex the fingers to promote blood flow.

    CAUTION: If you cannot obtain a reading, report to your supervisor promptly.
16. Record the time and your reading. The reading is written as a fraction, with systolic over diastolic. For example, BP 124/72 (or 124/80/72 if the change in sound is noted).
17. Remove the cuff. Expel any remaining air by squeezing the cuff. Use a disinfectant wipe to clean the stethoscope earpieces and diaphragm/bell. Replace all equipment.
18. Check patient for safety and comfort before leaving.
19. Wash hands.
20. 

    Record all required information on the patient's chart or enter it into the computer. For example: date, time, BP 126/74, your signature and title. Report any abnormal readings immediately to your supervisor.

(continues)

PROCEDURE 16:7 (CONT.)

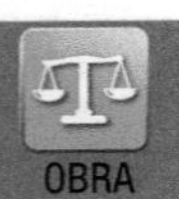

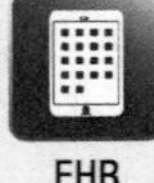

NOTE: In health care agencies using electronic health records (EHRs), also known as electronic medical records (EMRs), the information is entered directly into the patient's record on a computer.

PRACTICE: **Go to the workbook and use the evaluation sheet for 16:7, Measuring and Recording Blood Pressure, to practice this procedure. When you believe you have mastered this skill, sign the sheet and give it to your instructor for further action.**

FINAL CHECKPOINT: Using the criteria listed on the evaluation sheet, your instructor will grade your performance.

TODAY'S RESEARCH TOMORROW'S HEALTH CARE

An Artificial Heart That Eliminates the Need for Heart Transplants?

Artificial hearts have been in use for many years. They are used to keep a patient alive until a heart transplant can be found. The first artificial heart was used on Barney Clark, a Seattle dentist, in 1982. It was implanted by Dr. William DeVries. This heart, the Jarvik-7, was connected to an electrical generator the size of a refrigerator. Wires connected the heart with the generator. Barney Clark lived for 112 days connected to this device.

Now researchers have developed a new type of artificial heart. By using miniaturized electronics and high-capacity lithium batteries, scientists have created a heart that allows a patient to wear a battery pack on his or her waist. Electrical energy passes through the patient's skin to power the implanted heart. This allows the patient to resume many normal daily activities. The patient is no longer attached by wires to a power source. Patients have lived for many months with this type of heart while waiting for a suitable transplant.

One artificial heart that received FDA approval in 2010 is the Thoratec Heart-Mate II. This device was approved for patients who are waiting for a transplant and to extend the life of patients who are not candidates for a transplant. Another artificial heart that received FDA approval in 2011 is the Berlin Heart and it was approved for use in pediatric patients who are waiting for a transplant. Many other artificial heart devices are going through clinical studies for FDA approval.

Researchers are now working on an artificial heart that will work with or in place of a patient's damaged heart. This heart will have computerized intelligence to understand when additional blood is needed by the body. It will be able to respond to the demands of the body, and increase or decrease the heart rate as needed. It will be created from materials that will not cause a rejection reaction in the body. And finally, it will last for many years.

CHAPTER 16 SUMMARY

Vital signs are important indicators of health states of the body. The five main vital signs are temperature, pulse, respiration, blood pressure, and pain.

Temperature is a measurement of the balance between heat lost and heat produced by the body. It can be measured orally, rectally, aurally (by way of the ear), temporally, and between folds of skin, such as the axillary or groin area. An abnormal body temperature can indicate disease.

Pulse is the pressure of the blood felt against the wall of an artery as the heart contracts or beats. Pulse can be measured at various body sites, but the most common site is the radial pulse, which is at the wrist. The rate, rhythm, and volume (strength) should be noted each time a pulse is taken. An apical pulse is taken with a stethoscope at the apex of the heart. The stethoscope is used to listen to the heartbeat. Apical pulse is frequently taken on infants and small children with rapid pulse rates.

Respiration refers to the breathing process. Each respiration consists of an inspiration (breathing in) and an expiration (breathing out). The rate, rhythm, and character, or type, of respirations should always be noted.

Blood pressure is the force exerted by the blood against the arterial walls when the heart contracts or relaxes. Two measurements are noted: systolic and diastolic. An abnormal blood pressure can indicate disease.

Pain is an unpleasant sensation that is perceived by the nervous system when illness or injury occur. Pain can be acute or chronic and must be assessed frequently.

Vital signs are major indications of body function. The health care worker must use precise methods to measure vital signs so results are as accurate as possible. A thorough understanding of vital signs and what they indicate will allow the health care worker to be alert to any abnormalities so they can be immediately reported to the correct individual.

INTERNET SEARCHES

Use the search engines suggested in Chapter 12:9 in this text to search the Internet for additional information about the following topics:

1. **Organization:** Find the American Heart Association Web site to obtain information about the heart, pulse, arrhythmias, and blood pressure.
2. **Vital signs:** Research body temperature, pulse, respiration, blood pressure, pain, and apical pulse.
3. **Temperature scales:** Research Celsius (centigrade) versus Fahrenheit temperatures: try to locate conversion charts that can be used to compare the two scales.
4. **Diseases:** Research hypothermia, fever or pyrexia, hypertension, hypotension, and heart arrhythmias.

REVIEW QUESTIONS

1. List the five (5) main vital signs.
2. State the normal value or range for an adult for each of the following:
   a. oral temperature
   b. rectal or temporal temperature
   c. axillary or groin temperature
   d. pulse
   e. respiration
3. What three (3) factors must be noted about every pulse?
4. Why is an apical pulse taken?
5. What is the pulse deficit if an apical pulse is 112 and the radial pulse is 88?
6. Differentiate between hypertension and hypotension, and list the basic causes of each.
7. How does systolic pressure differ from diastolic pressure? What are the normal ranges for each?
8. If the systolic blood pressure is 132 and the diastolic pressure is 88, what is the pulse pressure?
9. Why does shock or dehydration decrease blood pressure?
10. Define each of the following:
    a. bradycardia
    b. arrhythmia
    c. dyspnea
    d. tachypnea
    e. rales
11. What is pain and how can it be assessed?

17 First Aid

CHAPTER OBJECTIVES

After completing this chapter, you should be able to:

- Demonstrate cardiopulmonary resuscitation for one-person rescue, two-person rescue, infants, children, and obstructed-airway victims.
- Describe first aid for:
  - Bleeding and wounds
  - Shock
  - Poisoning
  - Burns
  - Heat exposure
  - Cold exposure
  - Bone and joint injuries, including fractures
  - Specific injuries to the eyes, head, nose, ears, chest, abdomen, and genital organs
  - Sudden illness including heart attack, stroke, fainting, convulsions, and diabetic reactions
- Apply dressings and bandages, observing all safety precautions and using the circular, spiral, figure-eight, and recurrent, or finger wrap.
- Define, pronounce, and spell all key terms.

KEY TERMS

abration *(ah″-bray′-shun)*
amputation
avulsion *(ay″-vul′-shun)*
bandages
burn
cardiopulmonary resuscitation *(car′-dee-oh-pull′-meh-nah-ree re″-suh-sih-tay′-shun)*
cerebrovascular accident *(seh-ree′-bro-vass″-ku-lehr ax′-ih-dent)*
convulsion
diabetic coma
diaphoresis *(dy″-ah-feh-ree′-sis)*
dislocation
dressing
fainting
first aid
fracture
frostbite
heart attack
heat cramps
heat exhaustion
heat stroke

KEY TERMS (CONT.)

hemorrhage
hypothermia
incision
infection
insulin shock
laceration
poisoning
puncture
shock
sprain
strain
stroke
triage *(tree′-ahj)*
wound

Related Health Careers

Disaster Medicine Specialist
Emergency Medical Technician
Emergency Medicine Physician
First Responder
Paramedic

LEGAL ALERT

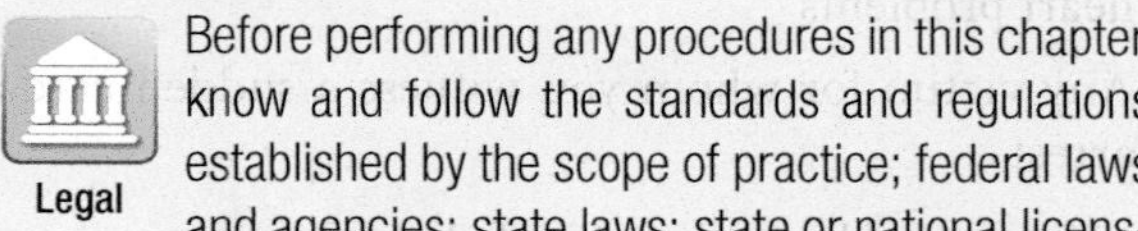

Legal

Before performing any procedures in this chapter, know and follow the standards and regulations established by the scope of practice; federal laws and agencies; state laws; state or national licensing, registration, or certification boards; professional organizations; professional standards; and agency policies.

It is your responsibility to learn exactly what you are legally permitted to do and to perform only procedures for which you have been trained.

17:1 Providing First Aid

Introduction

In every health care career, you may have experiences that require a knowledge of first aid. This section provides basic guidelines for all the first aid topics discussed in the remaining sections of this unit. *All students are strongly encouraged to take the First Aid Certification Course through their local Red Cross divisions to become proficient in providing first aid.*

First aid is not full and complete treatment. Rather, **first aid** is best defined as "immediate care that is given to the victim of an injury or illness to minimize the effect of the injury or illness until experts can take over." Application of correct first aid can often mean the difference between life and death, or recovery versus permanent disability. In addition, by knowing the proper first aid measures, you can help yourself and others in a time of emergency.

Basic Principles of First Aid

Comm

In any situation where first aid treatment is necessary, it is essential that you remain calm. Avoid panic. Evaluate the situation thoroughly. Always have a reason for anything you do. The treatment you provide will vary depending on the type of injury or illness, the environment, others present, equipment or supplies on hand, and the availability of medical help. Therefore, it is important for you to think about all these factors and determine what action is necessary.

The first step of first aid is to recognize that an emergency exists. Many senses can alert you to an emergency. Listen for unusual sounds such as screams, calls for help, breaking glass, screeching tires, or changes in machinery or equipment noises. Look for unusual sights such as an empty medicine container, damaged electrical wires, a stalled car, smoke or fire, a person lying motionless, blood, or spilled chemicals. Note any unusual, unfamiliar, or strange odors such as those of chemicals, natural gas, or pungent fumes. Watch for unusual appearances or behaviors in others such as difficulty in breathing, clutching of the chest or throat, abnormal skin colors, slurred or confused speech, unexplained confusion or drowsiness, excessive perspiration, signs of pain, and any symptoms of distress. Sometimes, signs of an emergency are clearly evident. An example is an automobile accident with victims in cars or on the street. Other times, signs are less obvious and require an alert individual to note that something is different or wrong. An empty medicine container and a small child with slurred speech, for example, are less obvious signs.

Safety

After determining that an emergency exists, the next step is to take appropriate action to help the victim or victims. Check the scene and make sure it

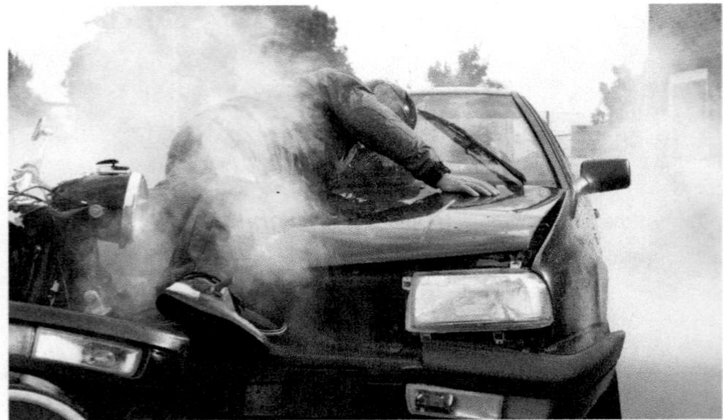

FIGURE 17–1 **Check the scene and make sure it is safe to approach before checking any accident victim.** © corepics/www.Shutterstock.com

is safe to approach (Figure 17–1). A quick glance at the area can provide information on what has occurred, dangers present, number of people involved, and other important factors. If live electrical wires are lying on the ground around an accident victim, for example, a rescuer could be electrocuted while trying to assist the victim. An infant thrown from a car during an automobile accident may be overlooked. A rescuer who pauses briefly to assess the situation will avoid such dangerous pitfalls and provide more efficient care. If the scene is not safe, call for medical help. Do not endanger your own life or the lives of other bystanders. Allow professionals to handle fires, dangerous chemicals, damaged electrical wires, and other life-threatening situations.

If the scene appears safe, approach the victim. Determine whether the victim is conscious. If the victim shows no sign of consciousness, tap him gently and call to him. If the victim shows signs of consciousness, try to find out what happened and what is wrong. Never move an injured victim unless the victim is in a dangerous area such as an area filled with fire and/or smoke, flood waters, or carbon monoxide or poisonous fumes, or one with dangerous traffic, where vehicles cannot be stopped. If it is necessary to move the victim, do so as quickly and as carefully as possible. Victims have been injured more severely by improper movement at the scenes of accidents, so avoid any unnecessary movement.

In an emergency, it is essential to call the emergency medical services (EMS) as soon as possible (Figure 17–2). The time factor is critical. Early access to the EMS system and advanced medical care increases the victim's chance of survival. Dial 911 on a telephone or cellular phone, or use a CB radio to contact any of the emergency medical services. Sometimes, it may be necessary to instruct others to contact EMS while you are giving first aid. Make sure that complete, accurate information is given to EMS. Describe the situation, actions taken, exact location, telephone number from which you are calling, assistance required, number of people involved, and the condition of the victim(s). Do not hang up the receiver or end the CB radio call until EMS has all the necessary information. If you are alone, call EMS immediately before providing any care to:

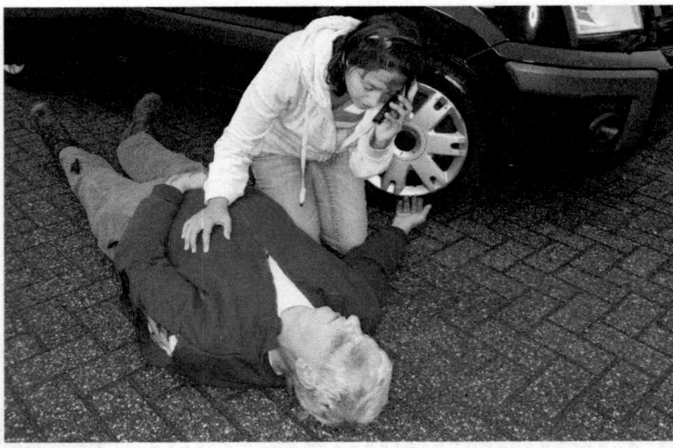

FIGURE 17–2 **Call for emergency medical services (EMS) as soon as possible.** © iStockphoto/Studio-Annika

- An unconscious adult
- An unconscious child who has reached puberty
- An unconscious infant or child with a high risk for heart problems
- Any victim for whom you witness a sudden cardiac arrest

If you are alone, shout for help and start cardiopulmonary resuscitation (CPR) if needed for:

- An unconscious infant or child from 1 year of age to puberty
- Any victim of submersion or near drowning
- Any victim with cardiac arrest caused by a drug overdose or trauma

If no one arrives to call EMS, continue providing care by giving five cycles of CPR (approximately 2 minutes). Then go to the nearest telephone, call for EMS, and return immediately to the victim.

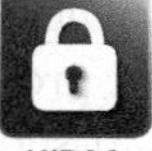

After calling for help, provide care to the victim. If possible, obtain the victim's permission before providing any care. Introduce yourself and ask if you can help. If the victim can respond, he or she should give you permission before you provide care. If the victim is a child or minor, and a parent is present, obtain permission from the parent. If the victim is unconscious, confused, or seriously ill and unable to consent to care, and no other relative is available to give permission, you can assume that you have permission. It is important to remember that every individual has the right to refuse care. If a person refuses to give consent for care, do not proceed. If possible, have someone witness the refusal of care. If a life-threatening emergency exists, call EMS, alert them to the situation, and allow the professionals to take over.

At times it may be necessary to **triage** the situation. Triage is a method of prioritizing treatment. If a victim has more than one injury or illness, the most severe injury or illness must be treated first. If two or more people are involved, triage also determines which person is treated first. Life-threatening emergencies must be treated first. Examples include:

- No breathing or difficulty in breathing
- No pulse
- Severe bleeding
- Persistent pain in the chest or abdomen
- Vomiting or passing blood
- Poisoning
- Head, neck, or spine injuries
- Open chest or abdominal wounds
- Shock
- Severe partial-thickness and all full-thickness burns

Proper care for these emergencies is described in the sections that follow. If the victim is conscious, breathing, and able to talk, reassure the victim and try to determine what has happened. Examine the victim thoroughly. Always have a sound reason for anything you do. Examples include:

- Ask the victim about pain or discomfort
- Check the victim for other types of injuries such as fractures (broken bones), burns, shock, and specific injuries
- Note any abnormal signs or symptoms
- Check vital signs
- Note the temperature, color, and moistness of the skin
- Check and compare the pupils of the eyes
- Look for fluids or blood draining from the mouth, nose, or ears
- Gently examine the body for cuts, bruises, swelling, and painful areas

Report any abnormalities noted to emergency medical services when they arrive at the scene.

Comm

Obtain as much information regarding the accident, injury, or illness as possible. This information can then be given to the correct authorities. Information can be obtained from the victim, other persons present, or by examination of items present at the scene. Emergency medical identification contained in a bracelet, necklace, medical card, or Vial-of-Life is an important source of information. Empty medicine containers, bottles of chemicals or solutions, or similar items also can reveal important information. Be alert to all such sources of information. Use this information to determine how you may help the victim.

Summary

Some general principles of care should be observed whenever first aid is necessary. Some of these principles are:

- Obtain qualified assistance as soon as possible. Report all information obtained, observations noted, treatment given, and other important facts to the correct authorities. It may sometimes be necessary to send someone at the scene to obtain help.
- Avoid any unnecessary movement of the victim. Keep the victim in a position that will allow for providing the best care for the type of injury or illness.
- Reassure the victim. A confident, calm attitude will help relieve the victim's anxiety.
- If the victim is unconscious or vomiting, do not give him or her anything to eat or drink. It is best to avoid giving a victim anything to eat or drink while providing first aid treatment, unless the specific treatment requires that fluids or food be given.
- Protect the victim from cold or chilling, but avoid overheating the victim.
- Work quickly, but in an organized and efficient manner.
- 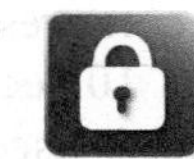 HIPAA Do *not* make a diagnosis or discuss the victim's condition with observers at the scene. It is essential to maintain confidentiality and protect the victim's right to privacy while providing treatment.
- Make every attempt to avoid further injury.

Legal

CAUTION: *Provide only the treatment that you are qualified to provide.*

STUDENT: Go to the workbook and complete the assignment sheet for 17:1, Providing First Aid.

17:2 Performing Cardiopulmonary Resuscitation

Introduction

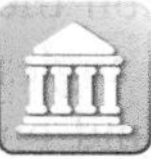
Legal

At some time in your life, you may find an unconscious victim who is not breathing. This is an emergency situation. Correct action can save a life. Students are strongly encouraged to take certification courses in cardiopulmonary resuscitation (CPR) offered by the American Red Cross and the American Heart Association. This section provides the basic facts about CPR for health care providers according to American Heart Association standards. *The information provided is not intended to take the place of an approved certification course.*

The word parts of **cardiopulmonary resuscitation** provide a fairly clear description of the procedure: cardio (the heart) plus pulmonary (the lungs) plus resuscitation (to remove from apparent death or unconsciousness). When you administer CPR, you breathe for the person *and* circulate the blood. The purpose is to keep oxygenated blood flowing to the brain and other vital body organs until the heart and lungs start working again, or until medical help is available.

Clinical death occurs when the heart stops beating and the victim stops breathing. *Biological death* refers to the death of the body cells. Biological death occurs 4–6 minutes after clinical death and can result in permanent brain damage, as well as damage to other vital organs. If CPR can be started immediately after clinical death occurs, the victim may be revived.

Components of CPR

Cardiopulmonary resuscitation is a life-saving technique used for people who have stopped breathing and have no pulse. The American Heart Association uses a CPR sequence of *CABD* (circulation, airway, breathing, defibrillation), with a major emphasis on chest compressions. The goal is to start compressions within 10 seconds of recognizing cardiac arrest. This sequence is used for adults, children, and infants and includes:

- *C stands for circulation.* By applying pressure to a certain area of the sternum (breastbone), the heart is compressed between the sternum and vertebral column. Blood is squeezed out of the heart and into the blood vessels. In this way, oxygen is supplied to body cells.
- *A stands for airway.* To open the victim's airway, use the *head-tilt/chin-lift* method (Figure 17–3). Put one hand on the victim's forehead and put the fingertips of the other hand under the bony part of the jaw, near the chin. Tilt the head back without closing the victim's mouth. This action prevents the tongue from falling back and blocking the air passage. If the victim has a suspected neck or upper spinal cord injury, try to open the airway by lifting the chin without tilting the head back. If it is difficult to keep the jaw lifted with one hand, use a *jaw-thrust maneuver* to open the airway. Assume a position at the victim's head and rest your elbows on the surface on which the victim is lying. Grasp the angles of the victim's lower jaw by positioning one hand on each side. Lift with both hands to move the lower jaw forward, making every attempt to avoid excessive backward tilting or side-to-side movement of the head.
- *B stands for breathing.* Breathing means that, while using a barrier device, you breathe into the victim's mouth or nose to supply needed oxygen or provide ventilations. Each breath should take about 1 second and the chest should rise. Rapid or forceful breaths should be avoided because they can force air into the esophagus and stomach, causing gastric distension (expansion of the stomach when air enters it). This can cause serious complications such as vomiting, aspiration of fluids into the lungs, and even pneumonia.

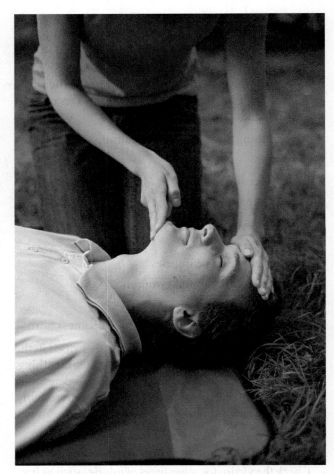

FIGURE 17–3 Open the airway by using the head-tilt/chin-lift method. © iStockphoto/JanekWD

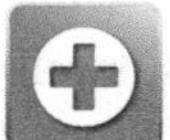

Precaution

CAUTION: *OSHA requires health care workers to use standard precautions in the workplace. This requires a barrier device for CPR. Use a CPR pocket face mask with a one-way valve to provide a barrier and prevent the transmission of disease (Figure 17–4). Special training is required for the use of this mask. Other protective barrier face shields are also available.*

- *D stands for defibrillation.* One of the most common causes of cardiac arrest is ventricular fibrillation, which is an arrhythmia, or abnormal electrical conduction pattern in the heart. When the heart is fibrillating, it does not pump blood effectively. A defibrillator is a machine that delivers an electric shock to the heart to try to restore the normal electrical pattern and rhythm. Automated external defibrillators (AEDs) are now available for use by trained first responders, emergency medical technicians, and even citizens (Figure 17–5). After electrode pads are positioned on the victim's

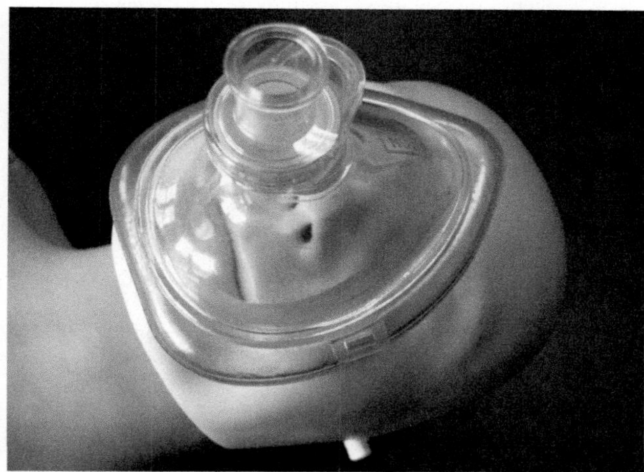

FIGURE 17–4 Use a CPR barrier mask to prevent transmission of disease while giving respirations. © Barbara J. Petrick/www.Shutterstock.com

chest, the AED determines the heart rhythm, recognizes abnormal rhythms that may respond to defibrillation, and sounds an audible or visual warning telling the operator to push a "shock" button. Some AEDs are fully automatic and even administer the shock. Anytime a shock is administered with an AED, it is essential to make sure no one is touching the victim. The rescuer should state "Clear the victim," and look carefully to make sure no one is in contact with the victim before pushing the shock button. Serious injuries, such as cardiac arrest, could occur in other rescuers if they are shocked by the AED.

Newer models of AEDs allow the rescuer to deliver either adult or child defibrillator shocks. By using smaller pediatric electrodes and/or a switch on the AED, the rescuer can deliver a smaller electrical shock. The pediatric dose is recommended for any child from 1–8 years of age. The adult defibrillator dose and adult electrodes should be used for any child 8 years or older. In addition, if an AED does not have the option of a pediatric dosage, the adult dosage and electrodes should be used on the child. For infants younger than 1 year, a manual defibrillator is preferred, but an AED with pediatric dosage can be used. Studies have shown that the sooner the defibrillation is provided, the greater the chances of survival are from a cardiac arrest caused by an arrhythmia. However, it is essential to remember that CPR is used until an AED is available. CPR will circulate the blood and prevent biological death.

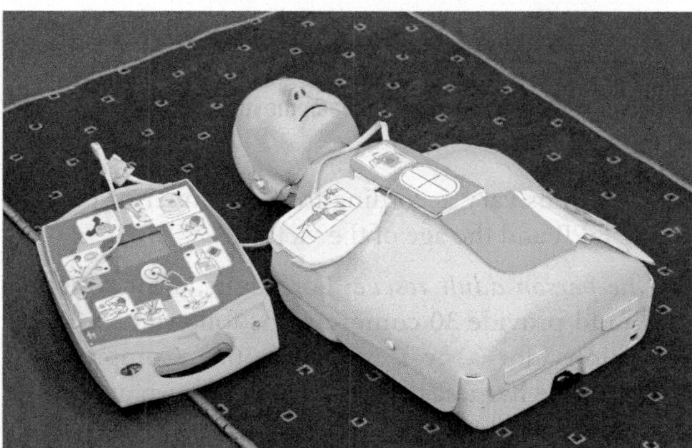

FIGURE 17–5 When cardiac arrest occurs, an automated external defibrillator (AED) can be used to analyze the electrical rhythm of the heart and to apply a shock to try to restore the normal heart rhythm. © Baloncici/www.Shutterstock.com

It is important to know and follow the *CABDs* in proper sequence while administering CPR.

Basic Principles of CPR

Extreme care must be taken to evaluate the victim's condition before CPR is started. The victim should be assessed for responsiveness and breathing first, and both assessments should be done at the same time. To determine if a victim is conscious, tap the victim gently and ask, "Are you OK?" If you know the victim, call the victim by name and speak loudly. If there is no response and the victim is unconscious and not breathing, or not breathing normally (gasping), call for help. The American Heart Association and the American Red Cross recommend a *"call first, call fast"* priority. If you are alone, *call first* before providing any care to:

- An unconscious adult
- An unconscious child who has reached puberty as defined by the presence of secondary sex characteristics
- An unconscious infant or child with a high risk for heart problems
- Any victim for whom you witness a sudden cardiac arrest

If you are alone, shout for help, and start CPR if needed for:

- An unconscious infant or child from 1 year of age to puberty
- Any victim of submersion or near drowning
- Any victim with cardiac arrest caused by a drug overdose or trauma

If no help arrives to call EMS, administer five cycles of CPR (about 2 minutes), and then *call fast* for EMS. Return to the victim immediately to continue providing care until EMS arrives.

After determining that a victim is unconscious and not breathing, or not breathing normally (gasping), position the victim on his or her back. If you must turn the victim, support the victim's head and neck, and keep the victim's body in as straight a line as possible while turning.

Check the carotid pulse in the neck to determine whether cardiac compression is needed. If you do not feel a pulse within 10 seconds, or you are not sure if you feel a pulse, start compressions.

Safety

CAUTION: *Cardiac compressions are not given if the pulse can be felt. If a person has stopped breathing but still has a pulse, it may be necessary to give only pulmonary respiration.*

Correct hand placement is essential before performing chest compressions. For adults, the hand is placed on the lower half of the sternum between the nipples. While kneeling alongside the victim, find the correct position by using the middle finger of your hand that is closest to the victim's feet to follow the ribs up to where the ribs meet the sternum, at the substernal notch (Figure 17–6A). Keep the middle finger on the notch and position the index finger above it so two fingers are on the sternum. Then place the heel of your opposite hand (the hand closest to the victim's head) on the sternum, next to the index finger (Figure 17–6B). Measuring in this manner minimizes the danger of applying pressure to the tip of the sternum, called the xiphoid process.

Safety

CAUTION: *The xiphoid process can be broken off quite easily and therefore should not be pressed.*

After positioning your hands on the sternum, straighten your arms and align your shoulders directly over your hands. To give compressions, push straight down on the victim's sternum with a hard, fast motion. On an adult, the sternum should be compressed at least 2 inches. After each compression, allow the chest to recoil completely. Deliver compressions at a rate of at least 100 to 120 compressions per minute and minimize interruptions in compressions. Proper administration of compressions will produce adequate blood flow and improve the victim's chances of survival.

Once 30 chest compressions are delivered, open the airway by using the head-tilt/chin-lift method or, if a neck or spinal cord injury is suspected, the jaw-thrust maneuver. This step will sometimes start the victim breathing. If the victim is not breathing, or not breathing normally (gasping), use a barrier device and give two breaths, each breath lasting approximately 1 second. Make sure the breaths are effective by watching for the victim's chest to rise. Do not give breaths too quickly or with too much force because this can cause gastric distension (stomach expansion due to air accumulation). Pause very briefly between breaths to allow air flow back out of the lungs. In addition, take a breath between the two breaths to increase the oxygen content of the rescue breath. After giving two breaths, immediately return to compressions.

CPR for Adults, Infants, and Children

Cardiopulmonary resuscitation can be performed on adults, children, and infants. In addition, it can be done by one person or two persons. Rates of ventilations and compressions vary according to the number of persons giving CPR and the age of the victim.

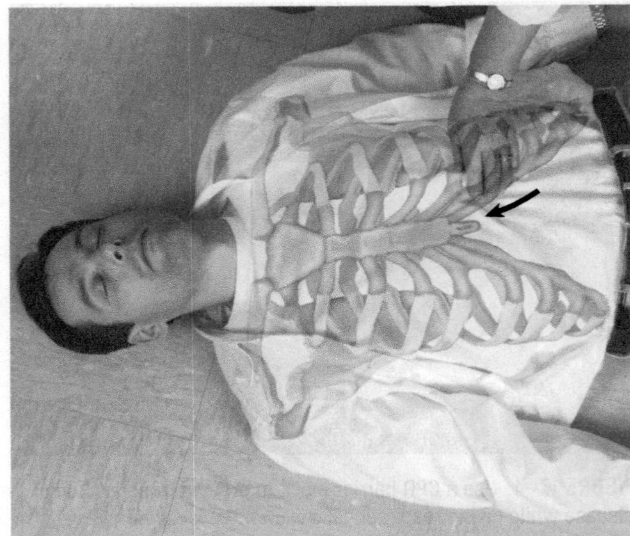

FIGURE 17–6A To position hands correctly for chest compressions, first use a finger to follow the ribs up to where they meet the sternum at the substernal notch.

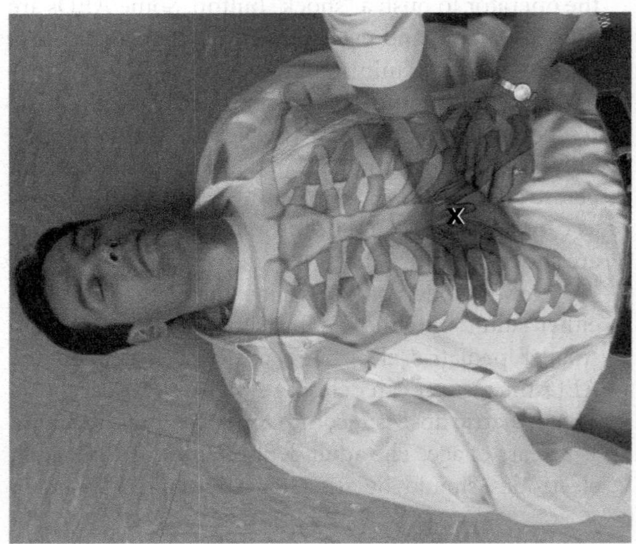

FIGURE 17–6B Place the heel of your opposite hand two fingers' width above the substernal notch. This should place the hand on the lower half of the sternum between the nipples.

- *One-person adult rescue:* For adults, a lone rescuer should provide 30 compressions followed by 2 ventilations, for a cycle ratio of 30:2. Compressions should be hard, fast, and deep, and given at the rate of at least 100 to 120 per minute. Five 30:2 cycles should be completed every 2 minutes. The hands should be positioned correctly on the sternum. The two hands should be interlaced and only the heel of the palm should rest on the sternum. Pressure should

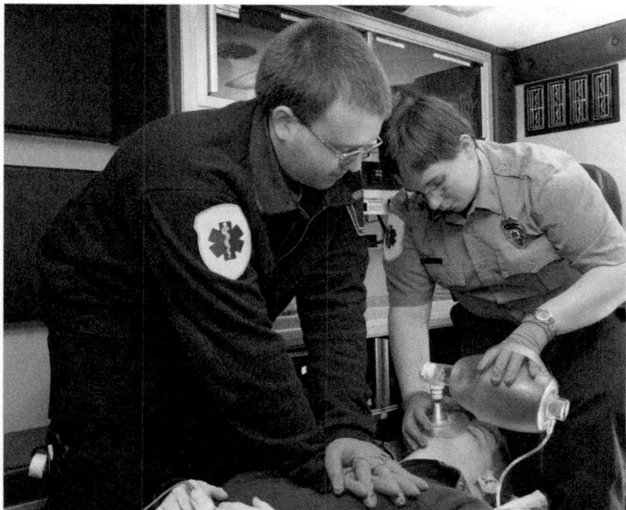

FIGURE 17–7 In a two-person rescue, one person gives breaths while the second person provides compressions. © iStockphoto/Nancy Louie

be applied straight down to compress the sternum at least 2 inches, or 5.0 centimeters (cm) but not more than 2.4 inches or 6 cm.

- *Two-person adult rescue:* Two people performing a rescue on an adult victim allows one person to give breaths while the second person provides compressions (Figure 17–7). During the rescue, the person giving breaths can check the effectiveness of the compressions by feeling for a carotid pulse while chest compressions are administered. One rescuer applies the compressions at the rate of at least 100 to 120 per minute. After every 30 compressions, the second rescuer provides 2 ventilations. Thus, there is a 30:2 ratio. The two rescuers should switch duties every 5 cycles, or about every 2 minutes. Switching should take less than 5 seconds.
- *Infants:* Cardiopulmonary resuscitation is given to any infant from birth to 1 year of age. It is different than that for an adult because of the infant's size. The brachial pulse site in the arm is used to check pulse (Figure 17–8). Compressions are given by placing two fingers on the lower half of the sternum just below an imaginary line drawn between the nipples. The sternum should be compressed at least ⅓ the depth of the chest, approximately 1½ inches or 4 centimeters. Compressions are given at a rate of at least 100 to 120 per minute. Once 30 compressions have been given, open the airway using the head-tilt/chin-lift method. The infant's head should not be tilted as far back as an adult's, because this can obstruct the infant's airway. Ventilations are given by using a barrier device and covering both the infant's nose and mouth. Breaths are given until the infant's chest visibly rises. Extreme care must be taken to avoid overinflating the lungs and/or forcing air into the stomach. A lone rescuer gives 30 compressions followed by 2 ventilations for a 30:2 ratio. The infant's back must be supported at all times when giving compressions. If two rescuers are available to perform CPR on an infant, a two-thumb technique can be used by one rescuer to perform compressions while the second rescuer gives breaths. The rescuer providing compressions stands at the infant's feet and places his or her thumbs next to each other on the lower half of the sternum just below the nipple line. The rescuer then wraps his or her hands around the infant to support the infant's back with the fingers. A ratio of 15 compressions to 2 ventilations is used by the two rescuers.

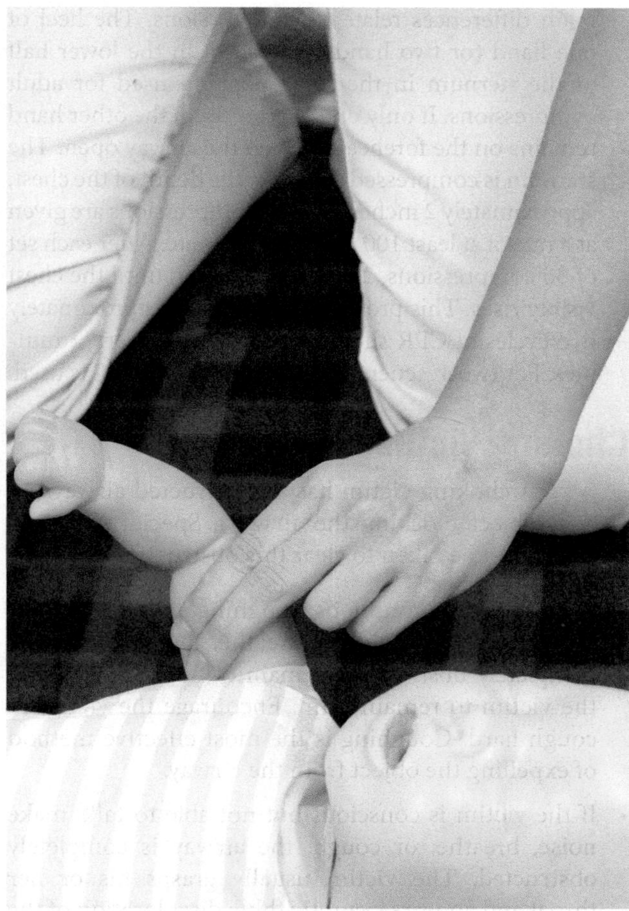

FIGURE 17–8 Use the brachial pulse site in the arm to check for a pulse in an infant. © pryzmat/www.Shutterstock.com.

- *Children:* Cardiopulmonary resuscitation for children depends on the size of the child. Health care providers should use child CPR methods for any child from 1 year of age to puberty (approximately 12 years of age). If a child shows signs of puberty, as evidenced by secondary sex characteristics, adult CPR methods should be used. The initial steps of CPR for a child are the same steps used in adult CPR, except that the head is not tilted as far back when the airway is opened. The main differences relate to compressions. The heel of one hand (or two hands) is placed on the lower half of the sternum in the same position used for adult compressions. If only one hand is used, the other hand remains on the forehead to keep the airway open. The sternum is compressed at least ⅓ the depth of the chest, approximately 2 inches (5 cm). Compressions are given at a rate of at least 100 to 120 per minute. After each set of 30 compressions, 2 breaths are given until the chest visibly rises. This provides a 30:2 ratio. Approximately five cycles of CPR should be completed every 2 minutes. For two-rescuer child CPR, a ratio of 15:2 is used.

Choking Victims

OBRA

A choking victim has an obstructed airway (an object blocking the airway). Special measures must be taken to clear this obstruction.

- If the victim is conscious, coughing, talking or making noise, and/or able to breathe, the airway is not completely obstructed. Remain calm and encourage the victim to remain calm. Encourage the victim to cough hard. Coughing is the most effective method of expelling the object from the airway.
- If the victim is conscious but not able to talk, make noise, breathe, or cough, the airway is completely obstructed. The victim usually grasps his or her throat and appears cyanotic (blue discoloration of the skin) (Figure 17–9). Immediate action must be taken to clear the airway. Abdominal thrusts, as described in Procedure 17:2E, are given to provide a force of air to push the object out of the airway.
- If the victim is unconscious and has an obstructed airway, administer adult CPR. Start with compressions (do not check for a pulse). Every time the airway is opened to give breaths, the rescuer should look in the victim's mouth for the object. If the object is visible, the rescuer should use a C-shaped or hooking motion to remove the object. If the object is not seen, the rescuer should try to administer breaths and then continue with chest compressions.
- If an infant (birth to 1 year old) has an obstructed airway, a different sequence of steps is used to remove the obstruction. The sequence includes five back blows; five chest thrusts; a check of the mouth; a finger sweep, if the object is seen; and an attempt to ventilate. The sequence, described in detail in Procedure 17:2F, is repeated until the object is expelled, ventilations are successful, or other qualified medical help arrives.
- If a child aged 1 to puberty (approximately age 12) has an obstructed airway, the same sequence of steps used for an adult is followed. A finger sweep of the mouth is *not* performed unless the object can be seen in the mouth.
- If the victim is pregnant or obese, perform chest thrusts.

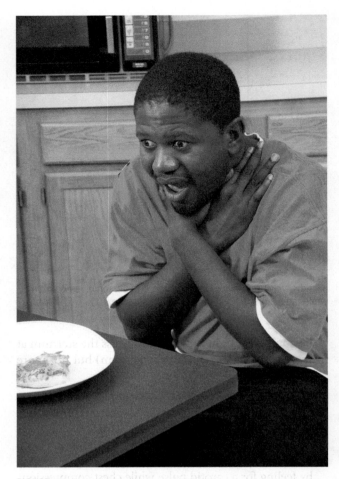
FIGURE 17–9 **A choking victim usually grasps his throat and appears cyanotic.**

Once CPR is started, it must be continued unless one of the following situations occur:

- The victim recovers and starts to breathe.
- Other qualified medical help arrives and takes over.
- A physician or other legally qualified person orders you to discontinue the attempt.
- The rescuer is so physically exhausted, CPR can no longer be continued.
- The scene suddenly becomes unsafe.
- You are given a legally valid do not resuscitate (DNR) order.

STUDENT: **Go to the workbook and complete the assignment sheet for 17:2, Performing Cardiopulmonary Resuscitation. Then return and continue with the procedures.**

PROCEDURE 17:2A

Performing CPR—One-Person Adult Rescue

Equipment and Supplies

CPR manikin, barrier device, alcohol or disinfecting solution, gauze sponges

Procedure

Safety

CAUTION: Only a CPR training manikin (Figure 17–10) should be used to practice this procedure. *Never* practice CPR on another person.

1. Assemble equipment. Position the manikin on a firm surface, usually the floor.

2. *Check for consciousness and breathing.* Shake the "victim" by tapping the shoulder. Ask, "Are you OK?" If the victim does not respond, activate EMS immediately. Follow the "call first, call fast" priority. Get an AED if available.

3. *Palpate the carotid pulse.* Kneeling at the victim's side, place the fingertips of your hand on the victim's voice box. Then slide the fingers toward you and into the groove at the side of the victim's neck, where you should find the carotid pulse. Take at least 5 seconds but not more than 10 seconds to feel for the pulse (Figure 17–11A). At the same time, watch for breathing, signs of circulation, and/or movement.

NOTE: The pulse may be weak, so check carefully.

4. *If the victim has a pulse but is not breathing, provide rescue breaths.* Give one breath every 5–6 seconds. Count, "One, one thousand; two, one thousand; three, one thousand; four, one thousand; and breathe," to obtain the correct timing. Recheck the pulse every 2 minutes to make sure the heart is still beating.

5. *If the victim does not have a pulse, or you are not sure if they have a pulse, administer chest compressions* as follows:

a. Locate the correct place on the sternum. While kneeling alongside the victim, use the middle finger of your hand

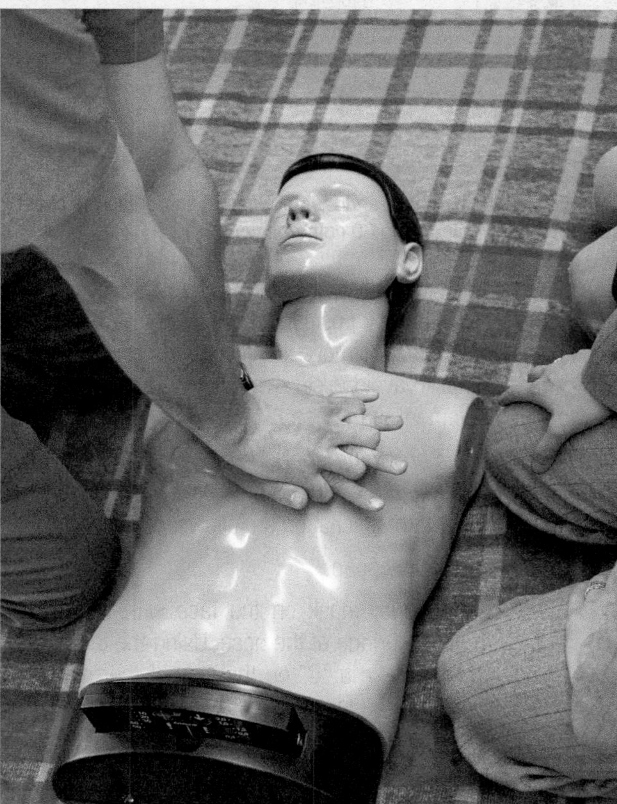

FIGURE 17–10 Use only training manikins while practicing CPR.

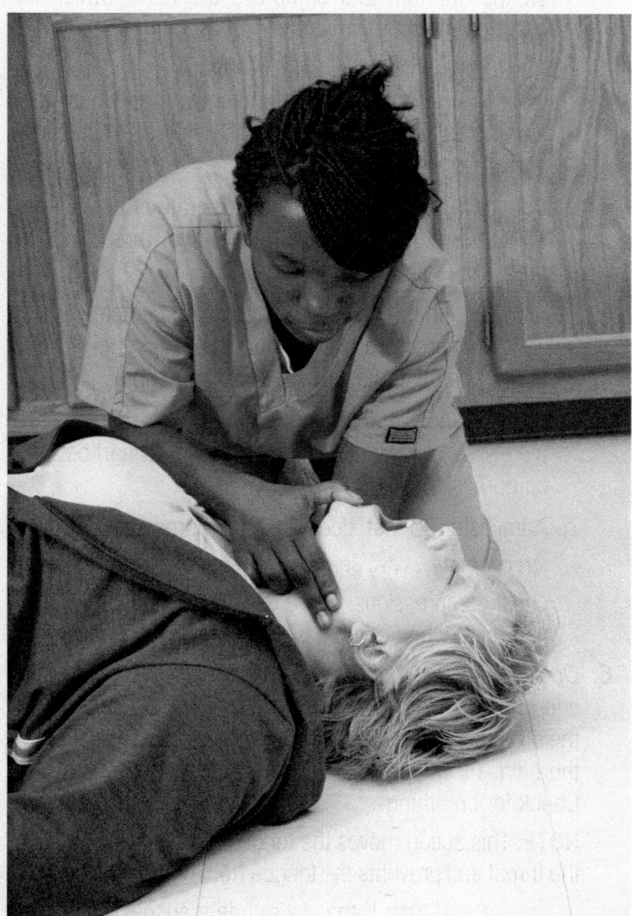

FIGURE 17–11A Palpate the carotid pulse for at least 5 but not more than 10 seconds to determine whether the heart is beating.

(continues)

PROCEDURE 17:2A (CONT.)

that is closest to the victim's feet to follow the ribs up to where the ribs meet the sternum, at the substernal notch. Keep the middle finger on the notch and position the index finger above it so two fingers are on the sternum. Then, place the heel of the opposite hand (the one closest to the victim's head) on the sternum, next to the index finger.

Safety

CAUTION: The heel of your hand should be in the center of the chest on the lower half of the sternum at the nipple line.

b. Place your other hand on top of the hand that is correctly positioned. Keep your fingers off the victim's chest. It may help to interlock your fingers.

c. Rise up on your knees so that your shoulders are directly over the victim's sternum. Lock your elbows and keep your arms straight.

NOTE: This position will allow you to push straight down on the sternum and compress the heart, which lies between the sternum and vertebral column.

d. Push down hard and fast to compress the chest at least 2 inches, or 5.0 centimeters but not more than 2.4 inches or 6 centimeters (Figure 17–11B). Use a smooth, even motion.

e. Administer 30 compressions at the rate of at least 100 to 120 per minute. Count, "One, two, three," and so forth, to obtain the correct rate.

f. Allow the chest to recoil or re-expand completely after each compression. Keep your hands on the sternum during the upstroke (chest relaxation period).

NOTE: When the chest recoils or re-expands completely, this allows more blood to refill the heart between compressions.

g. Administer 30 fast, deep chest compressions.

NOTE: Make every effort to minimize any interruptions to chest compressions. There is no blood flow to the brain and heart when compressions are not being performed.

6. *Open the airway.* Use the head-tilt/chin-lift method. Place one hand on the victim's forehead. Place the fingertips of the other hand under the bony part of the victim's jaw, near the chin. Tilt the head without closing the victim's mouth. Check for breathing.

NOTE: This action moves the tongue away from the back of the throat and prevents the tongue from blocking the airway.

Safety

CAUTION: If the victim has a suspected neck or upper spinal cord injury, use a jaw-thrust maneuver to open the airway. Assume a position on either side of the patient's head. Grasp the angles of the victim's lower jaw by positioning one hand on each side. Lift with both hands to move the lower jaw forward, making every attempt to avoid excessive backward tilting or side-to-side movement of the head.

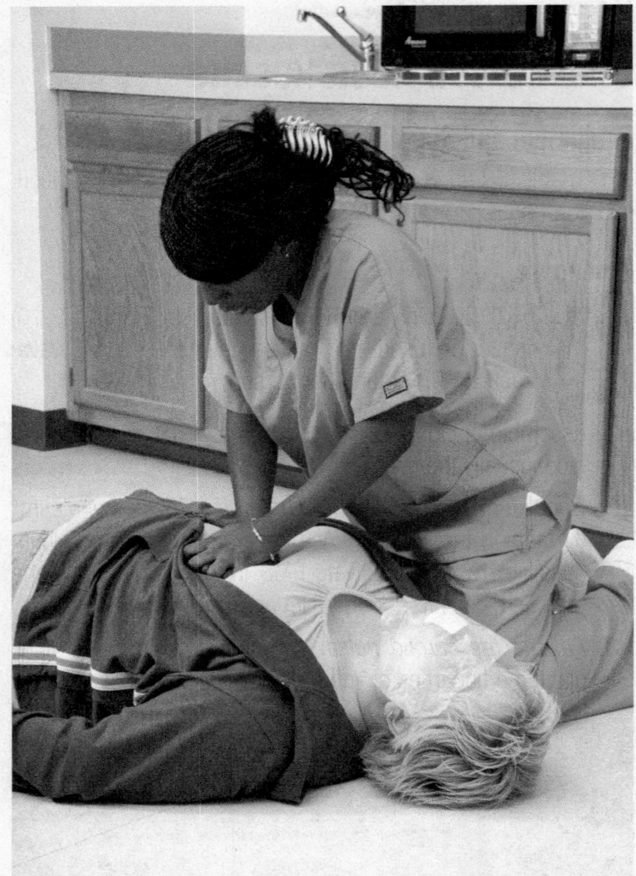

FIGURE 17–11B **Use hard and fast motions to compress the chest straight down while giving 30 compressions.**

7. *If the victim is breathing*, keep the airway open and obtain medical help. *If the victim is not breathing*, administer mouth-to-mouth resuscitation as follows:

a. Keep the airway open.

b. Place the barrier mask on the face with the narrow section on the bridge of the nose. Using the thumb and index finger, make a "C" on the side of the mask and press down on the face to create a seal.

c. Position your mouth on the barrier mask.

d. Give two breaths, each lasting approximately 1 second until the chest visibly rises (Figure 17–11C). Pause slightly between breaths. This allows air to flow out

PROCEDURE 17:2A (CONT.)

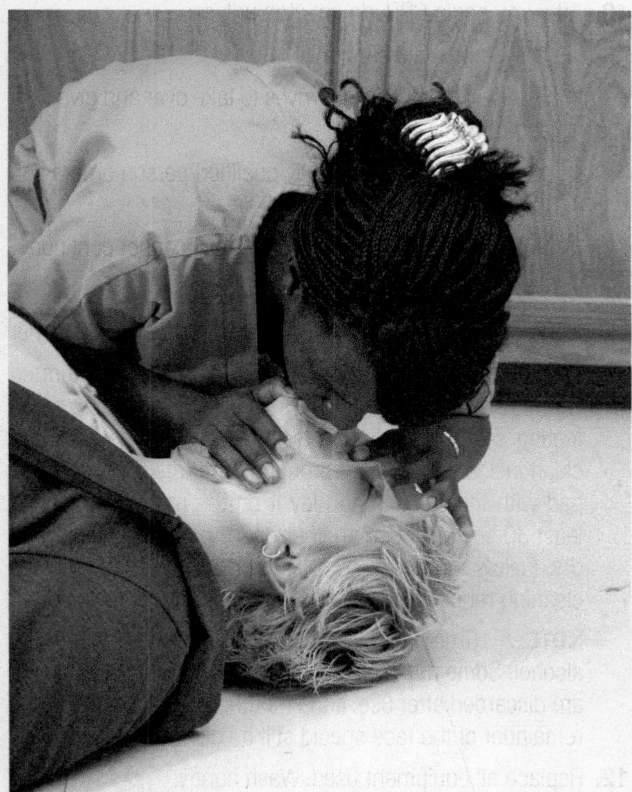

FIGURE 17–11C If the victim is not breathing, open the airway and use a barrier device to give two breaths. Watch for the chest to visibly rise.

and provides you with a chance to take a breath and increase the oxygen level for the second rescue breath.

e. Watch the chest for movement to be sure the air is entering the victim's lungs. Avoid overinflating the lungs and/or forcing air into the stomach.

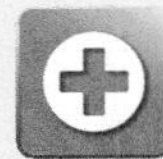

Precaution

CAUTION: Follow standard precautions. Use a CPR pocket face mask with a one-way valve to provide a barrier and prevent the transmission of disease.

Safety

CAUTION: Giving breaths too quickly or with too much force can cause gastric distention (bloating of the stomach when air enters it). This can lead to serious complications such as vomiting, aspiration (foreign material entering the lungs), and pneumonia.

8. Continue the cycles of 30 compressions followed by 2 ventilations until EMS providers take over, an AED arrives, or the victim recovers.

9. If an AED is available, give five cycles of CPR and then use the AED. Even though AEDs have different manufacturers and models, they all operate in basically the same way.

a. Position the AED at the victim's side next to the rescuer who is using it. If another person arrives to help, the second person can activate EMS (if this has not already been done) and then administer cycles of CPR on the victim's other side.

b. Open the case on the AED and turn on the power control.

NOTE: Some AEDs power on automatically when the case is opened.

c. Expose the victim's chest and attach the chest electrodes to bare skin. If the chest is covered with sweat or water, quickly wipe it dry. Choose the correct size electrode pad. Use adult size pads for any victim 8 years and older. Peel the backing off of the electrode pad. Place one pad on the upper right side of the chest, below the clavicle (collarbone) and to the right of the sternum (breastbone). Place the second electrode pad on the left side of the chest to the left of the nipple and a few inches below the axillae (armpit). If the victim has an implanted device such as a pacemaker, try to avoid putting the pads directly over the device. If possible, do not place the pads directly on a medication patch. If it does not delay shock, remove the patch and quickly wipe the area clean.

d. If necessary, attach the connecting cables of the electrodes to the electrode pad and AED. Some types of electrodes are preconnected.

e. Clearly state "Clear the victim." Look carefully to make sure no one is touching the victim. Push the analyze control to allow the AED to evaluate the heart rhythm (Figure 17–12). The analysis may take 5–15 seconds.

If the chest is very hairy and the AED is unable to analyze, press down firmly on the pads. If it still fails to analyze, pull the pads off and place new pads where the hair was pulled off by the previous pads.

f. Follow the recommendations of the AED. If the AED says NO SHOCK, resume CPR by giving 30 compressions followed by 2 ventilations.

g. If the AED says SHOCK, make sure the victim is clear. Loudly state "Clear victim," and look to make sure no one is touching the victim. Push the shock button.

Safety

CAUTION: If another rescuer is touching the victim, the rescuer will also receive the shock. This can cause a serious injury and/or a cardiac arrest.

(continues)

PROCEDURE 17:2A (CONT.)

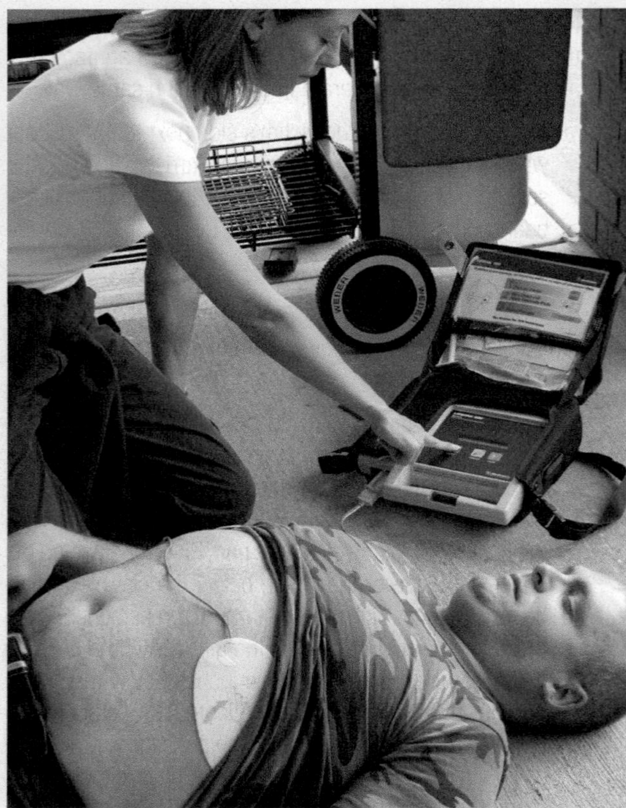

FIGURE 17–12 **"Clear" the victim before pushing the control to allow the automated external defibrillator (AED) to analyze the victim's heart rhythm.**

h. Begin cycles of CPR by starting with chest compressions immediately after the shock is delivered to the victim. After 2 minutes of CPR, most AEDs will prompt you to reanalyze the rhythm and deliver additional shocks if necessary.

10. After you begin CPR, do not stop unless:
    a. The victim recovers
    b. Qualified medical help arrives to take over and give CPR and/or apply an AED
    c. A physician or other legally qualified person orders you to discontinue the attempt
    d. You are so physically exhausted, you cannot continue
    e. The scene suddenly becomes unsafe
    f. You are given a legally valid do not resuscitate (DNR) order
11. After the practice session, use a gauze pad saturated with 70-percent alcohol or a 10-percent bleach disinfecting solution to clean the manikin. Wipe the face and clean inside the mouth thoroughly. Saturate a clean gauze pad with the solution and lay it on the mouth area for at least 30 seconds. Use another gauze pad to wipe the area dry. Follow manufacturer's instructions for any additional cleaning required.

    NOTE: A 10-percent bleach solution is more effective than alcohol. Some manikins have disposable mouthpieces that are discarded after use. If the mouthpiece is discarded, the remainder of the face should still be disinfected.
12. Replace all equipment used. Wash hands.

PRACTICE: **Go to the workbook and use the evaluation sheet for 17:2A, Performing CPR—One-Person Adult Rescue, to practice this procedure. When you believe you have mastered this skill, sign the sheet and give it to your instructor for further action.**

Check

FINAL CHECKPOINT: Using the criteria listed on the evaluation sheet, your instructor will grade your performance.

PROCEDURE 17:2B

Performing CPR— Two-Person Adult Rescue

Equipment and Supplies

CPR manikin, barrier device, alcohol or disinfecting solution, gauze sponges

Procedure

Safety

CAUTION: Only a CPR training manikin should be used to practice this procedure. *Never* practice CPR on another person.

1. Assemble equipment. Position the manikin on a firm surface, usually the floor.

PROCEDURE 17:2B (CONT.)

2. Check for consciousness and breathing. Gently shake the victim and ask, "Are you OK?"
3. If the victim is unconscious and not breathing, or not breathing normally, the first rescuer starts CPR. The second rescuer activates emergency medical services and obtains an AED if available.
4. Feel for the carotid pulse for at least 5 seconds and not more than 10 seconds.
5. *If there is no pulse*, or you are not sure if there is a pulse, give chest compressions. Locate the correct hand position on the sternum. Give 30 hard, fast, and deep compressions at a rate of at least 100 to 120 per minute.
6. Open the victim's airway using the head-tilt/chin-lift method. Place one hand on the victim's forehead. Place the fingertips of the other hand under the bony part of the victim's jaw, near the chin. Tilt the victim's head back without closing the victim's mouth. Check for breathing.
7. *If the victim is not breathing*, or not breathing normally (gasping), use a barrier device and give two breaths, each lasting approximately 1 second. Watch the chest for movement to be sure air is entering the victim's lungs. Avoid overinflating the lungs and/or forcing air into the stomach. Until the second rescuer returns, provide compressions and respirations as in a one-person rescue. Give 30 compressions for every 2 breaths.

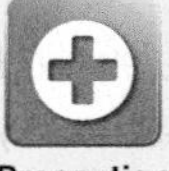
Precaution

CAUTION: Follow standard precautions. Use a CPR pocket face mask with a one-way valve to provide a barrier and prevent the transmission of disease.

8. When the second rescuer returns after calling for help, the first rescuer should complete the cycle of 30 compressions and 2 respirations.
9. The second rescuer should get into position for compressions and locate the correct hand placement while the first rescuer is giving the two breaths. The second rescuer should begin compressions at the rate of at least 100 to 120 per minute (Figure 17–13). The second rescuer should count out loud, "One, two, three, four, five. . . ." After each set of 30 compressions, the second rescuer should pause very briefly to allow the first rescuer to give 2 breaths. Rescue then continues with 2 breaths after each 30 compressions.
10. After every five cycles of CPR (approximately 2 minutes) the rescuers should change positions. The person giving compressions can provide a clear signal to change positions, such as, "Change, two, three, four. . . ." The compressor should complete a cycle of 30 compressions. The ventilator should give 2 breaths at the end of the 30 compressions. The ventilator should then move to the chest and locate the correct hand placement for compressions. The compressor should move to the head and open the airway. The new compressor should then give 30 hard, fast, and deep compressions at the rate of at least 100 to 120 per minute. The rescue should continue with 2 ventilations after each 30 compressions.

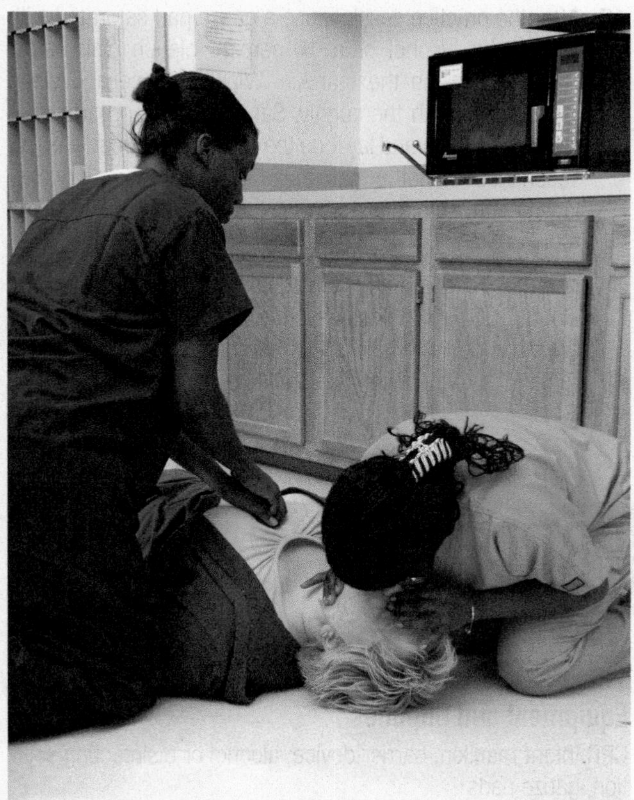

FIGURE 17–13 **In a two-person rescue, two breaths are given after every 30 compressions.**

11. If an AED is available, one rescuer should set up the AED while the other rescuer is giving cycles of CPR. When the AED is ready to analyze the heart rhythm, the rescuer operating the AED must make sure the other rescuer is clear of the victim. The steps for using the AED are discussed in detail in step 9 of Procedure 17:2A.
12. The rescuers should continue CPR until qualified medical help arrives, the victim recovers, a physician or other legally qualified person orders CPR discontinued, the scene suddenly becomes unsafe, or they are presented with a legally valid do not resuscitate (DNR) order.

(continues)

PROCEDURE 17:2B (CONT.)

13. After the practice session, use a gauze pad saturated with 70-percent alcohol or a 10-percent bleach disinfecting solution to clean the manikin. Wipe the face and clean inside the mouth thoroughly. Saturate a clean gauze pad with the solution and lay it on the mouth area for at least 30 seconds. Use another gauze pad to wipe the area dry. Follow manufacturer's instructions for any additional cleaning required.

    NOTE: A 10-percent bleach solution is more effective than alcohol. Some manikins have disposable mouthpieces that are discarded after use. If the mouthpiece is discarded, the remainder of the face should still be disinfected.

14. Replace all equipment used. Wash hands.

PRACTICE: Go to the workbook and use the evaluation sheet for 17:2B, Performing CPR—Two-Person Adult Rescue, to practice this procedure. When you believe you have mastered this skill, sign the sheet and give it to your instructor for further action.

Check

FINAL CHECKPOINT: Using the criteria listed on the evaluation sheet, your instructor will grade your performance.

PROCEDURE 17:2C

Performing CPR on Infants

Equipment and Supplies

CPR infant manikin, barrier device, alcohol or disinfecting solution, gauze pads

Procedure

Safety

CAUTION: Only a CPR training manikin should be used to practice this procedure. *Never* practice CPR on a human infant.

1. Assemble equipment.
2. Check for responsiveness and breathing. Gently shake the infant or tap the infant's foot (for reflex action) to determine consciousness. Call to the infant.

    NOTE: For CPR techniques, infants are usually considered to be under 1 year old.

3. If the infant is unconscious and not breathing, or not breathing normally (gasping), call aloud for help, and begin the steps of CPR. If no one arrives to call EMS, stop CPR after five cycles (approximately 2 minutes) to telephone for medical assistance. Resume CPR as quickly as possible.

    NOTE: If the infant is known to have a high risk for heart problems or a sudden collapse was witnessed, activate EMS and then begin CPR.

4. Check the pulse over the brachial artery. Place your fingertips on the inside of the upper arm and halfway between the elbow and shoulder (refer to Figure 17–8). Put your thumb on the posterior (outside) of the arm. Squeeze your fingers gently toward your thumb. Feel for the pulse for at least 5 but not more than 10 seconds.
5. *If a pulse is present, but the infant is not breathing*, provide ventilations by giving the infant 1 ventilation every 3 seconds (approximately 20 breaths per minute). Recheck the pulse every 2 minutes.
6. *If no pulse is present or if the heart rate is below 60 beats per minute with signs of poor circulation such as cyanosis*, administer cardiac compressions. Locate the correct position for compressions by drawing an imaginary line between the nipples. Place two fingers on the sternum just below this imaginary line. Give compressions at the rate of at least 100 to 120 per minute (Figure 17–14A). Make sure the infant is on a firm surface, or use one hand to support the infant's back while administering compressions. Press hard, fast, and deep enough to compress the infant's chest at least ⅓ the depth of the chest, approximately 1½ inches (4 cm). Give 30 compressions at the rate of at least 100 to 120 per minute. Allow the chest to recoil or re-expand completely between compressions.
7. Once 30 compressions are delivered, use the head-tilt/chin-lift method to open the infant's airway. Tip the head back gently, taking care not to tip it as far back as you would an adult's head.

Safety

CAUTION: Tipping the head too far will cause an obstruction of the infant's airway.

PROCEDURE 17:2C (CONT.)

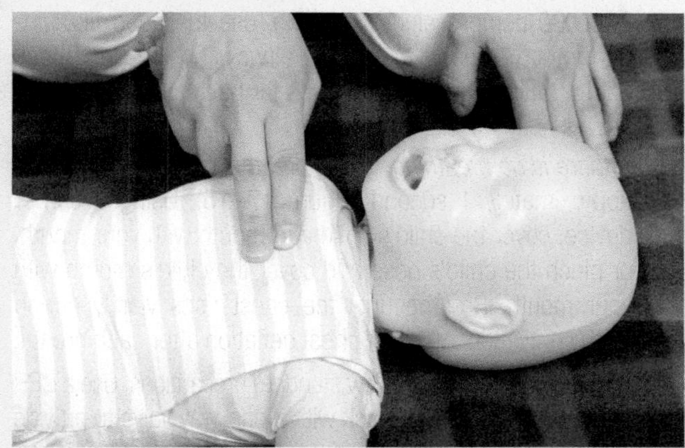

FIGURE 17–14A Use two fingers to give hard and fast compressions to the infant, at a rate of at least 100 to 120 compressions per minute. © pryzmat/www.Shutterstock.com

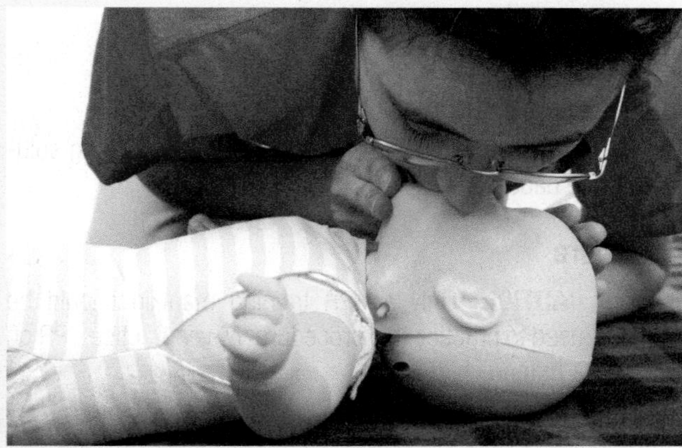

FIGURE 17–14B If the infant is not breathing, give 2 breaths. © pryzmat/www.Shutterstock.com

8. *If there is no breathing,* give 2 breaths, each breath lasting approximately 1 second (Figure 17–14B). Using a barrier device, cover the infant's nose and mouth with your mouth. Breathe until the chest rises visibly during each ventilation. Allow for chest deflation after each breath.

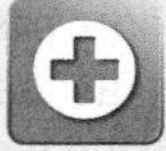

Precaution

CAUTION: Follow standard precautions. Use a CPR pocket face mask with a one-way valve to provide a barrier and prevent the transmission of disease.

9. After 2 breaths are given, administer 30 chest compressions.
10. Continue the cycle of 30 compressions followed by 2 ventilations. To establish the correct rate, count, "One, two, three, four, five . . . ."
11. If a second rescuer arrives to assist, the second rescuer should activate EMS if this has not been done. Then both rescuers can perform CPR on the infant.
    a. The first rescuer should finish a cycle of 30 compressions followed by 2 respirations.
    b. The second rescuer should stand at the infant's feet and place his or her thumbs next to each other on the lower half of the sternum just below the nipple line. The rescuer then wraps his or her hands around the infant to support the infant's back with the fingers, and uses the thumbs to administer 15 compressions.
    c. After 15 compressions, the person giving compressions pauses very briefly so the other rescuer can give 2 ventilations.

    NOTE: The ratio of compressions to ventilations is 15:2 for a two-person rescue on an infant.

    d. The rescuers should switch positions after every six to eight cycles (approximately 2 minutes) of CPR.
12. The rescuers should continue the cycles of CPR until qualified medical help arrives, the infant recovers, a physician or other legally qualified person orders CPR discontinued, or they are presented with a legally valid do not resuscitate (DNR) order (very rare for infants).
13. After the practice session, use a gauze pad saturated with 70-percent alcohol or a 10-percent bleach disinfecting solution to clean the manikin. Wipe the face and clean inside the mouth thoroughly. Saturate a clean gauze pad with the solution and lay it on the mouth area for at least 30 seconds. Use another gauze pad to wipe the area dry. Follow manufacturer's instructions for specific cleaning.

    NOTE: The 10-percent bleach solution is more effective than alcohol. Some manikins have disposable mouthpieces that are discarded after use. If the mouthpiece is discarded, the remainder of the face should still be disinfected.
14. Replace all equipment used. Wash hands.

PRACTICE: Go to the workbook and use the evaluation sheet for 17:2C, Performing CPR on Infants, to practice this procedure. When you believe you have mastered this skill, sign the sheet and give it to your instructor for further action.

Check

FINAL CHECKPOINT: Using the criteria listed on the evaluation sheet, your instructor will grade your performance.

PROCEDURE 17:2D

Performing CPR on Children

Equipment and Supplies

CPR child manikin, barrier device, alcohol or disinfecting solution, gauze pads

Procedure

Safety

CAUTION: Only a CPR training manikin should be used to practice this procedure. *Never* practice CPR on a human child.

1. Assemble equipment.
2. Check for responsiveness and breathing. Gently shake the child to determine consciousness. Call to the child.

   NOTE: Health care providers should use child CPR techniques on any child from 1 year of age to puberty, (approximately age 12) as evidenced by the development of secondary sex characteristics.
3. If the child is unconscious and not breathing call aloud for help, and begin the steps of CPR. If no one arrives to call EMS, stop CPR after five cycles (approximately 2 minutes) to telephone for medical assistance and obtain an AED if available. Resume CPR as quickly as possible.

   NOTE: If the child is known to have a high risk for heart problems or a sudden collapse was witnessed, activate EMS first and then begin CPR.
4. Check the pulse at the carotid pulse site. Feel for the pulse for at least 5 but not more than 10 seconds.
5. *If a pulse is present, but the child is not breathing,* provide ventilations by giving the child 1 ventilation every 3 seconds (approximately 20 breaths per minute). Recheck the pulse every 2 minutes.
6. *If no pulse is present or if the heart rate is below 60 beats per minute with signs of poor circulation such as cyanosis,* administer cardiac compressions. Place the heel of one hand on the lower half of the sternum just below a line drawn between the nipples or in the same position used for adult CPR. Keep the other hand on the child's forehead. If the child is larger, two hands can be positioned on the chest for compressions. Give compressions at the rate of at least 100 to 120 per minute. Make sure the child is on a firm surface, or use one hand to support the child's back while administering compressions. Press hard, fast, and deep enough to compress the child's chest at least ⅓ the depth of the chest, approximately 2 inches (5 cm). Give 30 compressions at the rate of at least 100 to 120 per minute. Allow the chest to recoil or re-expand completely between compressions.
7. Once 30 compressions are done, use the head-tilt/chin-lift method to open the child's airway. Tip the head back gently, taking care not to tip it as far back as you would an adult's head.
8. *If there is no breathing,* give 2 breaths, each breath lasting approximately 1 second (Figure 17–15). Using a barrier device, cover the child's nose and mouth with your mouth, or pinch the child's nose and cover the child's mouth with your mouth. Breathe until the chest rises visibly during each ventilation. Allow for chest deflation after each breath.

   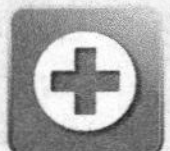
   Precaution

   CAUTION: Follow standard precautions. Use a CPR pocket face mask with a one-way valve to provide a barrier and prevent the transmission of disease.
9. Once 2 breaths are given, administer 30 compressions.
10. Continue the cycle of 30 compressions followed by 2 ventilations. To establish the correct rate, count, "One, two, three, four, five . . ."
11. If a second rescuer arrives to assist, the second rescuer should activate EMS if this has not been done. Then both rescuers can perform CPR on the child.
    a. The first rescuer should finish a cycle of 30 compressions followed by 2 respirations.
    b. The second rescuer should locate the proper position on the sternum for compressions. As soon as the first rescuer delivers the 2 respirations, the second rescuer should administer 15 compressions.
    c. After 15 compressions, the person giving compressions pauses very briefly so the other rescuer can give 2 ventilations.

       NOTE: The ratio of compressions to ventilations is 15:2 for a two-person rescue on a child.
    d. The rescuers should switch positions after every six to eight cycles (approximately 2 minutes) of CPR.

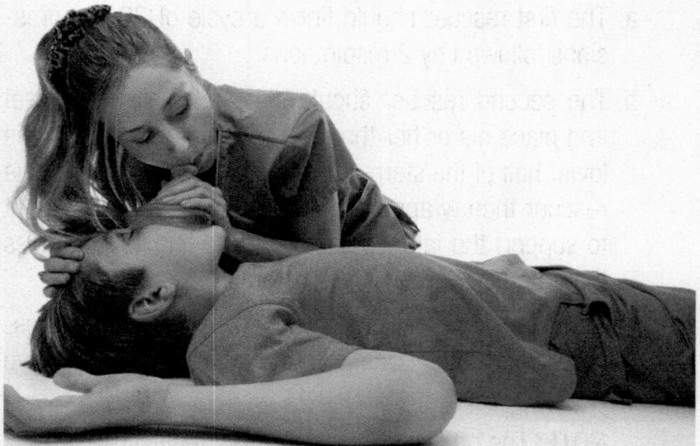

FIGURE 17–15 Using a barrier device, give 2 breaths. © iStockphoto/Leah-Anne Thompson

PROCEDURE 17:2D (CONT.)

12. If an AED is available, one rescuer should set up the AED while the other rescuer is giving cycles of CPR. When the AED is ready to analyze the heart rhythm, the rescuer operating the AED must make sure the other rescuer is clear of the victim. The steps for using the AED are discussed in detail in step 9 of Procedure 17:2A.

CAUTION: Adult electrode pads should be used on any child 8 years or older. Child or pediatric electrodes are used only on children from 1–8 years of age. In addition, if an AED does not have the option of a pediatric dosage, the adult dosage and electrodes should be used on the child.

13. The rescuers should continue the cycles of CPR until qualified medical help arrives, the child recovers, a physician or other legally qualified person orders CPR discontinued, or they are presented with a legally valid do not resuscitate (DNR) order.
14. After the practice session, use a gauze pad saturated with 70-percent alcohol or a 10-percent bleach disinfecting solution to clean the manikin. Wipe the face and clean inside the mouth thoroughly. Saturate a clean gauze pad with the solution and lay it on the mouth area for at least 30 seconds. Use another gauze pad to wipe the area dry. Follow manufacturer's instructions for specific cleaning.

    NOTE: The 10-percent bleach solution is more effective than alcohol. Some manikins have disposable mouthpieces that are discarded after use. If the mouthpiece is discarded, the remainder of the face should still be disinfected.
15. Replace all equipment used. Wash hands.

PRACTICE: **Go to the workbook and use the evaluation sheet for 17:2D, Performing CPR on Children, to practice this procedure. When you believe you have mastered this skill, sign the sheet and give it to your instructor for further action.**

FINAL CHECKPOINT: Using the criteria listed on the evaluation sheet, your instructor will grade your performance.

PROCEDURE 17:2E

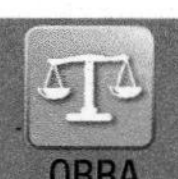

Performing CPR—Obstructed Airway on Conscious Adult or Child

Equipment and Supplies

CPR manikin or choking manikin and a barrier device

Procedure

CAUTION: Only a manikin should be used to practice this procedure. Do not practice on another person. Hand placement can be tried on another person, but the actual abdominal thrust should *never* be performed unless the person is choking.

1. Assemble equipment. Position the manikin in an upright position sitting on a chair.
2. Determine whether the victim has an airway obstruction. Ask, "Are you choking?" Check to see whether the victim can cough or speak.

CAUTION: If the victim is coughing forcefully, the airway is not completely obstructed. Encourage the victim to remain calm and cough hard. Coughing is usually very effective for removing an obstruction.

3. If the victim cannot cough, talk, make noise, or breathe, call for help.
4. Perform abdominal thrusts to try to remove the obstruction. Follow these steps:
    a. Stand behind the victim.
    b. Wrap both arms around the victim's waist.
    c. Make a fist of one hand (Figure 17–16A). Place the thumb side of the fist in the middle of the victim's abdomen, slightly above the navel (umbilicus) but well below the xiphoid process at the end of the sternum.
    d. Grasp the fist with your other hand.
    e. Use quick, upward thrusts to press into the victim's abdomen (Figure 17–16B).

(continues)

PROCEDURE 17:2E (CONT.)

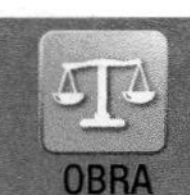

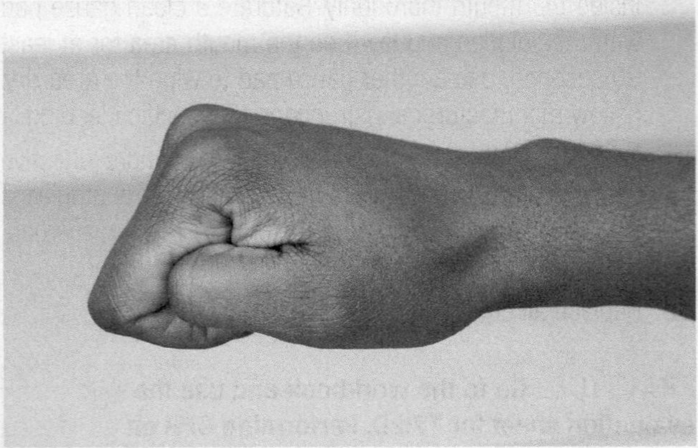

FIGURE 17–16A **Make a fist of one hand.**

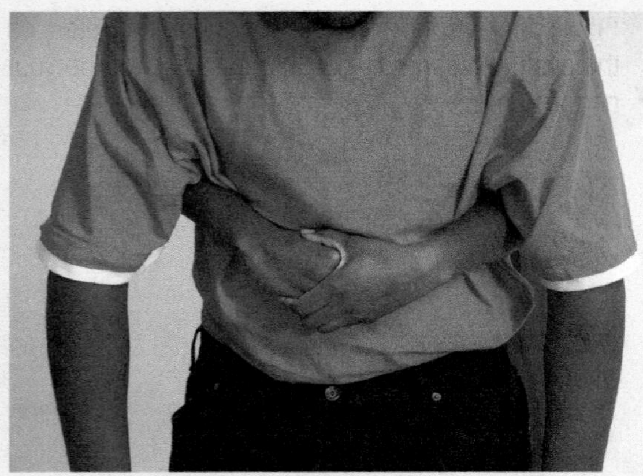

FIGURE 17–16B **Place the thumb side of the fist above the umbilicus but well below the xiphoid process at the end of the sternum. Grasp the fist with your other hand and use quick, upward thrusts to press into the victim's abdomen.**

NOTE: The thrusts should be delivered hard enough to cause a force of air to push the obstruction out of the airway.

CAUTION: Make sure that your forearms do not press against the victim's rib cage while the thrusts are being performed.

f. If you cannot reach around the victim to give abdominal thrusts (the victim is very obese), or if a victim is in the later stages of pregnancy, give chest thrusts. Stand behind the victim. Wrap your arms under the victim's axilla (armpits) and around to the center of the chest. Make a fist with one hand and place the thumb side of the fist against the center of the sternum but well above the xiphoid process. Grab your fist with your other hand and thrust inward.

g. Repeat the thrusts until the object is expelled or until the victim becomes unconscious.

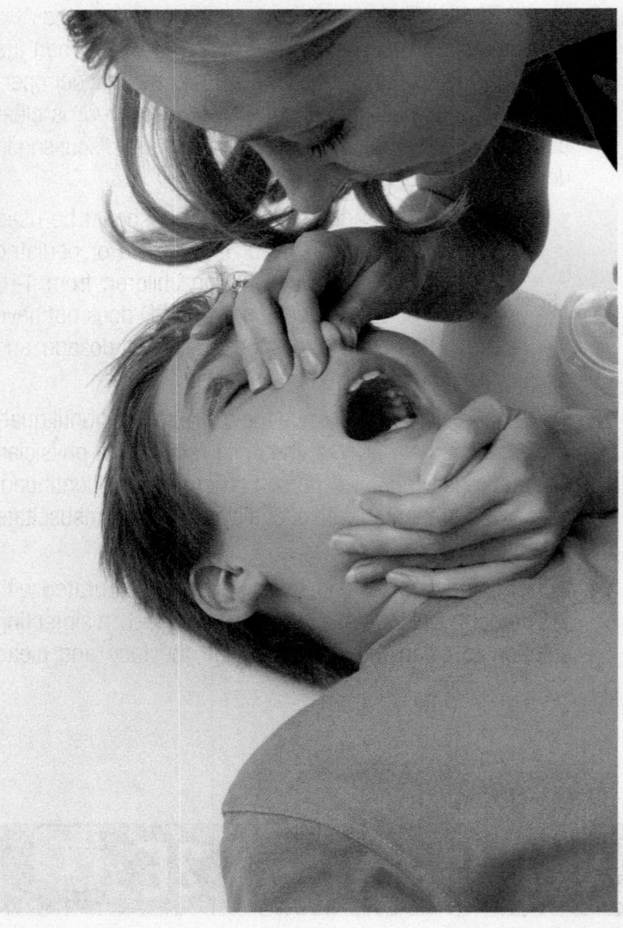

FIGURE 17–17 **Every time you open the airway, look in the mouth before giving breaths.** © iStockphoto/Leah-Anne Thompson

5. If the victim loses consciousness, begin CPR. Activate EMS if this has not already been done. Then start the cycle of CPR. Start with compressions—do not check for a pulse. Every time you open the airway you should look in the mouth before giving breaths (Figure 17–17). If you see an object, use a C-shaped or hooking motion to remove the object. Perform CPR.

a. Give 30 fast, deep chest compressions.

b. Open the airway.

c. Check the mouth for a foreign body. If you are able to see an object, use a hooking motion with your finger to try to remove it.

PROCEDURE 17:2E (CONT.)

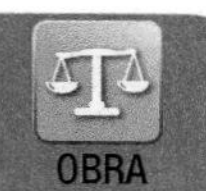

d. Using a barrier device, try to give 2 breaths.

e. Give 30 compressions and continue the cycle.

6. Do *not* stop CPR unless the victim recovers, qualified medical help arrives to take over, a physician or other legally qualified person orders you to discontinue the attempt, you are so physically exhausted you cannot continue, or the scene suddenly becomes unsafe.
7. Make every effort to obtain medical help for the victim as soon as possible.
8. After the practice session, replace all equipment used. Wash hands.

PRACTICE: **Go to the workbook and use the evaluation sheet for 17:2E, Performing CPR—Obstructed Airway on Conscious Adult or Child, to practice this procedure. When you believe you have mastered this skill, sign the sheet and give it to your instructor for further action.**

FINAL CHECKPOINT: Using the criteria listed on the evaluation sheet, your instructor will grade your performance.

PROCEDURE 17:2F

Performing CPR—Obstructed Airway on Conscious Infant

Equipment and Supplies

CPR infant manikin, barrier device, alcohol or disinfecting solution, gauze sponges

Procedure

CAUTION: Only an infant manikin should be used to practice this procedure. Do *not* practice on a real infant.

1. Assemble equipment. Kneel or sit with the infant in your lap.

   NOTE: An infant is any baby to 1 year of age. Health care providers should use the adult choking sequence for any child older than 1 year.

2. Shake the infant gently. Ask, "Are you OK?"
3. If the infant is conscious and coughing forcefully, allow the infant to cough. The airway is not completely obstructed and the coughing may expel the object.
4. If the infant cannot cry, make any sounds, is making a high-pitched noise while inhaling or no noise at all, is turning cyanotic, and does not appear to be breathing, the airway is completely obstructed. Activate EMS immediately.
5. Quickly bare the infant's chest to expose the sternum (breastbone).
6. Give five back blows. Hold the infant face down, with your arm supporting the infant's body and your hand supporting the infant's head and jaw. Position the head lower than the chest (Figure 17–18A). Use the heel of your other hand to give five firm back blows between the infant's shoulder blades.

CAUTION: When performing back blows on an infant, do not use excessive force.

7. Support the infant's head and neck to turn the infant face up. Hold the infant with your forearm resting on your thigh. Keep the infant's head lower than the chest.
8. Give five chest thrusts. Position two to three fingers on the sternum just below an imaginary line drawn between the nipples. Press straight down five times (Figure 17–18B), each with the intention of creating enough force to dislodge the obstruction.
9. Continue the cycle of five back blows followed by five chest thrusts until EMS arrives or the infant becomes unresponsive.
10. If the infant becomes unresponsive, place the infant on a firm surface. Open the airway and look for an object. If an object is visible, use a C-shaped or hooking motion to remove it. Then perform CPR starting with compressions—do not check for a pulse. Follow the normal procedure for an infant, except look in the mouth every time you are ready to give breaths.

    a. Give 30 fast, deep chest compressions.

    b. Open the airway.

(continues)

PROCEDURE 17:2F (CONT.)

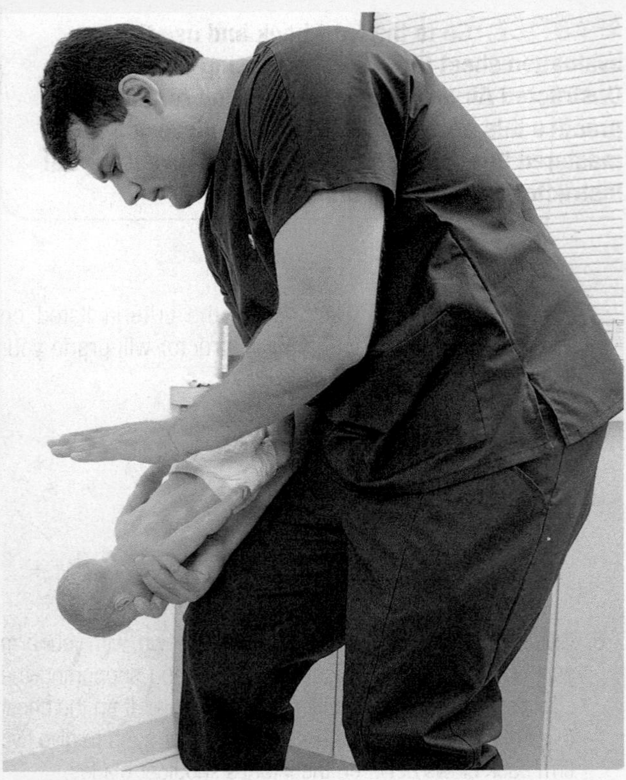

FIGURE 17–18A To give an infant five back blows, position the infant face down, with the head lower than the chest.

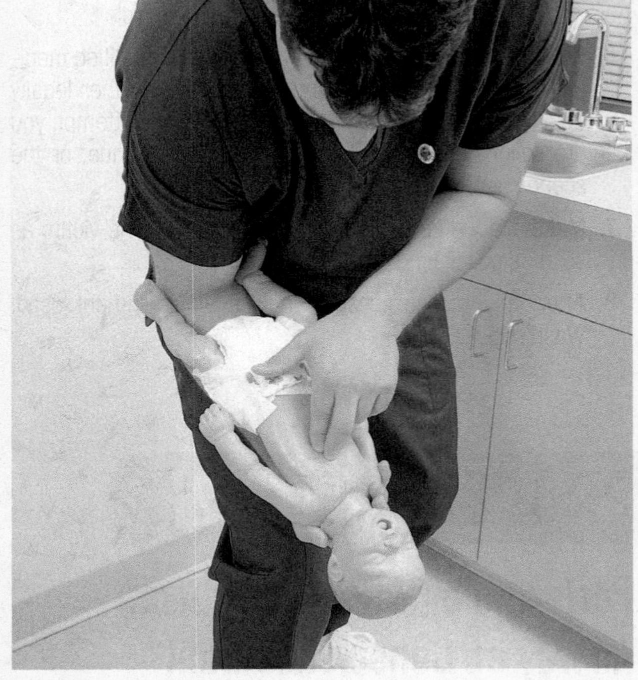

FIGURE 17–18B Give the infant five chest thrusts, keeping the head lower than the chest.

c. Check the mouth for a foreign body. If you are able to see an object, use a hooking motion with your finger to try to remove it.

d. Using a barrier device, try to give 2 breaths.

e. Give 30 compressions and continue the cycle.

11. Do *not* stop CPR unless the infant recovers, qualified medical help arrives to take over, a physician or other legally qualified person orders you to discontinue the attempt, you are so physically exhausted you cannot continue, or the scene suddenly becomes unsafe.

12. Make every effort to obtain medical help for the infant as soon as possible.

13. After the practice session, use a gauze pad saturated with 70-percent alcohol or a 10-percent bleach disinfecting solution to clean the manikin. Wipe the face and clean inside the mouth thoroughly. Saturate a clean gauze pad with the solution and lay it on the mouth area for at least 30 seconds. Use another gauze pad to wipe the area dry. Follow manufacturer's recommendations for specific cleaning or care.

NOTE: A 10-percent bleach solution is more effective than alcohol. Some manikins have disposable mouthpieces that are discarded after use. If the mouth-piece is discarded, the remainder of the face should still be disinfected.

14. Replace all equipment used. Wash hands.

PRACTICE: Go to the workbook and use the evaluation sheet for 17:2F, Performing CPR—Obstructed Airway on Conscious Infant, to practice this procedure. When you believe you have mastered this skill, sign the sheet and give it to your instructor for further action.

FINAL CHECKPOINT: Using the criteria listed on the evaluation sheet, your instructor will grade your performance.

17:3 Providing First Aid for Bleeding and Wounds

Introduction

In any health care career, as well as in your personal life, you may need to provide first aid to control bleeding or care for wounds. A **wound** involves injury to the soft tissues. Wounds are usually classified as open or closed. With an open wound, there is a break in the skin or mucous membrane. With a closed wound, there is no break in the skin or mucous membrane but injury occurs to the underlying tissues. An example of a closed wound is a bruise or hematoma. Wounds can result in bleeding, infection, and/or tetanus (lockjaw, a serious infection caused by bacteria). First aid care must be directed toward controlling bleeding before the bleeding leads to death, and toward either preventing or obtaining treatment for infection.

Types of Open Wounds

Open wounds are classified into types according to the injuries that occur. Some main types are abrasions, incisions, lacerations, punctures, avulsions, and amputations.

- **Abrasion**: With this type of wound the skin is scraped off. Bleeding is usually limited, but infection must be prevented because dirt and contaminants often enter the wound.
- **Incision**: This is a cut or injury caused by a sharp object such as a knife, scissors, or razor blade. The edges of the wound are smooth and regular. If the cut is deep, bleeding can be heavy and can lead to excessive blood loss. In addition, damage to muscles, nerves, and other tissues can occur (Figure 17–19A).
- **Laceration**: This type of wound involves tearing of the tissues by way of excessive force. The wound often has jagged, irregular edges (Figure 17–19B). Bleeding may be heavy. If the wound is deep, contamination may lead to infection.
- **Puncture**: This type of wound is caused by a sharp object such as a pin, nail, or pointed instrument. Gunshot wounds can also cause puncture wounds that are extremely dangerous because the damage is hidden under the skin and not visible. With all puncture wounds, external bleeding is usually limited, but internal bleeding can occur. In addition, the chance for infection is increased and tetanus may develop if tetanus bacteria enter the wound.

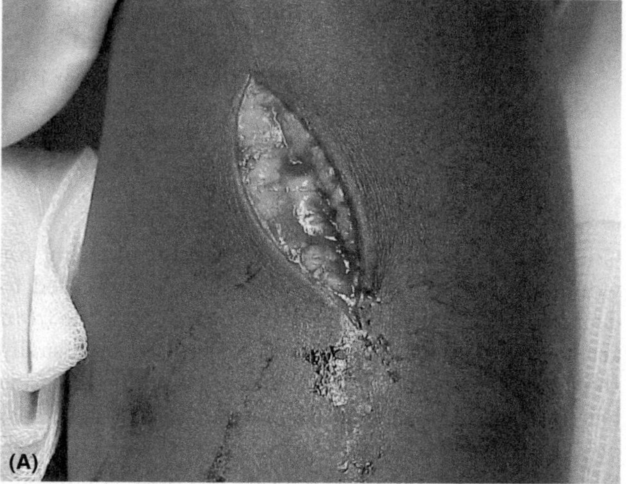

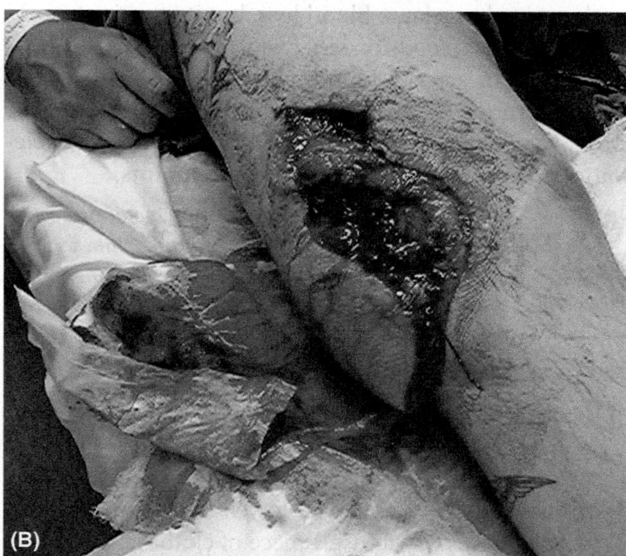

FIGURE 17–19 **Open wounds include (A) an incision that has smooth, regular edges, and (B) a laceration that has jagged irregular edges.** Courtesy of Ronald Stram, MD, Albany Medical Center, Albany, NY. Courtesy of Dr. Deborah Funk, Albany Medical Center

- **Avulsion**: This type of wound occurs when tissue is torn or separated from the victim's body. It can result in a piece of torn tissue hanging from the ear, nose, hand, or other body part. Bleeding is heavy and usually extensive. It is important to preserve the body part while caring for this type of wound, because a surgeon may be able to reattach it.
- **Amputation**: This type of injury occurs when a body part is cut off and separated from the body. Loss of a finger, toe, hand, or other body part can occur. Bleeding can be heavy and extensive. Care must be taken to preserve the amputated part because a surgeon may be able to reattach it. The part should be wrapped in a cool, moist dressing (use sterile water or

normal saline, if possible) and placed in a plastic bag. The plastic bag should be kept cool or placed in ice water and transported with the victim. The body part should never be placed directly on ice because ice can freeze the tissue.

Controlling Bleeding

Controlling bleeding is the first priority in caring for wounds, because it is possible for a victim to bleed to death in a short period of time. Bleeding can come from arteries, veins, and capillaries. *Arterial blood* usually spurts from a wound, results in heavy blood loss, and is bright red. Arterial bleeding is life-threatening and must be controlled quickly. *Venous blood* is slower, steadier, and dark red or maroon. Venous bleeding is constant and can lead to a large blood loss, but it is easier to control. *Capillary blood* "oozes" from the wound slowly, is less red than arterial blood, and clots easily. The four main methods for controlling bleeding are listed in the order in which they should be used: direct pressure, elevation, pressure bandage, and pressure points.

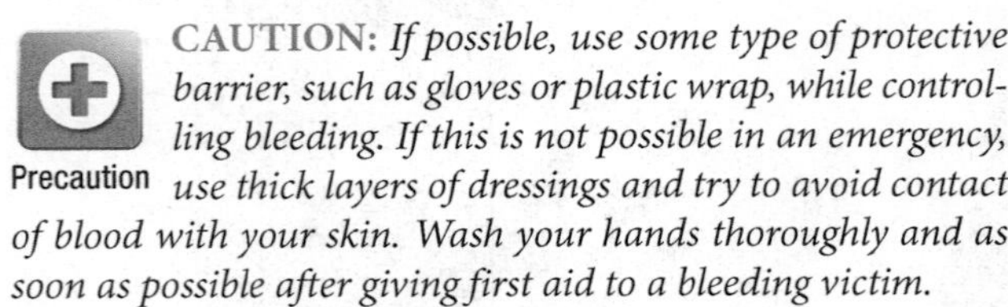

Precaution

CAUTION: *If possible, use some type of protective barrier, such as gloves or plastic wrap, while controlling bleeding. If this is not possible in an emergency, use thick layers of dressings and try to avoid contact of blood with your skin. Wash your hands thoroughly and as soon as possible after giving first aid to a bleeding victim.*

- *Direct pressure:* Using your gloved hand over a thick dressing or sterile gauze, apply pressure directly to the wound (Figure 17–20A). If no dressing is available, use a clean cloth or linen-type towel. In an emergency it may be necessary to use a piece of clothing or another material from the environment. Continue to apply pressure for 5–10 minutes or until the bleeding stops. If blood soaks through the dressing, apply a second dressing over the first and continue to apply direct pressure. Do *not* disturb blood clots once they have formed. Direct pressure will usually stop most bleeding.
- *Elevation:* Raise the injured part above the level of the victim's heart to allow gravity to aid in stopping the blood flow from the wound. Continue applying direct pressure while elevating the injured part (Figure 17–20B).

Safety

CAUTION: *If fractures (broken bones) are present or suspected, the part should not be elevated.*

- *Pressure bandage:* Apply a pressure bandage to hold the dressings in place. Maintain direct pressure and elevation while applying the pressure bandage. The procedure for applying a pressure bandage is described in step 4 of Procedure 17:3.

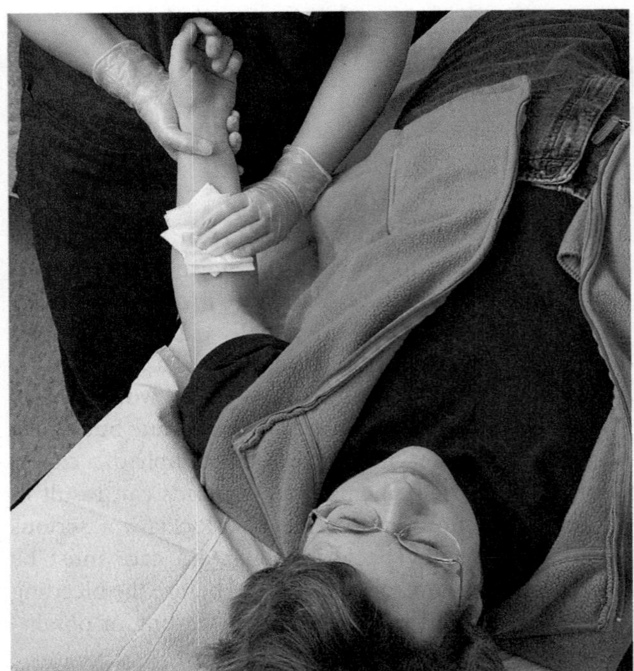

FIGURE 17–20A If possible, use some type of protective barrier, such as gloves or plastic wrap, while applying direct pressure to control bleeding.

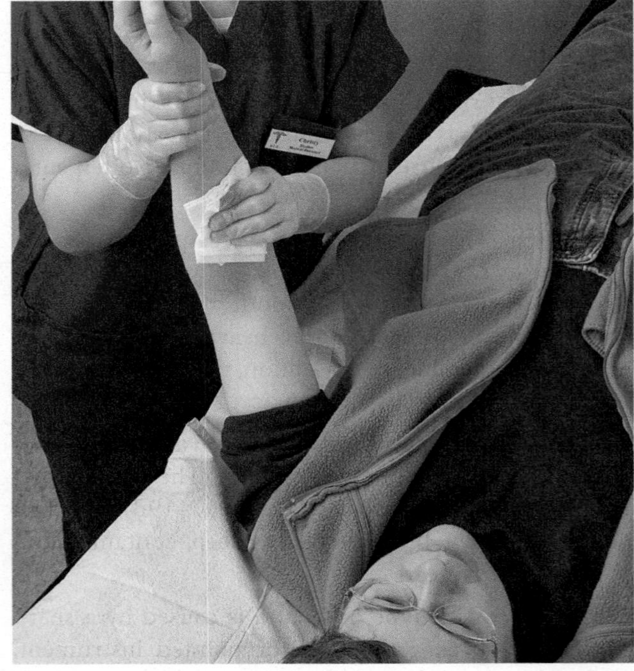

FIGURE 17–20B Continue to apply direct pressure while elevating the injured part above the level of the heart.

- *Pressure points:* If direct pressure, elevation, and the pressure bandage do not stop severe bleeding, it may be necessary to apply pressure to pressure points. By applying pressure to a main artery and pressing it against an

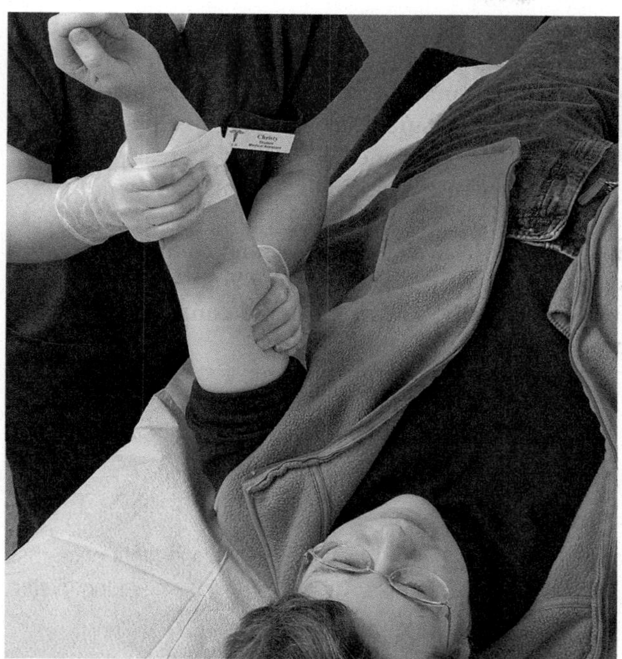

FIGURE 17–20C The main pressure point for the arm is the brachial artery. Pressure is applied to the artery only until the bleeding stops.

underlying bone, the main blood supply to the injured area can be cut off. However, because this technique also stops circulation to other parts of the limb, it should not be used any longer than is absolutely necessary. Direct pressure and elevation should also be continued while pressure is being applied to the pressure point.

The main pressure point for the arm is the brachial artery. It is located on the inside of the arm, approximately halfway between the armpit and the elbow (Figure 17–20C). The main pressure point for the leg is the femoral artery. The pulsation can be felt at the groin (the front middle point of the upper leg, in the crease where the thigh joins the body) (Figure 17–20D). When bleeding stops, slowly release pressure on the pressure point. Continue using direct pressure and elevation. If bleeding starts again, be ready to reapply pressure to the correct pressure point.

After severe bleeding has been controlled, obtain medical help for the victim. Do not disturb any blood clots or remove the dressings that were used to control the bleeding, because this may result in additional bleeding. Make no attempt to clean the wound, because this too is likely to result in additional bleeding.

Minor Wounds

In treating minor wounds that do not involve severe bleeding, prevention of infection is the first priority. Wash your hands thoroughly before treating the wound. Put on gloves to avoid contamination from blood or fluid draining from the wound. Use soap and water and sterile gauze, if possible, to wash the wound. Wipe in an outward direction, away from the wound. Discard the wipe after each use. Rinse the wound thoroughly with cool water. Use sterile gauze to gently blot the wound dry. Apply a sterile dressing or bandage. Watch for any signs of infection. Be sure to tell the victim to obtain medical help if any signs of infection appear.

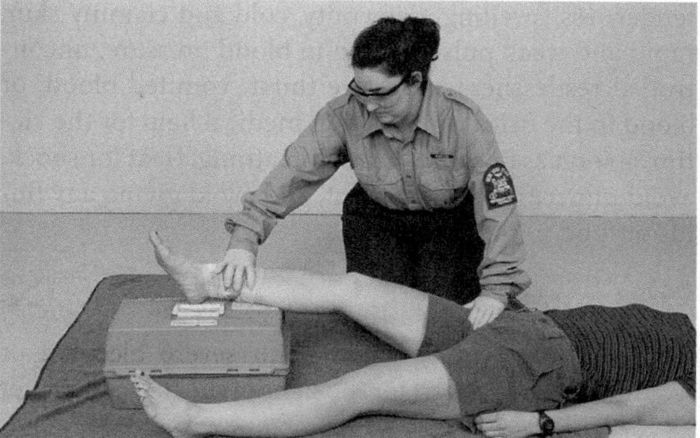

FIGURE 17–20D The main pressure point in the leg is the femoral artery. Pressure is applied while maintaining direct pressure to and elevation of the injured part.

Infection can develop in any wound. It is important to recognize the signs of infection and to seek medical help if they appear. Some signs and symptoms are swelling, heat, redness, pain, fever, pus, and red streaks leading from the wound. Prompt medical care is needed if any of these symptoms occur.

Tetanus bacteria can enter an open wound and lead to serious illness and death. Tetanus infection is most common in puncture wounds and wounds that involve damage to tissue underneath the skin. When this type of wound occurs, it is important to obtain information from the patient regarding his or her last tetanus shot and to get medical advice regarding protection in the form of a tetanus shot or booster.

With some wounds, objects can remain in the tissues or become embedded in the wound. Examples of such objects include splinters, small pieces of glass, small stones, and other similar objects. If the object is at the surface of the skin, remove it gently with sterile tweezers or tweezers wiped clean with alcohol or a disinfectant. Any objects embedded in the tissues should be left in the skin and removed by a physician.

Closed Wounds

Closed wounds (those not involving breaks in the skin) can occur anywhere in the body as a result of injury. If the wound is a bruise, cold applications can be applied to reduce swelling. Other closed wounds can be extremely serious and cause internal bleeding that may lead to death. Signs and symptoms may include pain, tenderness, swelling, deformity, cold and clammy skin, rapid and weak pulse, a drop in blood pressure, uncontrolled restlessness, excessive thirst, vomited blood, or blood in the urine or feces. Get medical help for the victim as soon as possible. Check breathing, treat for shock, avoid unnecessary movement, and avoid giving any fluids or food to the victim.

Summary

While caring for any victim with severe bleeding or wounds, always be alert for the signs of shock (see Chapter 17:4). Be prepared to treat shock while providing care to control bleeding and prevent infection in the wound.

Comm

At all times, remain calm while providing first aid. Reassure the victim. Obtain appropriate assistance or medical care as soon as possible in every case requiring additional care.

STUDENT: Go to the workbook and complete the assignment sheet for 17:3, Providing First Aid for Bleeding and Wounds. Then return and continue with the procedure.

PROCEDURE 17:3

Providing First Aid for Bleeding and Wounds

Equipment and Supplies

Sterile dressings and bandages, disposable gloves

Procedure

Severe Wounds

1. Follow the steps of priority care, if indicated:
   a. Check the scene. Move the victim only if absolutely necessary.
   b. Check the victim for consciousness and breathing.
   c. Call emergency medical services (EMS).
   d. Provide care to the victim.
2. To control severe bleeding, proceed as follows:
   a. 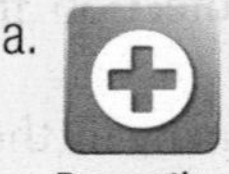 Precaution — Wear gloves or wrap your hands in plastic wrap to provide a protective barrier while controlling bleeding. If this is not possible in an emergency, use thick layers of dressings and try to avoid contact of blood with your skin.
   b. Using your hand over a thick dressing or sterile gauze, apply pressure directly to the wound.
   c. Continue to apply pressure to the wound for approximately 5–10 minutes. Do *not* release the pressure to check whether the bleeding has stopped.
   d. If blood soaks through the first dressing, apply a second dressing on top of the first dressing, and continue to apply direct pressure.

   NOTE: If sterile gauze is not available, use clean material or a bare hand.

Safety

CAUTION: Do *not* disturb blood clots once they have formed. This will cause the bleeding to start again.

3. Elevate the injured part above the level of the victim's heart unless a fracture or broken bone is suspected.

   NOTE: This allows gravity to help stop the blood flow to the area.

   NOTE: Direct pressure and elevation are used together. Do not *stop* direct pressure while elevating the part.
4. To hold the dressings in place, apply a pressure bandage. Maintain direct pressure and elevation while applying the pressure bandage. To apply a pressure bandage, proceed as follows:
   a. Apply additional dressings over the dressings already on the wound.
   b. Use a roller bandage to hold the dressings in place by wrapping the roller bandage around the dressings. Use overlapping turns to cover the dressings and to hold them securely in place.
   c. Tie off the ends of the bandage by placing the tie directly over the dressings (Figure 17–21).
   d. Make sure the pressure bandage is secure. Check a pulse site below the pressure bandage to make sure the bandage is not too tight. A pulse should be present and there should be no discoloration of the skin to indicate impaired circulation. If any signs of impaired circulation are present, loosen and replace the pressure bandage.
5. If the bleeding continues, it may be necessary to apply pressure to the appropriate pressure point. Continue using direct pressure and elevation, and apply pressure to the pressure point as follows:
   a. If the wound is on the arm or hand, apply pressure to the brachial artery. Place the flat surface of your

PROCEDURE 17:3 (CONT.)

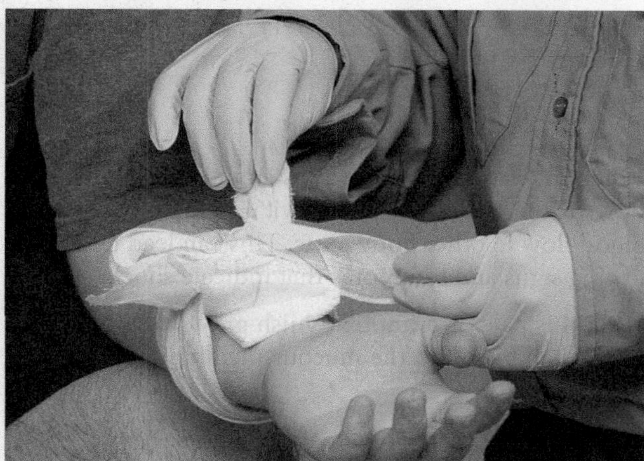

FIGURE 17–21 **Tie the ends of the bandage directly over the dressings to secure a pressure bandage.**

fingers (not your fingertips) against the inside of the victim's upper arm, approximately halfway between the elbow and axilla area. Position your thumb on the outside of the arm. Press your fingers toward your thumb to compress the brachial artery and decrease the supply of blood to the arm (refer to Figure 17–20C).

b. If the wound is on the leg, place the flat surfaces of your fingers or the heel of one hand directly over the femoral artery where it passes over the pelvic bone. The position is on the front, middle part of the upper thigh (groin) where the leg joins the body. Straighten your arm and apply pressure to compress the femoral artery and to decrease the blood supply to the leg (refer to Figure 17–20D).

6. When the bleeding stops, slowly release the pressure on the pressure point while continuing to use direct pressure and elevation. If the bleeding starts again, be ready to reapply pressure to the pressure point.
7. Obtain medical help for the victim as soon as possible. Severe bleeding is a life-threatening emergency.
8. While caring for any victim experiencing severe bleeding, be alert for the signs and symptoms of shock. Treat the victim for shock if any signs or symptoms are noted.
9. Comm — During treatment, constantly reassure the victim. Encourage the victim to remain calm by remaining calm yourself.
10. After controlling the bleeding, wash your hands as thoroughly and quickly as possible to avoid possible contamination from the blood. Wear gloves and use a disinfectant solution to wipe up any blood spills. Always wash your hands thoroughly after removing gloves.

Procedure

Minor Wounds

1. Wash hands thoroughly with soap and water. Put on gloves.
2. Use sterile gauze, soap, and water to wash the wound. Start at the center and wash in an outward direction. Discard the gauze after each pass.
3. Rinse the wound thoroughly with cool water to remove all of the soap.
4. Use sterile gauze to dry the wound. Blot it gently.
5. Apply a sterile dressing to the wound.
6. Caution the victim to look for signs of infection. Tell the victim to obtain medical care if any signs of infection appear.
7. If tetanus infection is possible (for example, in cases involving puncture wounds), tell the victim to contact a physician regarding a tetanus shot.

Safety

CAUTION: Do *not* use any antiseptic solutions to clean the wound and do not apply any substances to the wound unless specifically instructed to do so by a physician or your immediate supervisor.

8. Obtain medical help as soon as possible for any victim requiring additional care. Any victim who has particles embedded in a wound, risk for tetanus, severe bleeding, or other complications must be referred for medical care.
9. When care is complete, remove gloves and wash hands thoroughly.

PRACTICE: **Go to the workbook and use the evaluation sheet for 17:3, Providing First Aid for Bleeding and Wounds, to practice these procedures. When you believe you have mastered these skills, sign the sheet and give it to your instructor for further action.**

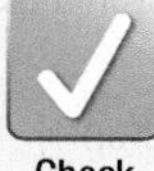
Check

FINAL CHECKPOINT: Using the criteria listed on the evaluation sheet, your instructor will grade your performance.

17:4 Providing First Aid for Shock

Introduction

Shock is a state that can exist with any injury or illness requiring first aid. It is important that you are able to recognize it and provide treatment.

Shock, also called *hypoperfusion*, can be defined as "a clinical set of signs and symptoms associated with an inadequate supply of blood to body organs, especially the brain and heart." If it is not treated, shock can lead to death, even when a victim's injuries or illness might not themselves be fatal. After just 4–6 minutes of hypoperfusion, brain cells are damaged irreversibly.

Causes of Shock

Many different things can cause the victim to experience shock: **hemorrhage** (excessive loss of blood); excessive pain; infection; heart attack; stroke; poisoning by chemicals, drugs, or gases; lack of oxygen; psychological trauma; and dehydration (loss of body fluids) from burns, vomiting, or diarrhea. The eight main types of shock are shown in Table 17–1. All types of shock impair circulation and decrease the supply of oxygen to body cells, tissues, and organs.

Signs and Symptoms

When shock occurs, the body attempts to increase blood flow to the brain, heart, and vital organs by reducing blood flow to other body parts. This can lead to the following signs and symptoms that indicate shock:

- Skin is pale or cyanotic (bluish gray) in color. Check the nail beds and the mucous membrane around the mouth.
- Skin is cool to the touch.
- **Diaphoresis**, or excessive perspiration, may result in a wet, clammy feeling when the skin is touched.
- Pulse is rapid, weak, and difficult to feel. Check the pulse at one of the carotid arteries in the neck.

TABLE 17–1 **Types of Shock**

Type of Shock	Cause	Description
Anaphylactic	Hypersensitive or allergic reaction to a substance such as food, medications, insect stings or bites, or snake bites	Body releases histamine causing vasodilation (blood vessels get larger) Blood pressure drops and less blood goes to body cells Urticaria (hives) and respiratory distress may occur
Cardiogenic	Damage to heart muscle from heart attack or cardiac arrest	Heart cannot effectively pump blood to body cells
Hemorrhagic	Severe bleeding or loss of blood plasma	Decrease in blood volume causes blood pressure to drop Decreased blood flow to body cells
Metabolic	Loss of body fluid from severe vomiting, diarrhea, or a heat illness Disruption in acid–base balance as occurs in diabetes	Decreased amount of fluid causes dehydration and disruption in normal acid–base balance of body Blood pressure drops and less blood circulates to body cells
Neurogenic	Injury and trauma to brain and/or spinal cord	Nervous system loses ability to control the size of blood vessels Blood vessels dilate and blood pressure drops Decreased blood flow to body cells
Psychogenic	Emotional distress such as anger, fear, or grief	Emotional response causes sudden dilation of blood vessels Blood pools in areas away from the brain Some individuals faint
Respiratory	Trauma to respiratory tract Respiratory distress or arrest (chronic disease, choking)	Interferes with exchange of oxygen and carbon dioxide between lungs and bloodstream Insufficient oxygen supply for body cells
Septic	Acute infection (toxic shock syndrome)	Poisons or toxins in blood cause vasodilation Blood pressure drops Less oxygen supply to body cells

- Respirations are rapid, shallow, and may be irregular.
- Blood pressure is very low or below normal, and may not be obtainable.
- Victim experiences general weakness. As shock progresses, the victim becomes listless and confused. Eventually, the victim loses consciousness.
- Victim experiences anxiety and extreme restlessness.
- Victim may experience excessive thirst, nausea, and/or vomiting.
- Victim may complain of blurred vision. As shock progresses, the victim's eyes may appear sunken and have a vacant or confused expression. The pupils may dilate or become large.

Treatment for Shock

It is essential to get medical help for the victim as soon as possible because shock is a life-threatening condition. Treatment for shock is directed toward (1) eliminating the cause of shock; (2) improving circulation, especially to the brain and heart; (3) providing an adequate oxygen supply; and (4) maintaining body temperature. Some of the basic principles for treatment include:

- Reduce the effects of or eliminate the cause of shock: control bleeding, provide oxygen if available, ease pain through position change, and/or provide emotional support.
- The position for treating shock must be based on the victim's injuries.

Safety

CAUTION: *If neck or spine injuries are suspected, the victim should not be moved unless it is necessary to remove him or her from danger.*

The best position for treating shock is usually to keep the victim lying flat on the back, because this improves circulation. Raising the feet and legs approximately 12 inches can also provide additional blood for the heart and brain. However, if the victim is vomiting or has bleeding and injuries of the jaw or mouth, the victim should be positioned on the side to prevent him or her from choking on blood and/or vomitus. If a victim is experiencing breathing problems, it may be necessary to raise the victim's head and shoulders to make breathing easier. If the victim has a head (not neck) injury and has difficulty breathing, the victim should be positioned lying flat or with the head raised slightly. It is important to position the victim based on the injury or illness involved.

- Cover the patient with blankets or additional clothing to prevent chilling or exposure to the cold. Blankets may also be placed between the ground and the victim. However, it is important to avoid overheating the victim. If the skin is very warm to the touch and perspiration is noted, remove some of the blankets or coverings.
- Avoid giving the victim anything to eat or drink. If the victim complains of excessive thirst, a wet cloth can be used to provide some comfort by moistening the lips and mouth.

Remember that it is important to look for signs of shock while providing first aid for any injury or illness. Provide care that will reduce the effect of shock. Obtain medical help for the victim as soon as possible.

STUDENT: **Go to the workbook and complete the assignment sheet for 17:4, Providing First Aid for Shock. Then return and continue with the procedure.**

PROCEDURE 17:4

Providing First Aid for Shock

Equipment and Supplies

Blankets, watch with second hand (optional), disposable gloves

Procedure

1. Follow the steps of priority care, if indicated:
   a. Check the scene. Move the victim only if absolutely necessary.
   b. Check the victim for consciousness and breathing.
   c. Call emergency medical services (EMS).
   d. Provide care to the victim.
   e. Control severe bleeding.

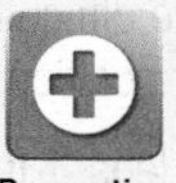
Precaution

CAUTION: Wear gloves or use a protective barrier while controlling bleeding.

(continues)

PROCEDURE 17:4 (CONT.)

2. Obtain medical help for the victim as soon as possible. Call or send someone to obtain help.

3. Observe the victim for any signs of shock. Look for a pale or cyanotic (bluish) color to the skin. Touch the skin and note if it is cool, moist, or clammy to the touch. Note diaphoresis, or excessive perspiration. Check the pulse to see if it is rapid, weak, or irregular. If you are unable to feel a radial pulse, check the carotid pulse. Check the respirations to see if they are rapid, weak, irregular, shallow, or labored. If equipment is available, check blood pressure to see if it is low. Observe the victim for signs of weakness, apathy, confusion, or consciousness. Note if the victim is nauseated or vomiting, complaining of excessive thirst, restless or anxious, or complaining of blurred vision. Examine the eyes for a sunken, vacant, or confused appearance, and dilated pupils.

4. Try to reduce the effects or eliminate the cause of shock.

a. Control bleeding by applying pressure at the site.

b. Provide oxygen, if possible.

c. Attempt to ease pain through position changes and comfort measures.

d. Give emotional support.

5. Position the victim based on the injuries or illness present.

a. If an injury of the neck or spine is present or suspected, do not move the victim.

b. If the victim has bleeding and injuries to the jaw or mouth, or is vomiting, position the victim's body on either side. This allows fluids, vomitus, and/or blood to drain and prevents the airway from becoming blocked by these fluids.

c. If the victim is having difficulty breathing, position the victim on the back, but raise the head and shoulders slightly to aid breathing.

d. If the victim has a head injury, position the victim lying flat or with the head raised slightly.

NOTE: Never allow the head to be positioned lower than the rest of the body.

e. If none of these conditions exist, position the victim lying flat on the back. To improve circulation, raise the feet and legs approximately 12 inches (Figure 17–22). If raising the legs causes pain or leads to difficult breathing, however, lower the legs to the flat position.

Safety

CAUTION: Do not raise the legs if the victim has head, neck, or back injuries, or if there are possible fractures of the hips or legs.

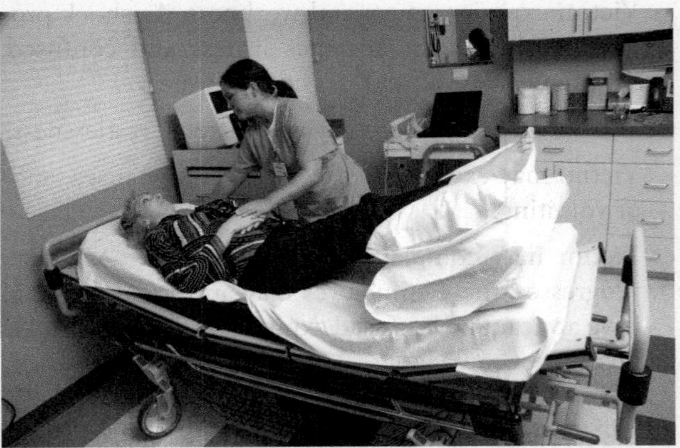

FIGURE 17–22 **Position a shock victim flat on the back and elevate the feet and legs approximately 12 inches. Do *not* use this position if the victim has a neck, spinal, head, or jaw injury, or if the victim is having difficulty breathing.**

f. If in doubt on how to position a victim according to the injuries involved, keep the victim lying down flat or in the position in which you found him or her. Avoid any unnecessary movement.

6. Place enough blankets or coverings on the victim to prevent chilling. Sometimes, a blanket can be placed between the victim and the ground. Avoid overheating the victim.

7. Do not give the victim anything to eat or drink. If the victim complains of excessive thirst, use a moist cloth to wet the lips, tongue, and inside of the mouth.

8. 
Comm

Constantly reassure the victim. Encourage the victim to remain calm by remaining calm yourself.

9. Observe and provide care to the victim until medical help is obtained.

10. Replace all equipment used. Wash hands.

PRACTICE: **Go to the workbook and use the evaluation sheet for 17:4, Providing First Aid for Shock, to practice this procedure. When you believe you have mastered this skill, sign the sheet and give it to your instructor for further action.**

Check

FINAL CHECKPOINT: Using the criteria listed on the evaluation sheet, your instructor will grade your performance.

17:5 Providing First Aid for Poisoning

Introduction

Poisoning can occur anywhere, anytime—not only in health care settings, but also in your personal life. **Poisoning** is a condition that occurs when contact is made with any chemical substance that causes injury, illness, or death. It can be caused by ingesting (swallowing) various substances, inhaling poisonous gases, injecting substances, or contacting the skin with poison. Any substance that causes a harmful reaction when applied or ingested can be called a poison. Anaphylactic shock is a common reaction to poisoning (refer to Table 17–1). Immediate action is necessary for any poisoning victim. Treatment varies depending on the type of poison, the injury involved, and the method of contact.

If the poisoning victim is unconscious, check for breathing. Provide artificial respiration if the victim is not breathing. Obtain medical help as soon as possible. If the unconscious victim is breathing, position the victim on his or her side so fluids can drain from the mouth. Obtain medical help quickly.

Ingestion Poisoning

If a poison has been swallowed, immediate care must be provided before the poison can be absorbed into the body. Basic steps of first aid include:

- Call a poison control center (PCC) or a physician immediately. If you cannot contact a PCC, call emergency medical services (EMS). Most areas have poison control centers that provide information on specific antidotes and treatment. Information can also be obtained at the American Association of Poison Control Centers at *www.aapcc.org*, or by calling 1-800-222-1222.
- Save the label or container of the substance taken so this information can be given to the PCC or physician.
- Calculate or estimate how much was taken and the time at which the poisoning occurred.
- If the victim vomits, save a sample of the vomited material.
- If the PCC tells you to induce vomiting, get the victim to vomit. To induce vomiting, tickle the back of the victim's throat or give the victim warm saltwater to drink.

CAUTION: *Vomiting must not be induced in unconscious victims, victims who swallowed an acid or alkali, victims who swallowed petroleum products, victims who are convulsing, or victims who have burns on the lips and mouth.*

- Activated charcoal may be recommended by the PCC to bind to the poison so it is not absorbed into the body. Activated charcoal should only be given to victims who are conscious and able to swallow. It is available in most drug stores. The directions on the bottle should be followed to determine the correct dosage.

Inhalation Poisoning

If poisoning is caused by inhalation of dangerous gases, the victim must be removed immediately from the area before being treated. A commonly inhaled poison is carbon monoxide. It is odorless, colorless, and very difficult to detect. If excessive amounts of gas or fumes are present, and the scene is not safe, do not enter the area. Wait for EMS to arrive. If a quick rescue can be achieved without inhaling the gases, the basic steps of first aid include:

- Before entering the danger area, take a deep breath of fresh air and do not breathe the gas while you are removing the victim from the area.
- After rescuing the victim, immediately check for breathing.
- Provide artificial respiration if needed.
- Obtain medical help immediately; death may occur very quickly with this type of poisoning.

Contact Poisoning

If poisoning is caused by chemicals or poisons coming in contact with the victim's skin, care for the victim includes:

- Use large amounts of water to wash the skin for at least 15–20 minutes to dilute the substance and remove it from the skin.
- Remove any clothing and jewelry that contain the substance.
- Call a PCC or physician for additional information.
- Obtain medical help as soon as possible for burns or injuries that may result from contact with the poison.

Contact with a poisonous plant such as poison ivy, oak, or sumac can cause a serious skin reaction if not treated immediately. Basic steps of first aid include:

- Wash the area thoroughly with soap and water.
- If a rash or weeping sores develop after 2–3 days, lotions such as Calamine or Caladryl, or a paste made from baking soda and water, may help relieve the discomfort.
- If the condition is severe and affects large areas of the body or face, obtain medical help.

Injection Poisoning

Injection poisoning occurs when an insect, spider, or snake bites or stings an individual. If an arm or leg is affected, position the affected area below the level of the heart. For an *insect sting*, first aid treatment includes:

- Remove any embedded stinger by scraping the stinger away from the skin with the edge of a rigid card, such as a credit card, or a tongue depressor. Do not use tweezers because tweezers can puncture the venom sac attached to the stinger, injecting more poison into body tissues.
- Wash the area well with soap and water.
- Apply a sterile dressing and a cold pack to reduce swelling.

If a *tick* is embedded in the skin, first aid treatment includes:

- Use tweezers to slowly pull the tick out of the skin.
- Wash the area thoroughly with soap and water.
- Apply an antiseptic.
- Watch for signs of infection.
- Obtain medical help if needed.

Ticks can cause Rocky Mountain spotted fever or Lyme disease, dangerous diseases if untreated.

For a *snakebite* or *spider bite*, first aid treatment includes:

- Wash the wound.
- Immobilize the injured area, positioning it lower than the heart, if possible.
- Do not cut the wound or apply a tourniquet.
- Monitor the breathing of the victim and give artificial respiration if necessary.
- Obtain medical help for the victim as soon as possible.

For any type of injection poisoning, watch for allergic reaction in all victims (Figure 17–23). Signs and symptoms of allergic reaction include redness and swelling at the site, itching, hives, pain, swelling of the throat, difficult or labored breathing, dizziness, and a change in the level of consciousness. Maintain respirations and

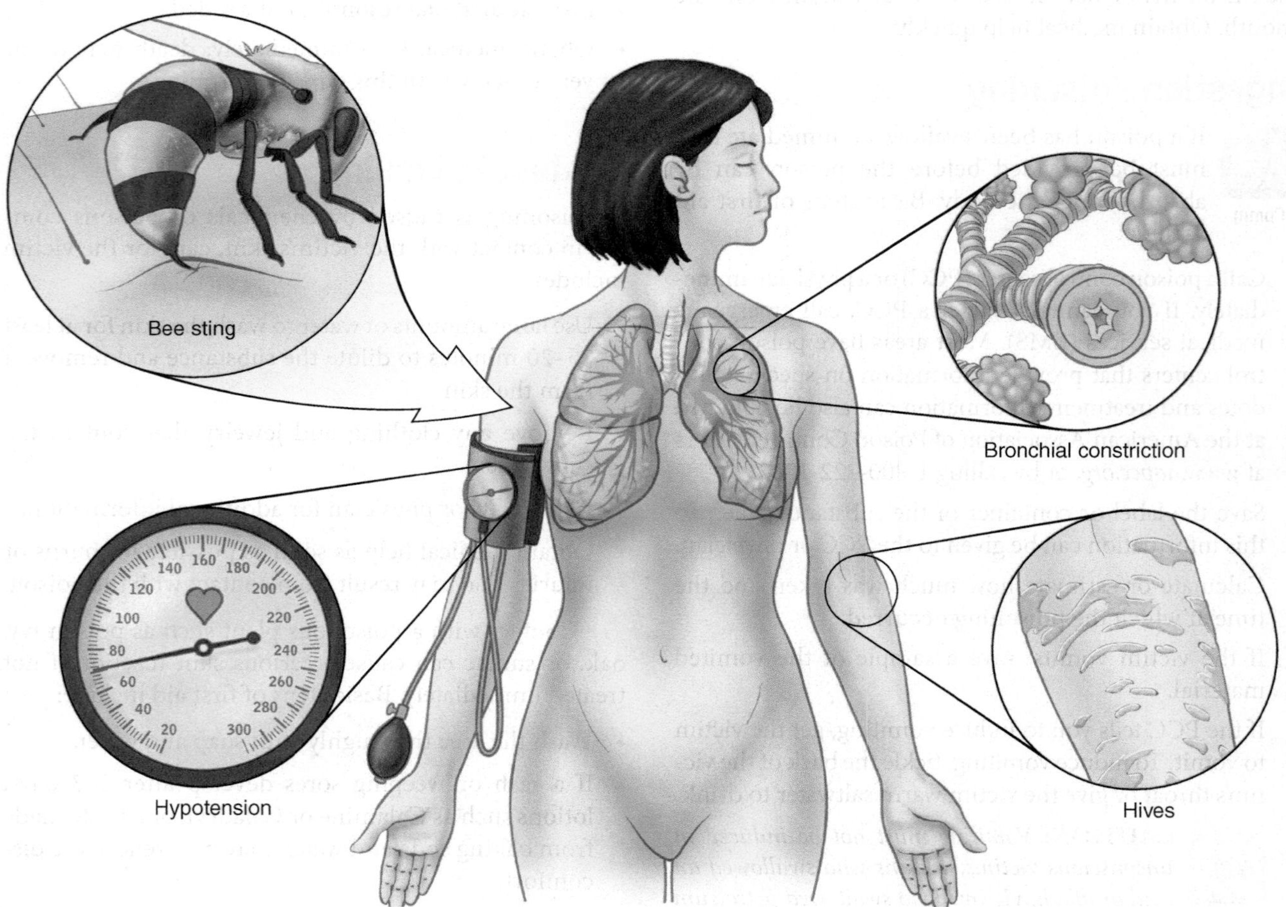

FIGURE 17–23 Watch for allergic reactions in all poisoning victims.

obtain medical help as quickly as possible for the victim who experiences an allergic reaction.

Summary

In all poisoning victims, observe for signs of anaphylactic shock. Treat the victim for shock, if necessary. Try to remain calm and confident while providing first aid for poisoning victims. Reassure the victim as needed. Act quickly and in an organized, efficient manner.

STUDENT: **Go to the workbook and complete the assignment sheet for 17:5, Providing First Aid for Poisoning. Then return and continue with the procedure.**

PROCEDURE 17:5

Providing First Aid for Poisoning

Equipment and Supplies

Telephone, disposable gloves

Procedure

1. Follow the steps of priority care, if indicated:
   a. Check the scene. Move the victim only if absolutely necessary.
   b. Check the victim for consciousness and breathing.
   c. Call emergency medical services (EMS).
   d. Provide care to the victim.
   e. Control severe bleeding.

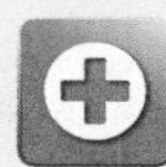

CAUTION: Wear gloves or use a protective barrier while controlling bleeding.

2. Check the victim for signs of poisoning. Signs may include burns on the lips or mouth, odor, a container of poison, or presence of the poisonous substance on the victim or in the victim's mouth. Information may also be obtained from the victim or from an observer.
3. If the victim is conscious, not convulsing, and has swallowed a poison:
   a. Try to determine the type of poison, how much was taken, and when the poison was taken. Look for the container near the victim.
   b. Call a poison control center (PCC) or physician immediately for specific information on how to treat the poisoning victim. Provide as much information as possible.
   c. Follow the instructions received from the PCC. Obtain medical help if needed.
   d. If the victim vomits, save a sample of the vomited material.
4. If the PCC tells you to get the victim to vomit, induce vomiting. Give the victim warm saltwater or tickle the back of the victim's throat.

CAUTION: Do *not* induce vomiting if the victim is unconscious or convulsing, has burns on the lips or mouth, or has swallowed an acid, alkali, or petroleum product.

5. If the PCC tells you to give the victim activated charcoal, follow the directions on the container. Make sure the victim is conscious and able to swallow before giving the charcoal.

   NOTE: Activated charcoal binds to the poison so it is not absorbed into the body.
6. If the victim is unconscious:
   a. Check for breathing. If the victim is not breathing, give artificial respiration and/or CPR as needed.
   b. If the victim is breathing, position the victim on his or her side to allow fluids to drain from the mouth.
   c. Call a PCC or physician for specific treatment. Obtain medical help immediately.
   d. If possible, save the poison container and a sample of any vomited material. Check with any observers to find out what was taken, how much was taken, and when the poison was taken.
7. If chemicals or poisons have splashed on the victim's skin, wash the area thoroughly with large amounts of water. Remove any clothing and jewelry containing the substance. If a large area of the body is affected, a shower, tub, or garden hose may be used to rinse the skin. Obtain medical help immediately for burns or injuries caused by the poison.
8. If the victim has come in contact with a poisonous plant such as poison ivy, oak, or sumac, wash the area of contact thoroughly with soap and water. Remove any contaminated clothing. If a rash or weeping sores develop in the next few days after exposure, lotions such as Calamine or Caladryl, or a paste made from baking soda and water, may help relieve the discomfort. If the condition is severe and affects large areas of the body or face, obtain medical help.

(continues)

PROCEDURE 17:5 (CONT.)

9. If the victim has inhaled poisonous gas, do not endanger your life by trying to treat the victim in the area of the gas. If excessive amounts of gas or fumes are present, and the scene is not safe, wait for EMS to arrive. If it is safe to enter the area, take a deep breath of fresh air before entering the area and hold your breath while you remove the victim from the area. When the victim is in a safe area, check for breathing. Provide artificial respiration and/or CPR as needed. Obtain medical help immediately.

10. If poisoning is caused by injection from an insect bite or sting or a snakebite, proceed as follows:

a. If an arm or leg is affected, position the affected area below the level of the heart.

b. For an *insect bite*, remove any embedded stinger by scraping it off with an object like a credit card. Wash the area well with soap and water. Apply a sterile dressing and a cold pack to reduce swelling.

c. If a *tick* is embedded in the skin, use tweezers to gently pull the tick out of the skin. Wash the area thoroughly with soap and water, and apply an antiseptic. Obtain medical help if needed.

d. For a *snakebite* or *spider bite*, wash the wound. Immobilize the injured area, positioning it lower than the heart if possible. Monitor the breathing of the victim and give artificial respiration if necessary. Obtain medical help for the victim as soon as possible.

e. Watch for the signs and symptoms of allergic reaction in all victims. Signs and symptoms of allergic reaction include redness and swelling at the site, itching, hives (Figure 17–24), pain, swelling of the throat, difficult or labored breathing, dizziness, and a change in the level of consciousness. Maintain respirations and obtain medical help as quickly as possible for the victim experiencing an allergic reaction.

11. Observe for signs of anaphylactic shock while treating any poisoning victim. Treat for shock as necessary.

12. Remain calm while treating the victim. Reassure the victim.

13. Comm — Always obtain medical help for any poisoning victim. Some poisons may have delayed reactions. Always keep the telephone numbers of a PCC and other sources of medical assistance in a convenient location so you will be prepared to provide first aid for poisoning.

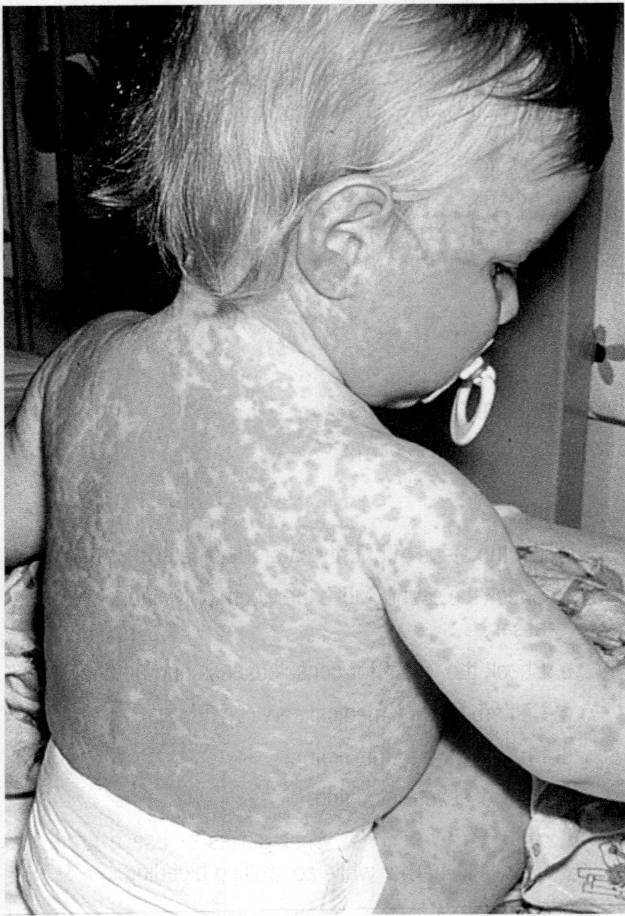

FIGURE 17–24 **Hives are a common sign of an allergic reaction.**
Courtesy of Robert A. Silverman, M.D., Clinical Associate Professor, Department of Pediatrics, Georgetown University

14. Wash hands thoroughly after providing care.

PRACTICE: **Go to the workbook and use the evaluation sheet for 17:5, Providing First Aid for Poisoning, to practice this procedure. When you believe you have mastered this skill, sign the sheet and give it to your instructor for further action.**

Check

FINAL CHECKPOINT: Using the criteria listed on the evaluation sheet, your instructor will grade your performance.

17:6 Providing First Aid for Burns

Types of Burns

A **burn** is an injury that can be caused by fire, heat, chemical agents, radiation, and/or electricity. Burns are classified as either superficial, partial thickness, or full thickness (Figure 17–25). Characteristics of each type of burn are as follows:

- *Superficial, or first-degree, burn:* This is the least severe type of burn. It involves only the top layer of skin, the epidermis, and usually heals in 5–6 days without permanent scarring. The skin is usually reddened or discolored. There may be some mild swelling, and the victim feels pain. Three common causes are overexposure to the sun (sunburn), brief contact with hot objects or steam, and exposure of the skin to a weak acid or alkali.
- *Partial-thickness, or second-degree, burn:* This type of burn involves injury to the top layers of skin, including both the epidermis and dermis. A blister or vesicle forms. The skin is red or has a mottled (blotchy with many shades of color) appearance. Swelling usually occurs, and the surface of the skin frequently appears to be wet. This is a painful burn and may take 3–4 weeks to heal. Frequent causes include excessive exposure to

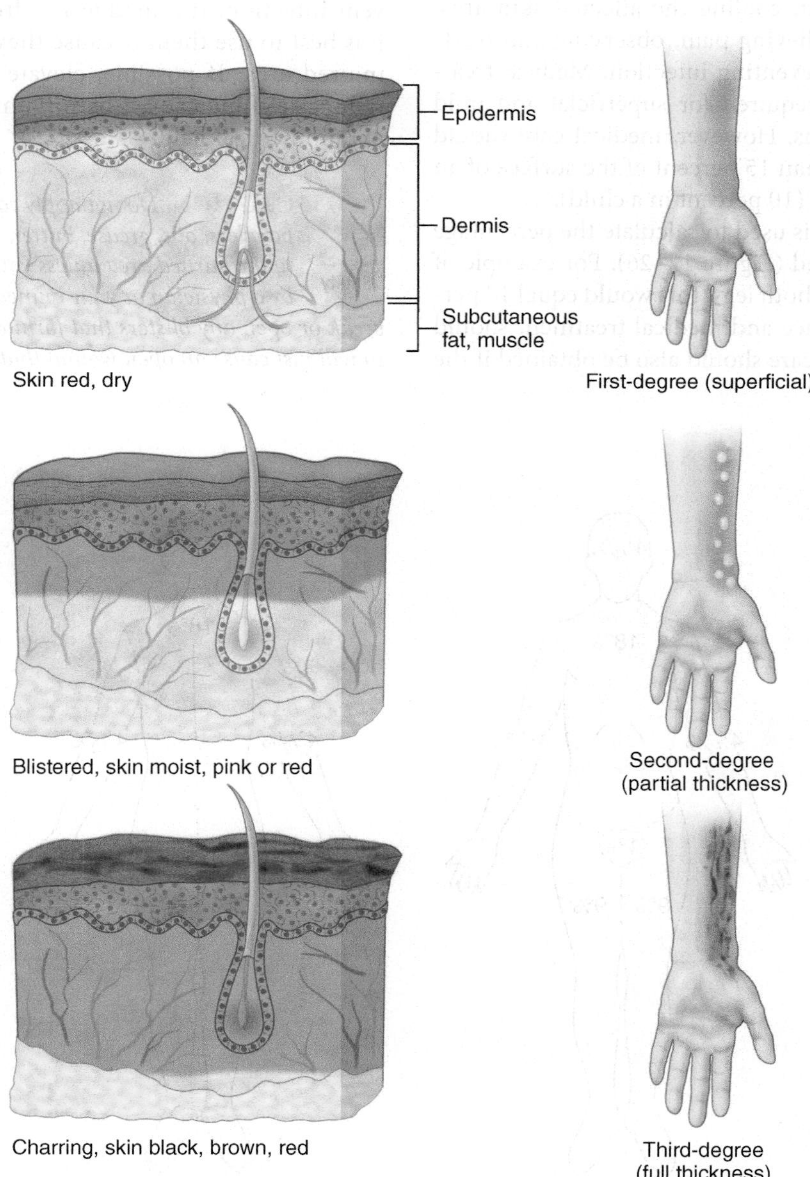

FIGURE 17–25 Types of burns.

the sun, a sunlamp, or artificial radiation; contact with hot or boiling liquids; and contact with fire.

- *Full-thickness, or third-degree, burn:* This is the most severe type of burn and involves injury to all layers of the skin plus the underlying tissue. The area involved has a white or charred appearance. This type of burn can be either extremely painful or, if nerve endings are destroyed, relatively painless. Third-degree burns can be life threatening because of fluid loss, infection, and shock. Frequent causes include exposure to fire or flames, prolonged contact with hot objects, contact with electricity, and immersion in hot or boiling liquids.

Treatment

First aid treatment for burns is directed toward removing the source of heat, cooling the affected skin area, covering the burn, relieving pain, observing and treating for shock, and preventing infection. Medical treatment is not usually required for superficial and mild partial-thickness burns. However, medical care should be obtained if more than 15 percent of the surface of an adult's body is burned (10 percent in a child).

The rule of nines is used to calculate the percentage of body surface burned (Figure 17–26). For example, if an adult has burns on both legs, this would equal 18 percent of the body surface and medical treatment should be obtained. Medical care should also be obtained if the burns affect the face or respiratory tract; if the victim has difficulty breathing; if burns cover more than one body part; if the victim has a partial-thickness burn and is under 5 or over 60 years of age; or if the burns resulted from chemicals, explosions, or electricity. All victims with full-thickness burns should receive medical care.

SUPERFICIAL AND MILD PARTIAL-THICKNESS BURNS

The main treatment for superficial and mild partial-thickness burns is to cool the area by flushing it with large amounts of cool water. Do *not* use ice or ice water on burns because doing so causes the body to lose heat. After the pain subsides, use dry, sterile gauze to blot the area dry. Apply a dry, sterile dressing to prevent infection. If nonadhesive dressings are available, it is best to use them because they will not stick to the injured area. If possible, elevate the affected part to reduce swelling caused by inflammation. If necessary, obtain medical help.

CAUTION: *Do not apply cotton, tissues, ointment, powders, oils, grease, butter, or any other substances to the burned area unless you are instructed to do so by a physician or your immediate supervisor. Do not break or open any blisters that form on burns because doing so will just cause an open wound that is prone to infection.*

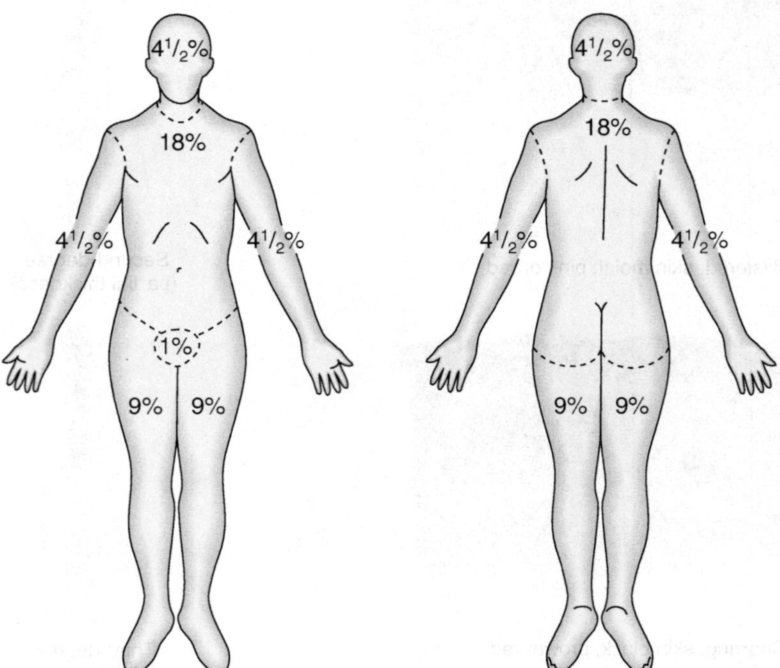

FIGURE 17–26 The *rule of nines* is used to calculate the percentage of body surface burned.

SEVERE PARTIAL-THICKNESS AND FULL-THICKNESS BURNS

Call for medical help immediately if the victim has severe partial-thickness or full-thickness burns. Cover the burned areas with thick, sterile dressings. Elevate the hands or feet if they are burned. If the feet or legs are burned, do *not* allow the victim to walk. If particles of clothing are attached to the burned areas, do *not* attempt to remove these particles. Watch the victim closely for signs of respiratory distress and/or shock. Provide artificial respiration and treatment for shock, as necessary. Watch the victim closely until medical help arrives.

CHEMICAL BURNS

For burns caused by chemicals splashing on the skin, use large amounts of water to flush the affected areas for 15–30 minutes or until medical help arrives. Gently remove any clothing, socks and shoes, or jewelry that contains the chemical to minimize the area injured. Continue flushing the skin with cool water and watch the victim for signs of shock until medical help can be obtained.

If the eyes have been burned by chemicals or irritating gases, flush the eyes with large amounts of water for at least 15–30 minutes or until medical help arrives. If only one eye is injured, be sure to tilt the victim's head in the direction of the injury so the injured eye can be properly flushed. Start at the inner corner of the eye and allow the water to run over the surface of the eye and to the outside. Continue flushing the eye with cool water and watch the victim for signs of shock until medical help can be obtained.

Safety

CAUTION: *Make sure that the water (or remaining chemical) does not enter the uninjured eye.*

Summary

Loss of body fluids (dehydration) can occur very quickly with severe burns, so shock is frequently noted in burn victims. Be alert for any signs of shock and treat the burn victim for shock immediately.

Comm

Remain calm while treating the burn victim. Reassure the victim. Obtain medical help as quickly as possible for any burn victim requiring medical assistance.

STUDENT: **Go to the workbook and complete the assignment sheet for 17:6, Providing First Aid for Burns. Then return and continue with the procedure.**

PROCEDURE 17:6

Providing First Aid for Burns

Equipment and Supplies

Water, sterile dressings, disposable gloves

Procedure

1. Follow the steps of priority care, if indicated:
   a. Check the scene. Move the victim only if absolutely necessary.
   b. Check the victim for consciousness and breathing.
   c. Call emergency medical services (EMS) if necessary.
   d. Provide care to the victim.
   e. Check for bleeding. Control severe bleeding.

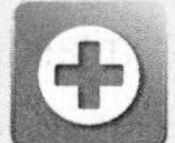
Precaution

CAUTION: Wear gloves or use a protective barrier while controlling bleeding.

2. Check the burned area carefully to determine the type of burn. A reddened or discolored area is usually a superficial, or first-degree, burn. If the skin is wet, red, swollen, painful, and blistered, the burn is usually a partial-thickness, or second-degree, burn (Figure 17–27A). If the skin is white or charred and there is destruction of tissue, the burn is a full-thickness, or third-degree, burn (Figure 17–27B).

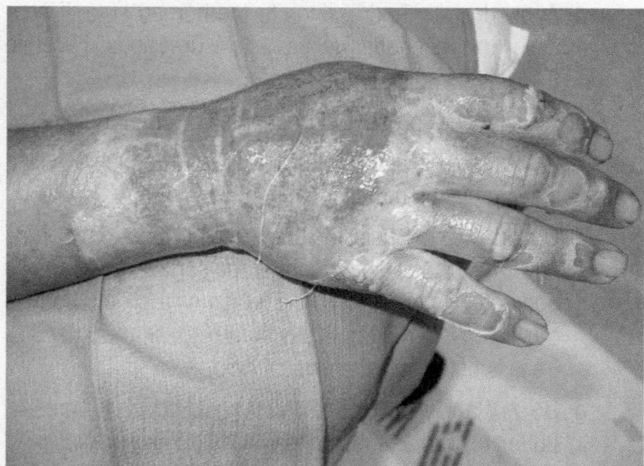
FIGURE 17–27A The skin is wet, red, swollen, painful, and blistered when a partial-thickness burn is present. The Victorian Adult Burns Service, Alfred Hospital, Melbourne, Australia

NOTE: Victims can have more than one type of burn at one time. Treat for the most severe type of burn present.

(continues)

PROCEDURE 17:6 (CONT.)

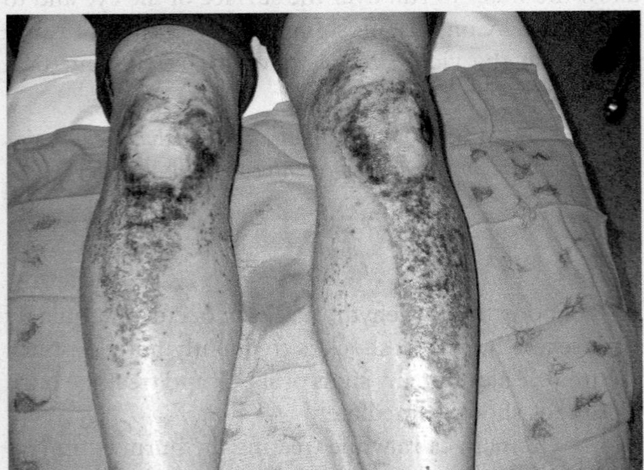

FIGURE 17–27B **A full-thickness burn destroys or affects all layers of the skin plus fat, muscle, bone, and nerve tissue. The skin is white or charred in appearance.** The Victorian Adult Burns Service, Alfred Hospital, Melbourne, Australia

3. For a superficial or mild partial-thickness burn:

a. Cool the burn by flushing it with large amounts of cool water. If this is not possible, apply clean or sterile cloths that are cold and wet. Continue applying cold water until the pain subsides.

b. Use sterile gauze to gently blot the injured area dry.

c. Apply dry, sterile dressings to the burned area. If possible, use nonadhesive (nonstick) dressings, because they will not stick to the burn.

d. If blisters are present, do *not* break or open them.

e. If possible, elevate the burned area to reduce swelling caused by inflammation.

f. Obtain medical help for burns to the face, or if burns cover more than 15 percent of the surface of an adult's body or 10 percent of the surface of a child's body. If the victim is having difficulty breathing, or any other distress is noted, obtain medical help.

g. Do *not* apply any cotton, ointment, powders, grease, butter, or similar substances to the burned area.

NOTE: These substances may increase the possibility of infection.

4. For a severe partial-thickness or any full-thickness burn:

a. Call for medical help immediately.

b. Use thick, sterile dressings to cover the injured areas.

c. Do *not* attempt to remove any particles of clothing that have stuck to the burned areas.

d. If the hands and arms or legs and feet are affected, elevate these areas.

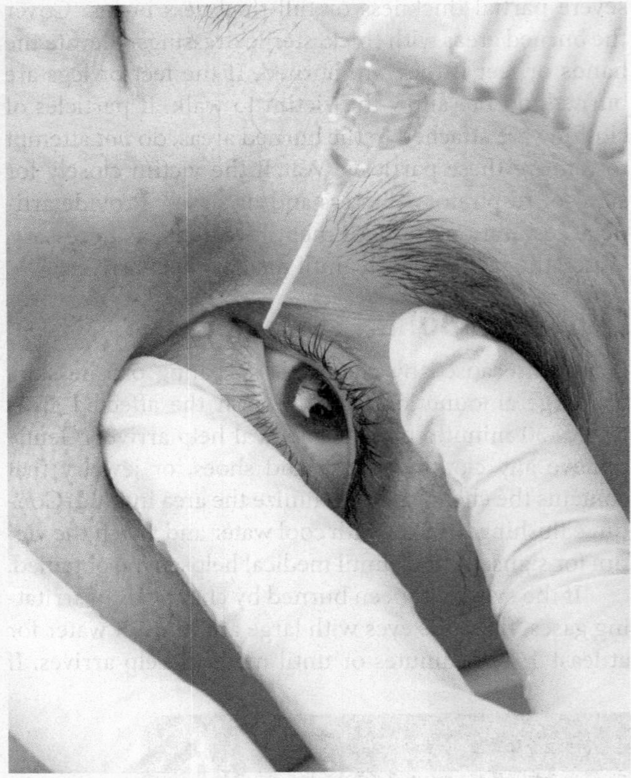

FIGURE 17–28 **To irrigate an eye, hold the eyelid open and irrigate from the inner part of the eye toward the outer part.**

e. If the victim has burns on the face or is experiencing difficulty in breathing, elevate the head.

f. Watch the victim closely for signs of shock and provide care if necessary.

5. For a burn caused by a chemical splashing on the skin:

a. Using large amounts of water, immediately flush the area for 15–30 minutes or until medical help arrives.

b. Remove any articles of clothing, socks and shoes, or jewelry contaminated by the substance.

c. Continue flushing the area with large amounts of cool water.

d. Obtain medical help immediately.

6. If the eye has been burned by chemicals or irritating gases:

a. If the victim is wearing contact lenses or glasses, ask him or her to remove them quickly.

b. Tilt the victim's head toward the injured side.

c. Hold the eyelid of the injured eye open. Pour cool water from the inner part of the eye (the part closest to the nose) toward the outer part (Figure 17–28).

PROCEDURE 17:6 (CONT.)

d. Use cool water to irrigate the eye for 15–30 minutes or until medical help arrives.

Safety

CAUTION: Take care that the water or chemicals do not enter the uninjured eye.

e. Obtain medical help immediately.

7. Observe for the signs of shock in all burn victims. Treat for shock as necessary.

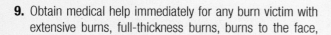

8. Reassure the victim as you are providing treatment. Remain calm and encourage the victim to remain calm.

Comm

9. Obtain medical help immediately for any burn victim with extensive burns, full-thickness burns, burns to the face, signs of shock, respiratory distress, eye burns, and/or chemical burns to the skin.

10. Wash hands thoroughly after providing care.

PRACTICE: Go to the workbook and use the evaluation sheet for 17:6, Providing First Aid for Burns, to practice this procedure. When you believe you have mastered this skill, sign the sheet and give it to your instructor for further action.

Check

FINAL CHECKPOINT: Using the criteria listed on the evaluation sheet, your instructor will grade your performance.

17:7 Providing First Aid for Heat Exposure

Excessive exposure to heat or high external temperatures can lead to a life-threatening emergency (Figure 17–29). Overexposure to heat can cause a chemical imbalance in the body that can eventually lead to death. Harmful reactions can occur when water or salt are lost through perspiration or when the body cannot eliminate excess heat.

Heat cramps are caused by exposure to heat. They are muscle pains and spasms that result from the loss of water and salt through perspiration. Firm pressure applied to the cramped muscle will provide relief from the discomfort. The victim should rest and move to a cooler area. In addition, small sips of water or an electrolyte solution, such as sport drinks, can be given to the victim.

Heat exhaustion occurs when a victim is exposed to heat and experiences a loss of fluids through sweating. Signs and symptoms include pale and clammy skin, profuse perspiration (diaphoresis), fatigue or tiredness, weakness, headache, muscle cramps, nausea and/or vomiting, and dizziness and/or fainting. Body temperature is about normal or just slightly elevated. It is important to treat heat exhaustion as quickly as possible. If it is not treated, it can develop into heat stroke. Treatment methods include moving the victim to a cooler area whenever possible; loosening or removing excessive clothing; applying cool, wet cloths; laying the victim down and elevating the victim's feet 12 inches;

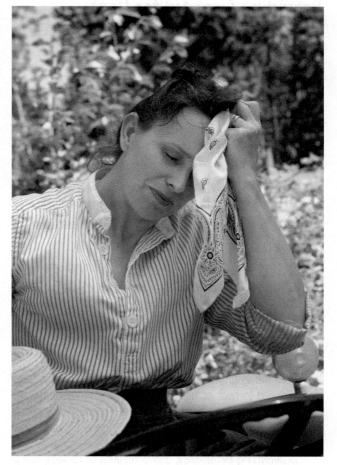

FIGURE 17–29 Excessive exposure to heat or high external temperatures can lead to a life-threatening emergency. © iStockphoto/Mike Rodriguez

and giving the victim small sips of cool water, approximately 4 ounces every 15 minutes if the victim is alert and conscious. If the victim vomits, develops shock, or experiences respiratory distress, medical help should be obtained immediately.

Heat stroke is caused by prolonged exposure to high temperatures. It is a medical emergency. The body is unable to eliminate the excess heat, and internal body temperature rises to 105°F (40.6°C) or higher. Normal body defenses such as the sweating mechanism no longer function. Signs and symptoms in addition to the high body temperature include red, hot, and dry skin. The pulse is usually rapid, but may remain strong. The victim may lose consciousness. Treatment is geared primarily toward ways of cooling the body quickly, because a high body temperature can cause convulsions and/or death in a very short period of time. The victim can be placed in a tub of cool water, or the skin can be sponged with cool water. Ice or cold packs can be placed on the victim's wrists, ankles, in each axillary (armpit) area, and in the groin. Be alert for signs of shock at all times. Obtain medical help immediately.

Comm

After victims have recovered from any condition caused by heat exposure, they must be warned to avoid abnormally warm or hot temperatures for several days. They should also be encouraged to drink sufficient amounts of water and/or electrolyte solutions.

STUDENT: **Go to the workbook and complete the assignment sheet for 17:7, Providing First Aid for Heat Exposure. Then return and continue with the procedure.**

PROCEDURE 17:7

Providing First Aid for Heat Exposure

Equipment and Supplies

Water, wash cloths or small towels

Procedure

1. Follow the steps of priority care, if indicated:
   a. Check the scene. Move the victim only if absolutely necessary.
   b. Check the victim for consciousness and breathing.
   c. Call emergency medical services (EMS) if necessary.
   d. Provide care to the victim.
   e. Check for bleeding. Control severe bleeding.

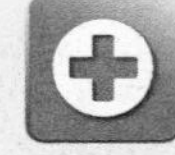
Precaution

CAUTION: Wear gloves or use a protective barrier while controlling bleeding.

2. Observe the victim closely for signs and symptoms of heat exposure. Information may also be obtained directly from the victim or from observers. If the victim has been exposed to heat or has been exercising strenuously, and is complaining of muscular pain or spasm, he or she is probably experiencing heat cramps. If the victim has close-to-normal body temperature but has pale and clammy skin, is perspiring excessively, and complains of nausea, headache, weakness, dizziness, or fatigue, he or she is probably experiencing heat exhaustion. If body temperature is high (105°F, or 40.6°C, or higher); skin is red, dry, and hot; and the victim is weak or unconscious, he or she is experiencing heat stroke.
3. If the victim has heat cramps:
   a. Use your hand to apply firm pressure to the cramped muscle(s). This helps relieve the spasms.
   b. Encourage relaxation. Allow the victim to lie down in a cool area, if possible.
   c. If the victim is alert and conscious and is not nauseated or vomiting, give him or her small sips of cool water or an electrolyte solution such as a sport drink. Encourage the victim to drink approximately 4 ounces every 15 minutes.
   d. If the heat cramps continue or get worse, obtain medical help.
4. If the victim has heat exhaustion:
   a. Move the victim to a cool area, if possible. An air-conditioned room is ideal, but a fan can also help circulate air and cool the victim.
   b. Help the victim lie down flat on the back. Elevate the victim's feet and legs 12 inches.
   c. Loosen any tight clothing. Remove excessive clothing such as jackets and sweaters.
   d. Apply cool, wet cloths to the victim's face.
   e. If the victim is conscious and is not nauseated or vomiting, give him or her small sips of cool water or

PROCEDURE 17:7 (CONT.)

an electrolyte solution such as a sport drink. Encourage the victim to drink approximately 4 ounces every 15 minutes.

f. If the victim complains of nausea and/or vomits, discontinue the water. Obtain medical help.

5. If the victim has heat stroke:

a. Immediately move the victim to a cool area, if at all possible.

b. Remove excessive clothing.

c. Sponge the bare skin with cool water, or place ice or cold packs on the victim's wrists, ankles, and in the axillary and groin areas. The victim can also be placed in a tub of cool water to lower body temperature.

Safety

CAUTION: Watch that the victim's head is not submerged in water. If the victim is unconscious, you may need assistance to place him or her in the tub.

d. If vomiting occurs, position the victim on his or her side. Watch for signs of difficulty in breathing and provide care as indicated.

e. Obtain medical help immediately. This is a life-threatening emergency.

6. Shock can develop quickly in all victims of heat exposure. Be alert for the signs of shock and treat as necessary.

Safety

CAUTION: Obtain medical help for heat cramps that do not subside, heat exhaustion with signs of shock or vomiting, and all heat stroke victims as soon as possible.

7. Reassure the victim as you are providing treatment. Remain calm.

Comm

8. Wash hands thoroughly after providing care.

PRACTICE: Go to the workbook and use the evaluation sheet for 17:7, Providing First Aid for Heat Exposure, to practice this procedure. When you believe you have mastered this skill, sign the sheet and give it to your instructor for further action.

Check

FINAL CHECKPOINT: Using the criteria listed on the evaluation sheet, your instructor will grade your performance.

17:8 Providing First Aid for Cold Exposure

Exposure to cold external temperatures can cause body tissues to freeze and body processes to slow. If treatment is not provided immediately, the victim can die. Factors such as wind velocity, amount of humidity, and length of exposure all affect the degree of injury.

Prolonged exposure to the cold can result in **hypothermia**, a condition in which the body temperature is less than 95°F (35°C). Elderly individuals are more susceptible to hypothermia than are younger individuals (Figure 17–30). Signs and symptoms include shivering, numbness, weakness or drowsiness, low body temperature, poor coordination, confusion, and loss of consciousness. If prolonged exposure continues, body processes will slow down and death can occur. Treatment consists of getting the victim to a warm area; removing wet clothing; slowly warming the victim by wrapping in blankets or putting on dry clothing; and, if the victim is fully conscious, giving warm nonalcoholic, noncaffeinated liquids by mouth. Avoid warming the victim too quickly, because rapid warming can cause dangerous heart arrhythmias.

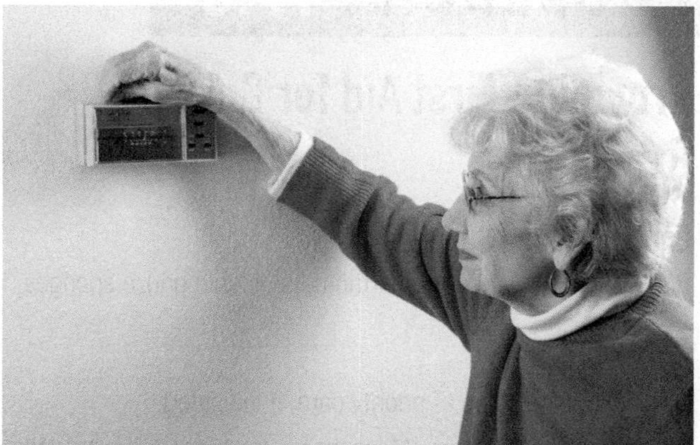

FIGURE 17–30 Elderly individuals are more susceptible to hypothermia than are younger individuals. © iStockphoto/David Sucsy

Frostbite is actual freezing of tissue fluids accompanied by damage to the skin and underlying tissues (Figure 17–31). It is caused by exposure to freezing or below-freezing temperatures. Early signs and symptoms include redness and tingling. As frostbite progresses, signs and symptoms include pale, glossy skin that is white or grayish yellow in color; blisters; skin that is cold to the touch; numbness; and sometimes, pain that

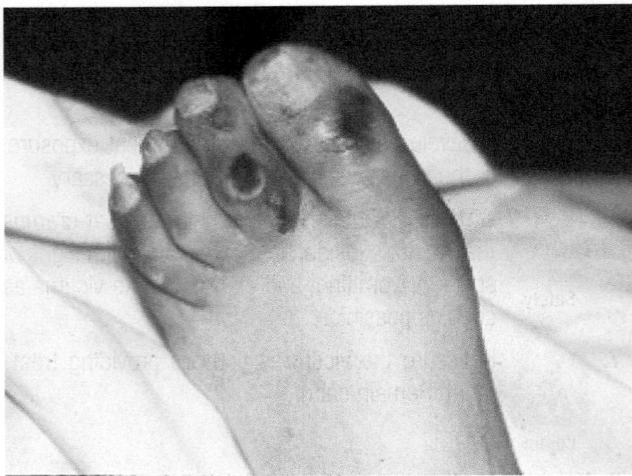

FIGURE 17–31 Frostbite is actual freezing of tissue fluids accompanied by damage to skin and underlying tissues. Courtesy of Dr. Deborah Funk, Albany Medical Center

gradually subsides until the victim does not feel any pain. If exposure continues, the victim may become confused, lethargic, and incoherent. Shock may develop followed by unconsciousness and death. First aid for frostbite is directed at maintaining respirations, treating for shock, warming the affected parts, and preventing further injury. Frequently, small areas of the body are affected by frostbite. Common sites include the fingers, toes, ears, nose, and cheeks. Extreme care must be taken to avoid further injury to areas damaged by frostbite. Because the victim usually does not feel pain, the part must be warmed carefully, taking care not to burn the injured tissue. The parts affected may be immersed in warm water at 100°F–104°F (37.8°C–40°C).

Safety

CAUTION: *Heat lamps, hot water above 104° F (40° C), or heat from a stove or oven should not be used. Furthermore, the parts should not be rubbed or massaged, because this may cause gangrene (death of the tissue). Avoid opening or breaking any blisters that form because doing so will create an open wound. Do not allow the victim to walk or stand if the feet, legs, or toes are affected. Dry, sterile dressings can be placed between toes or fingers to prevent them from rubbing and causing further injury. Medical help should be obtained as quickly as possible.*

Shock is frequently noted in victims exposed to the cold. Be alert for all signs of shock and treat for shock as necessary.

STUDENT: **Go to the workbook and complete the assignment sheet for 17:8, Providing First Aid for Cold Exposure. Then return and continue with the procedure.**

PROCEDURE 17:8

Providing First Aid for Cold Exposure

Equipment and Supplies

Blankets, bath water and thermometer, sterile gauze sponges

Procedure

1. Follow the steps of priority care, if indicated:
   a. Check the scene. Move the victim only if absolutely necessary.
   b. Check the victim for consciousness and breathing.
   c. Call emergency medical services (EMS) if necessary.
   d. Provide care to the victim.
   e. Check for bleeding. Control severe bleeding.

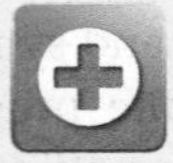
Precaution

CAUTION: Wear gloves or use a protective barrier while controlling bleeding.

2. Observe the victim closely for signs and symptoms of cold exposure. Information may also be obtained directly from the victim or observers. Note shivering, numbness, weakness or drowsiness, confusion, low body temperature, and lethargy. Check the skin, particularly on the toes, fingers, ears, nose, and cheeks. Suspect frostbite if any areas are pale, glossy, white or grayish yellow, and cold to the touch, and if the victim complains of any part of the body feeling numb or painless.
3. Move the victim to a warm area as soon as possible.
4. Immediately remove any wet or frozen clothing. Loosen any tight clothing that decreases circulation.
5. Slowly warm the victim by wrapping the victim in blankets or dressing the victim in dry, warm clothing. If a body part is affected by frostbite, immerse the part in warm water measuring 100°F–104°F (37.8°C – 40°C).

Safety

CAUTION: Warm a victim of hypothermia slowly. Rapid warming can cause heart problems or increase circulation to the surface of the body, which causes additional cooling of vital organs.

PROCEDURE 17:8 (CONT.)

Safety

CAUTION: Do *not* use heat lamps, hot water above the stated temperatures, or heat from stoves or ovens. Excessive heat can burn the victim.

6. After the body part affected by frostbite has been thawed and the skin becomes flushed, discontinue warming the area because swelling may develop rapidly. Dry the part by blotting gently with a towel or soft cloth. Gently wrap the part in clean or sterile cloths. Use sterile gauze to separate the fingers and/or toes to prevent them from rubbing together.

Safety

CAUTION: *Never* rub or massage the frostbitten area, because doing so can cause gangrene.

7. Help the victim lie down. Do not allow the victim to walk or stand if the legs, feet, or toes are injured. Elevate any injured areas.
8. Observe the victim for signs of shock. Treat for shock as necessary.
9. If the victim is conscious and is not nauseated or vomiting, give warm liquids to drink.

Safety

CAUTION: Do *not* give beverages containing alcohol or caffeine. Give the victim warm broth, water, or milk.

10. 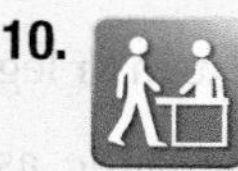 Comm Reassure the victim while providing treatment. Remain calm and encourage the victim to remain calm.
11. Obtain medical help as soon as possible.
12. Wash hands thoroughly after providing care.

PRACTICE: Go to the workbook and use the evaluation sheet for 17:8, Providing First Aid for Cold Exposure, to practice this procedure. When you believe you have mastered this skill, sign the sheet and give it to your instructor for further action.

Check

FINAL CHECKPOINT: Using the criteria listed on the evaluation sheet, your instructor will grade your performance.

17:9 Providing First Aid for Bone and Joint Injuries

Injuries to bones and joints are common in accidents and falls. A variety of injuries can occur to bones and joints. Such injuries sometimes occur together; other times, these injuries occur by themselves. Examples of injuries to bones and joints are fractures, dislocations, sprains, and strains.

Fractures

A **fracture** is a break in a bone. A closed, or simple, fracture is a bone break that is not accompanied by an external or open wound on the skin. A compound, or open, fracture is a bone break that is accompanied by an open wound on the skin. The types of fractures are discussed in Chapter 7:4 and shown in Figure 7–25.

Signs and symptoms of fractures can vary. Not all signs and symptoms will be present in every victim. Common signs and symptoms include:

- Deformity
- Limited motion or loss of motion
- Pain and tenderness at the fracture site
- Swelling and discoloration
- The protrusion of bone ends through the skin
- The victim heard a bone break or snap or felt a grating sensation (crepitation)
- Abnormal movements within a part of the body

Basic principles of treatment for fractures include:

- Maintain respirations
- Treat for shock
- Keep the broken bone from moving
- Prevent further injury
- Use devices such as splints and slings to prevent movement of the injured part
- Obtain medical help whenever a fracture is evident or suspected

Dislocations

A **dislocation** is when the end of a bone is either displaced from a joint or moved out of its normal position within a joint. This injury is frequently accompanied by a tearing or stretching of ligaments, muscles, and other soft tissue.

Signs and symptoms that may occur include:

- Deformity
- Limited or abnormal movement
- Swelling
- Discoloration
- Pain and tenderness
- A shortening or lengthening of the affected arm or leg

First aid for dislocations is basically the same as that for fractures. No attempt should be made to reduce the dislocation (that is, replace the bone in the joint). The affected part must be immobilized in the position in which it was found. Immobilization is accomplished by using splints and/or slings. Movement of the injured part can lead to additional injury to nerves, blood vessels, and other tissue in the area. Obtain medical help immediately.

Sprains

A **sprain** is an injury to the tissues surrounding a joint; it usually occurs when the part is forced beyond its normal range of movement. Ligaments, tendons, and other tissues are stretched or torn. Common sites for sprains include the ankles and wrists.

Signs and symptoms of a sprain include swelling, pain, discoloration, and sometimes, impaired motion. Frequently, sprains resemble fractures or dislocations. If in doubt, treat the injury as a fracture.

First aid for a sprain includes:

- Apply a cold application to decrease swelling and pain
- Elevate the affected part
- Encourage the victim to rest the affected part
- Apply an elastic bandage to provide support for the affected area but avoid stretching the bandage too tightly
- Obtain medical help if swelling is severe or if there is any question of a fracture

Strains

A **strain** is the overstretching of a muscle; it is caused by overexertion or lifting. A frequent site for strains is the back. Signs and symptoms of a strain include sudden pain, swelling, and/or bruising.

Basic principles of first aid treatment for a strain include:

- Encourage the victim to rest the affected muscle while providing support
- Recommend bed rest with a backboard under the mattress for a strained back
- Apply cold applications to reduce the swelling
- After the swelling decreases, apply warm, wet applications because warmth relaxes the muscles; different types of cold and heat packs are available (Figure 17–32)
- Obtain medical help for severe strains and all back injuries

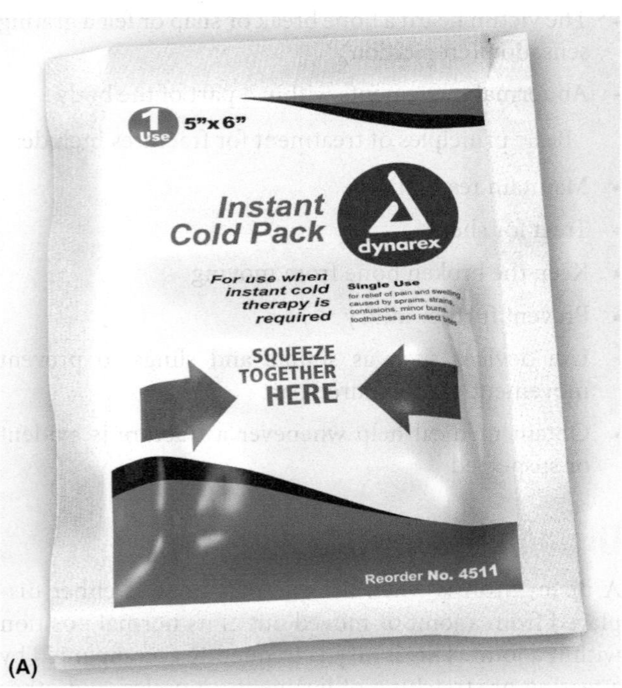

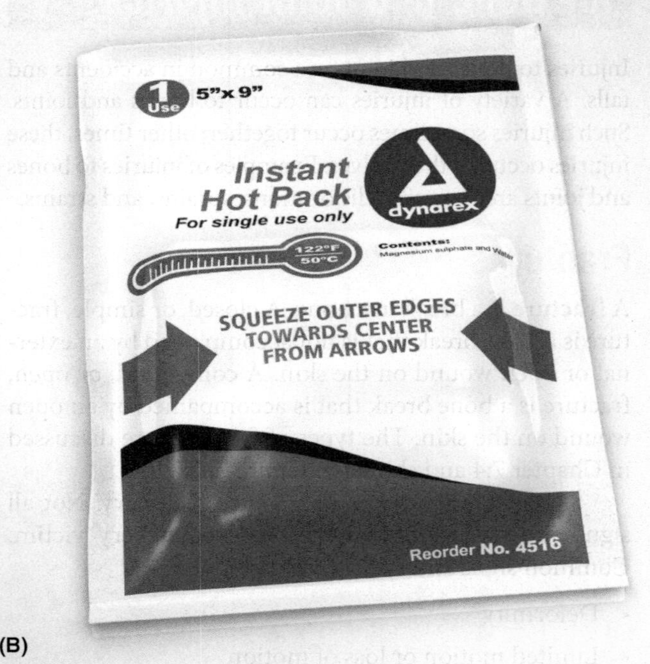

FIGURE 17–32 Disposable (A) cold and (B) heat packs contain chemicals that must be activated before using. Courtesy, Dynarex

Splints

Splints are devices that can be used to immobilize injured parts when fractures, dislocations, and other similar injuries are present or suspected. Many commercial splints are available, including inflatable, or air, splints; padded boards; and traction splints. Splints can also be made from cardboard, newspapers, blankets, pillows, boards, and other similar materials. Some basic principles regarding the use of splints are as follows:

- Splints should be long enough to immobilize the joint above and the joint below the injured area (Figure 17–33). By preventing movement in these joints, the injured bone or area is held in position and further injury is prevented.
- Splints should be padded, especially at bony areas and over the site of injury. Cloths, thick dressings, towels, and similar materials can be used as padding.
- Strips of cloth, roller gauze, triangular bandages folded into bands or strips, and similar materials can be used to tie splints in place.
- Splints must be applied so that they do not put pressure directly over the site of injury.
- If an open wound is present, use a sterile dressing to apply pressure and control bleeding.

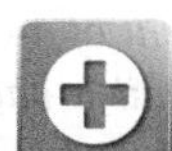
Precaution

CAUTION: *Wear gloves or use a protective barrier while controlling bleeding to avoid contamination from the blood.*

Safety

CAUTION: *Leave the dressing in place, and apply the splint in such a way that it does not put pressure on the wound.*

- *Never* make any attempt to replace broken bones or reduce a fracture or dislocation. Do *not* move the victim. Splint wherever you find the victim.
- *Pneumatic* splints are available in various sizes and shapes for different parts of the arms and legs. Care must be taken to avoid any unnecessary movement while the splint is being positioned. There are two main types of pneumatic splints: air (inflatable) and vacuum (deflatable).

  If an *air splint* is positioned over a fracture site, air pressure is used to inflate the splint. Some air splints have nozzles; these splints are inflated by blowing into the nozzles. Other air splints require the use of pressurized material in cans, while still others are inflated with cool air from a refrigerant solution. The coldness reduces swelling. Care must be taken to avoid overinflating air splints. To test whether the splint is properly inflated, use a thumb to apply slight pressure to the splint; an indentation mark should result.

  Vacuum pneumatic splints are deflated after being positioned over a fracture site. Air is removed from the splint with a hand pump or suction pump until the splint molds to the fracture site to provide support (Figure 17–34). Care must be taken to avoid overdeflation of the splint. A pulse site below the splint should be checked to make sure the splint is not applying too much pressure and cutting off circulation.
- Traction splints are special devices that provide a pulling or traction effect on the injured bone. They are frequently used for fractures of the femur, or thigh bone.

Legal

CAUTION: *Only persons specifically trained in the application of traction splints should apply them.*

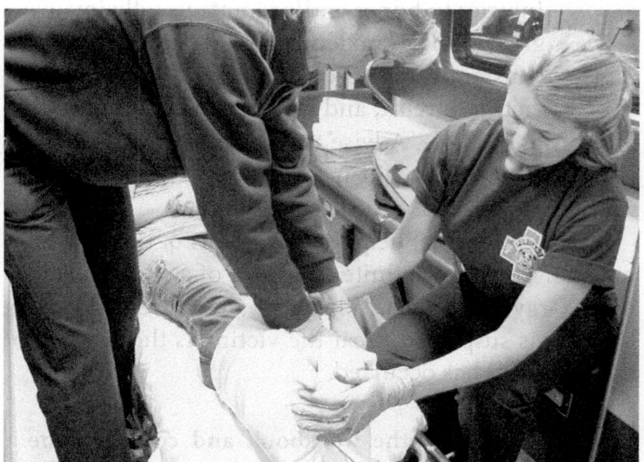

FIGURE 17–33 A pillow can be used to splint an ankle injury to immobilize the joint above and below the injured area. Courtesy of Larry Torrey, RN, EMT-P

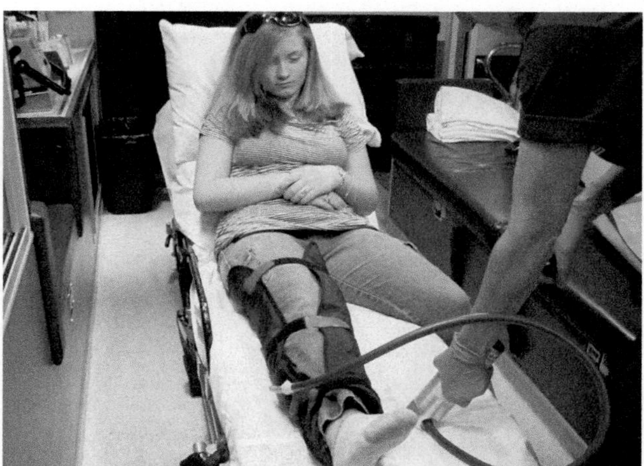

FIGURE 17–34 Vacuum pneumatic splints are deflated until the splint molds to the fracture site to provide support. Courtesy of Larry Torrey, RN, EMT-P

- After a splint is applied, it is essential to note the circulation and the effects on the nerve endings of the skin below the splint to make sure the splint is not too tight. Check skin temperature (it should be warm to the touch), skin color (pale or blue indicates poor circulation), swelling or edema, numbness or tingling, and pulse, if possible.

Safety

CAUTION: *If any signs of impaired circulation or impaired neurological status are present, immediately loosen the ties holding the splint.*

Slings

Slings are available in many different forms. Commercial slings usually have a series of straps that extend around the neck and/or thoracic (chest) region (Figure 17–35). A common type of sling used for first aid is the triangular bandage. Slings are usually used to support the arm, hand, forearm, and shoulder. They may be used when casts are in place. In addition, they are also used to provide immobility if a fracture of the arm or shoulder is suspected. Basic principles to observe with slings include:

- When a sling is applied to an arm, the sling should be positioned in such a way that the hand is higher than the elbow. The purpose of elevating the hand is to promote circulation, prevent swelling (edema), and decrease pain.
- Circulation in the limb and nerve supply to the limb must be checked frequently. Specifically, check for skin temperature (should be warm if circulation is good), skin color (blue or very pale indicates poor circulation), swelling (edema), amount of pain, and tingling or numbness. Nail beds can also be used to check circulation. When the nail beds are pressed slightly, they blanch (turn white). If circulation is good, the pink color should return to the nail beds immediately after the pressure is released.
- If a sling is being applied because of a suspected fracture to the bone, extreme care must be taken to move the injured limb as little as possible while the sling is being applied. The victim can sometimes help by holding the injured limb in position while the sling is slipped into place.
- If a triangular bandage is used, care must be taken so that the knot tied at the neck does not press against a bone. The knot should be tied to either side of the spinal column. Place gauze or padding under the knot of the sling to protect the skin.
- When shoulder injuries are suspected, it may be necessary to keep the arm next to the body. After a sling has been applied, another bandage can be placed around the thoracic region to hold the arm against the body.

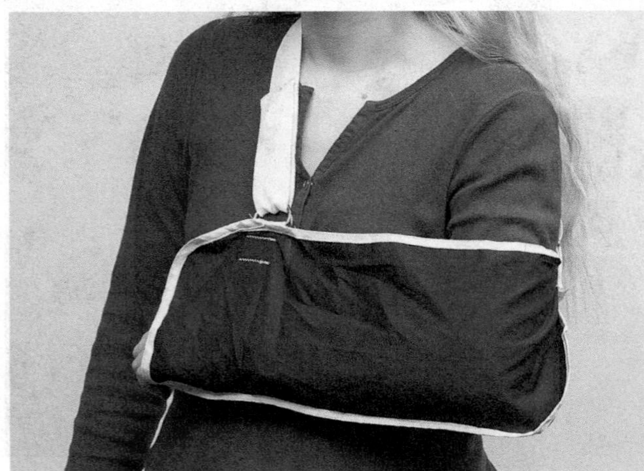

FIGURE 17–35 Commercial slings usually have a series of straps that extend around the neck and/or thoracic region.

Neck and Spine Injuries

Injuries to the neck or spine are the most dangerous types of injuries to bones and joints.

Safety

CAUTION: *If a victim who has such injuries is moved, permanent damage resulting in paralysis can occur. If at all possible, avoid any movement of a victim with neck or spinal injuries. Wait until a backboard, cervical collar, and adequate help for transfer is available.*

Summary

Victims with injuries to bones and/or joints also experience shock. Always be alert for signs of shock and treat as needed.

Comm

Injuries to bones and/or joints usually involve a great deal of anxiety, pain, and discomfort, so constantly reassure the victim. Encourage the victim to relax, and position the victim as comfortably as possible. Advise the victim that medical help is on the way. First aid measures are directed toward relieving the pain as much as possible.

Obtain medical help for all victims of bone or joint injuries. The only definite diagnosis of a closed fracture is an X-ray of the area. Whenever a fracture and/or dislocation is suspected, treat the victim as though one of these injuries has occurred.

STUDENT: Go to the workbook and complete the assignment sheet for 17:9, Providing First Aid for Bone and Joint Injuries. Then return and continue with the procedure.

PROCEDURE 17:9

Providing First Aid for Bone and Joint Injuries

Equipment and Supplies

Blankets, splints of various sizes, air or inflatable splints, triangular bandages, strips of cloth or roller gauze, disposable gloves

Procedure

1. Follow the steps of priority care, if indicated:
   a. Check the scene. Move the victim only if absolutely necessary. If the victim must be moved from a dangerous area, pull in the direction of the long axis of the body (that is, from the head or feet). If at all possible, tie an injured leg to the other leg or secure an injured arm to the body before movement.

Safety

CAUTION: If neck or spinal injuries are suspected, avoid any movement of the victim unless movement is necessary to save the victim's life.

   b. Check the victim for consciousness and breathing.
   c. Call emergency medical services (EMS) if necessary.
   d. Provide care to the victim.
   e. Control severe bleeding. If an open wound accompanies a fracture, take care not to push broken bone ends into the wound.

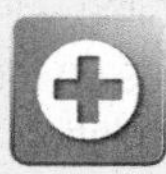
Precaution

CAUTION: Wear gloves or use a protective barrier while controlling bleeding.

2. Observe for signs and symptoms of a fracture, dislocation, or joint injury. Note deformities (such as a shortening or lengthening of an extremity), limited motion or loss of motion, pain, tenderness, swelling, discoloration, and bone fragments protruding through the skin. Also, the victim may state that he or she heard a bone snap or crack, or may complain of a grating sensation.
3. Immobilize the injured part to prevent movement.

Safety

CAUTION: Do *not* attempt to straighten a deformity, replace broken bone ends, or reduce a dislocation. Avoid any unnecessary movement of the injured part. If a bone injury is suspected, treat the victim as though a fracture or dislocation has occurred. Use splints or slings to immobilize the injury.

4. To apply splints:
   a. Obtain commercial splints or improvise splints by using blankets, pillows, newspapers, boards, cardboard, or similar supportive materials.
   b. Make sure that the splints are long enough to immobilize the joint both above and below the injury.
   c. Position the splints, making sure that they do *not* apply pressure directly at the site of injury. Two splints are usually used. However, if a pillow, blanket, or similar item is used, one such item can be rolled around the area to provide support on all sides.
   d. Use thick dressings, cloths, towels, or other similar materials to pad the splints. Make sure bony areas are protected. Avoid direct contact between the splint material and the skin.

   NOTE: Many commercial splints are already padded. However, additional padding is often needed to protect the bony areas.

   e. Use strips of cloth, triangular bandages folded into strips, roller gauze, or other similar material to tie or anchor the splints in place. The use of elastic bandage is discouraged because the bandage may cut off or interfere with circulation. If splints are long, three to five ties may be required. Tie the strips above and below the upper joint and above and below the lower joint. An additional tie should be placed in the center region of the splint.
   f. Avoid any unnecessary movement of the injured area while splints are being applied. If possible, have another individual support the area while you are applying the splints.
5. To apply air (inflatable) splints:
   a. Obtain the correct splint for the injured part.

   NOTE: Most air splints are available for full arm, lower arm, wrist, full leg, lower leg, and ankle/foot.

   b. Some air splints have zippers for easier application, but others must be slipped into position on the victim. If the splint has a zipper, position the open splint on the injured area, taking care to avoid any movement of the affected part. Use your hand to support the injured area. Close the zipper. If the splint must be slipped into position, slide the splint onto your arm first. Then hold the injured leg or arm and slide the splint from your arm to the victim's injured extremity. This technique prevents unnecessary movement.

(continues)

PROCEDURE 17:9 (CONT.)

c. Inflate the splint. Many splints are inflated by blowing into the nozzle. Others require the use of a pressure solution in a can. Follow instructions provided by the manufacturer of the splint.

d. Check to make sure that the splint is not overinflated. Use your thumb to press a section of the splint. Your thumb should leave a slight indentation if the splint is inflated correctly.

6. To apply a sling, follow the manufacturer's instructions for commercial slings. To use a triangular bandage for a sling (Figure 17–36), proceed as follows:

a. If possible, obtain the help of another individual to support the injured arm while the sling is being applied. Sometimes, the victim can hold the injured arm in place.

b. Place the long straight edge of the triangular bandage on the uninjured side. Allow one end to extend over the shoulder of the uninjured arm. The other end should hang down in front of the victim's chest. The short edge of the triangle should extend back and under the elbow of the injured arm.

CAUTION: Avoid excessive movement of the injured limb while positioning the sling.

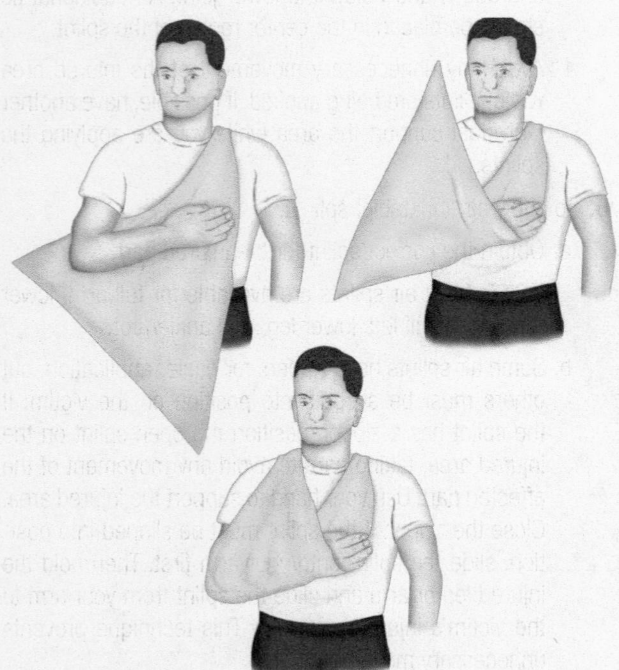

FIGURE 17–36 **Steps for applying a triangular bandage as a sling.**

c. Bring the long end of the bandage up and over the shoulder of the injured arm.

d. Use a square knot to tie the two ends together near the neck. Make sure the knot is not over a bone. Tie it to either side of the spinal column. Place gauze or padding between the knot and the skin. Make sure the hand is elevated 5–6 inches above the elbow.

e. The point of the bandage is now near the elbow. Bring the point forward, fold it, and pin it to the front of the sling. If no pin is available, coil the end and tie it in a knot.

CAUTION: If you use a pin, put your hand between the pin and the victim's skin while inserting the pin.

f. Check the position of the sling. The fingers of the injured hand should extend beyond the edge of the triangular bandage. In addition, the hand should be slightly elevated to prevent swelling (edema).

g. If a shoulder injury is suspected, it may be necessary to secure the arm close to the body. Apply a large bandage around the thoracic region to stabilize the shoulder joint (Figure 17–37).

7. After splints and/or slings have been applied, check for signs of impaired circulation. Skin color should be pink. A pale or cyanotic (bluish) color is a sign of poor circulation. The skin should be warm to the touch. Swelling can indicate poor circulation. If the victim complains of pain or pressure from the splints and/or slings, or of numbness or tingling in the area below the splints/sling, circulation may be impaired. Slightly press the nail beds on the foot or hand so they temporarily turn white. If circulation is good, the pink color will return to the nail beds immediately after pressure is released. If you note any signs of impaired circulation, loosen the splints and/or sling immediately.

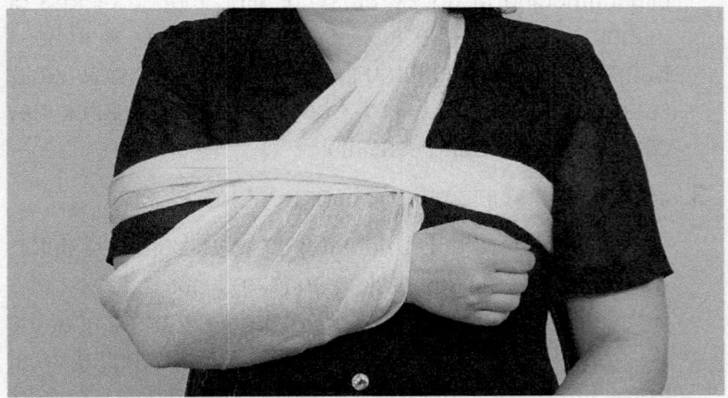

FIGURE 17–37 **If a shoulder injury is suspected, use a long bandage to secure the arm against the body to stabilize the shoulder joint.**

PROCEDURE 17:9 (CONT.)

8. Watch for signs of shock in any victim with a bone and/or joint injury. Remember, inadequate blood flow is the main cause of shock. Watch for signs of impaired circulation, such as a cyanotic (bluish) tinge around the lips or nail beds. Treat for shock, as necessary.
9. If medical help is delayed, cold applications such as cold compresses or an ice bag can be used on the injured area to decrease swelling.

Safety

CAUTION: To prevent injury to the skin, make sure that the ice bag is covered with a towel or other material.

10. Place the victim in a comfortable position, but avoid any unnecessary movement.

Safety

CAUTION: Avoid *any* movement if a neck or spinal injury is suspected.

11. 
Comm
Reassure the victim while providing first aid. Try to relieve the pain by carefully positioning the injured part, avoiding unnecessary movement, and applying cold.
12. Obtain medical help as quickly as possible.
13. Wash hands thoroughly after providing care.

PRACTICE: Go to the workbook and use the evaluation sheet for 17:9, Providing First Aid for Bone and Joint Injuries, to practice this procedure. When you believe you have mastered this skill, sign the sheet and give it to your instructor for further action.

Check

FINAL CHECKPOINT: Using the criteria listed on the evaluation sheet, your instructor will grade your performance.

17:10 Providing First Aid for Specific Injuries

Although treatment for burns, bleeding, wounds, poisoning, and fractures is basically the same for all regions of the body, injuries to specific body parts require special care. Examples of these parts are the eyes, ears, nose, brain, chest, abdomen, and genital organs.

Eye Injuries

Any eye injury always involves the danger of vision loss, especially if treated incorrectly. In most cases involving serious injury to the eyes, it is best *not* to provide major treatment. Obtaining medical help, preferably from an eye specialist, is a top priority of first aid care.

- *Foreign objects* such as dust, dirt, and similar small particles frequently enter the eye. These objects cause irritation and can scratch the eye or become embedded in the eye tissue. Signs and symptoms include redness, a burning sensation, pain, watering or tearing of the eye, and/or the presence of visible objects in the eye. If the foreign body is floating freely, prevent the victim from rubbing the eye, wash your hands thoroughly, and gently draw the upper lid down over the lower lid. This stimulates the formation of tears. The proximity of the lids also creates a wiping action, which may remove the particle. If this does not remove the foreign body, use your thumb and forefinger to grasp the eyelashes and gently raise the upper eyelid. Tell the victim to look down and tilt his or her head toward the injured side. Use water to gently flush the eye or use the corner of a piece of sterile gauze to gently remove the object.

Safety

CAUTION: *If this does not remove the object or if the object is embedded, make no attempt to remove it.*

Apply a dry, sterile dressing and obtain medical help for the victim. Serious injury can occur if any attempt is made to remove an object embedded in the eye tissue.

- *Blows to the eye* from a fist, accident, or explosion may cause contusions or black eyes as a result of internal bleeding and torn tissues inside the eye. Because this can lead to loss of vision, the victim should be examined as soon as possible by an eye specialist. Apply sterile dressings or an eye shield, keep the victim lying flat, and obtain medical help. It is sometimes best to cover both eyes to prevent involuntary movement of the injured eye.
- *Penetrating injuries* that cut the eye tissue are extremely dangerous.

Safety

CAUTION: *If an object is protruding from the eye, make no attempt to remove the object. Rather, support it by loosely applying dressings. A paper cup with a hole cut in the bottom can also be used to stabilize the object and prevent it from moving (Figure 17–38).*

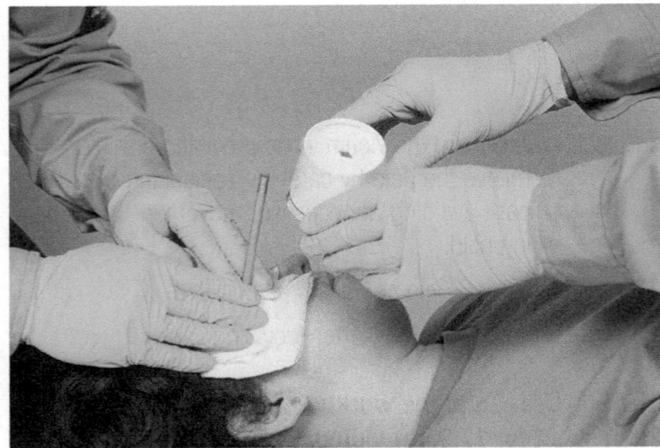

FIGURE 17–38 A cup can be used to stabilize an object impaled in the eye and to prevent it from moving.

Apply dressings to both eyes to prevent involuntary movement of the injured eye. Avoid applying pressure to the eye while applying the dressings. Keep the victim lying flat on his or her back to prevent fluids from draining out of the eye. Obtain medical help immediately.

Ear Injuries

Injuries to the ear can result in rupture or perforation of the eardrum. These injuries also require medical care. Treatment for specific types of ear injuries is as follows:

- Wounds of the ear frequently result in torn or detached tissue. Apply sterile dressings with light pressure to control bleeding.

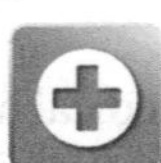

Precaution

CAUTION: *If possible, wear gloves or use a protective barrier while controlling bleeding.*

Save any torn tissue and wrap it in gauze moistened with cool sterile water or sterile normal saline solution. Put the gauze-wrapped tissue in a plastic bag to keep it cool and moist. Send the torn tissue to the medical facility along with the victim.

NOTE: *If sterile water is not available, use cool, clean water.*

- Keep the victim lying flat, but raise his or her head (if no other conditions prohibit raising the head).
- If the eardrum is ruptured or perforated, place sterile gauze loosely in the outer ear canal. Do *not* allow the victim to hit the side of the head in an attempt to restore hearing. Do *not* put any liquids into the ear. Obtain medical help for the victim.
- Clear or blood-tinged fluid draining from the ear can be a sign of a skull or brain injury. Allow the fluid to flow from the ear. Keep the victim lying down. If possible, turn the victim on his or her injured side and elevate the head and shoulders slightly to allow the fluid to drain. Obtain medical help immediately and report the presence and description of the fluid.

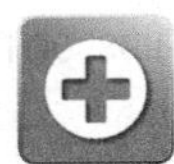

Precaution

CAUTION: *Wear gloves or use a protective barrier to avoid skin contact with fluid draining from the ear.*

Head or Skull Injuries

Wounds or blows to the head or skull can result in injury to the brain. Again, it is important to obtain medical help as quickly as possible for the victim.

- Signs and symptoms of brain injury include clear or blood-tinged cerebrospinal fluid draining from the nose or ears, loss of consciousness, headache, visual disturbances, pupils unequal in size, muscle paralysis, speech disturbances, convulsions, and nausea and vomiting.
- Keep the victim lying flat and treat for shock. If there is no evidence of neck or spinal injury, raise the victim's head slightly by supporting the head and shoulders on a small pillow or a rolled blanket or coat.
- Watch closely for signs of respiratory distress and provide artificial respiration as needed.
- Make *no* attempt to stop the flow of fluid. Loose dressings can be positioned to absorb the flow.

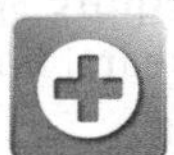

Precaution

CAUTION: *Wear gloves or use a protective barrier to avoid contamination from the cerebrospinal fluid.*

- Do *not* give the victim any liquids. If the victim complains of excessive thirst, use a clean, cool, wet cloth to moisten the lips, tongue, and inside of the mouth.
- If the victim loses consciousness, note how long the victim is unconscious and report this to the emergency rescue personnel.

Nose Injuries

Injuries to the nose frequently cause a nosebleed, also called an *epistaxis*. Nosebleeds are usually more frightening than they are serious. Nosebleeds can also be caused by change in altitude, strenuous activity, high blood pressure, and rupture of small blood vessels after a cold. Treatment for a nosebleed includes:

- Keep the victim quiet and remain calm.
- If possible, place the victim in a sitting position with the head leaning slightly forward.

- Apply pressure to control bleeding by pressing the bleeding nostril toward the midline. If both nostrils are bleeding, press both nostrils toward the midline.

  NOTE: *If both nostrils are blocked, tell the victim to breathe through the mouth.*

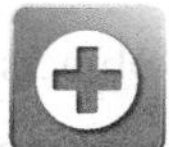
Precaution

CAUTION: *Wear gloves or use a protective barrier to avoid contamination from blood.*

- If application of pressure against the midline or septum does not stop the bleeding, insert a small piece of gauze in the nostril and then apply pressure on the outer surface of the nostril. Be sure to leave a portion of the gauze extending out of the nostril so that the packing can be removed later.

Safety

CAUTION: *Do not use cotton balls because the fibers will shed and stick.*

- Apply a cold compress to the bridge of the nose. A covered ice pack or a cold, wet cloth can be used.
- If the bleeding does not stop or a fracture of the nose is suspected, obtain medical assistance. If a person has repeated nosebleeds, a referral for medical attention should be made. Nosebleeds can indicate an underlying condition, such as high blood pressure, that requires medical care and treatment.

Chest Injuries

Injuries to the chest are usually medical emergencies because the heart, lungs, and major blood vessels may be involved. Chest injuries include sucking chest wounds, penetrating wounds, and crushing injuries. In all cases, obtain medical help immediately.

- *Sucking chest wound:* This is a deep, open chest wound that allows air to flow directly in and out with breathing. The partial vacuum that is usually present in the pleura (sacs surrounding the lungs) is destroyed, causing the lung on the injured side to collapse. Immediate medical help must be obtained. An air-tight dressing must be placed over the wound to prevent air flow into the wound. Aluminum foil, plastic wrap, or other nonporous material should be used to cover the wound. Tape or a bandage can be used to hold the nonporous material in place on three sides. The fourth side should be left loose to allow air to escape when the victim exhales. When the victim inhales, the negative pressure of inspirations will draw the dressing against the wound to create an air-tight seal. Maintain an open airway (through the nose or mouth) and provide artificial respiration as needed. If possible, position the victim on his or her injured side and elevate the head and chest slightly. This allows the uninjured lung to expand more freely and prevents pressure on the uninjured lung from blood and damaged tissue.

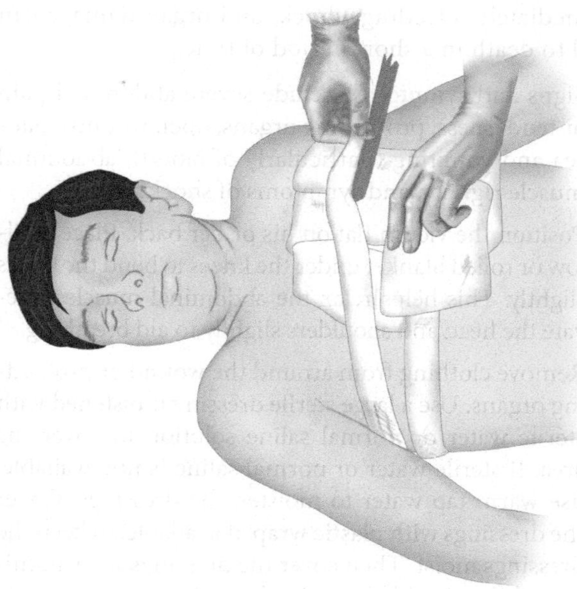

FIGURE 17–39 Immobilize an object protruding from the chest by placing dressings around the object and taping the dressings in place.

- *Penetrating injuries to the chest:* These injuries can result in sucking chest wounds or damage to the heart and blood vessels. If an object (for example, a knife) is protruding from the chest, do *not* attempt to remove the object. If possible, immobilize the object by placing dressings around it and taping the dressings in position (Figure 17–39). Place the victim in a comfortable position, maintain respirations, and obtain medical help immediately.
- *Crushing chest injuries:* These injuries are caused in vehicular accidents or when heavy objects strike the chest. Fractured ribs and damage to the lungs and/or heart can occur. Place the victim in a comfortable position and, if possible, elevate the head and shoulders to aid breathing. If an injury to the neck or spine is suspected, avoid moving the victim. Obtain medical help immediately.

Abdominal Injuries

Abdominal injuries can damage internal organs and cause bleeding in major blood vessels. The intestines and other abdominal organs may protrude from an open wound. Medical help must be obtained immediately; bleeding, shock, and organ damage can lead to death in a short period of time.

- Signs and symptoms include severe abdominal pain or tenderness, protruding organs, open wounds, nausea and vomiting (particularly of blood), abdominal muscle rigidity, and symptoms of shock.
- Position the victim flat on his or her back. Place a pillow or rolled blanket under the knees to bend the knees slightly. This helps relax the abdominal muscles. Elevate the head and shoulders slightly to aid breathing.
- Remove clothing from around the wound or protruding organs. Use a large sterile dressing moistened with sterile water or normal saline solution to cover the area. If sterile water or normal saline is not available, use warm tap water to moisten the dressings. Cover the dressings with plastic wrap, if available, to keep the dressings moist. Then cover the dressings with aluminum foil or a folded towel to keep the area warm.

Safety

CAUTION: *Make no attempt to reposition protruding organs.*

- Avoid giving the victim any fluids or food. If the victim complains of excessive thirst, use a cool, wet cloth to moisten the lips, tongue, and inside of the mouth.

Injuries to Genital Organs

Injuries to genital organs can result from falls, blows, or explosions. Zippers catching on genitals and other accidents sometimes bruise the genitals. Because injuries to the genitals may cause severe pain, bleeding, and shock, medical help is required. Basic principles of first aid include the following:

- Control severe bleeding by using a sterile (or clean) dressing to apply direct pressure to the area.

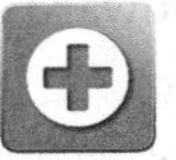
Precaution

CAUTION: *Wear gloves or use a protective barrier to avoid contamination from blood.*

- Treat the victim for shock.
- Do not remove any penetrating or inserted objects.
- Save any torn tissue and wrap it in gauze moistened with cool sterile water or sterile normal saline. Put the gauze-wrapped tissue in a plastic bag to keep it cool and moist. Send the torn tissue to the medical facility along with the victim.
- Use a covered ice pack or other cold applications to decrease bleeding and relieve pain.
- Obtain medical help.

Summary

Shock frequently occurs in victims with specific injuries to the eyes, ears, chest, abdomen, or other vital organs. Be alert for the signs of shock and immediately treat all victims.

Comm

Most of the specific injuries discussed in this section result in extreme pain for the victim. It is essential that you reassure the victim constantly and encourage the victim to relax as much as possible. Direct first aid care toward providing as much relief from pain as possible.

STUDENT: **Go to the workbook and complete the assignment sheet for 17:10, Providing First Aid for Specific Injuries. Then return and continue with the procedure.**

PROCEDURE 17:10

Providing First Aid for Specific Injuries

Equipment and Supplies

Blankets, pillows, dressings, bandages, tape, aluminum foil or plastic wrap, eye shields or sterile dressings, sterile water, disposable gloves

Procedure

1. Follow the steps of priority care, if indicated:
   a. Check the scene. Move the victim only if absolutely necessary.
   b. Check the victim for consciousness and breathing.
   c. Call emergency medical services (EMS), if necessary.
   d. Provide care to the victim.
   e. Check for bleeding. Control severe bleeding.

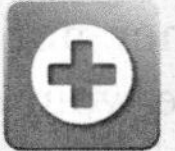
Precaution

CAUTION: Wear gloves or use a protective barrier while controlling bleeding.

2.  Comm Observe the victim closely for signs and symptoms of specific injuries. Do a systematic examination of the victim. Always have a reason for everything you do. Explain what you are doing to the victim and/or observers.

PROCEDURE 17:10 (CONT.)

3. If the victim has an eye injury, proceed as follows:

a. If the victim has a free-floating particle or foreign body in the eye, warn the victim *not* to rub the eye. Wash your hands thoroughly to prevent infection. Gently grasp the upper eyelid and draw it down over the lower eyelid. If this does not remove the object, use your thumb and forefinger to grasp the eyelashes and gently raise the upper eyelid. Tell the victim to look down and tilt his or her head slightly to the injured side. Use water to gently flush the eye or use the corner of a piece of sterile gauze to gently remove the object. If this does not remove the object or if the object is embedded, proceed to step b.

b. If an object is embedded in the eye, make *no* attempt to remove it. Rather, apply a dry, sterile dressing to loosely cover the eye. Obtain medical help.

c. If an eye injury has caused a contusion, a black eye, internal bleeding, and/or torn tissue in the eye, apply sterile dressings or eye shields to both eyes. Keep the victim lying flat. Obtain medical help.

NOTE: Both eyes are covered to prevent involuntary movement of the injured eye.

d. If an object is protruding from the eye, make *no* attempt to remove the object. If possible, support the object in position by loosely placing dressings around it. A paper cup with the bottom removed can also be used to surround and prevent any movement of the object. Apply dressings to the uninjured eye to prevent movement of the injured eye. Keep the victim lying flat. Obtain medical help immediately.

4. If the victim has an ear injury:

a. Control severe bleeding from an ear wound by using a sterile dressing to apply light pressure.

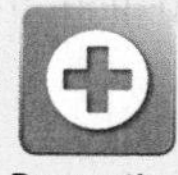
Precaution

CAUTION: Wear gloves or use a protective barrier to prevent contamination from the blood.

b. If any tissue has been torn from the ear, preserve the tissue by placing it in gauze moistened with cool, sterile water or normal saline solution. Place the gauze-wrapped tissue in a plastic bag. Send the torn tissue to the medical facility along with the victim.

NOTE: If sterile water is not available, use cool, clean water.

c. If a rupture or perforation of the eardrum is suspected or evident, place sterile gauze loosely in the outer ear canal. Caution the victim against hitting the side of the head to restore hearing. Obtain medical help.

d. If cerebrospinal fluid is draining from the ear, make no attempt to stop the flow of the fluid. If no neck or spinal injury is suspected, turn the victim on his or her injured side and slightly elevate the head and shoulders to allow the fluid to drain. A dressing may be positioned to absorb the flow. Obtain medical help immediately.

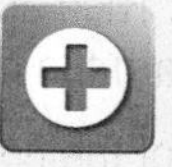
Precaution

CAUTION: Wear gloves or use a protective barrier to prevent contamination from the cerebrospinal fluid.

5. If the victim has a brain injury:

a. Keep the victim lying flat. Treat for shock. If there is no evidence of a neck or spinal injury, place a small pillow or a rolled blanket or coat under the victim's head and shoulders to elevate the head slightly.

Safety

CAUTION: Never position the victim's head lower than the rest of the body.

b. Watch closely for signs of respiratory distress. Provide artificial respiration if needed.

NOTE: Remove the pillow if artificial respiration is given.

c. If cerebrospinal fluid is draining from the ears, nose, and/or mouth, make no attempt to stop the flow. Position dressings to absorb the flow.

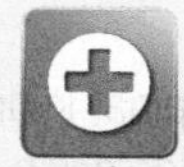
Precaution

CAUTION: Wear gloves or use a protective barrier to prevent contamination from the cerebrospinal fluid.

d. Avoid giving the victim any fluids by mouth. If the victim complains of excessive thirst, use a cool, wet cloth to moisten the lips, tongue, and inside of the mouth.

e. If the victim is unconscious, note for how long and report this information to the emergency rescue personnel.

f. Obtain medical help as quickly as possible.

6. If the victim has a nosebleed:

a. Try to keep the victim calm. Remain calm yourself.

b. Position the victim in a sitting position, if possible. Lean the head forward slightly. If the victim cannot sit up, slightly elevate the head.

c. Apply pressure by pressing the nostril(s) toward the midline. Continue applying pressure for at least 5 minutes and longer if necessary to control the bleeding.

NOTE: If both nostrils are bleeding and must be pressed toward the midline, tell the victim to breathe through the mouth.

(continues)

PROCEDURE 17:10 (CONT.)

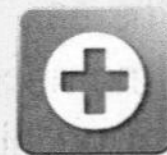
Precaution

CAUTION: Wear gloves or use a protective barrier to prevent contamination from the blood.

d. If application of pressure does not control the bleeding, insert gauze into the bleeding nostril, taking care to allow some of the gauze to hang out. Then apply pressure again by pushing the nostril toward the midline.

e. Apply cold compresses to the bridge of the nose. Use a cold, wet cloth or a covered ice bag.

f. If the bleeding does not stop, if a fracture is suspected, or if the victim has repeated nosebleeds, obtain medical help.

NOTE: Nosebleeds can indicate a serious underlying condition, such as high blood pressure, that requires medical attention.

7. If the victim has a chest injury:

a. If the wound is a sucking chest wound, apply a nonporous dressing. Use plastic wrap or aluminum foil to create an air-tight seal. Use tape on three sides to hold the dressing in place. Leave the fourth side loose to allow excess air to escape when the victim exhales (Figure 17–40).

b. Maintain an open airway. Constantly be alert for signs of respiratory distress. Provide artificial respiration as needed.

c. If there is no evidence of a neck or spinal injury, position the victim with his or her injured side down. Slightly elevate the head and chest by placing small pillows or blankets under the victim.

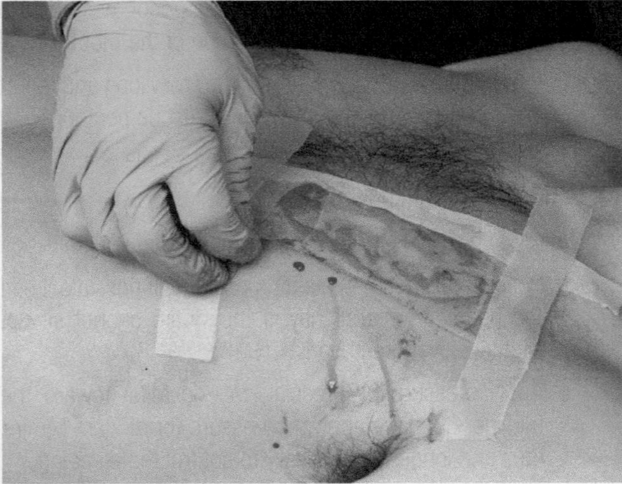

FIGURE 17–40 An air-tight dressing is used to cover a sucking chest wound. It is taped on three sides. The fourth side is left open to allow excess air to escape when the victim exhales.

d. If an object is protruding from the chest, make *no* attempt to remove it. If possible, immobilize the object with dressings, and tape around it.

e. Obtain medical help immediately for all chest injuries.

8. If the victim has an abdominal injury:

a. Position the victim flat on the back. Place a small pillow or a rolled blanket or coat under the victim's knees to flex them slightly. Elevate the head and shoulders to aid breathing. If movement of the legs causes pain, leave the victim lying flat.

b. If abdominal organs are protruding from the wound, make *no* attempt to reposition the organs. Remove clothing from around the wound or protruding organs. Use a sterile dressing that has been moistened with sterile water or normal saline solution to cover the area. If sterile water or normal saline is not available, use warm tap water to moisten the dressings.

c. Cover the dressing with plastic wrap, if available, to keep the dressing moist. Then apply a folded towel or aluminum foil to keep the area warm.

d. Avoid giving the victim any fluids or food. If the victim complains of excessive thirst, use a cool, wet cloth to moisten the lips, tongue, and inside of the mouth.

e. Obtain medical help immediately.

9. If the victim has an injury to the genital organs:

a. Control severe bleeding by using a sterile dressing to apply direct pressure.

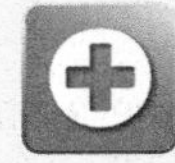
Precaution

CAUTION: Wear gloves or use a protective barrier to prevent contamination from the blood.

b. Position the victim flat on the back. Separate the legs to prevent pressure on the genital area.

c. If any tissue is torn from the area, preserve the tissue by wrapping it in gauze moistened with cool, sterile water or normal saline solution. Put the gauze-wrapped tissue in a plastic bag and send it to the medical facility along with the victim.

d. Apply cold compresses such as covered ice bags to the area to relieve pain and reduce swelling.

e. Obtain medical help for the victim.

PROCEDURE 17:10 (CONT.)

10. Be alert for the signs of shock in all victims. Treat for shock immediately.
11. Comm Constantly reassure all victims while providing care. Remain calm. Encourage the victim to relax as much as possible.
12. Always obtain medical help as quickly as possible. Shock, pain, and injuries to vital organs can cause death in a very short period of time.
13. Wash hands thoroughly after providing care.

PRACTICE: Go to the workbook and use the evaluation sheet for 17:10, Providing First Aid for Specific Injuries, to practice this procedure. When you believe you have mastered this skill, sign the sheet and give it to your instructor for further action.

Check

FINAL CHECKPOINT: Using the criteria listed on the evaluation sheet, your instructor will grade your performance.

17:11 Providing First Aid for Sudden Illness

The victim of a sudden illness requires first aid until medical help can be obtained. Sudden illness can occur in any individual. At times, it is difficult to determine the exact illness being experienced by the victim. However, by knowing the signs and symptoms of some major disorders, you should be able to provide appropriate first aid care. Information regarding a specific condition or illness may also be obtained from the victim, medical alert bracelets or necklaces, or medical information cards. Be alert to all of these factors while caring for the victim of a sudden illness.

Heart Attack

A **heart attack** is also called a *coronary thrombosis, coronary occlusion*, or *myocardial infarction*. It may occur when one of the coronary arteries supplying blood to the heart is blocked. If the attack is severe, the victim may die. If the heart stops beating, cardiopulmonary resuscitation (CPR) must be started. Main facts regarding heart attacks are as follows:

- Signs and symptoms of a heart attack may vary depending on the amount of heart damage. Severe, painful pressure under the breastbone (sternum) with pain radiating to the shoulders, arms, neck, and jaw is a common symptom (Figure 17–41). The victim usually experiences intense shortness of breath. The skin, especially near the lips and nail beds, becomes pale or cyanotic (bluish). The victim feels very weak but is also anxious and apprehensive. Nausea, vomiting, diaphoresis (excessive perspiration), and loss of consciousness may occur. The signs and symptoms of a heart attack in women are often more subtle. They may experience unusual fatigue and sleep disturbances for weeks prior to the attack. Cold sweats are common, as is pain in other areas than the chest, such as the arms, back, stomach, neck, and/or jaw. Heart attacks are often misdiagnosed in women.

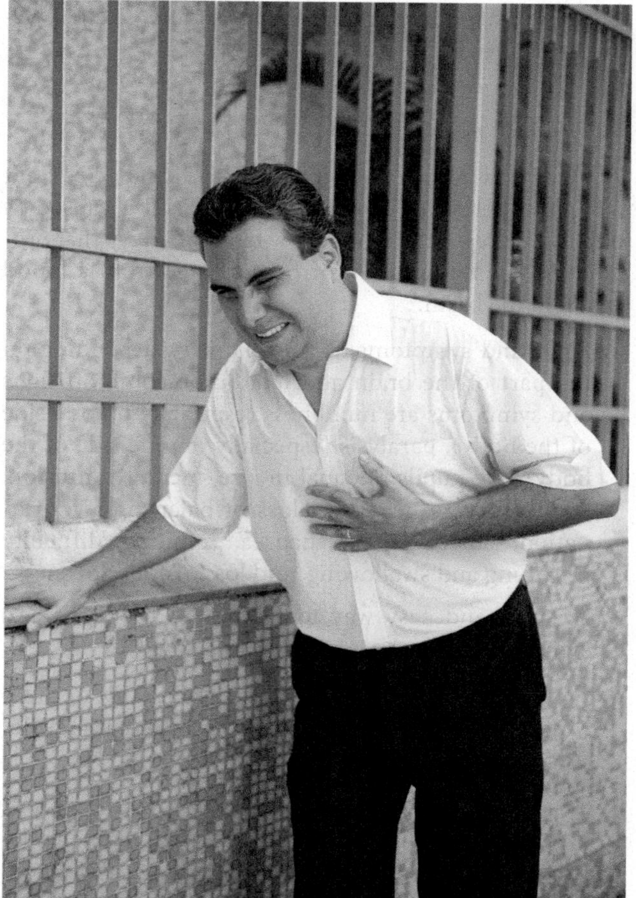

FIGURE 17–41 Severe pressure under the sternum with pain radiating to the shoulders, arms, neck, and jaw is a common symptom of a heart attack. © mangostock/www.Shutterstock.com

- First aid for a heart attack is directed toward encouraging the victim to relax, placing the victim in a comfortable position to relieve pain and assist breathing, and obtaining medical help. Shock frequently occurs, so provide treatment for shock. Prevent any unnecessary stress and avoid excessive movement because any activity places additional strain on the heart. Reassure the victim constantly, and obtain appropriate medical assistance as soon as possible.
- Legal After calling EMS, the American Heart Association recommends that patients who can should take an aspirin. Aspirin keeps platelets in the blood from sticking together to cause a clot. However, there are legal restrictions as to which health care providers can administer medications. Only qualified individuals should give the victim aspirin.

Cerebrovascular Accident or Stroke

A **stroke** is also called a **cerebrovascular accident** (CVA), apoplexy, or cerebral thrombosis. It is caused by either the presence of a clot in a cerebral artery that provides blood to the brain or hemorrhage from a blood vessel in the brain.

- Signs and symptoms of a stroke vary depending on the part of the brain affected. Some common signs and symptoms are numbness (especially on one side of the body), paralysis (especially on one side of the body), eye pupils unequal in size, mental confusion, sudden severe headache, loss of balance or coordination, slurred speech, nausea, vomiting, difficulty breathing and swallowing, and loss of consciousness.
- A quick and easy way to remember the signs and symptoms of stroke is to think *FAST*:

  F = *Face:* ask the person to smile. If one side of the face appears to be drooping or crooked, it may be a sign of stroke.

  A = *Arms:* ask the person to raise both of their arms. If they have difficulty lifting one, or keeping one raised, it may be a sign of stroke.

  S = *Speech:* ask the person to speak. If the words are slurred or they have difficulty speaking, it may be a sign of stoke.

  T = *Time:* if they have any of these symptoms, call 911 immediately.
- First aid for a stroke victim is directed toward maintaining respirations, laying the victim flat on the back with the head slightly elevated or on the side to allow secretions to drain from the mouth, and avoiding any fluids by mouth. Reassure the victim, prevent any unnecessary stress, and avoid any unnecessary movement.

Comm

NOTE: *Always remember that although the victim may be unable to speak or may appear to be unconscious, he or she may be able to hear and understand what is going on.*

- It is very important to know exactly when the symptoms started and to obtain medical help as quickly as possible. Immediate care during the first 3 hours can help prevent brain damage. If the CVA is caused by a blood clot, treatment with thrombolytic or "clot busting" drugs such as TPA (tissue plasminogen activator) or angioplasty of the cerebral arteries can dissolve a blood clot and restore blood flow to the brain. If the CVA is caused by a hemorrhage, thrombolytic therapy is not an option. In this case, treatment will depend on the cause of the bleed (hypertension, use of anticoagulants, trauma, etc.). In some cases, surgery can be done to stop the bleeding.

Fainting

Fainting occurs when there is a temporary reduction in the supply of blood to the brain. It may result in partial or complete loss of consciousness. The victim usually regains consciousness after being in a supine position (that is, lying flat on the back).

- Early signs of fainting include dizziness, extreme pallor, diaphoresis, coldness of the skin, nausea, and a numbness and tingling of the hands and feet.
- If early symptoms are noted, help the victim to lie down or to sit in a chair and position his or her head at the level of the knees.
- If the victim loses consciousness, try to prevent injury. Provide first aid by keeping the victim in a supine position. If no neck or spine injuries are suspected, use a pillow or blankets to elevate the victim's legs and feet 12 inches. Loosen any tight clothing and maintain an open airway. Use cool water to gently bathe the victim's face. Check for any injuries that may have been caused by the fall. Permit the victim to remain flat and quiet until color improves and the victim has recovered. Then allow the victim to get up gradually. If recovery is not prompt, if other injuries occur or are suspected, or if fainting occurs again, obtain medical help. Fainting can be a sign of a serious illness or condition that requires medical attention.

Convulsion

A **convulsion**, which is a type of *seizure*, is a strong, involuntary contraction of muscles. Convulsions may occur in conjunction with high body temperatures, head injuries, brain disease, and brain disorders such as epilepsy.

- Convulsions cause a rigidity of body muscles followed by jerking movements. During a convulsion, a person may stop breathing, bite the tongue, lose bladder and bowel control, and injure body parts. The face and lips may develop a cyanotic (bluish) color. The victim may lose consciousness. After regaining consciousness at the end of the convulsion, the victim may be confused and disoriented, and complain of a headache.
- First aid is directed toward preventing self-injury. Removing dangerous objects from the area, providing a pillow or cushion under the victim's head, and providing artificial respiration, as necessary, are all ways to assist the victim.
- Do *not* try to place anything between the victim's teeth. This can cause severe injury to your fingers, and/or damage to the victim's teeth or gums.
- Do *not* use force to restrain or stop the muscle movements; this only causes the contractions to become more severe.
- When the convulsion is over, watch the victim closely. If fluid, such as saliva or vomit, is in the victim's mouth, position the victim on his or her side to allow the fluid to drain from the mouth. Allow the victim to sleep or rest.
- Obtain medical help if the seizure lasts more than a few minutes, if the victim has repeated seizures, if other severe injuries are apparent, if the victim does not have a history of seizures, or if the victim does not regain consciousness.

Diabetic Reactions

Diabetes mellitus is a metabolic disorder caused by an insufficient production of insulin (a hormone produced by the pancreas). Insulin helps the body transport glucose, a form of sugar, from the bloodstream into body cells where the glucose is used to produce energy. When there is a lack of insulin, sugar builds up in the bloodstream. Insulin injections can reduce and control the level of sugar in the blood. Individuals with diabetes are in danger of developing two conditions that require first aid: diabetic coma and insulin shock (Figure 17–42).

- **Diabetic coma** or *hyperglycemia* is caused by an increase in the level of glucose in the bloodstream. The condition may result from an excess intake of sugar, failure to take insulin, or insufficient production of insulin. Signs and symptoms include confusion; weakness or dizziness; nausea and/or vomiting; rapid, deep respirations; dry, flushed skin; and a sweet or fruity odor to the breath. The victim will eventually lose consciousness and die unless the condition is treated. Medical assistance must be obtained as quickly as possible.
- **Insulin shock** or *hypoglycemia* is caused by an excess amount of insulin (and a low level of glucose) in the bloodstream. It may result from failure to eat the recommended amounts, vomiting after taking insulin, or taking excessive amounts of insulin. Signs and symptoms include muscle weakness; mental confusion; restlessness or anxiety; diaphoresis; pale, moist skin; hunger pangs; and/or palpitations (rapid, irregular heartbeats). The victim may lapse into a coma and develop convulsions. The onset of insulin shock is sudden, and the victim's condition can deteriorate quickly; therefore, immediate first aid care is required. If the victim is conscious, give him or her a drink containing sugar, such as sweetened orange juice. A cube or teaspoon of granulated sugar can also be placed in the victim's mouth. If the victim is confused, avoid giving hard candy. Unconsciousness could occur, and the victim could choke on the hard candy. Many individuals with diabetes use tubes of glucose that they carry with them (Figure 17–43). If the victim is conscious and can swallow and a glucose tube is available, it can be given to the victim.

The intake of sugar should quickly control the reaction. If the victim loses consciousness or convulsions start, provide care for the convulsions and obtain medical assistance immediately.

Comm

By observing symptoms carefully and obtaining as much information as possible from the victim, you can usually determine whether the condition is diabetic coma or insulin shock. Ask the victim, "Have you eaten today?" and "Have you taken your insulin?" If the victim has taken insulin but has not eaten, insulin shock is developing because there is too much insulin in the body. If the victim has eaten but has not taken insulin, diabetic coma is developing. In cases when you know that the victim is diabetic but the victim is unconscious and there are no definite symptoms of either condition, you may not be able to determine whether the condition is diabetic coma or insulin shock. In such cases, the recommendation is to put granulated sugar under the victim's tongue and activate emergency medical services (EMS). This is the lesser of two evils. If the patient is in diabetic coma, the blood sugar level can be lowered as needed when the victim is transported for medical care. If the victim is in insulin shock, however, brain damage can occur if the blood-sugar level is not raised immediately. Medical care cannot correct brain damage.

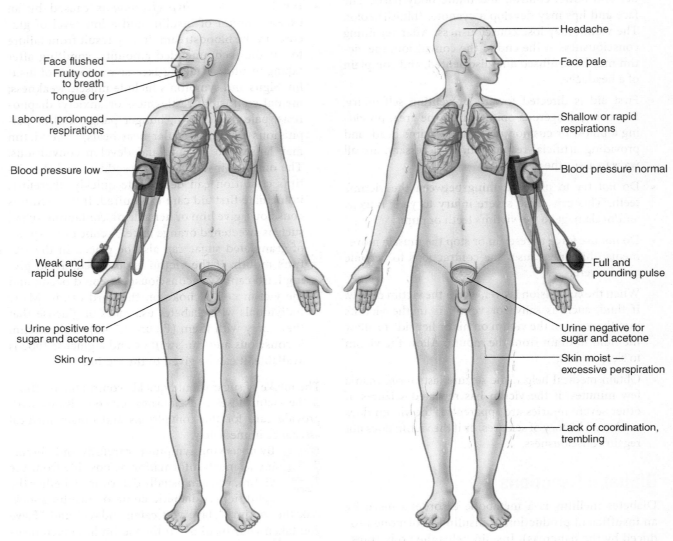

Diabetic coma (Hyperglycemia)
- Appears to be in stupor or coma
- High blood glucose levels

Face flushed
Fruity odor to breath
Tongue dry
Labored, prolonged respirations
Blood pressure low
Weak and rapid pulse
Urine positive for sugar and acetone
Skin dry

Insulin shock (Hypoglycemia)
- Excited, nervous, dizziness, confused, irritable, inappropriate responses
- Low blood glucose levels

Headache
Face pale
Shallow or rapid respirations
Blood pressure normal
Full and pounding pulse
Urine negative for sugar and acetone
Skin moist — excessive perspiration
Lack of coordination, trembling

FIGURE 17–42 Diabetic coma (hyperglycemia) versus insulin shock (hypoglycemia).

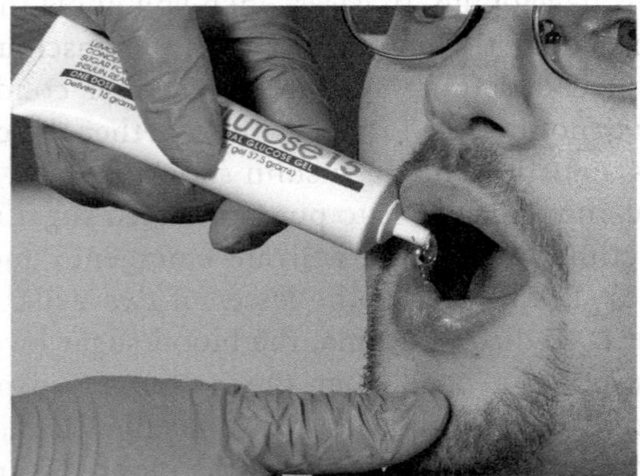

FIGURE 17–43 A victim experiencing insulin shock needs glucose or some form of sugar as quickly as possible.

Summary

In all cases of sudden illness, constantly reassure the victim and make every attempt to encourage the victim to relax and avoid further stress. Be alert for the signs of shock and provide treatment for shock to all victims. The pain, anxiety, and fear associated with sudden illness can contribute to shock.

STUDENT: Go to the workbook and complete the assignment sheet for 17:11, Providing First Aid for Sudden Illness. Then return and continue with the procedure.

PROCEDURE 17:11

Providing First Aid for Sudden Illness

Equipment and Supplies

Blankets, pillows, sugar, clean cloth, cool water, disposable gloves

Procedure

1. Follow the steps of priority care, if indicated.
   a. Check the scene. Move the victim only if absolutely necessary.
   b. Check the victim for consciousness and breathing.
   c. Call emergency medical services (EMS), if necessary.
   d. Provide care to the victim.
   e. Check for bleeding. Control severe bleeding.

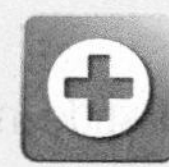
Precaution

CAUTION: Wear gloves or use a protective barrier while controlling bleeding.

2. 
Comm

Closely observe the victim for specific signs and symptoms. If the victim is conscious, obtain information about the history of the illness, type and amount of pain, and other pertinent details. If the victim is unconscious, check for a medical bracelet or necklace or a medical information card. Always have a reason for everything you do. Explain your actions to any observers, especially if it is necessary to check the victim's wallet for a medical card.

3. If you suspect the victim is having a heart attack, provide first aid as follows:
   a. Place the victim in the most comfortable position possible, but avoid unnecessary movement. Some victims will want to lie flat, but others will want to be in a partial or complete sitting position. If the victim is having difficulty breathing, use pillows or rolled blankets to elevate the head and shoulders.
   b. Obtain medical help for the victim immediately. Advise EMS that oxygen may be necessary.
   c. 
Comm

Encourage the victim to relax. Reassure the victim. Remain calm and encourage others to remain calm.

   d. Watch for signs of shock and treat for shock as necessary. Avoid overheating the victim.
   e. If the victim complains of excessive thirst, use a wet cloth to moisten the lips, tongue, and inside of the mouth. Small sips of water can also be given to the victim, but avoid giving large amounts of fluid.

Safety

CAUTION: Do *not* give the victim ice water or very cold water because the cold can intensify shock.

4. If you suspect that the victim has had a stroke:
   a. Place the victim in a comfortable position. Keep the victim lying flat or slightly elevate the victim's head and shoulders to aid breathing. If the victim has difficulty swallowing, turn the victim on his or her side to allow secretions to drain from the mouth and prevent choking on the secretions.
   b. 
Comm

Reassure the victim. Encourage the victim to relax.

   c. Avoid giving the victim any fluids or food by mouth. If the victim complains of excessive thirst, use a cool, wet cloth to moisten the lips, tongue, and inside of the mouth.
   d. Attempt to determine the exact time the symptoms started and obtain medical help for the victim as quickly as possible.

5. If the victim has fainted:
   a. Keep the victim in a supine position (that is, lying flat on the back). Raise the legs and feet 12 inches.
   b. Check for breathing. Provide artificial respiration, if necessary.
   c. Loosen any tight clothing.
   d. Use cool water to gently bathe the face.
   e. Check for any other injuries.
   f. Encourage the victim to continue lying down until his or her skin color improves.
   g. If no other injuries are suspected, allow the victim to get up slowly. First, elevate the head and shoulders. Then place the victim in a sitting position. Allow the victim to stand slowly. If any signs of dizziness, weakness, or pallor are noted, return the victim to the supine position.
   h. If the victim does not recover quickly, or if any other injuries occur, obtain medical care. If fainting has occurred frequently, refer the victim for medical care.

NOTE: Fainting can be a sign of a serious illness or condition.

(continues)

PROCEDURE 17:11 (CONT.)

6. If the victim is having a convulsion, provide first aid as follows:

a. Remove any dangerous objects from the area. If the victim is near heavy furniture or machinery that cannot be moved, move the victim to a safe area.

b. Place soft material such as a blanket, small pillow, rolled jacket, or other similar material under the victim's head to prevent injury.

c. Closely observe respirations at all times. During the convulsion, there will be short periods of apnea (cessation of breathing).

NOTE: If breathing does not resume quickly, artificial respiration may be necessary.

d. Do *not* try to place anything between the victim's teeth. This can cause injury to the teeth and/or gums.

e. Do *not* attempt to restrain the muscle contractions. This only makes the contractions more severe.

f. Comm Note how long the convulsion lasts and what parts of the body are involved. Be sure to report this information to the EMS personnel.

g. After the convulsion ends, closely watch the victim. Encourage the victim to rest.

h. Obtain medical assistance if the convulsion lasts more than a few minutes, if the victim has repeated convulsions, if other severe injuries are apparent, if the victim does not have a history of convulsions, or if the victim does not regain consciousness.

7. If the victim is in diabetic coma:

a. Place the victim in a comfortable position. If the victim is unconscious, position him or her on either side to allow secretions to drain from the mouth.

b. Frequently check respirations. Provide artificial respiration as needed.

c. Obtain medical help immediately so the victim can be transported to a medical facility.

8. If the victim is in insulin shock:

a. If the victim is conscious and can swallow, offer a drink containing sugar or oral glucose if a tube is available.

b. If the victim is unconscious, place a small amount of granulated sugar under the victim's tongue.

c. Place the victim in a comfortable position. Position an unconscious victim on either side to allow secretions to drain from the mouth.

d. If recovery is not prompt, obtain medical help immediately.

9. Observe all victims of sudden illness for signs of shock. Treat for shock as necessary.

10. Comm Constantly reassure any victim of sudden illness. Encourage relaxation to decrease stress.

11. Wash hands thoroughly after providing care.

PRACTICE: **Go to the workbook and use the evaluation sheet for 17:11, Providing First Aid for Sudden Illness, to practice this procedure. When you believe you have mastered this skill, sign the sheet and give it to your instructor for further action.**

Check

FINAL CHECKPOINT: Using the criteria listed on the evaluation sheet, your instructor will grade your performance.

17:12 Applying Dressings and Bandages

In many cases requiring first aid, it will be necessary for you to apply dressings and bandages. This section provides basic information on types of bandages and dressings and on application methods.

A **dressing** is a sterile covering placed over a wound or an injured part. It is used to control bleeding, absorb blood and secretions, prevent infection, and ease pain. Materials that may be used as dressings include gauze pads in a variety of sizes and compresses of thick, absorbent material (Figure 17–44). Fluff cotton should *not* be used

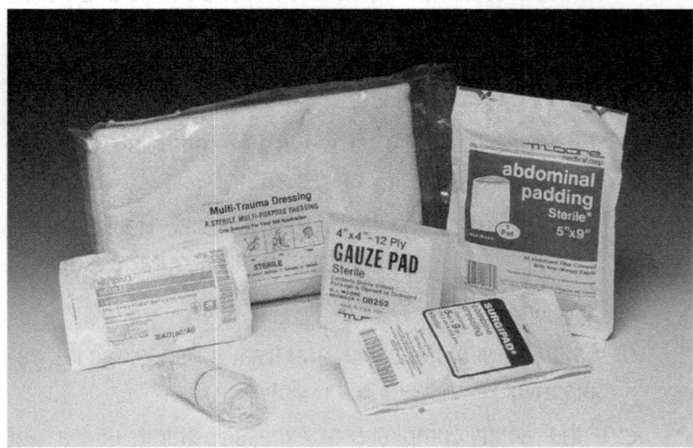

FIGURE 17–44 **Dressings to cover a wound are available in many different sizes.**

as a dressing because the loose cotton fibers may contaminate the wound. In an emergency when no dressings are available, a clean handkerchief or pillowcase may be used. The dressing is held in place with tape or a bandage.

Bandages are materials used to hold dressings in place, to secure splints, and to support and protect body parts. Bandages should be applied snugly enough to control bleeding and prevent movement of the dressing, but not so tightly that they interfere with circulation. Types of bandages include roller gauze bandages, triangular bandages, and elastic bandages (Figure 17–45).

- *Roller gauze bandages* come in a variety of widths, most commonly 1-, 2-, and 3-inch widths. They can be used to hold dressings in place on almost any part of the body.
- *Triangular bandages* can be used to secure dressings on the head/scalp or as slings. A triangular bandage is sometimes used as a covering for a large body part such as a hand, foot, or shoulder. By folding the triangular bandage into a band of cloth called a *cravat* (Figure 17–46), the bandage can be used to secure splints or dressings on body parts.
- *Elastic bandages* are easy to apply because they readily conform, or mold, to the injured part. However, they can be quite hazardous; if they are applied too tightly or are stretched during application, they can cut off or constrict circulation. Elastic bandages are sometimes used to provide support and stimulate circulation.

Several methods are used to wrap bandages. The method used depends on the body part involved. Some common wraps include the spiral wrap; the figure-eight wrap for joints; and the finger, or recurrent, wrap. The wraps are described in Procedure 17:12, immediately following this information section.

After any bandage has been applied, it is important to check the body part below the bandage to make sure the bandage is not so tight as to interfere with blood circulation. Signs that indicate poor circulation include swelling, a pale or blue (cyanotic) color to the skin, coldness to the touch, and numbness or tingling. If the bandage has been applied to the hand, arm, leg, or foot, press lightly on the nail beds to blanch them (that is, make them turn white [Figure 17–47A]). The pink color should return to the nail beds immediately after pressure is released (Figure 17–47B). If the pink

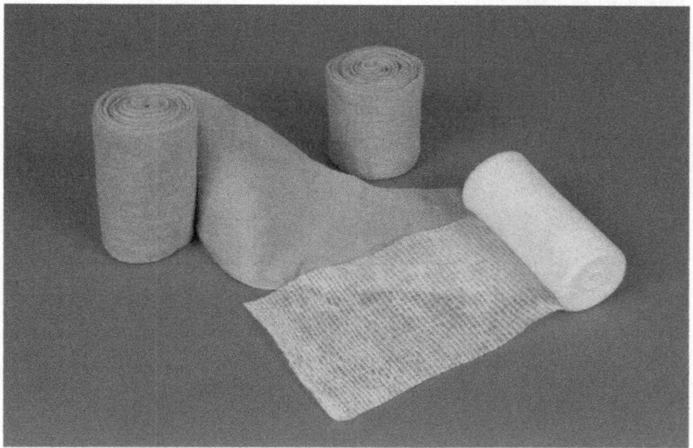

FIGURE 17–45 Roller gauze and elastic bandages can be used to hold dressings in place.

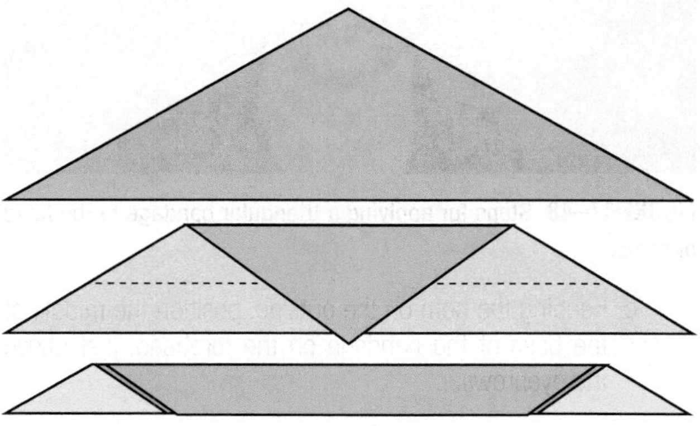

FIGURE 17–46 Folding a cravat bandage from a triangular bandage.

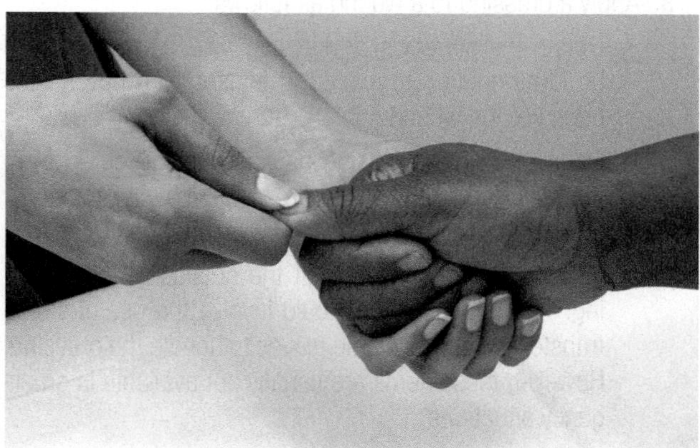

FIGURE 17–47A To check circulation, press lightly on the nail bed to blanch it or make it turn white.

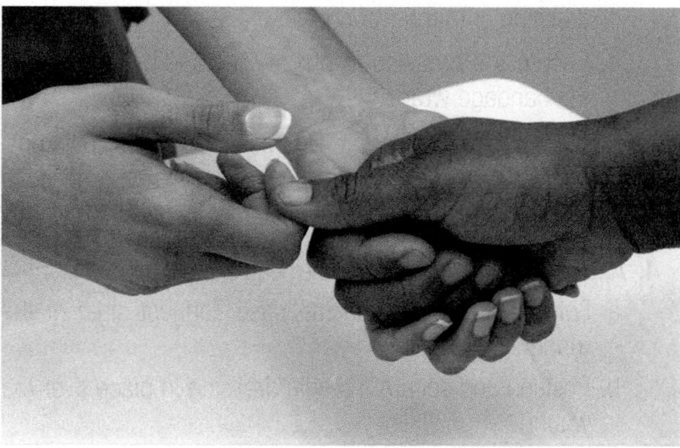

FIGURE 17–47B If the nail bed does not turn to pink immediately after pressure is released, circulation may be impaired.

color does not return or returns slowly, this is an indication of poor or impaired circulation. If any signs of impaired circulation are noted, loosen the bandages immediately.

STUDENT: **Go to the workbook and complete the assignment sheet for 17:12, Applying Dressings and Bandages. Then return and continue with the procedure.**

PROCEDURE 17:12

Applying Dressings and Bandages

Equipment and Supplies

Sterile gauze pads, triangular bandage, roller gauze bandage, elastic bandage, tape, disposable gloves

Procedure

1. Assemble equipment.
2. Precaution: Wash hands. Put on gloves if there is any chance of contact with blood or body fluids.
3. Apply a dressing to a wound as follows:
   a. Obtain the correct size dressing. The dressing should be large enough to extend at least 1 inch beyond the edges of the wound.
   b. Open the sterile dressing package, taking care not to touch or handle the sterile dressing with your fingers.
   c. Use a pinching action to pick up the sterile dressing so you handle only one part of the outside of the dressing. The ideal situation would involve the use of sterile transfer forceps or sterile gloves to handle the dressing. However, these items are usually not available in emergency situations.
   d. Place the dressing on the wound. The untouched (sterile) side of the dressing should be placed on the wound. Do *not* slide the dressing into position. Instead, hold the dressing directly over the wound and then lower the dressing onto the wound.
   e. Secure the dressing in place with tape or with one of the bandage wraps.

Safety

CAUTION: If tape is used, do not wrap it completely around the part. This can lead to impaired circulation.

4. Apply a triangular bandage to the head or scalp (Figure 17–48):
   a. Fold a 2-inch hem on the base (longest side) of the triangular bandage.
   b. Position and secure a sterile dressing in place over the wound.

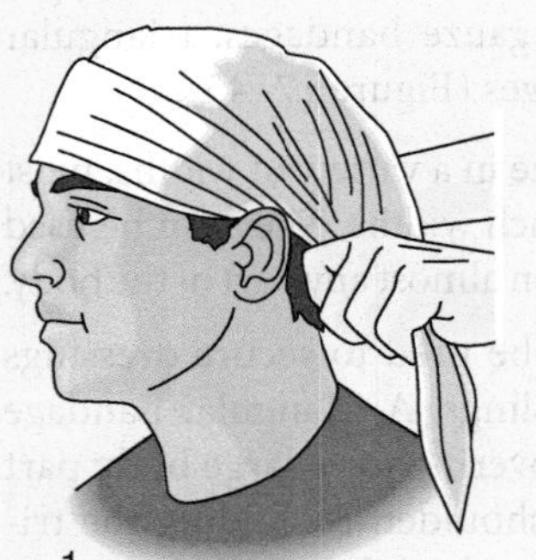

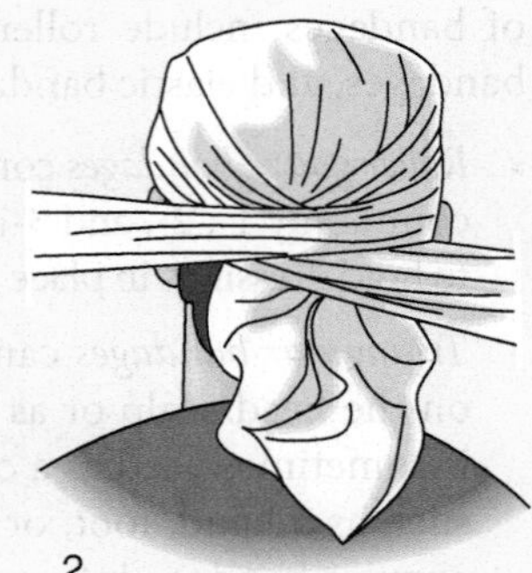

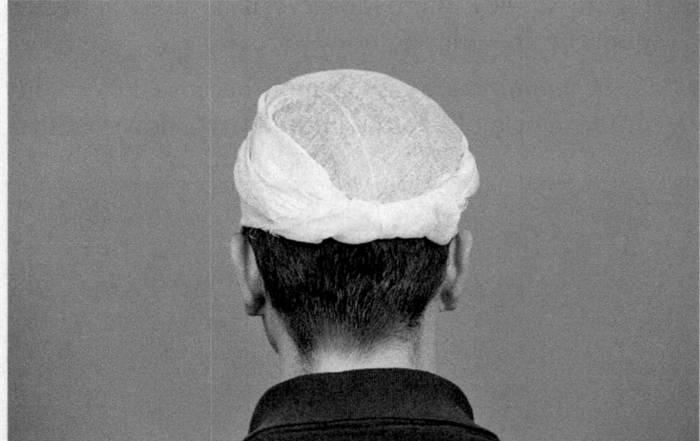

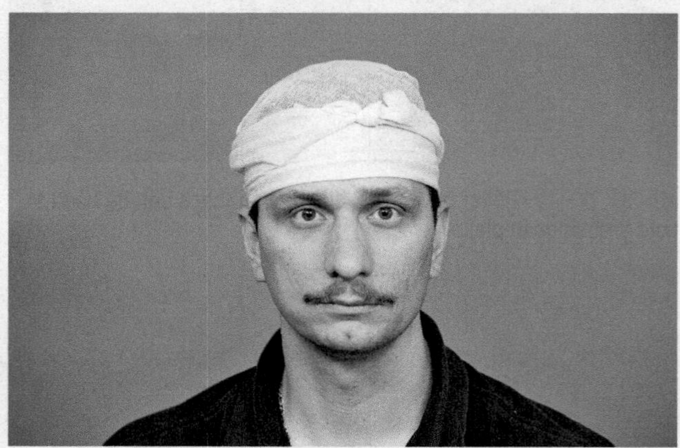

FIGURE 17–48 **Steps for applying a triangular bandage to the head or scalp.**

   c. Keeping the hem on the outside, position the middle of the base of the bandage on the forehead, just above the eyebrows.

PROCEDURE 17:12 (CONT.)

d. Bring the point of the bandage down over the back of the head.

e. Bring the two ends of the base of the bandage around the head and above the ears. Cross the ends when they meet at the back of the head. Bring them around to the forehead.

f. Use a square knot to tie the ends in the center of the forehead.

g. Use one hand to support the head. Use the other hand to gently but firmly pull down on the point of the bandage at the back of the head until the bandage is snug against the head.

h. Bring the point up and tuck it into the bandage where the bandage crosses at the back of the head.

5. Make a cravat bandage from a triangular bandage (review Figure 17–46):

a. Bring the point of the triangular bandage down to the middle of the base (the long end of the bandage).

b. Continue folding the bandage lengthwise until the desired width is obtained.

6. Apply a circular bandage with the cravat bandage (Figure 17–49):

a. Place a sterile dressing on the wound.

b. Place the center of the cravat bandage over the sterile dressing.

c. Bring the ends of the cravat around the body part and cross them when they meet.

d. Bring the ends back to the starting point.

e. Use a square knot to tie the ends of the cravat over the dressing.

Safety

CAUTION: Avoid tying or wrapping the bandage too tightly. This could impair circulation.

NOTE: Roller gauze bandage can also be used.

Safety

CAUTION: This type of wrap is *never* used around the neck because it could strangle the victim.

7. Apply a spiral wrap using roller gauze bandage or elastic bandage:

a. Place a sterile dressing over the wound.

b. Hold the roller gauze or elastic bandage so that the loose end is hanging off the bottom of the roll.

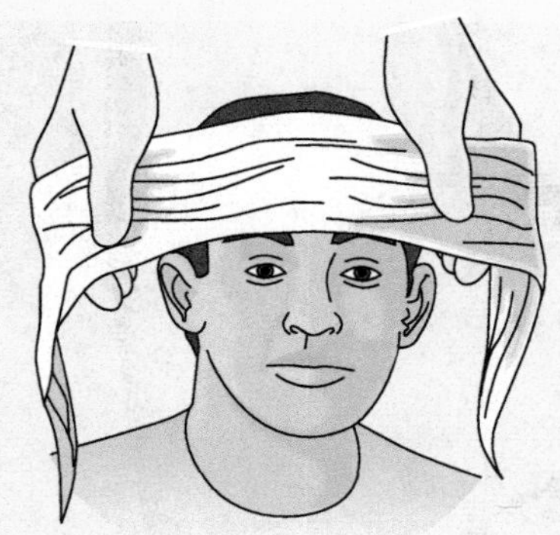

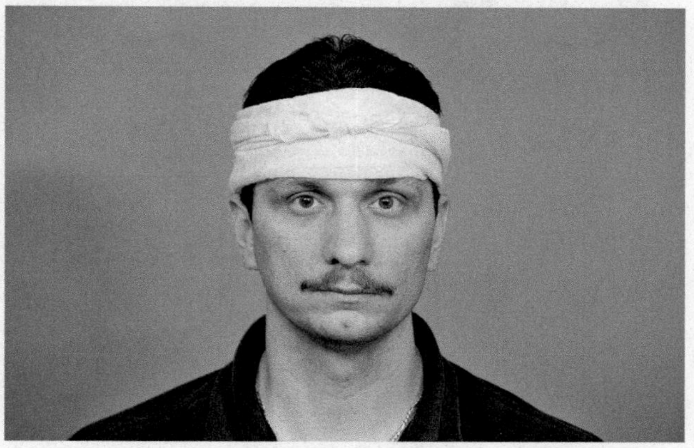

FIGURE 17–49 **Steps for applying a circular bandage with a cravat bandage.**

c. Start at the farthest end (the bottom of the limb) and move in an upward direction.

d. Anchor the bandage by placing it on an angle at the starting point. To do this, encircle the limb once, leaving a corner of the bandage uncovered. Turn down this free corner and then encircle the part again with the bandage (Figure 17–50A).

e. Continue encircling the limb. Use a spiral type motion to move up the limb. Overlap each new turn approximately half the width of the bandage.

f. Use one or two circular turns to finish the wrap at the end point.

g. Secure the end by taping, pinning, or tying. To avoid injury when pins are used, place your hand under the double layer of bandage and between the pin and the skin before inserting the pin (Figure 17–50B). The end of the bandage can also be cut in half and the two halves brought around opposite sides and tied into place.

(continues)

PROCEDURE 17:12 (CONT.)

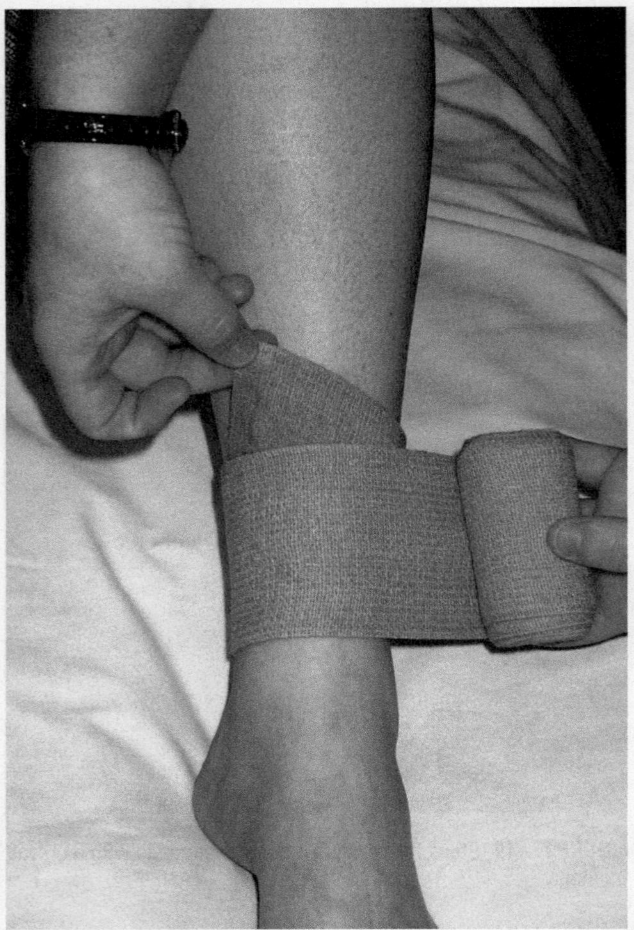

FIGURE 17–50A **Anchor the bandage by leaving a corner exposed. This corner is then folded down and covered when the bandage is circled around the limb.**

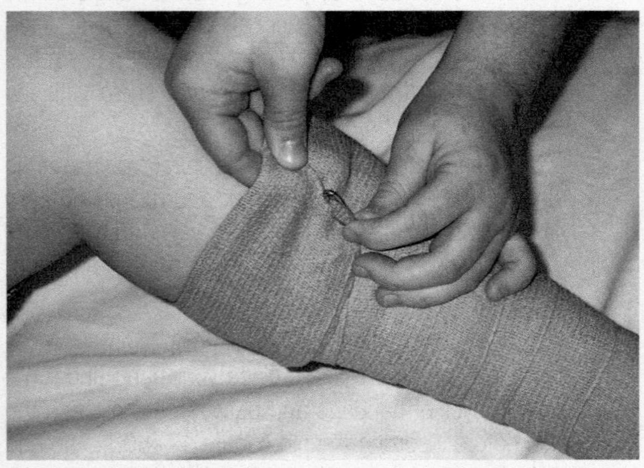

FIGURE 17–50B **Place your hand between the bandage and the victim's skin while inserting a pin.**

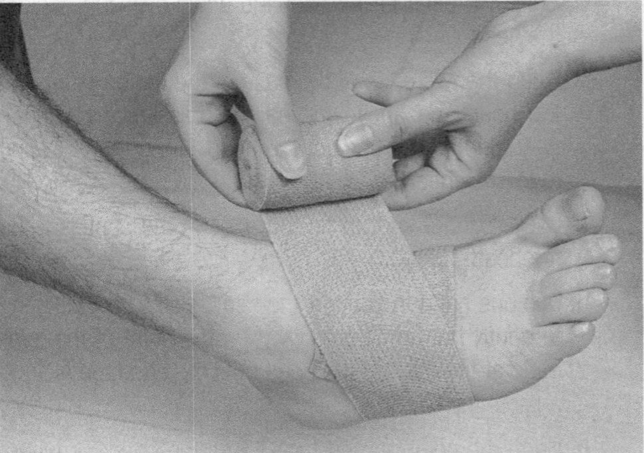

FIGURE 17–51A **Bring the bandage over the foot in a diagonal direction for the start of the figure-eight pattern.**

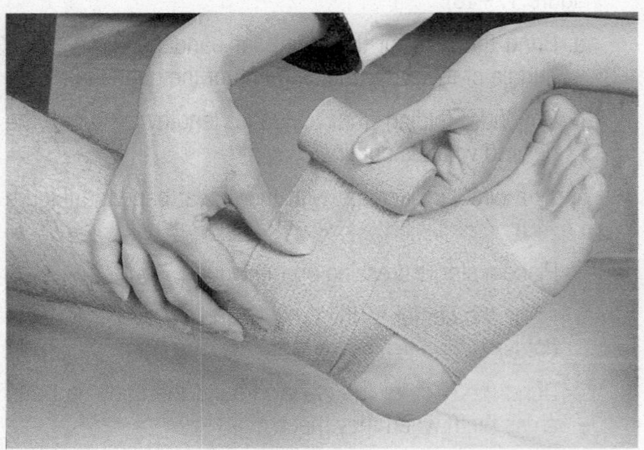

FIGURE 17–51B **Keep repeating the figure-eight pattern by moving downward and backward toward the heel with each turn.**

8. Use roller gauze bandage or elastic bandage to apply a figure-eight ankle wrap:

a. Position a dressing over the wound.

b. Anchor the bandage at the instep of the foot.

c. Make one or two circular turns around the instep and foot (Figure 17–51A).

d. Bring the bandage up over the foot in a diagonal direction. Bring it around the back of the ankle and then down over the top of the foot. Circle it under the instep. This creates the figure-eight pattern.

e. Repeat the figure-eight pattern. With each successive turn, move downward and backward toward the heel (Figure 17–51B). Overlap the previous turn by one-half to two-thirds the width of the bandage.

PROCEDURE 17:12 (CONT.)

NOTE: Hold the bandage firmly but do not pull it too tightly. If you are using elastic bandage, avoid stretching the material during the application.

f. Near completion, use one or two final circular wraps to circle the ankle.

g. Secure the bandage in place by taping, pinning, or tying the ends, as described in step 7g.

Safety

CAUTION: To avoid injury to the victim when pins are used, place your hand between the bandage and the victim's skin.

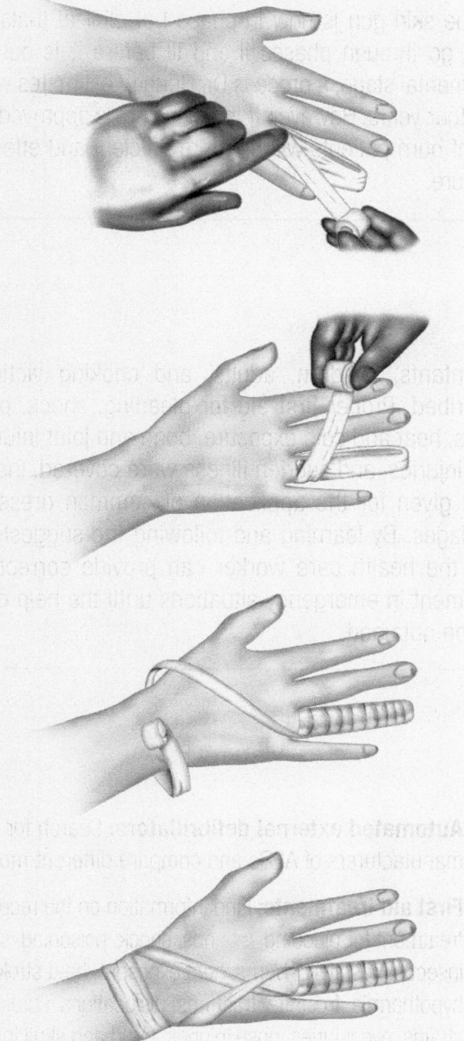

FIGURE 17–52 **Recurrent wrap for the finger.**

9. Use roller gauze bandage to apply a recurrent wrap to the fingers (Figure 17–52).

a. Place a sterile dressing over the wound.

b. Hold the roller gauze bandage so that the loose end is hanging off the bottom of the roll.

c. Place the end of the bandage on the bottom of the finger. Then bring the bandage up to the tip of the finger and down to the bottom of the opposite side of the finger. With overlapping wraps, fold the bandage backward and forward over the finger three or four times.

d. Start at the bottom of the finger and use a spiral wrap up and down the finger to hold the recurrent wraps in position.

e. Complete the bandage by using a figure-eight wrap around the wrist. Bring the bandage in a diagonal direction across the back of the hand. Circle the wrist at least two times. Bring the bandage back over the top of the hand and circle the bandaged finger. Repeat this figure-eight motion at least twice.

f. Secure the bandage by circling the wrist once or twice. Tie the bandage at the wrist.

10. After any bandage has been applied, check the circulation below the bandage at frequent intervals. If possible, check for a pulse at a site below the bandage. Note any signs of impaired circulation, including swelling, coldness, numbness or tingling, pallor or cyanosis, and poor return of pink color after nail beds are blanched by lightly pressing on them. If any signs of poor circulation are noted, loosen the bandages immediately.

11. Obtain medical help for any victim who may need additional care.

12. Remove gloves and wash hands.

PRACTICE: Go to the workbook and use the evaluation sheet for 17:12, Applying Dressings and Bandages, to practice this procedure. When you believe you have mastered this skill, sign the sheet and give it to your instructor for further action.

Check

FINAL CHECKPOINT: Using the criteria listed on the evaluation sheet, your instructor will grade your performance.

TODAY'S RESEARCH TOMORROW'S HEALTH CARE

A Skin Gun to Treat Burns?

Burns are a very common injury. Their intensity can range from a superficial burn, such as mild sunburn, to a partial-thickness burn that damages the top layers of skin, to a full-thickness burn that damages all layers of the skin and underlying tissue. Superficial burns usually heal by themselves in five to six days. For more severe burns, the major treatment is a skin graft, which involves taking skin from other parts of a patient's body or using sheets of artificial skin to cover the burn. The grafts can take weeks and even months to heal and are prone to infections. Frequently the grafted skin causes scars and disfigurement.

Now Dr. Jörg Gerlach and a team of researchers at the University of Pittsburgh's McGowan Institute for Regenerative Medicine have developed a skin gun that is similar to a paint spray gun or airbrush. The process begins with surgeons using a dermatome, a special knife that can remove a very thin layer of the patient's healthy skin. Skin stem cells are isolated from this layer of skin and put into a water solution for approximately 90 minutes. Then this mixture of cells and water is put into syringes and inserted into the nozzle of the gun. The gun is attached to a processor-controlled pneumatic (air) device that produces an even flow of solution. The skin cells are then sprayed directly onto the burn. The sprayed wound is covered with a specially created dressing that contains tubes connected to a source of nutrients and antibiotics that provide nourishment for the cells and help prevent infections. The entire process takes less than two hours for most patients. In clinical trials, the burns heal in just days instead of the weeks for skin grafts. In addition, there is less scarring of the tissue. At the present time, the skin gun can only be used on partial-thickness burns, but research continues to improve the method so it can be used to treat full-thickness burns.

The skin gun is now in phase I of clinical trials. It still has to go through phases II and III before it is out of the experimental stage, a process Dr. Gerlach estimates will take about four years. However, if the skin-gun is approved, treatment of burn patients will be more efficient and effective in the future.

CHAPTER 17 SUMMARY

First aid is defined as "the immediate care given to the victim of an injury or illness to minimize the effect of the injury or illness until experts can take over." Nearly everyone at some time experiences situations for which a proper knowledge of first aid is essential. It is important to follow correct techniques while administering first aid and to provide only the treatment you are qualified to provide.

The basic principles of first aid were presented in this unit. Methods of cardiopulmonary resuscitation (CPR) for infants, children, adults, and choking victims were described. Proper first aid for bleeding, shock, poisoning, burns, heat and cold exposure, bone and joint injuries, specific injuries, and sudden illness were covered. Instructions were given for the application of common dressings and bandages. By learning and following the suggested methods, the health care worker can provide correct first aid treatment in emergency situations until the help of experts can be obtained.

INTERNET SEARCHES

Use the search engines suggested in Chapter 12:9 in this text to search the Internet for additional information about the following topics:

1. **Organizations:** Find websites for the American Red Cross, the American Heart Association, Emergency Medical Services, and Poison Control Centers to learn services offered.
2. **CPR:** Look for sites that discuss the principles of cardiopulmonary resuscitation, abdominal thrusts, and cardiac emergencies.
3. **Automated external defibrillators:** Search for manufacturers of AEDs and compare different models.
4. **First aid treatments:** Find information on the recommended treatment for bleeding, wounds, shock, poisoning, snakebites, insect stings, ticks, burns, heat exposure, heat stroke, hypothermia, frostbite, fractures, dislocations, sprains, strains, eye injuries, nose injuries, head and skull injuries, spine injuries, chest injuries, abdominal injuries, myocardial infarction, cerebrovascular accident or stroke, fainting, convulsions or seizures, diabetic coma, and insulin shock.

REVIEW QUESTIONS

Review the following case histories. List the correct first aid care, in proper order of use, that should be used to treat each victim.

1. You are slicing carrots and cut off the end of your finger.
2. You find your 2-year-old brother in the bathroom. An empty bottle of aspirin tablets is on the floor. His mouth is covered with a white powdery residue.
3. You are watching television with your parents. Suddenly your father complains of severe pain in his chest and left arm. He is very short of breath and his lips appear cyanotic.
4. You are working in chemistry lab. Suddenly an experiment boils over and concentrated hydrochloric acid splashes into your lab partner's face and eyes. She starts screaming with pain.
5. You are driving and the car ahead of you loses control, goes off the road, and hits a tree. When you get to the car, the driver is slumped over the wheel. His arm is twisted at an odd angle. You notice a small fire at the rear of the car. In the back seat a small child in a car seat is crying.
6. You are playing tennis on a hot summer day with a friend. Suddenly your friend collapses on the tennis court. When you get to her, her skin is hot, red, and dry. She is breathing but she is unconscious.

For additional information on first aid and emergency care, write to:

- American Red Cross—contact your local chapter for First Aid and CPR courses and certification, or check the website at: *www.redcross.org*
- American Heart Association—contact your local chapter for CPR courses and certification or check the website at: *www.heart.org*
- Contact the National Highway Traffic Safety Administration, Office of Emergency Medical Services (NTI-140), 1200 New Jersey Avenue SE, Washington, DC 20590, or check the website at: *www.ems.gov*

CHAPTER 18

Basic Hospital Radiation Precautions

Basic Hospital Radiation Precautions

Introduction

Since the early 1900's, scientists have been aware of the beneficial as well as the destructive potential of ionizing radiation. By using the knowledge of radiation hazards that has been gained over the years and by employing effective methods to limit or eliminate those hazards, people can exercise greater control over the use of radiant energy. Various methods of radiation protection can be utilized to ensure additional safety for individuals employed in the radiation industries and the population at large.

Ionizing Radiation

It is the transfer of energy in matter caused by interaction of particles at the atomic level that produces positively and negatively charged particles called **ions**.

Incident electrons strike target, convert their tremendous kinetic energy to the atoms of the target material which in turn produces X-ray photons. The greater the mass or speed of the incident electron, the greater the quality and quantity of photons produced.

Radiation is measured in terms of Roentgen (Rem). There is 1000 millirem(millirad) in 1 Rem(rad). The average person in the United States receives about 360 millirems per year from natural sources. Health care professionals working in a hospital receive about 150 millirems more per year due to additional exposure to radiologic procedures. The National Council on Radiation Protection (NCRP) recommends that equivalent whole body limit of exposure of radiation workers to 5 Rems per year. For an ordinary individual, about one tenth or .5 Rems per year.

Sources of Ionizing Radiation

A. **Background or Natural**: Natural sources of ionizing radiation have always been a part of the environment. It has three components: **Terrestrial, cosmic and radionuclides**. Terrestrial sources pertain to the naturally occurring radioactive elements deposited in the earth such as uranium, radium and thorium. The quantity of terrestrial radiation present depends on the composition of the soil or rocks in the geographic area. By far, man's highest exposure to ionizing radiation from Terrestrial sources comes from **Radon Gas**, a heavy, colorless, odorless, tasteless gas that is a by-product of the decay of radium. Exposure to this radioactive gas is considered to be the largest contributor to human exposure to natural sources. It penetrates through the soil, walls and foundations of buildings but varies in concentration in a particular structure, from day to day and season to season. High indoor concentrations of radon gas have a potential for serious health conditions. When inhaled, this airborne, radioactive gas leaves alpha-emitting particles that remain in the lungs. As these products deteriorate, they give off radiation which can injure the lung tissue and subsequently increase the chances of developing lung cancer. In fact, it is considered to be the second leading cause of lung cancer in the United States, next to smoking. Accurate radon testing and appropriate structural repairs are essential to the reduction of lung cancer risks from radon. The rest of the terrestrial elements contribute about 8% of the background radiation. Cosmic rays are of extraterrestrial origin and are the result of nuclear interactions between the heavenly bodies particularly the sun and stars. The intensity of cosmic rays varies with altitude relative to the earth's surface. The greatest intensity occurs at higher altitudes and the lowest sea level. The average individual receives about 8% of the background radiation from cosmic rays including secondary cosmic sources such as alpha and gamma rays that accompany high energy electrons and protons. The human body contains naturally occurring radioactive nuclides such as Potassium-40, Hydrogen-3 and Strontium-90 that when an outside ray penetrates the tissues and bombard these elements, it generates positively and negatively charged particles such the term Radionuclide. About 11% of our exposure from background radiation is from these radionuclides.

B. **Man-made**: Ionizing radiation created or produced by humans for various uses are called man-made sources. It includes airport surveillance systems, television receivers, computer monitors, nuclear reactors, radioactive fallouts caused by nuclear explosions/detonations. Collectively, contributes to about 4% of human radiation exposure from commercial sources. In the earlier days of television and computer monitors, there was a substantial exposure to ionizing radiation when they were on but because of technological advances, it became almost negligible today. The advent of nuclear power generation of electricity lead to additional possibility of exposure, and when there is a nuclear accident like in Chernobyl and the Three Mile Island incidents, there was a great release of radioactive material in the atmosphere. This increases the unplanned amount of human and environment exposure to ionizing radiation. In the Medical/Dental fields, the greatest source of exposure to ionizing radiation comes from the use of X-ray machines and some Nuclear Medicine procedures. There has been an increase in the use of radiation in the healing arts. More and more health care providers are relying on radiologic diagnosis and treatment. Improving accuracy in radiologic diagnosis due to educational and technological advances make these usage inevitable. The increasing frequency of use of these equipment and procedures account for about 15% of our exposure from man-made sources.

Biological Effects of Ionizing Radiation

A. **Prompt**
Occur at high doses only (hundreds of Rems). Acute radiation sickness marked by burns, nausea, vomiting, extreme weakness, and death.

B. **Delayed**
Signs and symptoms occur many years after exposure, e.g. cancer induction.

C. **Genetic**
Abnormalities in the offspring like chromosomal changes.

D. **Prenatal**
The fetus is the most sensitive tissue in the body to ionizing radiation so exposure of the fetus or embryo during pregnancy can lead to abnormal head size, mental retardation, etc. It is therefore the main concern of health care providers to safeguard the fetus.

In the earlier years of using radiation in medicine, the "Ten-day Rule" was adopted as a safeguard to the unnecessary exposure of the fetus. It was based on the assumption that the probability of a woman of child-bearing age to be pregnant during the first "TEN" days of menstruation is almost negligible. Of course, this was repelled by the American Medical Association and therefore is no longer in existence but some of the practices under this rule are still being observed today, like the personal screening questions pertaining to pregnancy.

The question of whether to have therapeutic abortion due to ionizing radiation exposure of the fetus during pregnancy is answered by the National Council on Radiation Precaution with the statement "The risk is considered to be negligible at 5 Rems or less when compared to other risks of pregnancy, and the risk of malformations is significantly increased above control levels of 15 Rems, therefore, the decision to perform an abortion should not only be based on exposure as the sole reason for termination of pregnancy". Most medical procedures would result in fetal exposures of less than 1 Rem so the risk of abnormality is very small. It is the position of the American College of Radiology that "abdominal radiological examinations requested after full consideration of the clinical status of the patient including the possibility of pregnancy, need not be postponed or selectively scheduled". In other words, if the physician decides that the benefits of taking x-ray outweighs the risks to the fetus, the procedure should not be postponed. However, special efforts should be made to minimize the dose of radiation received by the patient's lower abdomen and pelvic region.

Radiation Precautions to minimize unnecessary exposure

1. Distance: It is the most effective means of protection from ionizing radiation. Personnel receive less exposure if they keep as much distance between them and the source. This is due to the inverse square law of distance which states that the intensity of radiation is inversely proportional to the square of the distance.
2. Time: The shorter time spent near the source of radiation, the smaller the received dose.
3. Shielding: Anyone around a source of ionizing radiation should be protected some kind of barrier. If no fixed barrier exists, appropriate protective devices such as lead aprons, gloves, vests should be worn. Protective eyeglasses, neck and thyroid shield should be considered.

4. Cleanliness: It includes good personal hygiene. It is imperative to have a clean and orderly environment in and around a source of radiation so as to minimize possible contamination as in the area of nuclear medicine that uses radioactive particles in procedures like teletherapy, brachiotherapy and Iodine therapy.

Above measures are to maintain exposures to ionizing radiation to as low as reasonably achievable (ALARA)

Conclusion

When ionizing radiation penetrates body tissues, it produces damage in the body primarily by ionizing at the atomic level, then in turn produce changes at the molecular level, which in turn cause cellular damage that may cause abnormal or loss of cell function. Humans are unable to control natural or background radiation exposures therefore, in order to minimize unnecessary exposures, we have to employ our efforts in trying to control radiation coming from man made sources.

CHAPTER 19

Venipuncture

Venipuncture

Venipuncture means the collection of blood by puncturing the vein. It is sometimes referred to as phlebotomy. Blood is the most common specimen obtained for laboratory analysis. The accuracy of result of the tests done on this blood specimen is greatly affected by the proper collecting technique to include the appropriate color of tubes used. Venipuncture is the most commonly used procedure to obtain that blood. The main goal of a phlebotomist is **patient safety and collection of quality sample.**

The most commonly used venipuncture system is the **evacuated tube system**. As a general rule of thumb, the most commonly used part of the body that blood is drawn from is the arm. The most commonly used part of the arm is the **antecubital space**. The most commonly used vein in this fossa is the **median cubital** because it is usually better anchored than the cephalic or basilic veins. The size of needle used depends on the size of the vein selected. The most commonly used is a 21 gauge, one and one half inch long needle that may or may not have a rubber sheath on the end of the short needle to prevent blood spillage when collecting more than one tube. The gauge, size, bore of the needle refers to the **inside diameter** of the needle, the higher the number, the smaller the bore. The most commonly used antiseptic is 70 percent isopropyl alcohol.

1. **Complications of Venipuncture:** Complications in performing venipuncture is not uncommon. Regardless of how it is done, there is always a possibility of occurrence. However, when done properly, complications can be minimized. Some common complications are:
    a. <u>Hyperventilation</u> – Increased anxiety speeds up breathing or respirations. Too fast of a respiration can produce tingling, numbness sensations. There is way no way to predict how each individual will react to the procedure, so it is best to always reassure patient and encourage them to relax. A phlebotomist should act calm and professional.
    b. <u>Fainting</u> – In some individuals, venipuncture procedure may provoke a psychogenic reaction that may cause them to faint. Always ask them if they have this problem in the past. If so, lay them down or in a low Fowler's position before proceeding.
    c. <u>Phlebitis</u> – Inflammation of the vein that may be caused by unnecessary trauma when trying to penetrate the vein. May include redness, pain and swelling at he puncture site or along the length of the vein. It is commonly caused by "fishing" for the vein. If first attempt to draw the blood fails, do not "dig around". Instead, withdraw the needle slowly. If no blood return, properly discontinue procedure and restart on another appropriate site with all new equipment and supplies.
    d. <u>Hematoma</u> – The collection of blood underneath the body tissue. The common cause is withdrawing the needle before the tourniquet is removed. Another cause is not applying pressure to the puncture site after the needle is withdrawn, long enough for the blood to clot. Another

common mistake is bending the elbow after the withdrawal of the needle. Extending the elbow after it has been kept bent for a short period of time may dislodge a formed clot at the puncture site and resulting in subcutaneous bleeding.

e. Infection – It is caused by introduction of bacteria into the puncture site. Surface of the skin contain some bacteria and if the site is not properly prepped with antiseptic swab, the bacteria may be introduced with the penetration of the needle. The puncture site should be wiped with an antiseptic like alcohol pad, starting from the center of the intended puncture site and circling outward, never touching the site again. If it is necessary to re-palpate the vein in the area, re-wipe the site again before proceeding.

2. Universal Precautions

The basic premise of universal precautions is that all body fluids including blood and blood products should be considered infectious and as such, health care providers potentially exposed to these fluids must take extra precautions by wearing personal protective equipment like gloves, gowns, shields as appropriate. Use extreme caution when disposing contaminated material particularly used needles. **Do not cut, bend or recap used needles**. Dispose of needles in the Sharps container.

If accidental needle stick occur, follow steps outlined by the institution and notify supervisor as soon as possible.

3. Preparation for Venipuncture

a. Obtain doctor's order. It specifies parameters, type of laboratory testing to be done which determines what type of tube to be used, and how much specimen is to be obtained.
b. Obtain necessary equipment and supplies. Needles, alcohol pads, gauze, tourniquet, band aid, vacutainer or needle holder, appropriate number and color of tubes.
c. Identification of the patient. A lot of emphasis is placed on properly performing venipuncture and too little attention is given to the importance of properly identifying the patient. Patient identification is crucial in insuring that the blood obtained is from the correct patient. The phlebotomist must identify the patient by asking their name and comparing it to the request form, or by checking ID bands. Any discrepancy should be clarified first before drawing blood specimen.
d. Reassuring the patient. The venipuncturist needs to gain the patient's confidence by a calm and professional attitude, always inform the patient of the procedure. Honestly answer any questions or concerns of the patient. Patients should never be told "this won't hurt" especially children.

e. Positioning the patient. Before starting the procedure, both the phlebotomist and the patient should be in a comfortable position, i.e. the patient sitting or lying down and the phlebotomist standing up. A comfortable position enables the venipuncturist to find the vein easily. Adequate lighting is important so that veins may be readily palpated, visualized and evaluated. Never try to draw blood on patients that are standing. They could faint and hurt themselves which could lead to lawsuits.

4. Performing Venipuncture

a. Wash your hands
b. Assemble all needed equipment. Open any packet that needs to be open.
c. Locate the appropriate vein. When locating the best vein for venipuncture, consider whether it is going to be short term or long term use. If the sole purpose is for routine venipuncture, the antecubital fossa is the best place to locate the appropriate vein. Median cubital vein is the most commonly used for venipuncture. If the needle or catheter is meant to remain in place for an extended period of time, avoid this area because it is difficult to maintain patency when the patient's arm is bent. The vein should feel spongy with resiliency, not hard or chord like. Examine the direction of the chosen vein to find out if it is tortuous. Avoid veins that are tortuous or non-resilient. Do not use veins that lay on arteries, bifurcating veins, repeatedly used veins, thin and superficial veins, veins in extremities that are paralyzed by stroke, veins compromised by surgery, veins in the areas of rash, scarring, bruises, cuts or infection. May apply the tourniquet about 3-4 inches superior to the intended puncture site but do not leave it on for longer than a minute. The tourniquet should only be tight enough to occlude venous blood flow and not arterial blood flow. If the patient's arm turns pale or ashy and patient complains of pain, it is too tight. Remove tourniquet and reapply properly.
d. Verify location of the vein and cleanse site. Cleanse intended puncture site with isopropyl alcohol or betadine swab in a circular outward motion starting from the center. Do not touch area again until needle is ready to enter the skin.
e. Put on gloves. Make sure they are the right size for you. Use latex gloves if not allergic to latex.
f. Puncture the vein. With the bevel of the needle facing up, enter the vein at about 15-30 degree angle quickly but smoothly until you feel a "give" or a "pop" through the vein. Deep veins require a steeper angle of entry. There is no need to push all the length of the needle. The needle should only puncture the upper wall of the vein.
g. Insert the proper tube in the needle holder. Minimize unnecessary movements by not exchanging hands to push the tube into the needle. The hand holding the needle should stay steady and firm. Blood should enter the tube and stops when vacuum is exhausted.

h. Release the tourniquet. Pull the looped end of the tourniquet to release it without jerking the arm. Disengage the tube from the needle. With a quick and smooth motion, withdraw the needle at the same angle that it was inserted. Do not apply pressure to site while withdrawing the needle. Wait until the needle is fully out before applying direct pressure to the puncture site.
i. Care for the puncture site. Apply pressure to puncture site for 3-5 minutes to ensure blood clot formation to the site. Do not allow the patient to bend elbow for about 3-5 minutes, instead, have patient elevate arm while applying pressure to the site. Apply band aid as necessary.
j. Properly label collected blood specimen. While the patient is holding pressure to the puncture site, properly label the specimen from the requisition form and according to institution policy.
k. Evaluate and release the patient. Insure all information is verified and that the patient safe and is well enough to be released.
l. Clean up. Properly discard used supplies to trash receptacle. Be extra cautious when handling used needles. Discard needles without recapping into the sharp's container.

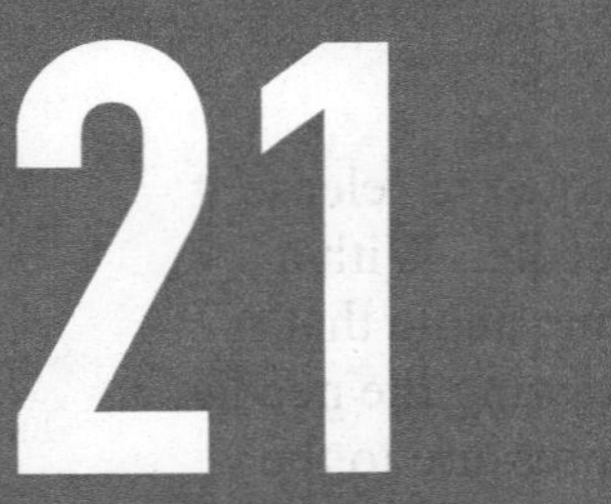
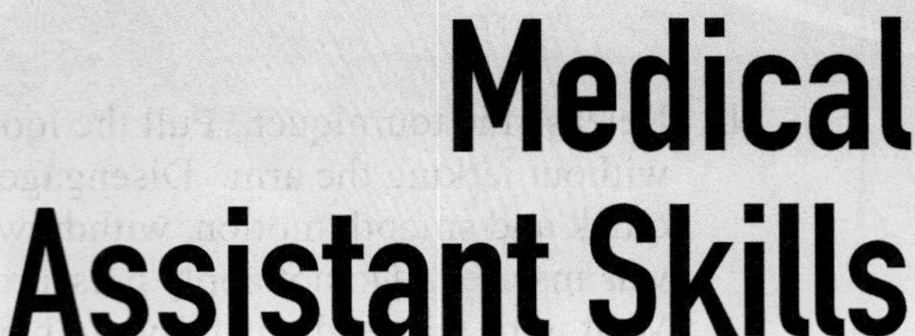
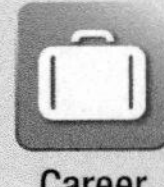

21 Medical Assistant Skills

CHAPTER OBJECTIVES

After completing this chapter, you should be able to:

- Measure and record height and weight.
- Position and properly drape a patient in horizontal recumbent, prone, Sims', knee–chest, Fowler's, lithotomy, dorsal recumbent, Trendelenburg, and jackknife positions.
- Use a Snellen chart to screen for vision problems.
- Prepare for and assist with an eye, ear, nose, and throat examination.
- Prepare for and assist with a gynecological examination.
- Prepare for and assist with a general physical examination.
- Set up a minor surgery tray without contaminating equipment or supplies.
- Set up a suture removal tray without contaminating equipment or supplies.
- Record and mount an electrocardiogram.
- Use the *Physicians' Desk Reference* (PDR) to find basic information about various drugs.
- Identify methods of administering medications and safety rules that must be observed.
- Define, pronounce, and spell all key terms.

KEY TERMS

auscultation *(oss"-kull-tay'-shun)*
Ayer blade *(a'-ur)(A as in "say")*
bandage scissors
cervical spatula
dorsal recumbent
electrocardiogram (ECG) *(ee-leck"-trow-car'-dee-oh-gram)*
Fowler's
hemostats *(hee'-mow"-stats)*
horizontal recumbent
hyperopia *(high"-puh-row'-pee-ah)*
jackknife (protologic)
knee–chest
laryngeal mirror *(lar"-ren-gee'-ul)*
leads
left lateral
lithotomy *(lith"-ought'-eh-me)*
medication
myopia *(my"-oh'-pee-ah)*
needle holder
observation
ophthalmoscope *(op-thayl'-mow-skope")*
otoscope *(oh'-toe-skope")*
palpation
Papanicolaou *(pah"-pan-ee'-cow-low)*
percussion

KEY TERMS (CONT.)

percussion (reflex) hammer
Physicians' Desk Reference (PDR)
prone
retractors
scalpels *(skal' -pelz)*
sigmoidoscope *(sig-moy' -doh-skope")*
Sims'
Snellen charts
speculum *(speck' -you-lum)*
sphygmomanometer
splinter forceps
stethoscope
supine *(sue-pine')*
surgical scissors
suture removal sets
sutures
tissue forceps
tongue blade/depressor
towel clamps
Trendelenburg *(Tren' -dell-en" -burg)*
tuning fork
visual acuity

career highlights

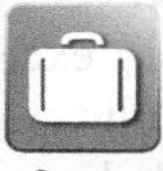

Medical assistants work under the supervision of physicians, and they are important members of the health care team. Educational requirements vary from state to state but can include on-the-job training (less frequent), 1- or 2-year health science education (HSE) programs, and/or an associate's degree. Certification can be obtained from the American Association of Medical Assistants (AAMA), and registered credentials can be obtained from the American Medical Technologists (AMT) Association, each of which has specific requirements. The duties of medical assistants vary depending on the size and type of practice, and on the legal requirements of the state in which they work. Duties are often classified as administrative or clinical. Administrative, or "front office," duties may include tasks such as answering telephones, greeting patients, scheduling appointments, maintaining records, handling correspondence, and bookkeeping. These duties are usually performed by medical administrative assistants who can obtain certification. Clinical, or "back office," duties may include taking medical histories, recording vital signs, preparing patients for and assisting with examinations and treatments, and performing basic laboratory tests. Some medical assistants perform both administrative and clinical duties; others specialize in either administrative or clinical work. The procedures discussed in this chapter represent clinical duties. Administrative duties are discussed in Chapter 24 of this textbook. In addition to the knowledge and skills presented in this chapter, medical assistants must also learn and master skills such as:

- Presenting a professional appearance and attitude
- Obtaining knowledge regarding health care delivery systems, organizational structure, and teamwork
- Meeting all legal responsibilities
- Communicating effectively
- Being sensitive to and respecting cultural diversity
- Comprehending human anatomy, physiology, and pathophysiology
- Learning medical terminology
- Observing all safety precautions
- Practicing all principles of infection control
- Taking and recording vital signs
- Performing CLIA-waived laboratory tests
- Administering first aid and cardiopulmonary resuscitation
- Promoting good nutrition and a healthy lifestyle to maintain health
- Using computer and technology skills
- Performing administrative duties such as answering the telephone, scheduling appointments, preparing correspondence, completing insurance forms, maintaining accounts, recording medical histories, and maintaining patient records
- Ordering and maintaining supplies and materials

LEGAL ALERT

Legal

Before performing any procedures in this chapter, know and follow the standards and regulations established by the scope of practice; federal laws and agencies; state laws; state or national licensing, registration, or certification boards; professional organizations; professional standards; and agency policies.

It is your responsibility to learn exactly what you are legally permitted to do and to perform only procedures for which you have been trained.

21:1 Measuring/Recording Height and Weight

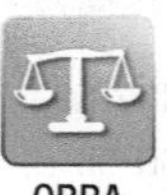
OBRA

Height and weight measurements are taken in many health care fields. Height and weight measurements are used to determine whether a patient is overweight or underweight. Either of these conditions can indicate disease. Height–weight charts are used as averages. A 10-percent deviation is usually considered normal. Height–weight measurements must be accurate. Always recheck your calculations.

Height–weight measurements are a part of the general physical examination in a physician's office. They are also usually done routinely when a patient is admitted to a hospital, long-term care facility, or other health care agency. In addition, the measurements provide necessary information in performing and evaluating certain laboratory tests and in calculating dosages of certain medications.

The height, weight, head circumference, and, at times, chest circumference measurements of infants and toddlers is monitored frequently because growth is rapid. Usually infants are checked every two months to detect any changes that may indicate problems with growth and development. The measurements are usually recorded on a National Center for Health Statistics (NCHS) growth graph (Figure 21–1). The graphed information allows the physician to check the child's growth and compare it to the average percentiles of other children the same age. Abnormal growth patterns may indicate nutritional deficiencies or genetic diseases.

The head circumference in infants can be an early indication of abnormal development of the brain. Any head circumference that measures above the 95th percentile usually indicates *hydrocephalus*, an accumulation of fluid around the brain. This leads to increased intracranial pressure and brain damage. Hydrocephalus can be caused by abnormal development of the ventricles in the brain, bacterial meningitis, and/or tumors. A below-normal value for head circumference can be an indication of *microencephaly*, or a small brain. This too can lead to mental retardation. Microencephaly can be caused by a congenital defect, infections during pregnancy, a premature closure of the fontanels in the brain, drug or alcohol abuse during pregnancy (fetal alcohol syndrome), and genetic defects.

Chest circumference is also measured in infants, especially if suspicion exists of overdevelopment or underdevelopment of the heart and/or lungs or a calcification of the rib cartilage. From birth to 1 year of age the head circumference is usually greater than the chest circumference. At about 1–2 years, the head and chest circumferences are equal. After that, the chest circumference is larger than the head circumference. Chest circumferences may also be measured in adults with chronic obstructive pulmonary diseases (COPDs) such as emphysema to determine the progression of the disease.

Frequent weight measurements to monitor excessive weight loss or gain are also done for adults with hormone disorders such as diabetes, thyroid disease, digestive disorders, and hypertension (high blood pressure) with fluid retention. Patients with cancer or patients receiving chemotherapy are weighed frequently to monitor weight loss. Daily weights are often ordered for patients with edema (swelling) due to heart, kidney, or other diseases. When taking daily weights, note the following points:

- Use the same scale each day.
- Make sure the scale is balanced before weighing the patient.
- Weigh the patient at the same time each day.
- If possible, weigh the patient early in the morning before any food or liquids have been consumed.
- Make sure the patient is wearing the same amount of clothing each day.
- Ask the patient to void to empty the bladder.

Height measurements are performed more frequently in older adults to check for *osteoporosis*, a degeneration of the spinal column caused by a deterioration of cartilage and bone. As the intervertebral disks between the vertebrae deteriorate, the individual will become shorter.

Safety

Careful consideration must be given to the safety of the patient while weight and height are being measured. Observe the patient closely at all times. Prevent falls from the scale and possible injury from the protruding height lever.

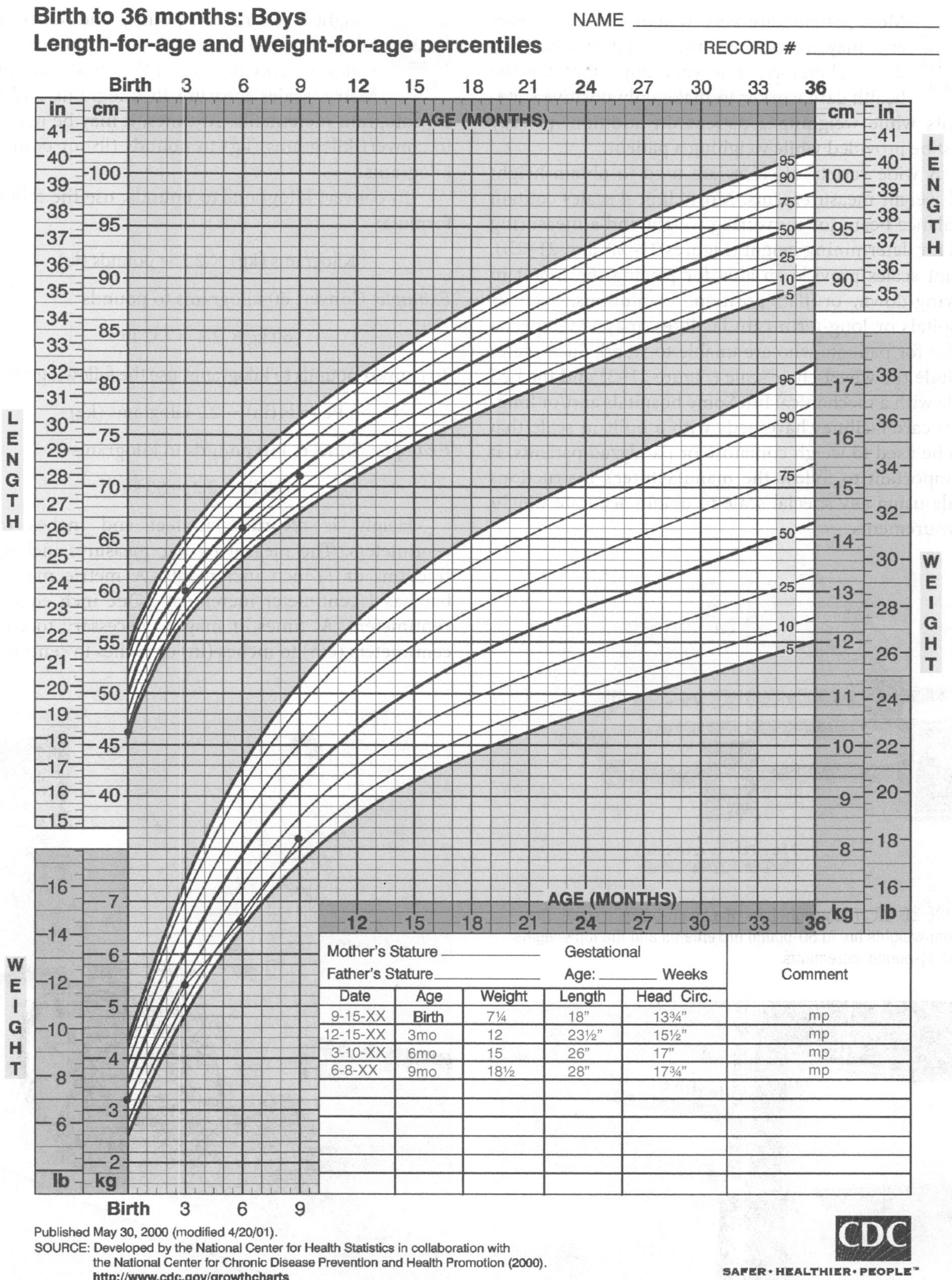

Date	Age	Weight	Length	Head Circ.	Comment
9-15-XX	Birth	7¼	18"	13¾"	mp
12-15-XX	3mo	12	23½"	15½"	mp
3-10-XX	6mo	15	26"	17"	mp
6-8-XX	9mo	18½	28"	17¾"	mp

FIGURE 21–1 The National Center for Health Statistics (NCHS) growth graph is used to monitor the growth and development of infants and toddlers. Source: Kuczmarski RJ, Ogden CL, Guo SS, et al. 2000 CDC growth charts for the United States: Methods and development. National Center for Health Statistics. Vital Health Stat 11(246), 2002.

Comm

Most patients are very weight conscious. Parents may worry about the weight of their children. Therefore, it is very important for the health care worker to make only positive statements while weighing a patient. In addition, privacy must be provided while weighing a patient.

A wide variety of scales are used to obtain height and weight measurements. Most clinical scales contain a balance beam for measuring weight and a measuring rod for determining height (Figures 21–2A and 21–2B). Infant scales provide an area for placing the infant in a lying-down, or flat, position. Institutions, such as hospitals or long-term care facilities, may have special scales for patients who are unable to stand. Such scales include the wheel-chair scale (Figure 21–3) and the bed scale with a mechanical lift. Some hospitals and/or long-term care facilities have beds with a built-in scale that can be used to weigh comatose or paralyzed patients. It is important to follow the manufacturer's instructions while using any special scale to obtain accurate weight measurements.

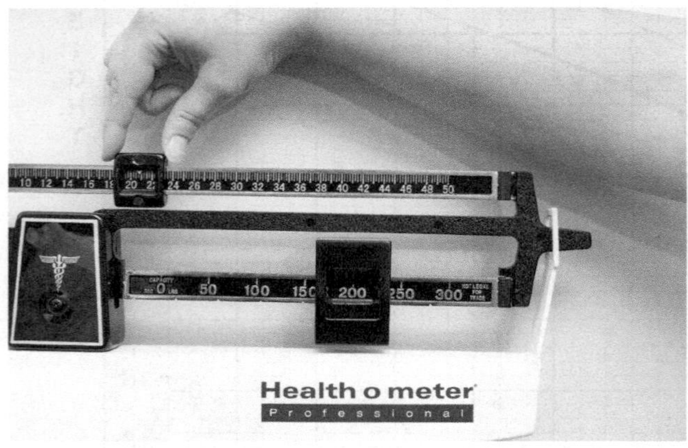

FIGURE 21–2A The weight bars of a beam-balance scale. The bottom weights are in 50-pound increments and the top weights are in ¼-pound increments.

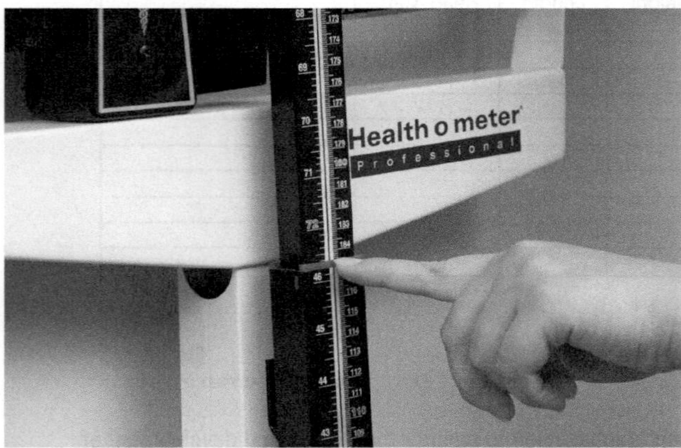

FIGURE 21–2B The height bar of a beam-balance scale. The height is read at the break point on the movable bar.

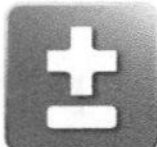
Math

Weight is recorded as pounds and ounces or as kilograms (1.0 kilogram = 2.2 pounds). Most scales measure pounds in ¼-pound increments. Metric scales measure in kilograms and have 0.1-kilogram increments. At times, it may be necessary to convert kilograms (kg) to pounds (lb) or pounds to kilograms.

To convert kilograms to pounds, use the following formula:

$$\text{Kilograms (kg)} \times 2.2 = \text{pounds (lb)}$$

Example: Convert 60 kilograms to pounds

$$60 \text{ kg} \times 2.2 = 132 \text{ lb}$$

To convert pounds to kilograms, use the following formula:

$$\text{Pounds (lb)} \div 2.2 \text{ kilograms (kg)}$$

Example: Convert 110 pounds to kilograms

$$110 \text{ lb} \div 2.2 = 50 \text{ kg}$$

Height is recorded as feet and inches or as centimeters. The measuring bar measures inches and fractions or ¼-inch increments. A metric measuring bar has 1-centimeter increments. One inch equals 2.5 centimeters. At times, it may be necessary to convert centimeters (cm) to inches (in) or inches to centimeters.

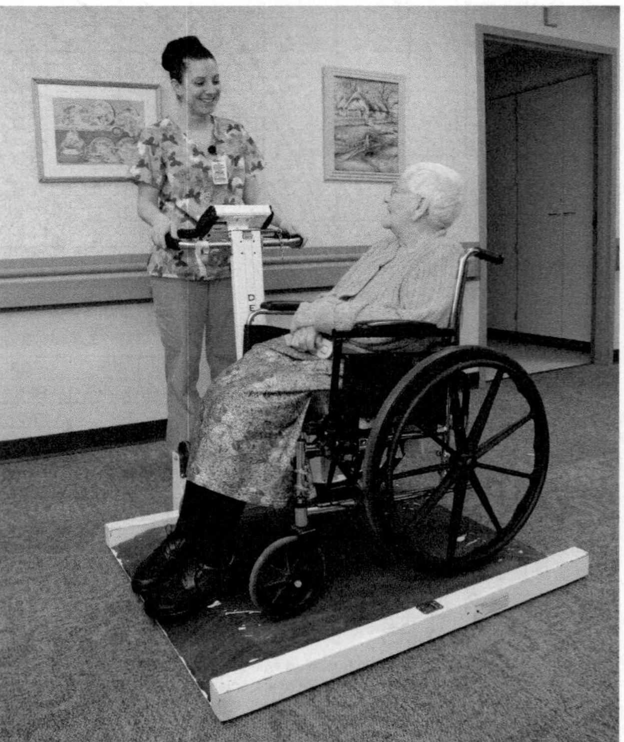

FIGURE 21–3 A wheelchair scale is a convenient scale for weighing a patient who may have difficulty standing on a beam-balance scale.

To convert centimeters to inches, use the following formula:

Centimeters (cm) ÷ 2.5 = inches (in)

Example: Convert 95 centimeters to inches

95 cm ÷ 2.5 = 38 in

To convert inches to centimeters, use the following formula:

Inches (in) × 2.5 = centimeters (cm)

Example: Convert 24 inches to centimeters

24 in × 2.5 = 60 cm

STUDENT: **Go to the workbook and complete the assignment sheet for 21:1, Measuring/Recording Height and Weight. Then return and continue with the procedures.**

PROCEDURE 21:1A

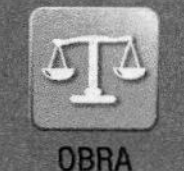

Measuring/Recording Height and Weight

Equipment and Supplies

Balance scale, paper towel, paper, pen and/or computer

Procedure

1. Assemble equipment.
2. Wash hands.
3. Prepare the scale. Place a paper towel on the foot stand of the scale (Figure 21–4A). Move both weights to the *zero* position. If the end of the balance bar swings freely, the scale is balanced. If the scale is *not* balanced, follow the manufacturer's instructions to balance the scale.

   NOTE: Most scales have a small screw by the end of the balance bar. By adjusting the screw, the scale can be balanced.

   NOTE: The paper towel prevents spread of disease.
4. 

   Introduce yourself. Identify the patient. Explain the procedure. Remember to make only positive statements.
5. Ask the patient to remove shoes, jackets, heavy outer clothing, purses, and heavy objects that may be in the pockets of clothing.

   NOTE: In a hospital or long-term care facility, the patient is usually weighed in a gown or in pajamas.
6. Assist the patient onto the scale (Figure 21–4B). The patient should stand unassisted, with his or her feet centered on the platform and slightly apart.

   CAUTION: Watch closely at all times to prevent falls.

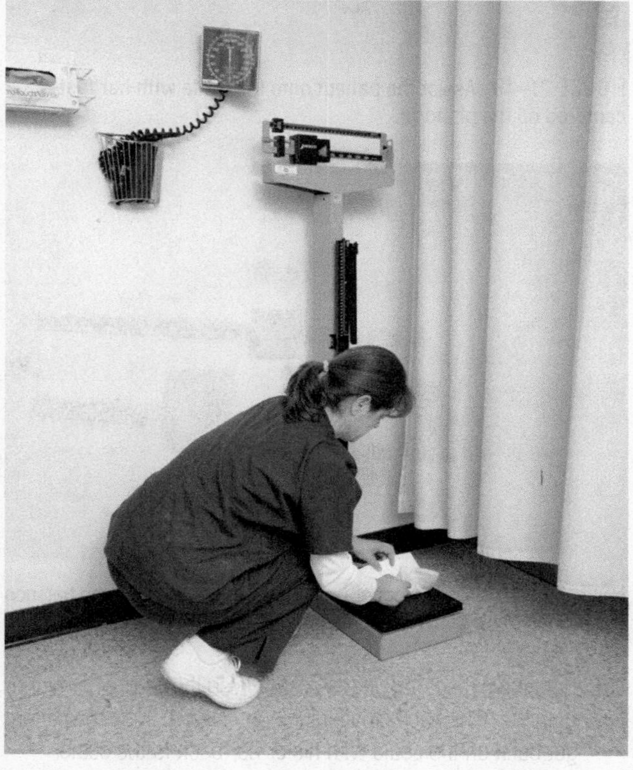

FIGURE 21–4A **Place a paper towel on the foot stand of the scale.**

7. 

   Move the large 50-pound weight to the right until the balance bar drops down on the lower guide. Then move this weight back one notch. Move the smaller ¼-pound weight until the balance bar swings freely halfway between the upper and lower guides (Figure 21–4C). Add the two weights together to determine the patient's correct weight. Recheck your reading. Record the weight correctly.

   Check **CHECKPOINT:** Your instructor will check your reading for accuracy.

(continues)

PROCEDURE 21:1A (CONT.)

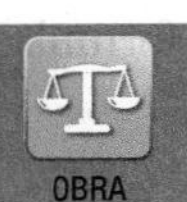

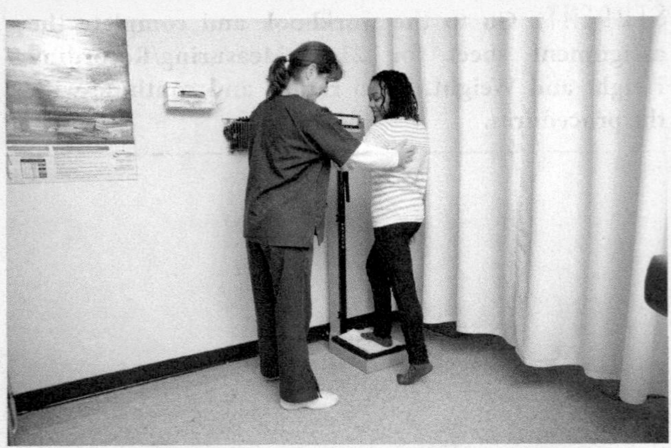

FIGURE 21–4B **Assist the patient onto the scale with her feet centered on the platform.**

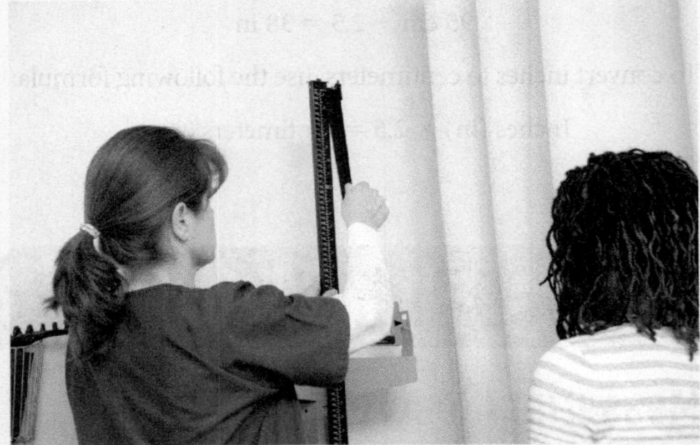

FIGURE 21–5A **Raise the height bar of the scale higher than the height of the patient.**

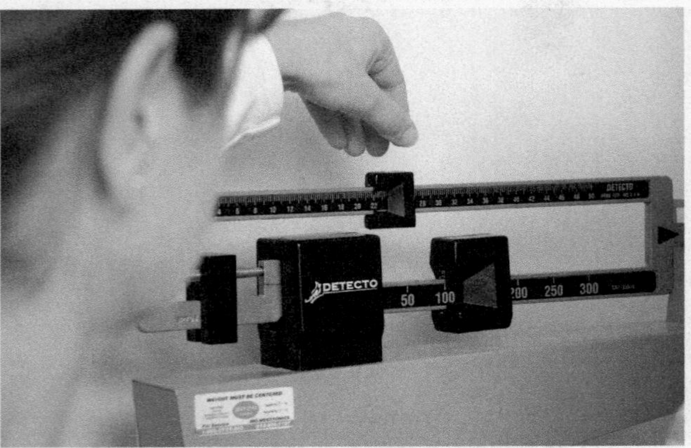

FIGURE 21–4C **Move the upper or smaller weight bar until the balance bar swings freely halfway between the upper and lower guides.**

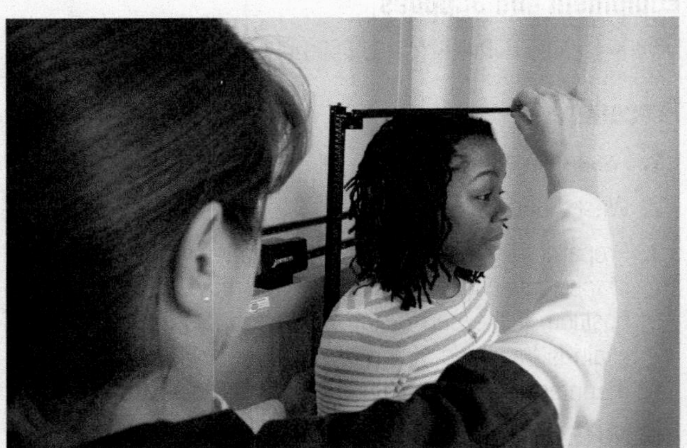

FIGURE 21–5B **Move the bar of the measuring scale down until it just touches the top of the patient's head.**

8. Help the patient get off the scale. Raise the height bar higher than the height of the patient (Figure 21–5A). Help the patient get back on the scale with his or her back to the scale.

Safety

CAUTION: Watch closely at all times to prevent falls.

9. Instruct the patient to stand as erect as possible. Ask the patient to look straight ahead to keep the head level.

10. Move the bar of the measuring scale down until it just touches the top of the patient's head (Figure 21–5B).

Safety

CAUTION: Move slowly. Do *not* hit the patient with the bar.

11. Read the measurement in inches or centimeters. Recheck your reading. Record the height correctly.

NOTE: If the height is difficult to read, assist the patient off the scale without moving the height bar. Then read the correct height measurement.

NOTE: If the reading is in inches, it can be converted to feet and inches after the patient is off the scale.

NOTE: If the height bar is extended above the break point of the movable bar, remember to read the height at the point of the break by reading in a downward direction on the upper bar (Figure 21–5C).

Check

CHECKPOINT: Your instructor will check your reading for accuracy.

12. Elevate the height bar.

13. Help the patient get off the scale.

Safety

CAUTION: Watch the patient closely to prevent fails.

14. Replace all equipment. Throw the paper towel in a waste can.

PROCEDURE 21:1A (CONT.)

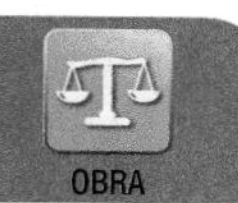

OBRA

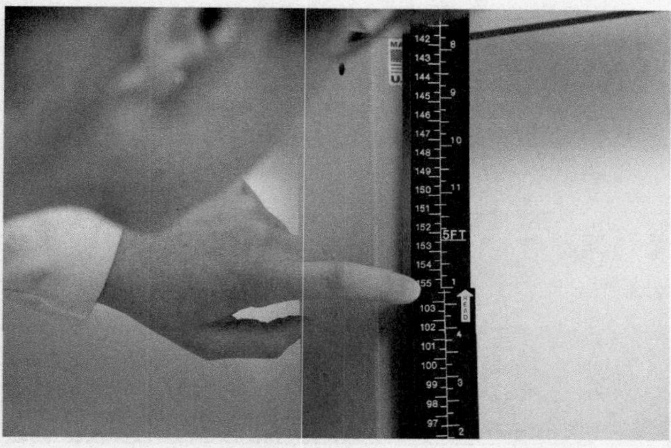

FIGURE 21–5C **Read the height at the point of the break by reading in a downward direction on the upper bar.**

15. Return both weight beams to the zero positions. Lower the measurement bar.
16. Math — Convert the inches to feet and inches by dividing by 12. For example, 64½ inches divided by 12 equals 5 feet, 4½ inches.

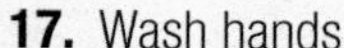

17. Wash hands.

18. Comm — Record all required information on the patient's chart or enter it into the computer. For example: date, time, Wt: 132½ lb, Ht: 5 ft, 4¼ in, and your signature and title.

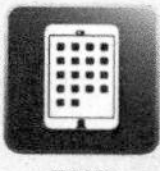

EHR — **NOTE:** In offices with electronic health records (EHRs), also called electronic medical records (EMRs), information is entered directly into the patient's record on a computer.

PRACTICE: **Go to the workbook and use the evaluation sheet for 21:1A, Measuring/Recording Height and Weight, to practice this procedure. When you believe you have mastered this skill, sign the sheet and give it to your instructor for further action.**

Check — **FINAL CHECKPOINT:** Using the criteria listed on the evaluation sheet, your instructor will grade your performance.

PROCEDURE 21:1B

Measuring/Recording Height and Weight of an Infant

Equipment and Supplies

Infant scale, towel or scale paper, tape measure, growth graph, patient's chart or paper, pen and/or computer

Procedure

1. Assemble equipment.
2. Wash hands.
3. Prepare the scale. Place a towel or scale paper on the scale to protect the infant from the shock of the cold metal and pathogens (germs). Then balance the scale. Move both weights to the *zero* position. If the end of the balance bar swings freely, the scale is balanced. If the scale is *not* balanced, follow the manufacturer's instructions to balance the scale.

   NOTE: Most scales have a small screw by the end of the balance bar. By adjusting the screw, the scale can be balanced.

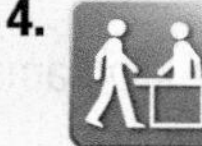

4. Comm — Introduce yourself. Explain the procedure to the parent. Identify the infant by asking the parent for the infant's name. Ask the parent to undress the infant.

   NOTE: An undershirt or pajama is sometimes left on the infant.
5. Pick up the infant. Use one arm to support the neck and shoulders and the other arm to support the back and hips.
6. Place the infant on the scale.

Safety — **CAUTION:** Watch closely at all times. To prevent falls, keep one hand over the infant while adjusting the scales (Figure 21–6).

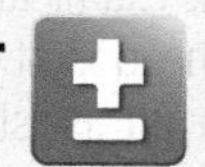

7. Math — Move the large weight to the right until the balance bar drops down on the lower guide. Then move this weight back one notch. Move the smaller weight until the balance bar swings freely halfway between the upper and lower guides. Add the two weights together to determine the infant's correct weight.

(continues)

PROCEDURE 21:1B (CONT.)

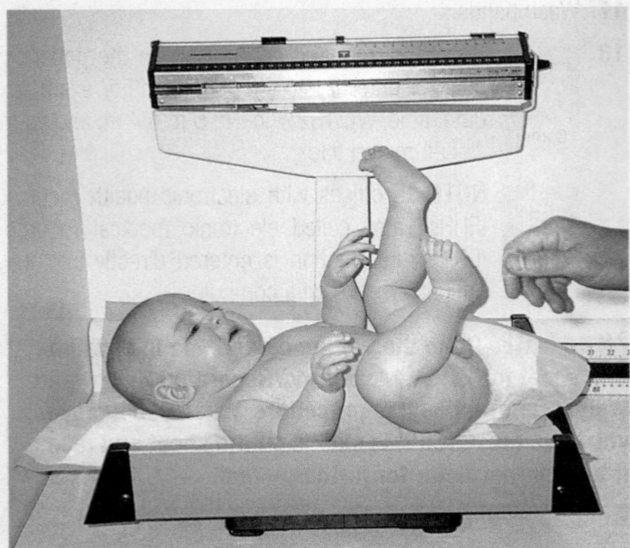

FIGURE 21–6 **Always keep one hand close to the infant to prevent the infant from falling off the scale.**

NOTE: If the infant scale contains only one bar and one weight, move the weight to the right until the balance bar swings freely halfway between the upper and lower guide. Read the weight on the bar.

NOTE: Many offices have scales with digital readouts. The weight is measured automatically when the infant is placed on the scale. However, it is important to make sure that you are not touching the infant when you read and record the weight.

8. Record the weight in pounds and ounces or in kilograms. Recheck your reading.

Check

CHECKPOINT: Your instructor will check your reading for accuracy.

9. Pick up and place the infant on a flat surface.

Safety

CAUTION: Watch closely at all times. Do not leave the infant unattended. If it is necessary to reach for anything nearby, use one hand to hold the infant and the other hand to reach.

10. Place the zero mark of the measuring tape or rod at the infant's head. If the measuring bar is a part of the examination table, position the infant so that the infant's head is at the zero mark (Figure 21–7A). Ask the parent or an assistant to hold the head at this mark. Gently straighten the infant's legs. If a measuring tape is used, measure to the infant's heel (Figure 21–7B). If a bar is used, position the heel on the bar while holding the leg straight.

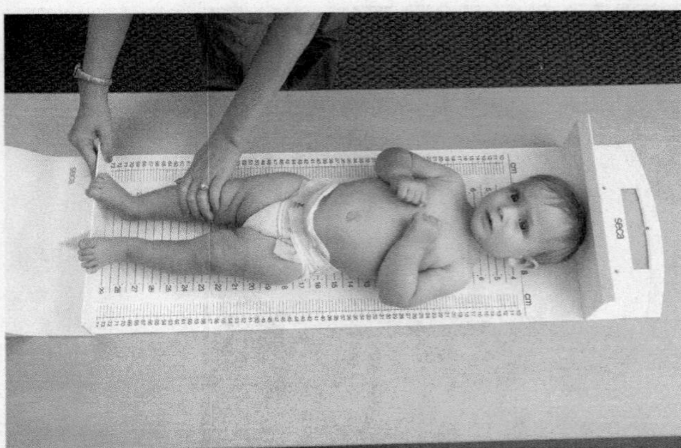

FIGURE 21–7A **Position the infant's head against the zero mark bar and gently straighten the legs to measure the infant's height.**

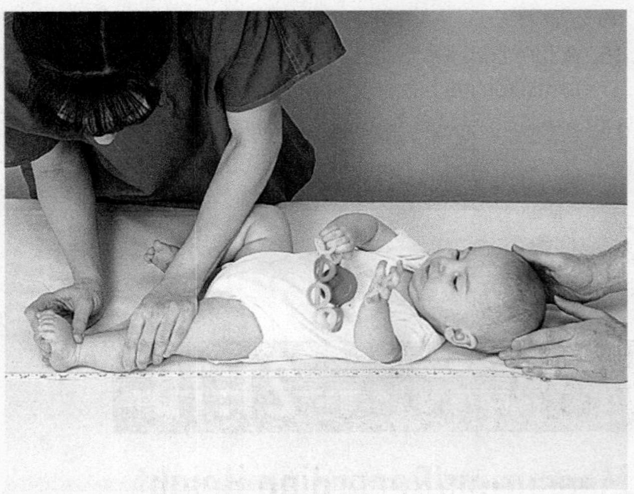

FIGURE 21–7B **Hold the tape measure in a straight line to measure an infant's height.**

NOTE: If the infant is lying on examining table paper, mark the paper at the infant's head and heel. Then measure the marked area.

11. Record the height correctly in inches or centimeters. Recheck your reading.

Check

CHECKPOINT: Your instructor will check your reading for accuracy.

12. The head circumference is frequently measured on an infant. To measure head circumference:
    a. Position the infant on the examination table or ask the parent to hold the infant.
    b. Use a thumb or finger to hold the zero mark of the tape measure against the infant's forehead just above the eyebrows.

PROCEDURE 21:1B (CONT.)

c. Use your other hand to bring the tape around the infant's head, just above the ears, over the occipital bone at the back of the head, and back to the forehead to meet the zero mark on the tape (Figure 21–8).

d. Pull the tape snug to compress the hair, but not too tight.

e. Read the tape measure to the nearest ½ inch or 0.1 centimeter.

f. Record the reading.

Check

CHECKPOINT: Your instructor will check your reading for accuracy.

13. To measure chest circumference of the infant:

a. Lay the infant flat on his or her back.

b. Use the thumb of one hand to hold the zero mark of the tape at the middle of the sternum.

c. Use your other hand to wrap the tape snugly under the axillary area and around the back to meet at the mid-sternal area (Figure 21–9).

d. Make sure the tape is at the nipple level of the chest and that it is not twisted.

e. Read the measurement after the infant has exhaled or during the resting phase between respirations.

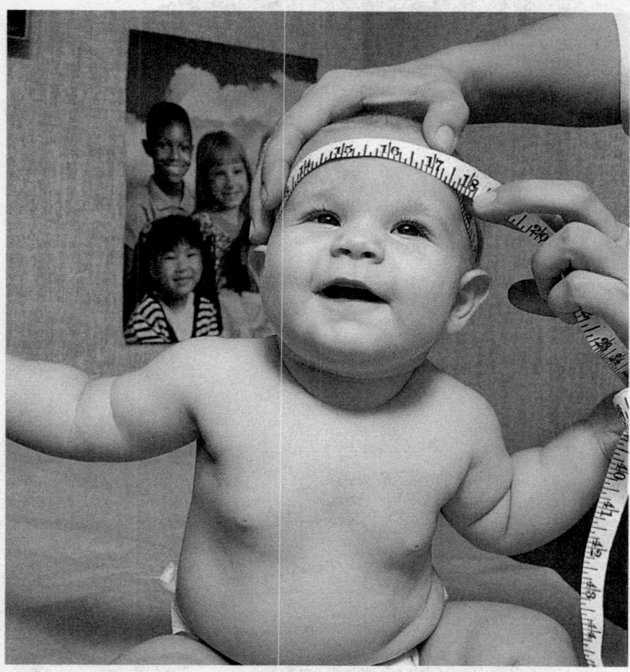

FIGURE 21–8 **To measure head circumference, bring the tape around the infant's head, just above the ears, and back to the forehead.**

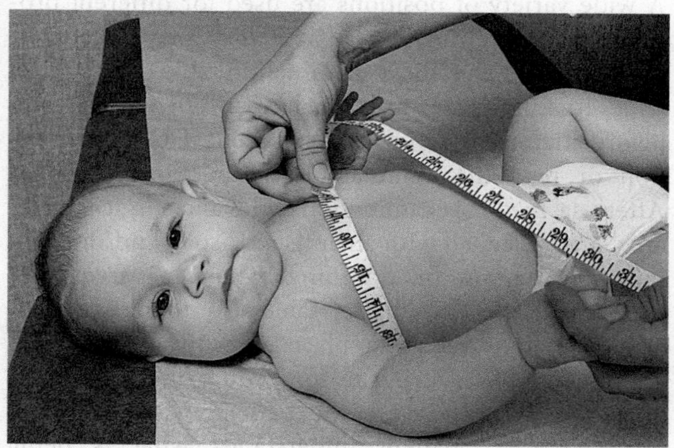

FIGURE 21–9 **To measure chest circumference, wrap the tape snugly around the chest and back at the nipple line.**

f. Read the tape measure to the nearest ½ inch or 0.1 centimeter.

Check

CHECKPOINT: Your instructor will check your reading for accuracy.

14. Return the infant to the parent.

15. Clean and replace all equipment. Use a disinfectant to wipe the scale. Set the weights at zero. Fold up the tape measure.

16. Wash hands.

17. 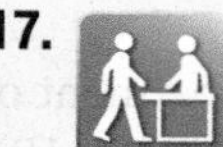
Comm

Record all required information on the infant's chart or enter it into the computer. For example: date, time, Wt: 9 lb 8 oz, Ht: 23½ in, Head circumference: 16¾ in, Chest circumference: 17¼ in, and your signature and title. The measurements should also be recorded on the infant's growth graph.

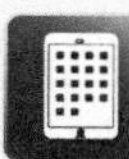
EHR

NOTE: In health care agencies using electronic health records (EHRs), also known as electronic medical records (EMRs), the information is entered directly into the patient's record on a computer.

PRACTICE: **Go to the workbook and use the evaluation sheet for 21:1B, Measuring/Recording Height and Weight of an Infant, to practice this procedure. When you believe you have mastered this skill, sign the sheet and give it to your instructor for further action.**

Check

FINAL CHECKPOINT: Using the criteria listed on the evaluation sheet, your instructor will grade your performance.

21:2 Positioning a Patient

A wide variety of positions are used for different procedures and examinations. The patient may need to be positioned on a medical examination table or a surgical table. It is important to know how to operate the table before attempting to position a patient. Obtain instruction or read the manufacturer's directions carefully. After use, medical examination tables and surgical tables are usually cleaned with an antiseptic soap and/or a disinfectant solution. In addition, table paper is frequently used to cover an examination table prior to the examination and is removed and replaced after the examination.

Comm

Safety

During any procedure or examination, reassure the patient. Make sure the patient understands what is being done and grants permission for the procedure. At all times, watch the patient closely for signs of distress. Observe all safety factors to prevent falls and injuries. Use correct body mechanics at all times to prevent injury to yourself.

It is also essential to make sure that the patient is not exposed during any examination or procedure. The door to the room should be closed, and the curtains, if present, should be drawn. Care must be taken to properly drape or cover the patient to avoid unnecessary exposure. At the same time, the drape must be applied so that the physician or technician has ready access to the area to be examined or treated.

Some of the most common examination positions are listed and described.

Horizontal Recumbent (Supine) Position

- This position is used for examination or treatment of the front, or anterior, part of the body (Figure 21–10).
- The patient lies flat on the back with the legs slightly apart.
- One small pillow is allowed under the head.
- The arms are flat at the side of the body.
- The drape is placed over the patient but left loose on all sides to facilitate examination or treatment.

Prone Position

- This position is used for examination or treatment of the back or spine (Figure 21–11).
- The patient lies on the abdomen and turns the head to either side. A small pillow may be placed under the head.
- The arms may be flexed at the elbows and positioned on either side of the head or positioned along the side of the body.
- One sheet or drape is placed over the patient but left loose on all sides to facilitate examination or treatment.

Sims' (Left Lateral) Position

- This position is used for simple rectal and sigmoidoscopic examinations, enemas, rectal temperatures, and rectal treatments (Figure 21–12).

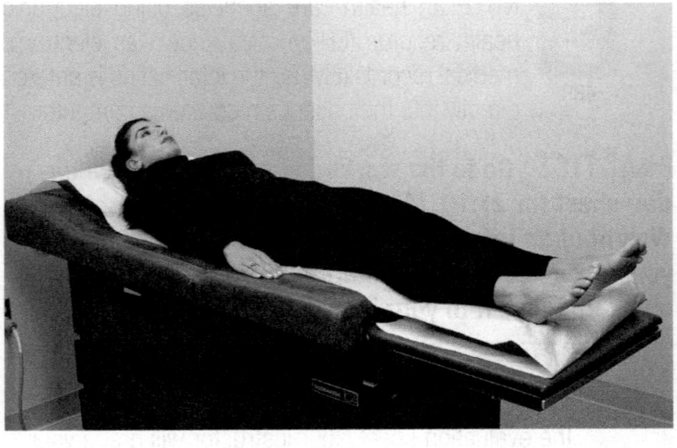

FIGURE 21–10 Horizontal recumbent (supine) position. Draping has been omitted for clarity.

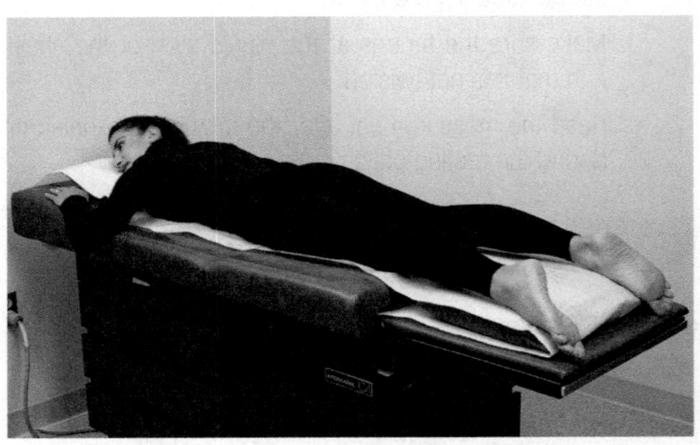

FIGURE 21–11 Prone position.

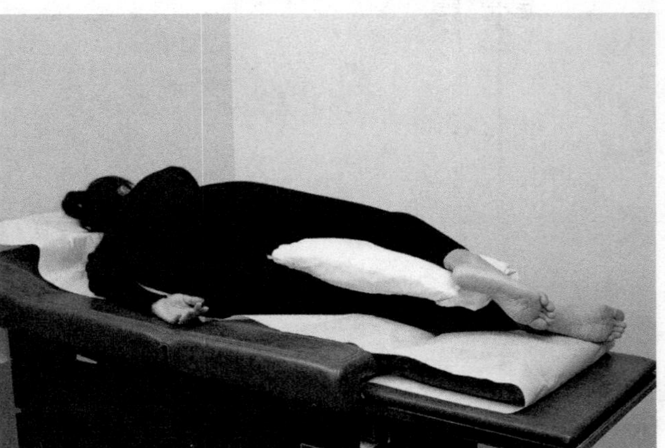

FIGURE 21–12 Sims' (left lateral) position.

- The patient lies on the left side.
- The left arm is extended behind the back.
- The head is turned to the side. A small pillow may be used.
- The right arm is in front of the patient, and the elbow is bent.
- The left leg is bent, or flexed, slightly.
- The right leg is bent sharply at the knee and brought up to the abdomen.
- Draping can be done with one large sheet or two small sheets that meet at the rectal area. A sheet with a hole at the examination site may also be used. All sheets hang free at the sides.

Knee–Chest Position

- This position is used for rectal examinations, usually a sigmoidoscopic examination (Figure 21–13). It is only used in rare circumstances when proctologic tables are not available.
- The patient rests the body weight on the knees and chest.
- The arms are flexed slightly at the elbows and are extended above the head.
- The knees are slightly separated, and the thighs are at right angles to the table.
- Draping can be done with one large sheet or two small sheets that meet at the rectal area. A large sheet with a hole at the rectal area can also be used. Sheets hang loose with no tucks.

Safety

CAUTION: *Do not place the patient in this position until the physician is ready to begin the examination.*

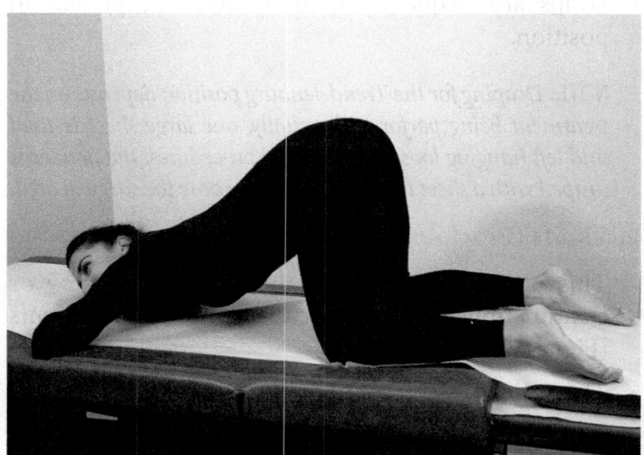

FIGURE 21–13 Knee–chest position.

Safety

CAUTION: *Never leave a patient alone in this position. This is a difficult position for the patient to maintain and should be used only as long as absolutely necessary.*

Fowler's Positions

- These positions are used to facilitate breathing, relieve distress, encourage drainage, and examine the head, neck, and chest.
- The patient lies on the back.
- The head is elevated to one of three main positions:
  - (1) *Low Fowler's:* the head is elevated to a 25-degree angle.
  - (2) *Semi-Fowler's:* the head is elevated to a 45-degree angle (the most frequently used position) (Figure 21–14A).
  - (3) *High Fowler's:* the head is elevated to a 90-degree angle (Figure 21–14B).
- The legs lie flat on the table but the knees are bent slightly and are sometimes supported on a pillow.

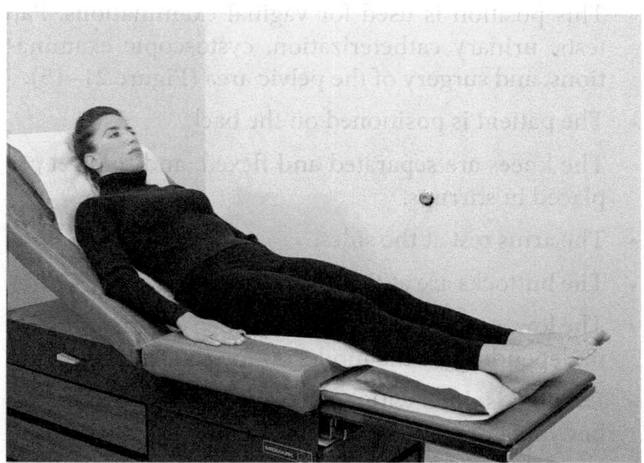

FIGURE 21–14A Semi-Fowler's (mid-Fowler's) position.

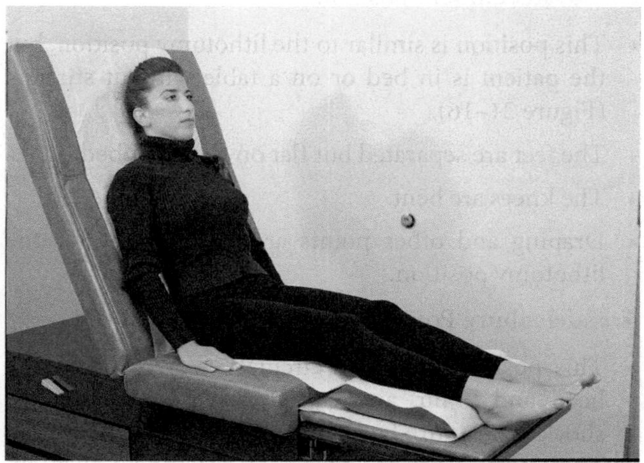

FIGURE 21–14B High Fowler's position.

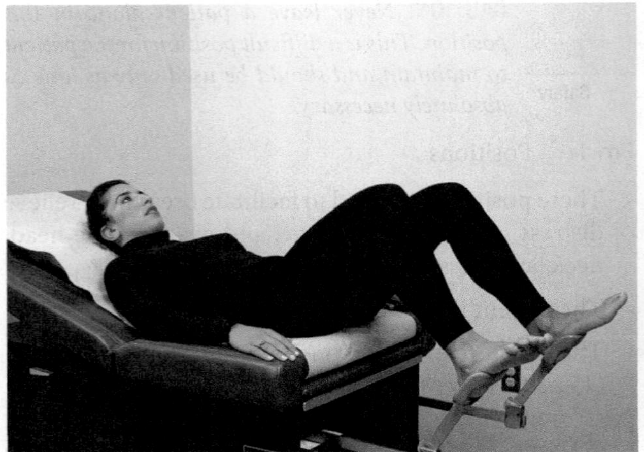

FIGURE 21–15 Lithotomy position.

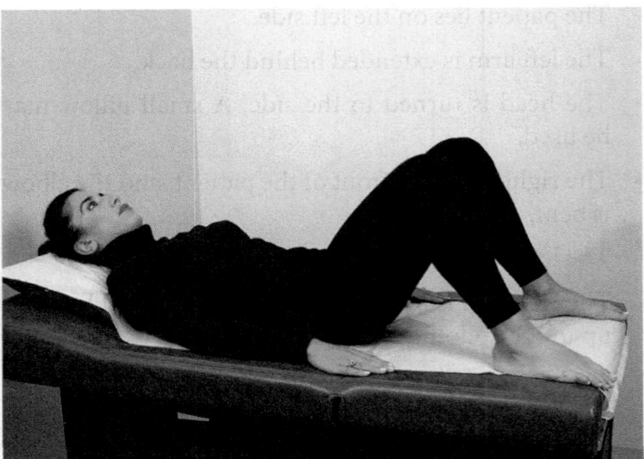

FIGURE 21–16 Dorsal recumbent position.

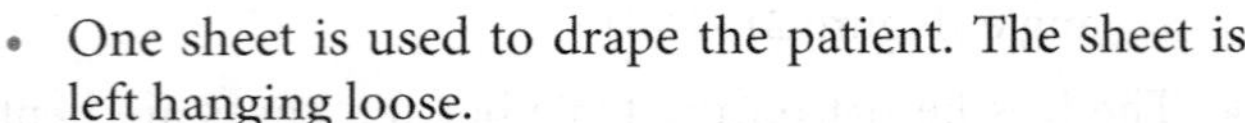

- One sheet is used to drape the patient. The sheet is left hanging loose.

Lithotomy Position

- This position is used for vaginal examinations, Pap tests, urinary catheterization, cystoscopic examinations, and surgery of the pelvic area (Figure 21–15).
- The patient is positioned on the back.
- The knees are separated and flexed, and the feet are placed in stirrups.
- The arms rest at the sides.
- The buttocks are at the lower end of the table.
- The lower end of the table is dropped down or pushed in depending on the model of the examination table.
- Draping is done with one large sheet placed over the body in a diamond shape. One corner is at the upper chest, and one corner hangs loose between legs. Each of the other two corners is wrapped around a foot.

Dorsal Recumbent Position

- This position is similar to the lithotomy position, but the patient is in bed or on a table without stirrups (Figure 21–16).
- The feet are separated but flat on the table/bed.
- The knees are bent.
- Draping and other points are the same as for the lithotomy position.

Trendelenburg Position

- This position increases circulation of blood to the head and brain, and can be used for circulatory shock. The entire bed or table is elevated at the feet. The patient lies in the horizontal recumbent position, with the head lower than the feet.

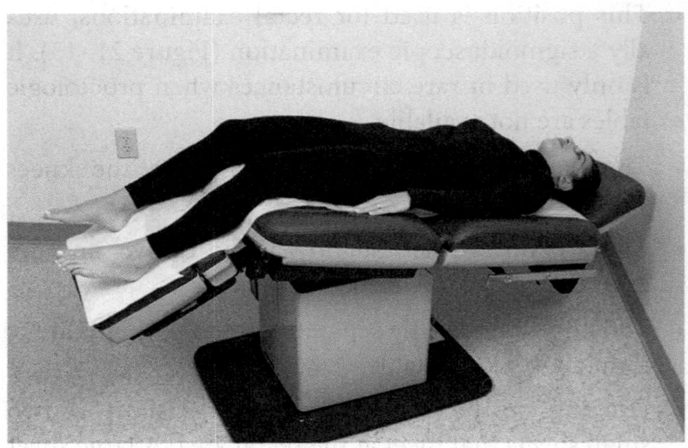

FIGURE 21–17 Surgical Trendelenburg position.

- The surgical Trendelenburg position (Figure 21–17) can be used for surgery on pelvic organs and for pelvic treatments. The patient is flat on the back. The table is lowered at a 45-degree angle to lower the head, and the feet and lower legs are inclined downward.
- Straps are frequently used to hold the patient in position.

NOTE: *Draping for the Trendelenburg position depends on the treatment being performed; usually, one large sheet is used and left hanging loose. For surgical procedures, the patient is draped with a sheet that has a hole to expose the surgical area.*

Jackknife (Proctologic) Position

- This position is used mainly for rectal surgery or examinations and for back surgery or treatments (Figure 21–18).
- The patient is in the prone position.
- The table is elevated at the center so that the rectal area is at a higher elevation. A special surgical table is required for this position.

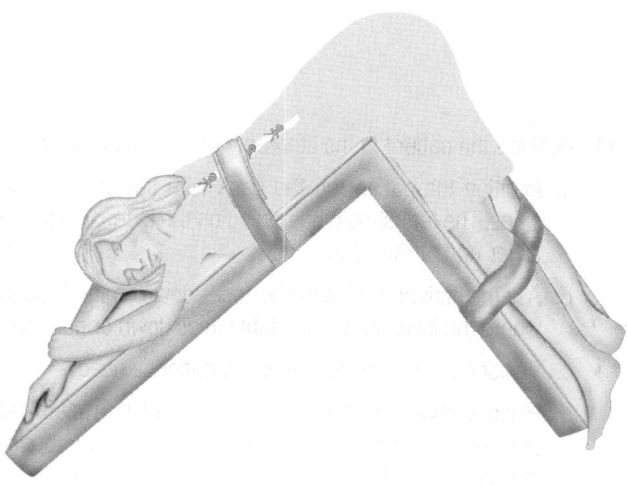

FIGURE 21–18 Jackknife (proctologic) position.

- The head and chest point downward. The feet and legs hang down at the opposite end of the table.
- The patient must be supported to prevent injury. Straps are used to hold the patient in position.
- Draping is done with a surgical sheet that has a hole to expose the surgical or treatment area. Two small sheets that meet at the surgical or treatment area can also be used.

Safety

CAUTION: *It is important to use good body mechanics while positioning the patient to protect both yourself and the patient.*

STUDENT: **Go to the workbook and complete the assignment sheet for 21:2, Positioning a Patient. Then return and continue with the procedure.**

PROCEDURE 21:2

Positioning a Patient

Equipment and Supplies

Two to three sheets or disposable drapes, examination table, patient gown, two small pillows, pen and/or computer

Procedure

1. Assemble equipment. Prepare the examination table by wiping it with a disinfectant and covering it with table paper.
2. Wash hands.
3. Introduce yourself. Identify the patient. Explain the procedure. Obtain the patient's consent.

   Comm
4. Instruct the patient to remove all clothing and to put on an examining gown. Instruct the patient to leave the opening in the front or the back depending on the examination to be performed. Ask the patient to void to prevent bladder discomfort during the examination or treatment.
5. Help the patient get on table.

   NOTE: Positioning of the patient will depend on the examination, treatment, or procedure to be performed.
6. Position the patient in the horizontal recumbent (supine) position as follows:
   a. Lay the patient flat on his or her back.
   b. Place a small pillow under the head.
   c. Rest the arms at the sides of the body.
   d. Position the legs flat and slightly separated.
   e. Use a large sheet or drape to drape the patient. Do *not* tuck the sheet in at the sides or bottom. It should hang loose.
7. Position the patient in the prone position as follows:
   a. Ask the supine patient to turn the body in your direction until lying on the abdomen. Hold the drape up while the patient is turning.

   Safety

   CAUTION: Watch the patient closely to make sure he or she does not roll off of the table. Do *not* leave the patient alone.

   b. Turn the head to either side to rest on a small pillow.
   c. Flex the arms at the elbows and place at the sides of the head.
   d. Use one large sheet or drape to drape the patient. Do *not* tuck in at the sides or bottom.
8. Position the patient in the Sims' (left lateral) position as follows:
   a. Ask the prone patient to turn on the left side.
   b. Extend the left arm behind the back.
   c. Rest the head on a small pillow.
   d. Bend the left leg slightly.
   e. Bend the right leg sharply to the abdomen.
   f. Place the right arm bent at the elbow in a comfortable position in front of the body.

(continues)

PROCEDURE 21:2 (CONT.)

g. Drape with one large sheet or drape. Do *not* tuck in at the sides or bottom. Draping can also be done with two small sheets. One sheet covers the upper part of the body and meets the second sheet, which covers the thighs and legs. A sheet with an opening at the rectal area may also be used.

9. Position the patient in the knee–chest position as follows:

a. Ask the patient to lie on the abdomen (that is, in the prone position).

b. Raise the buttocks and abdomen until the body weight is resting on the upper chest and knees.

Safety

NOTE: Do *not* place the patient in this position until the physician is ready to begin the examination. It is a difficult position for the patient to maintain.

c. Make sure the knees are slightly separated and the thighs are at right angles to the table.

d. Rest the head on a small pillow.

e. Flex the arms slightly and position on the sides of the head.

f. Drape with one large, untucked sheet or drape or two small sheets or drapes that meet at the rectal area. A drape with a hole at the rectal area can also be used.

Safety

CAUTION: *Never* leave the patient alone in the knee–chest position.

g. When the examination is complete, help the patient get into the prone position. Watch closely for signs of dizziness or discomfort and report any such signs immediately after being sure that the patient is in a comfortable, safe position.

10. Position the patient in the Fowler's positions as follows:

a. Place the patient in the horizontal recumbent position.

b. Place a small pillow under the patient's head.

c. Low Fowler's: elevate the head of the table/bed to a 25-degree angle.

d. Mid-, or semi-, Fowler's: elevate the head to a 45-degree angle.

e. High Fowler's: elevate the head to a 90-degree angle.

f. Place a second small pillow under the patient's knees after flexing them slightly.

g. Use a large sheet or drape to drape the patient. Do *not* tuck in the sides or end of the sheet or drape.

11. Position the patient in the lithotomy position as follows:

a. Position the patient on the back with the arms at the sides. The feet should be resting on the extension at the lower end of the table.

b. Ask the patient to slide the buttocks down on the table to where the lower end of the table folds down or pulls out.

c. Position a small pillow under the patient's head.

d. Place a sheet or drape over the patient in a diamond position. One corner should be at the chest, the opposite corner at the perineal area, or between the legs. Wrap each side corner around a foot.

e. Position the stirrups and lock them in place.

NOTE: Many tables have a knob at the side that is turned to lock the stirrups in position.

f. Flex and separate the knees.

g. Place the feet in the stirrups.

h. Drop the lower end of the table, or push in the extension.

i. To get the patient out of this position, first raise the end of the table or pull out the extension so that it is level. Lift the feet out of the stirrups and place them on the table. Ask the patient to move back up on the table.

12. Position the patient in the Trendelenburg positions as follows:

NOTE: These positions require a special bed or table and assistance. Care should be taken to prevent the patient from sliding off the table.

a. Put the patient in the horizontal recumbent position.

b. Operate the power table or electric bed to raise the foot of the table so that the patient's head is lower than the rest of the body. The lower frame of a bed is sometimes supported up on blocks.

c. For the surgical Trendelenburg position, lower the bottom end of the table so that the lower legs are inclined at a downward angle.

d. Use one large or two small sheets or drapes to drape the patient, or use a drape with a hole at the surgical site.

e. Use straps to secure the patient in position.

f. Remain with the patient at all times.

13. Position the patient in the jackknife or proctologic position as follows:

Safety

CAUTION: This position requires a special table and assistance (Figure 21–19). Care must be taken to prevent the patient from sliding off the table or being injured in any way.

PROCEDURE 21:2 (CONT.)

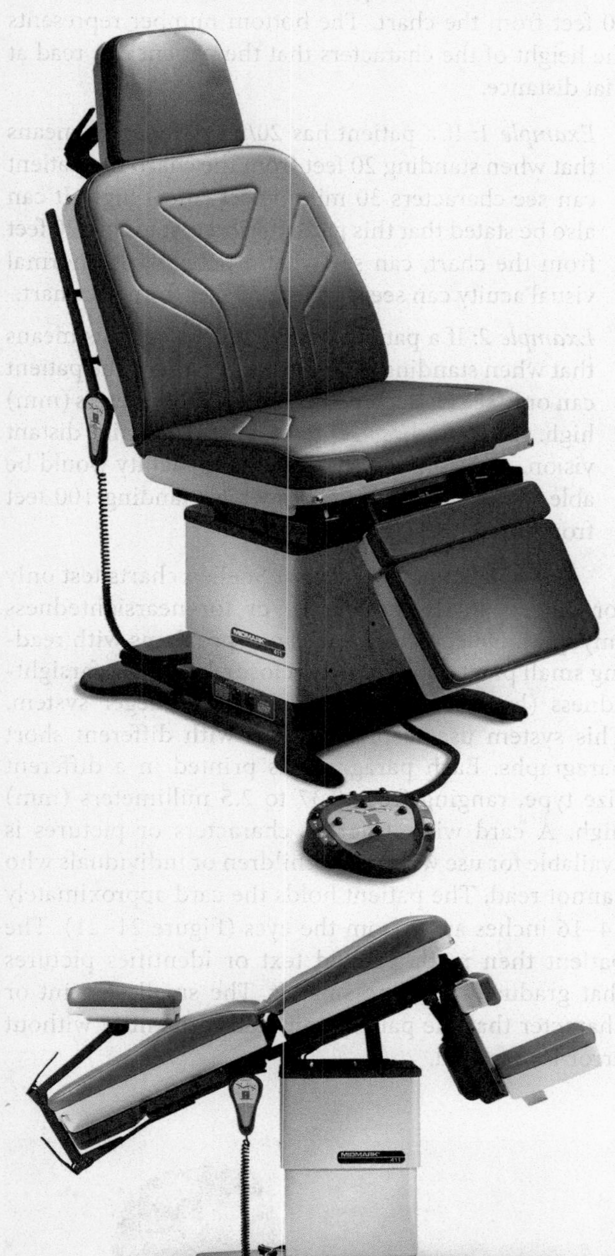

FIGURE 21–19 A special power table is required for the jackknife or proctologic position. Courtesy of Midmark Corp.

a. Position the patient in the prone position.

b. Secure the safety straps on the table.

c. Lower the top of the table so that the head and upper body are inclined at a downward angle.

d. Lower the bottom of the table so that the feet and legs are inclined at a downward angle.

e. Use a large sheet or special drape that has an opening in it to cover the patient. Place the opening over the rectal area. You may also use two small sheets that meet at the rectal area.

f. Remain with the patient at all times. Observe for any negative reactions to the position, such as dizziness, pain, or discomfort. Immediately report any such signs to your supervisor.

14. When the examination, treatment, or procedure is complete, allow the patient to sit up. Observe for signs of dizziness or weakness.

15. 
Comm

Help the patient get off the table. Ask the patient to get dressed or assist if necessary. Inform the patient of how and when he or she will be notified of test results (if tests were conducted during the examination).

Safety

CAUTION: Watch the patient closely and prevent falls.

16. Clean and replace all equipment.

17. Wash hands.

18. 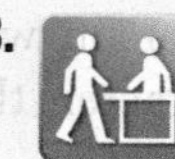
Comm

Record all required information on the patient's chart or enter it into the computer. For example: date, time, positioned in semi-Fowler's for comfort, appears to be resting well, and your signature and title.

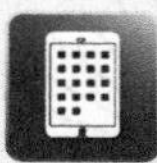
EHR

NOTE: In health care agencies using electronic health records (EHRs), also known as electronic medical records (EMRs), the information is entered directly into the patient's record on a computer.

PRACTICE: Go to the workbook and use the evaluation sheet for 21:2, Positioning a Patient, to practice this procedure. When you believe you have mastered this skill, sign the sheet and give it to your instructor for further action.

Check

FINAL CHECKPOINT: Using the criteria listed on the evaluation sheet, your instructor will grade your performance.

21:3 Screening for Vision Problems

Vision screening tests are given to measure an individual's **visual acuity**, or ability to perceive and comprehend the sense of sight. They are often given as part of a physical examination or to detect eye disease. Any test for visual acuity should be conducted in a well-lighted room. Natural daylight, with no direct sunlight, is preferred. During any test, it is important to watch the patient for squinting, leaning toward the eye chart, closing one eye when both eyes are being tested, excessive blinking, and/or watering of the eyes. If defects are noted on any test, the patient should be referred to an ophthalmologist for a more extensive examination.

One method of vision screening involves the use of Snellen charts. **Snellen charts** are used to test distant vision (Figure 21–20). They come in a variety of types. Some contain pictures for use with small children. Some contain the letter *E* in a variety of positions. The patient points in the direction that the *E* points. This type of chart is used for non-English-speaking people or nonreaders. Some contain letters of the alphabet. It is important to make sure the patient knows all the letters of the alphabet when using this type of chart.

Characters (that is, letters or pictures) on the Snellen chart have specific heights, ranging from small, on the bottom of the chart, to large, on the top of the chart. When standing 20 feet from the chart, a person with normal visual acuity should be able to see characters that are 20 millimeters high. Such a person is said to have 20/20 vision. When referring to 20/20 vision, the top number represents the distance the patient is from the chart. For this screening test, then, the patient is placed 20 feet from the chart. The bottom number represents the height of the characters that the patient can read at that distance.

- *Example 1:* If a patient has 20/30 vision, this means that when standing 20 feet from the chart, the patient can see characters 30 millimeters (mm) high. It can also be stated that this patient, who is standing 20 feet from the chart, can see what a patient with normal visual acuity can see standing 30 feet from the chart.
- *Example 2:* If a patient has 20/100 vision, this means that when standing 20 feet from the chart, the patient can only see characters that are 100 millimeters (mm) high. This finding represents a defect in distant vision. A person with normal visual acuity would be able to see the same figures while standing 100 feet from the chart.

It is important to note that Snellen charts test only for defects in distant vision, or for nearsightedness (myopia). Defects in close vision (problems with reading small print and seeing up close), known as farsightedness (hyperopia), are tested by the Jaeger system. This system uses a printed card with different short paragraphs. Each paragraph is printed in a different size type, ranging from 0.37 to 2.5 millimeters (mm) high. A card with different characters or pictures is available for use with small children or individuals who cannot read. The patient holds the card approximately 14–16 inches away from the eyes (Figure 21–21). The patient then reads printed text or identifies pictures that gradually become smaller. The smallest print or character that the patient can read or identify without error is recorded.

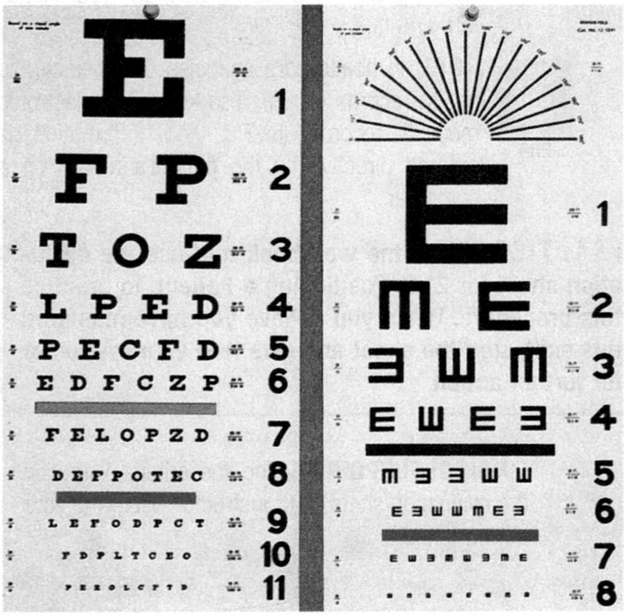

FIGURE 21–20 Snellen charts are used for vision screening.

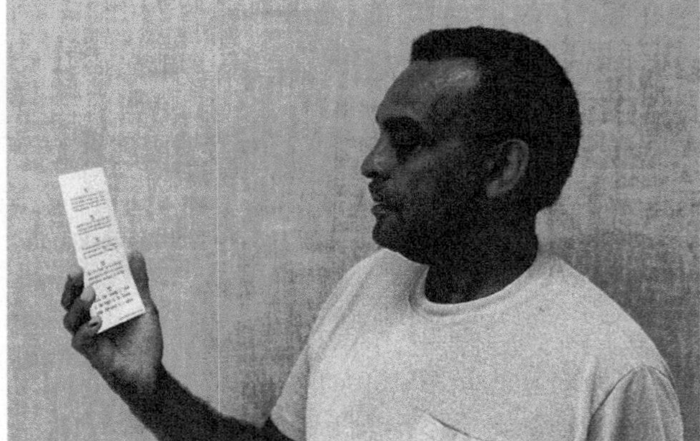

FIGURE 21–21 The patient holds the card 14–16 inches from the eyes when testing for defects in close vision.

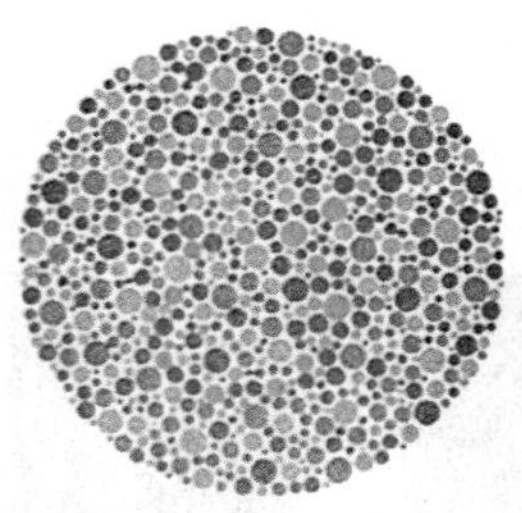
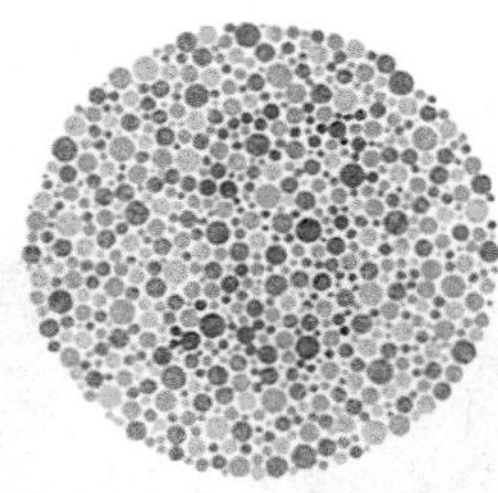

FIGURE 21–22 People with color blindness are not able to see the numbers in these Ishihara color plates.

Defects in color vision, or color blindness, are usually tested by the Ishihara method. The Ishihara book contains a series of numbers printed in colored dots against a background of dots in contrasting color (Figure 21–22). Patients with normal color vision are able to readily identify the numbers. Patients with color blindness either are unable to see the numbers or identify incorrect numbers. This test is most accurate when it is conducted in a room illuminated by natural daylight but not by bright sunlight.

When screening for visual acuity, there are some special terms or abbreviations to remember:

- ***OD***: abbreviation for *oculus dexter*, or right eye
- ***OS***: abbreviation for *oculus sinister*, or left eye
- ***OU***: abbreviation for *oculus uterque*, or each eye; both eyes
- **Myopia**: nearsightedness, defect in distant vision
- **Hyperopia**: farsightedness, defect in close vision
- ***Ophthalmoscope***: instrument for checking the eye
- ***Tonometer***: instrument to measure intraocular tension or pressure; increased pressure often indicates glaucoma

STUDENT: **Go to the workbook and complete the assignment sheet for 21:3, Screening for Vision Problems. Then return and continue with the procedure.**

PROCEDURE 21:3

Screening for Vision Problems

Equipment and Supplies

Snellen eye chart, Jaeger card, Ishihara book with color plates, pointer, tape, eye shield or occluder, paper, pen and/or computer

Procedure

1. Assemble equipment. Check the lighting in the room to make sure there is no glare. Natural daylight is preferred.

2. Attach the Snellen chart to the wall or place it in a lighted stand. Measure a distance of 20 feet directly away from the front of the chart. Place a piece of tape on the floor at the 20-foot mark.

NOTE: Most medical offices will have a mark on the floor to indicate the 20-foot distance.

NOTE: Vision screening devices that are calibrated for distance are also available. The patient looks through eyepieces to see the charts and identify letters. The device allows the operator to turn off the light in an eyepiece to test vision in either the right or left eye.

3. Wash hands.

4. 
Comm

Introduce yourself. Identify the patient. Explain the procedure.

NOTE: If using a chart with letters, make sure the patient knows the letters of the alphabet. If using a picture chart, make sure small children know what each picture represents.

5. Instruct the patient to stand facing the chart. Make sure the patient's toes are on the taped line; the patient's eyes will be 20 feet from the chart.

6. Point to various letters or pictures on the chart. Ask the patient to identify the letters or pictures. If the patient wears corrective lenses (glasses or contact lenses), check the vision with the corrective lenses first. Then ask the patient to remove the corrective lenses. Check the vision again. Record both readings. Observe the following points:

a. Start with the larger letters or pictures and proceed to the smaller ones.

b. Make sure the pointer you are using does not block the letters or pictures.

c. Select letters or pictures at random in each row. Do *not* start at one end of the row and go straight across the line. Patients may memorize order; random sampling makes the patient focus on individual letters or pictures.

(continues)

PROCEDURE 21:3 (CONT.)

NOTE: If you are sure the patient has not memorized the letters, you may ask the patient to read a row of letters. If the patient is able to read all letters correctly, proceed to a smaller row.

d. Watch to be sure the patient is not leaning forward or squinting to see the letters or pictures (Figure 21–23A). Note whether the patient is blinking excessively or if the eyes are watering.

NOTE: Some examiners do the left or right eye first, the opposite eye second, and both eyes last. Follow your agency's policy.

7. Ask the patient to correctly identify all the letters or pictures in the 20/20 line. If the patient is unable to do so, note the line that the patient *can* read with 100-percent accuracy.

8. Give the patient an eye shield or occluder with which to cover the left eye (Figure 21–23B). Warn the patient not to close the left eye while it is covered, because doing so can cause blurred vision. Repeat steps 6 and 7 to test the vision in the right eye (OD).

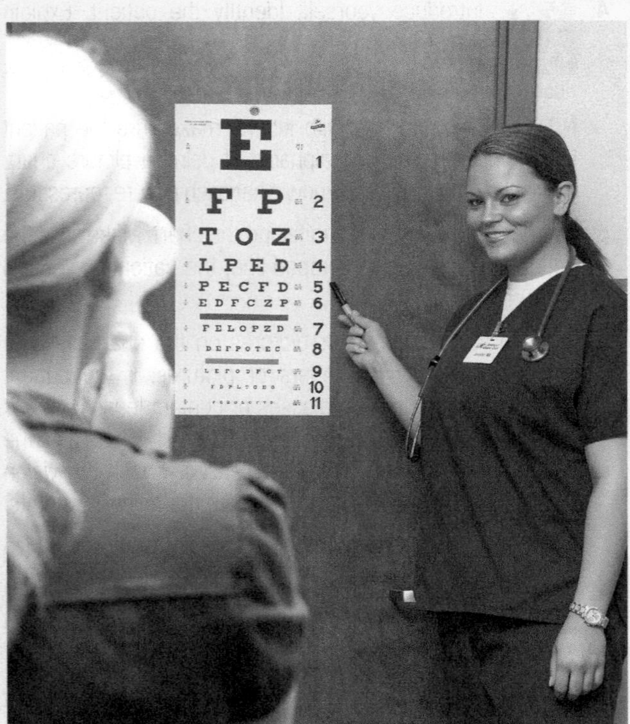

FIGURE 21–23A **Watch to make sure the patient is not leaning forward or squinting to see the letters.**

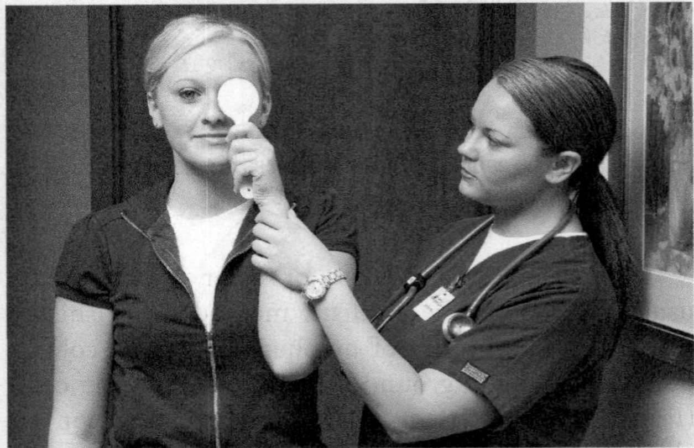

FIGURE 21–23B **The patient should keep the eye open while covering it with an eye shield or occluder.**

CAUTION: Warn the patient against pressing on the covered eye to avoid injuring the eye with the occluder or shield. Do *not* use the occluder or shield on another patient until it has been disinfected. Some occluders are disposable.

9. Ask the patient to cover the right eye. Repeat steps 6 and 7 to test the vision in the left eye (OS).

NOTE: Remind the patient to keep the right eye open while it is covered.

10. Record the test results for both eyes, the right eye, and the left eye. Use abbreviations of *OU, OD*, and *OS* and readings of *20/20, 20/30*, or the correct reading.

11. To test vision by the Jaeger system:

a. Seat the patient in a comfortable position.

b. Ask the patient to hold the Jaeger card 14–16 inches from the eyes.

c. Ask the patient to read the paragraphs out loud.

NOTE: If the patient cannot read, provide a Jaeger card that contains characters or pictures.

d. Record the smallest line of print the patient can read with both eyes.

e. Ask the patient to cover the right eye with an occluder and then to read the paragraphs out loud. Record the smallest line of print the patient can read with the left eye.

f. Ask the patient to cover the left eye with an occluder and then to read the paragraphs out loud. Record the smallest line of print the patient can read with the right eye.

PROCEDURE 21:3 (CONT.)

12. To test color vision with the Ishihara plates:
    a. Seat the patient in a comfortable position.
    b. Hold the plate approximately 30 inches from the patient's eyes.
    c. Ask the patient to read the number on the plate.

       NOTE: Some plates contain color lines in place of numbers. The patient is asked to trace the color line with a finger.
    d. Show the patient all of the plates. Record the number of plates the patient identifies correctly.
    e. Ask the patient to cover the right eye with an occluder and then to identify the numbers on the plates. Record the number of plates the patient identifies correctly with the left eye.
    f. Ask the patient to cover the left eye with an occluder and then to identify the numbers on the plates. Record the number of plates the patient identifies correctly with the right eye.
    g. Report any frame that the patient misses. This allows the physician to determine which type of color blindness the patient has.
13. Thank the patient for being cooperative.

    NOTE: These are only screening tests. Unfavorable results indicate the need for additional testing or referral to an eye specialist.
14. Clean and replace all equipment. If the eye shield is not disposable, wash it thoroughly and clean it with a disinfectant solution.
15. Wash hands.
16. 

Record all required information on the patient's chart or enter it into the computer. For example: date, time, vision screening with Snellen chart: OU 20/30, OD 20/40, OS 20/30, Jaeger card: OU #3 (0.62 m), OD #3 (0.62 m), OS #5 (1.00 m), Ishihara plates: 10 plates correct for OU, OD, and OS, and your signature and title.

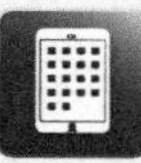

NOTE: In health care agencies using electronic health records (EHRs), also known as electronic medical records (EMRs), the information is entered directly into the patient's record on a computer.

PRACTICE: **Go to the workbook and use the evaluation sheet for 21:3, Screening for Vision Problems, to practice this procedure. When you believe you have mastered this skill, sign the sheet and give it to your instructor for further action.**

FINAL CHECKPOINT: Using the criteria listed on the evaluation sheet, your instructor will grade your performance.

21:4 Assisting with Physical Examinations

A large variety of physical examinations are performed. The methods used and the equipment available vary from physician to physician. However, there are some basic principles that apply to all examinations.

Three major kinds of examinations are:

- *EENT*: This is an eye, ear, nose, and throat examination. Special equipment should be available to examine these areas of the body.
- *GYN*: This is an examination of the female reproductive organs; that is, a gynecological examination. The physician usually examines the vagina, cervix, and other pelvic organs as well as the breasts. A Pap, or **Papanicolaou**, test frequently is done to detect cancer of the cervix or reproductive organs.
- *General*, or *complete*, *physical*: All areas of the body are examined. Blood and urine tests frequently are done. Radiographs and an electrocardiogram (ECG) may also be part of the examination. An EENT and/or GYN examination may be performed. Necessary equipment and tests are determined by the physician performing the examination.

Four main techniques used during the examination are observation, palpation, percussion, and auscultation.

- **Observation** (inspection): The physician looks at the patient carefully to observe things such as skin color, rash, growths, swelling, scars, deformities, body movements, condition of hair and nails, and general appearance (Figure 21–24).

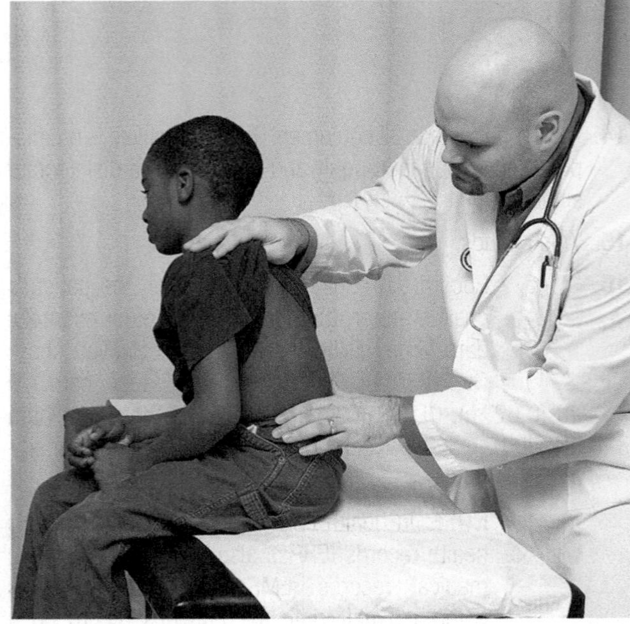

FIGURE 21–24 The physician uses observation to inspect the body for signs of disease.

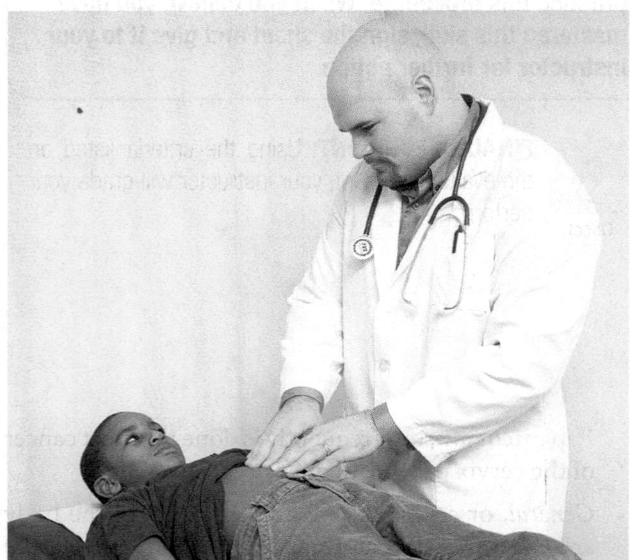

FIGURE 21–25 For palpation, the physician uses the hands and fingers to feel various parts of the body.

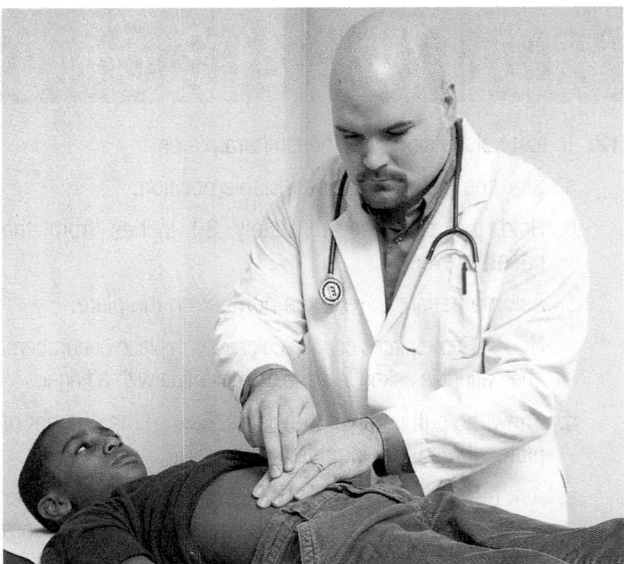

FIGURE 21–26 Percussion involves tapping on body parts and listening to sounds coming from body organs.

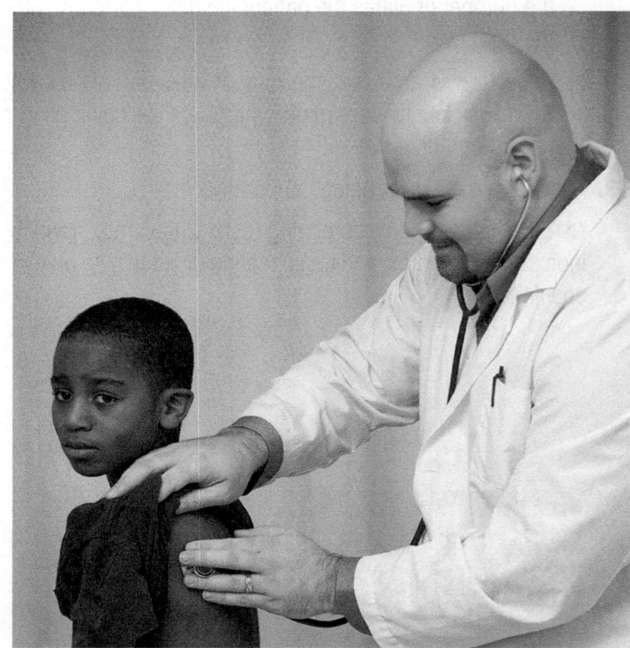

FIGURE 21–27 The physician is using a stethoscope and auscultation to listen to posterior lung and heart sounds.

- **Palpation**: The physician uses the hands and fingers to feel various parts of the body (Figure 21–25). The physician can determine whether a part of the body is enlarged, hard, out of place, or painful to the touch.
- **Percussion**: The physician taps and listens for sounds coming from various body organs (Figure 21–26). The physician may place one or several fingers of one hand on a part of the body, then use the fingers of the other hand to tap the body part. The sounds emitted allow a trained individual to determine the size, density, and position of underlying organs.
- **Auscultation**: The physician listens to sounds coming from within the patient's body (Figure 21–27). A stethoscope is used in most cases. The physician listens to sounds produced by the heart, lungs, intestines, and other body organs.

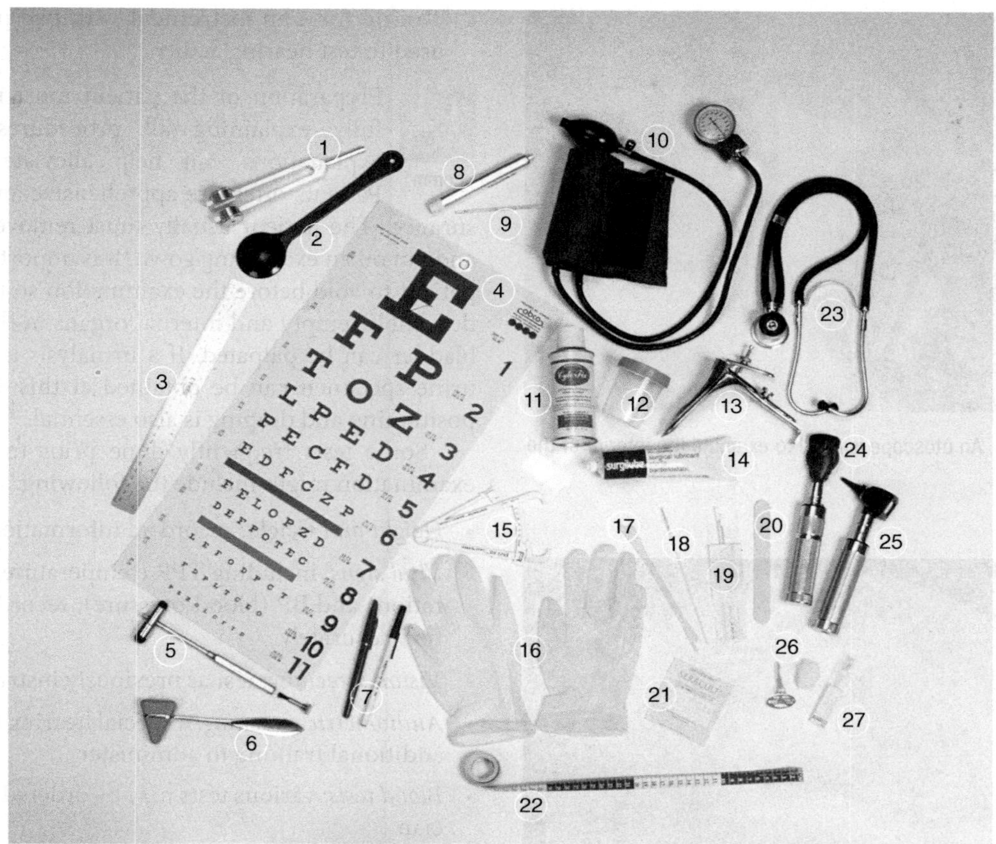

FIGURE 21–28 **Instruments and equipment for physical examinations: 1. Tuning fork. 2. Visual occluder. 3. Ruler. 4. Visual acuity chart. 5. Reflex hammer with brush. 6. Percussion hammer. 7. Pen and marking pen. 8. Penlight. 9. Thermometer. 10. Sphygmomanometer. 11. Slide and fixative. 12. Specimen cup. 13. Vaginal speculum. 14. Lubricant. 15. Goniometer to measure angles. 16. Gloves. 17. Cervical spatula (Ayer blade). 18. Cervical brush (cytobrush). 19. Cotton-tip applicator. 20. Tongue depressor. 21. Guaiac material for fecal occult blood. 22. Tape measure. 23. Stethoscope. 24. Ophthalmoscope. 25. Otoscope. 26. Neurological examination key and cotton ball. 27. Sterile needle.**

All necessary equipment should be assembled prior to the examination. The equipment needed will vary depending on the body areas to be examined. Try to anticipate what the physician will need, and assemble the items for convenient use. Some of the equipment and instruments used for different examinations (Figure 21–28) include:

- **Cervical spatula (Ayer blade)**: a wooden or plastic blade used to scrape cells from the cervix, or lower part of the uterus; it is usually a part of a Pap kit that also contains slides, swabs, and a cytology brush; used to perform a Pap test to check for cancer of the cervix
- **Laryngeal mirror**: an instrument with a mirror at one end; used to examine the larynx, or voice box, in the throat
- **Ophthalmoscope**: a lighted instrument used to examine the eyes (Figure 21–29)
- **Otoscope**: a lighted instrument used to examine the ears (Figures 21–30A and 21–30B)

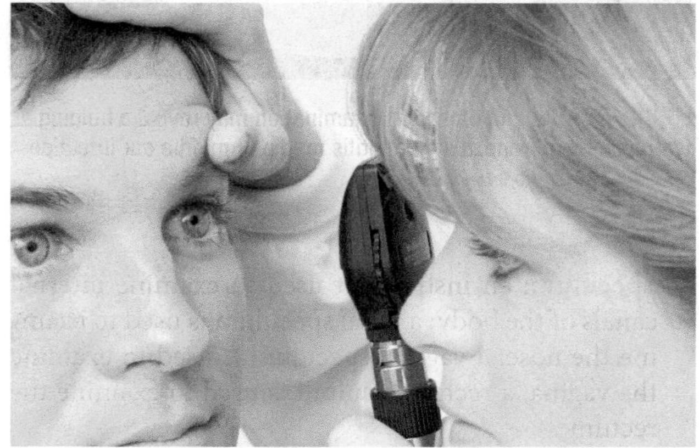

FIGURE 21–29 **An ophthalmoscope is used to examine the patient's eye.**

- **Percussion (reflex) hammer**: an instrument used to test tendon reflexes
- **Sigmoidoscope**: a lighted instrument used to examine the sigmoid colon, or inside of the lower part of the large intestine; used during sigmoidoscopic examinations

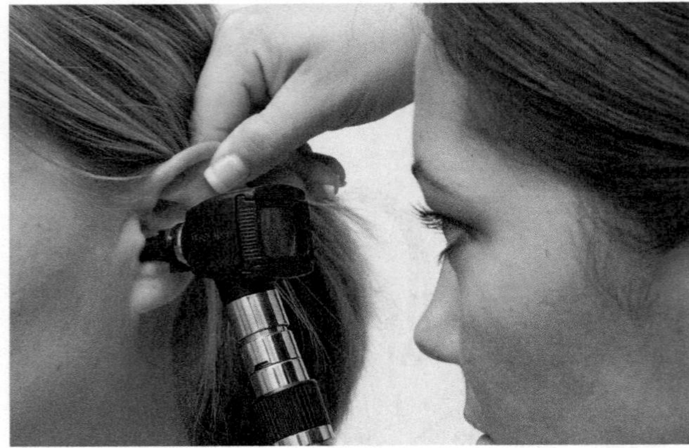

FIGURE 21–30A An otoscope is used to examine the interior of the patient's ear.

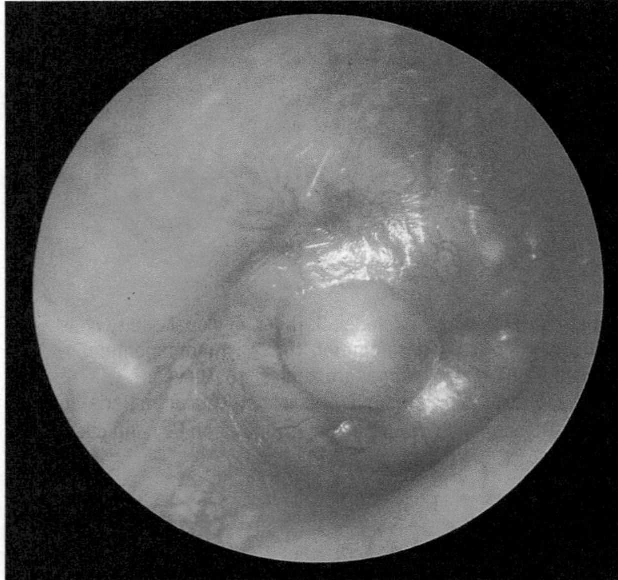

FIGURE 21–30B An otoscopic examination may reveal a bulging tympanic membrane, a sign of otitis media or middle ear infection.
Courtesy of Bruce Black, MD, Brisbane, Australia

- **Speculum**: an instrument used to examine internal canals of the body; a nasal speculum is used to examine the nose; a vaginal speculum is used to examine the vagina; a rectal speculum is used to examine the rectum
- **Sphygmomanometer**: an instrument used to measure blood pressure
- **Stethoscope**: an instrument used for listening to internal body sounds
- **Tongue blade/depressor**: a wood or plastic stick used to depress, or hold down, the tongue so that the throat can be examined
- **Tuning fork**: an instrument with two prongs that is used to test hearing acuity

Comm

Preparation of the patient must include carefully explaining all procedures. Thorough explanations can help alleviate some fear. Patients often are apprehensive and need reassurance. The patient usually must remove all clothing and put on an examining gown. It is important to tell the patient to void before the examination so that the bladder will be empty and internal organs in the area of the bladder can be palpated. If a urinalysis is ordered, the urine specimen can be obtained at this time. Correct positioning and draping is also essential.

Some tests frequently done prior to the physical examination might include the following:

- *Height and weight*: record all information accurately
- *Vital signs*: including TPR (temperature, pulse, respiration) and BP (blood pressure); record all information accurately
- *Vision screening*: test as previously instructed
- *Audiometric screening*: a special hearing test requiring additional training to administer
- *Blood tests*: various tests may be ordered by the physician
- *Electrocardiogram*: a test to check the electrical conduction pattern in the heart; performed if ordered by the physician

During the examination, be prepared to assist as necessary. Hand equipment to the physician as needed. Position the patient correctly for each part of the examination. Pay attention so that you are ready to help with each procedure.

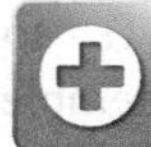
Precaution

Standard precautions (discussed in Chapter 15:4) must be followed at all times while assisting with physical examinations. Hands must be washed frequently, and gloves must be worn if contact with blood or body fluids is likely. If splashing or spraying of blood or body fluids is possible, other personal protective equipment (PPE) such as a mask, eye protection, and/or a gown must be worn. Any instruments or equipment contaminated by blood or body fluids must be correctly cleaned and disinfected or sterilized after use. The medical assistant must always be aware of and take steps to prevent the spread of infection.

STUDENT: **Go to the workbook and complete the assignment sheet for 21:4, Assisting with Physical Examinations. Then return and continue with the procedures.**

PROCEDURE 21:4A

Eye, Ear, Nose, and Throat Examination

NOTE: This is a basic guideline. Methods and equipment will vary from physician to physician.

Equipment and Supplies

Tray covered with a towel, basin lined with a paper towel, cotton-tipped applicators, ophthalmoscope, otoscope, tuning fork, nasal speculum, tongue blades or depressors, flashlight or penlight, Snellen chart, culture tubes and slides (as needed), disposable gloves, infectious-waste bag, patient's chart, lab requisition forms, pen and/or computer

Procedure

1. Assemble equipment. Arrange the instruments on a Mayo stand or tray.
2. Wash hands. Put on gloves for any procedure that involves contact with blood or body fluids.

   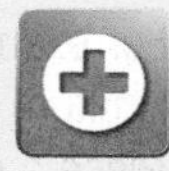
   Precaution

   CAUTION: Observe standard precautions at all times.
3. 
   Comm

   Introduce yourself. Identify the patient. Explain the procedure. Remember that this procedure has multiple steps.
4. Screen for visual acuity with a Snellen chart, Jaeger card, and/or Ishihara plates as required. Record all results accurately.
5. Place the patient in a sitting position.

   NOTE: If an eye, ear, nose, and throat examination (EENT) is the only examination being done, the patient can remain dressed.
6. Ask the patient to remove glasses and/or hearing aid(s). Tell the patient to place these items in a safe place.

   NOTE: Hearing aids are sometimes *not* removed until the actual ear examination. This is particularly true if the patient cannot hear questions without a hearing aid.
7. Notify the physician that the patient is ready. Have disposable gloves available for the physician to use. The physician may put the gloves on at the start of the examination or at the point during the examination when contact with body fluids may occur.
8. Eyes are usually examined first. The physician may use a penlight or flashlight to examine the eyes and check whether the pupils of the eyes are the same size and whether they react to light. Then, turn the ophthalmoscope light on and hand the ophthalmoscope to the physician. When the physician hands the ophthalmoscope back, turn the light off if the physician did not do so.

   NOTE: Some physicians want the room light turned off during the eye examination.
9. The nose is usually examined next. Have the nasal speculum and penlight ready for use. Also have cotton-tipped applicators ready. If a culture is taken, handle the culture stick correctly.

   NOTE: Refer to Procedure 20:2A, Obtaining a Culture Specimen, if necessary.
10. The ears are usually examined next. Pass the otoscope with its light on to the physician. Have a cotton-tipped applicator ready for use. When the examination is done, turn off the otoscope light. Place the otoscope tip in the towel-lined basin. If the physician wants to test hearing acuity, hand the physician the tuning fork. Hold the tuning fork in the middle so the physician can grasp it at the stem end. The physician will check auditory acuity (hearing) with the tuning fork (Figures 21–31A to 21–31C).
11. The mouth and throat are usually examined last. Pass the tongue blade or depressor by holding it in the center. Turn on the penlight and hand it to the physician, as needed.

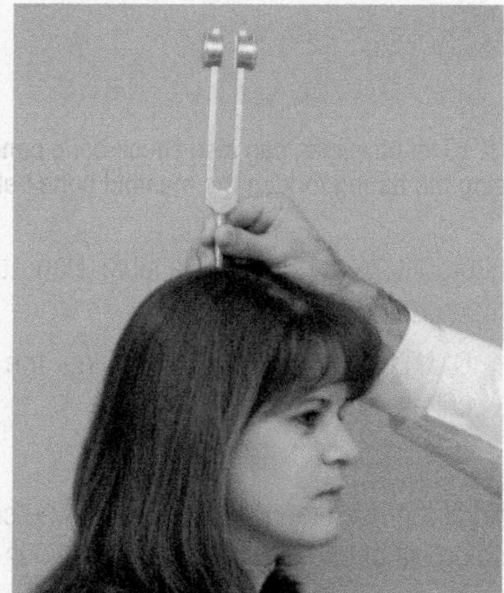

FIGURE 21–31A The physician places the vibrating tuning fork on the top of the head to ascertain whether both ears can hear the sound.

(continues)

PROCEDURE 21:4A (CONT.)

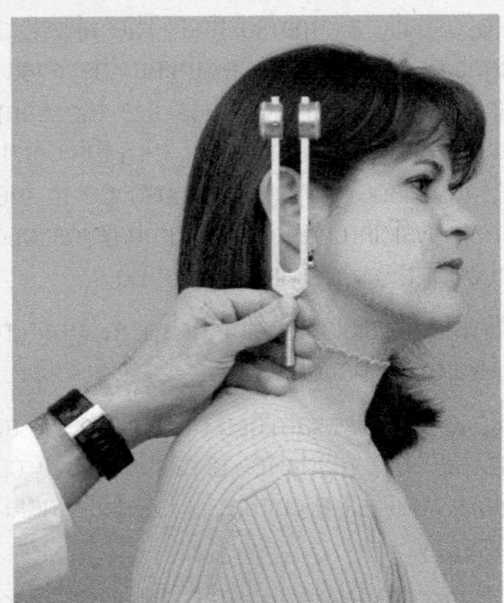

FIGURE 21–31B The physician can also test auditory acuity by placing the vibrating tuning fork about 1–2 inches away from each ear.

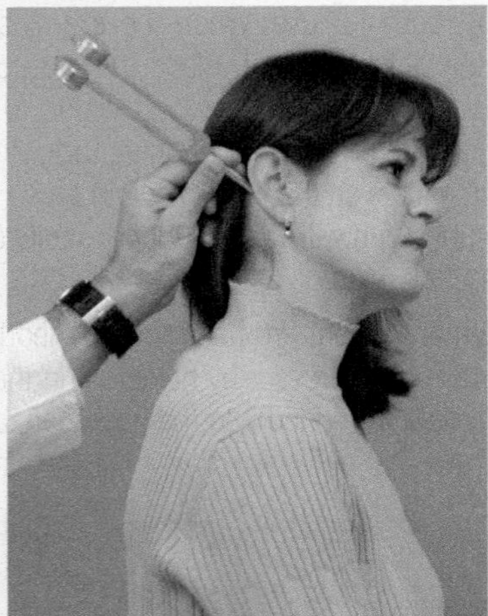

FIGURE 21–31C The physician can also check bone conduction of sound by placing the tuning fork on the mastoid bone behind the ear.

12. Have culture sticks and tubes available. Hand these to the physician correctly.

Safety

CAUTION: Avoid contaminating the tip of the culture stick.

13. Take hold of the used tongue depressor in the center. Without touching either end, place it in the infectious-waste bag.

14.  Comm When the examination is complete, help the patient replace glasses, hearing aid(s), and so forth. Help the patient get off the examination table. Inform the patient of how and when he or she will be notified of test results.

15.  Comm Label all specimens correctly with the patient's name, identification number, and physician's name. Print all information on the lab requisition form or use a computer-generated label. This might include date, time, patient's name, address, identification number, physician's name and identification number, type or site of specimen, and test ordered. Send all specimens to the laboratory as soon as possible.

16. 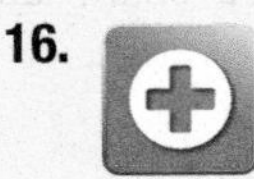 Precaution Clean and replace all equipment. Put on gloves while disinfecting and sterilizing contaminated instruments or equipment. Put all contaminated disposable supplies in the infectious-waste bag. Use a disinfectant to wipe any contaminated areas.

17. Remove gloves and discard in an infectious-waste bag. Wash hands.

18. 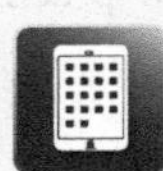 Comm Record all required information on the patient's chart or enter it into the computer. For example: date, time, EENT examination, throat culture sent to lab, and your signature and title. Place a copy of any lab requisitions in the patient's chart. The physician sometimes records the required information.

EHR

NOTE: In health care agencies using electronic health records (EHRs), also known as electronic medical records (EMRs), the information is entered directly into the patient's record on a computer.

PRACTICE: **Go to the workbook and use the evaluation sheet for 21:4A, Assisting with an Eye, Ear, Nose, and Throat Examination, to practice this procedure. When you believe you have mastered this skill, sign the sheet and give it to your instructor for further action.**

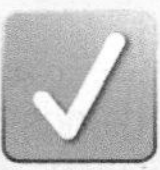
Check

FINAL CHECKPOINT: Using the criteria listed on the evaluation sheet, your instructor will grade your performance.

PROCEDURE 21:4B

Assisting with a Gynecological Examination

NOTE: The equipment and steps of this procedure can vary from physician to physician.

Equipment and Supplies

Tray covered with a towel, sheet or drape, patient gown, cotton-tipped applicators; sterile cotton-tipped applicators, gloves, lubricant, vaginal speculum, cervical spatulas (Ayer blades), cytology (cervical) brush or ThinPrep test kit, culture tubes, slides and fixative, examining light, cotton balls, basin lined with a paper towel, tissues, infectious-waste bag, patient's chart, lab requisition forms, pen and/or computer

Procedure

1. Assemble equipment and arrange on a tray or Mayo stand (Figure 21–32).
2. Wash hands. Put on gloves.

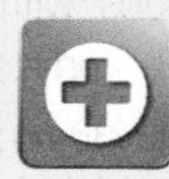
Precaution

CAUTION: Gloves must be worn when any contact with vaginal secretions is possible.

3. 
Comm

Introduce yourself. Identify the patient. Explain the procedure. Remember that this procedure has multiple steps.

4. Ask the patient to void. If a urinalysis is ordered, obtain the urine specimen at this time.

NOTE: An empty bladder makes it easier for the physician to palpate the uterus.

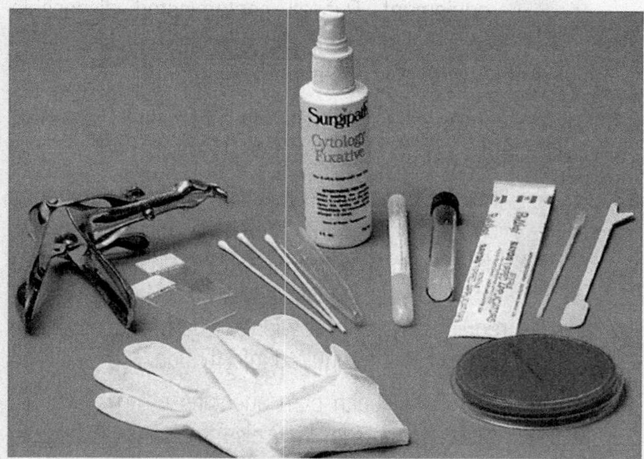

FIGURE 21–32 Basic equipment for a gynecological examination.

5. Ask the patient to remove all clothing and put on an examination gown. The gown is usually open in the front to facilitate the breast examination.
6. Make sure the extension of the examining table is pushed in or dropped down. Then assist the patient into a sitting position on the table. Use the drape to cover the patient's lap and legs.
7. Notify the physician that the patient is ready for examination.
8. The breasts are usually examined first. After the physician has examined the breasts, place the patient in the horizontal recumbent position. Drape correctly. The physician will usually complete the breast examination at this point.

Comm

NOTE: The patient should be taught how to do a breast self-examination, or BSE (refer to Figure 7–82). This can be done before or after the examination. Pamphlets describing the procedure, available from the American Cancer Society, can be given to the patient.

9. Place the patient in the lithotomy position. Drape correctly. Position the examining light for proper lighting.
10. Warm the vaginal speculum by placing it in warm water or rubbing it with a clean towel. Hand the speculum in the closed position to the physician. Have cotton-tipped applicators ready for use.

NOTE: Lubricant is not placed on the speculum because it can distort the shape of cervical cells for a Pap test and/or organisms if a culture is being obtained.

11. If a culture is to be taken, hand the sterile applicator to the physician. Take care to avoid contaminating the tip. Have the culture tube or slide available to receive the culture.
12. If a Pap test is to be done, hand the physician the cervical spatula (Ayer blade). Grasp the blade in the center and place the blunt end in the physician's hand. The V-shaped end is inserted in the patient by the physician.

NOTE: A cytology (cervical) brush may be used in place of or in addition to the cervical spatula. Again, grasp the brush in the center, with the brush end directed toward the patient, to hand the brush to the physician.

NOTE: If a ThinPrep Pap smear is being done, hand the physician the cytology (cervical) broom from the test kit (Figure 21–33).

NOTE: A Pap test is done to detect cancer of the cervix.

13. If a conventional Pap test is being performed:
    a. Have a slide ready for use. The physician will place the smear on the slide or hand the cervical spatula or cytology brush to you. If the latter, spread the smear evenly and moderately thin on the slide.

(continues)

PROCEDURE 21:4B (CONT.)

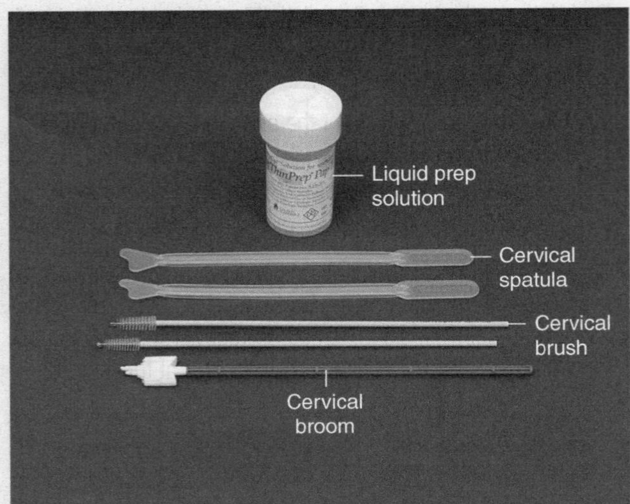

FIGURE 21–33 A cervical broom is usually used to perform a ThinPrep Pap smear, but some physicians use a cervical spatula.

NOTE: If the smear is too thick, the cells cannot be seen.

b. Put the cervical spatula or cytology brush in the infectious-waste bag.

c. Frequently, two or three slides are prepared: a cervical smear, a vaginal smear, and/or an endocervical smear. Label each slide with the patient's name and place a *C* on the cervical slide, a *V* on the vaginal smear, and an *E* on the endocervical smear.

d. Apply fixative to the slide(s). The fixative is usually a spray that is applied to the entire slide. Sometimes the entire slide is placed in a specimen jar containing fixative solution.

NOTE: Fixative makes the cells adhere (stick) to the slide until the slide is examined.

14. If a ThinPrep Pap test is being performed:

a. Grasp the cytology broom in the middle as the physician hands it to you.

b. Vigorously swish the cytology broom in the ThinPrep solution to wash the specimen off the brush.

NOTE: This suspends the entire specimen in the solution. At the laboratory, the solution will be processed to eliminate blood cells, mucus, and any other substances. The remaining cervical cells are then placed on a slide for examination. By eliminating other cells and debris, the slide can be read much more accurately by either a computerized or manual method.

c. Close the lid on the ThinPrep solution container.

d. Discard the cytology broom in an infectious-waste bag.

15. When the physician hands you the vaginal speculum, place it in the towel-lined basin. If it is disposable, place it in the infectious-waste bag.

16. The digital (finger) examination is usually done next. Place lubricant on the physician's gloved fingers without touching the gloves. The physician usually does a digital examination of both the vagina and rectum.

17. When the examination is complete, assist the patient out of the lithotomy position. Offer tissue to the patient to remove excess lubrication. Place the tissue in the infectious-waste bag. If no signs of weakness or dizziness are noted, help the patient get off the table.

Safety

CAUTION: Watch the patient closely to prevent falls.

18.  Comm

Inform the patient how and when she will be notified of test results. Ask the patient to get dressed or assist with dressing if necessary.

19.  Comm

Completely label all cultures and slides with the patient's name, identification number, and physician's name. Print all information on the lab requisition form or use a computer-generated label. This might include date, time, patient's name, address, identification number, physician's name and identification number, type or site of specimen, test ordered, date of last menstrual period, and information on any hormone therapy. Be sure you have all required information before the patient leaves the office.

20. Send all specimens to the laboratory as soon as possible.

21. Precaution

Wear gloves while cleaning and sterilizing the speculum and any contaminated instruments or equipment. Put all contaminated disposable supplies in the infectious-waste bag. Use a disinfectant to wipe any contaminated areas.

22. Remove gloves and discard in an infectious-waste bag. Wash hands.

23. Comm

Record all required information on the patient's chart or enter it into the computer. For example: date, time, GYN examination, Pap smear sent to lab, and your signature and title. Place a copy of any lab requisitions in the patient's chart. The physician sometimes records the required information.

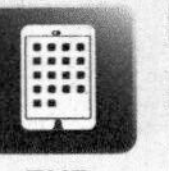
EHR

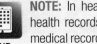

NOTE: In health care agencies using electronic health records (EHRs), also known as electronic medical records (EMRs), the information is entered directly into the patient's record on a computer.

PROCEDURE 21:4B (CONT.)

PRACTICE: **Go to the workbook and use the evaluation sheet for 21:4B, Assisting with a Gynecological Examination, to practice this procedure. When you believe you have mastered this skill, sign the sheet and give it to your instructor for further action.**

Check

FINAL CHECKPOINT: Using the criteria listed on the evaluation sheet, your instructor will grade your performance.

PROCEDURE 21:4C

Assisting with a General Physical Examination

NOTE: The equipment and steps of this procedure can vary from physician to physician.

Equipment and Supplies

Tray or Mayo stand and cover, patient gown, drape or sheet, basin lined with paper towels, tissues, scale, Snellen chart, thermometer, stethoscope, sphygmomanometer, ophthalmoscope, otoscope, nasal speculum, tuning fork, tongue depressors, percussion hammer, new safety pin or sensory wheel, rectal speculum or proctoscope, Pap test kit and vaginal speculum (female), culture tubes, slides, fixative solution, sterile applicators, lubricant, alcohol swabs, gloves, penlight or examining light, infectious-waste bag, patient's chart, lab requisition forms, pen, and/or computer

Procedure

1. Assemble equipment. Arrange equipment conveniently on the Mayo stand or tray (Figure 21–34).
2. Wash hands. Put on gloves or have gloves available for later use.

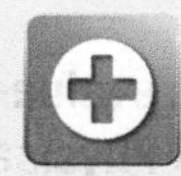

Precaution

CAUTION: Gloves must be worn anytime contact with blood or body fluids is possible. Observe standard precautions at all times.

3. 

Comm

Introduce yourself. Identify the patient. Explain the procedure. Remember that this procedure has multiple steps.

4. Ask the patient to remove all clothing and put on an examining gown. Ask the patient to void. If a urinalysis is ordered, collect the urine specimen at this time.

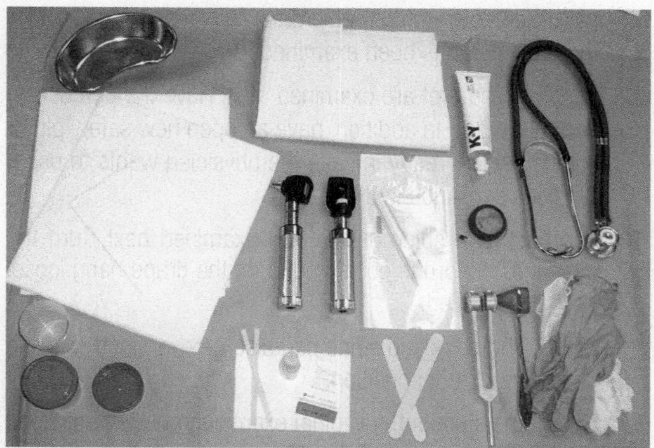

FIGURE 21–34 Equipment and supplies for a physical examination should be arranged in a convenient order.

5. Do any of the required following procedures:
   a. Record height and weight.
   b. Take and record TPR (temperature, pulse, respiration) and/or BP (blood pressure).
   c. Use a Snellen chart to test visual acuity; record results.
   d. Check visual acuity with a Jaeger card and/or Ishihara plates; record results.
   e. Perform an audiometric screening if ordered; record results.
   f. Run an electrocardiogram if ordered.
   g. Obtain all required blood samples for tests ordered.
6. Seat the patient on the examining table. Drape the patient correctly.
7. Notify the physician that the patient is ready.

(continues)

PROCEDURE 21:4C (CONT.)

8. Assist with eye, ear, nose, and throat examination as previously instructed.
9. Give the physician the stethoscope and/or sphygmomanometer. Remain quiet while the patient's heart and lungs are examined.

   NOTE: The physician may check the blood pressure.

   NOTE: The physician may also do an initial examination of the breasts, legs, and feet.
10. Place the patient in the horizontal recumbent or supine position. Drape correctly.
11. The physician will examine the chest and abdomen. Draw the drape down to the pubic area. Replace the drape after the abdomen has been examined.
12. The legs and feet are examined next. Have the percussion hammer ready. In addition, have an open new safety pin or sensory wheel ready in case the physician wants to use it to check sensation in the feet.
13. The back and spine are usually examined next. Turn the patient to the prone position and let the drape hang loose. Assist as needed.

    NOTE: The back and spine can also be examined with the patient in a sitting position.
14. On a female patient, a vaginal examination is usually done next. Put the patient in the lithotomy position. Drape correctly. Assist as taught for a gynecological examination. The male patient can be placed in the horizontal recumbent position for a genital organ examination.

    NOTE: Male patients should be taught how to do a testicular self-examination. This can be done at this point or at the end of the examination.
15. The rectal area is examined last in most cases. A female can be examined while still in the lithotomy position or in the Sims' position. A male is usually placed in the Sims' position. Hand gloves and lubricant to the physician, as needed. Have the rectal speculum or anoscope in a closed position ready for use. If the physician wants to check fecal occult blood, put on gloves. Hand guaiac paper to the physician.

    NOTE: The physician will place a small amount of fecal material on the guaiac paper. To test the paper, add one to two drops of hemoccult developing solution to the paper. A color change indicates the presence of blood in the stool.

    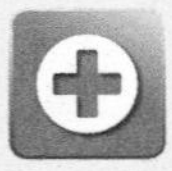
    Precaution

    CAUTION: Gloves must be worn any time contact with fecal material is possible.
16. 
    Comm

    When the examination is complete, assist the patient into a sitting position on the examination table. Allow the patient to rest for a few minutes. If no signs of weakness or dizziness are noted, help the patient get off the table. Inform the patient how and when he or she will be notified of test results. Ask the patient to get dressed or assist with dressing if necessary.

    Safety

    CAUTION: Watch closely to prevent falls.
17. 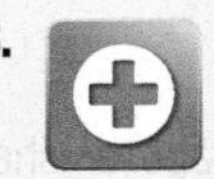
    Comm

    Label all specimens and cultures with the patient's name, identification number, and physician's name. Print all information on the lab requisition form(s) or use a computer-generated form. This might include date, time, patient's name, address, identification number, physician's name and identification number, type or site of specimen, and test ordered. Send specimens to the laboratory as soon as possible.
18. Precaution

    Wear gloves while cleaning and sterilizing any contaminated instruments or equipment. Put all contaminated disposable supplies in the infectious-waste bag. Use a disinfectant to wipe any contaminated areas.
19. Remove gloves and discard in an infectious-waste bag. Wash hands.
20. Comm

    Record all required information on the patient's chart or enter it into the computer. For example: date, time, physical examination, throat culture and Pap smear sent to laboratory, and your signature and title. Place a copy of any lab requisition forms in the patient's chart. The physician sometimes records the required information.

    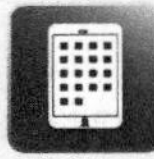
    EHR

    NOTE: In laboratories or offices using electronic health records (EHRs), also known as electronic medical records (EMRs), the information is entered into the patient's EHR on a computer.

PRACTICE: Go to the workbook and use the evaluation sheet for 21:4C, Assisting with a General Physical Examination, to practice this procedure. When you believe you have mastered this skill, sign the sheet and give it to your instructor for further action.

Check

FINAL CHECKPOINT: Using the criteria listed on the evaluation sheet, your instructor will grade your performance.

21:5 Assisting with Minor Surgery and Suture Removal

As a health care worker, you may be required to prepare for and assist with minor surgery or suture removal in a medical, dental, or health care facility. Minor surgery includes removing warts, cysts, tumors, growths, or foreign objects; performing biopsies of skin growths or tumors; suturing wounds; incising and draining body areas; and other similar procedures.

Instruments and equipment used depend on the type of surgery or procedure being done. Some basic instruments and supplies that may be used (Figure 21–35) include the following:

- **Scalpels**: instruments with a handle attached to knife blades; used to incise (cut) skin and tissue; disposable scalpels with a protective retractable blade to prevent sharps injuries are also available for use (Figure 21–36)
- **Surgical scissors**: special scissors with blunt ends or sharp points or a combination; identified as sharp-sharp, sharp-blunt, or blunt-blunt; used to cut tissue

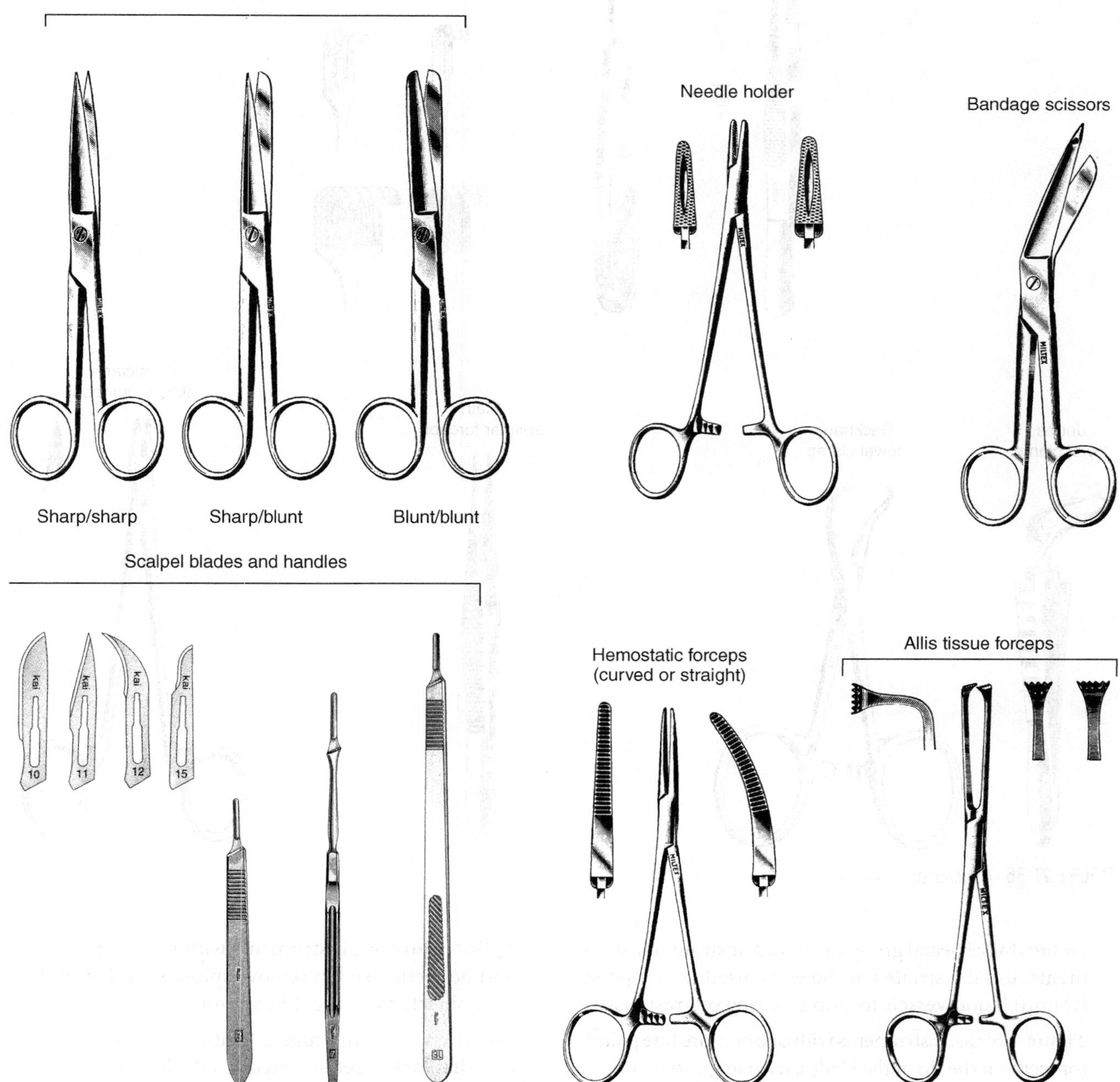

FIGURE 21–35 Some sample surgical instruments. *(continued)* Courtesy of Miltex, Inc.

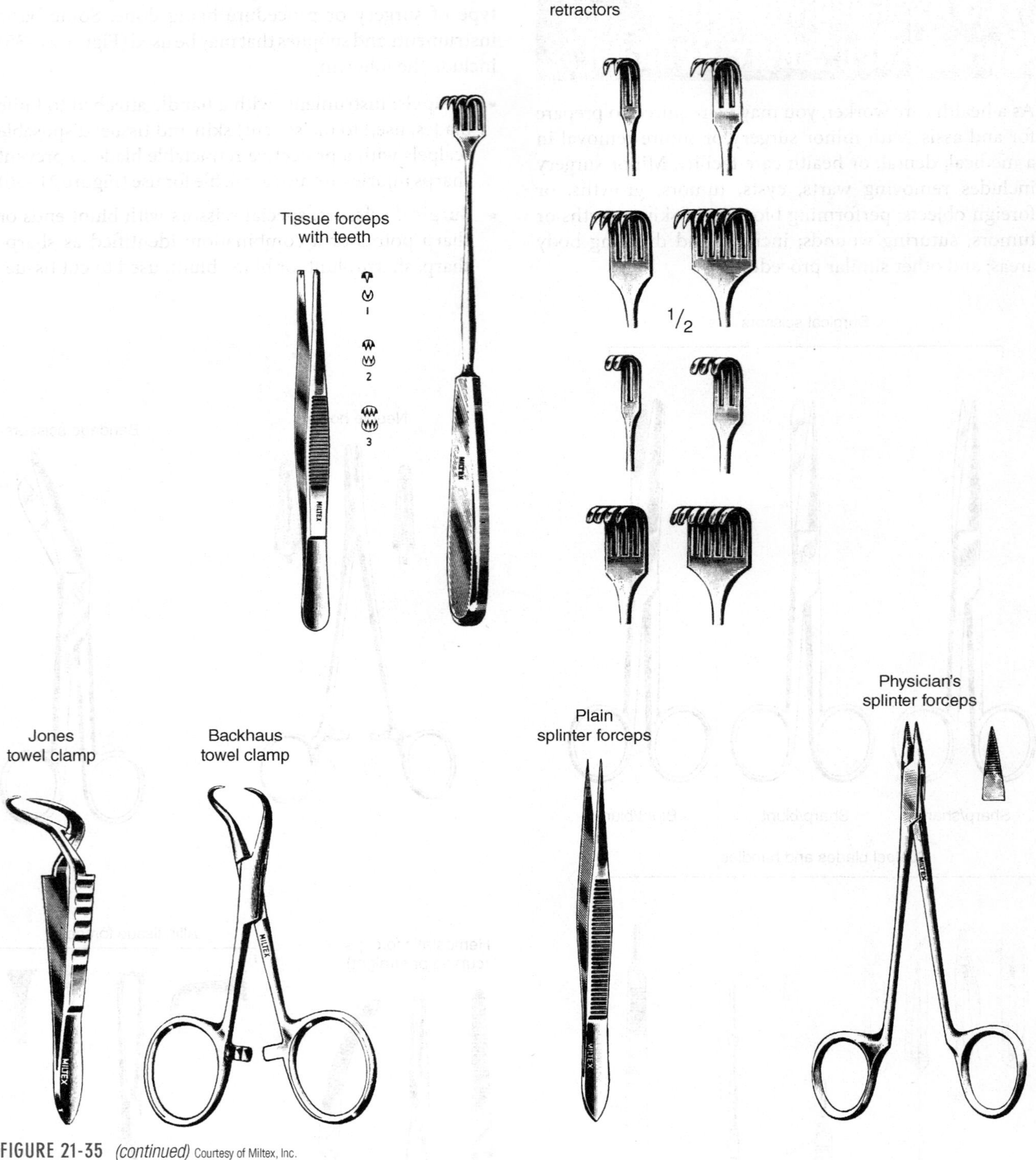

FIGURE 21-35 *(continued)* Courtesy of Miltex, Inc.

- **Hemostats**: special group of curved or straight instruments, usually striated at the ends; used to compress (clamp) blood vessels to stop bleeding or grasp tissue
- **Tissue forceps**: instruments with one or more fine points (or teeth) at the tip of the blades; used to grasp tissue
- **Splinter forceps**: instruments with fine-pointed ends and no teeth; used to remove splinters and other foreign objects from the skin and/or tissues
- **Towel clamps**: instruments with sharp points at the end that lock together; used to attach surgical drapes

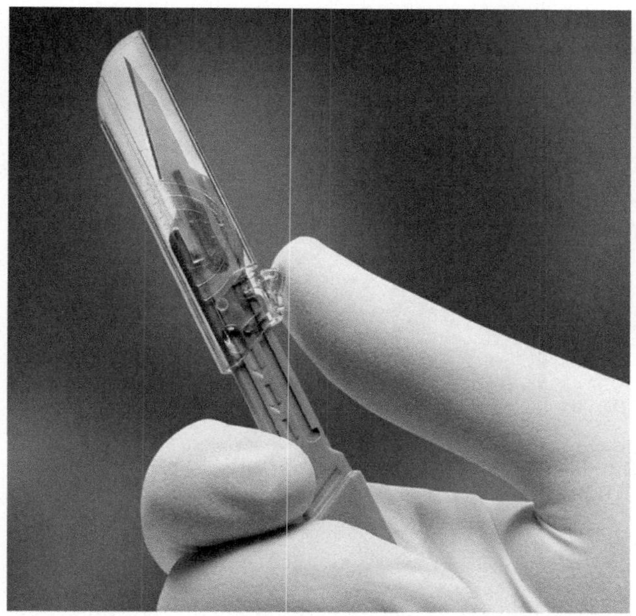

FIGURE 21–36 **Disposable scalpels with a protective retractable blade help prevent sharps injuries.** Photo reprinted courtesy of BD [Becton, Dickinson and Company]

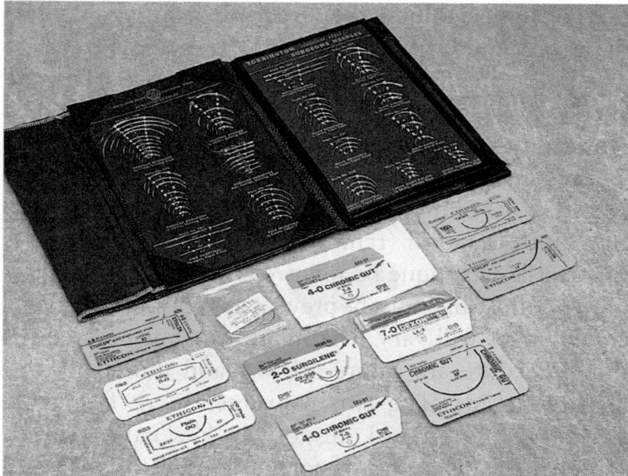

FIGURE 21–37 **A wide variety of suture materials and needles are available for minor surgeries.**

to each other; also used to clamp on to tissue that has been dissected (separated or cut into pieces)

- **Retractors**: instruments used to hold or draw back the lips, or sides, of a wound or incision; also called *skin hooks*
- *Suture materials:* special materials used for stitches (**sutures**); applied to hold a wound or incision closed; absorbable suture material such as surgical gut or vicryl is digested by tissue enzymes and absorbed by the body; nonabsorbable suture materials such as silk, nylon, Dacron, stainless steel, and metal skin clips or staples are removed after the tissue or skin has healed (Figure 21–37)
- **Needle holder**: special instrument used to hold or support the needle while sutures are being inserted
- *Needle:* pointed, slender instrument with an eye at one end; used to hold suture material while sutures are being inserted into an incision or wound; usually curved for easier insertion into the skin; *swaged* needles have the suture material attached to the needle as one unit
- **Bandage scissors**: special scissors with blunt lower ends; used to remove dressings and bandages; the blunt ends prevent injury to the skin directly next to the dressing material

Preparation of the surgical tray requires the use of strict sterile technique to prevent infection. Instruments and supplies must be sterilized. Care must be taken to avoid contaminating the instruments and supplies when they are placed on the tray. Complete sterile setups are also available in commercially prepared, disposable packages. Examples include setups for insertion of sutures and for removal of sutures. It is important to follow sterile technique (see Chapter 15:8) while opening the packages to maintain sterility of all materials in the package.

A skin prep is sometimes done before minor surgery. This means that the surgical site is cleansed thoroughly with an antiseptic soap. If the surgical area has excessive hair, the area may be shaved. Shaving the surgical area is controversial because shaving increases the risk for abrasions leaving open areas that are prone to infection. The person doing the skin prep should wear gloves. The entire surgical area must be washed thoroughly with an antiseptic soap. If the site is shaved, the skin is held taut while a disposable razor is used to shave in the direction of hair growth. It is important to avoid nicking the patient with the razor. The procedure is described in detail in Procedure 22:13A.

Before minor surgery, a local anesthetic is often administered by the physician. This numbs the surgical site and decreases pain. Before the injection of local anesthesia, the physician may apply a liquid or spray topical anesthetic to the surface of the skin to decrease the pain of the injection. Anesthetics must be available for use. They are usually placed on the side of the sterile tray. Sterile needles and syringes can be placed on the surgical tray or kept in their packages by the side of the tray.

During surgery, the medical assistant will be expected to assist as needed. The procedure will depend on the physician doing the surgery. Be alert to all points of the procedure and be ready to help as needed.

Sterile dressings must be available for use. These are usually placed directly on the surgical tray so that they are readily accessible. Some physicians prefer that sterile dressings be left in the original sterile wrappers and placed in the immediate area.

Suture removal (removal of stitches) also requires that sterile technique be followed. Infection is an ever-present threat and must be prevented. Again, instruments and supplies will vary. The main instruments used for this procedure are suture scissors and thumb forceps (Figure 21–38). The two instruments are frequently packaged in sterilized, disposable kits called **suture removal sets**. The thumb forcep is used to grasp and hold the suture. It is compressed with the thumb and forefinger. The suture scissors have a curved blade that is inserted under the suture material so that the stitch can be cut and removed. Basic guidelines are provided in Procedure 21:5B.

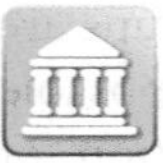
Legal

Before any minor surgery, the patient must sign a written consent form. The consent form must describe the procedure, cite alternative treatments, and list possible complications and/or risks of the surgery. If the patient is a minor or is incompetent, an authorized person must sign the form. Most offices also provide written preoperative and postoperative instructions.

Comm

Patients who are undergoing minor surgery or suture removal are often fearful and apprehensive. Reassure the patient to the best of your ability. Refer specific questions regarding the surgery or procedure to the physician.

Body tissues, abnormal growths, and other specimens removed during surgery are usually sent to a laboratory for examination. Each specimen must be placed in an appropriate container immediately to avoid loss. A biopsy specimen is usually placed in a formalin solution that preserves the specimen until it can be examined. Most laboratories will provide a health care facility with the required specimen containers. The containers must be labeled correctly, and the lab requisition form must be filled in completely. Many labs use computer generated forms. The specimens should be sent to the laboratory as soon as possible.

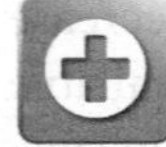
Precaution

Because contamination from blood and body fluids is possible during minor surgical procedures, standard precautions (discussed in Chapter 15:4) must be observed at all times. Hands must be washed frequently, and gloves must be worn. If splashing of blood or other body fluids is possible, a gown, mask, and eye protection must be worn. Instruments and equipment must be properly cleaned and sterilized after use. Contaminated areas must be wiped with a disinfectant. Contaminated disposable supplies must be placed in an infectious-waste bag prior to being disposed of according to legal requirements. Sharp objects such as scalpel blades (or disposable scalpels) and needles must be placed in a leakproof puncture-resistant sharps container immediately after use. The medical assistant must always be aware of and take steps to prevent the spread of infection.

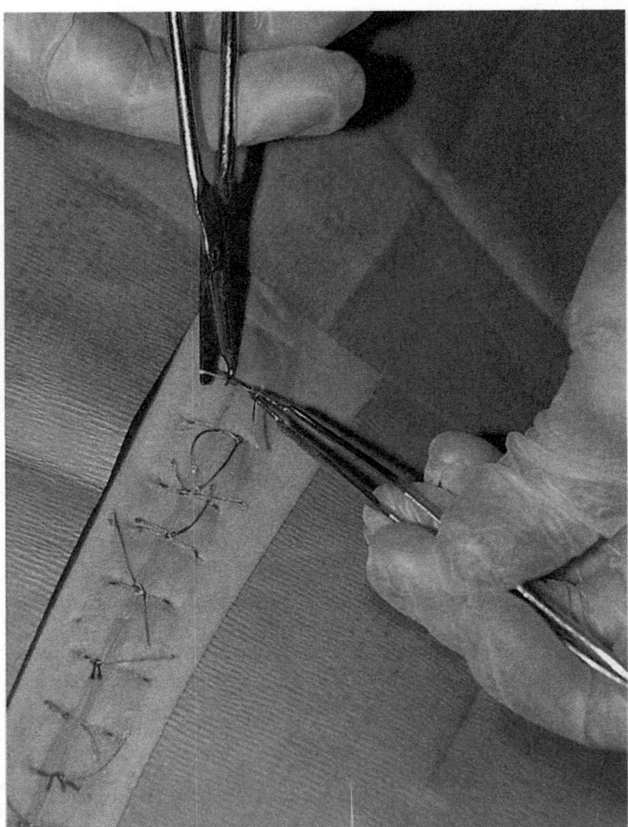

FIGURE 21–38 A suture removal set consists of suture scissors and thumb forceps.

STUDENT: **Go to the workbook and complete the assignment sheet for 21:5, Assisting with Minor Surgery and Suture Removal. Then return and continue with the procedures.**

PROCEDURE 21:5A

Assisting with Minor Surgery

NOTE: Instruments and procedures vary depending on the type of surgery and the physician.

Equipment and Supplies

Tray with cover or Mayo stand, infectious-waste bag, sharps container, personal protective equipment (disposable gloves, mask, eye protection, gown), tape, patient gown, patient's chart, lab requisition forms, pen and/or computer

NOTE: All the following equipment should be sterile: towels, drapes and towel clamps, two to three pairs of sterile gloves, needle and syringe, anesthetic medication, basin, antiseptic solution, gauze pads, scalpel and blades, surgical scissors, hemostat forceps (straight and curved), tissue forceps, retractors, needle holder, needle, suture material, and dressings (gauze and pads).

Procedure

1. Assemble equipment required.
2. Wash hands.
3. Check dates and sterilization indicators on all sterile supplies to make sure the supplies are still sterile. Make sure that the package has not been wet and that there are no tears or openings on the wrap.

   NOTE: Many sterile supplies are good for 1 month only.
4. Place the tray or stand in an area where there is freedom of movement and limited chance of contamination.
5. Open a sterile towel and place it on the tray so that the entire tray is covered.

   NOTE: Follow the correct procedure to avoid contamination (see Chapter 15:8).
6. Open the other sterile towels or drapes and place them on the tray.
7. Open a sterile basin. Place it on the tray. Put the sterile gauze in the basin. Obtain the correct antiseptic solution and pour a small amount of the solution in a sink or separate container to rinse the lip of the bottle. Then hold the solution bottle approximately 6 inches above the sterile basin and carefully pour the required amount of solution into the sterile basin.

   NOTE: Read the label three times to be sure you have the correct solution.

   Safety
   CAUTION: Avoid handling the inside of the solution bottle cap. If the cap is placed on a counter, make sure the open end, or inside, is facing up. This prevents contamination of the inside of the cap.

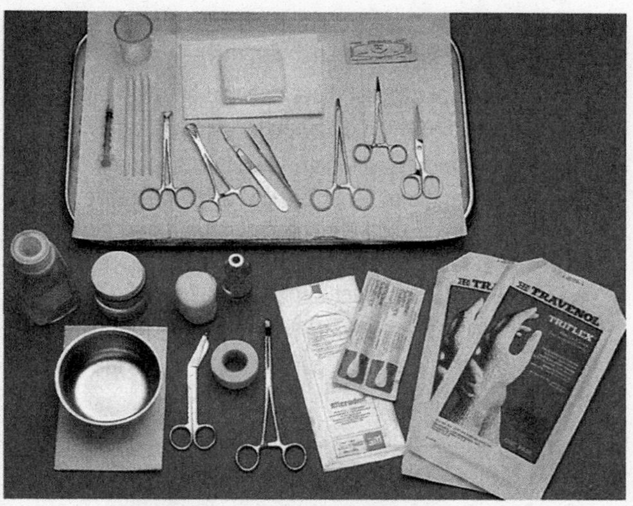

FIGURE 21–39 **Instruments and supplies for minor surgery should be arranged in a convenient order. Wrapped sterile items and nonsterile items are placed by the tray.**

Safety
CAUTION: Do *not* splash the solution onto the tray.

8. Open all wrapped instruments and place them on the tray in a convenient order, usually the order of use (Figure 21–39).

   NOTE: Number and type of instruments will depend on the type of surgery and the physician.
9. Open the needle and syringe and place it on the tray. Unless the physician has specified a certain size, have a variety of needles of different gauges available.
10. Open the suture packages. Place them on the tray. If specific sizes and types have not been requested by the physician, a variety of materials should be made available.
11. Place the sterile dressings on the tray. The outer dressings should be placed on the bottom of the pile. This way, the dressings are in the order of use.

    NOTE: In some offices the dressings and bandages are kept in their sterile wraps and placed to the side of the tray to be opened as needed at the end of the procedure.
12. Check the tray to be sure everything is present. Use a sterile towel to cover the tray.

Safety
CAUTION: Do *not* leave the tray unattended because contamination of the materials may occur.

(continues)

PROCEDURE 21:5A (CONT.)

13. Place the anesthetic solution, sterile gloves, tape, and infectious-waste bag close to the tray.

    NOTE: Several pairs of gloves should be available in case one pair becomes contaminated.

14. 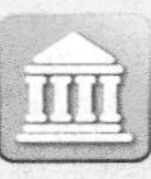 Comm Introduce yourself. Identify the patient. Confirm that the patient observed all preoperative instructions. Explain the procedure and preview postoperative orders. Ascertain that the patient has signed a written consent form.

     Legal **NOTE:** If the patient is a minor or is incompetent, an authorized person must sign the consent form.

15. Ask the patient to empty the bladder, remove clothing as necessary for the procedure, and put on a patient gown. Provide privacy for the patient or assist if necessary.
16. Take and record the patient's vital signs.
17. Position and drape the patient according to the surgery to be performed.
18. If necessary, prep the surgical site. Wash hands and put on gloves. Wash the site thoroughly with an antiseptic soap. If a skin shave has been ordered, hold the skin taut and use a disposable razor to shave in the direction of hair growth. Discard long hairs on a gauze pad or paper towel. Rinse the area and then pat it dry with gauze.

    Safety **CAUTION:** Be careful not to nick the skin.

    NOTE: Sometimes the physician prefers to do the skin prep before the surgery. Some minor surgeries will not require a skin prep.

    NOTE: The procedure for a skin prep is discussed in detail in Procedure 22:13A.

19. During the surgery, assist as needed:
    a. Uncover the tray when ready for use.
    b. Give the sterile gloves to the physician.

       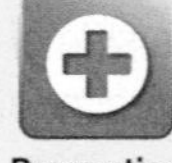 Precaution **CAUTION:** If splashing of blood or body fluids is possible, a gown, mask, and eye protection must be worn. Observe all standard precautions while performing or assisting with minor surgery.

    c. The physician will apply sterile drapes. Have towel clamps ready for the physician to use to hold the drapes in position. The physician may cleanse the surgical site with an antiseptic.
    d. When the physician is ready to inject the anesthetic, use a gauze pad saturated with alcohol to clean the top of the anesthetic solution vial. Hold the vial in a convenient position so the physician can fill the syringe (Figure 21–40). The physician will then inject the anesthetic. The needle and syringe should be discarded immediately into a sharps container.
    e. If required, put on sterile gloves and assist as needed. Hold retractors, hand instruments, and assist with the procedure.
    f. If tissue or a biopsy specimen is removed, open the lid of the specimen container. Hold the container close to the physician so the specimen can be placed into the container (Figure 21–41). Immediately close the lid on the container.
    g. Get additional supplies or equipment as needed.

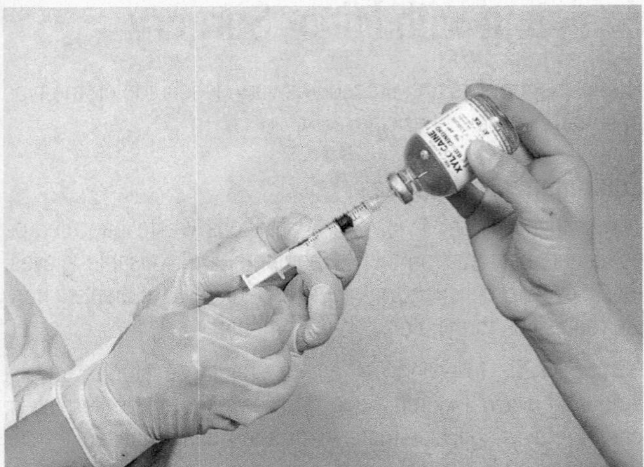

FIGURE 21–40 **Hold the anesthetic solution in a convenient position so the physician can fill the syringe without contaminating the needle.**

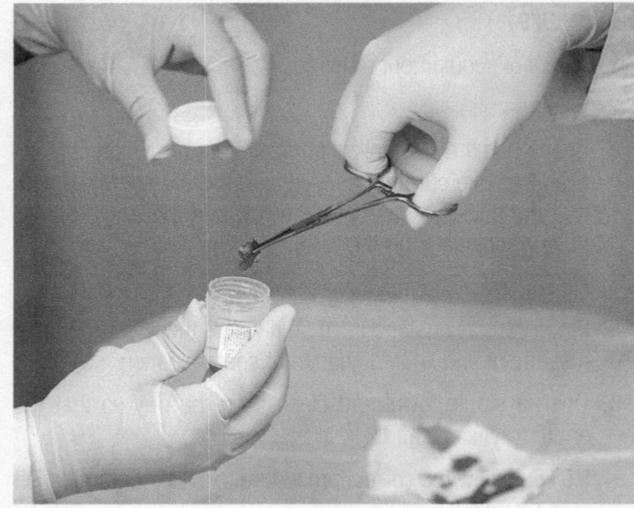

FIGURE 21–41 **Tissue or biopsy specimens removed during minor surgery must be placed in the correct type of specimen container so they can be examined by a pathologist.**

PROCEDURE 21:5A (CONT.)

20. 
Comm
After the surgery, assist as needed with placement of dressings and bandages. Observe for any signs of distress. If no signs of weakness or dizziness are noted, help the patient get off the table. Review postoperative orders with the patient. Provide the patient with a written copy of postoperative orders if this is office policy. Inform the patient how and when he or she will be notified of test results.

21. 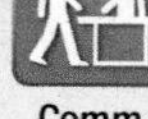
Comm
Label all specimens correctly with the patient's name, identification number, and physician's name or use a computer-generated label. Print all information on the lab requisition form. This might include date, time, patient's name, address, identification number, physician's name and identification number, type or site of specimen, and test ordered. Make sure each specimen is in the correct specimen container or bottle. Check the lids on the containers to make sure they are closed securely. Send specimens to the laboratory as soon as possible.

NOTE: Pathologists will provide special containers for most health care facilities.

22. 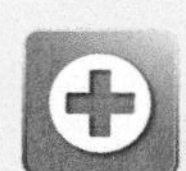
Precaution
Wear gloves to clean and sterilize all instruments and equipment. Put sharp objects such as the needle and syringe and scalpel blade (or disposable scalpel) in the sharps container immediately after use. Put contaminated disposable supplies in the infectious-waste container. Use a disinfectant to wipe any contaminated areas. Put all equipment in its correct place.

23. Remove gloves and discard in an infectious-waste bag. Wash hands.

24. 
Comm
Record all required information on the patient's chart or enter it into the computer. For example: date, time, surgical removal of tumor on right forearm, specimen sent to pathology lab, verbal and written postoperative instructions given to patient, and your signature and title. Place a copy of any lab requisitions in the patient's chart. The physician sometimes records the required information.

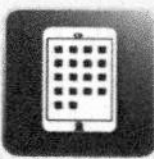
EHR
NOTE: In health care agencies using electronic health records (EHRs), also known as electronic medical records (EMRs), the information is entered directly into the patient's record on a computer.

PRACTICE: **Go to the workbook and use the evaluation sheet for 21:5A, Assisting with Minor Surgery, to practice this procedure. When you believe you have mastered this skill, sign the sheet and give it to your instructor for further action.**

Check
FINAL CHECKPOINT: Using the criteria listed on the evaluation sheet, your instructor will grade your performance.

PROCEDURE 21:5B

Assisting with Suture Removal

NOTE: The procedure for suture removal varies according to the physician. The following serves as a basic guideline only.

Equipment and Supplies

Tray or Mayo stand, suture removal set, sterile towel, sterile gloves, drapes (as needed), dressings (as indicated), sterile basin, sterile gauze, antiseptic solution, tape, infectious-waste bag, sharps container, patient gown if needed, patient's chart, pen and/or computer

Procedure

1. Assemble required equipment.
2. Wash hands.
3. Check the dates and sterilization indicators on all sterile supplies to make sure the supplies are still sterile. Make sure that the package has not been wet and that there are no tears or openings on the wrap.
4. Place a sterile towel on the tray.

   NOTE: Follow the correct procedure for unwrapping and placing all supplies. Refer to Chapter 15:8.
5. Place a sterile basin on the tray. Put gauze and antiseptic solution in the basin.
6. Place dressings on the tray. Outer dressings should be on the bottom. This way, dressings are in order of use.

(continues)

PROCEDURE 21:5A (CONT.)

NOTE: In some offices the dressings and bandages are kept in their sterile wraps and placed to the side of the tray to be opened as needed at the end of the procedure.

7. Place the sterile suture removal set on the tray.
8. Place a sterile towel or needed drapes on the tray.
9. Check the tray to be sure all equipment is present (Figure 21–42).

Safety

CAUTION: Do *not* leave the tray unattended.

10. Put the infectious-waste bag, tape, and sterile gloves near the tray.
11. Introduce yourself. Identify the patient. Explain the procedure. Obtain the patient's consent.

Comm

12. If necessary, ask the patient to remove clothing and put on a patient gown. Position and drape according to location of sutures. Reassure the patient as needed.
13. Assist the physician as necessary during the procedure.

NOTE: Frequently, medical assistants are trained and authorized to remove sutures.

14. When the sutures have been removed, place a clean dressing and bandages on the wound. Use dressing forceps or wear sterile gloves to apply a sterile dressing to the site (Figure 21–43A). Then apply roller gauze and/or tape to anchor the dressing in place (Figure 21–43B).

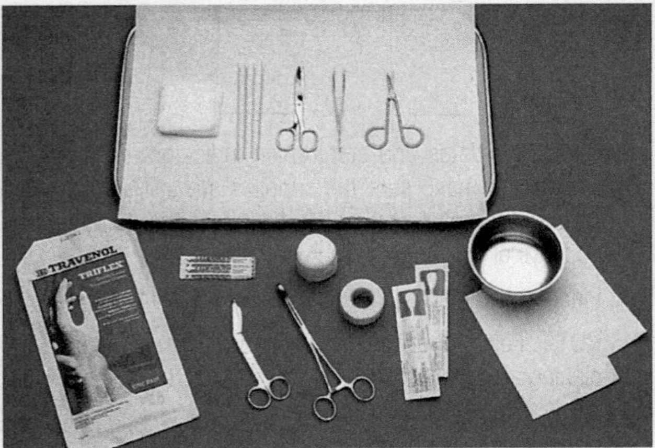

FIGURE 21–42 A sample suture removal tray setup.

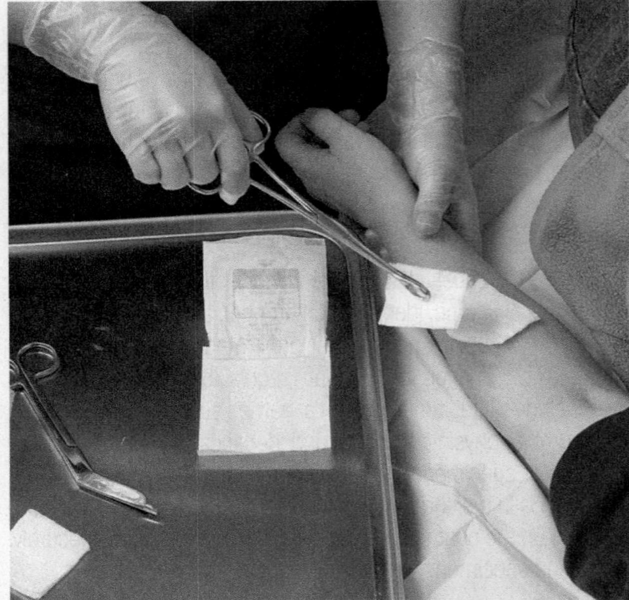

FIGURE 21–43A **Use dressing forceps or wear sterile gloves to apply a sterile dressing to the site.**

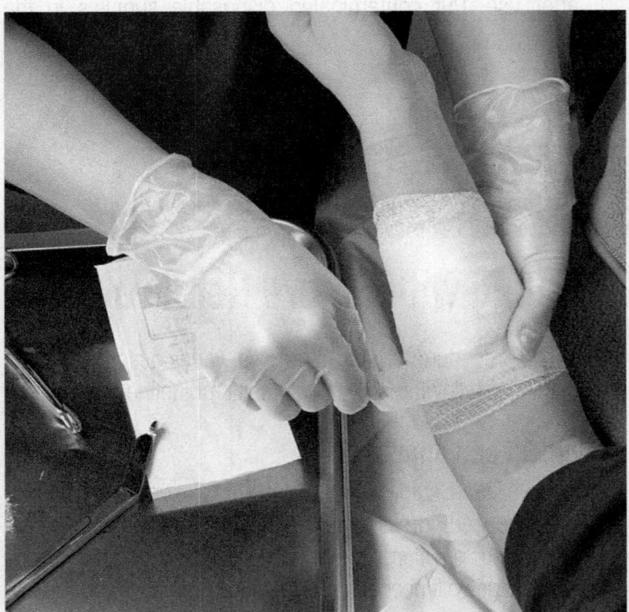

FIGURE 21–43B **Anchor the dressing in place with roller gauze and/or tape.**

PROCEDURE 21:5A (CONT.)

15.  Comm Instruct the patient on wound care and provide written instructions if this is office policy. Watch closely for signs of distress. If no signs of weakness or dizziness are noted, help the patient get off the table.

16. 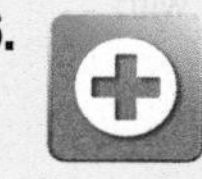 Precaution Wear gloves to clean and sterilize all instruments. If the suture set is disposable, place it in a sharps container. Put all contaminated disposable supplies in the infectious-waste bag. Use a disinfectant to wipe any contaminated areas.

17. Remove gloves and discard in an infectious-waste bag. Wash hands.

18. 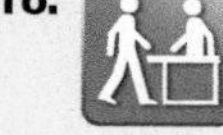 Comm Record all required information on the patient's chart or enter it into the computer. For example: date, time, sutures removed from right forearm, sterile dressing applied, and your signature and title. The physician sometimes records the required information.

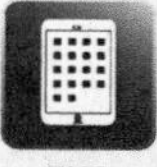 EHR **NOTE:** In laboratories or offices using electronic health records (EHRs), also known as electronic medical records (EMRs), the information is entered into the patient's EHR on a computer.

PRACTICE: **Go to the workbook and use the evaluation sheet for 21:5B, Assisting with Suture Removal, to practice this procedure. When you believe you have mastered this skill, sign the sheet and give it to your instructor for further action.**

 Check **FINAL CHECKPOINT:** Using the criteria listed on the evaluation sheet, your instructor will grade your performance.

21:6 Recording and Mounting an Electrocardiogram

 Science In order to understand an **electrocardiogram (ECG)**, it is essential to understand the electrical conduction pattern in the muscles of the heart (Figure 21–44). The contraction of the heart muscles is controlled by electrical impulses within the heart. The electrical impulse originates in the *sinoatrial (SA) node* of the heart, located near the top of the right atrium. The impulse moves through the atria, causing the muscles of the atria to contract. The impulse next travels to the *atrioventricular (AV) node*, through a band of fibers called the *bundle of His*, and then through the *right and left bundle branches* to the final branches, called the *Purkinje fibers*. The Purkinje fibers distribute the impulse to the muscles of the right and left ventricles, which then contract.

The movement of the electrical impulse is recorded by an electrocardiograph machine as a series of waves known as a *PQRST complex*. The P wave occurs as the impulse originates in the SA node and travels through the atria. The QRS wave represents the movement of the impulse through the AV node, bundle of His, bundle branches, and Purkinje fibers. The T wave represents the *repolarization* of the ventricles, or the period of recovery in the ventricles before another contraction occurs.

The pattern of electrical current in the heart is recorded by an electrocardiograph machine as an ECG. Each PQRST pattern represents the electrical activity that occurs during each contraction of the heart muscle; thus, each PQRST complex represents one heartbeat. Because an abnormal pattern of the electrical impulses will be evident on an ECG, the ECG can be used to diagnose disease and/or damage to the muscles of the heart.

Using special electrodes, the electrical activity is recorded from different angles, called **leads**. The different leads give the physician a more complete picture of the heart. By noting an electrical disturbance in any of the leads, the physician can determine which parts of the heart are diseased or malfunctioning.

A complete ECG normally consists of 12 leads. Electrodes are placed at specific locations on the body to pick up the voltage present. Connections between the various electrodes create the various leads. The leads are labeled as 1 (I), 2 (II), 3 (III), aVR, aVL, aVF, V_1, V_2, V_3, V_4, V_5, and V_6. There are three classifications: standard, augmented, and chest leads (Figure 21–45).

- *Standard*, or *limb, leads:* Include leads 1 (I), 2 (II), and 3 (III) (Figure 21–46). Each records the voltage between two extremities.

  Lead 1 (I) connects the right arm and the left arm.

  Lead 2 (II) connects the right arm and the left leg.

  Lead 3 (III) connects the left arm and the left leg.

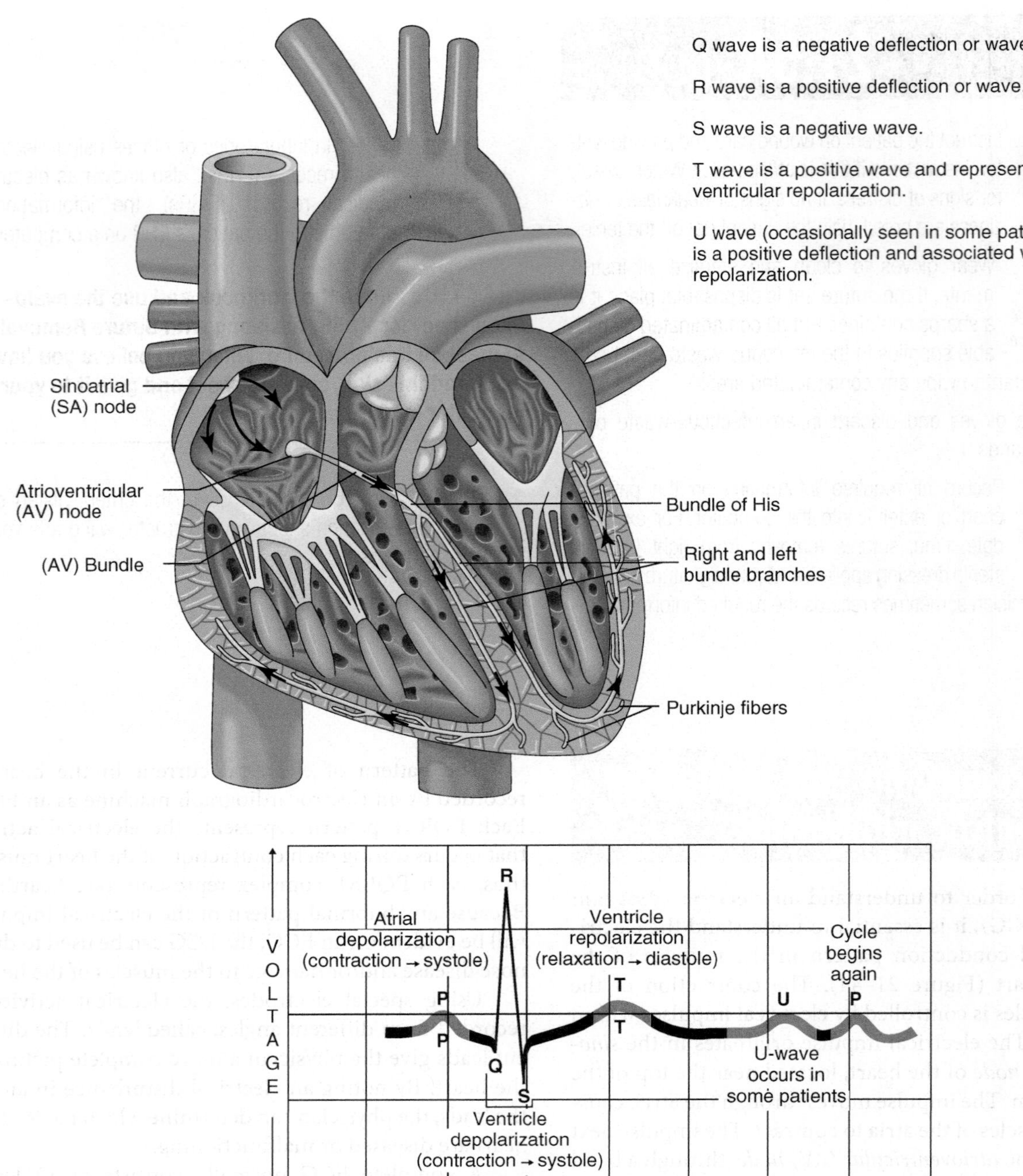

FIGURE 21–44 As the electrical impulse passes through the conduction pathway in the heart, it creates a pattern recorded as an electrocardiogram.

- *Augmented voltage leads:* Include aVR, aVL, and aVF. They are different angles of the standard leads 1 (I), 2 (II), and 3 (III). The aVR stands for augmented voltage right arm, aVL stands for augmented voltage left arm, and aVF stands for augmented voltage left foot.
- *Chest leads:* The six chest, or precordial, leads record angles of the electrical impulse from a central point within the heart to specific sites on the front of the chest (refer to Figure 21–46). Chest electrodes are placed at six specific locations on the chest to obtain these angles (refer back to Figure 21–45).

V_1: fourth intercostal (between ribs) space on the right side of the sternum (breastbone)

V_2: fourth intercostal space on the left side of the sternum

V_3: midway between the V_2 and V_4 positions

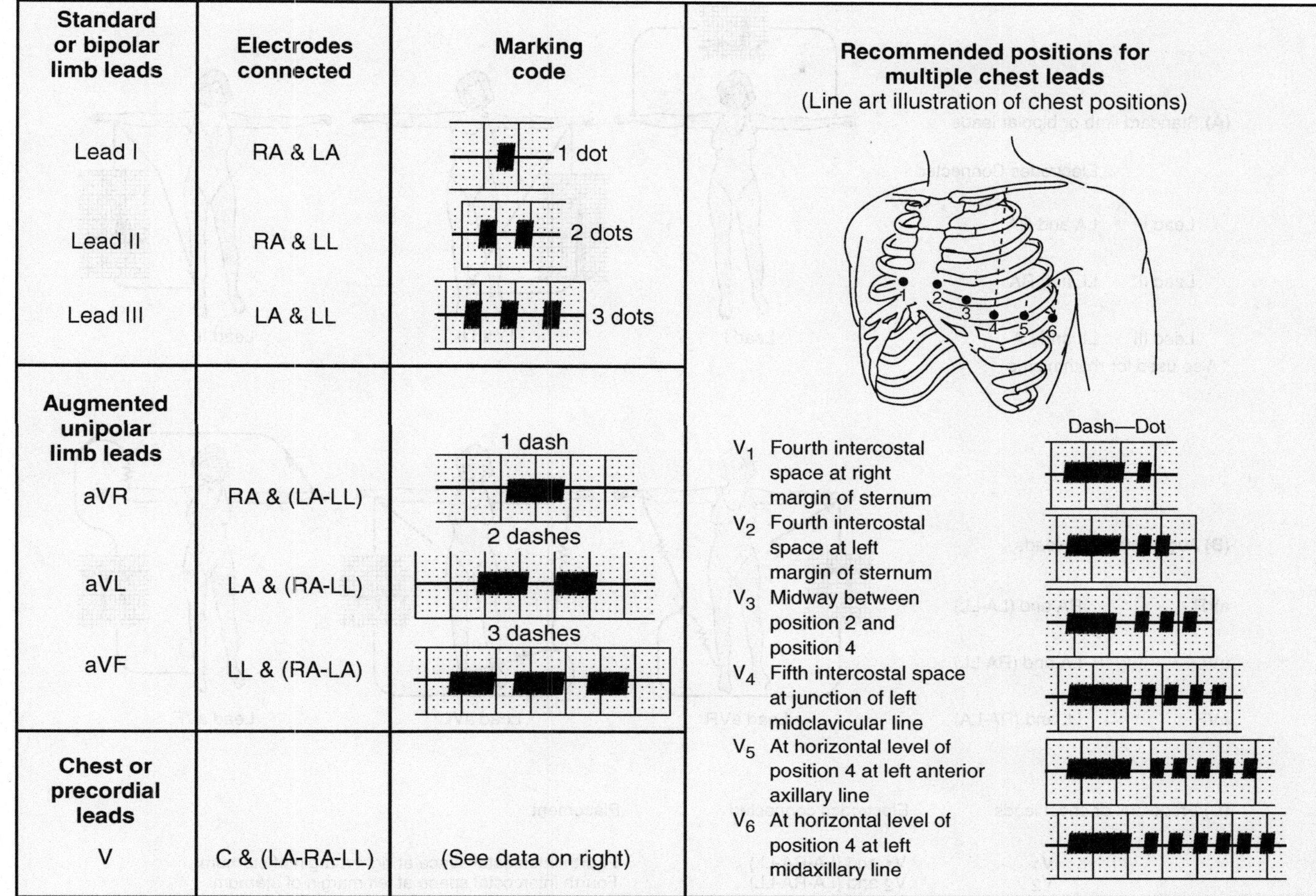

Standard or bipolar limb leads	Electrodes connected	Marking code	Recommended positions for multiple chest leads (Line art illustration of chest positions)
Lead I	RA & LA	1 dot	
Lead II	RA & LL	2 dots	
Lead III	LA & LL	3 dots	
Augmented unipolar limb leads			Dash—Dot
aVR	RA & (LA-LL)	1 dash	V_1 Fourth intercostal space at right margin of sternum
aVL	LA & (RA-LL)	2 dashes	V_2 Fourth intercostal space at left margin of sternum
aVF	LL & (RA-LA)	3 dashes	V_3 Midway between position 2 and position 4
			V_4 Fifth intercostal space at junction of left midclavicular line
Chest or precordial leads			V_5 At horizontal level of position 4 at left anterior axillary line
V	C & (LA-RA-LL)	(See data on right)	V_6 At horizontal level of position 4 at left midaxillary line

FIGURE 21–45 The lead arrangement and coding for a standard electrocardiogram. Courtesy of Quinton Cardiology, Inc.

V_4: fifth intercostal space at the junction of the midclavicular line (line drawn from the middle of the clavicle)

V_5: same level as 4 but at left anterior axillary line

V_6: same level as 4 but at left midaxillary line

Electrodes are placed on various parts of the body to record these 12 leads. The electrodes are coded so that each is put in the proper place. Codes are as follows:

- *RA* for right arm: Placed on the fleshy outer area of the upper part of the right arm
- *LA* for left arm: Placed on the fleshy outer area of the upper part of the left arm
- *RL* for right leg: Placed on the fleshy part of the lower right leg; does not record a lead but serves as a ground for electrical interference
- *LL* for left leg: Placed on the fleshy part of the lower left leg
- *C* or *V* for chest: Placed at six different locations on the chest (refer to Figure 21–45)

The ECG paper is marked with a code so that the physician knows which lead is being recorded. Most machines record this code automatically, but others must be coded manually. The code for each lead is as follows:

. Lead 1 (I)	—. V_1
. . Lead 2 (II)	—. . V_2
. . . Lead 3 (III)	—. . . V_3
– aVR	—. . . . V_4
– – aVL	—. . . . . V_5
– – – aVF	—. . . . . . V_6

Most newer ECG machines print the name of the lead (I, II, AVR, etc.) on the paper instead of using the codes.

Electrocardiograph machines vary slightly, but most have the same basic parts. It is important to read the specific manufacturer's instructions with each machine. There are two main classes of electrocardiographs: single channel and multiple channel. The single-channel electrocardiograph produces a narrow strip of

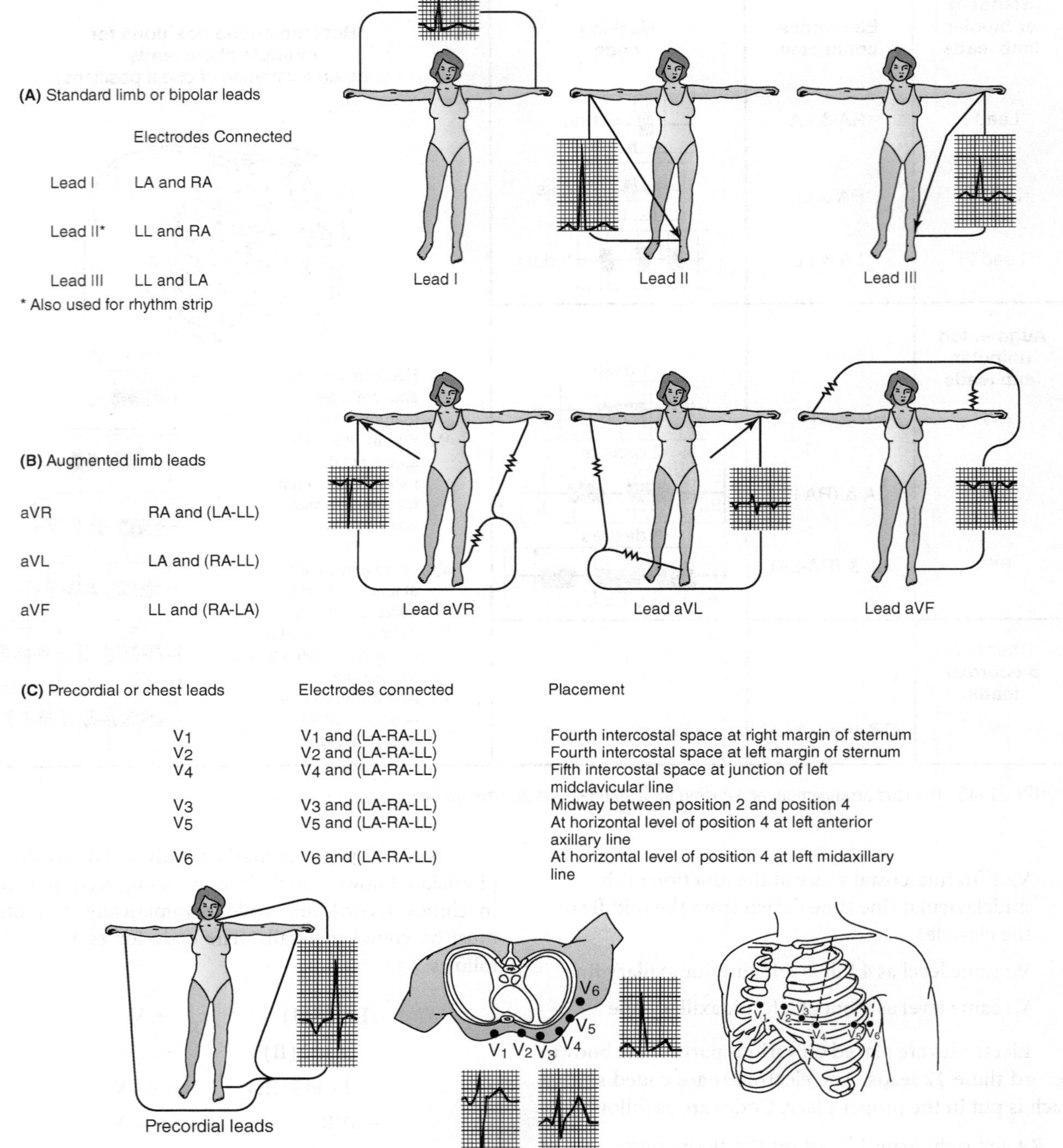

FIGURE 21–46 **Lead types, connections, and placement. (A) Standard limb leads. (B) Augmented voltage (AV) leads. (C) Precordial or chest leads.**

paper showing one lead at a time. The multiple-channel electrocardiograph produces a full sheet of paper showing all 12 leads (Figure 21–47). All electrocardiograph machines have most of the following basic parts:

- *Main switch:* Turns the machine on and off.
- *Pilot light:* A red light that indicates that the machine is on. On newer, computerized machines, this may be indicated by a *Ready* signal on the computer readout.
- *ST'D (standard control):* Used to perform a quality-control check and to ensure that the machine is calibrated correctly to record electrical impulses. One millivolt electrical input should cause the stylus (recording needle) to move 10 millimeters on the graph (10 small squares or 2 large squares on the paper) (Figure 21–48). If the standard is not the correct height during the standard check, the ST'D must be adjusted. Follow the manufacturer's instructions to adjust the standard to the proper height. Many of

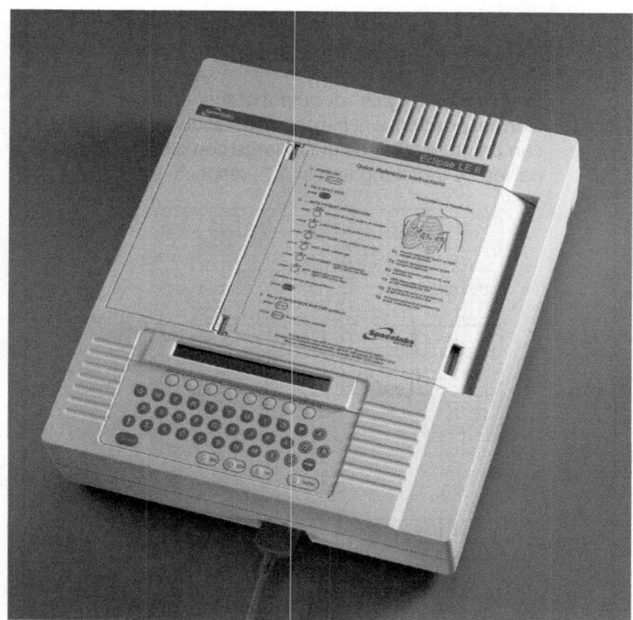

FIGURE 21–47 A multiple-channel electrocardiograph produces a full sheet of paper showing all 12 leads. Courtesy of Spacelabs Medical, Inc.

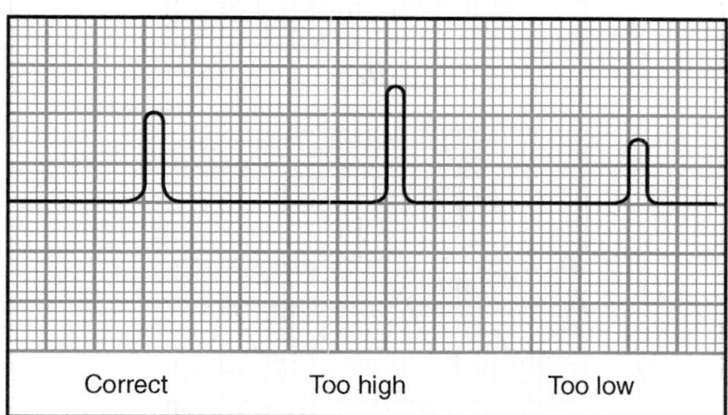

FIGURE 21–48 Standardization: correct, too high, too low.

the newer ECG machines perform an automatic standardization when the machine is turned on.

- *Stylus heat control:* Used to adjust stylus temperature (Figure 21–49). The heat from the stylus melts the plastic coating on the ECG paper, forming the black or blue line. At the same time, the coating lubricates the stylus. If the tracing is too light, the heat must be increased. If the tracing is too dark, the heat must be decreased. Follow the manufacturer's instructions to adjust the heat.
- *Stylus position control:* Used to move the recording up and down on the paper. In most cases, this control should be adjusted to center the ECG on the paper.
- *Record, or speed, control:* Has three or four separate functions to control the amplifier and paper drive, or the speed.
  (1) Amp off: The unit remains inactive; used when changing chest lead positions.

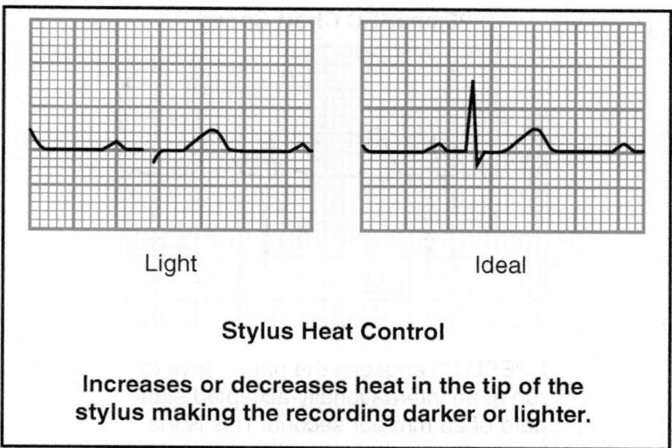

Light
Ideal
Stylus Heat Control
Increases or decreases heat in the tip of the stylus making the recording darker or lighter.

FIGURE 21–49 Stylus heat control: light and ideal.

  (2) Amp on: The amplifier is activated, causing the stylus to move, but the paper remains stationary. This position is useful for chest leads. After the chest electrode is in position, turn the machine to amp on, allow the stylus to stabilize or settle, and turn to Run 25.
  (3) Run 25: The position normally used when recording an ECG. The paper moves at a rate of 25 millimeters per second (Figure 21–50).
  (4) Run 50: The position used when the complexes of the ECG are so close together that they are difficult to examine. It increases the speed of the paper to 50 millimeters per second, stretching the ECG out on the paper. Often used for extremely fast tachycardias (pulse rate above 100). To make the physician aware of the increased speed, "Run 50" must be written on the paper with a pen or pencil (if not recorded automatically by the machine).
- *Lead coding marker:* Places a mark or code on the paper to identify the lead being recorded. On most electrocardiograph machines, this is done automatically. On some machines, the lead mark is recorded manually at the start of each lead recording. Many of the multiple-channel ECG machines print the name of the lead on the paper instead of the code.
- *Lead selector switch:* Allows selection of the lead to be run. It has a position for checking the standard and other positions for running each of the 12 leads of a standard ECG. This switch is not necessary on a multiple-channel ECG because all 12 leads are run at the same time.
- *Sensitivity switch:* Controls amplification (Figure 21–51). It is usually set at position 1. In position 1, the standard is 10 small blocks or 2 large blocks high. Other positions are as follows:
  (1) Position 2: Increases the size of the complex, making it twice as large. The standard will then be 20 small blocks or 4 large blocks high. Used when the PQRST pattern is too small to be easily seen.

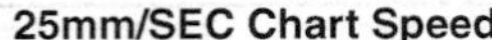

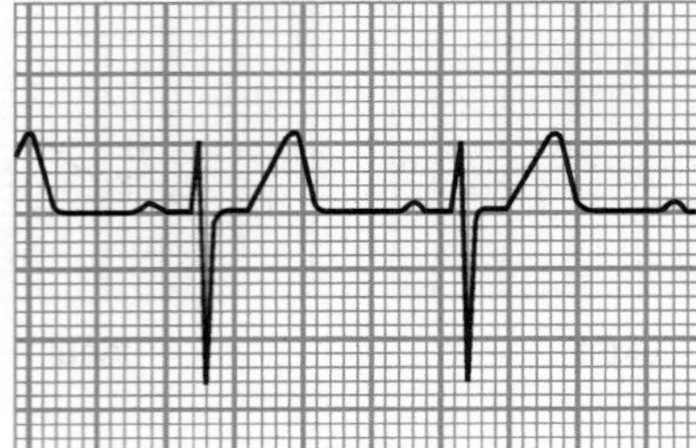

SPEED 25 engages the paper drive to run at an internationally-accepted standard of 25 mm per second. This is the "normal" speed for recording.

50mm/SEC Chart Speed

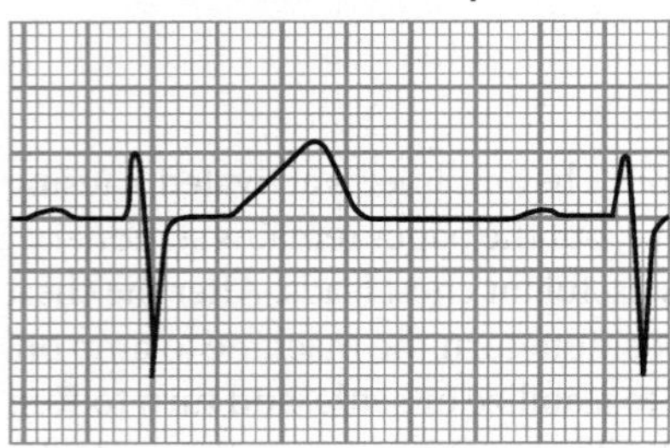

SPEED 50 doubles the speed of the paper to 50 mm per second. Useful when heart rate is rapid or when certain segments of a complex are close together, since it extends the recording to twice its normal width.

FIGURE 21–50 Speed settings for an electrocardiogram.

(2) Position ½: Decreases the size of the complex to one-half its normal size. The standard will then be five small blocks or one large block high. Used when the PQRST pattern is too large.

Many patients are frightened or apprehensive about having an ECG taken. It is important to explain this procedure to the patient. Stress that it is not a painful or uncomfortable test. Position the patient comfortably with all body parts supported. Encourage the patient to relax and to avoid moving while the ECG is being taken. Muscle movement can cause electrical interference and will be displayed on the ECG recording. Nervous tension can also interfere with the recording.

After all the ECG leads have been recorded, a section of each recorded lead is mounted. Most newer multiple-channel machines produce complete mounts. These mounts are sometimes attached to firmer backings using self-stick tape. For ECGs from single-channel machines, many different types of mounts are used. Some contain slots for inserting the individual leads. Some contain tape or self-stick areas for placement of each of the leads. Others utilize clamps. The final mount should be neat, with each lead in the correct area on the mount. The mount should be labeled with the patient's name and address, physician's name, date, and any other pertinent information.

Sensitivity Control

Regulates the "gain" or output of the amplifier. Normal position is 1. Height of small complexes can be doubled or height of large complexes halved by switching to 2 or 1/2, respectively.

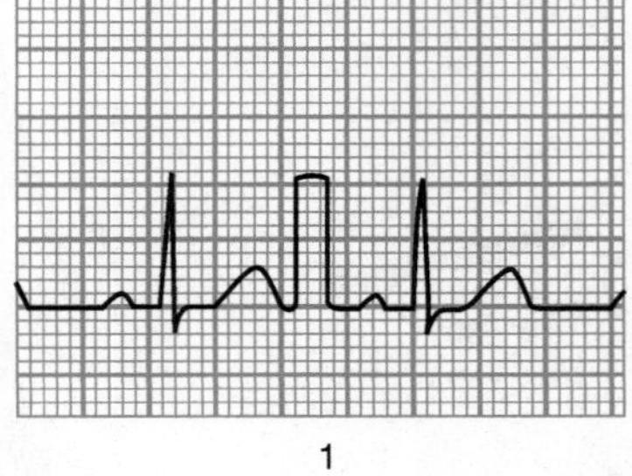

1

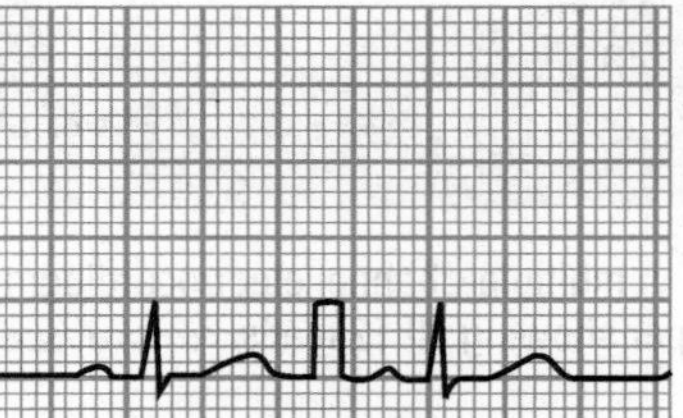

1/2

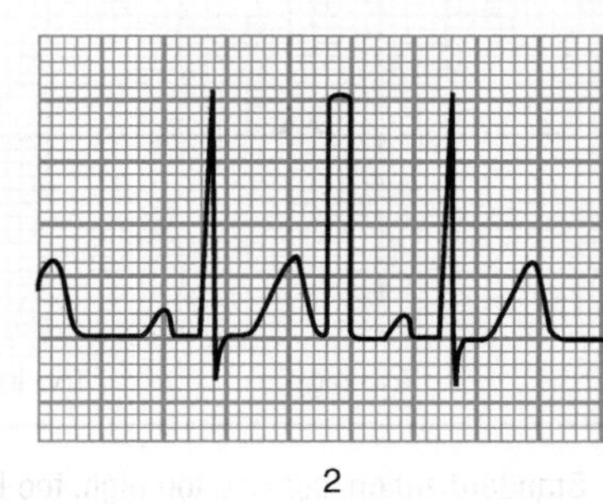

2

FIGURE 21–51 Sensitivity control on an electrocardiogram.

Computerized ECG machines will retain the ECG in the computer memory so it can be viewed on the screen. Most computerized ECG machines will also provide a printed copy of an ECG. Follow the manufacturer's instructions to save the ECG correctly in the patient's electronic health record (EHR), also called an electronic medical record (EMR).

STUDENT: Go to the workbook and complete the assignment sheet for 21:6, Recording and Mounting an Electrocardiogram. Then return and continue with the procedure.

PROCEDURE 21:6

Recording and Mounting an Electrocardiogram

NOTE: This procedure provides basic information about recording and mounting an electrocardiogram (ECG). It is important to read the specific operating instructions provided with each electrocardiograph machine.

Equipment and Supplies

Electrocardiograph machine, electrodes, electrocardiograph cables and cords, examination gown, drape, gauze pads and/or tongue depressors, pen and/or computer

Procedure

1. Assemble required equipment.
2. Wash hands.
3. 
Comm
Introduce yourself. Identify the patient. Explain the procedure. Reassure the patient. Tell the patient that you will be recording the activity of the heart. Stress that the patient will not feel any discomfort from the procedure. Explain that the patient must lie perfectly still because muscle movement will interfere with the recording.
4. Ask the patient to remove clothing and put on an examination gown. The gown is usually open in the front for easy placement of the chest electrodes.

   NOTE: In some offices, the patient is asked to remove clothing from the waist up and to uncover the lower legs.
5. Position the patient. Patient should be lying on a firm bed or examination table. A small pillow can be placed under the head. Use the drape to cover the patient.
6. Position the machine in a convenient location. It may be easier to work from the left side because this is where most of the chest leads are positioned.
7. Connect the power cord to the machine. Do *not* let the power cord pass under the bed or examination table. Plug it in so that it is pointing away from the patient.

   Safety
   CAUTION: Check the three prongs and the cord before using the power cord. Never use a defective cord for any procedure.

   NOTE: Positioning the power cord away from the patient helps reduce electrical interference.
8. Obtain a package of disposable electrodes (Figure 21–52A). Apply the four limb electrodes. The arm electrodes are placed on the fleshy outer areas of the upper arms. The leg electrodes are placed on fleshy parts of the lower legs. Avoid bony areas. Use a tongue depressor or gauze pad to vigorously rub the site to stimulate circulation. If the patient's skin is oily, wipe the electrode area with alcohol and allow it to air-dry. Then, separate the electrode from the protective backing to uncover the sticky surface. Apply the electrode to the correct site using a smooth, even motion to make sure all parts of the electrode adhere to the skin. The disposable electrodes can only be used with ECG machines that have an alligator clip attached to the ends of the cable wires (Figure 21–52B).

   NOTE: If the skin surface is hairy, it may be necessary to shave small areas at the application sites to allow for better attachment and conduction of the electrodes.

   NOTE: Alligator clip attachments can be purchased for older ECG cable wires.
9. Apply the chest electrodes. Refer to Figure 21–45 for the exact location for each electrode. Use a tongue depressor or gauze pad to vigorously rub the site to stimulate circulation.

FIGURE 21–52A **A disposable electrode has a sticky surface that allows the electrode to adhere to the skin.** Courtesy of Spacelabs Medical, Inc.

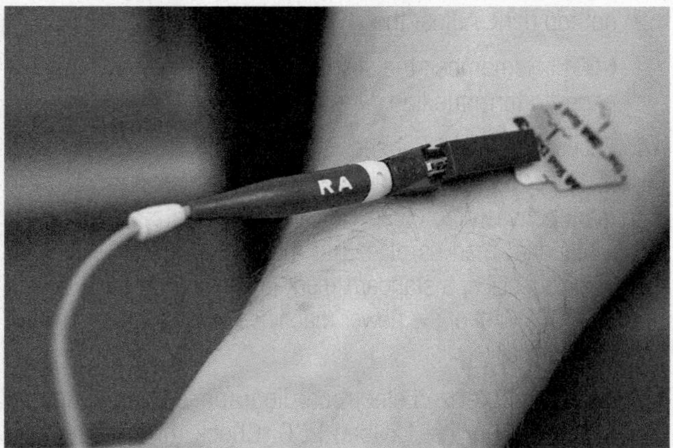

FIGURE 21–52B **An alligator clip on the end of the electrocardiograph cable wire attaches to the disposable electrode.**

(continues)

PROCEDURE 21:6 (CONT.)

If the patient's skin is oily, wipe the electrode area with alcohol and allow it to air-dry. Then, separate the electrode from its protective backing to uncover the sticky surface. Apply the electrode to the site using a smooth, even motion to make sure all parts of the electrode adhere to the skin. Position all six chest electrodes in the correct locations.

NOTE: If the skin surface is very hairy, it may be necessary to shave small areas at the application sites to allow for better attachment and conduction of the electrodes.

10. Connect the cable wires to the electrodes. The lead wires should follow body contour (Figures 21–53A and 21–53B). If there is excess wire, coil it in a loop and fasten with tape or a band. Pay particular attention to the labels and color codes to connect the cable ends to the correct electrodes. Make sure all connections are tight and in the same direction.

    NOTE: Labels are as follows: RA for right arm; LA for left arm; RL for right leg; LL for left leg; and C or V for chest.

    NOTE: Color codes are as follows: white for RA, black for LA, green for RL, red for LL, and brown or multicolored for chest or V depending on the model of the ECG machine.

11. Turn on the main switch. If a computerized ECG machine is being used, enter the required patient information. The machine will print this information on the ECG.
12. Check standardization of the machine. Put the lead selector in the ST'D position. Set the record switch to Run 25. Make sure sensitivity is set at 1. Center the stylus. Momentarily press the ST'D button. Check the standard. It should be 10 small blocks or 2 large blocks high.

    NOTE: If the standard is not correct, adjust it to the correct height by following the manufacturer's instructions. Newer machines may perform an automatic standardization check.

13. Check the color of the line. It should be clearly visible but not too dark. Adjust the stylus heat control, if necessary.

    NOTE: Remember, the stylus heat melts the coating on the paper to form the line.

14. Record the leads. Set sensitivity at 1. Put the record switch at Run 25. Record several complexes. Insert a standard mark between the complexes, if required. In some agencies, a standard mark is placed at the beginning of the ECG. In other agencies, a standard mark is centered in each lead of the ECG. Most of the newer machines insert a standard mark automatically.
15. On a computerized electrocardiograph, set the control to Auto and run the 12-lead ECG. Check the ECG recording carefully as the leads are being run (Figure 21–54). When all 12 leads are complete, proceed to step 17 of this procedure. On a manual electrocardiograph, set the

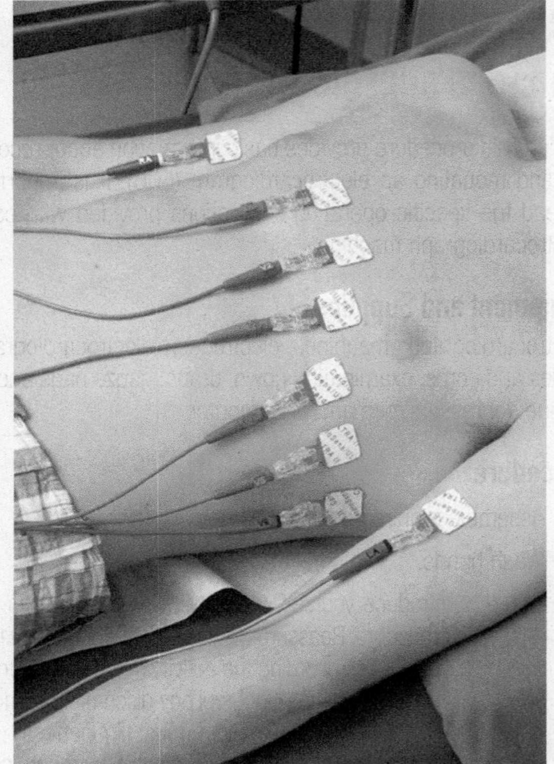

A

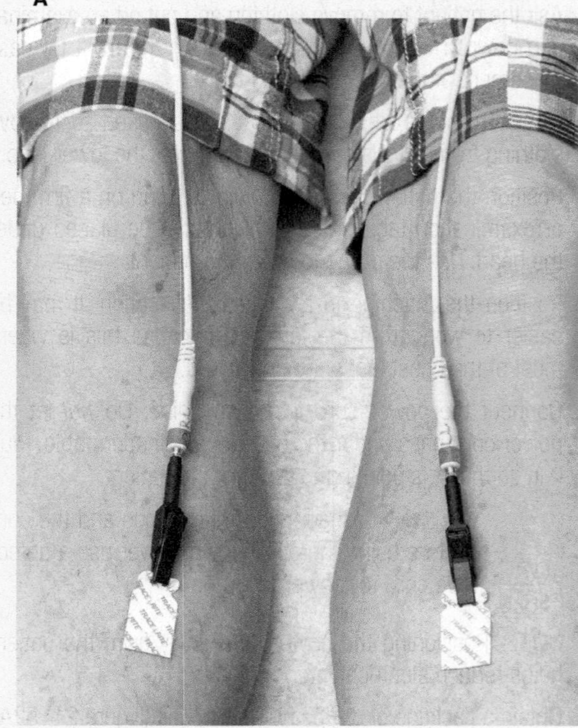

B

FIGURE 21–53 The lead cables should follow body contour when they are connected to the electrodes: (A) chest and arm leads and (B) leg leads.

PROCEDURE 21:6 (CONT.)

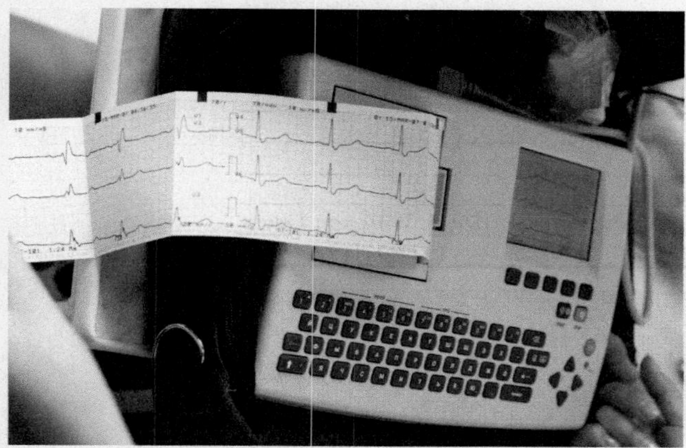

FIGURE 21–54 **Check the ECG recording carefully as the leads are being run.** © Kiselev Andrey Valerevich/www.Shutterstock.com

lead selector switch to each lead and allow the machine to record an adequate amount for each lead. While running the leads, make sure the following points are noted:

a. The recording should be centered on the paper.

b. Record a sufficient amount for each lead. Leads 1, 2, and 3 each usually require 8–10 inches. Each of the remaining leads usually require 5–6 inches.

c. An ST'D mark is in the center of each lead or at the start, depending on agency or physician preference.

d. Make sure that the amplitude of the complexes is correct. If complexes are too small, set sensitivity to 2. If complexes are too large, set sensitivity to ½. If the sensitivity is changed, be sure to insert a standard in the lead. A standard that is five small blocks or one large block high indicates a sensitivity setting of ½. A standard that is 20 small blocks or 4 large blocks high indicates a sensitivity setting of 2.

e. Make sure complexes are not too close together. For severe tachycardias, it is often necessary to increase the speed to Run 50. Alert the physician by marking "Run 50" on the paper with pen or pencil.

f. Make sure that no electrical interference or artifact is present. Watch patient movement. Use a ground wire, as needed.

16. Run all of the leads as instructed in step 15. There is no need to turn off the machine between leads. Simply move the lead selector switch to the next position.

NOTE: Most machines code each lead automatically; others require manual coding when leads are run; and some newer machines record the name of the lead instead of the code.

17. When all 12 leads have been run, turn the lead selector to the standard position. Allow all of the recording to run out of the machine. Then turn the record switch to Off.

NOTE: Make sure that all of the recording is out of the machine's window before stopping the movement of the machine.

18. Turn the power button off. Remove the electrodes from the patient and discard. Use warm water to wash the patient's skin. Dry the skin thoroughly. Help the patient get off the examination table or bed.

19. Coil all wires and replace in the proper area. Coil power cord and replace in the proper area.

NOTE: If wires are bent, they will break.

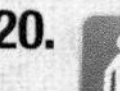

20.  Comm

Write the patient's name, the date, and the physician's name on the ECG if the machine does not do this. If the ECG has been recorded with all 12 leads on one sheet of paper, it may be necessary to attach it to a self-stick mount. Follow the manufacturer's instructions. This type of ECG is sometimes simply placed in the patient's chart without mounting. If the ECG is one long roll, cut into leads and attach to a mount. It is important to follow instructions provided with the mounts, and to make sure that the length for each lead is cut correctly. Look for the lead marking code to determine the lead represented. Use scissors or an ECG cutter to cut a section of the lead to the correct length. Attach the lead to the correct area of the mount. Make sure you match the lead markings on the ECG strip with those on the mount to place each section in its correct location (Figure 21–55). Most mounts have adhesive backs for easy attachment. When all 12 leads are mounted in their correct areas, recheck the ECG. Make sure it is neat and labeled correctly.

NOTE: Some physicians prefer to read the strip before it is mounted to mark specific areas or arrhythmias to mount.

21. Wash hands.

22.  Comm

Record all required information on the patient's chart or enter it into the computer. For example: date, time, ECG recorded, and your signature and title.

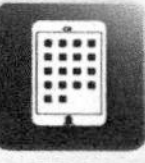 EHR

NOTE: In health care agencies using electronic health records (EHRs), also known as electronic medical records (EMRs), the information is entered directly into the patient's record on a computer.

PRACTICE: **Go to the workbook and use the evaluation sheet for 21:6, Recording and Mounting an Electrocardiogram, to practice this procedure. When you believe you have mastered this skill, sign the sheet and give it to your instructor for further action.**

 Check

FINAL CHECKPOINT: Using the criteria listed on the evaluation sheet, your instructor will grade your performance.

(continues)

PROCEDURE 21:6 (CONT.)

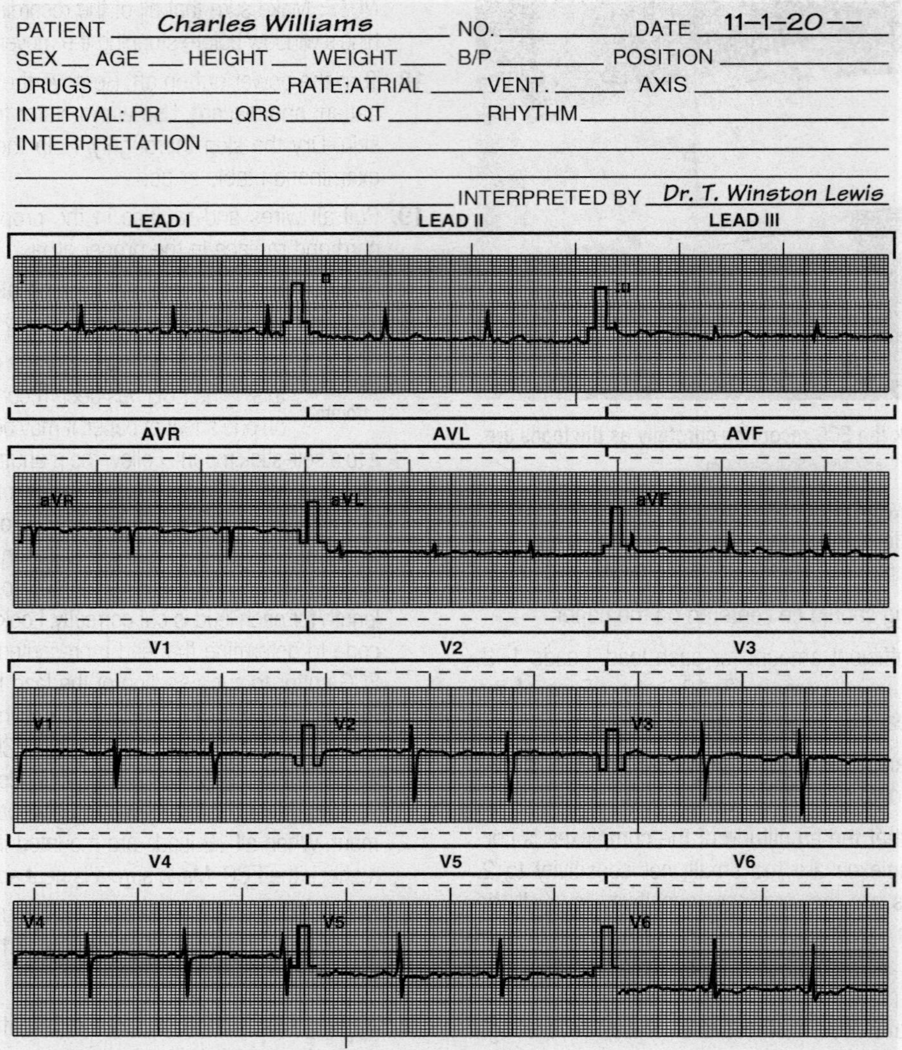
PATIENT Charles Williams NO. ____ DATE 11-1-20--
SEX ___ AGE ___ HEIGHT ___ WEIGHT ___ B/P ____ POSITION ____
DRUGS ____ RATE:ATRIAL ____ VENT. ____ AXIS ____
INTERVAL: PR ____ QRS ____ QT ____ RHYTHM ____
INTERPRETATION ____
____ INTERPRETED BY Dr. T. Winston Lewis

FIGURE 21–55 A mounted single-channel electrocardiogram.

21:7 Using the Physicians' Desk Reference (PDR)

The **Physicians' Desk Reference**, or **PDR**, is a book that provides essential information about drugs and medications currently in use. It is published yearly and has periodic supplements that provide up-to-date information on new products available. It is also available in an online electronic version and a DVD. The *Physicians' Desk Reference for Nonprescription Drugs* is another resource that can be used to obtain information about over-the-counter (OTC) medications that can be purchased without a prescription.

The *PDR* contains six main sections. Each section has a specific purpose and provides certain types of information. The main sections are as follows:

- *Manufacturers' index:* This is the initial white section. Major drug manufacturers in the United States are listed in alphabetical order. Company names, addresses, telephone numbers, and departments to contact are listed. A partial list of each manufacturer's products is also included.

- *Brand and generic names:* The second main section, this is usually pink. It provides an alphabetical listing of products by *brand* name or *generic (chemical)* name. All drugs listed by generic name are followed by a list of brand names. The manufacturer's name is given in parentheses after each product. In addition, if drug information is found in a later section, the page number for the information is provided.
- *Product classification, or category, index:* The third main section is blue. It is a quick-reference section for drugs available for various conditions. For example, if a patient has an infection, a physician can readily find a long list of drugs that can be used to treat the condition by looking under the heading *antibiotics.* Drugs in each group are listed by brand names, with the manufacturers in parentheses. If additional information on the drug is provided in a later section, the page number is listed.
- *Product identification guide:* The next main section provides color, actual-size pictures of a variety of drugs. Drugs shown are listed alphabetically by manufacturers. Identification numbers may be given for some drugs, but these numbers may be changed by the manufacturer.
- *Product information:* This is the largest section in the book and is white. It contains a detailed list of drugs and information on the chemical nature, indications for use, contraindications, warnings, adverse reactions, recommended dosage, and administration routes for each drug. Drugs are listed by manufacturers. All page number references in preceding sections refer to this section.
- *Diagnostic product information section:* This green section lists all diagnostic products, such as radiographic (X-ray) dyes, by manufacturers.

Several smaller information sections can be found in the back of the *PDR*. These include:

- *Poison control centers:* a list of certified poison control centers arranged alphabetically by state
- *Discontinued products:* an alphabetical listing of products withdrawn from the market during the past year
- *U.S. Food and Drug Administration (FDA) telephone directory:* the numbers for key reporting programs and information services
- *Key to FDA Use-in-Pregnancy ratings:* describes how drugs are rated for use during pregnancy

It is important to check the *PDR* for information regarding actions, dosages, side effects, and other vital facts for any medication. You must be familiar with this reference and be able to use it readily. In addition, other references available for pharmaceutical product information should be available for use. Examples of these include the *National Formulary*, the *Pharmacopoeia of the United States of America* (USP), and packet inserts that are found in medication packages.

STUDENT: **Read Procedure 21:7, Using the *Physicians' Desk Reference* (*PDR*). Then go to the workbook and complete the three assignment sheets for 21:7, Using the *Physicians' Desk Reference* (*PDR*) by following the guidelines in Procedure 21:7.**

PROCEDURE 21:7

Using the Physicians' Desk Reference (PDR)

Equipment and Supplies

Physicians' Desk Reference or online version, pen, and/or computer

Procedure

1. Read information section 21:7 on the *PDR*. Locate the various sections in the *PDR* while you are reading this section. Become familiar with each section and what it contains.
2. Think of the name of a major drug manufacturer. Turn to the manufacturers' index and find this name. Note the address of the company, the telephone number, and the department to contact.
3. Think of the common brand name of a drug with which you are familiar. Turn to the brand and generic name index (pink section) and locate this drug. If it refers to a page number, turn to that page in the product information section and read the information provided on the drug.
4. Think of the generic, or chemical, name of a drug. You may want to look in journals for some examples. Locate the name of this drug in the brand and generic name index. If a list of brand names appears, choose one or two of the names. Refer to the noted page number in the product information section to read about the properties of these drugs. Note how they are alike and how they might differ.

(continues)

PROCEDURE 21:7 (CONT.)

5. Think of any type of illness or disease. Find this disease in the blue product classification, or category, index. Note the list of drugs available to treat the condition. Look up product information on several of the drugs listed.

6. Glance through the product identification guide. Note the pictures of the many drugs listed. Pay particular attention to size, manufacturers' marks such as numbers or letters, and coloring. These signs might help you identify a drug for which you do not know the name. After finding a drug that looks interesting, look up the name in the brand and generic name index, where an alphabetical list is provided. This list provides a page number in the product information section, where more information about the drug can be obtained. Turn to the correct page and read the product information provided.

7. Go to the workbook and complete the first assignment sheet for 21:7, Using the *Physicians' Desk Reference* (*PDR*). Use information section 21:7 and the steps in this procedure to complete the assignment sheet. When you are done, give the assignment sheet to your instructor.

PRACTICE: **Your instructor will grade Assignment Sheet #1. Note any changes or corrections. Then complete Assignment Sheet #2. Give this sheet to your instructor for grading. Note any changes or corrections. Repeat this process for Assignment Sheet #3.**

Check

FINAL CHECKPOINT: After reviewing your completed assignment sheets for 21:7, Using the *Physicians' Desk Reference* (PDR), your instructor will grade your performance.

21:8 Working with Medications

Legal

A **medication** is a drug used to treat or prevent a disease or condition. The following discussion provides only basic information about the preparation and administration of medications. Even so, it should make you aware of the need for extreme care in handling all medications. It is important to remember that *only authorized persons can administer medications.*

Medications are available in various forms, usually liquids, solids, or semi-solids.

- ***Liquids:***
  (1) Aqueous suspension: medication is dissolved in water
  (2) Suspension: solid form of a medication is mixed with solution; usually must be shaken well before use to resuspend the medication in the solution
  (3) Syrup: concentrated solution of sugar, water, and medication
  (4) Tincture: medication dissolved in alcohol

  NOTE: *Liquid medications must be poured at eye level to ensure that the dosage is exact (Figure 21–56).*

- ***Solids*** (Figure 21–57):
  (1) Capsule: gelatin-like shell with medication inside
  (2) Pill: powdered medication mixed with a cohesive substance and molded into shape
  (3) Tablet: compressed or molded preparation
  (4) Troche or lozenge: large, flat disc that is dissolved in the mouth
  (5) Enteric coated: medication with a special coating that does not dissolve until the substance reaches the small intestine

- ***Semi-solids:***
  (1) Ointment: medication in a fatty base
  (2) Paste: ointment with an adhesive substance
  (3) Cream: medication with water-soluble base

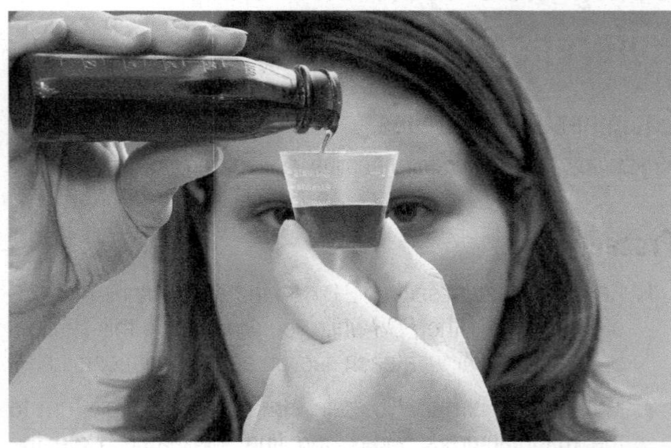

FIGURE 21–56 **Liquid medications must be poured at eye level to ensure the dosage is correct.**

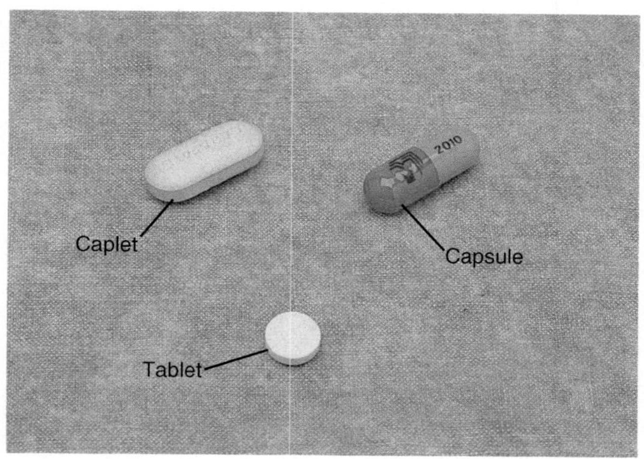

FIGURE 21–57 Types of solid medications.

(4) Suppository: medication mixed with substances that melt at body temperature; cocoa butter is often the base material; usually inserted into the rectum, vagina, or urethra

Medications may be given in a variety of ways. Some of the routes of administration are:

- *Oral:* given by mouth; for liquid and solid forms
- *Rectal:* given in the rectum; liquids and suppositories
- *Injections:* given with a needle and syringe; often called "parenteral," which means any route other than the alimentary canal (digestive tract) (Figure 21–58).
  (1) Subcutaneous (subQ): injected into the layer of tissue just under the skin
  (2) Intramuscular (IM): injected into a muscle
  (3) Intravenous (IV): injected into a vein
  (4) Intradermal: injected just under the top layer of skin; the skin tests for allergies and tuberculosis (TB) are examples
- *Topical or local:* applied directly to the top of the skin; ointments, sprays, liquids, and adhesive patches; transdermal adhesive patches applied to the skin can be used to provide a continuous dosage of medication for motion sickness, heart disease, hormonal imbalance, and nicotine withdrawal (for individuals who are trying to stop smoking) (Figures 21–59A and 21–59B)
- *Inhalation:* inhaled, or breathed in, by way of sprays, inhalers, or special machines
- *Sublingual:* given under the tongue

There are six main points to watch each and every time a medication is given. These can be called the "six rights."

- Right medication
- Right dose, or amount
- Right patient
- Right time
- Right method or mode of administration
- Right documentation

Certain safety rules must be observed when giving medication.

- Read the order carefully. Note all six *rights*.
- Check for patient allergies before administering any medication.

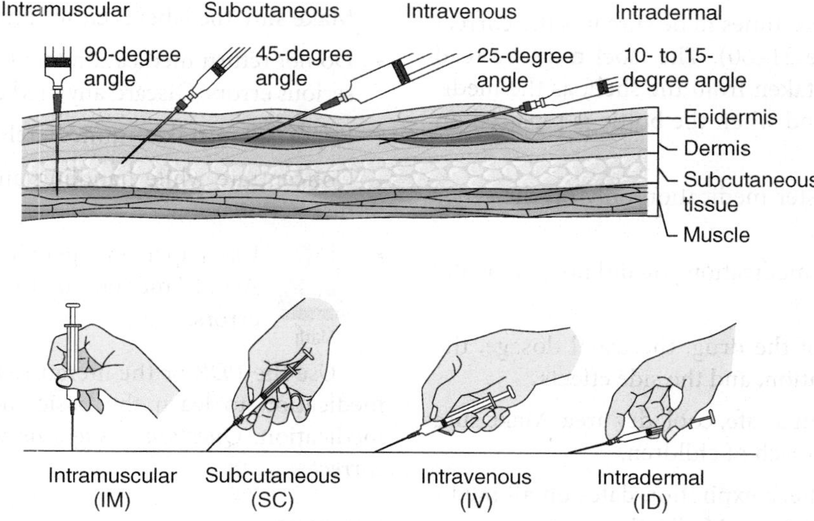

FIGURE 21–58 Types of injections and the correct angles for administration of parenteral medications.

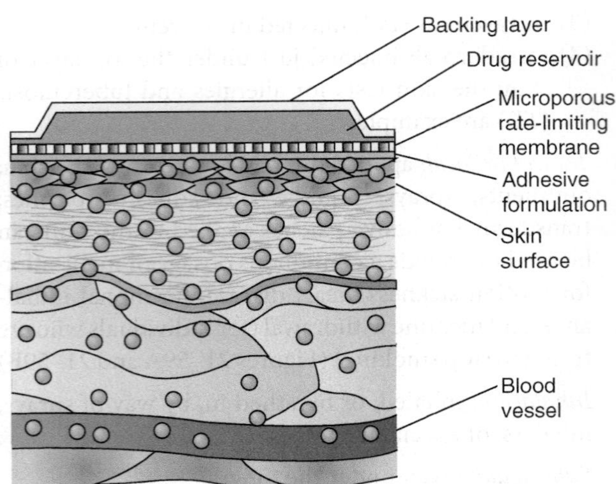

FIGURE 21–59A The layers of a transdermal patch allow the medication to be absorbed into the bloodstream over a period of time, frequently 24 hours.

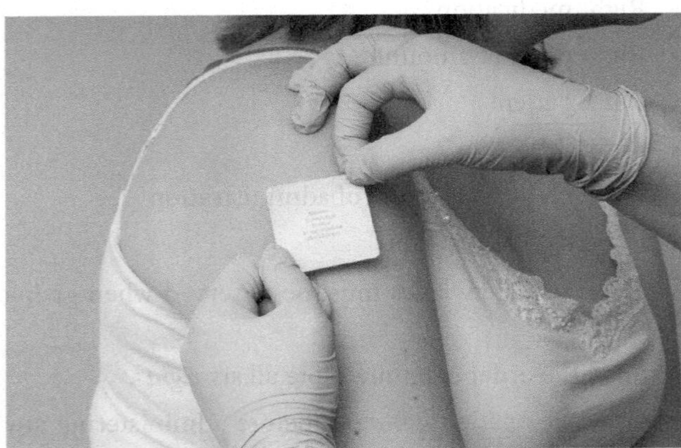

FIGURE 21–59B A transdermal patch is applied to the skin.

- Check the label three times to be sure it is the correct medication (Figure 21–60). The label must be read when the bottle is taken from the shelf, as the medication is poured, and when the bottle is replaced on the shelf.
- Prepare or administer medication only on the order of a physician.
- *Never* administer a medication you did not personally prepare.
- Know the action of the drug, the usual dosage, the route of administration, and the side effects.
- Store medications in a safe, cool, dry area. Make sure they are out of the reach of children.
- 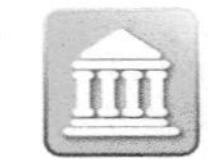 Legal  Comm Check expiration dates on all medications. Medications must *never* be used beyond the expiration date and expired medications must be destroyed. Follow agency policy and federal and state laws to dispose of medications. If the policies/laws call for destruction of the medications, many states have prescription drug drop boxes at specific pharmacies or law enforcement agencies. The medications are destroyed following recommendations of the Food and Drug Administration (FDA) and the Environmental Protection Agency (EPA). Record all required information regarding the destruction of the medication according to agency policy. Expired controlled substances, such as narcotics, *must* be returned to the pharmacy as required by law. Make sure you complete all required documentation when you return expired controlled substances to the pharmacy. If a partial amount of a unit dose (single dose package) of a controlled substance is used because of the dosage ordered, witnesses must cosign when the remaining medication is destroyed.

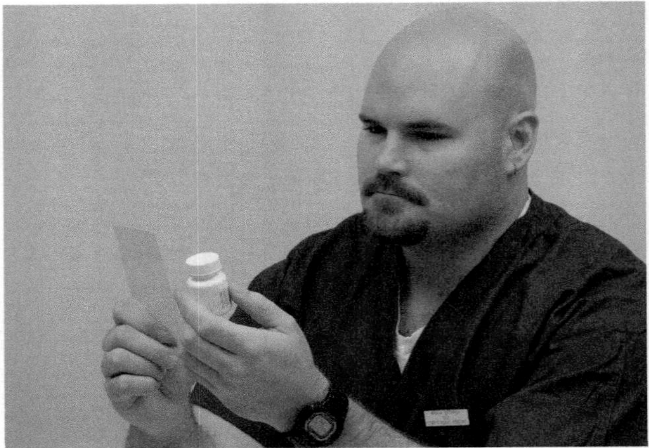

FIGURE 21–60 Check the label of any medication at least three times.

- *Never* use medication from an unmarked bottle. Make sure the label is clear. If in doubt, throw it out.
- Do *not* return medication to a bottle. This can lead to serious errors. Discard any medication that is *not* used.
- Report all mistakes immediately.
- Concentrate while handling any medication. Avoid distractions.
- 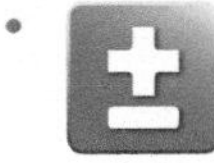 Math Use paper and pencil to calculate dosages. Avoid "mental" math because it can cause errors.

Use the *PDR* or the literature that comes with each medication to learn the basic information about the medication. *Question dosages or uses that do not seem correct.*

STUDENT: Go to the workbook and complete the assignment sheet for 21:8, Working with Medications.

TODAY'S RESEARCH TOMORROW'S HEALTH CARE

The Nose Knows Cancer?

The American Cancer Society estimates that each year in the United States over 1.5 million people will be diagnosed with some type of cancer and more than 500,000 people will die. Even though treatment for cancer has improved and many lives have been saved, some types of cancers are extremely difficult to detect at an early stage when cure is most likely. Examples include stomach, bone, kidney, pancreatic, and ovarian cancer.

Now scientists all over the world are researching the possibility of a "smell test" for cancer. Initially, researchers at the Pine Street Foundation, a nonprofit cancer research institute in California, trained five different dogs to smell breast and lung cancer on a patient's breath. The dogs were able to identify breast cancer 88 percent of the time and lung cancer 99 percent of the time. A group of researchers in Germany trained four dogs, three shepherds and a Lab, to detect lung cancer using breath samples from 100 patients with lung cancer. When the dogs were given 400 other samples from individuals without lung cancer, the dogs only had an 8 percent false positive rate. In addition, the dogs were able to distinguish between patients with cancer and patients with chronic obstructive lung disease. In Japan, scientists trained a black Lab to detect colorectal cancer. The Lab correctly identified 98 percent of the positive samples, a rate much better than the fecal occult (hidden blood in the feces) test which has a high rate of false positives. Researchers think the dogs were able to smell the cancers by sensing minute amounts of volatile organic compounds (VOCs) that are exhaled in the breath. In fact, as many as 4,000 different VOCs have been identified in human breath. Estimates are that a dog's sense of smell can be 10,000 to 100,000 times superior to a human's sense of smell, so the dogs can detect minute quantities of the VOCs. Does that mean that in the future every medical facility or physician's office will have a cancer-sniffing dog on staff? Of course not, but this research has created a unique way of developing tests that will detect cancer in its early stages.

Currently, many researchers are working to identify and isolate the chemical compounds associated with different types of cancers. This is very challenging because the smell of cancer is probably made up of many different chemicals. In fact, each type of cancer might have a very unique chemical combination. At the same time, researchers are trying to develop artificial noses that will be able to detect specific chemical compounds. Doctors at Ohio's Cleveland Clinic have developed an instrument that uses color changes to analyze breath chemicals. The initial attempt was 66 percent accurate in diagnosing lung cancer. Scientists at California's Brain Mapping Foundation (BMF) are trying to determine if the electronic "nose" developed by NASA and used in the International Space Station can be used to identify signs of brain cancer in tissue samples. The NASA electronic nose, or e-nose, has an array of non-specific chemical sensors. After being calibrated to a baseline of clean air, the e-nose sends an alert when a large quantity or variety of contaminants is noted in the air. Once the compounds associated with cancer are identified, it may be possible to modify the e-nose to detect them. Eventually, it is very possible that a simple noninvasive breath test could lead to early detection of cancer. Man's best friend may have started research that will save many lives.

CHAPTER 21 SUMMARY

A basic knowledge of the main skills used by medical assistants is beneficial for many health care workers, because many of these skills are used in other health care areas.

Height and weight measurements are important in evaluating basic health status of patients. Thus, knowing how to correctly measure height and weight is important for every health care worker.

Proper positioning of patients for examinations and other procedures is another skill needed by the medical assistant. By following correct techniques, the medical assistant can properly prepare patients, as well as provide patients with comfort and privacy.

A knowledge of the basic instruments used and procedures performed during physical examinations, minor surgery, and suture removal is essential. This knowledge allows the medical assistant to work with the physician to provide quality health care to the patient in an efficient manner. Understanding the basic principles of electrocardiography allows the medical assistant to efficiently perform an electrocardiogram.

A knowledge of how to find information on medications and of correct techniques for dispensing medications is also an important responsibility of the medical assistant. By mastering these basic skills, the medical assistant can become an important part of the medical office team.

INTERNET SEARCHES

Use the search engines suggested in Chapter 12:9 in this text to search the Internet for additional information about the following topics:

1. **Organizations:** Find websites for the American Medical Association, American Association of Medical Assistants, American Society of Podiatric Medical Assistants, Registered Medical Assistants of the American Medical Technologists, and the American Optometric Association to research medical assisting careers and duties.
2. **Vision:** Search for information about Snellen charts, Ishihara color plates, the Jaeger system, myopia, hyperopia, and ophthalmic and optometric treatments and care.
3. **Electrocardiogram:** Research electrocardiographs, myocardial infarctions, and cardiac arrhythmias.
4. **Medications:** Research the *Physicians' Desk Reference*, other medication references, prescription medications, and websites of drug manufacturers.
5. **Suppliers:** Research medical and pharmaceutical suppliers to evaluate the types of supplies and equipment available for medical offices; compare and contrast different types of ECG machines; and locate online pharmacies to determine services available.

REVIEW QUESTIONS

1. Why are height and weight measurements important?
2. Identify at least six (6) different positions that can be used for examinations and/or treatments. For each position, list at least two (2) types of treatments or examinations that are performed when a patient is in the position.
3. Differentiate between a Snellen chart, Jaeger card, and an Ishihara plate by stating the type of eye defects evaluated with each method.
4. Interpret or define each of the following:
   a. OU
   b. OS
   c. OD
   d. myopia
   e. hyperopia
5. Name the areas of the body examined and the type of tests performed during each of the following examinations:
   a. EENT
   b. gynecological
   c. general physical
6. Explain at least five (5) standard precautions that must be observed while assisting with minor surgery and/or suture removal.
7. What is the difference between a hemostat and a needle holder? What is the function of each instrument?
8. Name the twelve (12) leads for an electrocardiogram and the code that is used for each lead.
9. List the six (6) "rights" that must be observed while administering any medication.
10. Use a *Physicians' Desk Reference* to find the medication Celebrex. List the main action of this drug, suggested dosage, route of administration, and warnings/side effects.

For additional information on medical assisting careers, contact the following associations:

- American Association of Medical Assistants
  20 North Wacker Drive, Suite 1575
  Chicago, Illinois 60606
  Internet address: *www.aama-ntl.org*
- American Medical Technologists Association (AMT)
  10700 West Higgins Road, Suite 150
  Rosemont, IL 60018
  Internet address: *www.americanmedtech.org*

Career OBRA

Nurse Assistant Skills 22

CHAPTER OBJECTIVES

After completing this chapter, you should be able to:

- Admit, transfer, or discharge a patient, demonstrating proper care of the patient's belongings.
- Position a patient in correct alignment and with no bony prominences exposed.
- Move and turn a patient in bed, using correct body mechanics.
- Perform the following transfer techniques (using correct body mechanics): dangling, wheelchair, chair, and stretcher.
- Transfer a patient by way of a mechanical lift and observe all safety points.
- Make closed, open, and occupied beds, using correct body mechanics.
- Administer routine, denture, and special oral hygiene.
- Administer hair care and nail care.
- Administer a backrub, using the five major movements.
- Shave a patient using a safety or an electric razor, observing all safety precautions.
- Change a patient's bedclothes.
- Administer a partial bed bath and a complete bed bath with perineal care.
- Help a patient take a tub bath or shower, observing all safety points.
- Measure and record intake and output.
- Assist a patient with eating; feed a patient.
- Administer a bedpan or urinal.
- Provide catheter care.
- Empty a urinary-drainage unit without contaminating the catheter or unit.
- Provide ostomy care.
- Collect urine and stool specimens.
- Administer tap-water, soap-solution, disposable, and oil-retention enemas.
- Insert a rectal tube.
- Apply restraints, observing all safety precautions.
- Administer preoperative care as directed.
- Shave an operative site, observing all safety precautions.
- Prepare a postoperative unit with all equipment in the correct position.

CHAPTER OBJECTIVES (CONT.)

- Apply surgical (elastic) hose.
- Apply binders.
- Safely administer oxygen with an oxygen mask, nasal cannula, or tent.
- Give postmortem care.
- Define, pronounce, and spell all key terms.

KEY TERMS

alignment *(ah-line′ -ment)*
anesthesia *(an-es-thee′ -sha)*
bed cradle
binders
catheter
closed bed
colostomy
complete bed bath (CBB)
contracture *(kon-track′ -tyour″)*
dangling
defecate *(deaf′ -eh-kate″)*
dehydration *(dee″ -high-dray′ -shun)*
edema *(eh-dee′ -mah)*
enema
fanfolding
ileostomy
impaction
intake and output (I&O)
mechanical lifts
micturate *(mick′ -chur-rate″)*
midstream (clean catch) specimen
mitered corners *(my′ -terd corn″ -urz)*
Montgomery straps
occult blood *(ah-kult′)*
occupied bed
open bed
operative care
oral hygiene
ostomy
partial bed bath
personal hygiene
postmortem care
postoperative care
preoperative care
pressure (decubitus) ulcer *(deh-ku′ -beh-tuss uhl″ -sir)*
rectal tube
restraints
sequential compression device (SCD)
stoma
stool specimen
suppository *(sup-poz′ -ih-tor-ee)*
surgical (elastic) hose
surgical shave
24-hour urine specimen
ureterostomy
urinary-drainage unit
urinate
urine specimen
void
wound VAC

career highlights

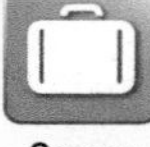

Nurse assistants, also called nurse aides, nurse technicians, patient care technicians (PCTs), patient care assistants (PCAs), and orderlies, work under the supervision of registered nurses or licensed practical/vocational nurses. They are important members of the health care team. Educational requirements vary with states, but many assistants obtain training through health science education (HSE) programs. Assistants who work in long-term care facilities or home health must complete a minimum of 75 to 120 hours in a mandatory state-approved program and pass a written and/or competency examination to obtain certification or registration. Additional educational requirements include continuing education, periodic evaluation of performance, and retraining if the assistant is not employed for two or more years.

Geriatric aides or assistants provide care for patients in environments such as extended care facilities, nursing homes, retirement or assisted-living centers, and adult day care agencies.

careerhighlights (CONT.)

Home health assistants or aides perform many of the duties of nurse assistants, but they provide care in the patient's home, usually for an extended period. Examples of patients who require home care include patients who have just been discharged from a hospital or long-term care facility, patients who have a disability, elderly patients who require assistance, and patients receiving hospice care. In addition to performing many of the personal care duties of the nurse assistant, home health assistants may also shop for food and prepare meals, maintain and clean the home environment, wash laundry, and accompany patients on shopping trips or to medical appointments. Throughout this chapter, special notes are provided to help a home health assistant adapt the procedure to home care.

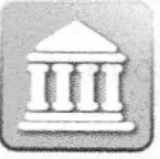
Legal

The duties of nurse assistants vary depending on the facility in which they work and on the nursing practice laws of the state in which they work. *Every nurse assistant must know and follow the legal requirements of the state in which he or she is employed.* In addition to the knowledge and skills presented in this chapter, nurse assistants must also learn and master skills such as:

- Presenting a professional appearance and attitude
- Obtaining knowledge regarding health care delivery systems, organizational structure, and teamwork
- Meeting all legal responsibilities
- Communicating effectively
- Being sensitive to and respecting cultural diversity
- Comprehending anatomy, physiology, and pathophysiology
- Learning medical terminology
- Observing all safety precautions
- Practicing all principles of infection control
- Taking and recording vital signs
- Administering first aid and cardiopulmonary resuscitation
- Promoting good nutrition and a healthy lifestyle to maintain health
- Measuring and recording height and weight
- Positioning patients for and assisting with examinations and treatments
- Administering basic physical therapy including range-of-motion exercises, ambulation with assistive devices, and warm or cold applications
- Performing basic laboratory tests such as monitoring glucose or testing urine with reagent strips
- Using computer and technology skills
- Recording information on patient records

LEGAL ALERT

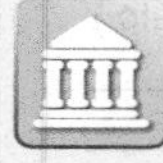
Legal

Before performing any procedures in this chapter, know and follow the standards and regulations established by the scope of practice; federal laws and agencies; state laws; state or national licensing, registration, or certification boards; professional organizations; professional standards; and agency policies.

It is your responsibility to learn exactly what you are legally permitted to do and to perform only procedures for which you have been trained.

22:1 Admitting, Transferring, and Discharging Patients

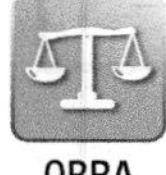
OBRA

As a health care worker in a hospital or long-term care facility, one of your responsibilities may be to admit, transfer, and discharge patients or residents. Although these procedures vary slightly in different facilities, basic principles apply in all facilities.

Comm

Admission to a health care facility can cause anxiety and fear in many patients and their families. Even a transfer from one room or unit in a facility to another room or unit can cause anxiety because the individual has to adjust to another new environment. It is essential for the health care worker to create a positive first impression. By being courteous, supportive, and kind, the health care worker can do much to alleviate fear and anxiety. Giving clear instructions about how to operate equipment and the type of routine to expect, such as mealtimes, helps the patient or resident become familiar with the environment. It is also important not to rush while admitting, transferring, or discharging a patient. Allow the individual to ask questions and express concerns. If you do not know the answers to specific questions, refer these questions to your immediate supervisor.

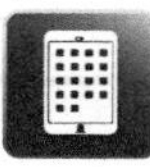
EHR

Most facilities have specific forms that are used during an admission, transfer, or discharge. A sample admission form is shown in Figure 22–1.

PATIENT PREFERS TO BE ADDRESSED AS: ______________________

FROM: ❑ E.R. ❑ E.C.F. ❑ Home ❑ M.D.'s Office

MODE OF TRANSPORTATION:
❑ Ambulatory ❑ Other ________ Smoker: Y❑ N❑
❑ Wheelchair
❑ Stretcher

COMMUNICATES IN ENGLISH: ❑ Well ❑ Minimal ❑ Not At All ❑ Other Language (Specify) ________

❑ INTERPRETER (Name Person) ________ ❑ None

Home Telephone No. ( ) ________

Work Telephone No. ( ) ________

ORIENTATION TO ENVIRONMENT:

❑ Armband Checked
❑ Bed Control
❑ TV Control
❑ Bathroom
❑ Personal Property Policy
❑ Call Light
❑ Phone
❑ Side Rail Policy
❑ Visitation Policy
❑ Smoking Policy

PERSONAL BELONGINGS: (Check and Describe)

❑ Clothing ________
❑ Jewelry ________
❑ Money ________
❑ Walker ________
❑ Wheelchair ________
❑ Cane ________
❑ Other ________

DENTURES:
❑ Upper ❑ Partial
❑ Lower ❑ None

CONTACT LENSES:
❑ Hard ❑ LT ❑ RT
❑ Soft

GLASSES: ❑ Y ❑ N **HEARING AID:** ❑ Y ❑ N

PROSTHESIS: ❑ Y ❑ N

(Describe) ________

DISPOSITION OF VALUABLES:

❑ Patient Given To: ________
❑ Home Relationship: ________
❑ Placed in Safe ________ (Claim No.)

IN CASE OF EMERGENCY NOTIFY:

Name: ________
Relationship: ________
Home Telephone No. ( ) ________
Work Telephone No. ( ) ________

VITAL SIGNS:

TEMP: ________ ❑ Oral ❑ Rectal ❑ Axillary
PULSE: ________ ❑ Radial ❑ Apical Respiratory Rate ________
B/P: ________ ❑ RT ❑ LT ❑ Standing ❑ Sitting ❑ Lying
HEIGHT: ________ WEIGHT: ________ ❑ Bedside ❑ Standing

ALLERGIES:

Medications: ❑ None Known
❑ Penicillin
❑ Sulfa
❑ Iodine
❑ Aspirin
❑ Morphine
❑ Demerol
❑ Tape
❑ Other (List)

Food: ❑ None Known
(Shellfish, Eggs, Milk, etc.)

MEDICATIONS: (Prescription/ Non-Prescription)	Dose/Frequency	Last Dose (Date/Time)
1.		
2.		
3.		
4.		
5.		
6.		

DISPOSITION OF MEDICATIONS:
❑ None Brought to Hospital
❑ Sent Home
With ________
❑ To Pharmacy: (List)

ADMITTING DIAGNOSIS: ________

NURSE'S SIGNATURE: ________ RN/LVN Date ________ Time ________

FIGURE 22–1 A sample admission form.

In many facilities, the forms are computerized, and a laptop or tablet computer is used to enter patient information. Patient records are stored electronically and are called electronic health records (EHRs) or electronic medical records (EMRs). However, all of the forms list the procedures that must be performed and will vary slightly from facility to facility. It is important for the health care worker to become familiar with the information required on such forms. Much of the information on an admission form is used as a basis for the nursing care plan. Therefore, this information must be complete and accurate. If the patient is unable to answer the questions, a relative or the person responsible for the patient is usually able to provide the information. In some facilities, questions regarding medications and allergies are the responsibility of the nurse. Follow agency policy regarding these sections on the form.

When a patient is admitted to a facility, certain procedures are performed. These usually include vital signs, height and weight measurements, and collection of a routine urine specimen. Follow correct techniques while performing these procedures.

A personal inventory list is made of the patient's clothing, valuables, and personal items to protect his or her possessions. In a hospital, a family member frequently will take clothing home. Any clothing or personal items (such as radios and cell phones) kept in the room should be noted on the list. The list should be checked and signed by both the health care worker and the patient (or the person responsible for the patient). At the time of transfer or discharge, the personal inventory list of clothing and personal items should be checked to make sure that the patient has all belongings.

If the family does not take valuables home, these should be put in a safe place. Most facilities require that they be kept in a safe or sent to security. A description of the valuables is usually written on a valuables envelope, and the items are placed inside. Care should be taken when describing valuables. For example, record "a yellow colored band with a white colored stone," instead of "a gold band with a diamond." If money is left in the patient's wallet, it should be counted, and the exact amount recorded on the envelope. Both the health care worker and the patient (or the person responsible for the patient) should check the items and sign the valuables envelope. The valuables are then put in the safe or sent to security, and a receipt is given to the patient or put on the patient's chart. If a patient is transferred or discharged, the valuables are taken from the safe and checked by both the health care worker and the patient. Again, both individuals sign the envelope to indicate that valuables have been returned to the patient.

Comm

Patients and family members should be oriented to the facility. Instructions about how to operate the call signal, bed controls, television remote control (if present), telephone, and other similar equipment should be provided. Visiting hours, location of lounges, smoking regulations, availability of services such as religious services and activities, mealtimes, and other rules or routines in the facility should be explained. Many facilities give patients and family members pamphlets or papers listing such information, but it is still important to explain the main information.

Transfers are done for a variety of reasons. A transfer is sometimes related to a change in the patient's condition. For example, a person may be transferred from or to an intensive care unit. Other times, a transfer is made at the patient's request, such as a request to be moved to a private room. Agency policy must be followed during any transfer. The reason for the transfer should be explained to the patient and family. This is usually the responsibility of the physician or nurse. The new room or unit must be ready to receive the patient. Clothing, personal items, certain equipment, and medications must be transferred with the patient. The health care worker should also find out how to transport the patient. Wheelchairs, stretchers, and even the patient's bed can be used for the transfer. An organized and efficient transfer helps prevent fear and anxiety in the patient.

A physician's order is usually required before a patient or resident can be discharged from a facility. If an individual plans to leave the facility without permission, report this immediately to your supervisor. Facilities have special policies that must be followed when a person leaves against medical advice (AMA). When an order for discharge has been received, the health care worker must check and pack the patient's belongings. The personal inventory list completed at the time of admission must be checked to ascertain that all of the patient's belongings have been packed. A careful check of the unit, including any drawers, closets, and storage areas, helps ensure that all items are found. Most facilities require that a staff member accompany the individual to a car. Some facilities allow patients to walk, but many prefer to transport patients by wheelchair. If a patient is to be transferred by ambulance, the ambulance attendants will bring a stretcher to the room. In this case, it is important for the health care worker to have the patient's belongings ready for the transport. Again, most agencies have forms or checklists that are used during discharge to ensure that all procedures are followed.

STUDENT: **Go to the workbook and complete the assignment sheet for 22:1, Admitting, Transferring, and Discharging Patients. Then return and continue with the procedures.**

PROCEDURE 22:1A

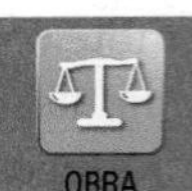

Admitting the Patient

Equipment and Supplies

Admission form and personal inventory list, valuables envelope, admission kit (if used), thermometer, stethoscope, sphygmomanometer, watch with second hand, scale, urine-specimen container, patient gown (if needed), paper and pen or computer

Procedure

1. Obtain orders from your immediate supervisor or check orders to obtain permission for the procedure.
2. Wash hands.
3. Assemble equipment. Prepare the room for the admission. Fanfold the top bed linen down to open the bed. If an admission kit is used, unpack the kit and place the items in the bedside stand or table. The admission kit usually includes a water pitcher, cup, soap dish, bar of soap, lotion, toothbrush, toothpaste, and mouthwash (Figure 22–2). Place a bedpan and/or urinal, bath basin, and emesis basin in the bedside stand. Check the room to be sure all equipment and supplies are in their proper places.
4. You may be required to go to the admissions office to get the new patient or resident, or the patient may be brought to the room by other personnel.
5. 

Greet and identify the patient. Ask the patient if he or she prefers to be called by a particular name. Introduce yourself by name and title to the patient and to any family members present. If another patient is in the room, introduce the new patient. Explain the procedure and obtain consent.

   NOTE: Be friendly and courteous at all times. Do not rush or hurry the patient.
6. Ask the family or visitors to wait in the lounge or lobby while you complete the admission process, if this is facility policy.

   NOTE: If a patient is not able to answer questions, a family member or other person responsible for the patient can remain in the room to complete the admission process.
7. Close the door and pull the curtain for privacy (Figure 22–3). Ask the patient to change into a gown or pajamas. Assist the patient as necessary.

   NOTE: In long-term care facilities, residents usually wear street clothes during the day. In this case, gowns or pajamas are not used.
8. Position the patient comfortably in the bed or in a chair.

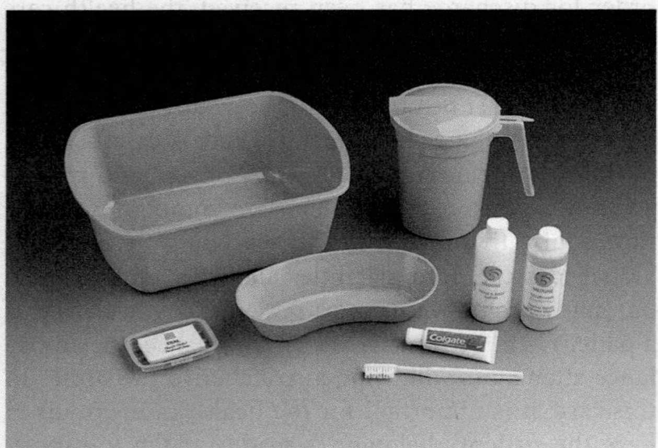

FIGURE 22–2 A sample admission kit. Courtesy of Medline Industries Inc., 1-860-MEDLINE

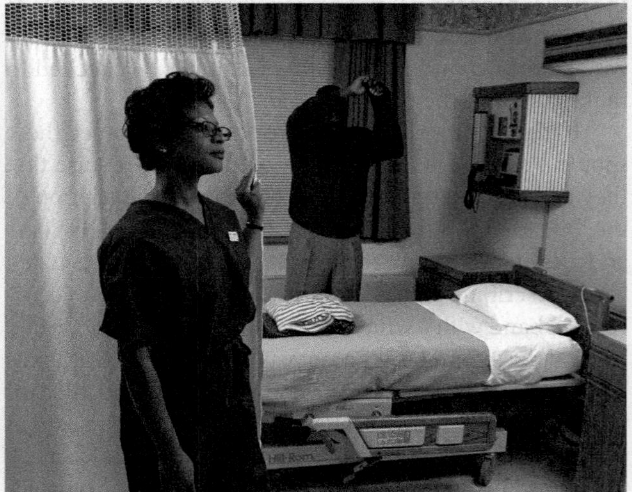

FIGURE 22–3 Close the door and pull the curtain to provide privacy while the patient undresses.

PROCEDURE 22:1A (CONT.)

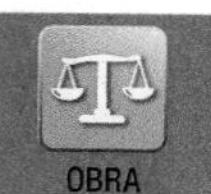

9. 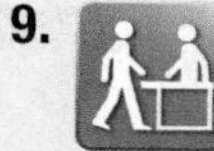

Complete the admission form. Ask questions slowly and clearly. Provide time for the patient to answer the questions.

NOTE: Observe the patient carefully during the admission process. Record all observations noted. If the patient expresses certain concerns, be sure to record and report these concerns.

10. Measure and record vital signs. Follow the procedures outlined in Chapter 16.
11. Weigh and measure the patient. Follow Procedure 21:1A. Record the information on the admission form.
12. Complete a personal inventory list. Be sure to list all personal items that will be kept in the patient's unit such as clothing, shoes, clocks, radios, cell phones, religious items, and books. Make sure the patient or a responsible individual checks and signs the list. Assist the patient as necessary in hanging up clothing or putting away personal items.
13. Complete a valuables list. If a family member takes the valuables home, be sure to obtain a signature on the proper form. If the valuables are to be placed in a safe or sent to security, fill out the form and obtain the patient's or a relative's signature. Follow agency policy for securing valuables.
14. Obtain a routine urine specimen if ordered. Follow Procedure 22:10A.
15. Orient the patient to the facility by demonstrating or explaining the following:
    a. Call signal or light
    b. Bed controls
    c. Television remote control and/or television rental policy
    d. Telephone
    e. Bathroom facilities and special call signal in bathroom
    f. Visiting hours
    g. Mealtimes and menu selections
    h. Activities or services available
    i. Health care facility regulations

    NOTE: Many health care facilities provide pamphlets or printed forms with the required information. However, it is still important to explain the main information to the patient and family.
16. Fill the water pitcher, if the patient is allowed to have liquids.
17. Observe all checkpoints before leaving the patient. Make sure the patient is comfortable and in good body alignment; the siderails are up, if indicated; the bed is at its lowest level; the call signal and supplies are in easy reach; and the area is neat and clean.
18. Clean and replace all equipment.
19. Wash hands.
20. When the admission process is complete, allow family members to return to the unit. Answer any questions they may have regarding facility policies. If you do not know the answers to their questions, obtain the correct answers from your immediate supervisor.
21. Comm Record all required information on the patient's chart or enter it into the computer. For example, date, time, admission form complete, valuables placed in safe (or sent to security), patient tolerated procedure well, and your signature and title. Report any abnormal observations to your immediate supervisor.

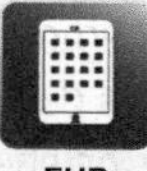

NOTE: In health care agencies using electronic health records (EHRs), also known as electronic medical records (EMRs), the information is entered directly into the patient's record on a computer.

PRACTICE: Go to the workbook and use the evaluation sheet for 22:1A, Admitting the Patient, to practice this procedure. When you believe you have mastered this skill, sign the sheet and give it to your instructor for further action.

FINAL CHECKPOINT: Using the criteria listed on the evaluation sheet, your instructor will grade your performance.

PROCEDURE 22:1B

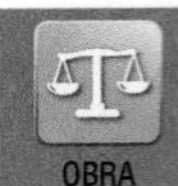

OBRA

Transferring the Patient

Equipment and Supplies

Transfer checklist (if used), personal inventory list, valuables list, cart (if needed), wheelchair or stretcher, gloves, paper and pen or computer

Procedure

1. Obtain permission from your immediate supervisor or check orders to obtain permission for the procedure. Find out the new unit or room number. Check to be sure that the unit is ready or ask your immediate supervisor to check. Check the method of transport to be used and obtain a wheelchair or stretcher, or use the patient's bed.
2. Assemble equipment.
3.  Comm Knock on the door and pause before entering. Introduce yourself. Identify the patient. Explain the procedure to the patient and obtain consent.

   NOTE: Reassure the patient as necessary. Patients are often apprehensive.
4. Wash hands.
5. Collect the patient's clothing and personal items. Check all items against the admission personal inventory list to be sure all items are present. Put the items in a bag or place them on a cart for transport. If the patient wears dentures, glasses, and/or a hearing aid, make sure he or she has these items.
6. Put any bedside equipment to be transferred onto a cart. This may include items such as the water pitcher, cup, soap dish, soap, emesis basin, bedpan, and bath basin. Check whether special equipment or medications are to be transferred. Follow agency policy regarding transfer of equipment.
7. If valuables are to be transferred, they must be checked and signed for by both the patient and the health care worker. The valuables are usually kept in the facility safe or with security, and the room or unit number of the patient is changed on the valuables bag when the patient is transferred.
8. Assist the patient into a wheelchair or stretcher depending on his or her condition. Follow the appropriate procedure as outlined in Chapter 22:2.
9. Transport the patient and the cart of supplies to the new unit or room (Figure 22–4). If help is not available, the patient may be taken to the new room first and the belongings taken afterward.

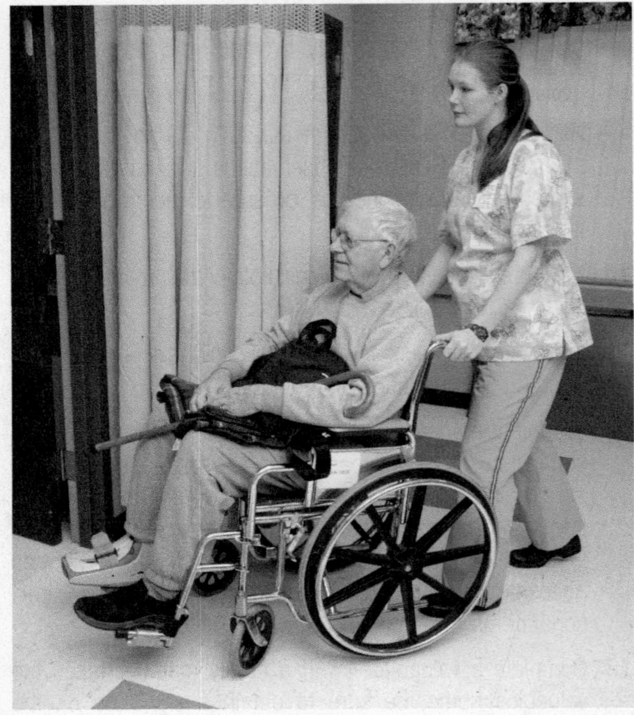

FIGURE 22–4 **If the patient's condition permits, use a wheelchair to transfer the patient to the new room or unit.**

 Safety **CAUTION:** Observe all safety precautions while transporting the patient.

10.  Comm Introduce the patient to the new staff members. Assist the staff members in getting the patient positioned comfortably in bed or in a chair. If another patient is in the room, introduce the patient. Orient the patient to the new room or unit by explaining or demonstrating the use of the equipment and supplies.

    NOTE: The staff members of the new unit may orient the patient.
11. Check the patient's belongings with the new staff member. Use the personal inventory and valuables checklist as needed. Be sure to obtain correct signatures according to agency policy.
12. Help put away the patient's clothing and personal items.
13. Observe all checkpoints before leaving the patient. Make sure the patient is comfortable and in good body alignment, the siderails are up (if indicated), the bed is at its lowest level, the call signal and supplies are in easy reach, and the area is neat and clean.

PROCEDURE 22:1B (CONT.)

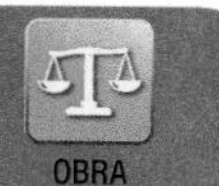

14. Replace all equipment.
15. Wash hands.
16.  Complete the transfer checklist. Record all required information on the patient's chart or enter it into the computer. For example, date, time, transferred to room 239-A by wheelchair, patient tolerated procedure well, transfer checklist completed, and your signature and title.
17. Return to the patient's previous room. Put on gloves. Strip the bed and remove any equipment that was not transferred. Follow agency policy for cleaning the room.

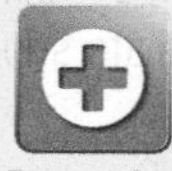

CAUTION: Wear gloves and observe standard precautions. Contact with body fluids, secretions, or excretions is possible.

NOTE: This may be the responsibility of the housekeeping department. If so, notify housekeeping that the patient has been transferred.

18. Remove gloves. Wash hands.
19.  Report to your immediate supervisor that the transfer has been completed.

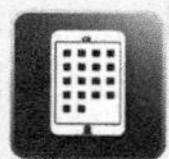

NOTE: In health care agencies using electronic health records (EHRs), also known as electronic medical records (EMRs), the information is entered directly into the patient's record on a computer.

PRACTICE: Go to the workbook and use the evaluation sheet for 22:1B, Transferring the Patient, to practice this procedure. When you believe you have mastered this skill, sign the sheet and give it to your instructor for further action.

FINAL CHECKPOINT: Using the criteria listed on the evaluation sheet, your instructor will grade your performance.

PROCEDURE 22:1C

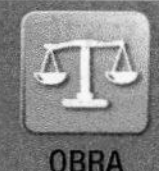

Discharging the Patient

Equipment and Supplies

Discharge checklist (if used), personal inventory list, valuables list, wheelchair (if needed), cart (if needed), gloves, paper and pen or computer

Procedure

1. Obtain orders from your immediate supervisor or check orders to obtain permission for the procedure. Check with the patient to determine when relatives or other individuals will be there to discharge the patient.

   NOTE: If the patient is to be discharged to another facility by ambulance, determine the time the ambulance will arrive.

2. Assemble equipment.
3. Knock on the door and pause before entering. Introduce yourself. Identify the patient. Explain the procedure and obtain consent.
4. Wash hands.
5. Close the door and pull the curtain for privacy. Help the patient dress, if assistance is needed.
6. Assemble all of the patient's personal belongings. If the patient wears dentures, glasses, and/or a hearing aid, make sure he or she has these items. Check drawers, closets, the bedside stand or table, and storage areas. Check all items against the personal inventory list to be sure everything is present. Obtain the patient's signature according to agency policy.
7. Assemble any equipment that is to be given to the patient. Examples include the supplies in the admission kit, such as the pitcher and cup.
8.  Check to make sure that the patient has received final instructions from the nurse and/or physician. These may include discharge instructions and prescriptions.
9. Obtain the patient's valuables, if they are in a safe or with security. Check the valuables with the patient. Obtain

(continues)

PROCEDURE 22:1C (CONT.)

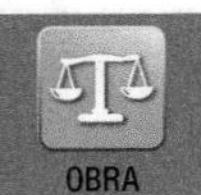

the correct signature to indicate that the valuables were returned to the patient.

NOTE: In some agencies, the patient or a responsible person obtains the valuables directly from the safe or security. In such a case, tell the patient how to obtain the valuables.

10. Complete a discharge checklist, if one is used, to be sure all procedures are complete.

11. Place all of the patient's belongings on a cart, if needed. Packed items sometimes are taken to the car by a relative.

12. Assist the patient into a wheelchair. Follow Procedure 22:2F

NOTE: Most facilities require the use of wheelchairs to transport patients. Some facilities allow patients to walk, but health care workers must accompany patients. Follow agency policy.

13. Transport the patient to the exit area. Help the patient into the car.

NOTE: If a cart is used to transfer the patient's belongings, another staff member should take the cart to the car.

CAUTION: Observe all safety factors while transporting the patient.

14. Help put the patient's belongings in the car.

15. Say good-bye to the patient.

16. Return to the unit. Put on gloves. Strip the bed and remove any equipment in the unit. Follow agency policy for cleaning the unit. Replace equipment.

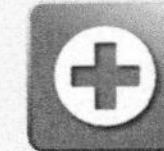

CAUTION: Wear gloves and observe standard precautions. Contact with body fluids, secretions, or excretions is possible.

NOTE: In some facilities, this is the responsibility of the housekeeping department. If so, notify housekeeping that the patient has been discharged.

17. Remove gloves. Wash hands.

18. Comm Record all required information on the patient's chart or enter it into the computer. For example, date, time, patient discharged, taken to husband's car by wheelchair, tolerated procedure well, and your signature and title. Report to your immediate supervisor that the discharge has been completed.

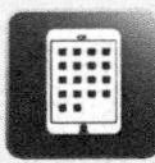

NOTE: In health care agencies using electronic health records (EHRs), also known as electronic medical records (EMRs), the information is entered directly into the patient's record on a computer.

PRACTICE: Go to the workbook and use the evaluation sheet for 22:1C, Discharging the Patient, to practice this procedure. When you believe you have mastered this skill, sign the sheet and give it to your instructor for further action.

FINAL CHECKPOINT: Using the criteria listed on the evaluation sheet, your instructor will grade your performance.

22:2 Positioning, Turning, Moving, and Transferring Patients

OBRA

As a health care worker, you may be responsible for positioning, turning, moving, and transferring many patients. If these procedures are done correctly, you will provide the patient with optimum comfort and care. In addition, you will prevent injury to yourself and the patient.

Legal

It is essential to remember that improper moving, turning, or transferring of a patient can result in serious injuries to the patient or health care worker. Some patients cannot be moved safely without special assistance or mechanical devices. Other patients who have had back, neck, or hip surgeries can only be turned certain ways. If a patient has restrictions for moving or transferring, the restrictions should be posted outside the door. If you are not sure whether a patient can be moved or transferred safely, *always* ask your supervisor before attempting any procedure. Remember, you are *legally* responsible for the safety and well-being of the patient.

Correct body mechanics are required for all procedures discussed here. Review and practice all of the rules of correct body mechanics as outlined in Chapter 14:1. If you are unable to move or turn a patient by yourself, always get help.

Alignment

Patient care must be directed toward maintaining normal body alignment. **Alignment** is defined as positioning body parts in relation to each other to maintain correct body posture. Benefits of proper alignment include:

- *Prevent fatigue*: Correct alignment helps the patient feel more comfortable and prevents fatigue.
- Science *Prevent* **pressure ulcers**: A pressure ulcer, also called a **decubitus ulcer**, pressure sore, or bedsore, is caused by prolonged pressure on an area of the body that interferes with circulation. Pressure ulcers are common in areas where bones are close to the skin, such as the tailbone, or coccygeal area; hips; knees; ankles; heels; and elbows. The tissue breakdown of a pressure ulcer occurs in four stages:
  (1) Stage I: a red or blue-gray discoloration appears on the intact skin (Figure 22–5A). The discoloration does not disappear after the pressure has been relieved.
  (2) Stage II: abrasions, bruises, and/or open sores develop as a result of tissue damage to the top layers of the skin (epidermis and dermis) (Figure 22–5B).
  (3) Stage III: a deep open crater forms when all layers of the skin are destroyed and fat and muscle tissues are exposed (Figure 22–5C).
  (4) Stage IV: damage extends into the muscle, tendon, and bone tissues (Figure 22–5D).

  It is easier to prevent pressure ulcers than it is to treat them. In addition, if pressure ulcers are detected in early stages, immediate treatment can help prevent further damage. Effective ways to prevent pressure ulcers include providing good skin care; using moisturizing lotions on dry skin; prompt cleaning of urine and feces from the skin; massaging in a circular motion around a reddened area; frequent turning (at

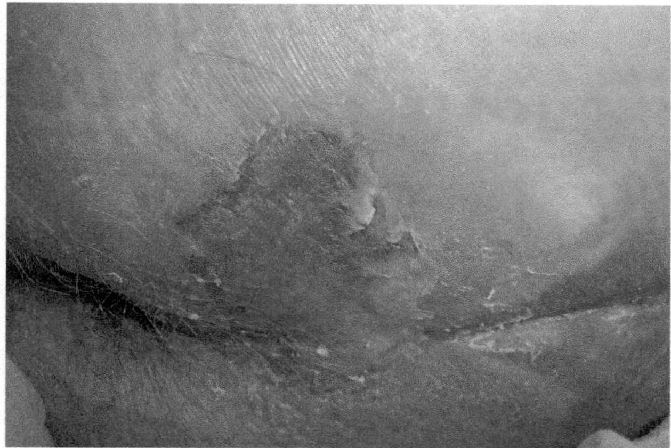

FIGURE 22–5B A stage II pressure ulcer is characterized by abrasions, bruises, and/or open sores as a result of tissue damage to the top layers of skin. Used with permission of the National Pressure Ulcer Advisory Panel 2012

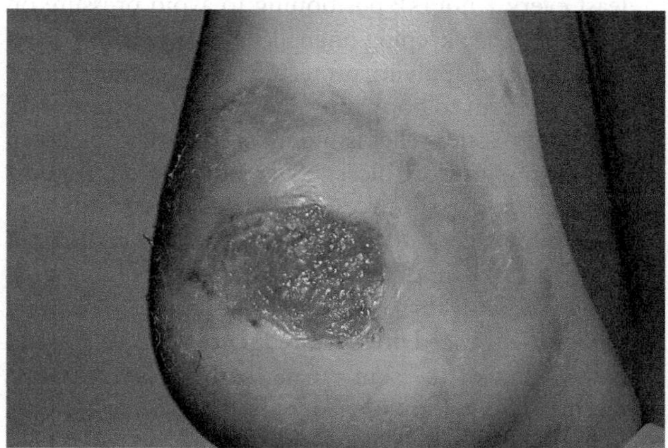

FIGURE 22–5C In a stage III pressure ulcer, a deep open crater forms when all layers of the skin are destroyed. Used with permission of the National Pressure Ulcer Advisory Panel 2012

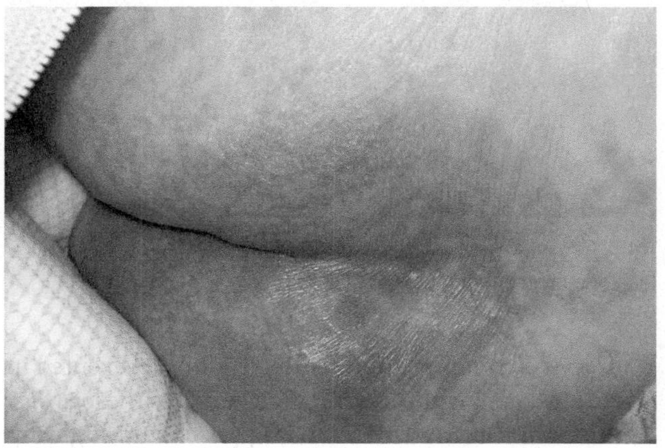

FIGURE 22–5A A stage I pressure ulcer has a red or blue-gray discoloration that does not disappear after pressure has been relieved. Used with permission of the National Pressure Ulcer Advisory Panel 2012

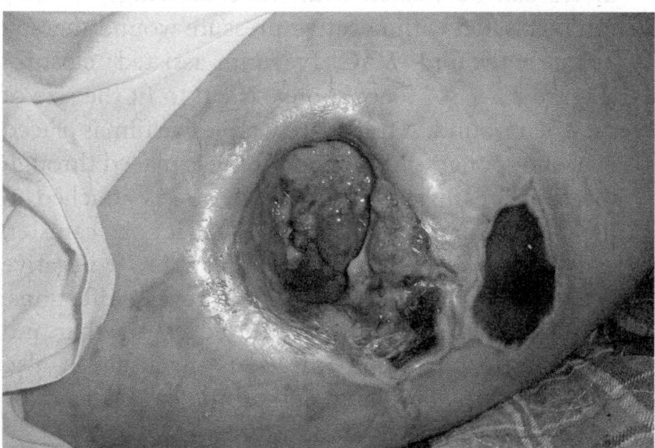

FIGURE 22–5D In a stage IV pressure ulcer, damage extends into the muscle, tendon, and bone tissues. Used with permission of the National Pressure Ulcer Advisory Panel 2012

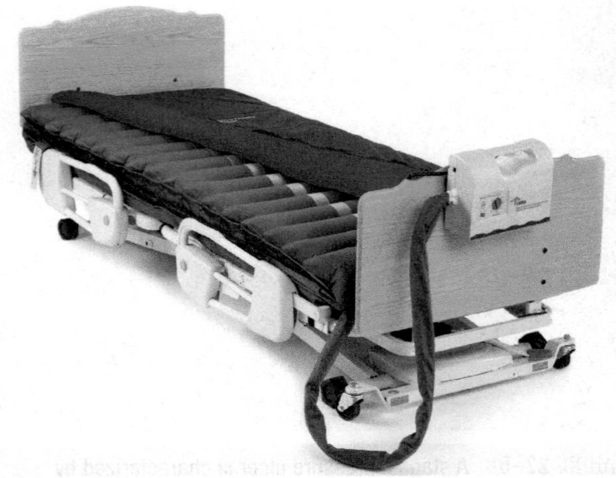

FIGURE 22–6 **An alternating air pressure mattress constantly changes the pressure points against a patient's skin.** Courtesy of Medline Industries Inc., 1-860-MEDLINE

least every 2 hours); positioning to avoid pressure on irritated areas; keeping linen clean, dry, and free from wrinkles; and applying protectors of sheepskin, lamb's wool, or foam to bony prominences such as heels and elbows. Pressure relief is the most important factor in preventing pressure ulcers. Over 100 different support surfaces or pressure-reducing products are available to prevent ulcers. Alternating air pressure mattresses (Figure 22–6) and continuous lateral rotation beds (that constantly turn the patient side to side) are among the most advanced pressure-reducing surfaces. Careful observation of the skin during bathing or turning is essential. If a pale, reddened, or blue-gray area is noted, this should be reported and documented immediately.

- *Treatment of pressure ulcers*: Stage I and stage II pressure ulcers are often treated with special foam or hydrocolloid dressings along with frequent turning to keep pressure off the ulcer. Stage III and stage IV ulcers can be treated with these dressings, or they can be treated with negative-pressure wound therapy using a wound VAC (vacuum-assisted closure) (Figure 22–7). A foam sponge is cut to fit the size of the open wound. A transparent adhesive film is placed over the sponge and suction tubing is placed through the film dressing. The suction tubing is attached to the suction and a disposable collection canister. This device seals the wound and applies a negative pressure to promote healing and prevent infections. It works by drawing the wound edges together and removing exudate and infectious materials. It also reduces edema (swelling) and promotes perfusion by forcing the flow of fluid in the area.
- *Prevent contractures*: A **contracture** (Figure 22–8) is a tightening or shortening of a muscle usually caused by lack of movement or usage of the muscle. Foot drop is a common contracture. It can be prevented in part by keeping the foot at a right angle to the leg (Figure 22–9). Footboards, foot supports, and high-top tennis shoes can be used to keep the foot in this position. Range-of-motion (ROM) exercises, discussed in Chapter 23:1, also help prevent contractures.

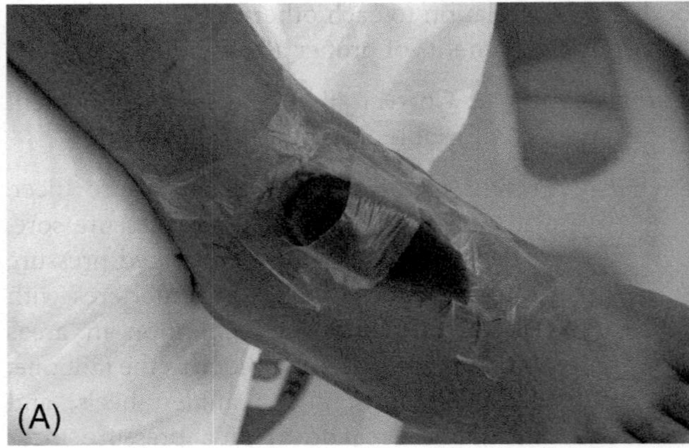

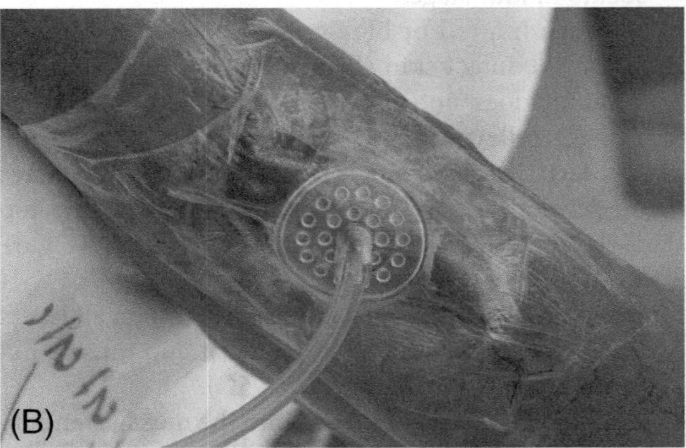

FIGURE 22–7 **(A) After a pressure ulcer or wound is covered with a gauze or foam dressing, (B) the wound VAC is attached to apply negative pressure to the area to promote healing.**

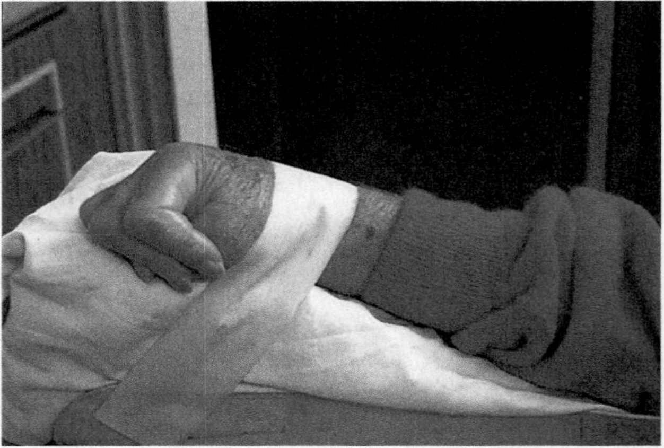

FIGURE 22–8 **A contracture is a tightening of a muscle caused by lack of movement or usage of the muscle.**

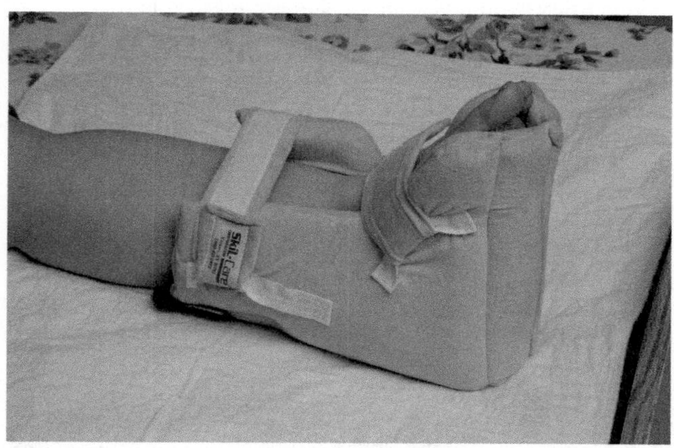

FIGURE 22–9 Foot supports can be used to hold the feet at right angles and prevent foot drop, a common contracture.

Turning

The patient confined to bed must be turned frequently. The patient's position should be changed at least every 2 hours, if permitted by the physician. Some agencies post a turning position schedule by the patient's bed. For example: 6 AM: Right side; 8 AM: Back; 10 AM: Left side; and 12 Noon: Abdomen. Frequent turning provides exercise for the muscles. It also stimulates circulation, decreases pulmonary congestion, helps prevent pressure ulcers and contractures, and provides comfort to the patient. Correct turning procedures must be followed to prevent injury to both the patient and the health care worker.

Dangling

If a patient has been confined to bed for a period of time, the patient is frequently placed in a dangling position before being transferred from the bed. **Dangling** means sitting with the legs hanging down over the side of the bed. This allows the patient some time to adjust to the sitting position. The pulse rate is checked at least three times during this procedure: before, during, and after the dangling period. It is taken just before the patient is moved to the dangling position; this pulse rate serves as a control, or resting, rate. The pulse rate is checked again immediately after positioning the patient in the dangling position. The third check occurs after the patient is returned to a lying-down (supine) position in the bed. By noting changes in the pulse rate, the health care worker can determine how well the patient tolerates the procedure. Blood pressure can also be checked to determine a patient's tolerance of the procedure. The blood pressure is taken while lying down, sitting, and standing. A patient might experience a drop in blood pressure with position changes, a condition called *orthostatic hypotension*. In addition to taking the pulse and blood pressure, observe the patient's respiratory rate, balance (the patient may complain of vertigo or dizziness), amount of perspiration, color, and other similar characteristics. If the pulse rate shows an abnormal increase, the blood pressure drops measurably, respirations become labored, color becomes pale, increased perspiration is noted, or the patient gets dizzy or very weak, the patient should be returned immediately to the supine, resting position.

Transfers

Patients are frequently transferred to wheelchairs, chairs, or stretchers. Again, correct procedures must be followed to prevent injury to both the patient and the worker. Many different models of wheelchairs and stretchers are available. It is important to read the manufacturer's instructions regarding the operation of any given piece of equipment. If no instructions are available, ask your immediate supervisor to demonstrate the correct operation of a particular wheelchair or stretcher.

Mechanical lifts are frequently used to transfer weak or paralyzed patients. Again, it is important to read the operating instructions provided with the lift. Straps, clasps, and the sling should be checked carefully for any defects. Smooth, even movements must be used while operating the lift. Patients are often frightened of the lift and must be reassured that it is safe.

In home care situations, it is important to move unnecessary furniture out of the way during transfers. If the bed does not raise or lower, it is essential for the health care worker to observe correct body mechanics and to bend at the hips and knees instead of the waist. It is possible to rent hospital beds, wheelchairs, mechanical lifts, and other similar items for home care.

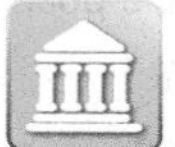
Legal

Before a patient is moved or transferred, the health care worker must obtain approval or orders from his or her immediate supervisor. Never move or transfer a patient without proper authorization.

Safety

During any move or transfer, it is important to watch the patient closely. Note changes in pulse rate, blood pressure, respirations, and color. Observe for signs of weakness, dizziness, increased perspiration, or discomfort. If you note any abnormal changes, return the patient to a safe and comfortable position and check with your immediate supervisor. The supervisor will determine whether the move or transfer should be attempted.

STUDENT: **Go to the workbook and complete the assignment sheet for 22:2, Positioning, Turning, Moving, and Transferring Patients. Then return and continue with the procedures.**

PROCEDURE 22:2A

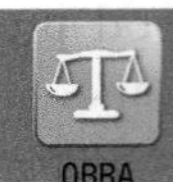

Aligning the Patient

Equipment and Supplies

Three pillows, two or three bath blankets, two or three large towels, two or three washcloths or small towels, protectors for bony prominences, footboard, gloves, paper and pen or computer

Procedure

1. Obtain orders from your immediate supervisor or check orders to obtain permission for the procedure.
2. Assemble equipment.
3. 

Knock on the door and pause before entering. Introduce yourself. Identify the patient. Explain the procedure and obtain consent.
4. Provide privacy. Close the door and pull the curtain.
5. Wash hands. Put on gloves.

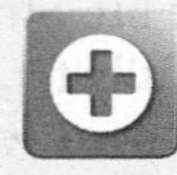

CAUTION: Wear gloves and observe standard precautions. Contact with body fluids, secretions, or excretions is possible.

6. Lock the wheels on the bed. Elevate the bed to a comfortable height. If siderails are elevated, lower the bedrail or siderail on the side of the bed where you are working.

CAUTION: If the bed does not raise to a working height, use correct body mechanics and bend from the hips and knees, not the waist, to get close to the patient.

7. Align the patient who is lying on the back in a supine position as follows (Figure 22–10):
   a. Position the head in a straight line with the spine.
   b. Place pillow under the head and neck to provide support.
   c. A pillow or rolled blanket may be placed under the lower legs, from the knees to 2 inches above the heels to provide support and keep the heels off the bed.
   d. Protector pads may be placed on the heels or elbows (Figure 22–11).
   e. Toes should point upward. You may place a footboard, pillow, or rolled blanket against the soles of the feet to achieve this. High-top tennis shoes can also be placed on the feet to keep them at this angle.

   NOTE: Check the patient for comfort, safety, and support before leaving. Make sure no bony prominences are exposed and all body parts are supported.

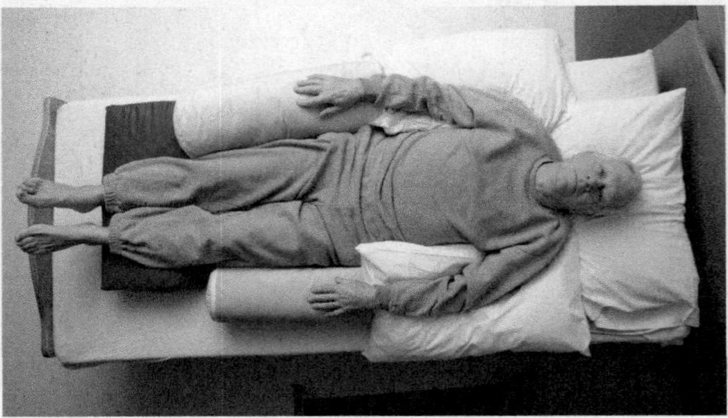

FIGURE 22–10 **Correct alignment for a patient positioned on the back in the horizontal recumbent or supine position.**

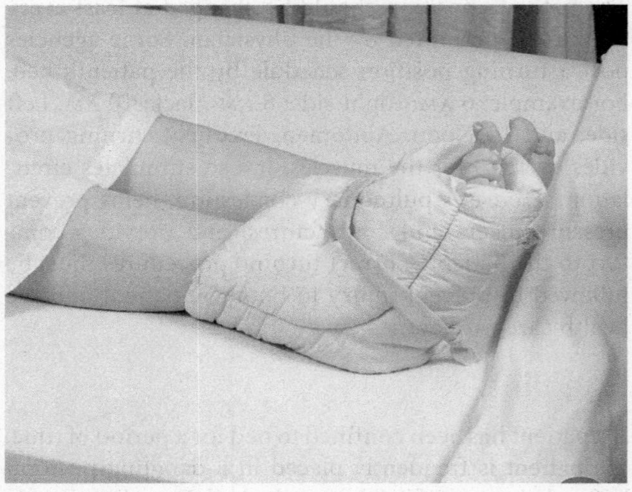

FIGURE 22–11 **Foot protectors can help prevent pressure ulcers on the heels.**

8. Align the patient who is lying on the side (Figure 22–12) as follows:
   a. Place a small pillow under the head and neck for support.
   b. Flex the lower arm at the elbow. It can be placed in line with the face.
   c. Support the upper arm, flexed at the elbow, on a pillow or rolled blanket.
   d. Flex both knees slightly. Place a firm pillow or rolled blanket between the legs. The pillow should extend from the upper leg to the ankle.

PROCEDURE 22:2A (CONT.)

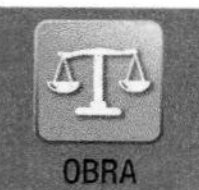
OBRA

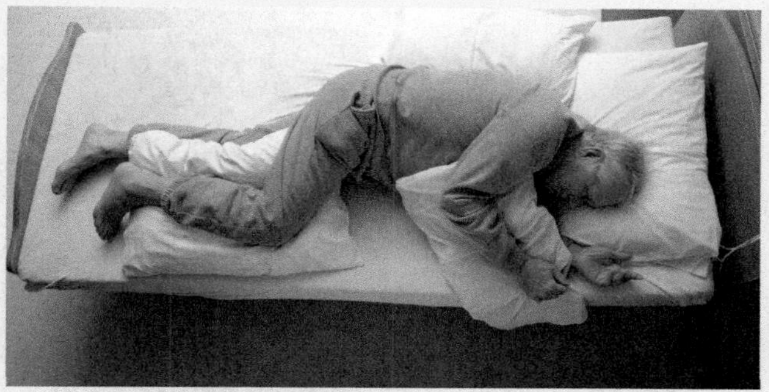

FIGURE 22–12 **Correct alignment for a patient positioned on the side.**

e. Use a footboard, pillow, rolled blanket, or high-top tennis shoes to keep the feet at right angles (90 degrees) to the legs.

f. Rolled washcloths or foam rubber balls may be placed in paralyzed hands to prevent contractures.

g. Use pillows to support the back and abdomen.

h. Protector pads may be placed on the ankles, heels, and elbows.

Safety

CAUTION: Make sure that the patient's body is not twisted and that any one body part is not applying direct pressure on any other body part.

NOTE: Check all aspects of the patient's position before leaving.

9. Align the patient who is lying on the abdomen (in the prone position) as follows:

a. Place the head in a direct line with the spine.

b. Turn the head to one side. It may be supported with a small pillow. Placing the pillow at an angle will keep it away from the patient's face.

c. A small pillow may be placed under the waist for support.

d. Place a firm pillow under the lower legs. This will slightly flex the knees.

e. The feet can be extended over the end of the mattress so that they will remain at right angles to the legs. They can also be supported in this position by pillows or rolled blankets (Figure 22–13).

f. Place the arms in line on either side of the head. Use pads to protect the elbows. Flex the elbows slightly for comfort.

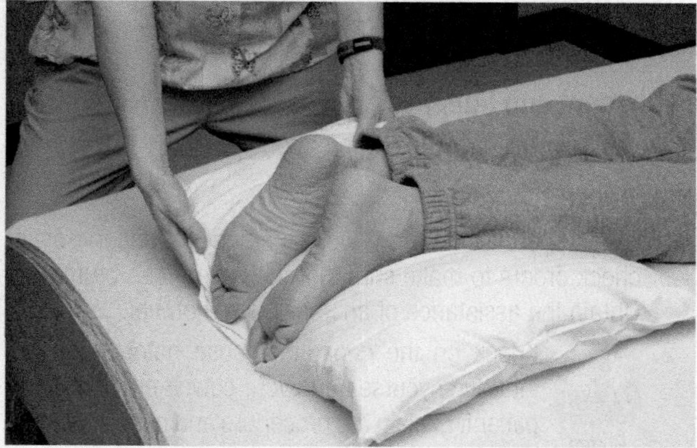

FIGURE 22–13 **A large pillow can be used to support the feet when the patient is lying in the prone position.**

NOTE: Check all aspects of position, comfort, and safety before leaving the patient.

10. Observe all checkpoints before leaving the patient. Make sure the siderails are elevated (if indicated), the bed is at its lowest level, the call signal and supplies are in easy reach, the patient is comfortable and in good body alignment, and the area is neat and clean.

11. Properly replace all equipment not being used.

12. Remove gloves. Wash hands.

13. 
Comm

Report that the procedure is complete or record all required information on the patient's chart or enter it into the computer. For example, date, time, positioned on left side in correct alignment, patient appears to be resting comfortably, and your signature and title. Note any unusual observations.

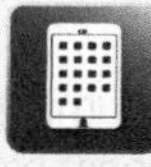
EHR

NOTE: In health care agencies using electronic health records (EHRs), also known as electronic medical records (EMRs), the information is entered directly into the patient's record on a computer.

PRACTICE: **Go to the workbook and use the evaluation sheet for 22:2A, Aligning the Patient, to practice this procedure. When you believe you have mastered this skill, sign the sheet and give it to your instructor for further action.**

Check

FINAL CHECKPOINT: Using the criteria listed on the evaluation sheet, your instructor will grade your performance.

PROCEDURE 22:2B

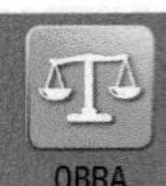
OBRA

Moving the Patient Up in Bed

Equipment and Supplies

Lift sheet, gloves, paper and pen or computer

Procedure

1. Obtain permission from your immediate supervisor or check orders to make sure that the patient can be moved. Obtain the assistance of another team member.
2. 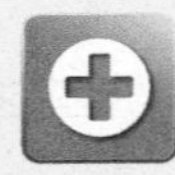 Comm — Knock on the door and pause before entering. Introduce yourself and your coworker. Identify the patient. Explain the procedure and obtain consent.
3. Provide privacy. Close the door and pull the curtain.
4. Wash hands. Put on gloves.

    Precaution — **CAUTION:** Wear gloves and observe standard precautions. Contact with body fluids, secretions, or excretions is possible.
5. One person should be on each side of the bed. Lock the bed (usually by way of wheel locks) to prevent movement of the bed. Elevate the bed to a comfortable height. Lower the siderails, if elevated.

   NOTE: Locks and siderails on beds vary. If you do not know how to lock a bed or operate siderails, check with your immediate supervisor.
6. Lower the head of the bed. Remove all pillows. One pillow can be placed against the headboard of the bed to prevent injury to the patient's head while moving the patient up in bed.

   NOTE: Observe the patient for respiratory distress.

   Safety — **CAUTION:** If any breathing difficulty is noted, immediately raise the head of the bed. Check with your supervisor before proceeding.
7. Position the lift sheet under the patient by turning the patient to one side (Figure 22–14A). The lift sheet can be fanfolded to the center of the bed. Make sure it extends under the patient's head, shoulders, hips, and thighs. Turn the patient to the opposite side and unfold the lift sheet so it covers the entire bed. Turn the patient on his or her back.

   NOTE: Use proper body mechanics throughout the procedure. Use the weight of your body to move the patient. Avoid back strain.
8. Two people should use the lift sheet to move the patient.
   a. One person stands on each side of the bed. Each person positions one hand on the lift sheet by the patient's shoulders and the other hand by the patient's hips.
   b. Each person faces the head of the bed and gets a broad base of support by putting one foot ahead of the other. Each person should be close to the patient and the bed.

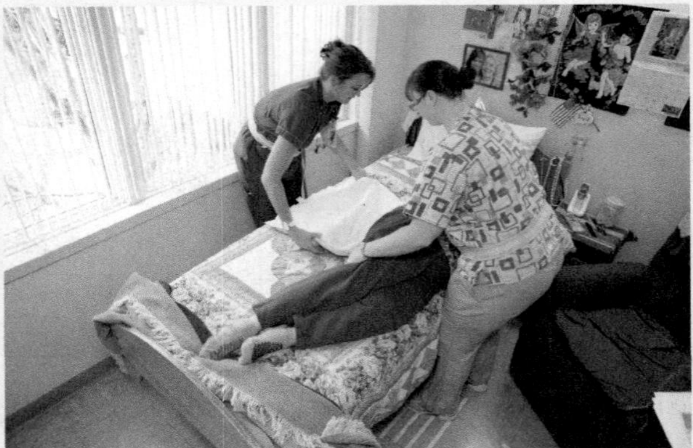

FIGURE 22–14A Turn the patient to one side to position the lift sheet under the patient.

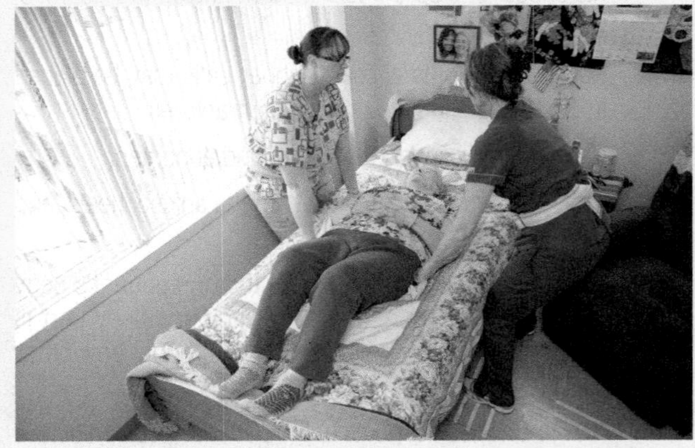

FIGURE 22–14B Both health care workers should roll the edges of the lift sheet inward close to both sides of the patient's body.

   c. If the patient's condition permits, ask the patient to flex his or her knees and brace both feet firmly on the bed.
   d. Each person rolls the edges of the lift sheet inward close to both sides of the patient's body (Figure 22–14B).
   e. At a given signal, such as *one-two-lift,* the two health care workers lift the sheet and patient, and move the patient to the head of the bed (Figure 22–14C).

   NOTE: Shift your weight from the rear leg to the forward leg at the same time that you slide the patient.
   f. After the patient is positioned, each worker tucks the lift sheet back into the side of the bed.
9. Leave the patient in good body alignment. Make sure the patient is comfortable.
10. Elevate the siderails (if indicated). Place the call signal and any needed supplies within easy reach of the patient. Lower the bed to its lowest level.
11. Replace all equipment. Make sure the area is neat and clean.

PROCEDURE 22:2B (CONT.)

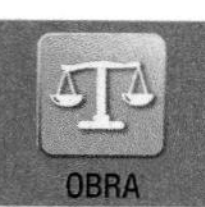

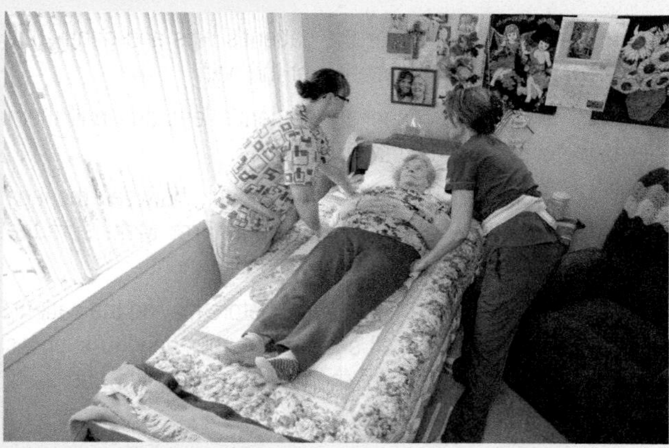

FIGURE 22–14C At a given signal, the workers lift and move the sheet and patient to the head of the bed.

12. Remove gloves. Wash hands.
13. 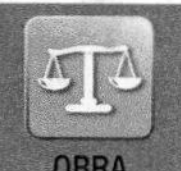 Report that the patient has been moved up in bed and/or record all required information on the patient's chart or enter it into the computer. For example, date, time, moved to head of bed, tolerated procedure well, and your signature and title. Note any unusual observations.

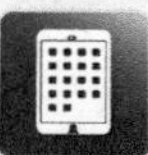

NOTE: In health care agencies using electronic health records (EHRs), also known as electronic medical records (EMRs), the information is entered directly into the patient's record on a computer.

PRACTICE: **Go to the workbook and use the evaluation sheet for 22:2B, Moving the Patient Up in Bed, to practice this procedure. When you believe you have mastered this skill, sign the sheet and give it to your instructor for further action.**

FINAL CHECKPOINT: Using the criteria listed on the evaluation sheet, your instructor will grade your performance.

PROCEDURE 22:2C

OBRA

Turning the Patient Away to Change Position

Equipment and Supplies

Paper and pen or computer, gloves

Procedure

1. Obtain permission from your immediate supervisor or check orders to make sure that the patient can be turned.
2. Comm Knock on the door and pause before entering. Introduce yourself. Identify the patient. Explain the procedure and obtain consent.
3. Provide privacy. Close the door and pull the curtain.
4. Wash hands. Put on gloves.

   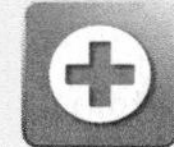

   CAUTION: Wear gloves and observe standard precautions. Contact with body fluids, secretions, or excretions is possible.
5. Lock wheels to prevent movement of the bed. Elevate the bed to a comfortable height.
6. If siderails are present and elevated, lower the siderail nearest to you. Make sure the opposite siderail is raised and locked securely.
7. The patient should be lying on the side of the bed close to you. If so, proceed to step 8. If the patient is at the center or close to the far side of the bed, move the patient as follows:
   a. Place one hand under the patient's head and neck. Place your other hand under the patient's upper back. Slide the upper part of the patient's body toward you.
   b. Place both hands under the patient's hips. Slide the hips toward you.
   c. Place both hands under the patient's upper and lower legs. Slide the legs toward you.

   CAUTION: If you are not able to move the patient, get help.

   CAUTION: Check the opposite siderail. Make sure it is up before proceeding.
8. Ask the patient to place his or her arms across the chest and move the proximal leg (the one closest to you) over the other leg.

   NOTE: This will make it easier to turn the patient and helps prevent injury.

(continues)

PROCEDURE 22:2C (CONT.)

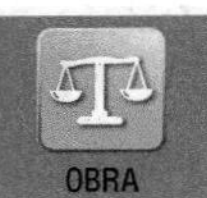

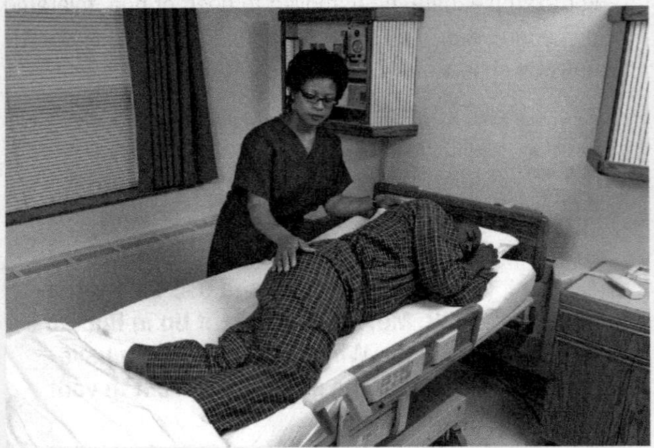

FIGURE 22–15 **Put one hand under the patient's shoulder and the other hand under the patient's hip. Then use a smooth, even motion to roll the patient away from you.**

CAUTION: Do not cross the legs if the patient had hip replacement surgery.

9. Get close to the patient by bending your knees and keeping your back straight. Position your feet to provide a broad base of support. Place one arm under the patient's shoulders. Place your opposite hand under the patient's hips.
10. Use a smooth, even motion to roll the patient away from you and onto his or her side (Figure 22–15).

NOTE: Explain what you are doing to the patient.

11. Place your hands under the patient's head and shoulders. Draw the head and shoulders back toward the center of the bed.
12. Place your hands under the patient's hips and gently pull them back toward the center of the bed.
13. Place your hands under the patient's legs and pull them back toward the center of the bed.
14. Place a pillow behind the patient's back, between the legs to align the hips, and under the upper arm. Make sure the patient is comfortable and in good alignment.
15. Elevate the siderails (if indicated) before leaving the patient. Make sure that the call signal and other needed supplies are within easy reach of the patient. Lower the bed to its lowest level.
16. Replace all equipment. Leave the area neat and clean.
17. Remove gloves. Wash hands.
18. 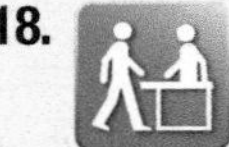 Report that patient has been turned and/or record all required information on the patient's chart or enter it into the computer. For example, date, time, turned on left side and positioned in correct alignment, and your signature and title. Note any unusual observations.

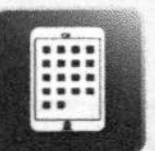

NOTE: In health care agencies using electronic health records (EHRs), also known as electronic medical records (EMRs), the information is entered directly into the patient's record on a computer.

PRACTICE: **Go to the workbook and use the evaluation sheet for 22:2C, Turning the Patient Away to Change Position, to practice this procedure. When you believe you have mastered this skill, sign the sheet and give it to your instructor for further action.**

FINAL CHECKPOINT: Using the criteria listed on the evaluation sheet, your instructor will grade your performance.

PROCEDURE 22:2D

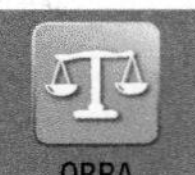

Turning the Patient Inward to Change Position

Equipment and Supplies

Paper and pen or computer, gloves

Procedure

1. Obtain permission from your immediate supervisor or check orders to make sure that the patient can be turned.
2.  Knock on the door and pause before entering. Introduce yourself. Identify the patient. Explain the procedure and obtain consent.
3. Provide privacy. Close the door and pull the curtain.
4. Wash hands. Put on gloves.

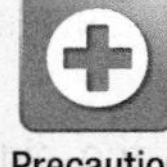

CAUTION: Wear gloves and observe standard precautions. Contact with body fluids, secretions, or excretions is possible.

5. Lock the wheels of the bed to prevent movement. Elevate the bed to a comfortable height.

PROCEDURE 22:2D (CONT.)

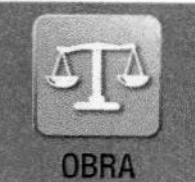

OBRA

6. Lower the siderail nearest to you, if present and elevated.
7. If the patient is too close to the near side of the bed, move him or her to the opposite side as follows:
   a. Place one hand under the patient's head and shoulders and the other hand under the patient's back. Slide the upper part of the body toward the opposite side of the bed.
   b. Place both hands under the patient's hips. Slide the hips toward the opposite side of the bed.
   c. Place both hands under the patient's legs. Slide the legs toward the opposite side of the bed.
8. Instruct the patient to cross his or her arms on the chest. Place the patient's leg that is farthest from you on top of the leg that is nearest to you.

   NOTE: This prevents injury to the patient's arms and legs.

Safety

CAUTION: Do not cross the legs if the patient has had hip replacement surgery.

9. Get close to the patient by bending your knees and keeping your back straight. Position your feet to provide a broad base of support. Place your hand that is closest to the head of the bed on the patient's far shoulder. Place your other hand behind the patient's hip (Figure 22–16A). Use your knee to brace your body against the side of the bed. Use a gentle, smooth motion to roll the patient toward you (Figure 22–16B).
10. A lift sheet can also be used by one or two health care workers to turn the patient. The workers grasp the edges of the lift sheet and roll the edges inward close to the patient's body (Figure 22–16C). At a given signal, the workers use a smooth, even motion to turn the patient inward (Figure 22–16D).

Safety

CAUTION: Observe proper body mechanics at all times.

11. Raise and secure the siderail, if indicated. Go to the opposite side of the bed and lower the siderail, if present and elevated.
12. Place your hands under the patient's head and shoulders and draw the head and shoulders back toward the center of the bed.
13. Place your hands under the patient's hips and draw them toward the center of the bed.
14. Place your hands under the patient's legs and draw them toward the center of the bed.

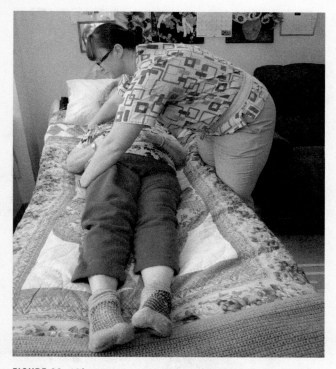

FIGURE 22–16A Position your hands on the patient's far shoulder and hip.

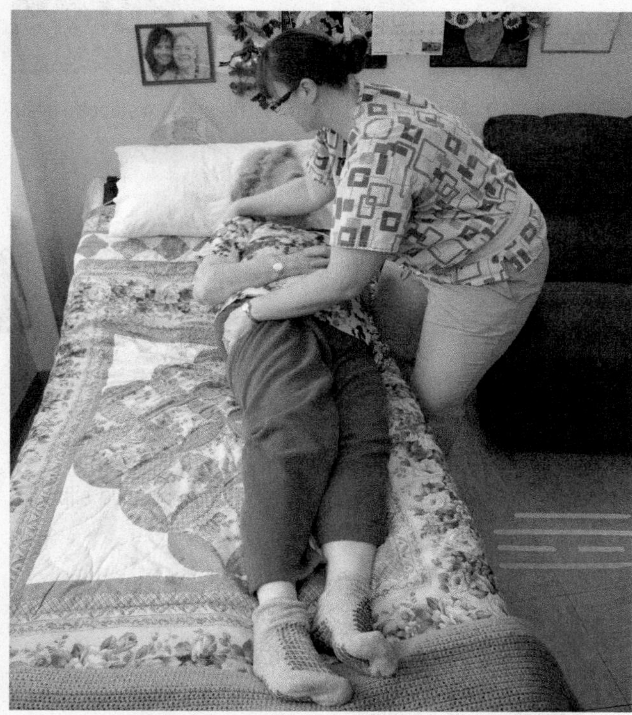

FIGURE 22–16B Use a gentle, smooth motion to roll the patient toward you.

(continues)

PROCEDURE 22:2D (CONT.)

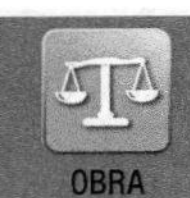

OBRA

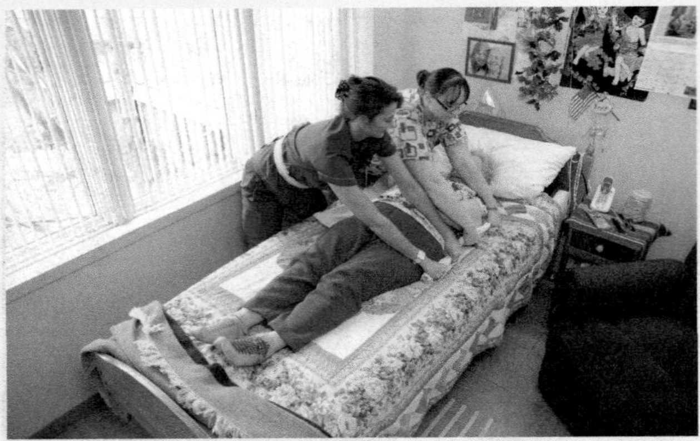

FIGURE 22–16C A lift sheet can also be used by one or two health care workers to turn the patient.

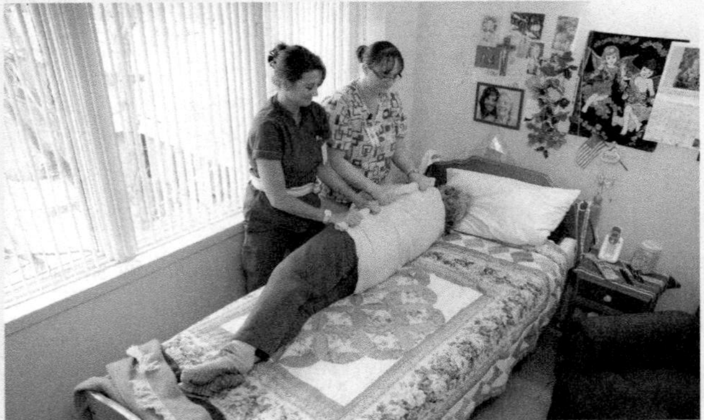

FIGURE 22–16D At a given signal, the workers use a smooth, even motion to turn the patient inward.

15. Place pillows behind the patient's back, between the legs, and under the upper arm to position the patient in good body alignment. Make sure that the patient is comfortable.
16. Elevate the siderail, if indicated. Place the call signal and other necessary supplies within easy reach of the patient. Lower the bed to its lowest level.
17. Replace all equipment. Leave the area neat and clean.
18. Remove gloves. Wash hands.
19.  Comm Report that patient has been turned and/or record all required information on the patient's chart or enter it into the computer. For example, date, time, turned on right side and positioned in correct alignment, and your signature and title. Note any unusual observations.

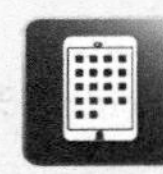 EHR **NOTE:** In health care agencies using electronic health records (EHRs), also known as electronic medical records (EMRs), the information is entered directly into the patient's record on a computer.

PRACTICE: **Go to the workbook and use the evaluation sheet for 22:2D, Turning the Patient Inward to Change Position, to practice this procedure. When you believe you have mastered this skill, sign the sheet and give it to your instructor for further action.**

 Check **FINAL CHECKPOINT:** Using the criteria listed on the evaluation sheet, your instructor will grade your performance.

PROCEDURE 22:2E

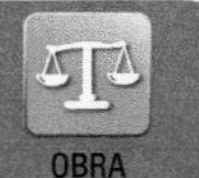

OBRA

Sitting Up to Dangle

Equipment and Supplies

Footstool (if needed), bath blanket, robe and non-skid slippers, gloves, paper and pen or computer

Procedure

1. Check orders or obtain authorization from your immediate supervisor. Orders usually state the length of time the patient should dangle.
2. Assemble equipment.
3. 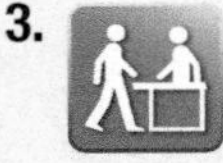 Comm Knock on the door and pause before entering. Introduce yourself. Identify the patient. Explain the procedure and obtain consent.
4. Provide privacy. Close the door and pull the curtain.
5. Wash hands. Put on gloves.

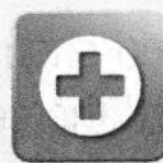 Precaution **CAUTION:** Wear gloves and observe standard precautions. Contact with body fluids, secretions, or excretions is possible.

6. Lock the bed wheels to prevent movement of the bed.
7. Lower the bed to its lowest level. If siderails are present and elevated, lower the siderail on the side where the patient is to dangle.

PROCEDURE 22:2E (CONT.)

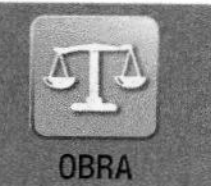

8. Check the patient's radial pulse. This reading will serve as a guideline on how the patient tolerates the procedure.

   NOTE: Blood pressure may also be checked at this time. Follow agency policy.

9. Slowly elevate the head of the bed to a sitting position. Provide time for the patient to adjust to this position.

10. Get close to the patient by bending your knees and keeping your back straight. Position your feet to provide a broad base of support. Place your arm that is nearest to the head of the bed around the patient's shoulders. Place your other arm under the patient's knees (Figure 22–17A). Slowly and smoothly rotate the patient toward the side of the bed (Figure 22–17B).

    Safety

    CAUTION: Use proper body mechanics at all times.

    Safety

    CAUTION: Stand in front of the patient to prevent falls.

11. Put a robe on the patient. Prevent unnecessary exposure.

12. Use the bath blanket to cover the patient's lap and legs. Put non-skid slippers on the patient. Rest the patient's feet on a footstool (if necessary).

13. Check the patient's radial pulse. Note any signs of distress, such as pale color, increased perspiration, labored respirations, weakness, dizziness, or nausea.

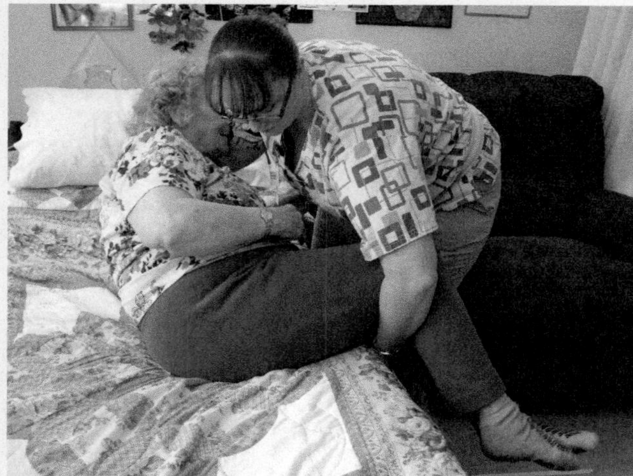

FIGURE 22–17A **Place one arm around the patient's shoulders and the other arm under the patient's knees.**

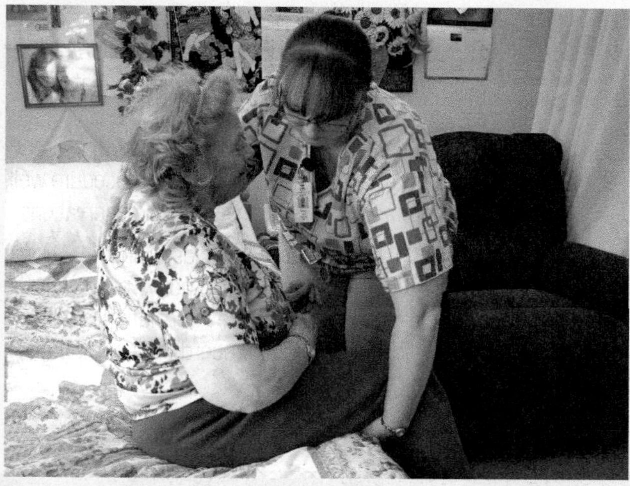

FIGURE 22–17B **Slowly rotate the patient toward the side of the bed.**

   NOTE: Blood pressure may also be checked at this time. Follow agency policy.

   Safety

   CAUTION: If any of these signs are noted, go immediately to step 17 and return the patient to the original position in bed.

14. Instruct the patient to flex and extend the legs and feet. This increases circulation to the area and stimulates the muscles.

15. Have the patient dangle for the time ordered or as the patient's condition permits.

16. When the time is up, remove the patient's robe, slippers, and the bath blanket.

17. Place one arm around the patient's shoulders and your other arm under the patient's knees. Gently and slowly return the patient to the bed.

    Safety

    CAUTION: Use correct body mechanics.

18. Slowly lower the head of the bed.

19. Position the patient in good alignment.

20. Check the patient's radial pulse. Note any major changes. Report any changes immediately.

21. Observe all checkpoints before leaving the patient. Make sure the siderails are elevated (if indicated), the bed is at its lowest level, the call signal and other supplies are within easy reach, and the area is neat and clean.

22. Remove gloves. Wash hands.

(continues)

PROCEDURE 22:2E (CONT.)

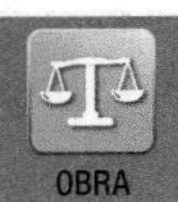
OBRA

23. 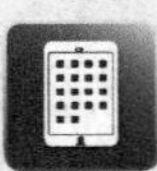 Comm Report that the patient has dangled and/or record all required information on the patient's chart or enter it into the computer. For example, date, time, sat on side of bed for 15 minutes, P 72 strong and regular at start of procedure, P 78 strong and regular at end, knees and legs flexed and extended, tolerated procedure well, and your signature and title. Note any unusual observations.

 EHR **NOTE:** In health care agencies using electronic health records (EHRs), also known as electronic medical records (EMRs), the information is entered directly into the patient's record on a computer.

PRACTICE: **Go to the workbook and use the evaluation sheet for 22:2E, Sitting Up to Dangle, to practice this procedure. When you believe you have mastered this skill, sign the sheet and give it to your instructor for further action.**

 Check **FINAL CHECKPOINT:** Using the criteria listed on the evaluation sheet, your instructor will grade your performance.

PROCEDURE 22:2F

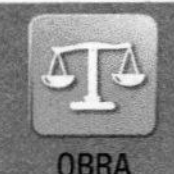
OBRA

Transferring a Patient to a Chair or Wheelchair

NOTE: Wheelchairs vary slightly. Read the manufacturer's instructions or ask your immediate supervisor to demonstrate correct operation of the footrests, wheel locks, and other parts.

Equipment and Supplies

Wheelchair or chair, bathrobe, transfer belt, one to two bath blankets, non-skid slippers, gloves, paper and pen or computer

Procedure

1. Obtain orders from your immediate supervisor or check physician's orders to obtain authorization.
2. Assemble equipment.
3.  Comm Knock on the door and pause before entering. Introduce yourself. Identify the patient. Explain the procedure and obtain consent.
4. Close the door and pull the curtain to provide privacy for the patient.
5. Wash hands. Put on gloves if needed.

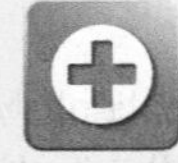 Precaution **CAUTION:** Wear gloves and observe standard precautions. Contact with body fluids, secretions, or excretions is possible.

6. Position the wheelchair or chair. It can be placed at the head of the bed facing the foot or at the foot of the bed facing the head. Positioning often depends on other equipment in the room.

NOTE: Whenever possible, the chair should be positioned so that it is secure against a wall or solid furniture and will not slide backward.

7. Securely lock the wheels of the wheelchair. Raise the footrests so that they are out of the way (Figure 22–18A).

Safety **CAUTION:** Double-check the locks on the wheelchair.

NOTE: For additional comfort and warmth, a bath blanket can be folded lengthwise and placed in the chair or wheelchair.

8. Lock the bed to prevent movement. Lower the bed to its lowest level.
9. Slowly elevate the head of the bed.

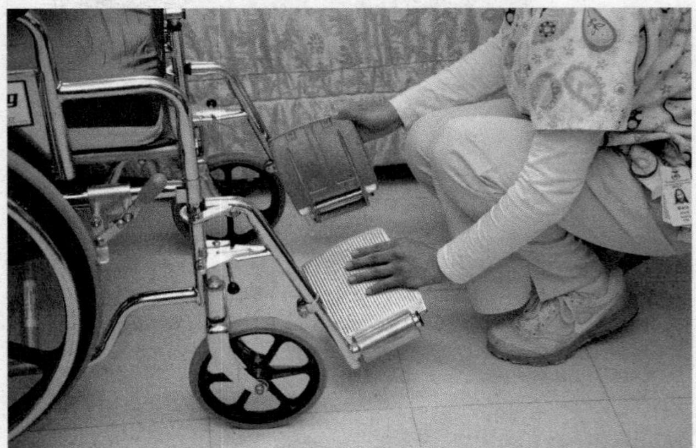

FIGURE 22–18A **Lock the wheels and elevate the footrests before moving a patient to a wheelchair.**

PROCEDURE 22:2F (CONT.)

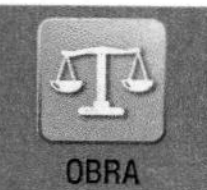

OBRA

10. If siderails are present and elevated, lower the siderail on the side that the patient is to exit from the bed. Fanfold the bed linen to the foot of the bed.

NOTE: Avoid exposing the patient during this procedure.

11. Assist the patient to a sitting position on the side of the bed with his or her feet flat on the floor. Observe for any signs of distress. Note color, pulse rate, breathing, and other similar signs. Put socks and shoes or slippers with non-slip soles on the patient. Put a transfer (gait) belt on the patient following Procedure 23:2A.

NOTE: Refer to Procedure 22:2E on dangling.

Safety

CAUTION: If the patient is weak or too heavy, get help.

Safety

CAUTION: If distress is noted, return the patient to bed immediately.

Safety

CAUTION: Use proper body mechanics.

12. If the patient needs a robe, put the robe on the patient.

13. Keep your back straight. Place one hand on each side of the belt using an underhand grasp. Face the patient and stand close to the patient. Position your feet to provide a broad base of support. If the patient has a weak leg, support the leg by positioning your knee against the patient's knee or by blocking the patient's foot with your foot.

NOTE: If the use of a transfer belt is contraindicated, place your hands under the patient's arms and around to the back of the shoulders to provide support.

14. 

Comm

Arrange a signal with the patient, such as counting to three. Instruct the patient to push against the bed with his or her hands to rise to a standing position.

15. At the given signal, assist the patient to a standing position. Lift up on the belt while the patient pushes up from the bed (Figure 22–18B). Place your knees and feet firmly against the patient's knees and feet to provide support.

16. Allow the patient to adjust to the upright position. Then keeping your hands in the same position, help the patient turn by using several pivot steps until the backs of his or her legs are touching the seat of the chair (Figure 22–18C).

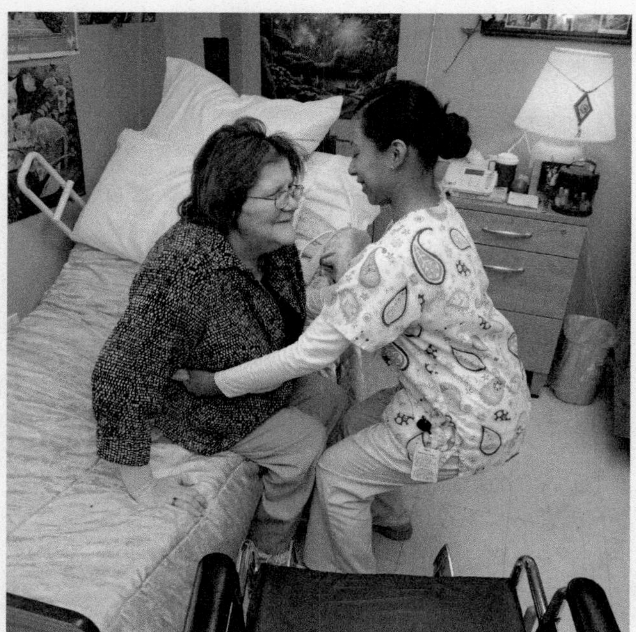

FIGURE 22–18B **Lift up on the belt while the patient pushes up from the bed.**

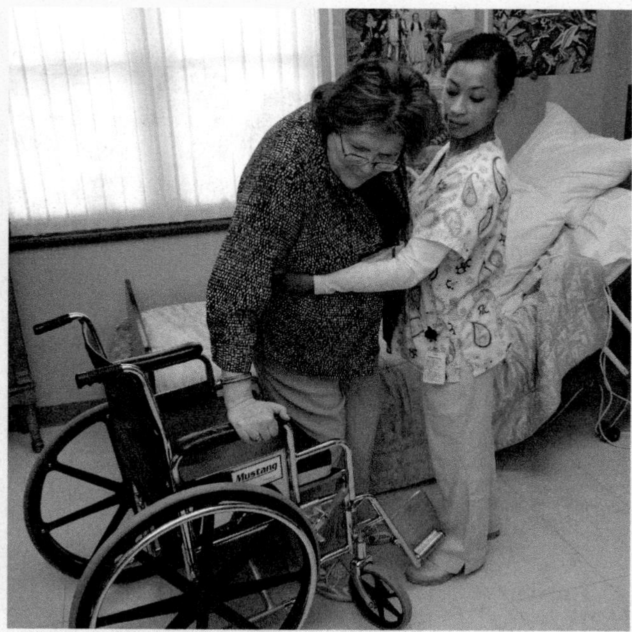

FIGURE 22–18C **Help the patient turn until the backs of her legs are touching the seat of the chair.**

(continues)

PROCEDURE 22:2F (CONT.)

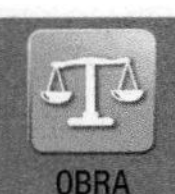

OBRA

17. Ask the patient to place his or her hands on the armrests and to bend at the knees as you gradually and slowly lower the patient to a sitting position in the chair (Figure 22–18D).

Safety

CAUTION: Bend at the hips and knees and keep your back straight.

18. Position the patient comfortably. Remove the transfer belt. Use a bath blanket to cover the patient's lap and legs. Lower the footrests on the wheelchair, taking care not to hit the patient's feet (Figure 22–18E).

    NOTE: Observe for any signs of distress.

19. Remain with the patient until you are sure there are no problems. If you leave the patient seated in a wheelchair or chair, make sure that the call signal and other supplies are within easy reach. Leave the area neat and clean. Check on the patient at frequent intervals.
20. If you are transporting the patient in the wheelchair, observe the following rules:
    a. Walk on the right side of the hall or corridor.
    b. Slow down and look for other traffic at doorways and intersections.
    c. To enter an elevator, turn the chair around and back into the elevator.
    d. To go down a steep ramp, turn the chair around and back down the ramp.
    e. Use the weight of your body to push the chair. Stand close to the chair.
    f. Watch the patient closely for signs of distress while transporting.
21. To return the patient to bed, reverse the procedure, beginning by putting a transfer belt on the patient and raising the footrests (step 18).

Safety

CAUTION: Be sure the wheels are locked before helping the patient out of the wheelchair. Lock the bed to prevent movement.

22. Position the patient in good body alignment after returning him or her to bed.
23. Observe all checkpoints before leaving the patient: elevate the siderails (if indicated), lower the bed to its lowest level, and place the call signal and other supplies within easy reach of the patient.
24. Replace all equipment used. Wipe the wheelchair with a disinfectant and return it to its proper place. Leave the area neat and clean.
25. Remove gloves if worn. Wash hands.

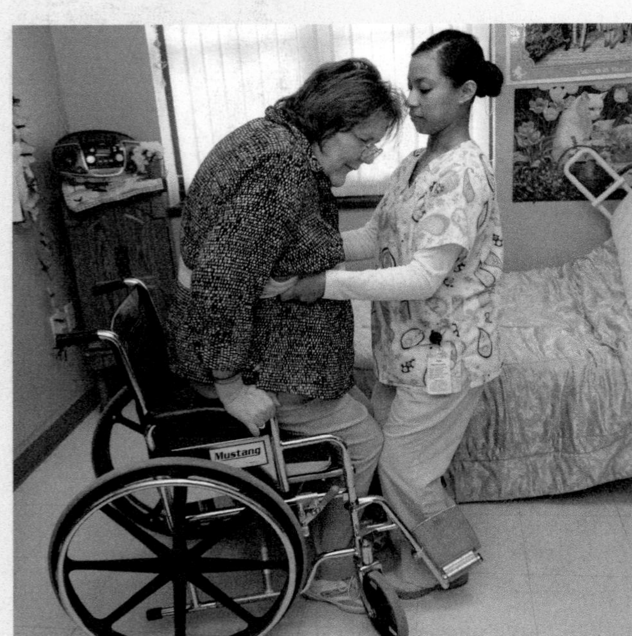

FIGURE 22–18D **Gradually and slowly lower the patient to a sitting position in the chair.**

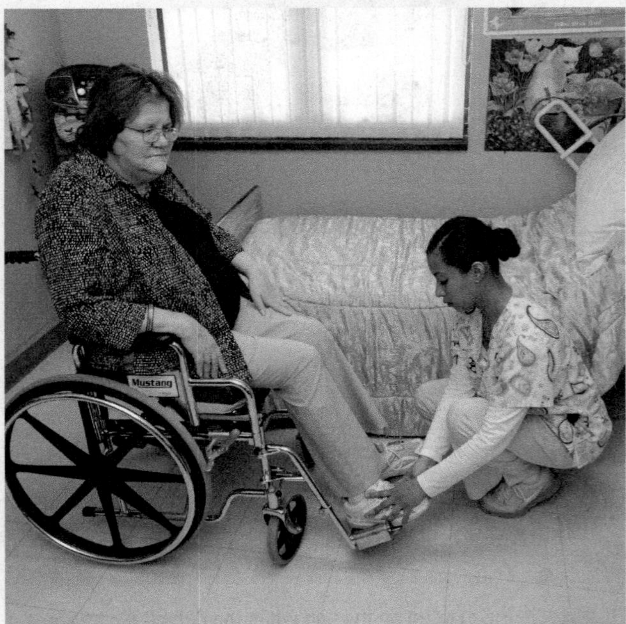

FIGURE 22–18E **Lower the footrests of the wheelchair and position the patient's feet on the footrests.**

PROCEDURE 22:2F (CONT.)

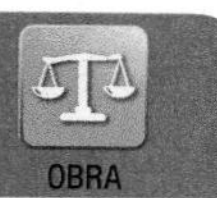

26.  Comm Report that the patient was transferred to a wheelchair and/or record all required information on the patient's chart or enter it into the computer. For example, date, time, transferred to chair, sat in chair for 30 minutes, tolerated well, and your signature and title. Note any unusual observations.

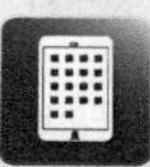 EHR **NOTE:** In health care agencies using electronic health records (EHRs), also known as electronic medical records (EMRs), the information is entered directly into the patient's record on a computer.

PRACTICE: **Go to the workbook and use the evaluation sheet for 22:2F, Transferring a Patient to a Chair or Wheelchair, to practice this procedure. When you believe you have mastered this skill, sign the sheet and give it to your instructor for further action.**

 Check **FINAL CHECKPOINT:** Using the criteria listed on the evaluation sheet, your instructor will grade your performance.

PROCEDURE 22:2G

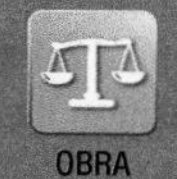

Transferring a Patient to a Stretcher

Equipment and Supplies

Stretcher with siderails and safety belt(s), bath blanket, gloves, paper and pen or computer

NOTE: Because this procedure requires more than one person, it is best to determine what tasks each of the assistants will perform before beginning the procedure.

Procedure

1. Check physician's orders or obtain authorization from your immediate supervisor for the transfer.
2. Assemble equipment. Cover the stretcher with a clean sheet.
3. Comm Knock on the door and pause before entering. Introduce yourself. Identify the patient. Explain the procedure and obtain consent.
4. Provide privacy. Close the door and pull the curtain.
5. Wash hands. Put on gloves if needed.

   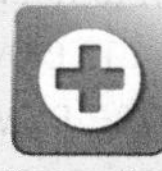 Precaution **CAUTION:** Wear gloves and observe standard precautions. Contact with body fluids, secretions, or excretions is possible.
6. Elevate the bed to the level of the stretcher. Lock the bed wheels to prevent movement of the bed. If siderails are present and elevated, lower the siderail on the side of the transfer.
7. Place a bath blanket over the patient. Fold bed linen to the foot of the bed.

   NOTE: Avoid exposing the patient.
8. Place the stretcher next to the bed. The bed and the stretcher should be parallel.
9. Lock the wheels of the stretcher.

   Safety **CAUTION:** In addition to the locks, use the weight of your body to hold the stretcher against the bed during this procedure.

    Safety **CAUTION:** Use correct body mechanics at all times.
10. If the patient is conscious and capable of moving unassisted, proceed as follows:
    a. Reach across the stretcher and hold up the bath blanket.
    b. Ask the patient to slide from the bed to the stretcher. Hold the stretcher against the bed (Figure 22–19).
    c. If the patient needs assistance, help by moving first the patient's head and shoulders, then the patient's hips, and finally the patient's legs and feet.

     Safety **CAUTION:** Make sure that the bed and stretcher wheels are locked and stabilized while the patient is being moved toward you.

     Safety **CAUTION:** If the patient is too heavy or unable to assist with the move, obtain help.
11. If the patient is very weak, paralyzed, semiconscious, or unconscious, proceed as follows:
    a. Obtain the assistance of three or four other people.

(continues)

PROCEDURE 22:2G (CONT.)

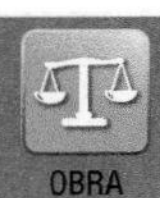

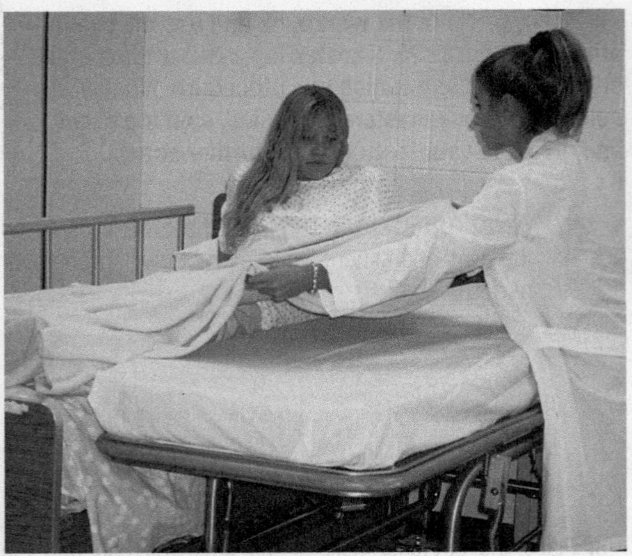

FIGURE 22–19 **Hold up the bath blanket and use the weight of your body to hold the stretcher against the bed while the patient is moving to the stretcher.**

b. Position a lifting sheet or blanket under the patient extending from the patient's head and neck to the feet.

c. Position two or three people by the stretcher and two or three people on the open side of the bed.

d. Roll the sides of the lifting sheet or blanket close to the patient's body.

e. Using overhand grasps, one assistant should grasp the sheet by the patient's head and waist. The second assistant should grasp the sheet by the hip and leg. The assistants on the open side of the bed should grasp the sheet in the same areas (Figure 22–20A). If a third assistant is available for one or both sides, they should be positioned so the patient's weight is equally distributed among the three.

f. At a given signal, all assistants should lift the sheet slightly to gently slide the patient from the bed to the stretcher (Figure 22–20B).

NOTE: Some facilities use slider boards instead of a lifting sheet or blanket.

12. Position the patient comfortably on the stretcher.

13. Lock the safety belt(s). Raise both siderails of the stretcher.

14. To transport the patient, two persons should direct the stretcher (one at the head and one at the foot).

a. Unlock the wheels of the stretcher. Move slowly.

b. The stretcher patient always travels feet first.

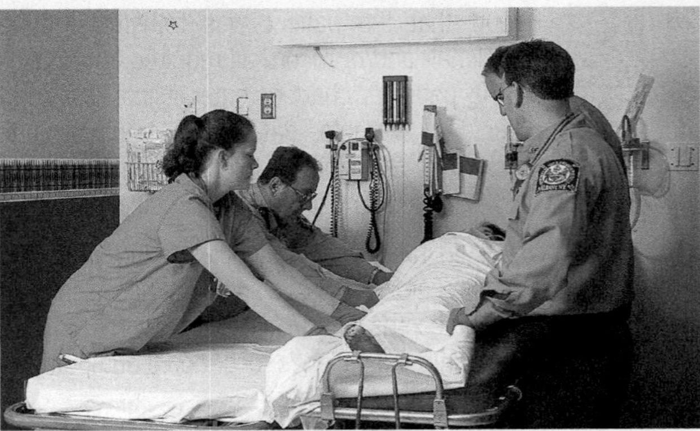

FIGURE 22–20A **Team members on both sides of the stretcher should roll the sides of the lift sheet close to the patient and position themselves so all parts of the patient's body are supported.**

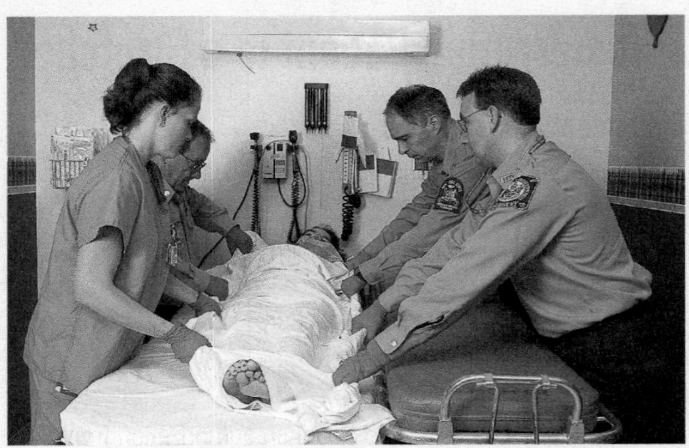

FIGURE 22–20B **At a given signal, all assistants should lift the sheet slightly to gently slide the patient from the stretcher to the bed.**

c. Walk on the right side of the hall.

d. Watch for cross traffic at doorways and intersections.

e. When going down an incline, the person at the foot of the stretcher should go backward and use body weight to control the stretcher.

f. To enter an elevator, push the correct button to keep the elevator door open. Back the stretcher into the elevator so that the head end enters first. To leave the elevator, push the button to keep the door open, and push the stretcher out feet end first.

15. To return the patient to bed, reverse the procedure, beginning with locking the wheels of the stretcher and bed and unlocking the safety belt(s) (see step 13).

CAUTION: Always check the wheel locks before transferring patients.

PROCEDURE 22:2G (CONT.)

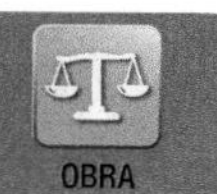

16. Observe all checkpoints before leaving the patient: position the patient in correct alignment, elevate the siderails (if indicated), lower the bed to its lowest level, place the call signal and other supplies within easy reach of the patient, and leave the area neat and clean.
17. Remove the sheet from the stretcher and place the sheet in a linen hamper. Use a disinfectant to wipe the stretcher. Replace all equipment used. Leave the area neat and clean.
18. Remove gloves if worn. Wash hands.
19.  Report that the patient was transferred to a stretcher and/or record all required information on the patient's chart or enter it into the computer. For example, date, time, transferred to stretcher and transported to radiology department, tolerated procedure well, and your signature and title. Note any unusual observations.

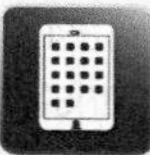

NOTE: In health care agencies using electronic health records (EHRs), also known as electronic medical records (EMRs), the information is entered directly into the patient's record on a computer.

PRACTICE: **Go to the workbook and use the evaluation sheet for 22:2G, Transferring a Patient to a Stretcher, to practice this procedure. When you believe you have mastered this skill, sign the sheet and give it to your instructor for further action.**

FINAL CHECKPOINT: Using the criteria listed on the evaluation sheet, your instructor will grade your performance.

PROCEDURE 22:2H

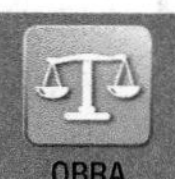

Using a Mechanical Lift to Transfer a Patient

NOTE: Mechanical lifts vary slightly. Read the manufacturer's instructions or ask your immediate supervisor to demonstrate the correct operation of the lift.

CAUTION: The manufacturer will indicate the weight limits for the mechanical lift. Do not use the mechanical lift if the patient weighs more than the weight limit.

Equipment and Supplies

Mechanical lift with straps and sling, bath blanket, chair or wheelchair, gloves, paper and pen or computer

NOTE: If the lift is being used to transfer a patient to a bathtub or shower area, a chair or wheelchair is not required.

CAUTION: Most facilities require that two health care providers perform this procedure. One person operates the lift while the second person guides the movements of the patient. Follow agency policy for this procedure.

Procedure

1. Obtain orders from your immediate supervisor or check physician's orders to obtain authorization.
2. Assemble equipment. Read the operating instructions provided with the mechanical lift or ask your immediate supervisor to demonstrate operation of the lift. Check the straps, sling, and any clasps to make sure there are no defects. Check the hydraulic unit and look for evidence of oil leaks.

CAUTION: Do not use the lift if straps or sling are torn or defective, if clasps are not secure, or if oil is leaking from the hydraulic unit. Serious injury may result. Label the defective mechanical lift with a warning or lock-out and notify your supervisor immediately.

3.  Obtain the assistance of another team member. Knock on the door and pause before entering. Introduce yourself and your coworker. Identify the patient. Explain the procedure and obtain consent. Reassure the patient, as needed.

NOTE: Patients are often apprehensive about being transferred by lift. It is important that they be as relaxed as possible for the transfer. Constant reassurance and encouragement are necessary.

4. Close the door and pull the curtain for privacy during the transfer.
5. Wash hands. Put on gloves if needed.

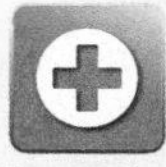

CAUTION: Wear gloves and observe standard precautions. Contact with body fluids, secretions, or excretions is possible.

6. Position the chair or wheelchair next to the foot of the bed, with the open seat facing the head of the bed. Lock the wheels of the wheelchair. Raise the footrests to the upright position.

(continues)

PROCEDURE 22:2H (CONT.)

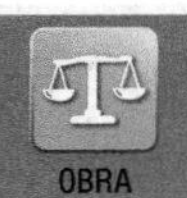

7. Lock the wheels of the bed. If siderails are present and elevated, lower the siderail on the side of the transfer.

8. Turn or move the patient to position the sling under the patient. The sling should be positioned under the shoulders, buttocks, and thighs. Make sure that the sling is smooth and that the center is near the center of the patient's back (Figure 22–21A).

9. Position the mechanical lift over the bed (Figure 22–21B). Open the base of the lift to its widest position to provide a broad base of support.

10. Attach the suspension straps to the sling. Insert the hooks from the inside of the sling to the outside to keep the open end of the hooks away from the patient's body. Make sure that the straps are not tangled or twisted. If clasps are present on the hooks, make sure they are secure.

11. Attach the straps to the frame of the lift (Figure 22–21C). Check to make sure that the suspension straps are locked to the frame or attached securely. Make sure that the straps are not tangled or twisted. Position the patient's arms inside the straps. Encourage the patient to keep his or her arms folded across the chest to keep the arms inside the straps.

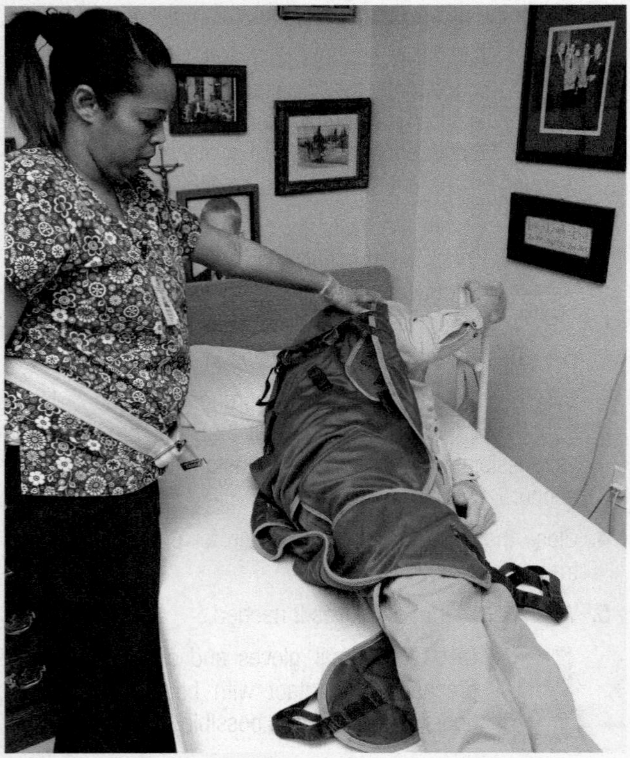

FIGURE 22–21A Position the sling under the patient's shoulders, buttocks, and thighs.

12. 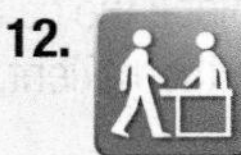

Tell the patient that he or she will be lifted from the bed. Constantly reassure the patient.

13. Turn the crank or use the hydraulic control to slowly raise the patient slightly above the bed. Check the straps, sling, and position of the patient to be sure that the patient is suspended securely by the lift. Then continue to raise the patient as needed until you can slowly turn the lift to move the patient away from the bed and into position over the chair or wheelchair. Keep all movements as smooth and even as possible (Figure 22–21D).

CAUTION: Move slowly to prevent jerking motions that may frighten the patient.

14. Slowly lower the lift to position the patient in the chair or wheelchair. Guide the patient's legs into position on the chair (Figure 22–21E).

15. Unhook the suspension straps from the sling (Figure 22–21F). Remove the sling from under the patient (Figure 22–21G). At times, the sling is left in position under the patient. Carefully move the lift away from the patient.

CAUTION: Be careful not to injure the patient with the straps or lift while moving the lift away from the chair.

16. Use the blanket to cover the patient. Lower the footrests of the wheelchair and position the patient's feet in a comfortable position. Slippers or shoes and socks can be put on the patient's feet.

17. To return the patient to bed, reverse the procedure. Begin by making sure the wheels of the chair and bed are locked. Attach the suspension straps securely to the sling.

18. Observe all checkpoints before leaving the patient: position the patient in correct alignment, elevate the siderails (if indicated), lower the bed to its lowest level, place the call signal and other supplies within easy reach of the patient, and leave the area neat and clean.

19. Use a disinfectant to wipe the mechanical lift. Properly replace all equipment used. Leave the area neat and clean.

20. Remove gloves if worn. Wash hands.

21. 

Report that the patient was transferred to a chair or wheelchair using a mechanical lift and/or record all required information on the patient's

PROCEDURE 22:2H (CONT.)

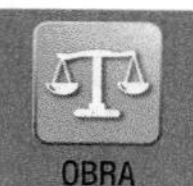

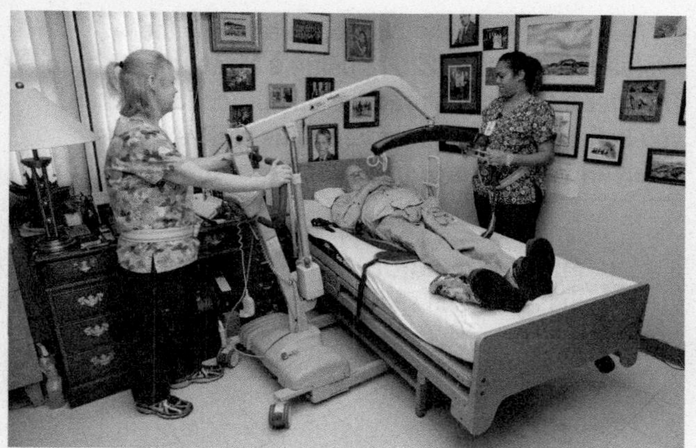

FIGURE 22–21B Position the mechanical lift over the bed.

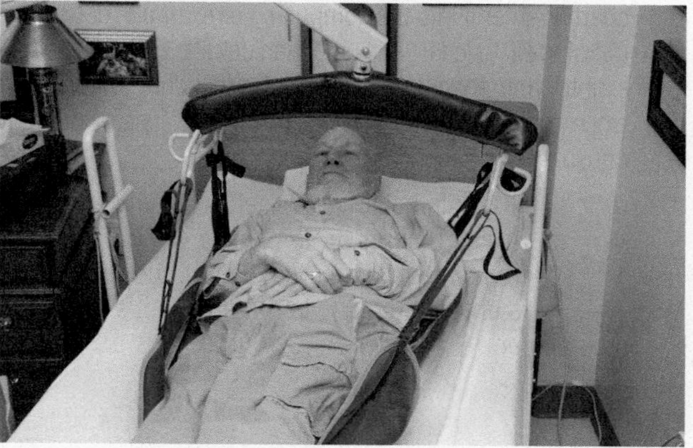

FIGURE 22–21C Attach the suspension straps of the frame to the lift, and make sure they are locked to the frame or attached securely.

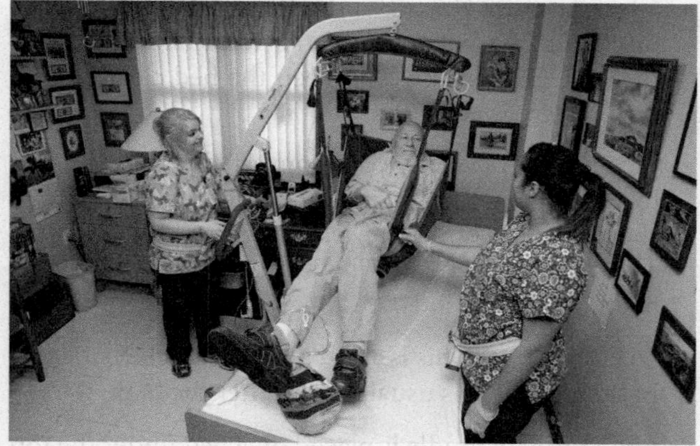

FIGURE 22–21D Use a smooth motion to lift the patient out of the bed.

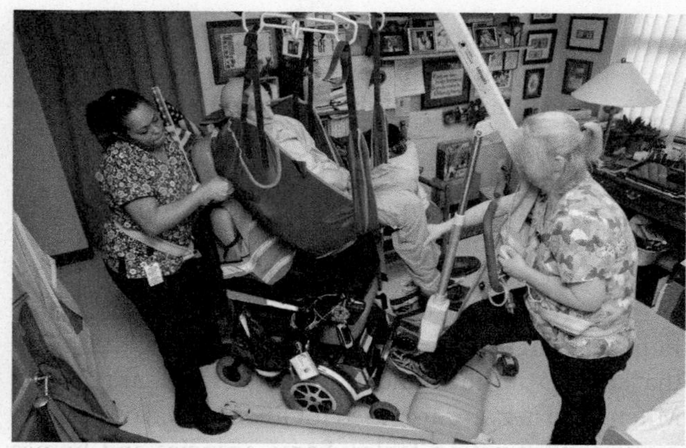

FIGURE 22–21E Lower the lift slowly to position the patient in the wheelchair.

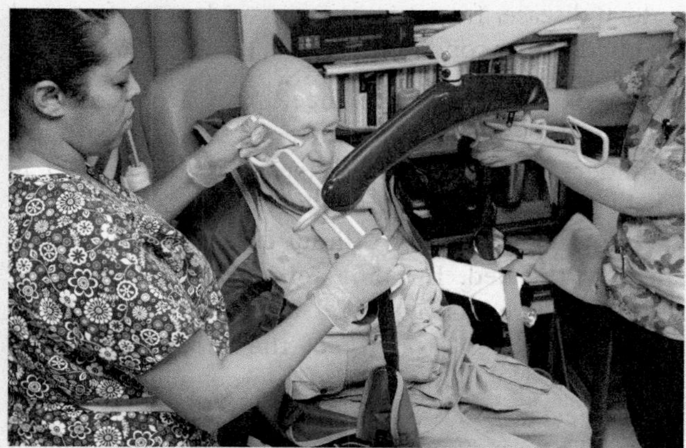

FIGURE 22–21F Unhook the suspension straps from the sling.

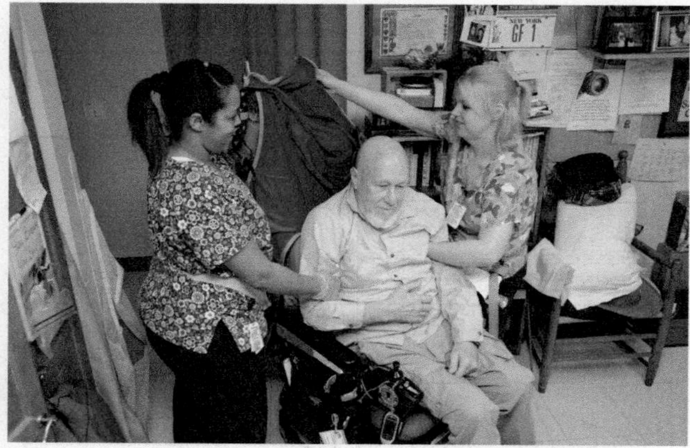

FIGURE 22–21G Remove the sling from under the patient.

(continues)

PROCEDURE 22:2H (CONT.)

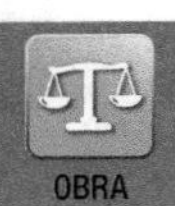

chart or enter it into the computer. For example, date, time, transferred to chair with mechanical lift, patient seemed slightly apprehensive at start of procedure but relaxed while in chair, and your signature and title. Note any unusual observations.

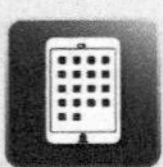

NOTE: In health care agencies using electronic health records (EHRs), also known as electronic medical records (EMRs), the information is entered directly into the patient's record on a computer.

PRACTICE: Go to the workbook and use the evaluation sheet for 22:2H, Using a Mechanical Lift to Transfer a Patient, to practice this procedure. When you believe you have mastered this skill, sign the sheet and give it to your instructor for further action.

FINAL CHECKPOINT: Using the criteria listed on the evaluation sheet, your instructor will grade your performance.

22:3 Bedmaking

Making beds correctly is a task that must be performed by many health care workers. A correctly made bed provides comfort and protection for the patient confined to bed for long periods. Therefore, care must be taken when beds are made. The bed linen must be free of all wrinkles. Wrinkles cause discomfort and can lead to the formation of pressure ulcers.

Mitered corners are used to hold the linen firmly in place. Mitering corners is a special folding technique that secures the linen under the mattress (Figure 22–22). Mitered corners are also used for linen placed on stretchers and examination tables. Some agencies and homes use fitted contour sheets for bottom sheets. Mitered corners would not be used with these sheets, but would be used with top sheets.

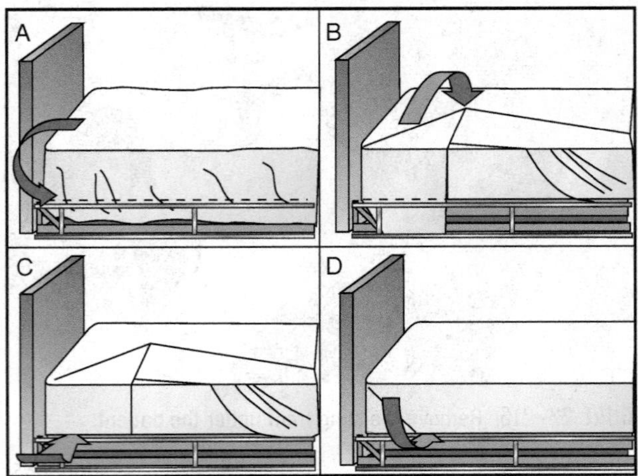

FIGURE 22–22 Steps for making a mitered corner.

Following are examples of the types of beds that you may be required to make:

- **Closed bed**: This is a bed made following the discharge of a patient and after terminal cleaning of the unit. Its purpose is to keep the bed clean until a new patient is admitted.
- **Open bed**: A closed bed is converted to an open bed by **fanfolding** (folding like accordion pleats) the top sheets. This is done to "welcome" a new patient. It is also done for patients who are ambulatory or out of bed for short periods.
- **Occupied bed**: This is a bed made while the patient is in the bed. This is usually done after the bath.
- **Bed cradle**: A cradle is placed on a bed under the top sheets to prevent bed linen from touching parts of the patient's body. A cradle frequently is used for patients with burns, skin ulcers, lesions, blood clots, circulatory disease, fractures, surgery on legs or feet, and other similar conditions.

Draw sheets are half sheets that are frequently used on beds. A draw sheet extends from the patient's shoulders to the patient's knees. The draw sheet is used to protect the mattress. If soiled, the draw sheet can be changed readily without changing the bottom sheet of the bed. In some settings, disposable bed protectors, frequently called underpads, are placed under the patient to protect the sheets instead of using draw sheets. Draw sheets are sometimes used as lift sheets.

To prevent injury to yourself, you must observe correct body mechanics while making beds. It is also important to conserve time and energy. Keeping linen arranged in the order of use is one way to conserve time and energy. In addition, most beds are made completely first on one side and then on the other side. This limits unnecessary movement from one side of the bed to the opposite side.

It is also important to limit the movement of organisms and, therefore, the spread of infection while making beds. Wear gloves to handle dirty or soiled linen. Roll dirty or soiled linen while removing it from the bed. Hold dirty linen away from your body and place it in a linen hamper, cart, or bag immediately. Never place dirty linen on the floor. Some facilities do not allow linen hampers or carts in a patient's room. The hamper or cart is left in the hall. Soiled linen is placed in a pillowcase or plastic bag, carried to the hall, and placed in the hamper or cart. Remove the gloves and wash your hands after handling dirty linen and before handling clean linen. Clean linen should be stored in a closed closet or on a covered linen cart. Never allow clean linen to contact your uniform. Never bring extra linen to the patient's room because it is then considered contaminated and cannot be used for another patient. Avoid shaking clean sheets. Unfold them gently. Place the open end of the pillowcase away from the door. This looks neater and also helps prevent the entrance of organisms from the hall.

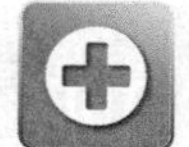
Precaution

Linen may be contaminated by blood, body fluids, secretions, excretions, urine, or feces. Observe standard precautions (discussed in Chapter 15:4). Wash your hands frequently and wear gloves while handling linen. Gloves must be worn while removing dirty linen. Before handling clean linen, the contaminated gloves should be removed, and the hands should be washed. If there is any chance of contamination in the room, clean gloves should be applied before handling clean linen. Follow agency policy for proper disposal of linen. Many agencies have special self-dissolving plastic laundry bags that dissolve during the washing process. The contaminated linen is placed in the bag, and the bag is sealed. The bag is then placed inside another plastic bag and labeled before being sent to the laundry department. The second bag is necessary because wet linen may dissolve the water-soluble bag before it reaches the laundry department. The health care worker must be alert at all times to prevent the spread of infection by contaminated linen.

STUDENT: **Go to the workbook and complete the assignment sheet for 22:3, Bedmaking. Then return and continue with the procedure.**

PROCEDURE 22:3A

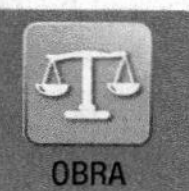

Making a Closed Bed

Equipment and Supplies

Two large sheets (or one large sheet and one fitted sheet); draw sheet (if used); spread; pillow; pillowcase; blanket (as necessary); linen hamper, cart, or bag; gloves

Procedure

1. Assemble equipment.
2. Wash hands. Put on gloves.

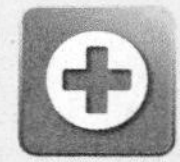
Precaution

CAUTION: Wear gloves and observe standard precautions. Contact with body fluids, secretions, or excretions is possible.

3. Arrange the clean linen on a chair in the order in which the linen is to be used.

NOTE: This simplifies the procedure and prevents excessive handling of linen.

4. Elevate the bed to a comfortable height. Lock the wheels to prevent movement.
5. Remove dirty linen from the bed. Roll it into a compact bundle. Hold the linen away from your body. Place it in the linen hamper, bag, or cart. After disposing of the dirty linen, remove the gloves and wash your hands. If there is any chance of contamination in the room, put on clean gloves.

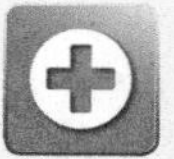
Precaution

CAUTION: Prevent the spread of organisms and infection by wearing gloves and observing standard precautions. Linen may be contaminated with blood, body fluids, secretions, or excretions.

If the mattress is soiled, wipe it with a disinfectant. After removing contaminated linen, remove the gloves and wash your hands before handling clean linen.

Safety

CAUTION: Never place dirty linen on the floor.

NOTE: Some facilities do not allow linen hampers or carts in a patient's room. The hamper or cart is left in the hall. Soiled linen is placed in a pillowcase or plastic bag, carried to the hall, and placed in the hamper or cart.

6. Unfold the bottom sheet right side up. Place the small hem even with the foot of the mattress (Figure 22–23A). The center fold should be at the center of the bed. The wide hem should be at the head of the bed.

Safety

CAUTION: Avoid shaking the sheet because doing so spreads germs.

(continues)

PROCEDURE 22:3A (CONT.)

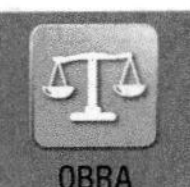

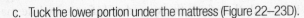

NOTE: If a fitted sheet is used, it is positioned on the bed, with the contour corners positioned at the head and foot of the mattress. Fit one contour corner smoothly around the foot of the mattress. Then fit the contour corner around the head of the mattress.

NOTE: Complete one side of the bed entirely before going to the opposite side. This saves time and energy.

7. Tuck 12–18 inches of the sheet under the mattress at the head of the bed (Figure 22–23B).

8. Make a mitered corner as follows:

a. Pick up the sheet approximately 12 inches from the head of the bed.

b. Form a triangle with a 45-degree angle on top of the mattress (Figure 22–23C).

c. Tuck the lower portion under the mattress (Figure 22–23D).

d. Hold the fold with one hand and bring the triangle down to the side of the bed with the other (Figure 22–23E).

e. Tuck the folded part under the mattress (Figure 22–23F).

f. The mitered corner will help hold the sheet securely in place (Figure 22–23G).

9. Tuck in the side of the sheet by working from the head to the foot of the bed.

CAUTION: Avoid injury. Use correct body mechanics. Work close to the bed and with a broad base of support.

10. Place a draw sheet, if used, in the center of the bed, approximately 14–16 inches from the head of the bed. Tuck the draw sheet in at the side of the bed.

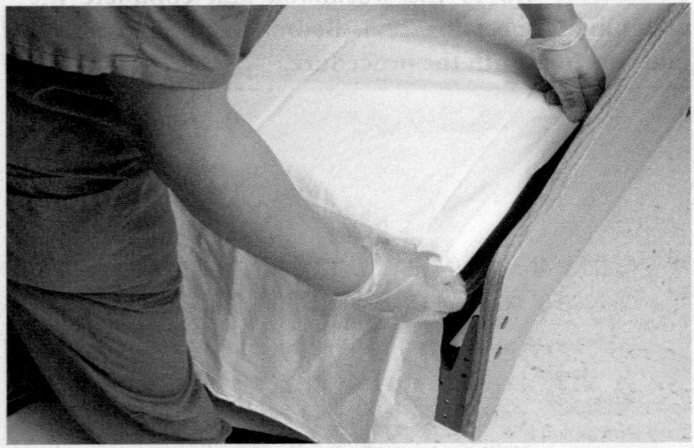

FIGURE 22–23A Position the small hem of the bottom sheet even with the foot of the mattress.

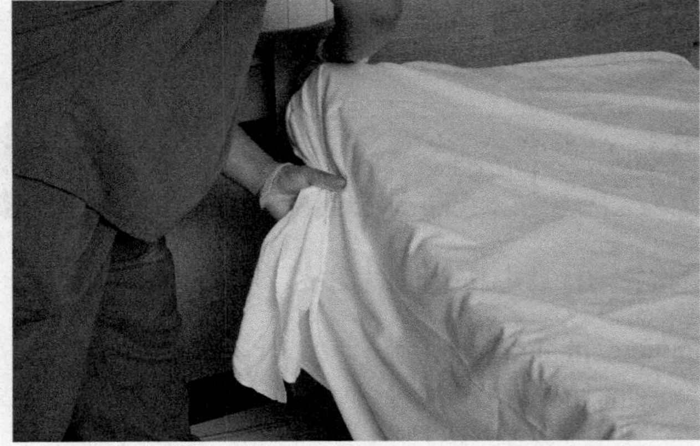

FIGURE 22–23B Tuck 12–18 inches of the sheet under the mattress at the head of the bed.

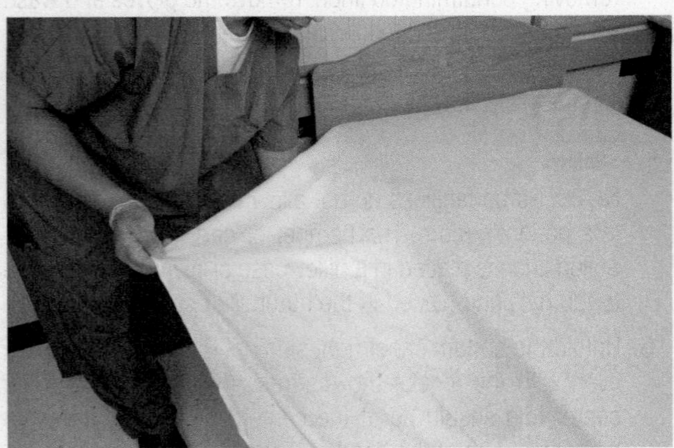

FIGURE 22–23C To make a mitered corner, pick up the sheet approximately 12 inches from the head of the bed and form a triangle with a 45-degree angle.

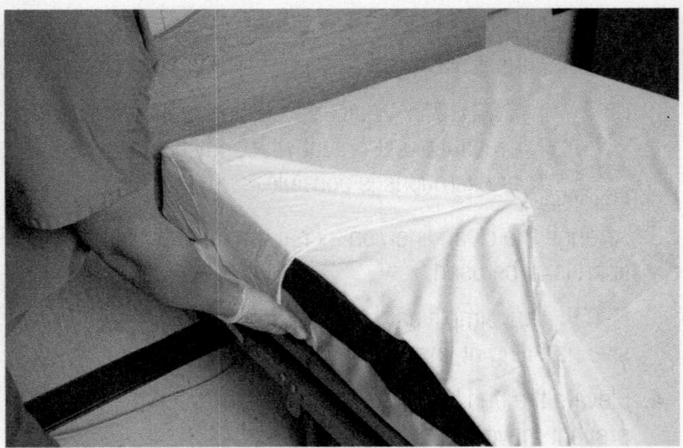

FIGURE 22–23D Tuck the bottom part of the triangle under the mattress.

PROCEDURE 22:3A (CONT.)

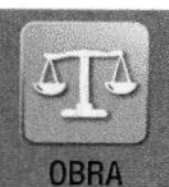

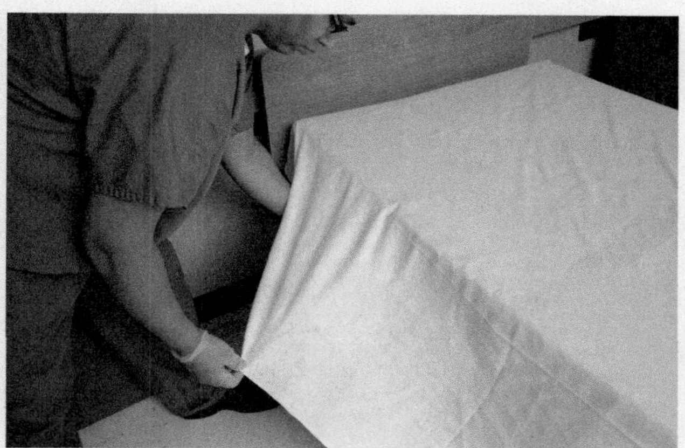

FIGURE 22–23E **Bring the triangle down to the side of the bed.**

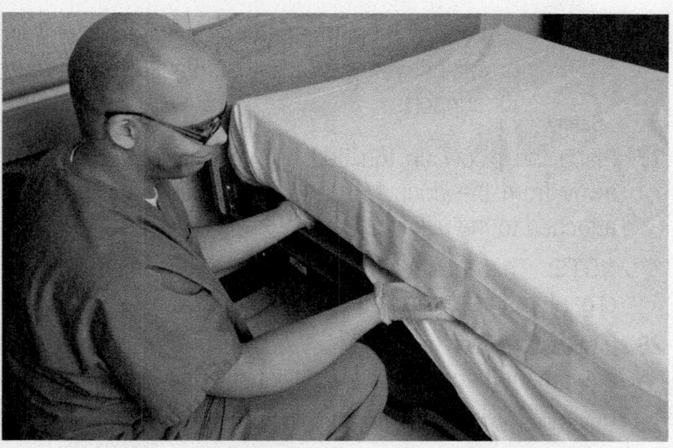

FIGURE 22–23F **Tuck the sheet firmly under the mattress to finish the mitered corner.**

NOTE: Make sure the tucks are secure and as far under the mattress as possible. This helps hold the sheets in place.

NOTE: Not all agencies use draw sheets. Underpads may be placed on the bed to prevent soiling of the linen.

11. Place the top sheet on the bed, wrong side up. Use the center fold to center the sheet. The wide hem should be even with the top edge of the mattress.
12. Tuck the top sheet over the foot of the mattress.
13. Make a mitered corner as previously instructed.
14. Tuck the side of the sheet under the mattress to the center of the bed only.
15. If a blanket is used, it can be placed on the bed in the same manner as the top sheet. The top sheet and blanket can be tucked in at the same time.

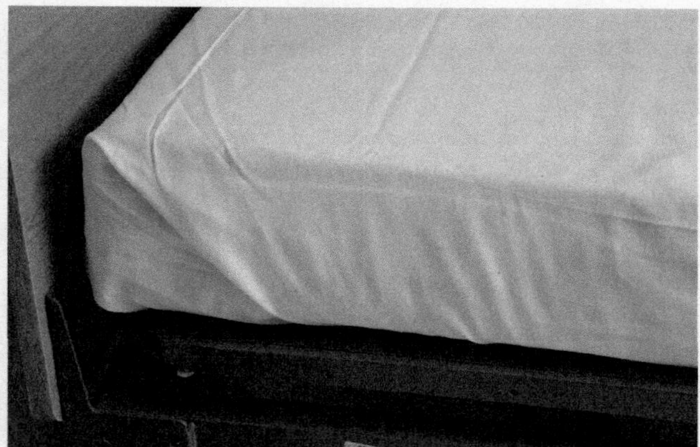

FIGURE 22–23G **The finished mitered corner will help hold the sheet securely in position.**

16. Place the spread on the bed right side up. The top edge should be even with the top edge of the mattress. Use the center fold to center the spread.
17. Tuck the spread under the mattress at the foot of the bed.

    NOTE: The top sheet, blanket, and spread can all be placed on the bed at the same time. They are then tucked in as one unit at the bottom of the bed, and a mitered corner is made with all of the linen (Figure 22–23H).
18. Make a mitered corner but do not tuck the final end under the side of the mattress. Let the triangle hang loose (Figure 22–23I).
19. Go to the opposite side of the bed. From the side, fanfold the top covers to the center of the bed so you can work with the bottom sheet.
20. Tuck the bottom sheet under the head of the mattress. Make a mitered corner.
21. Work from the head of the bed to the foot to tuck in the side of the sheet. Pull the sheet gently to remove all wrinkles before tucking in the side.
22. Grasp the draw sheet in the center. Pull gently to remove wrinkles. Tuck in firmly at the side.
23. Tuck in the top sheet (and blanket) at the foot of the bed. Make a mitered corner. Remove all wrinkles and tuck in at the side up to the center of the bed only.
24. Tuck in the spread at the foot of the bed. Make a mitered corner but do not tuck in the final fold. Let it hang.
25. Line up all sheets so they are smooth and free of wrinkles. If a blanket is used, the top sheet can be folded back over the blanket, making a cuff. This protects the patient from the edge of the blanket.

(continues)

PROCEDURE 22:3A (CONT.)

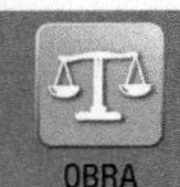

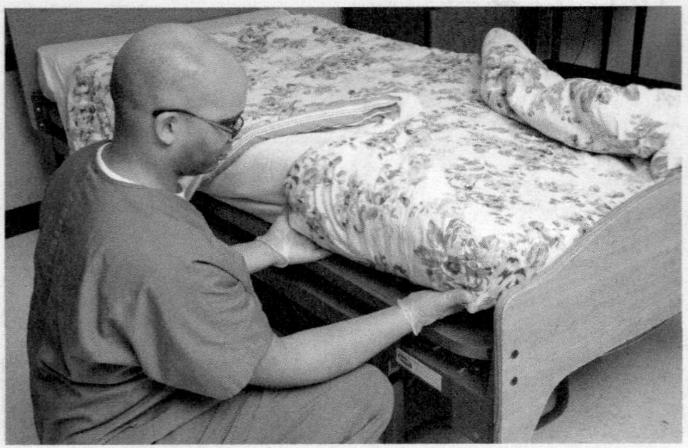

FIGURE 22–23H **The top sheet, blanket, and spread can be tucked under the mattress as one unit and secured with a single mitered corner.**

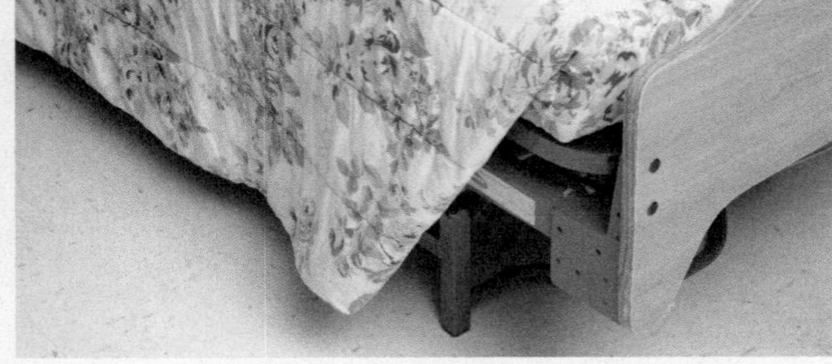

FIGURE 22–23I **After making a mitered corner, allow the top sheet, blanket, and spread to hang free on the side of the mattress.**

26. Insert the pillow into the pillowcase as follows:

a. Place hands in the clean pillowcase and loosen the corners.

b. Use one hand to grasp the center of the end seam on the outside. Turn the case back over the hand and lower arm (Figure 22–24A).

c. Using the hand that is covered by the case, grab the end of the pillow at the center of the pillow (Figure 22–24B).

d. Using your free hand, unfold the case over the pillow (Figure 22–24C).

e. Adjust the end corners of the pillow into the corners of the case.

f. Adjust the pillowcase on the pillow. It may be necessary to make a lengthwise pleat for a better fit.

CAUTION: Do not hold the pillow under your chin or against your body. Rather, place it on the bed for support.

27. Place the pillow on the bed, with the open end pointed away from the door. Make sure the call signal is firmly attached to the pillow or bed (Figure 22–24D).

NOTE: This position looks neater and allows fewer organisms from the hall to enter the pillow.

28. Lower the bed to its lowest position. Replace all other equipment (bedside table, call signal, chair, etc.).

29. Before leaving the area, check to make sure it is neat and clean.

30. Remove gloves if worn. Wash hands.

31. Comm Record or report that a closed bed was made.

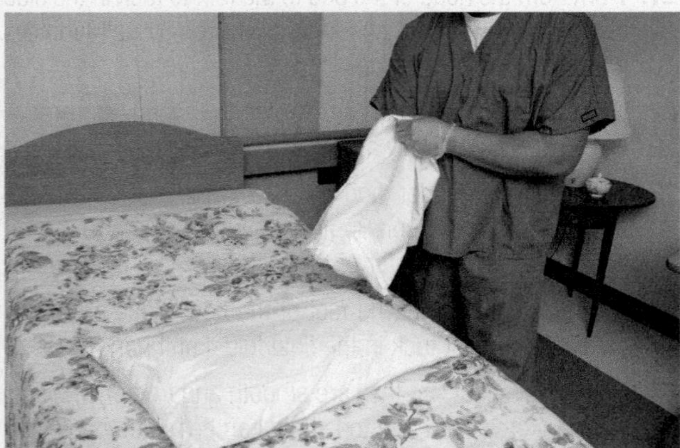

FIGURE 22–24A **Grasp the center of the end seam on the pillowcase and turn the case back over the hand and lower arm.**

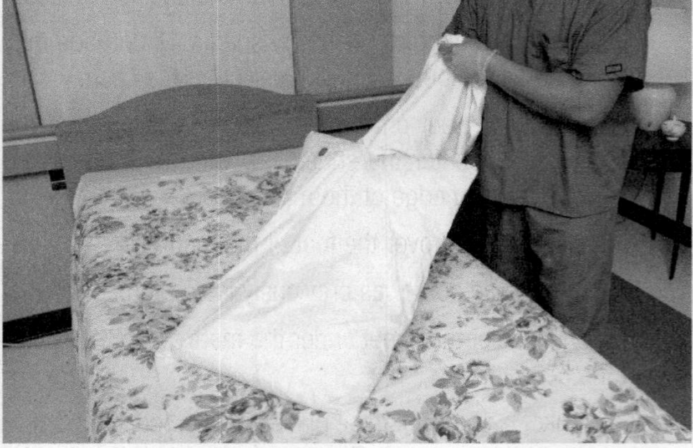

FIGURE 22–24B **Using the pillowcase-covered hand, grab the end of the pillow.**

PROCEDURE 22:3A (CONT.)

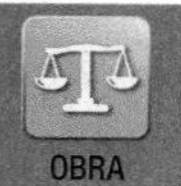
OBRA

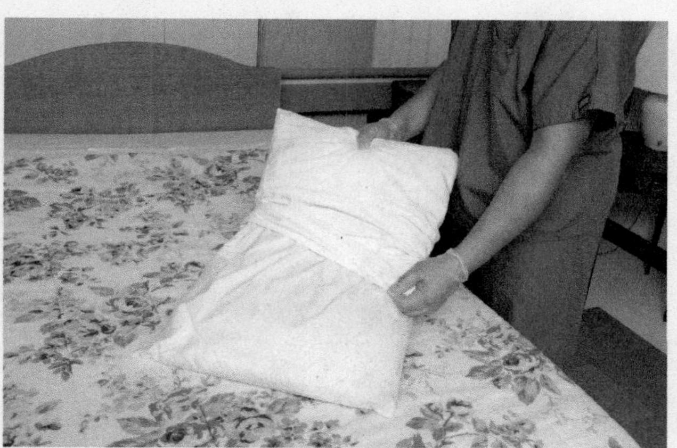
FIGURE 22–24C **Unfold the pillowcase over the pillow.**

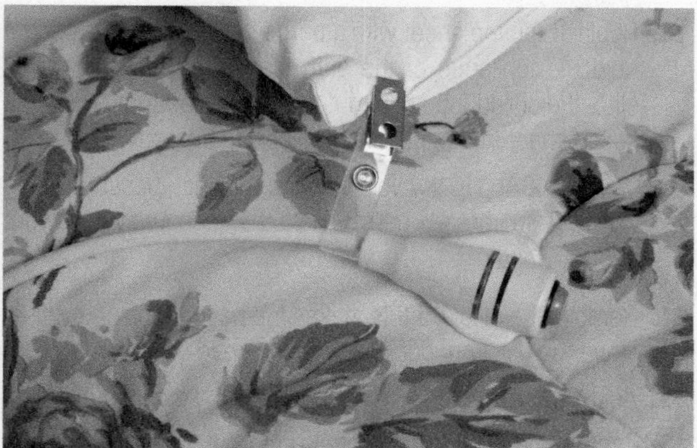
FIGURE 22–24D **Make sure the call signal is firmly attached to the pillow or bed.**

PRACTICE: **Go to the workbook and use the evaluation sheet for 22:3A, Making a Closed Bed, to practice this procedure. When you believe you have mastered this skill, sign the sheet and give it to your instructor for further action.**

Check

FINAL CHECKPOINT: Using the criteria listed on the evaluation sheet, your instructor will grade your performance.

PROCEDURE 22:3B

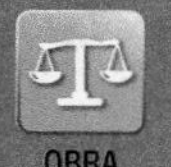
OBRA

Making an Occupied Bed

Equipment and Supplies

Laundry hamper, cart, or bag; two large sheets (or one large sheet and one fitted sheet); draw sheet (if used); spread; pillow; pillowcase; blanket (if needed); bath blanket; disposable protective pads; gloves; paper and pen or computer

Procedure

1. Assemble equipment.
2. Comm — Knock on the door and pause before entering. Introduce yourself. Identify the patient. Explain the procedure and obtain consent.
3. Close the door and pull the curtain for privacy.
4. Wash hands. Put on gloves.

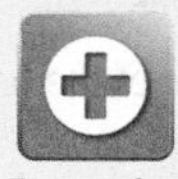
Precaution

CAUTION: Put on gloves and observe standard precautions. Linen on the bed may be contaminated with blood, body fluids, secretions, or excretions.

5. Arrange the clean linen on a chair in the order in which the linen will be used.
6. Lock the wheels of the bed. Elevate the bed to a comfortable working position.
7. Lower the headrest and footrest so that the bed is flat, if permissible.

   NOTE: Make sure the patient can tolerate this position before continuing with the procedure.
8. If siderails are present and elevated, lower the siderail on the side where you are working.

Safety

CAUTION: Make sure the siderail on the opposite side is elevated.

9. Loosen the top bedclothes at the bottom of the mattress. Remove the spread and blanket. If they are to be reused, fold and place them over the chair.

(continues)

PROCEDURE 22:3B (CONT.)

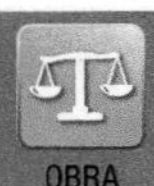
OBRA

10. Replace the top sheet with a bath blanket. Have the patient hold the top edge of the bath blanket, if able, while you slide the soiled top sheet out from top to bottom. Place the soiled sheet in the linen hamper, cart, or bag.

Safety

CAUTION: Avoid shaking the linen because doing so spreads germs. Hold the linen away from your body.

11. Remove the pillow. If this makes the patient uncomfortable, leave the pillow under the patient's head.

12. Assist the patient in turning to the opposite side of the bed.

13. Fanfold the cotton draw sheet up to the patient's body.

14. Fanfold the bottom sheet up to and under the draw sheet (Figure 22–25A). Make sure all of the sheets are as close to the patient as possible.

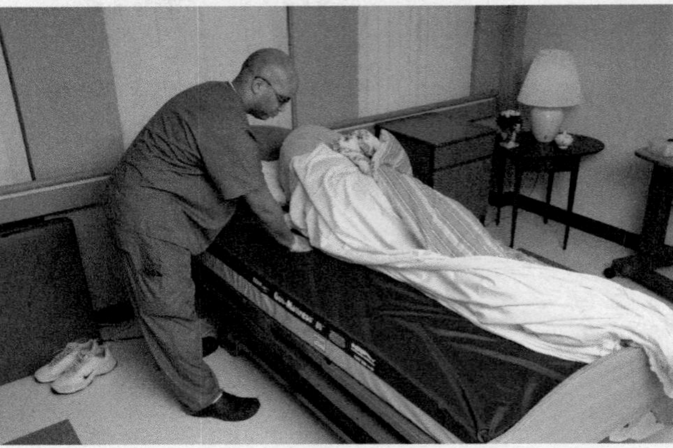

FIGURE 22–25A Fanfold the bottom sheet to the center of the bed.

15. Place the clean bottom sheet on the bed right side up. Place the narrow hem even with the foot of the bed. Center using the center fold. Fanfold the opposite side close to patient.

Safety

CAUTION: Avoid injury. Use correct body mechanics, including a broad base of support.

16. Tuck in the clean bottom sheet at the head of the bed. Make a mitered corner. Working from the head to the foot of the bed, tuck in the entire side (Figure 22–25B).

NOTE: If a fitted sheet is used, it is positioned on the bed with the contour corners positioned at the head and foot of the mattress.

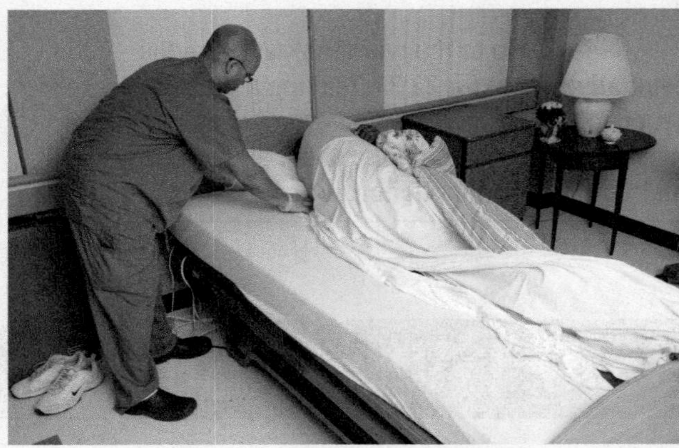

FIGURE 22–25B Position the clean bottom sheet on the bed, fanfold it at the center of the bed, make a mitered corner at the top edge, and tuck in the side of the sheet.

17. Place the clean draw sheet on the bed. Center using the draw sheet's center fold. Fanfold the opposite half close to the patient. Tuck the draw sheet firmly under the mattress at the side (Figure 22–25C).

18. Comm — Turn the patient toward you. Caution the patient that he or she will be turning over the top of the fanfolded linen. Elevate the siderail, if indicated.

19. Go to the opposite side of the bed. Lower the siderail, if elevated.

20. Remove the soiled bottom sheet and draw sheet (Figure 22–25D). Place in the linen hamper, cart, or bag.

21. Pull the clean bottom sheet into place. Tuck it under the mattress at the head of the bed. Make a mitered corner.

22. Pull gently to remove all wrinkles. Tuck the side of the sheet under the mattress, working from top to bottom.

23. Pull the clean draw sheet into place (Figure 22–25E). Remove all wrinkles and tuck it firmly under the side of the mattress.

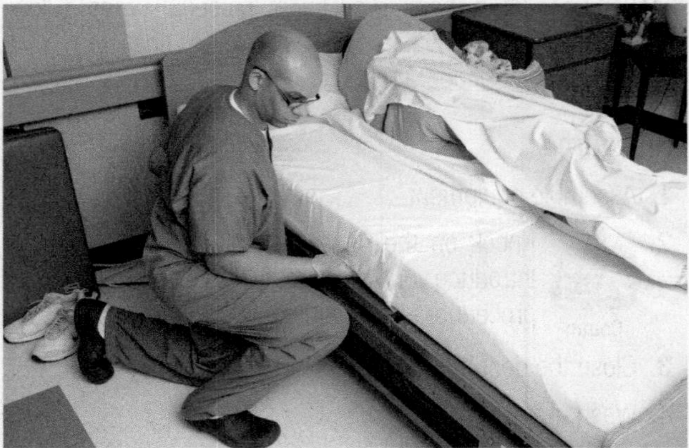

FIGURE 22–25C Fanfold the draw sheet at the center of the bed and tuck it into the side of the bed.

PROCEDURE 22:3B (CONT.)

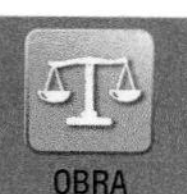

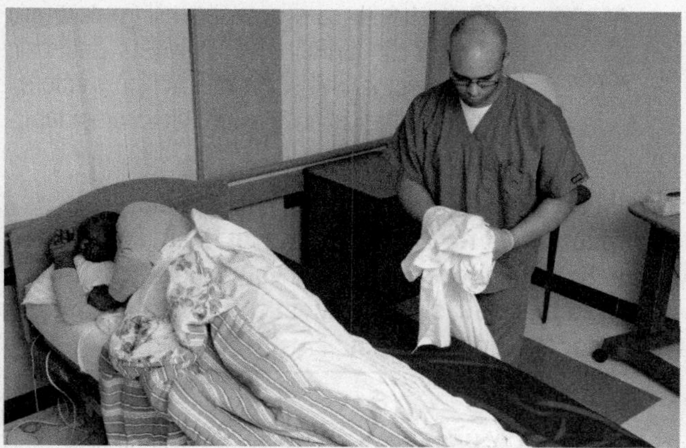

FIGURE 22–25D **Go to the opposite side of the bed and remove the soiled draw sheet and bottom sheet.**

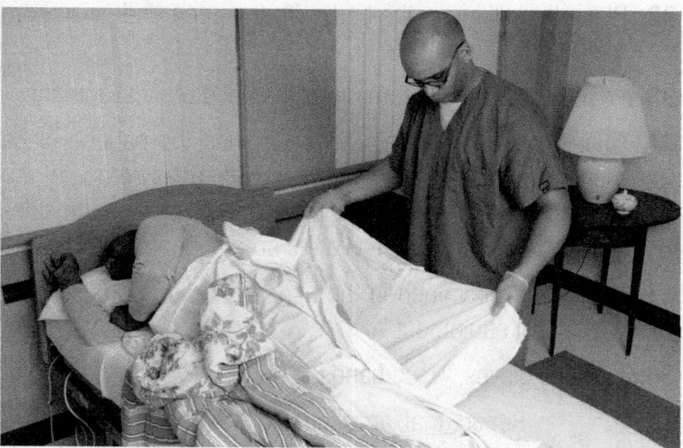

FIGURE 22–25E **Pull the clean draw sheet into place and tuck it under the side of the mattress.**

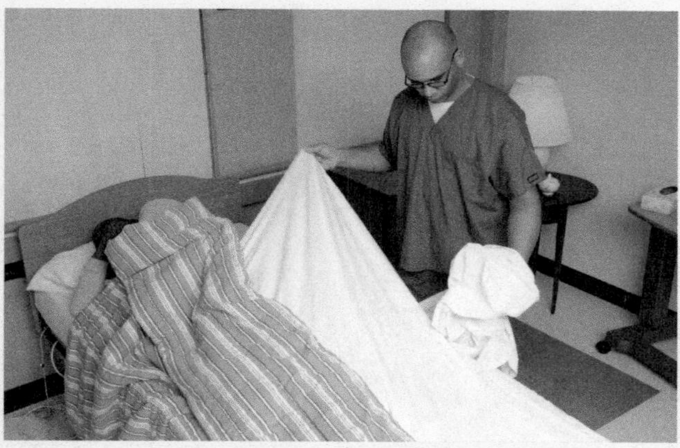

FIGURE 22–25F **Position a clean top sheet on the patient and remove the bath blanket, if used, or the soiled top sheet.**

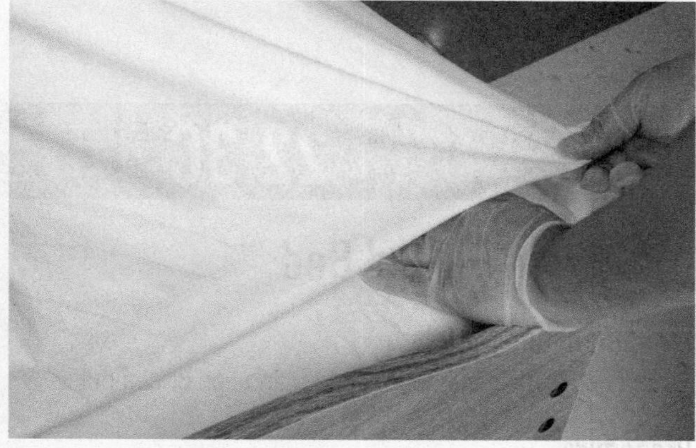

FIGURE 22–25G **Make a toe pleat in the top linen to provide more room for the patient's feet and toes.**

24. Assist the patient to turn onto his or her back in the center of the bed.

25. Place the top sheet, wrong side up, over the bath blanket. Center using the sheet's center fold. Ask the patient to hold the top edge of the clean sheet. Remove the bath blanket by pulling it from the top to the bottom of the bed (Figure 22–25F).

CAUTION: Avoid exposing the patient during this procedure.

26. If a blanket is to be used, place it over the top sheet.

27. Place the spread on top, right side up. Center it on the bed.

28. Tuck the top sheet, blanket, and spread into the bottom of the mattress. Make a mitered corner. Before tucking in the final fold, form a toe pleat by making a 3-inch fold in the top of the linen (Figure 22–25G). The fold should be made toward the foot of the bed. Complete the mitered corner.

NOTE: The toe pleat provides more room for the patient's feet and toes and prevents pressure on the toes from the sheets.

29. Raise the siderail, if indicated, and go to the opposite side of the bed. Lower the siderail, if elevated, and complete the top sheets on the opposite side of the bed.

30. Fold the top edge of the spread over and under the top of the blanket. Bring the top sheet over the top of the spread and blanket, and make a 6- to 8-inch cuff.

31. Insert the pillow into a clean pillowcase as instructed in Procedure 22:3A.

(continues)

PROCEDURE 22:3B (CONT.)

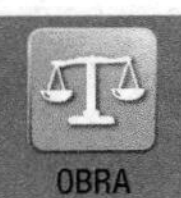
OBRA

32. Place the pillow on the bed, with the open end away from the door.
33. Position the patient comfortably in good body alignment.
34. Observe all checkpoints before leaving the patient: place the call signal and other supplies within easy reach of the patient, lower the bed to its lowest level, elevate the siderails (if indicated), and leave the area neat and clean.
35. Dispose of dirty linen in the appropriate location. Properly replace all equipment.
36. Remove gloves. Wash hands.
37. 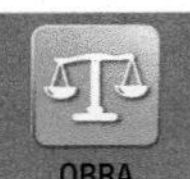 Comm Report that an occupied bed was made and/or record all required information on the patient's chart or enter it into the computer. For example, date, time, occupied bed made, and your signature and title. Note any unusual observations.

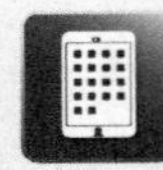 EHR **NOTE:** In health care agencies using electronic health records (EHRs), also known as electronic medical records (EMRs), the information is entered directly into the patient's record on a computer.

PRACTICE: **Go to the workbook and use the evaluation sheet for 22:3B, Making an Occupied Bed, to practice this procedure. When you believe you have mastered this skill, sign the sheet and give it to your instructor for further action.**

 Check **FINAL CHECKPOINT:** Using the criteria listed on the evaluation sheet, your instructor will grade your performance.

PROCEDURE 22:3C

OBRA

Opening a Closed Bed

Equipment and Supplies

Closed bed with linen in place, paper and pen or computer

Procedure

1. Wash hands.
2. Check the closed bed to be sure it was made correctly. Lock the wheels and elevate the height of the bed to a comfortable working position.

   NOTE: For an ambulatory patient, the bed is made as a closed bed and then converted to an open bed.
3. Place the pillow on a chair or overbed table.
4. Go to the head of the bed and work from its side. Fold the top edge of the spread over and under the blanket. Fold the top sheet down over the blanket and spread to form a cuff.
5. Face the foot of the bed. Hold the upper edge of the top layers of linen (spread, blanket, and sheet) with both hands.
6. Fanfold the linen into three even layers down to the foot of the bed (Figure 22–26).

   NOTE: The top of the fold should be facing the head of the bed. In this manner, the patient will be able to pull the top covers up more readily after getting into the bed.

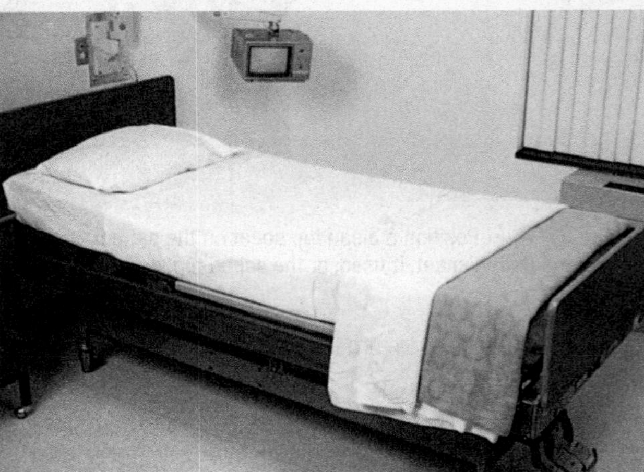

FIGURE 22–26 **In an open bed, the top sheets are fanfolded to the foot of the bed.**

7. Place the pillow back at the head of the bed. Make sure the open end is away from the door.
8. Observe all checkpoints before leaving the area: place the call signal within easy reach of the bed, lower the bed to its lowest level, lock the bed wheels, correctly position all equipment, and leave the area neat and clean.
9. Wash hands.

PROCEDURE 22:3C (CONT.)

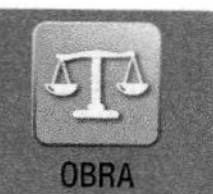

10.  Report that an open bed was made and/or record all required information on the patient's chart or enter it into the computer. For example, date, time, open bed made, and your signature and title.

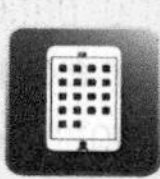 **NOTE:** In health care agencies using electronic health records (EHRs), also known as electronic medical records (EMRs), the information is entered directly into the patient's record on a computer.

PRACTICE: Go to the workbook and use the evaluation sheet for 22:3C, Opening a Closed Bed, to practice this procedure. When you believe you have mastered this skill, sign the sheet and give it to your instructor for further action.

 **FINAL CHECKPOINT:** Using the criteria listed on the evaluation sheet, your instructor will grade your performance.

PROCEDURE 22:3D

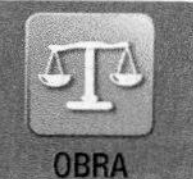

Placing a Bed Cradle

Equipment and Supplies

Laundry hamper, cart, or bag; bed cradle; two large sheets (or one large sheet and one fitted sheet); draw sheet (if used); spread; pillow; pillowcase; blanket (if needed); bath blanket; gloves; paper and pen or computer

Procedure

1. Assemble equipment
2. 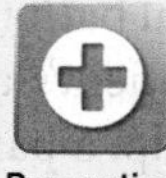 Knock on the door and pause before entering. Introduce yourself. Identify the patient. Explain the procedure and obtain consent.
3. Close the door and pull the curtain to provide privacy.
4. Wash hands. Put on gloves.

   CAUTION: Wear gloves and observe standard precautions. Linen may be contaminated with blood, body fluids, secretions, or excretions.
5. Lock the bed wheels. Elevate the bed to a comfortable working height. If siderails are present and elevated, lower the siderail on the side of the bed where you are working.

    **CAUTION:** If siderails are present, check the opposite siderail to make sure it is raised and secured.
6. Use a bath blanket to cover the patient. Remove soiled top linen and place it in the linen hamper, cart, or bag.
7. Turn the patient toward the opposite side of the bed.
8. Loosen the bottom sheet and draw sheet, and fanfold them to the center of the bed.
9. Place the clean bottom sheet and draw sheets on the bed as described in Procedure 22:3B, Making an Occupied Bed. Finish changing bottom linen on both sides of the bed.
10. Position the patient in the center of the bed and on his or her back.
11. Place the bed cradle into position (Figure 22–27).

     **CAUTION:** To prevent injury, make sure the cradle is not touching any part of the patient's skin.
12. Tie or anchor the cradle to the bed as necessary. Many bed cradles have metal clamps that attach to the mattress or bed frame. If no clamps are present, roller gauze or straps can be attached to the cradle and then fastened to the bedframe under the mattress.

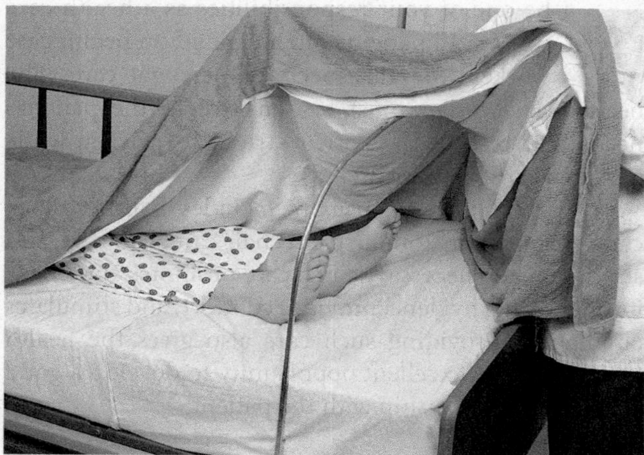

FIGURE 22–27 **A bed cradle supports the top linen and prevents the linen from coming into contact with the patient's legs and feet.**

(continues)

PROCEDURE 22:3D (CONT.)

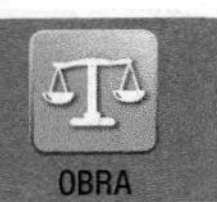

NOTE: A restless or confused patient may knock the cradle off of the bed. The cradle should be clamped or tied in place to prevent this.

13. Place the top sheet, blanket, and spread over the top of the cradle and patient. Remove the bath blanket. Tuck in the top sheets at the foot of the bed.
14. Miter the corners and tuck them into place. A larger fold can be made near the lower edge of the cradle to form a neater mitered corner.
15. Make a cuff by folding the top sheet over the blanket and spread.
16. Insert the pillow into a clean pillowcase. Position the pillow on the bed, with the open end away from the door.
17. Observe all checkpoints before leaving the patient: the patient is safe, comfortable, and in good body alignment; the call signal and other supplies are within easy reach of the patient; the siderails are elevated (if indicated); the bed is at its lowest level; and the area is neat and clean.
18. Check placement of the bed cradle at the end of the procedure and at intervals afterward. Make sure it keeps the bed linen away from the patient. Make sure it is securely in place.
19. Replace all equipment.
20. Wash hands.
21.  Report that a bed with cradle was made and/or record all required information on the patient's chart or enter it into the computer. For example, date, time, bed with cradle made, and your signature and title. Note any unusual observations.

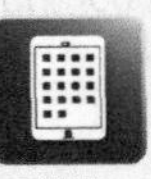

NOTE: In health care agencies using electronic health records (EHRs), also known as electronic medical records (EMRs), the information is entered directly into the patient's record on a computer.

PRACTICE: **Go to the workbook and use the evaluation sheet for 22:3D, Placing a Bed Cradle, to practice this procedure. When you believe you have mastered this skill, sign the sheet and give it to your instructor for further action.**

FINAL CHECKPOINT: Using the criteria listed on the evaluation sheet, your instructor will grade your performance.

22:4 Administering Personal Hygiene

Administering personal care and hygiene may be one of your responsibilities as a health care worker. Ill patients often depend on health care workers for all aspects of personal care. The health care worker must be sensitive to the patient's needs and respect the patient's right to privacy while personal care is administered.

Personal hygiene usually includes bathing, back care, perineal care, oral hygiene, hair care, nail care, and shaving, when necessary. Such care promotes good habits of personal hygiene, provides comfort, and stimulates circulation. Providing such care also gives the health care worker an excellent opportunity to develop a good and caring relationship with the patient.

Types of Baths

Different types of baths are given to patients. The type of bath depends on the patient's condition and ability to help.

- **Complete bed bath (CBB)**: The health care worker bathes all parts of the patient's body and also provides oral hygiene, back care, hair care, nail care, and perineal care. A complete bath is usually given to the patient who is confined to bed and is too weak or ill to bathe.
- **Partial bed bath**: The health care worker bathes some parts of the patient's body. The term partial bath (PB) has two meanings, both related to the patient's ability to help. If the patient is too weak to help, a partial bath means that only the face, arms, hands, back, and perineal area are bathed by the health care worker. If the patient is able to wash most of his or her body, a partial bath means that the health care worker completes the bath, usually bathing the patient's legs and back. In both types of partial baths, the health care worker prepares the supplies needed by the patient (Figure 22–28).
- *Tub bath or shower*: Some patients are allowed to take tub baths or showers. The health care worker helps as needed by providing towels and supplies, preparing the tub or shower area, and assisting the patient as much as the situation demands.

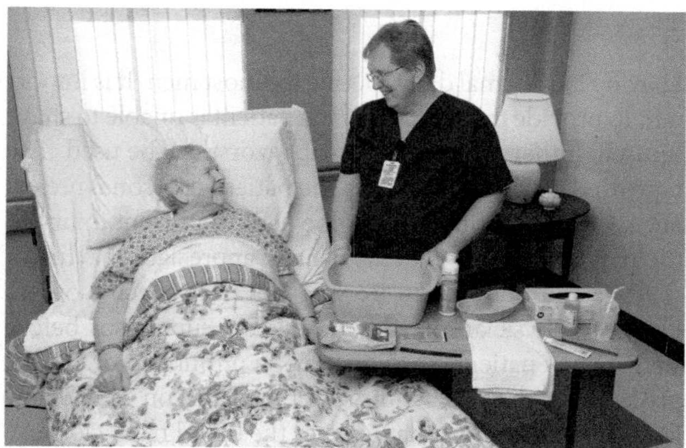

FIGURE 22–28 Position supplies conveniently when assisting a patient with a partial bath.

- *Waterless bath*: Some facilities are using prepackaged disposable cleansing cloths instead of basins of water for baths (Figure 22–29). The cleansing cloths contain a rinse-free cleanser and moisturizer, and are warmed in a microwave (follow package instructions) or in a special warmer. Most packages contain from 8–10 cloths. Usually one cloth is used for the face, neck, and ears; one for each arm and each leg; one for the chest and abdomen; one for the perineum; and one for the back and buttocks. The solution dries quickly on the skin, but a towel can be used to gently remove excess moisture. Extreme care must be taken to avoid overheating the cloths. Read and follow manufacturer's instructions.

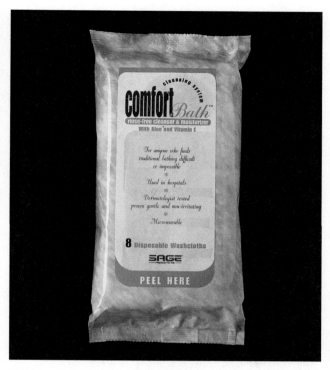

FIGURE 22–29 Packages of cleansing cloths containing a rinse-free cleaner and moisturizer can be used to give a waterless bath.
Courtesy of Sage Products, Inc.

Oral Hygiene

Oral hygiene means care of the mouth and teeth. Oral hygiene should be administered at least three times a day. If the patient's condition requires frequent oral care, it should be administered more often, usually at least every 2 hours. Proper oral hygiene prevents disease and dental caries, stimulates the appetite, and provides comfort. In addition, it aids in the prevention of halitosis (bad breath).

- *Routine oral hygiene* refers to regular, everyday toothbrushing and flossing. Many times, patients are able to provide their own care. In such cases, the health care worker provides all of the necessary equipment and supplies. In other cases, the worker helps the patient brush and care for the teeth and mouth.
- *Denture care* is necessary when a patient has dentures or artificial teeth. In such cases, the health care worker must help clean the dentures. Patients may be sensitive about dentures. Therefore, it is important that the health care worker provide privacy and reassure the patient. Extreme care must also be taken to prevent damage to the dentures.
- *Special oral hygiene* is usually provided for the unconscious or semiconscious patient. Because many of these patients breathe through their mouths, extra care must be taken to clean all parts of the mouth. Special supplies are used for this procedure.

Hair Care

Hair care is an important aspect of personal care that is, unfortunately, frequently neglected. Patients confined to bed often have tangles and knots in their hair. Tangles or knots can be removed by combing a small section of hair at a time and working from the ends toward the scalp. Conditioners can help prevent tangles. Braiding long hair after the tangles are removed also helps reduce the number of tangles and knots. Brushing stimulates circulation to the scalp and helps prevent scalp disease. Brushing also removes dirt and/or lint, and helps keep the hair shiny and attractive.

It is also important to observe the condition of the hair and scalp. Signs of disease, redness, scaling, scalp irritation, or any other conditions should be reported.

Shampooing must be approved by the physician. Various types of dry or fluid shampoos are available for patients confined to bed. Read all instructions carefully before using any of these products. Special devices are also available for use while giving a shampoo to a patient confined to bed (Figure 22–30).

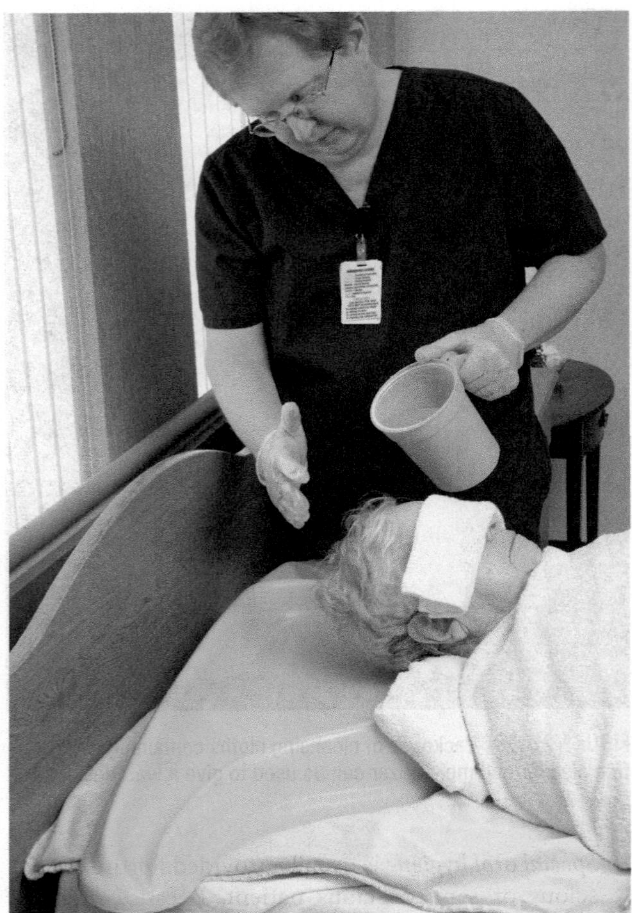

FIGURE 22–30 Special devices are available for use when shampooing the hair of a patient confined to bed.

Nail Care

Nail care is another often-neglected area in the personal care of the patient. Nails harbor dirt, which can lead to infection and disease. In addition, rough or sharp nails can cause injury. It is important that nail care be included as a part of the daily personal care provided to the patient. However, nails should never be cut unless you receive specific orders to do so from the physician or your immediate supervisor. Cutting nails may cause injury. In some facilities, only licensed or advanced practice personnel are allowed to cut fingernails. If you are permitted to cut fingernails, use nail clippers, not scissors, and clip the nails straight across. *Never* cut below the tips of the fingers. Clip slowly and carefully to avoid accidentally damaging the skin around the nail. Then file the nails straight across to remove rough edges. *Never* cut toenails because injuries to the feet are prone to infection and slow healing. File toenails straight across. Learn and follow your agency policy on nail care.

Shaving

Shaving is a normal daily routine for most men. It is important to provide this care when the patient is unable to shave himself. Either regular or electric razors may be used. The type used usually depends on the patient's personal preference. Correct technique must be used to prevent injury to the patient. Female patients usually appreciate shaving of the legs and underarms. Be sure you have specific orders from the physician or your immediate supervisor before shaving any patient. Shaving may be prohibited or special precautions may be required for patients on anticoagulants, or medications that prevent the blood from clotting.

Back Rub

Unless contraindicated by the patient's condition, a back rub is given as part of the daily bath. It can also be given at other times during the day and should be done at least once every 8 hours for a patient confined to bed. A good back rub takes at least 4–7 minutes and stimulates circulation, prevents pressure ulcers, and leads to relaxation and comfort. It is important that the health care worker's nails be short to prevent injury.

Changing a Gown or Clothing

Changing a patient's gown or pajamas is also important. Most patients prefer to wear their own gowns or pajamas. However, hospital gowns are frequently used on very ill patients or on patients with limited movement. These gown usually open down the back and are easier to position and remove. If the patient has a weak or injured arm, or if an intravenous solution is being infused in one arm, the gown or pajama top must be positioned with care. Usually, the sleeve of the soiled gown or pajama top is removed from the uninjured or untreated arm first. This allows more freedom of movement while removing the sleeve from the injured or treated arm. Likewise, the sleeve of the clean gown or pajama top is placed on the affected arm first and then is placed on the unaffected arm. It is sometimes necessary to leave one arm out of the gown and place the sleeve on the unaffected arm only. Some agencies have gowns with openings at the shoulders. Such a gown can be placed over a treated arm and then closed with snaps, ties, or Velcro strips at the shoulder area.

In home care, gowns or pajama tops can be opened at the arm seam for easy application. Velcro strips or ties can then be applied so that the gown or pajama top can be closed after being put on the patient. In long-term care facilities, most residents wear regular clothing during the day. It is important to help the resident as needed in choosing and dressing in appropriate clothing. If a resident has difficulty moving one side or is paralyzed, always put the clothing on the affected side first and remove it from the affected side last.

Summary

When administering personal hygiene, it is important that the health care worker be alert for any signs that might be unusual. When performing any personal hygiene procedure, watch for and report any unusual observations, including the following:

- *Sores, cuts, injuries*: Any injuries noted on the skin, mouth, or scalp must be reported.
- *Rashes:* Any type of rash should be reported. Many times, a rash is the first sign of an allergic reaction to a medication.
- *Color*: Any unusual color should be noted. Redness (erythema) of the skin is often the first sign of a pressure sore, or decubitus ulcer. A blue color (cyanosis) is a sign of poor circulation. A yellow color (jaundice) is a sign of liver disease, bile obstruction, or destruction of red blood cells.
- *Swelling, or edema*: This can indicate poor circulation or disease and should be reported immediately. Pay particular attention to the hands, feet, ankles, and toes.
- *Other signs of distress*: Difficult breathing (dyspnea), dizziness (vertigo), unusual weakness, excessive perspiration (diaphoresis), extreme pallor, or abnormal drowsiness or sluggishness (lethargy) should be reported immediately.

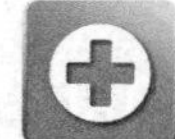
Precaution

When administering personal hygiene, standard precautions (described in Chapter 15:4) must be observed at all times. Hands must be washed frequently, and gloves must be worn. Contact with blood, body fluids, secretions, or excretions is possible. A gown must be worn if contamination of a uniform or clothing is likely. A mask and protective eyewear, or a face shield, must be worn if droplets of blood or body fluids are present, such as when a patient is coughing excessively. Health care workers with cuts, sores, or dermatitis on their hands must wear gloves for all patient contact. Preventing the spread of infection is a major responsibility of the health care provider.

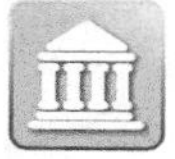
Legal

Always be sensitive to the patient's feelings and respect the patient's rights. Knock on the door and pause before entering a patient's or resident's room. Provide privacy during procedures by closing the door and pulling the curtain. Avoid exposing the patient when administering personal hygiene. Explain all procedures and reassure the patient as needed. Observe professional ethics at all times.

STUDENT: **Go to the workbook and complete the assignment sheet for 22:4, Administering Personal Hygiene. Then return and continue with the procedures.**

PROCEDURE 22:4A

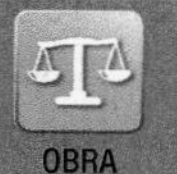
OBRA

Providing Routine Oral Hygiene

Equipment and Supplies

Toothbrush, toothpaste or powder, mouthwash solution (if used) in cup, cup of water, straw, emesis basin, bath towel, tissues, dental floss, plastic bag or plastic-lined waste can, disposable gloves, paper and pen or computer

Procedure

1. Obtain proper authorization and assemble equipment.
2. 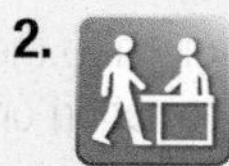
Comm
Knock on the door and pause before entering. Introduce yourself. Identify the patient. Explain the procedure and obtain consent.
3. Wash hands. Put on gloves. If spraying or splashing of oral fluids is possible, wear a face mask and eye protection.

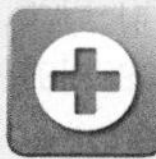
Precaution

CAUTION: Observe standard precautions. Contamination by body fluids is possible.

4. Position the patient comfortably. Close the door and pull the curtain to provide privacy. Raise the head of the bed, if permitted. Elevate the bed to a comfortable working height. If siderails are present and elevated, lower the siderail on the side where you are working. Position the overbed table containing all equipment in a convenient location (Figure 22–31A).

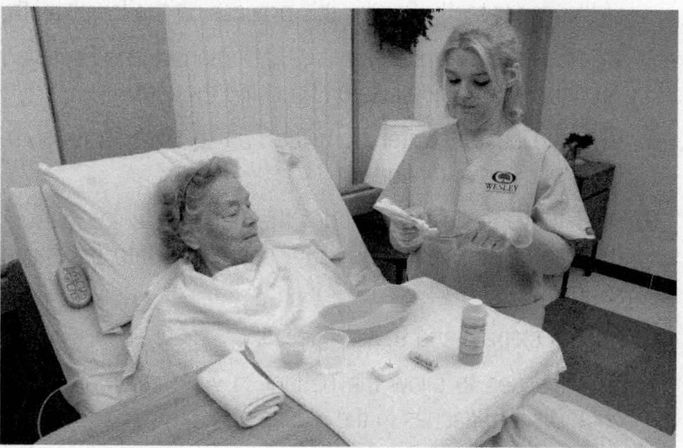

FIGURE 22–31A Position all supplies in a convenient location when assisting a patient with routine oral hygiene.

(continues)

PROCEDURE 22:4A (CONT.)

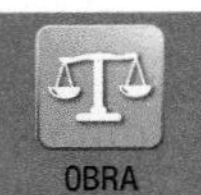

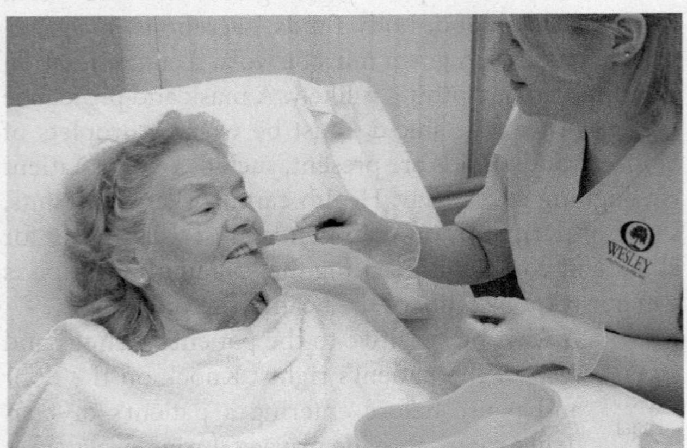

FIGURE 22–31B **Assist the patient with brushing the teeth if needed.**

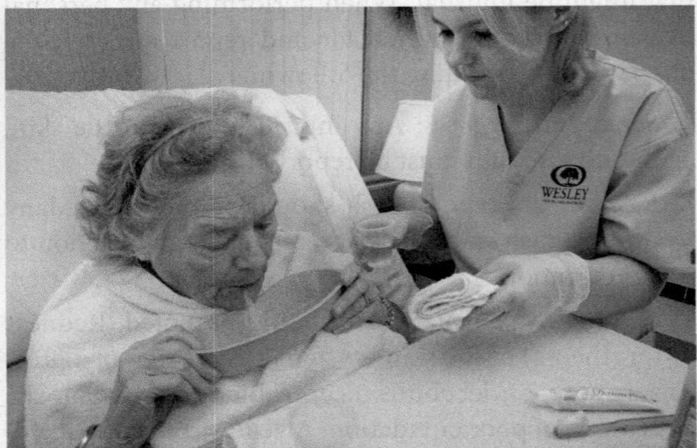

FIGURE 22–31C **Instruct the patient to expectorate (spit) into the emesis basin.**

NOTE: If the patient can brush his or her own teeth, the overbed table is usually positioned over the patient's lap.

5. Place the bath towel on the bedclothes and over the patient's shoulders.

   NOTE: A disposable bed protector can also be used to drape the patient.

6. Put water on the toothbrush. Add toothpaste. Give the brush to the patient.

   NOTE: Before adding the toothpaste, ask how much the patient uses.

7. If the patient cannot brush, brush the patient's teeth (Figure 22–31B). Carefully insert the brush into the patient's mouth. Start at the rear of the upper teeth. Place the brush at a slight angle to the gum, rotate gently, and then use a slight vibrating motion to thoroughly clean all of the upper teeth. Repeat this process on the lower teeth.

   NOTE: Refer to Procedure 19:9A, Demonstrating Brushing Technique, for guidelines on brushing the teeth.

8. Give the patient water from the cup to rinse the mouth. Provide a straw, if needed.
9. Hold the emesis basin under the patient's chin. Instruct the patient to expel the mouth secretions into the basin (Figure 22–31C).
10. Repeat steps 8 and 9, as necessary.
11. Offer tissues to allow the patient to wipe the mouth and chin. Discard tissues in the plastic bag.
12. Provide dental floss. Allow the patient to floss the teeth. Assist as needed. If the patient is not able to floss, obtain a piece of floss about 12–18 inches long. Gently insert the floss between the teeth. Curve the floss into a C-shape. Use a gentle up-and-down motion to clean the sides of the teeth. Repeat for both sides of every tooth.

    NOTE: Refer to Procedure 19:9B, Demonstrating Flossing Technique, for guidelines on flossing the teeth.

13. Provide mouthwash, if desired by the patient. Mouthwash is sometimes diluted to a proportion of half mouthwash to half water. Use the emesis basin and tissues, as necessary, to allow the patient to expectorate the mouthwash.
14. Remove all equipment. Position the patient comfortably. Be sure the patient is in good body alignment.
15. Observe all checkpoints before leaving the patient: elevate the siderails (if indicated), place the call signal and other supplies within easy reach of the patient, lower the bed to its lowest level, and leave the area neat and clean.
16. Rinse the toothbrush thoroughly. Use cool water and towels to clean the emesis basin. Properly replace all equipment.
17. Remove gloves. Remove mask and eye protection, if worn. Wash hands.
18. Comm Report that routine oral hygiene was given to the patient and/or record all required information on the patient's chart or enter it into the computer. For example, date, time, oral hygiene given, and your signature and title. Note any unusual observations.

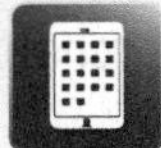

NOTE: In health care agencies using electronic health records (EHRs), also known as electronic medical records (EMRs), the information is entered directly into the patient's record on a computer.

PROCEDURE 22:4A (CONT.)

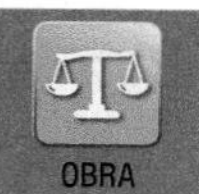

PRACTICE: Go to the workbook and use the evaluation sheet for 22:4A, Providing Routine Oral Hygiene, to practice this procedure. When you believe you have mastered this skill, sign the sheet and give it to your instructor for further action.

FINAL CHECKPOINT: Using the criteria listed on the evaluation sheet, your instructor will grade your performance.

PROCEDURE 22:4B

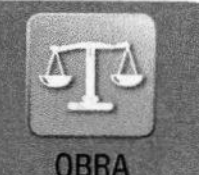

Cleaning Dentures

Equipment and Supplies

Toothbrush and toothpaste or denture brush and denture cleaner, denture cup, tissues, cup with mouthwash (if used), straw, applicators, bath towel, paper towels, emesis basin, plastic bag or plastic-lined waste can, disposable gloves, paper and pen or computer

Procedure

1. Obtain proper authorization and assemble equipment.
2. Knock on the door and pause before entering. Introduce yourself. Identify the patient. Explain the procedure and obtain consent.

   NOTE: The patient may be sensitive about dentures. Provide privacy and reassurance.
3. Close the door and pull the curtain for privacy.
4. Wash hands. Put on gloves.

   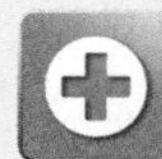

   CAUTION: Observe standard precautions. Contamination by body fluids is possible.
5. Elevate the bed to a comfortable working height. Raise the head of the bed, if permitted. If siderails are present and elevated, lower the siderail on the side where you are working.
6. Offer tissues to the patient. Ask the patient to remove the dentures. If the patient is unable to do so, use tissues or a gauze sponge to grasp the dentures between your thumb and index finger (Figure 22–32A). Gently apply downward and forward pressure to loosen and remove the top denture. Remove the lower denture by grasping it with your thumb and forefinger and turning it slightly to lift it out of the mouth.

   CAUTION: Never force dentures loose. They can break.
7. Carefully place the dentures in a denture cup. If indicated, raise the siderails for patient safety. Carry the dentures to the sink.
8. Line the sink with paper towels.

   NOTE: This provides a protective cushion for the dentures should they be dropped.

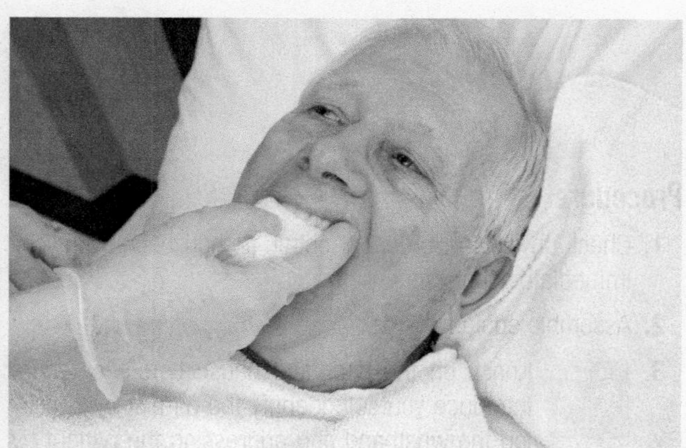

FIGURE 22–32A **Use tissues or a gauze sponge to grasp the dentures and ease them down and forward to remove them from the mouth.**

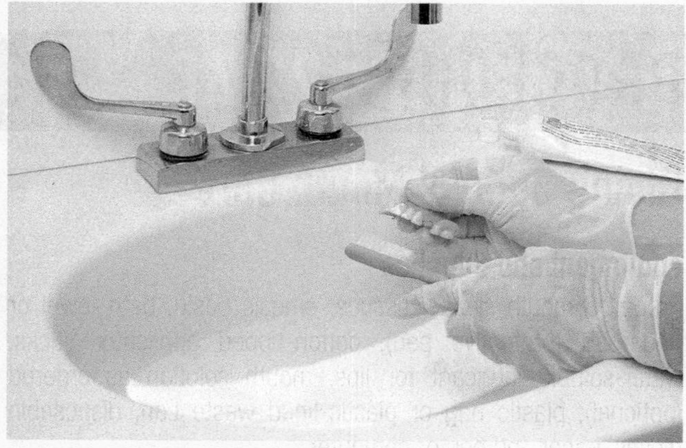

FIGURE 22–32B **Hold the dentures securely while brushing all surfaces.**

(continues)

PROCEDURE 22:4B (CONT.)

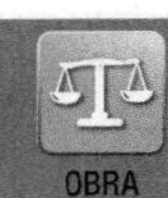

9. Put toothpaste or powder on the toothbrush. Place the dentures in the palm of one hand. Holding them under a gentle stream of cool or lukewarm water, brush all surfaces thoroughly (Figure 22–32B).

CAUTION: Do *not* use hot water. This can cause breakage.

NOTE: Clean all parts of the dentures, not just the teeth.

NOTE: Dentures can be soaked in a solution containing a cleansing tablet prior to brushing.

10. Rinse dentures thoroughly in cool water.

CAUTION: Do *not* use very cold water. This can also cause breakage.

11. Put clean, cool water in the denture cup. Place the cleaned dentures in the cup.
12. Return to the patient's bedside. If siderails are elevated, lower the siderail on the side where you will be working.
13. Help the patient to rinse the mouth with cool water and/or mouthwash. Use the emesis basin and tissues. Place used tissues in the plastic bag.

NOTE: Some patients want to brush their gums with a soft toothbrush or applicator moistened with mouthwash before inserting clean dentures. Assist the patient, as necessary.

14. Hand the dentures to the patient. Help the patient insert the dentures, as needed. The upper denture is inserted first.

NOTE: If the patient desires adhesive, line the palates (the sections holding the teeth) of the dentures with denture adhesive.

NOTE: If dentures are not immediately returned to the patient, they should be stored inside the denture cup in a safe area (such as a drawer) and labeled with the patient's name and room number. At times, a denture cleansing or soaking tablet is placed in the water when dentures are stored.

15. Observe all checkpoints before leaving the patient: position the patient in correct body alignment; elevate the siderails (if indicated); lower the bed to its lowest level; place the call signal, tissues, water, and supplies within easy reach of the patient; clean and replace all equipment; and leave the area neat and clean.
16. Remove gloves. Wash hands thoroughly.
17.  Report that denture care was given and/or record all required information on the patient's chart or enter it into the computer. For example, date, time, dentures cleaned, and your signature and title. Note any unusual observations.

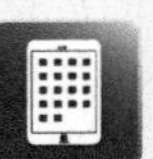

NOTE: In health care agencies using electronic health records (EHRs), also known as electronic medical records (EMRs), the information is entered directly into the patient's record on a computer.

PRACTICE: **Go to the workbook and use the evaluation sheet for 22:4B, Cleaning Dentures, to practice this procedure. When you believe you have mastered this skill, sign the sheet and give it to your instructor for further action.**

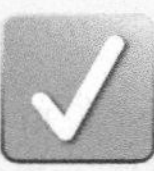

FINAL CHECKPOINT: Using the criteria listed on the evaluation sheet, your instructor will grade your performance.

PROCEDURE 22:4C

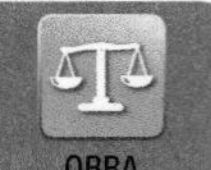

Giving Special Mouth Care

Equipment and Supplies

Prepared mouth swabs, tissues, emesis basin, bath towel or underpad (protective pad), cotton-tipped applicator sticks, water-soluble lubricant for lips, mouth solution as ordered (optional), plastic bag or plastic-lined waste can, disposable gloves, paper and pen or computer

Procedure

1. Check physician's orders or obtain authorization from your immediate supervisor.
2. Assemble equipment.
3.  Knock on the door and pause before entering. Introduce yourself. Identify the patient by checking the wristband and addressing the patient by name. Explain the procedure and obtain consent.

PROCEDURE 22:4C (CONT.)

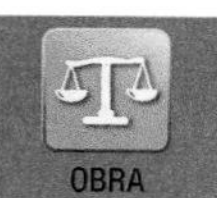

OBRA

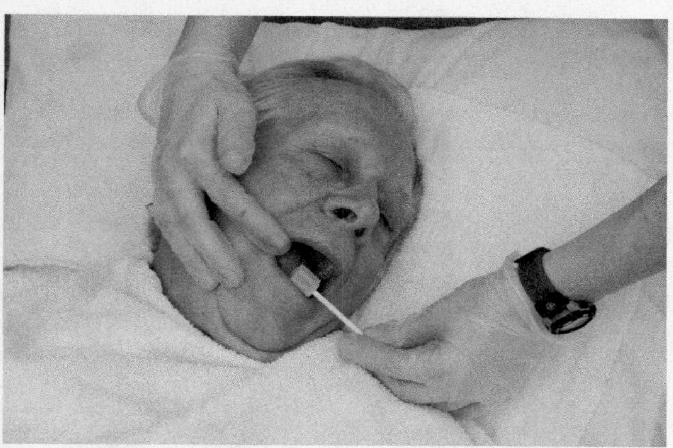

FIGURE 22–33 **Use a prepared swab to cleanse all parts of the patient's mouth while providing special oral hygiene.**

NOTE: Semiconscious or unconscious patients can sometimes hear.

4. Close the door and pull the curtain for privacy.
5. Wash hands. Put on gloves.

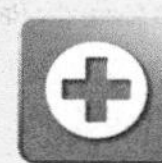

Precaution

CAUTION: Observe standard precautions. Contamination by body fluids is possible.

6. Elevate the bed to a comfortable working height. Raise the head of the bed if permissible. If siderails are present and elevated, lower the siderail on the side where you are working.
7. Turn the patient's head to the side toward you. Place the bath towel or underpad under the patient's head and chin.
8. Open the package of prepared mouth swabs.

   NOTE: Toothettes are a common brand name of mouth swabs.

   NOTE: Prepared mouth swabs may contain lemon and glycerine, hydrogen peroxide, or sodium bicarbonate.
9. Use the prepared swab to cleanse all parts of the patient's mouth (Figure 22–33). Cleanse the teeth, gums, tongue, and roof of the mouth thoroughly. Work from the gums to the cutting edges of the teeth. Use a gentle motion.
10. Discard used swabs in the plastic bag. Use fresh swabs until the entire mouth is clean.
11. If the patient is able to help, have him or her rinse the mouth with mouthwash, if allowed. Then follow with a freshwater rinse. If the patient is unconscious, use clean applicators moistened with clear water to rinse the patient's mouth. Use a soft towel to dry the area around the mouth.

Safety

CAUTION: Never give an unconscious or semiconscious patient mouthwash or any other liquids.

12. Use the cotton-tipped applicator sticks to apply water-soluble lubricant lightly to the tongue and lips.

    NOTE: This keeps the tissues soft and moist.
13. Reposition the patient in correct body alignment.
14. Replace all equipment used. A tray with supplies for special mouth care is sometimes kept at the bedside. If so, restock the supplies on the tray so it is always ready for use.
15. Observe all checkpoints before leaving the patient: elevate the siderails (if indicated), place the call signal within easy reach of the patient, lower the bed to its lowest level, and leave the area neat and clean.
16. Remove gloves. Wash hands.
17. Report that special mouth care was given and/or record all required information on the patient's chart or enter it into the computer. For example, date, time, special mouth care given, lips appear dry and chapped, and your signature and title. Immediately report any problems noted, including sores, irritated areas in the mouth, bleeding gums, or cuts.

Comm

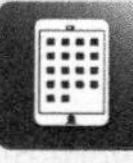

EHR

NOTE: In health care agencies using electronic health records (EHRs), also known as electronic medical records (EMRs), the information is entered directly into the patient's record on a computer.

PRACTICE: **Go to the workbook and use the evaluation sheet for 22:4C, Giving Special Mouth Care, to practice this procedure. When you believe you have mastered this skill, sign the sheet and give it to your instructor for further action.**

Check

FINAL CHECKPOINT: Using the criteria listed on the evaluation sheet, your instructor will grade your performance.

PROCEDURE 22:4D

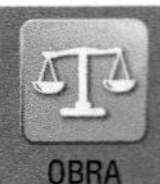
OBRA

Administering Daily Hair Care

Equipment and Supplies

Comb and/or brush, towel, alcohol or baby oil, gloves, paper and pen or computer

Procedure

1. Obtain proper authorization and assemble equipment.
2. 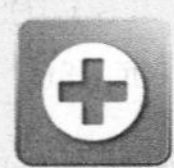 Comm — Knock on the door and pause before entering. Introduce yourself. Identify the patient. Explain the procedure and obtain consent.
3. Close the door and pull the curtain to provide privacy.
4. Wash hands. Put on gloves if needed.

    Precaution

   CAUTION: Wear gloves and observe standard precautions if the scalp has open sores or infected areas. Some health care facilities require that gloves be worn while providing hair care. Follow agency policy.
5. Elevate the bed to a comfortable working height. Raise the head of the bed, if permissible. If siderails are present and elevated, lower the siderail on the side where you are working.
6. Cover the pillow with the towel.
7. Ask the patient to move to the side of the bed nearest you. Assist as necessary.

   Safety

   CAUTION: Use proper body mechanics, including a broad base of support. Bend from hips.
8. Part or section the hair. Start at one side and work around to the other side.
9. Comb or brush the hair thoroughly. Keep the fingers of your hand between the scalp and comb whenever possible (Figure 22–34). If the hair is not tangled or knotted, begin at the scalp and work toward the ends of the hair.

   NOTE: This prevents pulling and decreases discomfort.
10. Do each section completely. To do the back of the head, turn the patient or lift the head slightly.
11. If the hair is very tangled or knotted, do the following:
    a. Spray a small amount of water on the hair. Comb or brush the hair gently starting at the ends and working toward the scalp to remove the knots and tangles. If the patient has conditioner, spraying a small amount of conditioner on the hair may also help remove the knots and tangles.

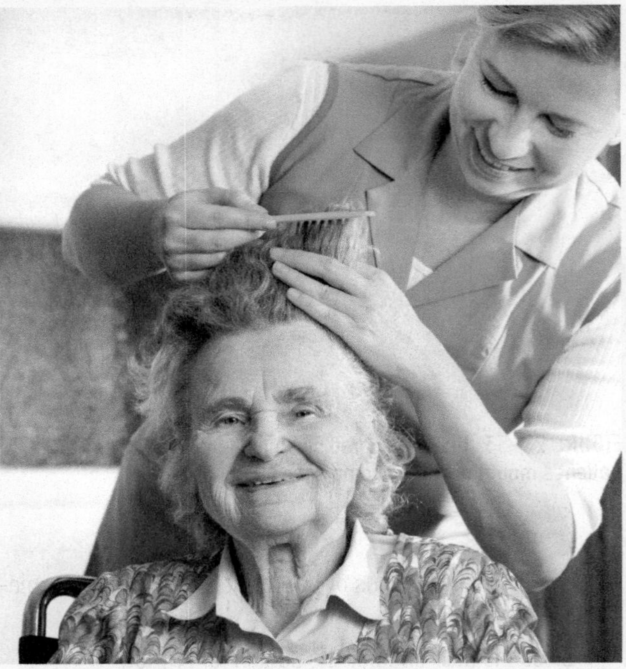

FIGURE 22–34 Keep the fingers of your hand between the patient's scalp and the comb while combing the hair. © Alexander Raths/ Shutterstock.com

    b. For very dry hair, put a very small amount of baby oil on your hands and rub it into the hair. Then comb or brush gently. Start at the ends of the hair and work toward the scalp.
    c. For very oily hair, put a small amount of alcohol on your hands and apply it to the hair. Comb or brush.

     Safety

    CAUTION: Be careful not to get alcohol near the patient's eyes.
12. When all areas of the hair have been brushed or combed, arrange the hair attractively according to the patient's preference. After obtaining the patient's permission, braid long hair to prevent tangling.

    NOTE: Hair bands or hairpins can be used to hold the hair in place. Take care that they will not injure the scalp. Avoid the use of rubber bands whenever possible because they can break and damage the hair.
13. Throughout the entire procedure, closely observe the condition of the scalp and hair. Report any abnormal conditions immediately.
14. Observe all checkpoints before leaving the patient: position the patient in correct body alignment, elevate the siderails

PROCEDURE 22:4D (CONT.)

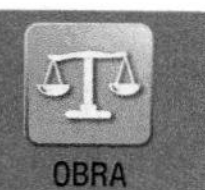

(if indicated), lower the bed to its lowest level, and place the call signal and supplies within easy reach of the patient.

15. Clean and replace all equipment used. It is sometimes necessary to remove hair from the brush and comb. Wash the comb and brush in a mild, soapy solution. Rinse thoroughly. Leave the area neat and clean.
16. Remove gloves if worn. Wash hands.
17.  Report that hair care was given and/or record all required information on the patient's chart or enter it into the computer. For example, date, time, hair combed and braided, and your signature and title. Note any unusual observations.

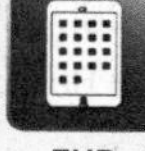

NOTE: In health care agencies using electronic health records (EHRs), also known as electronic medical records (EMRs), the information is entered directly into the patient's record on a computer.

PRACTICE: **Go to the workbook and use the evaluation sheet for 22:4D, Administering Daily Hair Care, to practice this procedure. When you believe you have mastered this skill, sign the sheet and give it to your instructor for further action.**

FINAL CHECKPOINT: Using the criteria listed on the evaluation sheet, your instructor will grade your performance.

PROCEDURE 22:4E

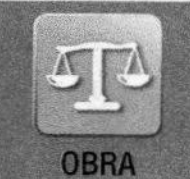

Providing Nail Care

Equipment and Supplies

Orange stick, emery board, nail clippers (if permitted), water and mild detergent in basin, towel, plastic bag, gloves, paper and pen or computer

CAUTION: In some facilities, only licensed or advance practice personnel are permitted to cut fingernails. In addition, cutting nails may be prohibited for some patients, such as patients who have diabetes. It is important to learn and follow agency policy regarding nail care.

Procedure

1. Check physician's orders or obtain authorization from your immediate supervisor.
2. Assemble equipment.
3.  Knock on the door and pause before entering. Introduce yourself. Identify the patient. Explain the procedure and obtain consent.
4. Close the door and pull the curtain to provide privacy.
5. Wash hands. Put on gloves.

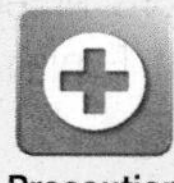

CAUTION: Wear gloves and observe standard precautions. Contact with nonintact skin or body fluids is possible.

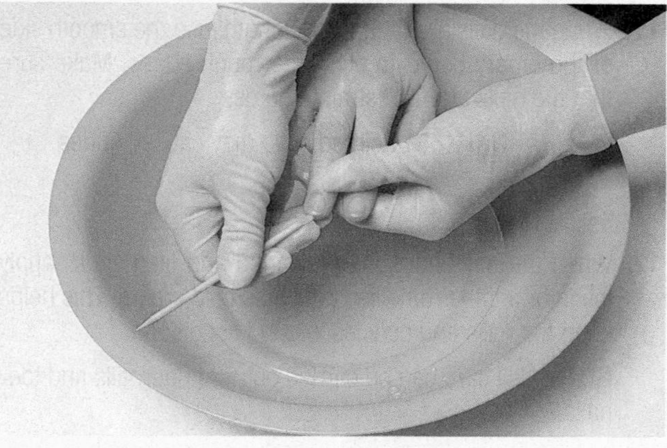

FIGURE 22–35 **After soaking the nails, use the blunt edge of an orange stick to remove any dirt from under the nails.**

6. Elevate the bed to a comfortable working height. If siderails are present and elevated, lower the siderail on the side where you are working.
7. Clean the nails by soaking them for 5–10 minutes in a solution of mild detergent and water at a temperature of 105°F–110°F (40.6°C–43.3°C). This loosens the dirt in the nail beds.

   NOTE: Oil is sometimes used instead of detergent.
8. Use the slanted or blunt edge of the orange stick to clean dirt out of the nail beds under the nails (Figure 22–35). A nail

(continues)

PROCEDURE 22:4E (CONT.)

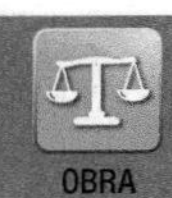
OBRA

brush can also be used to clean the nails. Carefully check the nails and surrounding skin while cleaning the nails.

Safety

CAUTION: Using the pointed edge of the orange stick can result in a puncture wound.

NOTE: If any redness, excessive dryness, or cracking of the skin is noted, report this to your supervisor immediately.

9. Use the emery board to file the nails and shorten them. Use short strokes. Work from the side of the nail to the top of the nail. Repeat for the opposite side.

   NOTE: Do *not* use a back-and-forth motion. Such a motion can split the nails.

10. If the fingernails are very long, and you are allowed to cut them, use nail clippers to cut the nails straight across. Be careful not to injure the skin around the nail. *Never* cut toenails. File them straight across.

Safety

CAUTION: Do *not* use scissors. They can cut the patient.

11. When the nails are the correct length, use the smooth side of the emery board to eliminate rough edges. Make sure that the nails are filed straight across.

Safety

CAUTION: Pointed nails may cause injuries.

12. When the nails have been cleaned and filed short, apply lotion or another emollient, such as cold cream. This helps keep the nails and cuticles in good condition.

    NOTE: Nail care can be carried out for fingernails and toenails.

13. Apply lotion to the hands and feet. Do *not* apply lotion between the toes because this promotes the growth of fungus.
14. Position the patient in correct body alignment.
15. Observe all checkpoints before leaving the patient: elevate the siderails (if indicated); place the call signal, water, and tissues within easy reach of the patient; lower the bed to its lowest level; and leave the area neat and clean.
16. Clean and properly replace all equipment used.
17. Remove gloves. Wash hands.
18. 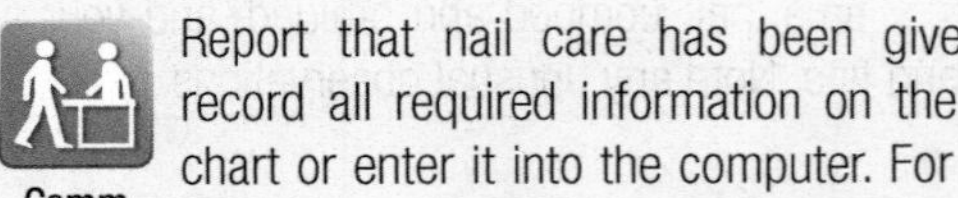
    Comm

    Report that nail care has been given and/or record all required information on the patient's chart or enter it into the computer. For example, date, time, nail care given to fingers and toes, and your signature and title. Report any observations that may signify problems.

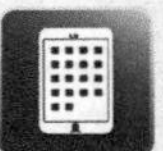
EHR

NOTE: In health care agencies using electronic health records (EHRs), also known as electronic medical records (EMRs), the information is entered directly into the patient's record on a computer.

PRACTICE: **Go to the workbook and use the evaluation sheet for 22:4E, Providing Nail Care, to practice this procedure. When you believe you have mastered this skill, sign the sheet and give it to your instructor for further action.**

Check

FINAL CHECKPOINT: Using the criteria listed on the evaluation sheet, your instructor will grade your performance.

PROCEDURE 22:4F

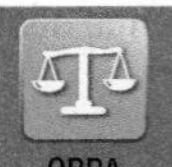
OBRA

Giving a Backrub

Equipment and Supplies

Lotion, bath towel, washcloth, soap and water, disposable gloves (if needed), basin, paper and pen or computer

Procedure

1. Obtain authorization from your immediate supervisor or check physician's orders.

   NOTE: Some patients *cannot* receive a backrub because of heart or lung disease or blood clots. Other patients with burns, back injuries, back surgeries, and similar conditions may not be able to tolerate a backrub.

2. Assemble equipment.
3. 
   Comm

   Knock on the door and pause before entering. Introduce yourself. Identify the patient. Explain the procedure and obtain consent.
4. Close the door and pull the curtain to provide privacy.

PROCEDURE 22:4F (CONT.)

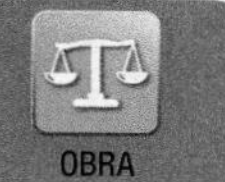

OBRA

5. Wash hands. Put on gloves if contact with nonintact skin is possible.

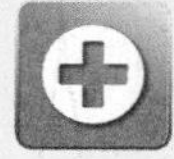

Precaution

CAUTION: Wear gloves and observe standard precautions. Contact with nonintact skin or body fluids is possible.

6. Elevate the bed to a comfortable working height. If siderails are present and elevated, lower the siderail on the side where you are working.
7. Position the patient. The patient can lie on the abdomen (prone), or, if this is not comfortable, on his or her side, facing away from you.
8. Place a bath towel lengthwise next to the patient's body.
9. Fill the basin with water at a temperature of 105°F–110°F (40.6°C–43.3°C). Wash the patient's back thoroughly. Rinse and dry the back.

   NOTE: If the patient has had a bed bath, this step is not necessary because the back has already been washed.

   NOTE: Be alert for any abnormal condition of the skin. Note any red areas, rash, sores, or cuts. Pay particular attention to bony parts.
10. Rub a small amount of lotion into your hands (Figure 22–36A).

    NOTE: This warms the solution slightly. The container of lotion can also be placed in a basin of warm water before use.
11. Begin at the base of the spine. Rub up the center of the back to the neck, around the shoulders, and down the sides of the back. Rub down over the buttocks, around, and circle back to the starting point. Use long, soothing strokes (Figure 22–36B). Use firm pressure on the upward strokes and gentle pressure on the downward strokes (Figure 22–37A). Repeat this step four times.

Safety

CAUTION: Long nails may scratch the patient. File your nails short before giving a backrub.

Safety

CAUTION: Use proper body mechanics. Get close to the patient by bending at your hips and knees, and keep your back straight. Position your feet to provide a broad base of support.

12. Repeat the long, upward strokes, but on the downward strokes, use a circular motion (Figure 22–37B). Pay particular attention to bony prominences. Repeat this motion four times.

Safety

CAUTION: Take care not to rub skin tags as this might cause them to bleed. Also avoid massaging directly over reddened areas. Massage around these areas. Report the presence of these areas to your supervisor immediately.

13. Repeat the long, upward strokes, but on the downward strokes, use very small circular motions (Figure 22–37C). Use the palm of your hand to apply firm pressure. Pay particular attention to the bony prominences. Do this motion one time.
14. Repeat the long, soothing strokes used initially (Figure 22–37D). Do this for 3–5 minutes.
15. End the backrub with up-and-down motions over the entire back (Figure 22–37E). Do this for 1–2 minutes. This provides relaxation after stimulation.

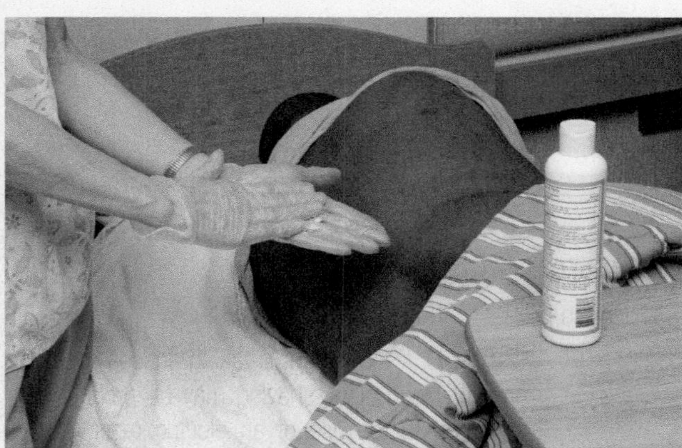

FIGURE 22–36A Rub a small amount of lotion into your hands.

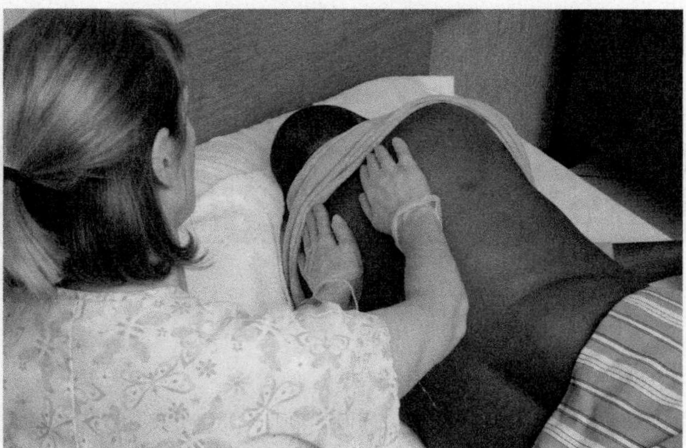

FIGURE 22–36B Use long, smooth strokes and firm pressure when giving a backrub.

(continues)

PROCEDURE 22:4F (CONT.)

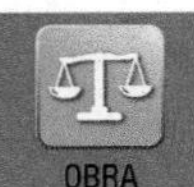

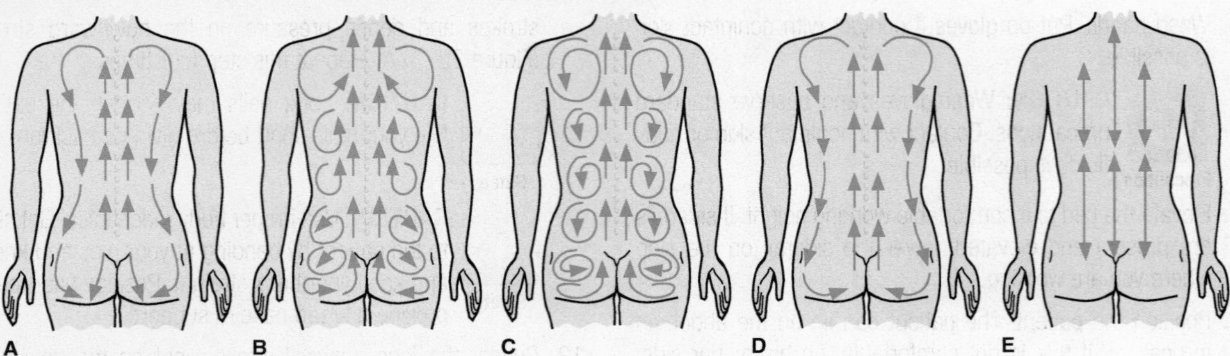

FIGURE 22–37 **Motions for a backrub.**

16. Dry the back thoroughly with the towel.
17. Straighten the bed linen. Change the patient's gown, if necessary.
18. Position the patient in good body alignment.
19. Observe all checkpoints before leaving the patient: elevate the siderails (if indicated); lower the bed to its lowest level; and place the call signal, water, and tissues within easy reach of patient.
20. Clean and replace all equipment. Leave the area neat and clean.
21. Remove gloves if worn. Wash hands.
22.  Comm Report that a backrub was given and/or record all required information on the patient's chart or enter it into the computer. For example, date, time, back massage given, patient states he feels very relaxed, and your signature and title. Report any abnormal observations immediately.

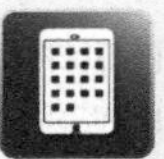 EHR

NOTE: In health care agencies using electronic health records (EHRs), also known as electronic medical records (EMRs), the information is entered directly into the patient's record on a computer.

PRACTICE: Go to the workbook and complete the evaluation sheet for 22:4F, Giving a Backrub, to practice this procedure. When you believe you have mastered this skill, sign the sheet and give it to your instructor for further action.

 Check

FINAL CHECKPOINT: Using the criteria listed on the evaluation sheet, your instructor will grade your performance.

PROCEDURE 22:4G

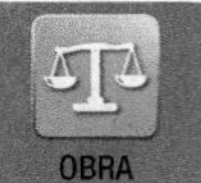

Shaving a Patient

Equipment and Supplies

Razor with blade, shaving lather, gauze pad, basin with water, towel, washcloth, mirror, electric razor (for some patients), aftershave lotion (optional), disposable gloves, sharps container, paper and pen or computer

Procedure

1. Obtain proper authorization.

 Safety

CAUTION: If the patient is taking anticoagulants to prevent blood clots, shaving may be prohibited or restricted to the use of an electric razor. Always check with your immediate supervisor to confirm whether a patient is on anticoagulants before shaving a patient.

PROCEDURE 22:4G (CONT.)

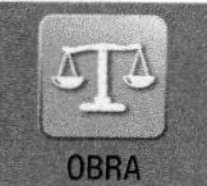

2. Assemble equipment. Examine the razor blade closely. Make sure there are no nicks or damaged edges. Carefully rub the razor blade over a folded gauze pad to check for damage.
3. 

Knock on the door and pause before entering. Introduce yourself. Identify the patient. Explain the procedure and obtain consent.
4. Close the door and pull the curtain to provide privacy.
5. Wash hands. Put on gloves.

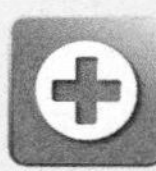

CAUTION: Observe standard precautions. A razor can nick the skin and cause bleeding.

6. Elevate the bed to a comfortable working height. Raise the head of the bed. If siderails are present and elevated, lower the siderail on the side where you are working. Put the patient in a comfortable position. Arrange all needed equipment on the overbed table.

NOTE: Allow the patient to help as much as possible.

7. Place a towel over the patient's chest and near the patient's shoulders.
8. Fill the basin with water at a temperature of 105°F–110°F (40.6°C–43.3°C). Use the washcloth to moisten the face (Figure 22–38A).
9. Apply lather. Put it on your fingers first and then apply it to the patient's cheek (Figure 22–38B).

NOTE: It is usually best to do one area of the face at a time.

10. Start in front of the ear. Hold the skin taut (stretched tightly) to prevent cuts (Figure 22–38C). Bring the razor down over the cheek and toward the chin.

CAUTION: Always shave in the direction of hair growth.

11. Rinse the razor after each stroke. Repeat until the lather is removed and the area is shaved.
12. Repeat steps 9 to 11 for the opposite cheek, the chin and neck area, and under the nose. When shaving the chin and under the nose, instruct the patient to hold the skin taut. Use firm, short strokes. Rinse the razor frequently.

CAUTION: If the skin is accidentally nicked, use a gauze pad to apply pressure directly over the area. Then apply an antiseptic or follow the policy of your agency. Be sure to report the incident to your immediate supervisor.

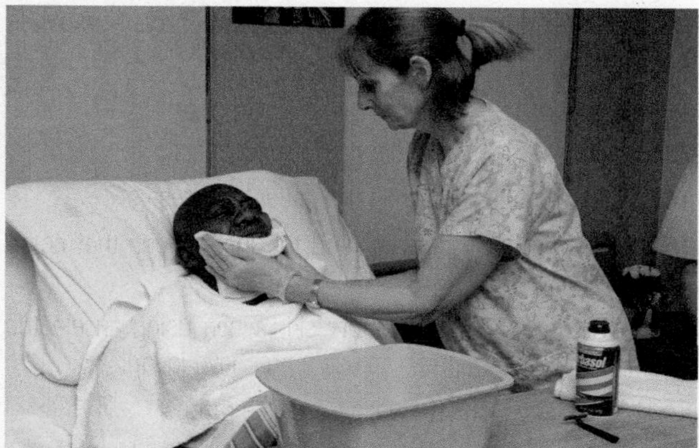

FIGURE 22–38A **Use the washcloth to moisten the face.**

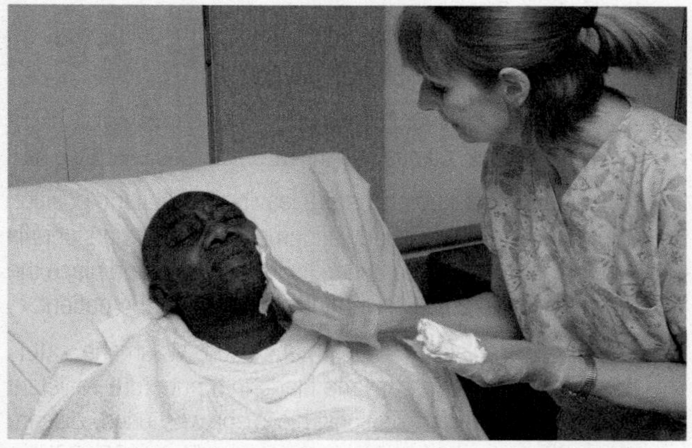

FIGURE 22–38B **Use your fingers to apply lather to the patient's cheek.**

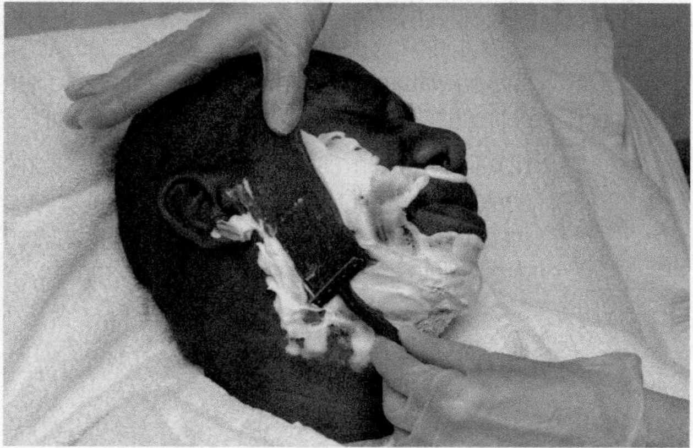

FIGURE 22–38C **Hold the skin taut and shave in the direction of hair growth while shaving the patient.**

(continues)

PROCEDURE 22:4G (CONT.)

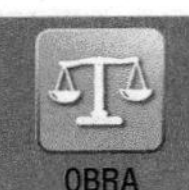

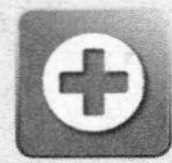

CAUTION: Observe standard precautions when controlling bleeding.

13. Wash and thoroughly dry the face and neck.
14. Apply aftershave lotion, if the patient desires.
15. To use an electric razor, read the instructions that come with the razor.
    a. Some patients prefer dry skin when using an electric razor. Others prefer to use a preshave lotion.
    b. Hold the skin taut while using the razor.
    c. Some razors require short, circular strokes. Others require short strokes in the direction of hair growth.
    d. Shave all areas of the face.
    e. Wash and dry the face thoroughly when done.
    f. Apply aftershave lotion, if desired.
    g. Clean the razor thoroughly after use. Use a small brush (which usually comes with the razor) to clean out all the hair.
16. Observe all checkpoints before leaving the patient: position the patient in correct body alignment, elevate the siderails (if indicated), lower the bed to its lowest level, and place the call signal and supplies within easy reach of the patient.
17. Clean and replace all equipment used. Wash the safety razor thoroughly. Discard the blade in a puncture-resistant sharps container. If a disposable razor was used, discard the entire razor in the sharps container (Figure 22–38D).
18. Remove gloves. Wash hands.
19. Comm: Report that the patient was shaved and/or record all required information on the patient's chart or enter it into the computer. For example, date, time, shaved with electric razor, and your signature and title. Report any observations that may signify problems.

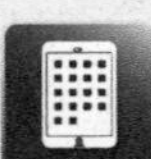

NOTE: In health care agencies using electronic health records (EHRs), also known as electronic medical records (EMRs), the information is entered directly into the patient's record on a computer.

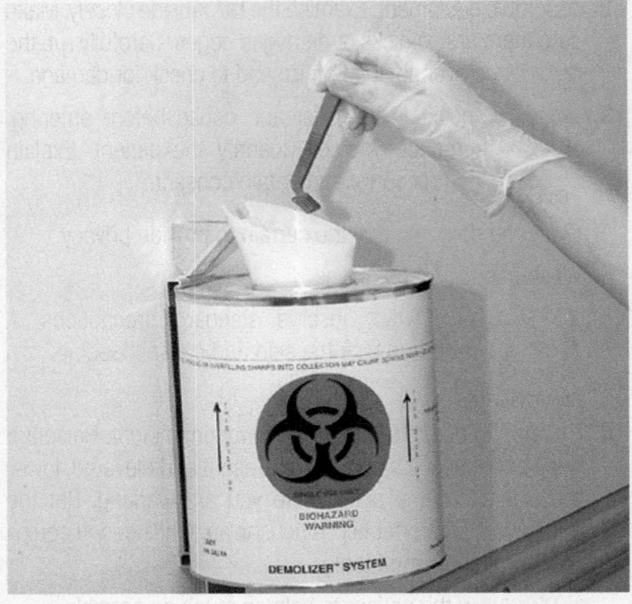

FIGURE 22–38D Discard the disposable razor in a sharps container.

NOTE: Female patients sometimes want facial, underarm, and/or leg hair shaved. Obtain proper authorization before doing any of these procedures. Follow the same steps: check the razor, moisten the area, apply lather or a soapy solution, hold the skin taut, shave in the direction of hair growth, rinse the area, do small sections at a time, and finish by thoroughly washing and drying the areas shaved.

PRACTICE: **Go to the workbook and use the evaluation sheet for 22:4G, Shaving a Patient, to practice this procedure. When you believe you have mastered this skill, sign the sheet and give it to your instructor for further action.**

FINAL CHECKPOINT: Using the criteria listed on the evaluation sheet, your instructor will grade your performance.

PROCEDURE 22:4H

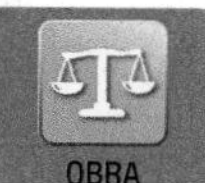
OBRA

Changing a Patient's Gown or Pajamas

Equipment and Supplies

Gown or pajamas; towel or bath blanket; linen hamper, cart, or bag; disposable gloves; paper and pen or computer

Procedure

1. Obtain proper authorization and assemble equipment.
2. Comm Knock on the door and pause before entering. Introduce yourself. Identify the patient. Explain the procedure and obtain consent.
3. Close the door and pull the curtain to provide privacy.
4. Wash hands. Put on gloves.

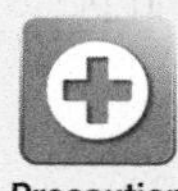
Precaution

CAUTION: Wear gloves and observe standard precautions. The gown may be contaminated with blood, body fluids, secretions, or excretions, such as drainage from an incision.

5. Elevate the bed to a comfortable working height. If siderails are present and elevated, lower the siderail on the side where you are working.

   NOTE: It is easier to change the patient's clothing if you first fold the bed covers to the foot of the bed and cover the patient with a bath blanket.
6. Loosen the patient's bedclothes:
   a. If the patient is wearing a hospital gown, untie the strings by having the patient turn on his or her side or by reaching under the neck. Then gently pull out any part of the gown that is under the patient.
   b. If the patient is wearing a gown of her own, loosen any buttons or ties. Gently ease the gown upward from the hemline to the neck. Prevent unnecessary exposure by using the towel or bath blanket, as necessary.
   c. If the patient is wearing pajamas, first untie or unbutton the pants at the waist. Gently ease the pants down over the legs and feet. Use the towel or bath blanket to drape the patient. Avoid exposing the patient. Unbutton the pajama top.
7. Take off the soiled clothing, one sleeve at a time. Gently grasp the edge of the sleeve near the shoulder. Ease the arm out. Do the far arm first. If the patient has an affected arm (injured, paralyzed, weak, etc.) or is receiving an intravenous (IV) infusion, remove the sleeve from the unaffected arm first and from the affected arm or arm with the IV second. Place the soiled clothing on a chair or in the laundry hamper.

   NOTE: If an IV is in place, ease the sleeve off of the upper arm, taking care not to disturb the infusion site, where the needle is inserted. Then gently ease the sleeve over the tubing by keeping your hand and arm in the sleeve holding the solution bottle above the infusion site, and passing the container through the sleeve (Figures 22–39A and 22–39B).

   NOTE: Many facilities use gowns that open at the shoulder when a patient has an IV. The gown is positioned over the shoulder and closed with snaps, ties, or Velcro strips.
8. Unfold the clean gown or pajama top and place it over the patient.
9. Put the patient's arms into the sleeves one at a time. Gather the sleeve of the gown or pajama top into your hands. Then put your arm through the sleeve, take the patient's hand in yours, and slip the sleeve up the patient's wrist and arm and to the shoulder.

   NOTE: If one arm is affected or has an IV, do this arm first. This places less strain on the arm. For an IV, pass the solution container and tubing through the sleeve first. Keep the solution container above the level of the infusion site at all times.

Safety

CAUTION: Sometimes, a sleeve cannot be placed because of an IV infusion machine, bulky dressing, or other similar problem. If this is the case,

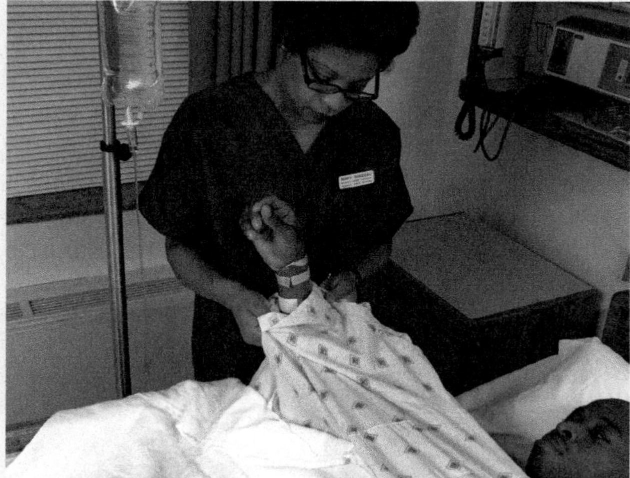

FIGURE 22–39A After removing the gown from the unaffected arm, gather the gown together on the arm with the IV infusion site.

(continues)

PROCEDURE 22:4H (CONT.)

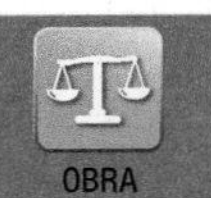

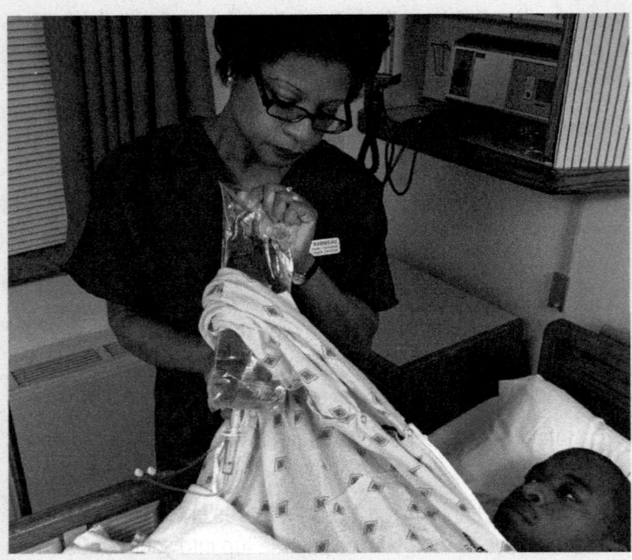

FIGURE 22–39B **Keeping the IV container above the level of the infusion site, pass the IV container through the arm of the gown.**

leave the sleeve off of the one arm, or use a gown that opens at the shoulders.

10. Pull the body of the gown down over the patient or position the pajama top correctly. Make sure that the gown or top is smooth and free from wrinkles or folds.

11. Tie the strings on the gown, or button the buttons on the pajama top. Make sure that the tied knot is not on a bony prominence.

CAUTION: Knots or wrinkles can lead to pressure ulcers.

NOTE: Avoid exposing the patient during the procedure. Continue to use the towel or bath blanket to drape the patient.

12. If the patient is wearing pajamas, put on the pants after the pajama top. Gently ease the pants over the feet and up the legs. Adjust them into position at the waist. Use the towel or bath blanket to cover the patient during this procedure. Tie or button the pants. Make sure the pants are smooth and free from wrinkles or folds.

13. Observe all checkpoints before leaving the patient: position the patient comfortably and in good body alignment; elevate the siderails (if indicated); place the call signal, water, and supplies within easy reach of the patient; lower the bed to its lowest level; and leave the area neat and clean.

14. Place a soiled hospital gown in the laundry hamper or bag. Place a soiled personal gown or pajamas in a drawer, the closet, or other location specified by the patient.

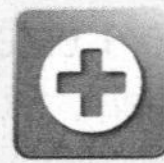

CAUTION: If the gown is contaminated with blood or body fluids, follow agency policy for handling contaminated linen.

NOTE: In long-term care facilities, the patient's soiled clothing is usually washed by the facility. Make sure the clothing is labeled with the patient's name and place it in the proper laundry hamper or bag.

15. Remove gloves. Wash hands thoroughly.

16. Report that the patient's gown has been changed and/or record all required information on the patient's chart or enter it into the computer. For example, date, time, pajamas changed, and your signature and title. Report any observations that may signify problems.

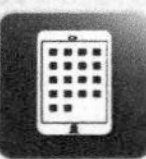

EHR

NOTE: In health care agencies using electronic health records (EHRs), also known as electronic medical records (EMRs), the information is entered directly into the patient's record on a computer.

PRACTICE: **Go to the workbook and use the evaluation sheet for 22:4H, Changing a Patient's Gown or Pajamas, to practice this procedure. When you believe you have mastered this skill, sign the sheet and give it to your instructor for further action.**

FINAL CHECKPOINT: Using the criteria listed on the evaluation sheet, your instructor will grade your performance.

PROCEDURE 22:41

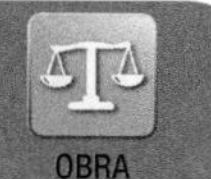

OBRA

Giving a Complete Bed Bath

Equipment and Supplies

Bed linen (complete set); laundry hamper, bag, or cart; bath blanket; two or three washcloths; face towel; one or two bath towels; soap and soap dish; basin; bath thermometer; clean gown or pajamas; supplies for hair care; supplies for nail care; shaving supplies; oral hygiene supplies; lotion; disposable gloves; paper and pen or computer

NOTE: When packaged cleansing cloths are available, they can be used in place of the washcloths, towels, soap, and basin.

Procedure

1. Obtain authorization from your immediate supervisor or check physician's orders to obtain authorization for the procedure.
2. Assemble equipment.
3.  Comm — Knock on the door and pause before entering. Introduce yourself. Identify the patient. Explain the procedure and obtain consent.
4. Close all doors, windows, and curtains. Eliminate drafts. Adjust the thermostat to a comfortable room temperature, if possible.
5. Wash hands. Put on gloves.

   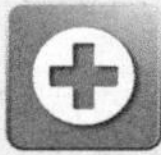 Precaution — **CAUTION:** Wear gloves and observe standard precautions. Contact with blood, body fluids, secretions, or excretions is possible.
6. Arrange all equipment conveniently. Put linen on the chair in the order of use. Position the laundry bag, hamper, or cart conveniently.

   NOTE: Proper preparation saves time and energy.
7. Elevate the bed to a comfortable working height. If siderails are present and elevated, lower the siderail on the side where you are working.
8. Replace the top linen with a bath blanket. If the same linen is to be reused, fanfold it to the bottom of the bed. If the linen is to be replaced, remove it and place it in the hamper.
9. Provide oral hygiene as previously instructed.
10. Shave the male patient, if necessary.

    NOTE: Some patients prefer to be shaved after the face is washed.
11. Fill the basin approximately two-thirds full with warm water at a temperature of 105°F–110°F (40.6°C–43.3°C). Check the temperature with a bath thermometer.

    NOTE: If cleansing cloths are used, remove them from the warmer or heat them according to instructions.
12. Help the patient move to the side of the bed nearest to you. Remove the patient's bedclothes as previously instructed.
13. Place a towel over the upper edge of the bath blanket.
14. With the washcloth, form a mitten around your hand. Tuck in the loose edges (Figure 22–40A–C).

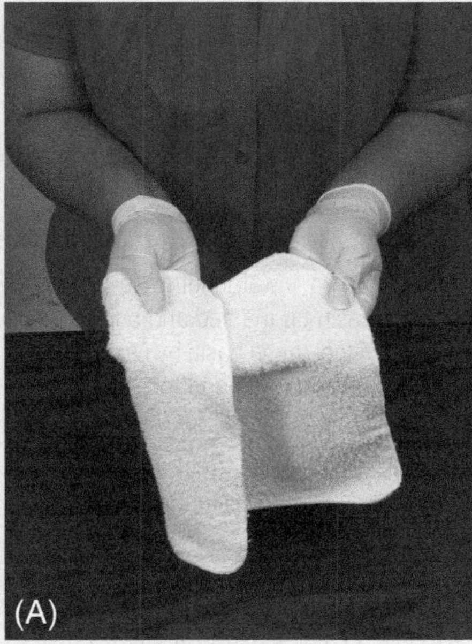

(A)

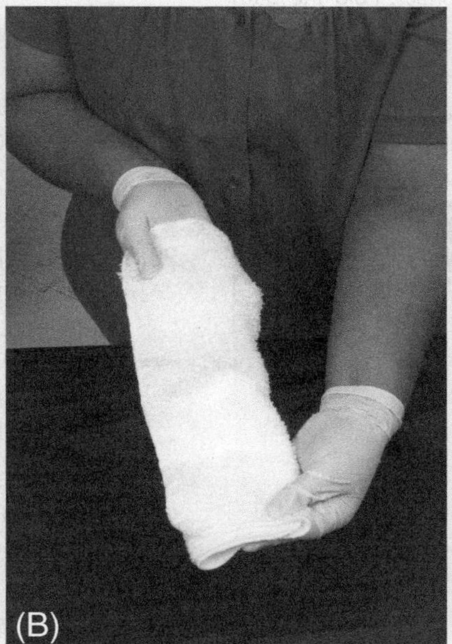

(B)

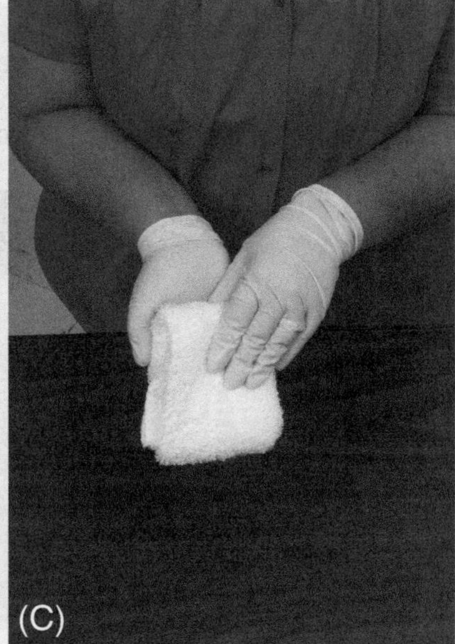

(C)

FIGURE 22–40A–C Fold the washcloth to form a bath mitten around your hand.

(continues)

PROCEDURE 22:41 (CONT.)

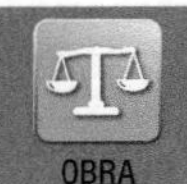

NOTE: This prevents the loose edges of the cloth from striking the patient as you work. It also keeps water from dripping on the patient and the bed.

15. Wet the washcloth and squeeze out excess water. Wash the patient's eyes first (Figure 22–41A). Start at the inner area and wash to the outside of the eye. Use a different section of the cloth when you wash the second eye.

NOTE: If using cleansing cloths, use one for the face and neck, one for the arms, one for the legs, one for the chest and abdomen, one for the back and buttocks, and one for the perineal area.

16. Rinse the washcloth. Ask whether the patient uses soap on the face and use soap if desired. Wash the face, neck, and ears. Rinse. Dry well.

17. Place a bath towel lengthwise under the patient's arm that is farthest from you. Place the basin of water on the bed and on the towel, at the lower end. Put the patient's hand and nails into the water. Wash, rinse, and dry the arm, from the axilla to the hand (Figure 22–41B). Repeat for the other arm.

NOTE: If the patient desires deodorant, it can be applied after the axillae are clean and dry.

18. Provide nail and hand care as previously instructed.

19. Elevate the siderail, if indicated. Discard the bath water and fill the basin with clean water at a temperature of 105°F–110°F.

20. Return to the bedside and lower the siderail, if elevated. Put a bath towel over the patient's chest. Fold the bath blanket down to the patient's waist.

21. Wash, rinse, and dry the chest and breasts (Figure 22–41C). Pay particular attention to the areas under a female patient's breasts. Dry these areas thoroughly.

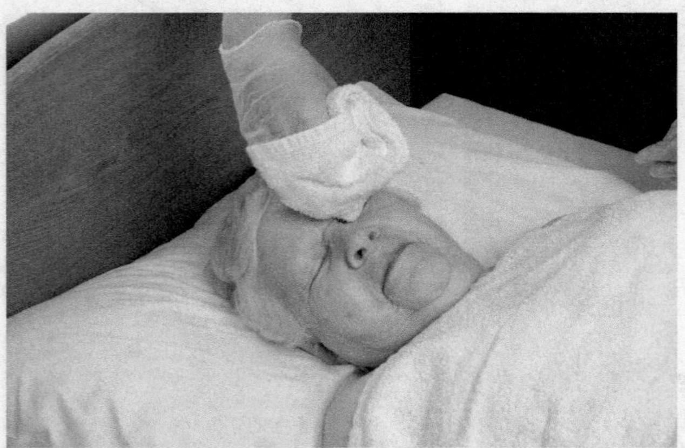

FIGURE 22–41A **Wash the eyes first, starting at the inner area and moving to the outside of the eye.**

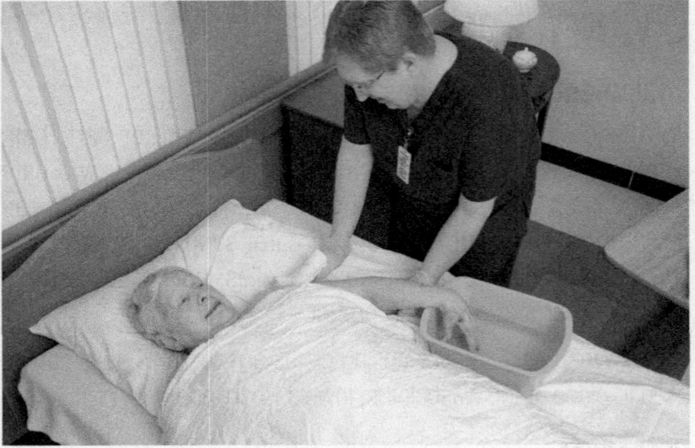

FIGURE 22–41B **With the hand in the basin, wash and rinse the arm from the axilla to the hand.**

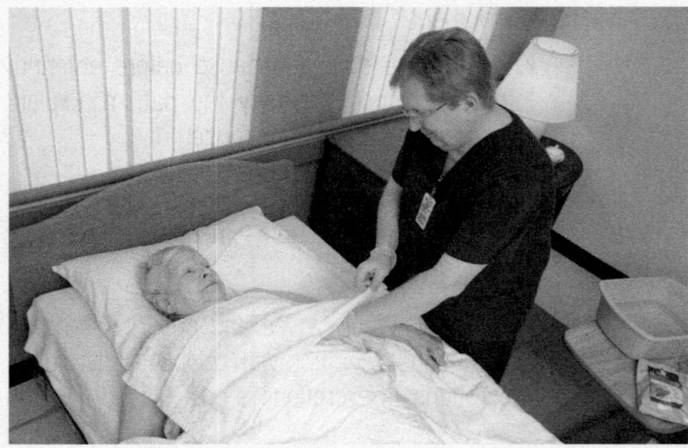

FIGURE 22–41C **Avoid exposing the patient when washing the breasts.**

22. Turn the bath towel lengthwise to cover the patient's chest and abdomen. Fold the bath blanket down to the pubic area. Wash, rinse, and dry the abdomen. Replace the bath blanket. Remove the towel.

23. Fold the bath blanket up to expose the patient's leg that is farthest from you. Place a towel lengthwise under the leg and foot. Place the basin on the bed and on top of the towel. Place the patient's foot in the basin by flexing the leg at the knee. Wash and rinse the leg and foot, remove the basin, and dry the leg and foot. Repeat for the other leg.

NOTE: Support the patient's leg and foot with your hand and lower arm when moving the foot in and out of the basin (Figure 22–41D).

24. Provide nail care to the toes, as needed. *Never* cut the toenails. File them straight across. Apply lotion to the feet, if the skin is dry. *Never* put lotion between the toes because this promotes the growth of fungus.

PROCEDURE 22:41 (CONT.)

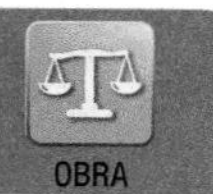

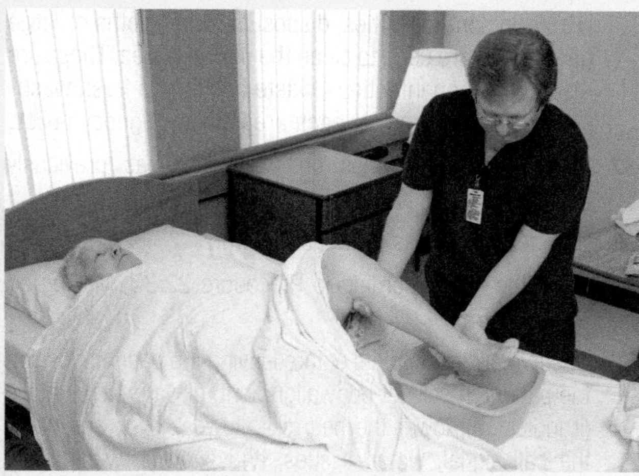

FIGURE 22–41D **Support the leg when placing the patient's foot in the basin.**

CAUTION: Observe for any color changes or irritated areas that may signify problems.

25. Elevate the siderail, if indicated. Change the water in the basin.

    NOTE: Water should always be changed at this point in the bath. However, it can be changed anytime it becomes too cool, dirty, or soapy.

26. Lower the siderail, if elevated.
27. Turn the patient on his or her side or into the prone position. Place the towel lengthwise on the bed and along the patient's back. Wash, rinse, and dry the entire back (Figure 22–41E).

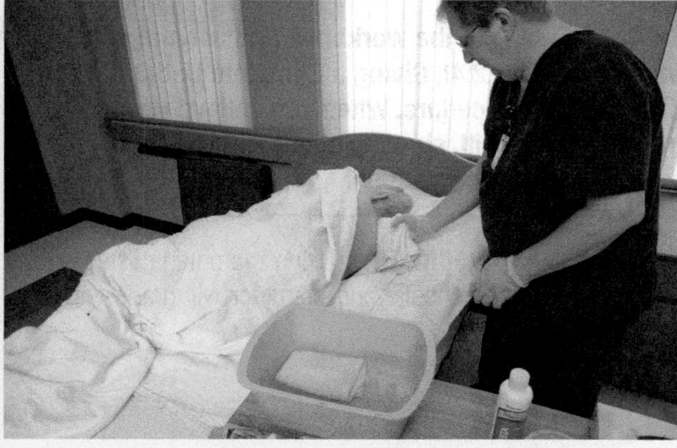

FIGURE 22–41E **Turn the patient onto his or her side to wash, rinse, and dry the back.**

CAUTION: Observe the back closely for any changes that may signify problems. Pay particular attention to bony areas and abnormal skin color. Report any abnormality to your supervisor.

28. Give a backrub as previously instructed.
29. Help the patient turn onto his or her back. Keep the patient draped with the bath blanket.
30. If the patient is able to wash the perineal area, place the basin with water, the soap, the washcloth, the towel, and the call signal within easy reach. Raise the siderail and wait outside the unit while the patient completes this procedure.
31. If the patient is not able to wash the perineal area, put on gloves. Drape and position the patient in the dorsal recumbent position. Put a towel or disposable underpad under the patient's buttocks and upper legs.
    a. For a female patient, always wash from the front to the back, or rectal, area. Separate the labia, or lips, and cleanse the area thoroughly with a front-to-back motion (Figure 22–42). Use a clean area of the washcloth or rinse the cloth between each wipe.
    b. For a male patient, cleanse the tip of the penis using a circular motion and starting at the urinary meatus and working outward. Cleanse the penis from top to bottom (Figure 22–43A). If a male patient is not circumcised, gently draw the foreskin back to wash the area (Figure 22–43B). After rinsing and drying the area, gently return the foreskin to its normal position. Wash the scrotal area, taking care to clean under the scrotum. To wash the rectal area, turn a male patient on his side.

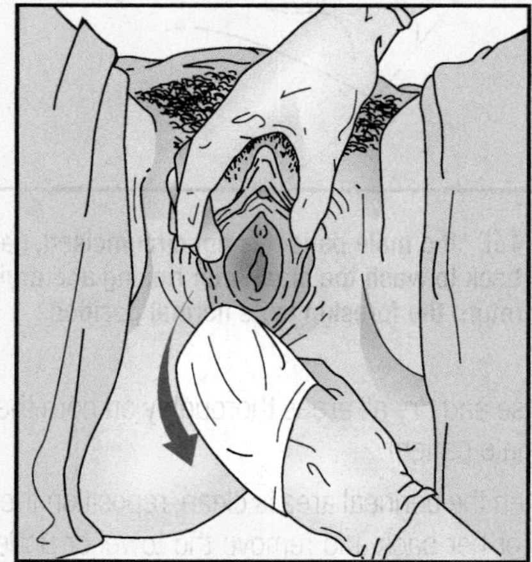

FIGURE 22–42 **To provide perineal care to a female patient, separate the labia and cleanse the area with a front-to-back motion.**

(continues)

PROCEDURE 22:4I (CONT.)

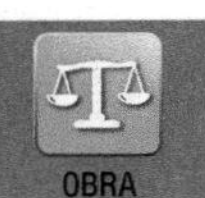

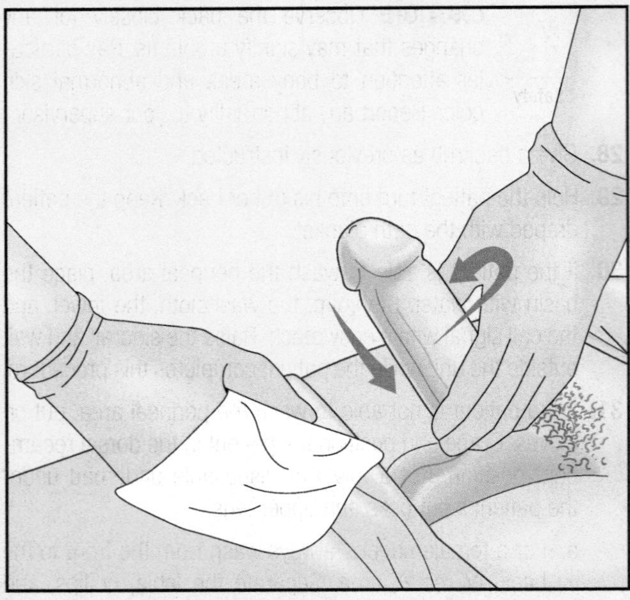

FIGURE 22–43A **Use a circular motion to cleanse the penis from the top to the base.**

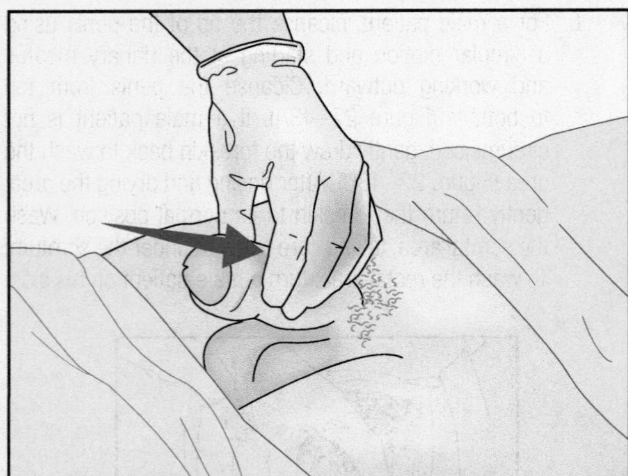

FIGURE 22–43B **If a male patient is not circumcised, gently draw the foreskin back to wash the area. After rinsing and drying the area, gently return the foreskin to its normal position.**

c. Rinse and dry all areas thoroughly on both the male and female patient.

d. When the perineal area is clean, reposition the patient on his or her back and remove the towel or underpad from under the buttocks. Remove gloves and wash hands.

NOTE: In some facilities, disposable washcloths or large gauze pads are used to clean the perineal area. These are discarded in an infectious-waste bag, and a fresh washcloth or pad is used for each area. Follow agency policy.

32. Place clean bedclothes on the patient as previously instructed.

33. Provide hair care as previously taught.

34. Make the bed according to Procedure 22:3B, Making an Occupied Bed.

35. Observe all checkpoints before leaving the patient: position the patient in correct body alignment; elevate the siderails (if indicated); lower the bed to its lowest level; and place the call signal, water, tissues, and supplies within easy reach of the patient.

36. Clean and replace all equipment. Wash the emesis basin and bath basin thoroughly.

37. Put the bag or hamper of dirty linen in the proper area or send it to the laundry according to agency policy. Replace all remaining equipment.

38. Remove gloves, if worn. Wash hands.

39. 

Report that a complete bed bath was given and/or record all required information on the patient's chart or enter it into the computer. For example, date, time, complete bed bath given, occupied bed made, patient stated he was tired at end of procedure, and your signature and title. Report any observations that may signify problems.

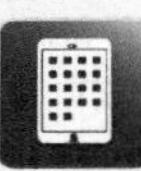

NOTE: In health care agencies using electronic health records (EHRs), also known as electronic medical records (EMRs), the information is entered directly into the patient's record on a computer.

PRACTICE: **Go to the workbook and use the evaluation sheet for 22:4I, Giving a Complete Bed Bath, to practice this procedure. When you believe you have mastered this skill, sign the sheet and give it to your instructor for further action.**

FINAL CHECKPOINT: Using the criteria listed on the evaluation sheet, your instructor will grade your performance.

PROCEDURE 22:4J

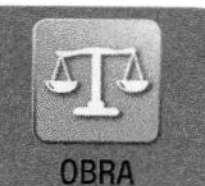
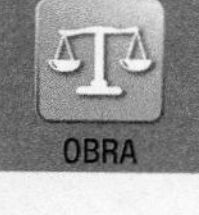

Helping a Patient Take a Tub Bath or Shower

Equipment and Supplies

Washcloth, two or three towels, soap and soap dish, bathmat, rubber mat, bath thermometer, chair or stool (placed in bath area), bedclothes, robe, slippers, disposable gloves, paper and pen or computer

Procedure

1. Check physician's orders or obtain authorization from your immediate supervisor. A physician's order is generally required before a tub bath or shower is allowed, unless the patient is considered able to take care of this need (for example, in the case of a totally ambulatory patient).
2. Assemble equipment.
3. 

Knock on the door and pause before entering. Introduce yourself. Identify the patient, explain the procedure, and obtain consent. Also, check to make sure the time is appropriate for taking a shower or bath.

   NOTE: If the patient has visitors or is receiving another treatment, time and energy would be wasted in preparing the tub or shower.
4. Wash hands. Put on gloves.

   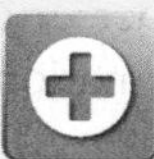

CAUTION: Wear gloves and observe standard precautions. Contact with blood, body fluids, secretions, or excretions is possible.
5. Take the supplies to the bath or shower area. Make sure the tub or shower is clean. If it is dirty, put on gloves to clean the tub or shower. Wipe it with a disinfectant. When the tub or shower is clean, remove the gloves and wash your hands. If nonskid strips are not present, put a rubber mat in the tub or shower to prevent the patient from slipping. Place the bathmat on the floor. Fill the tub half full with water at a temperature of 105°F (40.6°C).

   NOTE: Many health care facilities have shower or tub chairs that are used for patients who cannot stand in a shower or climb into a tub (Figure 22–44). The shower chair must be cleaned and disinfected before and after every use.
6. Help the patient put on a robe and slippers. Take the patient to the bath or shower area.

CAUTION: Use a wheelchair, if necessary.

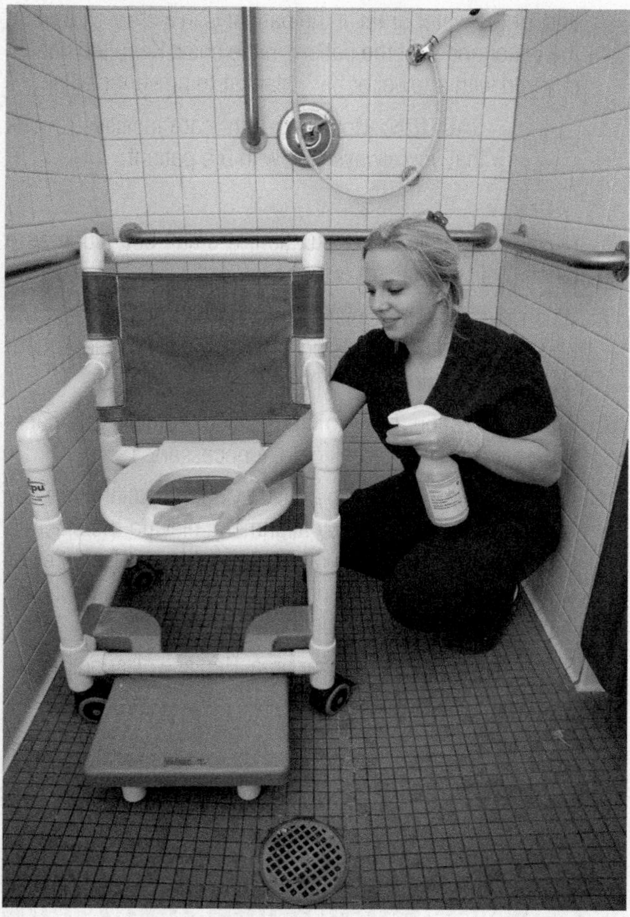

FIGURE 22–44 A shower chair is often used for patients who cannot stand in the shower or climb into a tub. It must be disinfected before and after it is used.

7. If necessary, help the patient undress. Help the patient into the tub or shower. If a shower chair is used, transfer the patient to the chair. Make sure the wheels on the chair are locked before transferring the patient.

CAUTION: Before the patient enters the shower, adjust the temperature of the shower water.
8. If necessary, remain with the patient and assist with the bath or shower. If the patient can manage without assistance, explain how to use the emergency call signal, leave the room, and check on the patient at frequent intervals.

CAUTION: If the patient shows any signs of weakness or dizziness, use the call button to get help. If the patient is in a tub, remove the plug

(continues)

PROCEDURE 22:4J (CONT.)

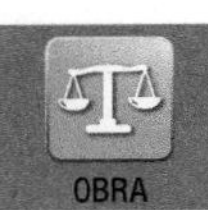

and let the water drain. If the patient is in a shower, turn off the water and seat the patient in the chair. Keep the patient covered with a towel or bath blanket to prevent chilling.

CAUTION: Most long-term care facilities require that you always stay with the patient.

NOTE: In a home care situation, a small bell (such as a dinner bell) can be left with the patient.

9. When the patient is finished bathing, help as needed. Dry all areas of the patient's body thoroughly. Put clean bedclothes or clothing on the patient.
10. Assist the patient back to the bedside. Administer a backrub. Help with hair or nail care, if necessary.
11. Observe all checkpoints before leaving the patient: position the patient in correct body alignment, elevate the siderails (if indicated), lower the bed to its lowest level, place the call signal and supplies within easy reach of the patient, and leave the area neat and clean.
12. Return to the bath or shower area. Replace all supplies and equipment used. Put on gloves. Clean the tub or shower thoroughly and wipe with a disinfectant.

    NOTE: If a shower chair was used, clean and disinfect the chair.
13. Remove gloves. Wash hands.
14. 

Report that a tub bath or shower was given and/or record all required information on the patient's chart or enter it into the computer. For example, date, time, assisted with tub bath, patient tolerated procedure well, and your signature and title. Report any observations that may signify problems.

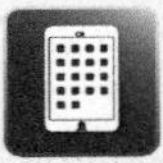

NOTE: In health care agencies using electronic health records (EHRs), also known as electronic medical records (EMRs), the information is entered directly into the patient's record on a computer.

PRACTICE: **Go to the workbook and use the evaluation sheet for 22:4J, Helping a Patient Take a Tub Bath or Shower, to practice this procedure. When you believe you have mastered this skill, sign the sheet and give it to your instructor for further action.**

FINAL CHECKPOINT: Using the criteria listed on the evaluation sheet, your instructor will grade your performance.

22:5 Measuring and Recording Intake and Output

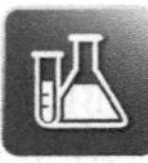

A record of how much fluid is taken in and eliminated by a patient often helps a physician provide care to the patient. A large part of the body is fluid, so there must be a balance between the amount of fluid taken into the body and the amount lost from the body. In a healthy individual, the fluid balance is usually maintained by the body structures. However, if an individual has heart or kidney disease, or loses large amounts of fluids through vomiting, diarrhea, excessive perspiration, or bleeding, the fluid balance may be abnormal. If excessive fluid is retained by the body, swelling, or **edema**, results. If excessive fluid is lost from the body, **dehydration** occurs. Either condition can lead to death if not treated. In such cases, physicians may order that a record be kept of all fluids taken in and discharged from the body. This record is usually called an intake and output (I&O) record.

An **intake and output (I&O)** record is a means of recording all fluids a person takes in and eliminates during a certain period. Each agency has its own paper or computerized form, but most contain similar information.

Intake

Intake refers to all fluids taken in by the patient. The following routes and liquids must be considered:

- *Oral* is intake by way of the mouth. Liquids taken in orally include water, coffee, tea, milk, juices, and other beverages. In addition, soups, gelatin, ice cream, and other similar foods that are liquid at room temperature also qualify. The nurse assistant often measures and records or reports these amounts.
- *Tube feedings, or enteral feedings*, are recorded as oral intake or in a special column. They are used for patients who are unable to swallow, who are unconscious or comatose, or who have certain digestive diseases. The solution given contains all of the nutrients required by the body and is more nourishing than an intravenous (IV) feeding. Enteral feedings may be administered through a nasogastric tube, orogastric tube, or a gastrostomy tube. A *nasogastric (NG) tube* is a tube inserted through the nose, down the esophagus, and

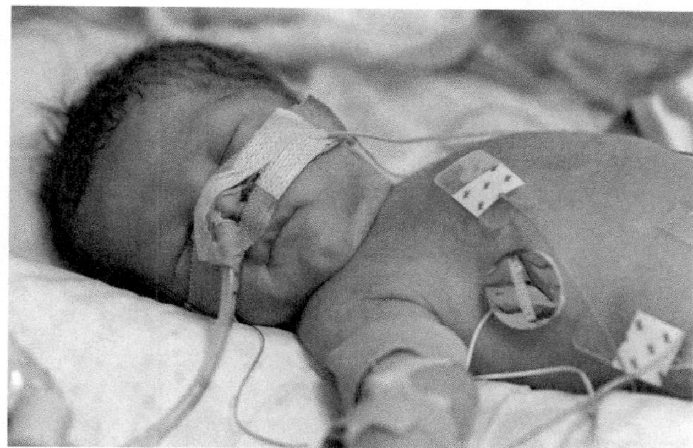

FIGURE 22–45 A nasogastric tube is inserted through the nose, down the esophagus, and into the stomach. © Steve Lovegrove/Shutterstock.com

into the stomach (Figure 22–45). An *orogastric (OG) tube* takes the same route but enters through the mouth. A syringe can be used to instill food or medication into the NG or OG tube (Figure 22–46). A *gastrostomy tube* is surgically inserted through the abdominal skin into the stomach (Figure 22–47). A feeding pump is

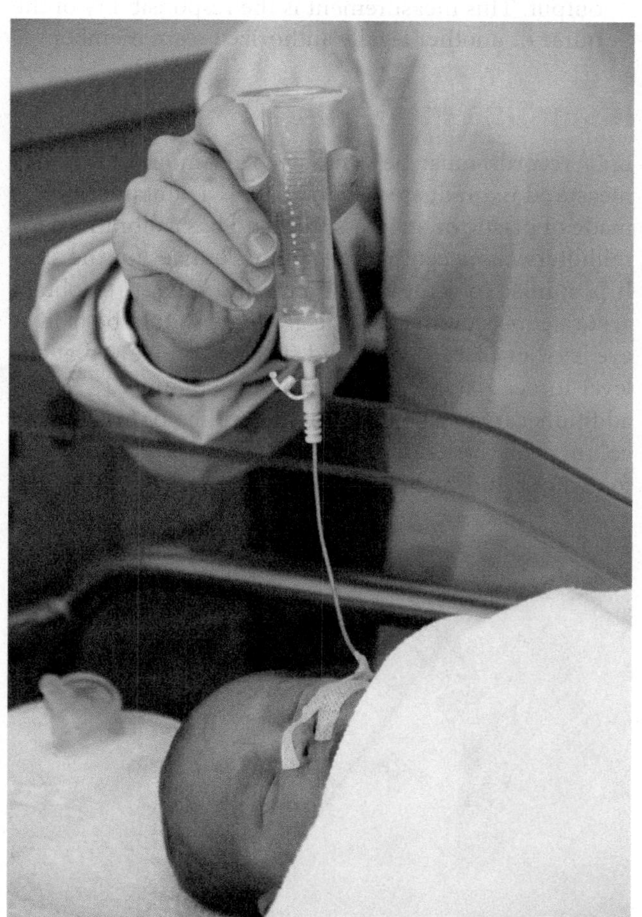

FIGURE 22–46 A syringe can be used to instill food or medication into the nasogastric (NG) tube. © andesign101/Shutterstock.com

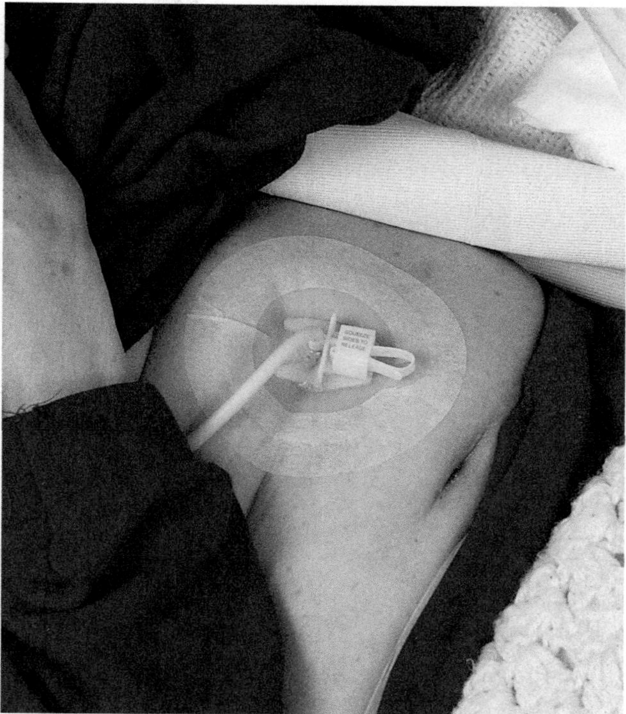

FIGURE 22–47 A gastrostomy tube is surgically inserted through the abdominal skin into the stomach.

usually used to administer the solution (Figure 22–48). A nurse or another legally authorized team member will administer the enteral feeding. The nurse assistant must keep the patient's head elevated 30–45 degrees during the feeding and for approximately 30–60 minutes after the feeding; make sure there are no kinks in the tubing; use extreme caution when turning or positioning the patient to avoid dislodging the tubing; provide frequent oral hygiene; and notify the nurse immediately if the alarm sounds on the feeding pump, if the solution is not flowing through the tubing, or if the solution container is low or empty.

- *Intravenous (IV)* refers to fluids given into a vein. Blood units, IV medications, and other intravenous (IV) solutions are measured. This measurement is the responsibility of the nurse or another legally authorized team member.
- 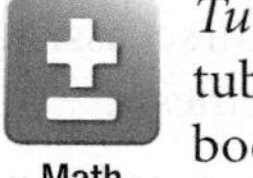 *Tubes and drains* refers to fluid placed into tubes or drains that have been inserted in the body. In some agencies, any fluid removed is not considered to be intake and is not recorded. For example, if a nasogastric tube is irrigated with 80 milliliters (mL) of solution and the same exact amount is immediately drawn back out of the tube, this is not recorded as intake. However, if 60 mL is withdrawn, the intake is recorded as 20 mL (80 minus 60 equals 20). In other agencies, any fluid

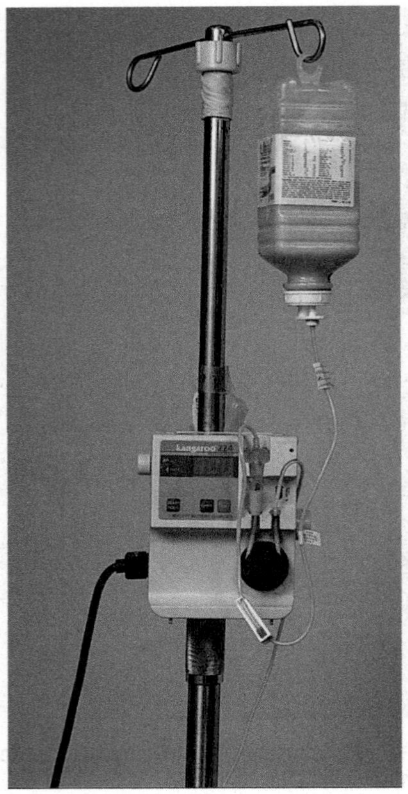

FIGURE 22–48 A feeding pump is usually used to administer tube or enteral feedings.

that is instilled is recorded under intake, and anything that comes out is output. Follow your agency policy. This measurement is also the responsibility of the nurse or another legally authorized team member.

Output

Output refers to all fluids eliminated by the patient. The following routes and liquids must be considered:

- *Bowel movement (BM)*: Liquid bowel movements are usually measured and recorded. A solid or formed BM is usually noted in the remarks column or described under feces. The nurse assistant may measure and record or report this elimination.
- *Emesis:* Anything that is vomited is measured and recorded. Color, type, and other facts are usually noted in the remarks column. The nurse assistant often measures and records or reports emesis.
- *Urine:* All urine voided or drained via a catheter is measured and recorded. This measurement may be the responsibility of the nurse assistant. A urine output of less than 30 milliliters (mL) per hour must be reported.
- *Tubes and drains*: Any irrigation or suction drainage, including drainage from nasogastric tubes, hemovacs, chest tubes, and other drainage tubes, is measured (Figure 22–49). The type, amount, color, and other facts are noted in the remarks column. If an irrigating solution is injected into a tube and more solution returns, the excess amount is considered output. This measurement is the responsibility of the nurse or another legally authorized team member.

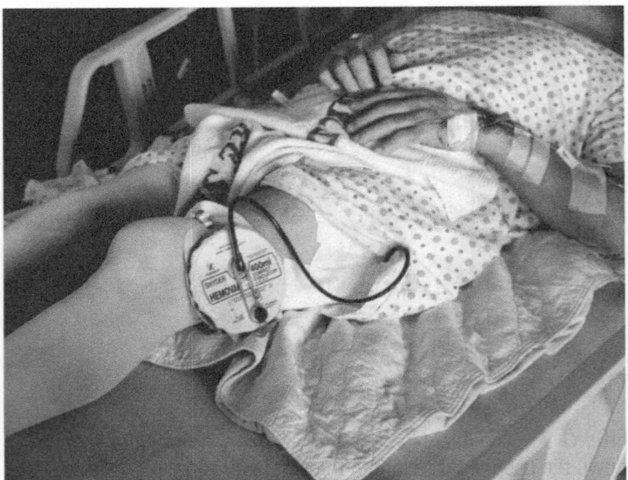

FIGURE 22–49 Suction drainage from a hemovac, one type of wound drainage system, is recorded as irrigation output on an intake and output (I&O) record.

Recording Intake and Output (I&O)

I&O records must be accurate. All amounts must be measured in graduates. A graduate is a container that is made of plastic or stainless steel and has calibrations for milliliters/cubic centimeters and/or ounces on the side. It is similar to a measuring cup and is used to obtain accurate measurements. The graduate should be held at eye level or placed on a solid surface and viewed at eye level to accurately record amounts (Figure 22–50). In addition, care must be taken when adding or totaling the columns on the I&O record. Most records contain totals for 8-hour and 24-hour periods. (See Figure 22–51 and

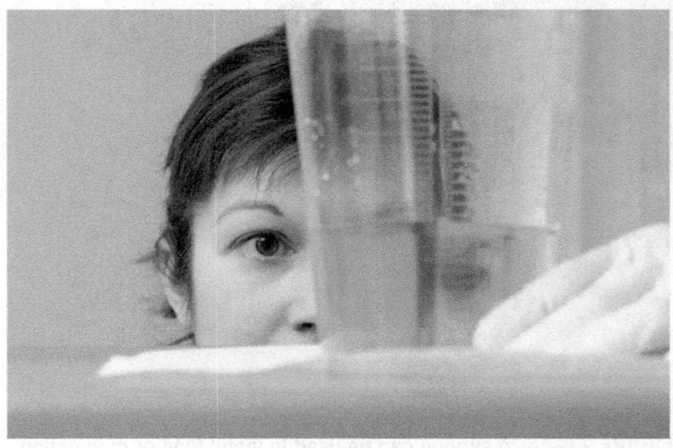

FIGURE 22–50 Place the graduate on a flat surface and obtain the reading at eye level to get an accurate measurement.

INTAKE AND OUTPUT RECORD

Family Name	First Name	Attending Physician	Room No.	Hosp. No.
JOHNSON, ROBERT		DR. MIKE SMITH	238	54-3201

Date 9/30	INTAKE				OUTPUT					OTHER				REMARKS
TIME	Oral	I.V.	Blood		Urine	Tube	Emesis	Feces						
7 - 8 AM	100													
8 - 9 AM	320						200							EMESIS– GREEN LIQUID
9 - 10 AM					420									
10 - 11 AM	100													
11 - 12 Noon				10										NG IRRIGATION NS
12 - 1 PM	240				310									
1 - 2 PM		850				200								NASOGASTRIC GOLD–BROWN
2 - 3 PM	60													
8 HOUR TOTAL	820	850		10	730	200	200							
3 - 4 PM														
4 - 5 PM	320	150						120						BROWN LIQUID
5 - 6 PM					280									
6 - 7 PM	180													
7 - 8 PM														
8 - 9 PM	100													
9 - 10 PM		500				240								NASOGASTRIC BROWNISH
10 - 11 PM					310									
8 HOUR TOTAL	600	650			590	240		120						
11 - 12 PM														
12 - 1 AM				10										NG IRRIGATION NS
1 - 2 AM	180				420									
2 - 3 AM														
3 - 4 AM							650							EMESIS– GREEN LIQUID
4 - 5 AM														
5 - 6 AM		600				180								NASOGASTRIC GOLD–BROWN
6 - 7 AM	100				380									
8 HOUR TOTAL	280	600		10	800	180	650							
24 HOUR TOTAL	1700	2100		20	2120	620	850	120						
	TOTAL INTAKE			3820	TOTAL OUTPUT			3170						

FIGURE 22–51 A sample intake and output (I&O) record.

study it carefully.) Some agencies use 12-hour periods for intake and output totals.

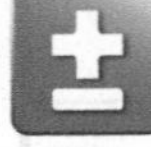
Math

For I&O records, fluids are measured in metric units called milliliters (mL). Approximate equivalents for units of the metric system are as follows:

Metric		Household
1 mL	=	15 gtts (drops)
5 mL	=	1 tsp (teaspoon)
15 mL	=	1 tbsp (tablespoon)
30 mL	=	1 oz (ounce)
240 mL	=	1 cup (8 oz)
500 mL	=	1 pt (pint) (16 oz)
1,000 mL	=	1 qt (quart) (32 oz)

NOTE: A few measurement devices might use cubic centimeters (cc). However, 1 milliliter (mL) and 1 cubic centimeter (cc) are the same amount. Therefore, 30 mL equals 30 cc.

Various agencies have different policies for recording I&O. In some agencies, the I&O record is kept at the bedside. Team members note the I&O of the patient and record the measurements on the record. At times, the patient is even taught to measure and write down the amounts. In other agencies, the I&O record is kept on the patient's chart. Measurements are noted on a slip of paper and reported. The nurse, medical secretary, health unit coordinator, or an authorized team member then records the information on the chart's I&O form. With computerized charting, totals are entered directly into the computer by the nurse or nursing assistant. Most computerized programs automatically add all columns. Ascertain and follow the policy of your agency.

Comm

Patients should be given careful instructions when an I&O record is being kept. The patient must inform health care providers when he or she drinks fluids not provided by the health care team. Sometimes, the patient records how many glasses of water or other liquids are consumed. Other times, the health care worker fills a water pitcher and then checks the quantity remaining before refilling the pitcher. The worker then subtracts this quantity from the total amount originally in the pitcher and records the difference as water intake. To avoid missing any amounts of oral intake, the health care worker must also think about fluid intake every time a glass, cup, or water pitcher is removed from the unit. If visitors bring milkshakes or other liquids, the amounts of these must also be recorded.

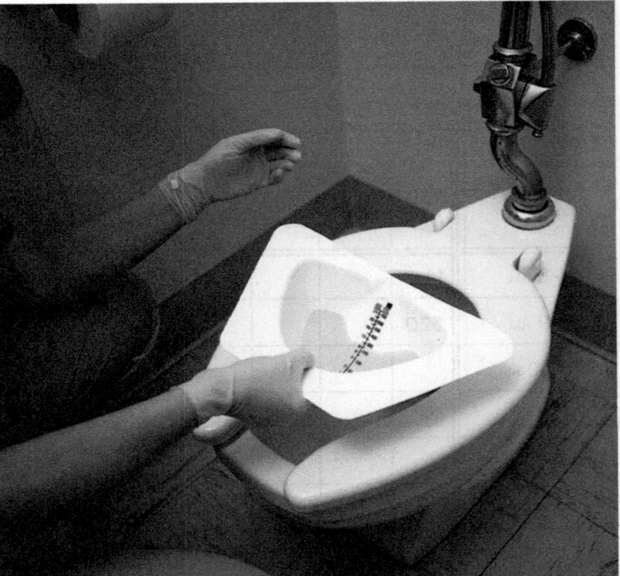

FIGURE 22–52 A specimen collector to collect urine can be placed under the seat of the toilet.

Female patients should be asked to urinate in a bedpan or to use a special urine collector that can be placed under the seat of the toilet (Figure 22–52). Female patients must be told not to place toilet tissue or expel a bowel movement into the bedpan or urine collector. Male patients can be told to use a urinal. If patients are given correct instructions, they can cooperate and accurate records can be maintained.

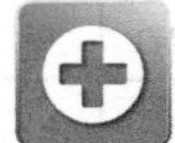
Precaution

Standard precautions (discussed in Chapter 15:4) must be followed at all times when body fluids such as urine, emesis, liquid bowel movements, and drainage are measured. Gloves must be worn while the fluids are being measured and discarded. Hands must be washed frequently and must always be washed immediately after gloves are removed. If splashing or spraying of fluids is possible, a mask, eye protection, and gown must be worn. The graduate or measuring device for monitoring a patient's output must be used for that patient only. It should be discarded or sterilized according to agency policy when output is no longer measured. Any areas contaminated by body fluids when measurements are being obtained must be wiped with a disinfectant. The health care provider must constantly take steps to prevent the spread of infection.

STUDENT: **Go to the workbook and complete the assignment sheet for 22:5A, Measuring Intake and Output. Then return and continue with the procedure.**

PROCEDURE 22:5

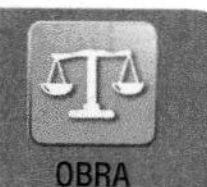

Recording Intake and Output

NOTE: Competency will be evaluated by way of successful completion of several assignment sheets rather than by way of the usual evaluation sheet. Follow the procedure steps to complete the assignment sheets.

Equipment and Supplies

Assignment sheets for this topic (Assignment sheets 1 to 5 for 22:5B), scrap paper and pen or computer, calculator (if permitted)

Procedure

1. Review the preceding information section, Figure 22–51, and your completed assignment sheet for 22:5A, Measuring Intake and Output.
2. Assemble equipment.
3. Go to the workbook and carefully read Assignment Sheet #1 for 22:5B, Recording Intake and Output. *It will be part of this procedure.* After reading it through once, do the assignment based on the following guidelines and instructions.
4. Use a pen to record all information or follow the software instructions on a computerized program to make entries.
   a. Find the correct time line on the intake and output (I&O) record.
   b. Find the correct column: for example, *oral intake* or *urine output.*
   c. Record the amounts stated on the assignment sheet in the correct block. Number of milliliters (mL) for a coffee cup and other containers are at the top of the I&O sheet.
5. When the information on the assignment sheet has been recorded in the appropriate places on the I&O record, recheck all areas of the record.
6. Make sure you have entered observations about color, type, and other facts in the remarks columns. Make sure the observations are on the right time lines by checking the times against the assignment sheet.
7. 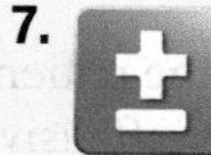 Under *intake*, add each column for 8-hour totals. For example, add all of the amounts for oral intake between 7 AM and 3 PM. Do the same for each of the other columns for all three 8-hour periods.

    **CAUTION:** Recheck your addition. The totals must be accurate.
8. 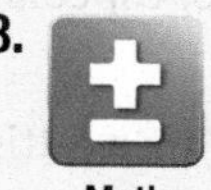 Now add the three 8-hour totals together for each column (7 AM to 6 AM) to get the 24-hour total at the bottom of the page. Do this for each column in intake and each column in output.

   NOTE: You should have a 24-hour total for oral intake and another total for IV intake.
9. Recheck all work.

   NOTE: If you make an error, draw one red line through the error. Place your initials in red by the error line. Then use a blue or black pen to write the correct information on the record. With computerized charting, you can modify your work and it will be marked as such. You will still be able to see what the original entry was. Follow the instructions on the computer software.
10. Give the paper to your instructor for grading. Replace all equipment used.

    NOTE: The record must be neat and legible. All figures must be recorded in metric units.

PRACTICE: Your instructor will grade Assignment Sheet #1 for 22:5B, Recording Intake and Output. When it is returned to you, note all comments or corrections. Then complete Assignment Sheet #2 for 22:5B, Recording Intake and Output. Give it to your instructor to grade. Again note comments or corrections. Repeat the process for Assignment Sheets #3, #4, and #5.

FINAL CHECKPOINT: Using the criteria listed on the evaluation sheet, your instructor will grade your performance.

22:6 Feeding a Patient

Good nutrition is an important part of a patient's treatment. It may be one of your responsibilities to make mealtimes as pleasant as possible for the patient. Mealtimes are often regarded as a time for social interaction. Most people prefer to eat with others. People who eat alone often have poor appetites and poor nutrition. In long-term care facilities, patients are encouraged to eat in the dining room. This provides an opportunity for social interaction with others. If a patient is confined to bed, it is important to talk with the patient while serving the food tray or feeding the patient.

Proper mealtime preparation is important. If the patient is ready to eat when the tray arrives, mealtime is likely to be more pleasant. Preparation before the tray is delivered includes:

- Offering the bedpan or urinal or assisting the patient to the bathroom; clearing the room of any offensive odors by using a deodorizer or opening a window
- Allowing the patient to wash his or her hands and face, if desired (Figure 22–53A)
- Providing oral hygiene, if desired; many individuals want to brush their teeth before meals, especially before breakfast
- Positioning the patient comfortably and in a sitting position, if possible
- Clearing the overbed table and positioning it for the tray
- Removing objects such as an emesis basin or bedpan from the patient's view; place such objects in the bedside stand, if they will not be needed

If a meal will be delayed because of radiographs (X-rays) or other treatments, be sure to explain this to the patient.

Check the tray carefully against the patient's name and room number and the type of diet ordered (Figure 22–53B). If anything seems out of place (for example, a salt shaker provided with a salt-free diet, or sugar with a diabetic diet), check with your immediate supervisor or the dietitian. Never add any food to the tray without checking the diet order first.

Allow patients to feed themselves whenever possible. If necessary, assist by cutting meat, opening beverage cartons, and buttering bread (Figure 22–53C). If a patient is blind or visually impaired, tell the patient what food is on the plate by comparing the plate to a clock. For example, say, "Swiss steak is at 12 o'clock, peas and carrots are at 4 o'clock, and mashed potatoes are at 9 o'clock." Make sure all food and utensils are conveniently placed.

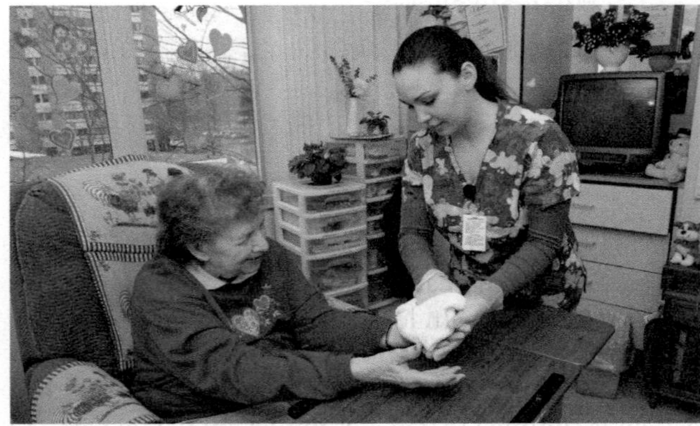

FIGURE 22–53A Allow the patient to wash her hands.

Before feeding any patient, test the temperature of all hot foods. A small amount can be placed on your wrist to check temperature. Never blow on hot food to cool it.

Points to observe when feeding a patient include:

- Alternate the foods by giving sips of liquids between solid foods.
- Use straws for liquids unless the patient has dysphagia (difficulty in swallowing). Straws can force liquids down the throat faster and cause choking. A food thickener can be added to liquids to solidify them

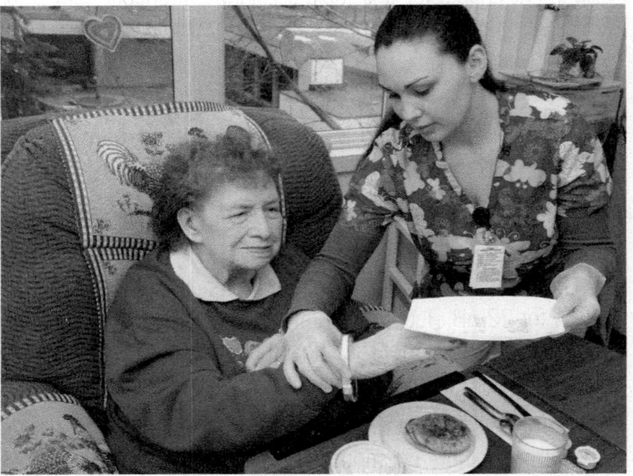

FIGURE 22–53B Check the food tray carefully against the patient's name, room number, and type of diet ordered.

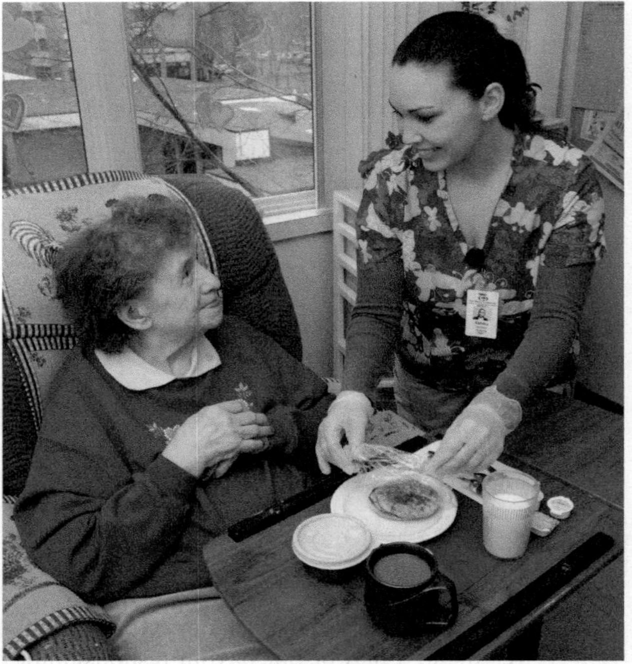

FIGURE 22–53C Assist the patient by cutting meat, opening beverage cartons, and positioning the food conveniently.

slightly and make them easier to swallow. A physician or dietitian must approve the use of this product.

- Offer only small bites of food at one time. Fill the spoon or fork one-third to one-half full.
- Hold the spoon or fork at right angles to the patient's mouth so you are feeding the patient from the tip of the utensil.
- Encourage the patient to eat as much as possible.
- Provide a relaxed, unhurried atmosphere.
- Give the patient sufficient time to chew the food.

Comm

Observe how much the patient eats so that a record of nutritional intake can be kept. If the patient does not like certain foods on the tray, ask your immediate supervisor or the dietitian whether a substitute can be provided. Record intake if an intake and output (I&O) record is being kept for the patient.

Safety

CAUTION: Always be alert to signs of choking while feeding a patient. Take every effort to prevent choking by feeding small quantities, allowing sufficient time for the patient to chew and swallow, and providing liquids to keep the mouth moist and make chewing and swallowing easier. If the patient coughs or chokes frequently when swallowing, the feeding should be stopped to prevent aspiration of food. Notify your supervisor immediately. If a patient had a stroke, one side of the mouth may be affected. As you feed the patient, direct food to the unaffected side. Watch the patient's throat to check swallowing. Watch for food that may be lodged in the affected side of the mouth. If a patient chokes on food, be prepared to provide abdominal thrusts as described in Procedure 17:2E, Performing CPR—Obstructed Airway on Conscious Adult or Child.

STUDENT: **Go to the workbook and complete the assignment sheet for 22:6, Feeding a Patient. Then return and continue with the procedure.**

PROCEDURE 22:6

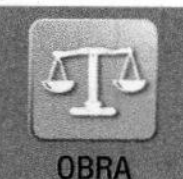
OBRA

Feeding a Patient

Equipment and Supplies

Food tray with diet card, flex straws, towel, gloves, paper and pen or computer

Procedure

1. Obtain proper authorization and assemble equipment.
2. Comm — Knock on the door and pause before entering. Introduce yourself. Identify the patient. Explain that it is almost time to eat and obtain consent. Close the door and pull the curtain to provide privacy.
3. Wash hands. Put on gloves.

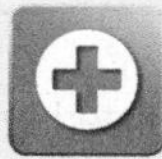
Precaution

CAUTION: Wear gloves and observe standard precautions. Contact with body fluids, secretions, or excretions is possible.

4. Prepare the patient for mealtime. Provide oral hygiene, if desired. Help the patient use the bedpan, as needed. Position the patient in a sitting position, if permitted. Allow the patient to wash his or her hands and face. Position the overbed table and remove unnecessary articles.

   NOTE: Make sure the patient is not scheduled for radiographs or any other treatment requiring the tray to be withheld.
5. Check the tray. Match the name on the diet card with the patient's identification band if one is worn. Check the type of diet ordered to make sure the food on the tray is correct. Do not add anything to the tray without first checking with your supervisor.

   NOTE: If any foods seem to be incorrect for the diet ordered, check immediately with your supervisor.
6. Place the tray on the overbed table. Place a towel or napkin under the patient's chin.
7. If the patient can feed himself or herself, arrange all food and silverware conveniently. Cut meat, butter bread, and open beverage cartons.
8. To feed a patient, proceed as follows:
   a. Follow the patient's preference for the order of foods eaten.
   b. Test hot liquids on your wrist before giving them to the patient. Wipe away any food placed on your wrist.

   NOTE: *Never* blow on the food to cool it. *Never* taste the patient's food. This can transmit infection.

   c. Use drinking straws for liquids unless the patient has dysphagia. Use a separate straw for each liquid offered. Give the patient a drink of water to wet the palate and make swallowing easier.

(continues)

PROCEDURE 22:6 (CONT.)

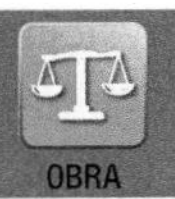
OBRA

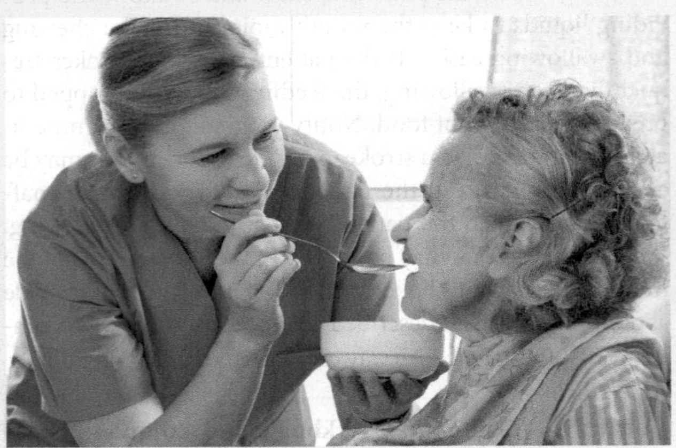

FIGURE 22–54 Hold utensils at a right angle to the mouth to feed the patient from the tip of the utensil. © Alexander Raths/Shutterstock.com

d. Hold utensils at a right angle (90-degree angle) to the patient's mouth (Figure 22–54). Feed the patient from the tip of the utensil.

e. Place a small amount of food on the utensil. Fill the spoon or fork about one-third to one-half full.

f. Tell the patient what he or she is eating.

g. If the patient had a stroke, place food in the unaffected side of the mouth. Watch the throat to make sure the patient is swallowing.

h. Allow sufficient time for the patient to chew. Do not hurry the patient.

i. Alternate foods, but don't mix foods together. Provide liquids at intervals to keep the mouth moist and make chewing and swallowing easier.

j. Allow the patient to hold bread and to help to the extent that he or she is able.

k. Use a towel or napkin to wipe the patient's mouth, as necessary.

Safety

CAUTION: Be alert at all times to signs of dysphagia or choking. If the patient coughs or chokes frequently when swallowing, stop the feeding to prevent aspiration of food. Notify your supervisor immediately.

9. Encourage the patient to eat as much as possible.

NOTE: If the patient does not like a particular food, check with your immediate supervisor or the dietitian about substitute foods.

10. When the meal is complete, allow the patient to wash his or her hands. Provide oral hygiene. Position the patient comfortably and in correct body alignment.

11. Observe all checkpoints before leaving the patient: elevate the siderails, if indicated; lower the bed to its lowest level; place the call signal and supplies within easy reach of the patient; and leave the area neat and clean.

12. Note how much food was eaten. Record amounts on the I&O record, if one is being kept.

NOTE: In many health care facilities, the supervisor must be notified if the patient refuses food and/or liquids or eats less than 25 percent of the food.

13. Clean and replace all equipment. Place the tray in the correct area.

14. Remove gloves. Wash hands.

15. 
Comm

Report that the patient has been fed and/or record all required information on the patient's chart or enter it into the computer. For example, date, time, fed breakfast, ate everything except one-half slice toast, and your signature and title.

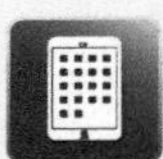
EHR

NOTE: In health care agencies using electronic health records (EHRs), also known as electronic medical records (EMRs), the information is entered directly into the patient's record on a computer.

PRACTICE: **Go to the workbook and use the evaluation sheet for 22:6, Feeding a Patient, to practice this procedure. When you believe you have mastered this skill, sign the sheet and give it to your instructor for further action.**

Check

FINAL CHECKPOINT: Using the criteria listed on the evaluation sheet, your instructor will grade your performance.

22:7 Assisting with a Bedpan/Urinal

Regular elimination of body wastes contributes to good health. Patients confined to bed must rely on the health care worker's help in meeting this important physical need.

Elimination of body wastes is essential. Death will occur if wastes are not eliminated. The following terms are used in reference to elimination:

- **Urinate**, **micturate**, or **void**: These terms refer to emptying the bladder, which stores the liquid waste, or urine, produced by the kidney. A urinal is used by male patients when they need to urinate, micturate,

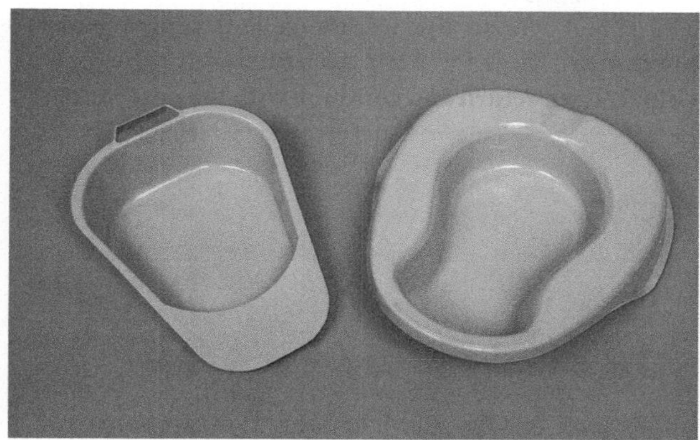

FIGURE 22–55 Two types of bedpans: the fracture, or orthopedic, bedpan (at left) and the standard bedpan (at right).

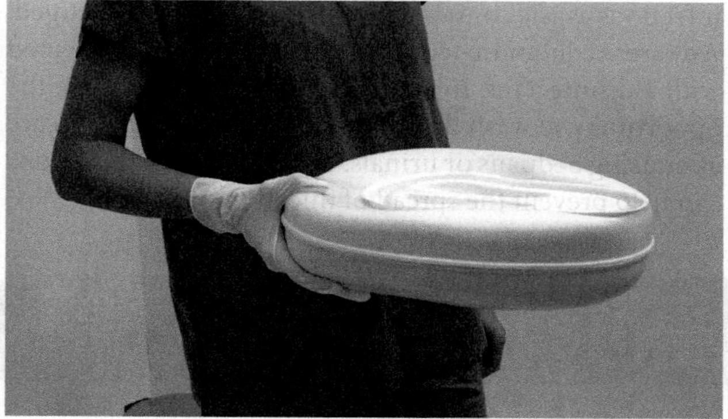

FIGURE 22–56 A one-glove technique can be used to carry a contaminated bedpan, leaving the other hand free to perform other tasks without contaminating the environment.

or void; a bedpan is used by female patients. Two main types of bedpans are the fracture, or orthopedic, bedpan and the standard bedpan (Figure 22–55).

- **Defecate**: This refers to having a bowel movement, or BM; the discharge of the waste through the rectum. The material is called feces or stool.

Many patients are sensitive about using bedpans or urinals. It is important that the health care worker provide privacy by closing the door, privacy curtain, and window curtain. Make the patient as comfortable as possible during this procedure. It is also important to provide the bedpan or urinal immediately when the patient requests it. In addition, a bedpan or urinal should be offered frequently to any patient confined to bed.

Accurate observations of the frequency, amount, and appearance of urine and stool are important. Abnormalities in any of these factors may indicate disease or complications. Any abnormality must be reported immediately, and a specimen must be saved for examination.

Before emptying a bedpan or urinal, it is the health care worker's responsibility to check whether specimens are needed. In addition, amounts must be measured and recorded if an intake and output (I&O) record is being kept for the patient. Check with your immediate supervisor or note physician's orders for this information.

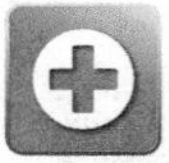
Precaution

Standard precautions must be observed when handling urine or feces. Hands must be washed frequently, and gloves must be worn. Eye protection must be worn if splashing or spraying is possible while emptying the bedpan. Some health care facilities require a one-glove technique to protect the environment while assisting with bedpans or urinals (Figure 22–56). Two gloves are worn to remove the bedpan or urinal. The bedpan or urinal is covered and placed on top of an underpad or bed protector that has been placed on a chair. The bedpan or urinal should never be placed on the overbed table or bedside stand. One glove is removed and held in the gloved hand. The ungloved hand is used to elevate the siderails, open doors, and turn on faucets. A paper towel can also be used with a gloved hand to prevent contact with items in the environment. It is important to protect environmental surfaces from contamination with substances on gloved hands.

Some agencies have special spray units in the bathrooms to rinse and clean bedpans and urinals (Figure 22–57). After rinsing, the bedpan or urinal must be disinfected. It must be used for only one patient. After the patient is discharged, it must be sterilized according to agency policy before being used for another patient. Some bedpans are disposable and are discarded in an

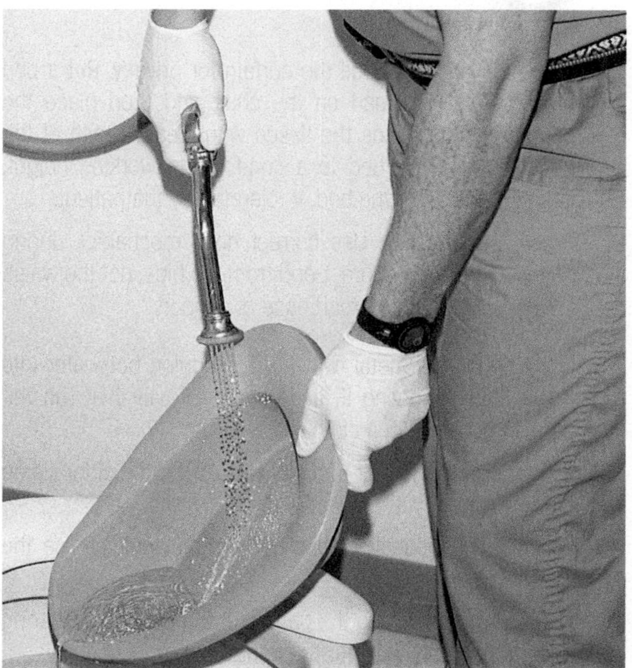

FIGURE 22–57 Some agencies have special spray units in the bathrooms to rinse and clean bedpans and urinals.

infectious-waste container when the patient is discharged. Any areas contaminated with urine or feces must be wiped with a disinfectant. In addition, patients should have the opportunity to wash their hands and receive perineal care after using bedpans or urinals. Taking proper precautions can help prevent the spread of infection.

STUDENT: Go to the workbook and complete the assignment sheet for 22:7, Assisting with a Bedpan/Urinal. Then return and continue with the procedures.

PROCEDURE 22:7A

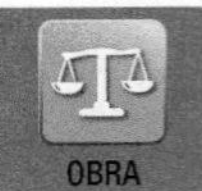

Assisting with a Bedpan

Equipment and Supplies

Bedpan with cover, bed protector or underpad, toilet tissue, basin, soap, washcloth, towel, disposable gloves, plastic waste bag, paper and pen or computer

NOTE: If cleansing cloths are available, they can be used in place of the basin, soap, and washcloth.

Procedure

1. Obtain proper authorization and assemble equipment.
2. Knock on the door and pause before entering. Introduce yourself. Identify the patient. Explain the procedure and obtain consent.

   Comm

3. Wash hands. Put on gloves.

   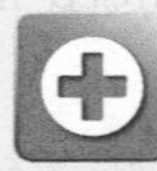

   CAUTION: Observe standard precautions when handling urine or feces.

4. Close the door and pull the curtain for privacy. Put a bed protector or underpad on the chair and then place the bedpan on top. Place the tissue within easy reach of the patient. Raise the bed to a comfortable working height. Lower the head of the bed, if tolerated by the patient.

   CAUTION: Use correct body mechanics during this procedure. Bend from the hips, not the waist. Maintain a broad base of support.

5. If the bedpan is metal, warm it by running hot water into it and then emptying it. If no water is available, rub the bedpan briskly with a cloth.
6. If siderails are present and elevated, lower the siderails on the side where you are working.
7. Fold the top bedcovers back at a right angle. Raise the patient's gown.

   NOTE: Avoid exposing the patient. If the patient is wearing pajama pants, help lower the pants.

   NOTE: The patient can also be covered with a bath blanket. The top sheets are then fanfolded to the foot of the bed.

8. 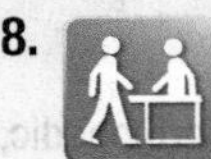

   Ask the patient to flex the knees and rest his or her weight on the heels, if able. Discuss a signal such as, "On the count of three, raise up."

9. At the signal, assist the patient to raise his or her hips by putting one of your hands under the small of the patient's back.

   CAUTION: If the patient is too heavy, get help.

10. With your other hand, slide the bedpan under the patient's hips. The narrow end should face the foot of bed. Adjust to the correct placement.

    NOTE: The patient's buttocks should rest on the rounded portion of the pan.

11. The patient who is too weak to get on the pan may be rolled away from the health care worker and onto his or her side. The bedpan can then be placed against the patient's buttocks (Figure 22–58). The patient is then rolled back onto the bedpan. The bedpan must be held in place during this procedure.

    NOTE: Lower bedpans, called *fracture* (or orthopedic) *bedpans*, can also be used by patients who are unable to help (refer again to Figure 22–55).

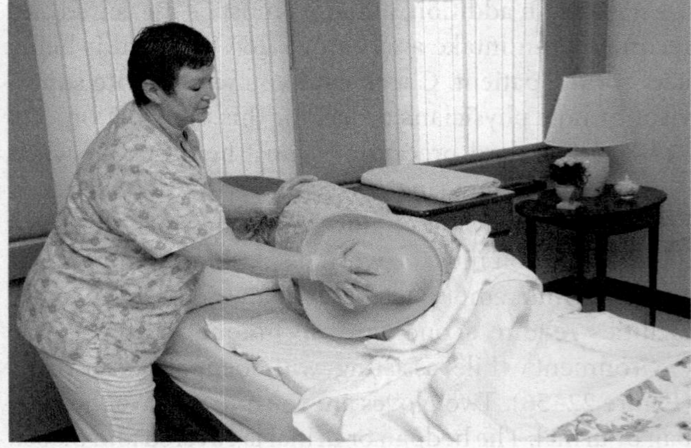

FIGURE 22–58 The patient can also turn onto his or her side so that the bedpan can be positioned. The patient then rolls back onto the bedpan.

PROCEDURE 22:7A (CONT.)

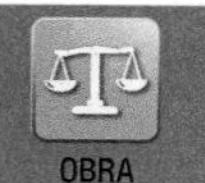

12. Remove gloves and place them in the plastic waste bag.
13. Replace the top bedcovers. Position the patient in a comfortable position. Raise the head of the bed, as needed.
14. Place the call signal and tissue within easy reach of the patient.

    NOTE: If a urine specimen is needed or the patient is on Intake and Output, instruct the patient not to put toilet tissue in the pan. Provide a small plastic bag for discarding the soiled tissue.
15. If indicated, raise the siderail before leaving the patient.
16. Wash hands thoroughly.
17. Answer the patient's call signal immediately.
18. Wash hands.
19. Fill the bath basin with water at a temperature of 105°F–110°F. Place the basin on the overbed table or bedside stand. Position soap, a washcloth, and towel by the basin.

    NOTE: Cleansing cloths can be used for this step if they are available.
20. Put on gloves.
21. If elevated, lower the siderail. Ask the patient to flex the knees and put his or her weight on the heels. Place one hand under the small of the patient's back. Assist in raising the patient's buttocks off the pan. With your other hand, remove the bedpan carefully.
22. Cover the bedpan and place it on the underpad on top of the chair.

    NOTE: If a bedpan cover is not available, cloth, paper bags, or tissue paper can be used to cover the bedpan.
23. If the patient is unable to assist in getting off the bedpan, it may be necessary to get help. Roll the patient off the bedpan and onto his or her side while holding the bedpan firmly in place with one hand. Cover the bedpan and place it on the underpad on top of the chair.
24. Clean the genital area, as necessary. Wipe from front to back. Drop the soiled tissue into the bedpan, unless a specimen is needed or output is being measured. In these situations, temporarily place the tissue in a plastic bag until you can discard it in the toilet or trash can in the utility room.
25. Wash the patient's perineal area, if necessary, or assist the patient as needed.
26. Remove gloves and place them in the plastic bag.
27. Replace the bedcovers. Elevate the siderails, if necessary.
28. Wash hands thoroughly.
29. Empty the bath basin and refill it with warm water or offer a clean cleansing cloth. Allow the patient to wash his or her hands.
30. Observe all checkpoints before leaving the patient: position the patient in correct body alignment; elevate the siderails (if indicated); lower the bed to its lowest level; and place the call signal, water, and tissues within easy reach of the patient.
31. Put on gloves. Take the bedpan to the bathroom. Note the contents. Check amount, color, type. If an I&O record is being kept for the patient, measure and record the amount.

    NOTE: Check to see whether a specimen is needed before emptying the bedpan.

    CAUTION: Save a sample of the contents if there are any abnormalities.
32. Empty the bedpan. Use a paper towel to cover your gloved hand while turning on the faucet or flushing the toilet. Put on eye protection if spraying or splashing is possible. Rinse the bedpan with cold water and a disinfectant. Rinse and dry.

    NOTE: Follow your agency's policy for cleaning bedpans.
33. Return the covered pan to the patient's unit. Use a paper towel on the gloved hand or remove one glove. Replace all equipment used.
34. Remove gloves. Wash hands thoroughly.
35. 

    Report and/or record all required information on the patient's chart or enter it into the computer. For example, date, time, used bedpan, voided 250 mL of straw yellow urine, and your signature and title. Always report unusual observations immediately.

    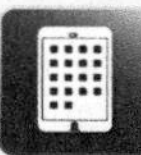

    NOTE: In health care agencies using electronic health records (EHRs), also known as electronic medical records (EMRs), the information is entered directly into the patient's record on a computer.

PRACTICE: **Go to the workbook and use the evaluation sheet for 22:7A, Assisting with a Bedpan, to practice this procedure. When you believe you have mastered this skill, sign the sheet and give it to your instructor for further action.**

FINAL CHECKPOINT: Using the criteria listed on the evaluation sheet, your instructor will grade your performance.

PROCEDURE 22:7B

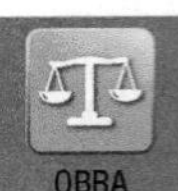

Assisting with a Urinal

Equipment and Supplies

Urinal with cover, bed protector or underpad, basin, soap, washcloth, towel, toilet tissue, disposable gloves, plastic waste bag, paper and pen or computer

NOTE: If cleansing cloths are available, they can be used in place of the basin, soap, and washcloth.

Procedure

1. Obtain proper authorization and assemble equipment. Make sure the urinal has a lid or cover of some type (Figure 22–59).
2. Knock on the door and pause before entering. Introduce yourself. Identify the patient. Explain the procedure and obtain consent.

   Comm

3. Wash hands. Put on gloves.

   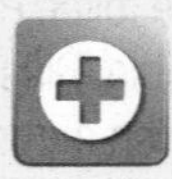

   CAUTION: Observe standard precautions when handling urine or feces.

4. Close the door and pull the curtain for privacy. Elevate the bed to a comfortable working height. If siderails are present and elevated, lower the siderail on the side where you are working.
5. If the patient is weak or helpless, lift the top bedcovers and help the patient grasp the handle and position the urinal.
6. Make sure the call signal and toilet tissue are within easy reach of the patient. Leave the patient alone, if possible, to ensure privacy. Remove one glove. If necessary, elevate the siderail with the ungloved hand before leaving.
7. Remove gloves and wash hands.

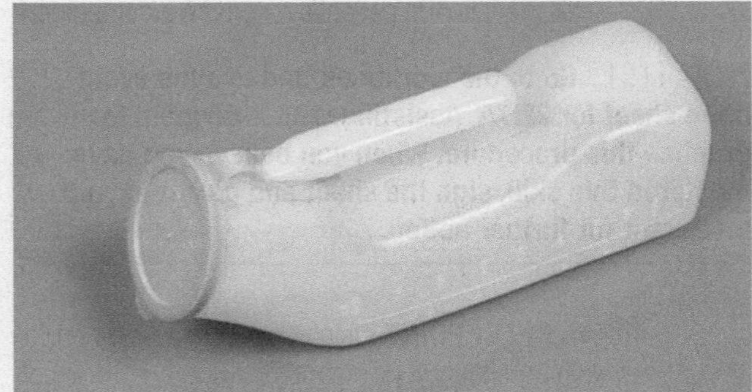

FIGURE 22–59 **A urinal should have a lid or cover.**

8. Answer the patient's call signal immediately.
9. Wash hands.
10. Fill the bath basin with water at a temperature of 105°F–110°F. Place the basin on the overbed table or bedside stand. Position soap, a washcloth, and towel by the basin.

    NOTE: If cleansing clothes are available, they can be used for this step.

11. Put on gloves.
12. Ask the patient to hand you the urinal. If the patient needs assistance, reach under the covers and take hold of the urinal handle. Close the lid or cover the top of the urinal and place it on top of the underpad on the chair.

    NOTE: Avoid exposing the patient.

13. Wash the patient's perineal area, if necessary, or assist the patient, as needed.
14. Remove gloves and place them in the plastic waste bag.
15. Replace the bedcovers. Elevate the siderails, if necessary.
16. Wash hands thoroughly.
17. Empty the basin and refill it with warm water or offer a clean cleansing cloth. Allow the patient to wash his hands or assist as needed.
18. Observe all checkpoints before leaving the patient: position the patient in correct body alignment, elevate the siderails, if indicated; lower the bed to its lowest level; and place the call signal and supplies within easy reach of the patient.
19. Put on gloves.
20. Take the urinal to the bathroom. Observe the contents. Measure and record the amount if an I&O record is being kept for the patient.

    NOTE: Check to see whether a specimen is needed before emptying the urinal.

    CAUTION: Save a specimen if there are any abnormalities. Report unusual observations immediately to your supervisor.

21. Empty the urinal. Use a paper towel to cover your gloved hand while turning on the faucet or flushing the toilet. Put on eye protection if spraying or splashing is possible. Rinse the urinal with cold water and a disinfectant. Rinse and dry.

    NOTE: Follow agency policy for cleaning the urinal.

22. Return the urinal to the patient's unit. Use a paper towel on the gloved hand or remove one glove. Place it in the bedside stand or in the urinal holder on the bed.
23. Remove gloves. Wash hands thoroughly.

PROCEDURE 22:7B (CONT.)

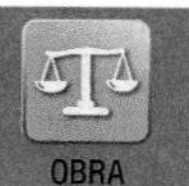

24. 

Report and/or record all required information on the patient's chart or enter it into the computer. For example, date, time, used urinal, voided 250 mL of straw yellow urine, and your signature and title. Always report unusual observations immediately.

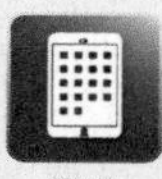

NOTE: In health care agencies using electronic health records (EHRs), also known as electronic medical records (EMRs), the information is entered directly into the patient's record on a computer.

PRACTICE: **Go to the workbook and use the evaluation sheet for 22:7B, Assisting with a Urinal, to practice this procedure. When you believe you have mastered this skill, sign the sheet and give it to your instructor for further action.**

FINAL CHECKPOINT: Using the criteria listed on the evaluation sheet, your instructor will grade your performance.

22:8 Providing Catheter and Urinary-Drainage Unit Care

Some patients are unable to urinate, or void. In these cases, a catheter may be inserted into the bladder to drain the urine. The catheter is usually connected to a drainage unit to collect the urine.

A **catheter** is a hollow tube, usually made of soft rubber or plastic. There are different kinds of catheters. A urethral, or straight, catheter is inserted into the bladder to drain urine but is not left in the bladder (Figure 22–60A). It is usually used to collect a sterile urine specimen. A Foley catheter (also called an *indwelling*, or *retention*, catheter) is usually used to drain the bladder over an extended period. It has a small balloon on the end that is inserted into the bladder (Figure 22–60B). Once the catheter is inserted, the balloon is inflated with sterile water to keep the catheter in place. The catheter must be kept sterile at all times. Insertion of a catheter is a sterile technique performed by a nurse, physician, or other authorized person. If a male patient requires urinary drainage, external condom catheters may be used (Figure 22–60C). The condom catheters eliminate the need for an internal catheter and decrease the chance of urinary infection. The condom catheter is placed on the penis and attached to the urinary-drainage tubing and collection bag. The condom must be removed at least every 24 hours, and the skin must be checked for any signs of irritation.

A **urinary-drainage unit** or bag is attached to the catheter to collect drained urine (Figure 22–61A). This is usually a closed unit to keep microorganisms from entering the catheter and, therefore, prevent infection. The unit consists of plastic or rubber tubing attached to the catheter and extending to a bag in which the urine is collected. Patients who are ambulatory may

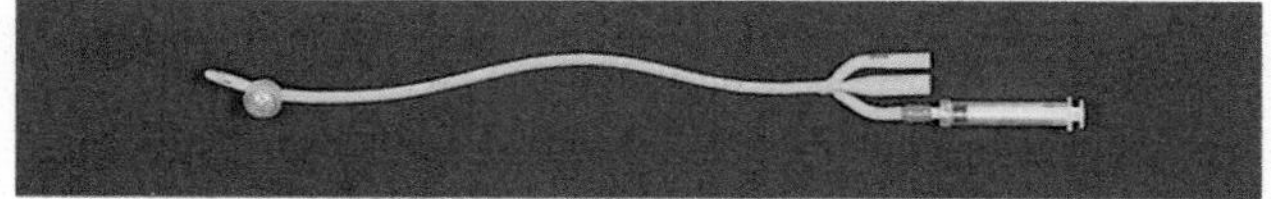

FIGURE 22–60B A Foley catheter has a small balloon on the end that is inserted into the bladder. The balloon is inflated with sterile water to hold the catheter in place.

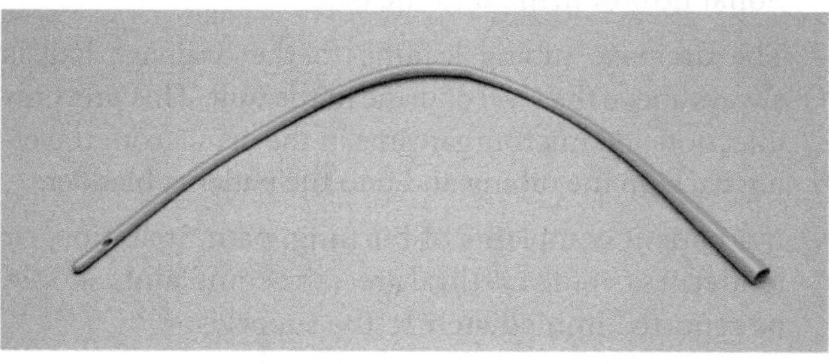

FIGURE 22–60A A straight catheter is inserted into the bladder to drain urine but is not left in the bladder.

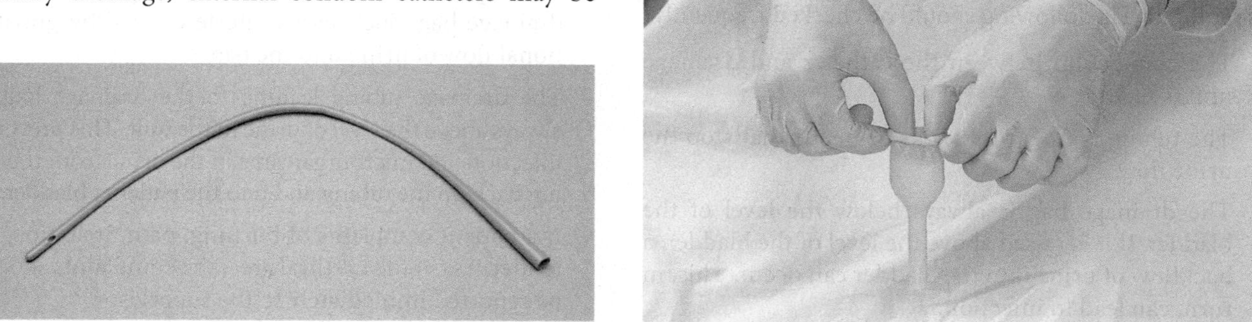

FIGURE 22–60C Condom catheters are used to provide an external urinary-drainage system for male patients.

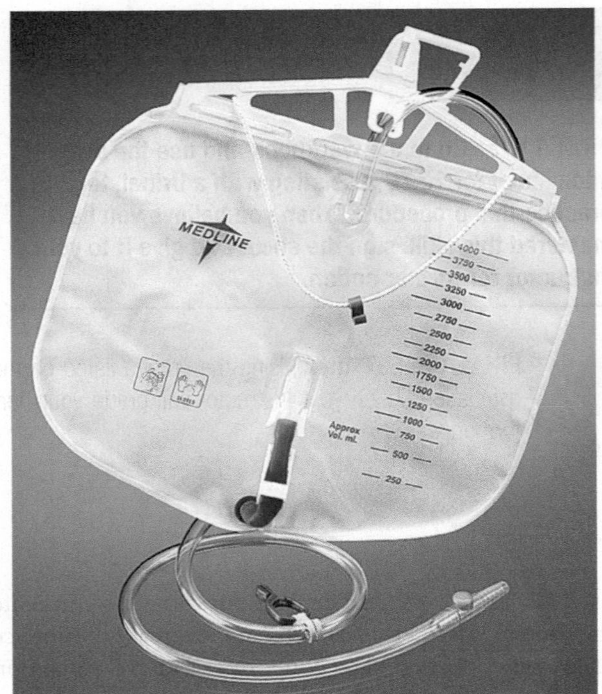

FIGURE 22–61A **The urinary-drainage bag is connected to the catheter and attached to the bed frame below the level of the bladder to collect the drained urine.** Courtesy of Medline Industries Inc., 1-860-MEDLINE

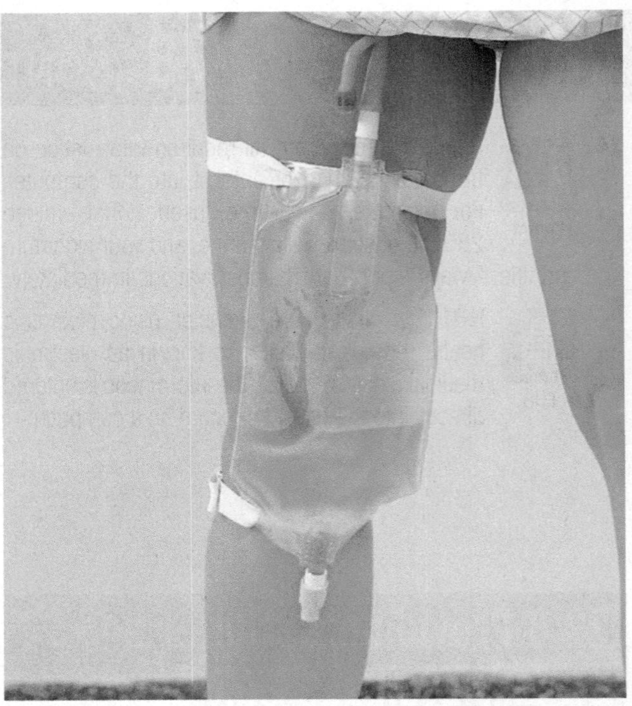

FIGURE 22–61B **A leg bag may be used for ambulatory patients to collect urine drained through a catheter. It is usually attached to the leg with Velcro straps.**

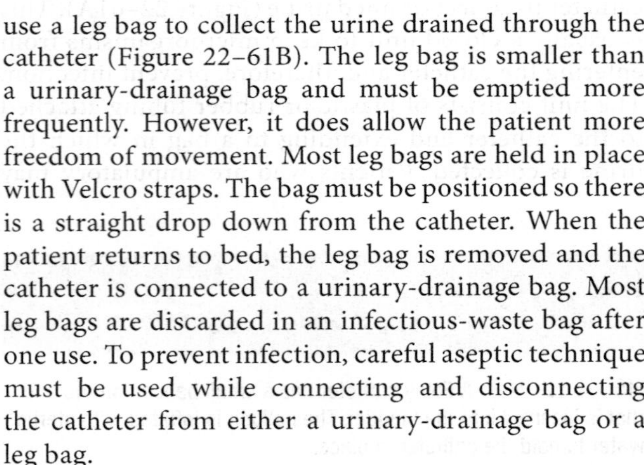

use a leg bag to collect the urine drained through the catheter (Figure 22–61B). The leg bag is smaller than a urinary-drainage bag and must be emptied more frequently. However, it does allow the patient more freedom of movement. Most leg bags are held in place with Velcro straps. The bag must be positioned so there is a straight drop down from the catheter. When the patient returns to bed, the leg bag is removed and the catheter is connected to a urinary-drainage bag. Most leg bags are discarded in an infectious-waste bag after one use. To prevent infection, careful aseptic technique must be used while connecting and disconnecting the catheter from either a urinary-drainage bag or a leg bag.

Careful observation of the catheter and drainage unit is required. The following should be checked frequently:

- The connection between the catheter and drainage unit is secure.
- The tubing is free from kinks or bends that stop the urine flow.
- The drainage bag is always below the level of the bladder. If it is raised above the level of the bladder, a backflow of urine into the bladder can occur. This, in turn, can lead to infection.
- The urine is flowing freely into the drainage bag. The system usually relies on gravity for drainage. Therefore, the drainage bag should be kept low enough to make use of the force of gravity.
- The catheter is secured to the patient's leg using a catheter stabilization device, or it can be taped or strapped onto the leg. This prevents pull on the catheter, which might dislodge it or cause irritation.
- The drainage unit is emptied frequently. Stagnant urine encourages the growth of microorganisms. The units are usually emptied every 8 hours, but they may be emptied more frequently, if required.
- The drainage bag and/or tubing are not lying on the floor. The drainage bag should be attached to the bed frame.
- No loops of the drainage tube are hanging below the drainage bag. Such loops interfere with the gravitational flow of urine into the bag.
- The drainage tubing leading to the drainage bag is always above the level of urine in the unit. This prevents infection and microorganisms in the urine from traveling back up the tubing and into the patient's bladder.
- If a patient complains of burning, pain, irritation, or tenderness in the urethral area, the complaints should be reported immediately to the supervisor.

When a catheter and urinary-drainage unit is in place, it is preferable to never disconnect the drainage unit. However, it may sometimes be necessary to disconnect the catheter from the unit. For example, if a patient uses a leg bag during ambulation, the catheter is disconnected from the urinary-drainage unit and attached to the leg bag. If a urine-collection area is not present on the drainage unit, and a sterile or fresh urine specimen is required (because the urine in the bag is not fresh and is contaminated), the drainage unit must be disconnected. In either instance, careful sterile technique must be followed to prevent infection. Both the catheter and top connection of the drainage unit must be kept sterile. Special clamps, plugs, and other equipment are available for disconnecting the catheter (Figure 22–62A). Follow agency policy for disconnecting the catheter. Usually, the catheter is clamped to prevent leakage of urine. The health care worker wears gloves to disconnect the catheter from the tubing, taking care to avoid touching the ends of the catheter or tubing to any surface. A plug is inserted into the catheter, and a cap is placed on the end of the drainage tubing (Figure 22–62B). The drainage tubing is attached to the bed frame so it cannot touch the floor or become contaminated before it is reconnected.

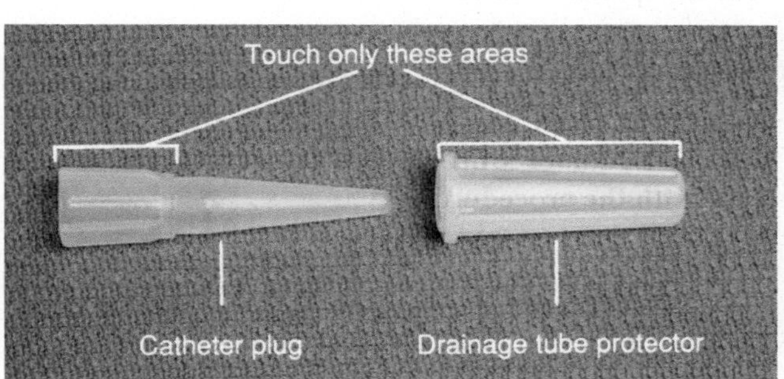

FIGURE 22–62A A sterile catheter plug and protective cap.

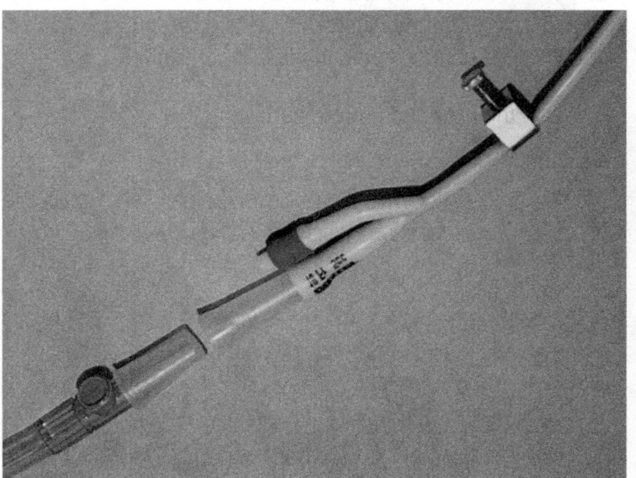

FIGURE 22–62B A catheter disconnected from the drainage tube and protected with the catheter plug. Note the protective cap on the drainage tube.

Most drainage units have special urine-collection areas on the tubing. The catheter does not have to be disconnected when a specimen is obtained from this type of unit. Follow the specific instructions provided with the unit or follow agency policy to maintain sterility during this procedure. A clamp is usually placed on the tubing below the collection unit to allow urine to collect in the tubing and/or bladder. The collection unit is wiped with a disinfectant, and a sterile syringe is inserted into the needleless port of the drainage tubing to obtain the urine specimen (Figures 22–63A and 22–63B). A few health care facilities use units without needleless ports. A syringe with a sterile needle is inserted in this type of port to obtain the specimen. The urine is then placed in a specimen container. Gloves must be worn during this procedure, and the contaminated syringe (and needle if one is used) must be placed in a sharps container immediately after use.

When a Foley, or indwelling, catheter is in place, the urinary meatus must be kept clean and free of secretions to help prevent bladder and kidney infections.

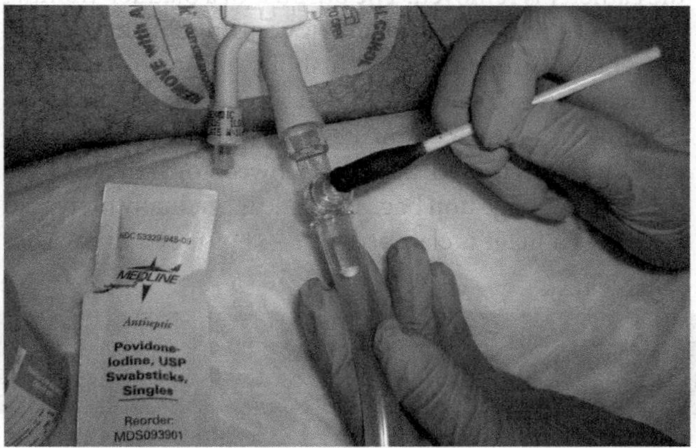

FIGURE 22–63A The urine-collection area is first wiped with a disinfectant.

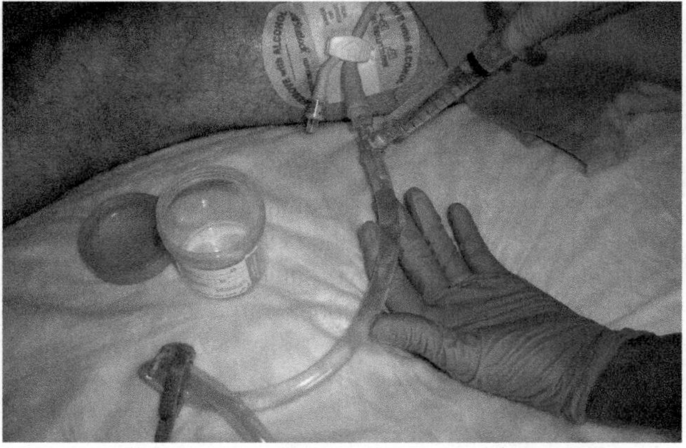

FIGURE 22–63B A sterile syringe is inserted into the port to obtain the urine specimen.

Catheter care is provided for this purpose, and it should be administered at least once every 8 hours, and more frequently if ordered. This care is usually provided during the bath and as part of perineal care. Disposable catheter-care kits containing applicators and antiseptic solution are used in many agencies. Other agencies use soap and water. Some kits also contain disposable bed protectors or underpads and gloves. Follow the instructions provided with the kit or the procedure recommended by your agency. Procedure 22:8A describes one method of catheter care.

Comm

Careful observations of the urine drained should be made. The amount, color, type, presence of other substances, and other observations should be noted. Unusual observations should be reported immediately.

Correct procedure must be followed when emptying the drainage unit to prevent contamination and infection. Procedure 22:8B describes one way of emptying a drainage unit.

If a patient has had an indwelling catheter in place for a time, a *bladder-training program* may be instituted before the catheter is removed. The purpose of a bladder-training program is to develop voluntary control of urination and prevent incontinence, or the inability to control urination. At first, the catheter is clamped for 1–2 hours at a time to allow urine to accumulate in the bladder. The clamp is then released, and urine is allowed to drain into the urinary-drainage unit bag. The time is gradually increased until the catheter is clamped for 3–4 hours at a time. After the catheter is removed, the patient is encouraged to void every 3–4 hours or whenever necessary to regain bladder control. Bladder-training programs can also be used for incontinent patients who do not have indwelling catheters in place. This type of program encourages the patient to attempt to void at regularly scheduled intervals. A record is kept of times of incontinence to establish when the patient should be encouraged to void. Staff members then assist the patient to the bathroom or offer the bedpan or urinal before the expected time of incontinence. The support, understanding, and cooperation of all staff members is important when a bladder-training program is used for a patient.

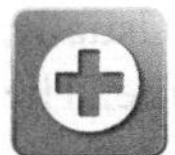
Precaution

Standard precautions (discussed in Chapter 15:4) must be observed at all times when handling urine. Gloves must be worn when providing catheter care, obtaining urine specimens from a urine-collection unit, and emptying a urinary-drainage unit. Hands must be washed frequently and immediately after removing gloves. If splashing or spraying of body fluids is possible, eye protection must be worn. Any areas contaminated with urine must be wiped with a disinfectant. Taking proper precautions helps prevent the spread of infection.

STUDENT: Go to the workbook and complete the assignment sheet for 22:8, Providing Catheter and Urinary-Drainage Unit Care. Then return and continue with the procedures.

PROCEDURE 22:8A

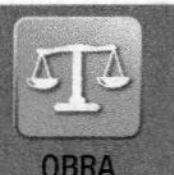
OBRA

Providing Catheter Care

Equipment and Supplies

Catheter-care kit (or sterile applicators, bowl, and antiseptic solution or soap and water), bath blanket, disposable underpad or bed protector, catheter stabilization device, catheter strap or tape (if needed), disposable gloves, infectious-waste bag, paper and pen or computer

NOTE: Catheter care is usually administered after the perineal area has been washed and cleaned during the bath. If administered at a different time, equipment must be obtained to wash and clean the perineal area before providing catheter care.

Procedure

1. Obtain proper authorization and assemble equipment.
2.  Comm — Knock on the door and pause before entering. Introduce yourself. Identify the patient. Explain the procedure and obtain consent.
3. Close the door and pull the curtain for privacy.
4. Wash hands. Put on gloves.

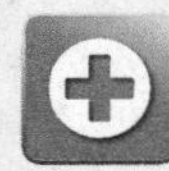
Precaution

CAUTION: Wear gloves and observe standard precautions when providing catheter care.

5. Elevate the bed to a comfortable working height. If siderails are present and elevated, lower the siderail on the side where you are working.
6. Cover the patient with a bath blanket. Without exposing the patient, fanfold the top bed linen to the foot of the bed.
7. Place the disposable underpad or bed protector under the patient's buttocks and upper legs.

PROCEDURE 22:8A (CONT.)

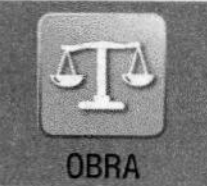

8. Position the patient in the dorsal recumbent position, if possible, with the legs separated and knees bent. Drape the patient so that only the perineal area is exposed.
9. Open the catheter-care kit and place it on the overbed table. Position the infectious-waste bag conveniently.
10. If sterile gloves are required, remove disposable gloves, wash hands, and put on sterile gloves.

    NOTE: Sterile gloves are required by some agencies. Follow agency policy.
11. Obtain a sterile applicator (usually a cotton ball or gauze pad) moistened with antiseptic solution or soap and water.

    NOTE: Some kits contain premoistened sterile applicators. Other kits contain containers of antiseptic solution that must be poured into small bowls provided with the kits. The sterile applicator is then placed in the antiseptic.
12. For a female patient:
    a. Use the thumb and forefinger of one hand to gently separate the labia, or lips, and expose the urinary meatus (opening).
    b. Wipe from front to back with the sterile applicator.
    c. Place the used applicator in the infectious-waste bag.
    d. Using a clean sterile applicator each time, continue to wipe from front to back until the area is clean.
13. For a male patient:
    a. Gently grasp the penis and draw the foreskin back.
    b. Use the sterile applicator to wipe from the meatus down the shaft.
    c. Place the used applicator in the infectious-waste bag.
    d. Using a clean sterile applicator each time, continue to wipe from the meatus down the shaft until the area is clean.
    e. After the area is clean, gently return the foreskin to its normal position.
14. Without pulling on the catheter, use a sterile applicator to clean the catheter from the meatus down approximately 4 inches. Place the used applicator in the infectious-waste bag. Repeat as necessary, using a fresh applicator for each stroke.
15. Observe the area carefully for any signs of irritation, abnormal discharge, or crusting.
16. Remove the bed protector or underpad and place it in the infectious-waste bag.
17. Remove gloves and discard in the infectious-waste bag. Wash hands.
18. Check the catheter to be sure it is secured to the leg. Tape or a strap may be used if a catheter stabilization device is not available (Figures 22–64A, 22–64B, and 22–64C).

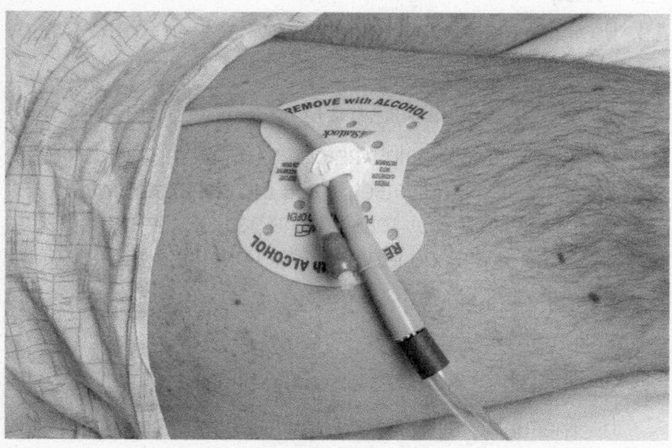

FIGURE 22–64A A catheter stabilization device can be used to secure the catheter to the leg.

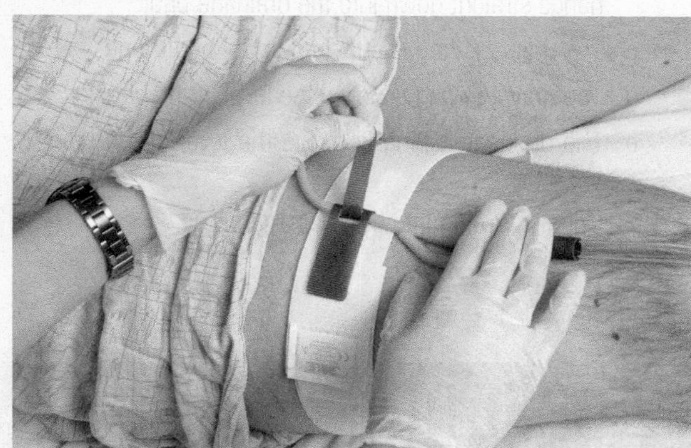

FIGURE 22–64B A strap can also be used to secure the catheter to the leg.

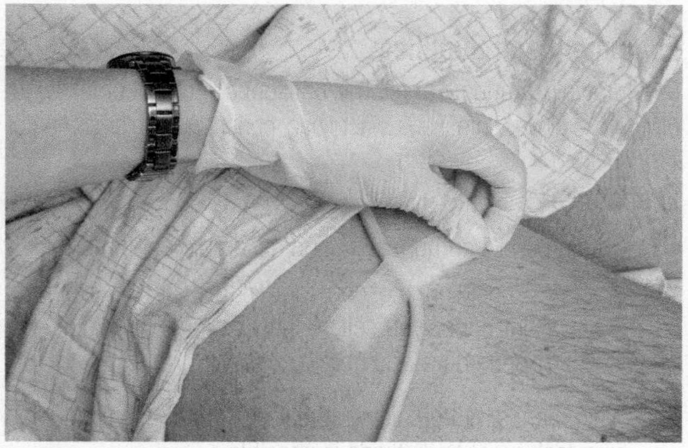

FIGURE 22–64C The catheter may also be taped to the leg. If possible, use hypoallergenic tape.

(continues)

PROCEDURE 22:8A (CONT.)

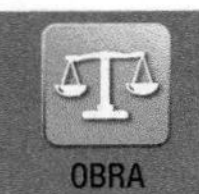

CAUTION: Make sure there is no strain or pull on the catheter.

19. Position the patient comfortably and in correct body alignment.
20. Replace the top bed linen and remove the bath blanket.
21. Observe all checkpoints before leaving the patient: elevate the siderails (if indicated); place the call signal, water, and supplies within easy reach of the patient; lower the bed to its lowest level; and leave the area neat and clean.
22. Perform a final check of the catheter and drainage unit to ensure the following:
    a. The tubing is free of kinks and bends.
    b. The tubing is positioned to allow for proper flow of urine. Do *not* allow excess tubing to hang below the drainage bag. Coil the excess tubing on the bed so the tubing hangs straight down into the drainage bag.
    c. The drainage bag is attached to the bed frame.
    d. The drainage bag is below the level of the bladder.
    e. The drainage tubing is above the level of the urine in the bag.
    f. Urine is flowing into the drainage bag.
23. Place all disposable supplies in the infectious-waste bag. Seal properly and dispose of in the correct area. Clean and properly replace any other equipment used.
24. Wash hands thoroughly.
25.  Report and/or record all required information on the patient's chart or enter it into the computer. For example, date, time, catheter care given, urine flowing into drainage bag, and your signature and title. Report any unusual observations immediately.

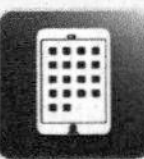

NOTE: In health care agencies using electronic health records (EHRs), also known as electronic medical records (EMRs), the information is entered directly into the patient's record on a computer.

PRACTICE: Go to the workbook and use the evaluation sheet for 22:8A, Providing Catheter Care, to practice this procedure. When you believe you have mastered this skill, sign the sheet and give it to your instructor for further action.

FINAL CHECKPOINT: Using the criteria listed on the evaluation sheet, your instructor will grade your performance.

PROCEDURE 22:8B

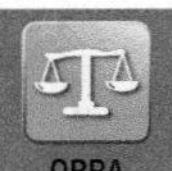

Emptying a Urinary-Drainage Unit

Equipment and Supplies

Paper towels, graduate or pitcher, antiseptic or disinfectant swab, disposable gloves, infectious-waste bag, paper and pen or computer

Procedure

1. Obtain proper authorization and assemble equipment.
2. 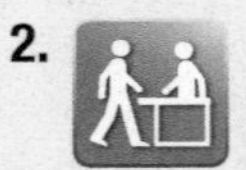 Knock on the door and pause before entering. Introduce yourself. Identify the patient. Explain the procedure and obtain consent.
3. Wash hands. Put on gloves. Wear eye protection if spraying or splashing of body fluids is possible.

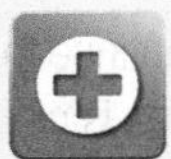

CAUTION: Observe standard precautions when measuring urine.

4. Place paper towels on the floor. Place the graduate on top of the towels.
5. Remove the drainage outlet from the drainage bag. Place the end of the outlet in the measuring pitcher or graduate.

CAUTION: Do not allow the end of the outlet to touch the graduate.

6. Release the clamp to allow the urine to drain. Empty all the urine (Figure 22–65A).

NOTE: If necessary, tilt the bag to remove all the urine.

PROCEDURE 22:8B (CONT.)

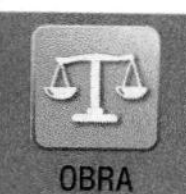

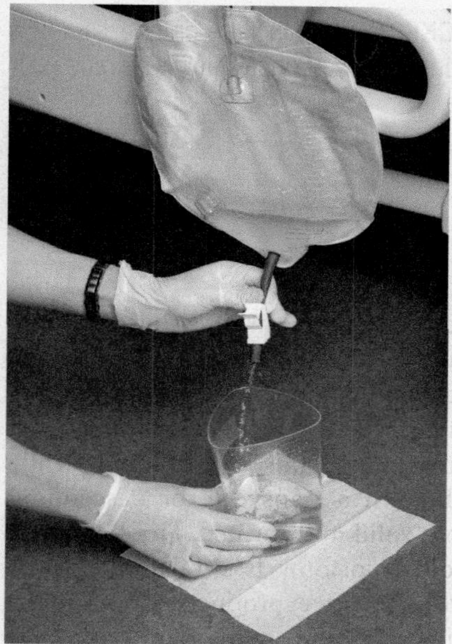

FIGURE 22–65A **Drain the urine from the urinary-drainage unit.**

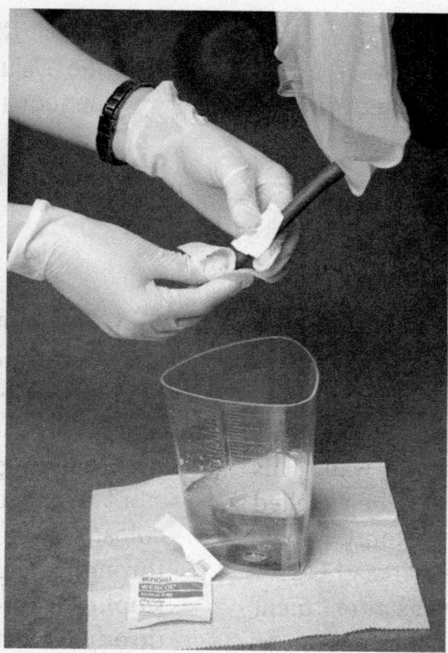

FIGURE 22–65B **Wipe the drainage outlet with a disinfectant.**

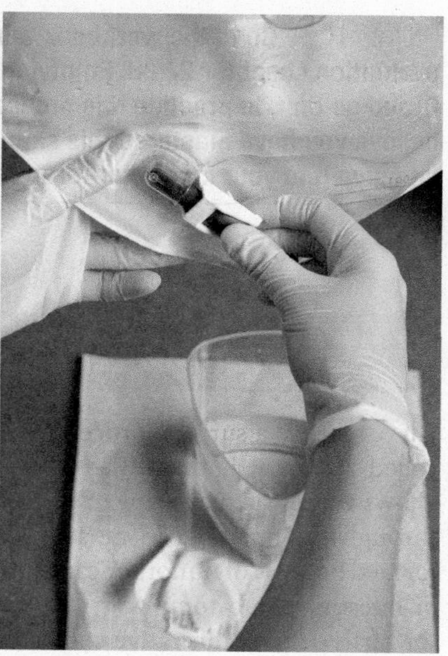

FIGURE 22–65C **Replace the drainage tube in the drainage unit.**

7. Clamp the drainage tube. Wipe the drainage outlet with an antiseptic or disinfectant swab (Figure 22–65B). Discard the antiseptic wipe in the infectious-waste bag. Replace the tube in the unit (Figure 22–65C).
8. Observe all checkpoints before leaving the patient: position the patient comfortably and in correct body alignment, elevate the siderails (if indicated), lower the bed to its lowest level, place the call signal and supplies within easy reach of the patient, and leave the area neat and clean.
9. Perform a final check of the catheter and unit to ensure the following:
   a. The catheter is secured to the patient's leg with a stabilization device, strap, or tape.
   b. The tubing is free of kinks and bends.
   c. The tubing does not loop down below the drainage bag. Do *not* allow excess tubing to hang below the drainage bag. Coil the excess tubing on the bed so the tubing hangs straight down into the drainage bag.
   d. The drainage bag is attached to the bed frame.
   e. The drainage bag is below the level of the bladder.
   f. The drainage tubing is above the level of the urine in the bag.
   g. Urine is flowing into the bag.
10. Pick up the graduate and paper towel. Discard the paper towel in the infectious-waste bag.
11. Take the graduate to the patient's bathroom. Place the graduate on a paper towel on a counter and read the measurement at eye level. Record the amount and color of urine in the graduate. Record any unusual observations and report such observations immediately.

    NOTE: Save a specimen if needed, or if anything unusual is noted about the urine.
12. Empty the graduate into the toilet. Rinse it with cold water. Wash with soap and warm water. Clean with a disinfectant. Rinse and dry. Return to its proper place.

    NOTE: The graduate is usually kept in the patient unit. It should be used for one patient only. Most agencies use disposable graduates. If the graduate is not disposable, it should be sterilized according to agency policy before being used for another patient.
13. Remove gloves. Wash hands.
14. Comm — Report and/or record all required information on the patient's chart or enter it into the computer. For example, date, time, emptied urinary-drainage unit, 580 mL of light yellow urine, and your signature and title. Report any unusual observations immediately.

    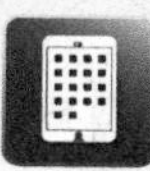

    NOTE: In health care agencies using electronic health records (EHRs), also known as electronic medical records (EMRs), the information is entered directly into the patient's record on a computer.

(continues)

PROCEDURE 22:8B (CONT.)

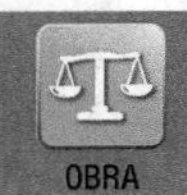

OBRA

PRACTICE: **Go to the workbook and use the evaluation sheet for 22:8B, Emptying a Urinary-Drainage Unit, to practice this procedure. When you believe you have mastered this skill, sign the sheet and give it to your instructor for further action.**

Check

FINAL CHECKPOINT: Using the criteria listed on the evaluation sheet, your instructor will grade your performance.

22:9 Providing Ostomy Care

An **ostomy** is a surgical procedure in which an opening, called a **stoma**, is created in the abdominal wall. This allows wastes such as urine or stool (feces) to be expelled through the opening. In most cases, an ostomy is performed because of tumors or cancer in the urinary bladder or intestine. An ostomy may also be done as a treatment for birth defects, ulcerative colitis, bowel obstruction, or injury. At times, an ostomy is permanent. At other times, an ostomy is temporary and is repaired when the injury heals or the condition necessitating the ostomy improves. There are different types of ostomies including:

Science

- **ureterostomy**: A ureterostomy is an opening into one of the two ureters that drain urine from the kidney to the bladder. The ureter is brought to the surface of the abdomen, and urine drains from the stoma, or opening.
- **ileostomy**: An ileostomy is an opening into the ileum, a section of the small intestine. A loop of the ileum is brought to the surface of the abdomen. Because the entire large intestine is bypassed, the stools expelled are frequent and liquid, and contain digestive enzymes that irritate the skin.
- **colostomy**: A colostomy is an opening into the large intestine, or colon. There are different kinds of colostomies, depending on the area of large intestine involved (Figure 22–66). Stool expelled through an ascending colostomy tends to be liquid, while stool expelled through a transverse or descending colostomy is more solid and formed. Stool expelled through a sigmoid colostomy is similar to normal stool, because the digestive products have moved through most of the intestine, and water and other substances have been reabsorbed.

Most patients with ostomies wear a bag or pouch over the stoma to collect the drainage (Figure 22–67). The pouch is held in place with a belt or an adhesive seal. Problems that can occur include leakage, odor, and irritation of the skin surrounding the stoma. The pouch must be emptied frequently. Many pouches have areas that can be opened to allow urine or stool to drain. The drainage end of the bag is placed in a bedpan (Figure 22–68). If the patient is ambulatory, the patient can sit on the toilet and position the drainage end of the bag over the toilet. The clamp at the drainage end of the bag is opened to allow the stool or urine to drain. The drainage end is then cleaned to prevent odors and the clamp is resealed. Some pouches are disposable and are removed and replaced. Used bags should be discarded in an infectious-waste bag.

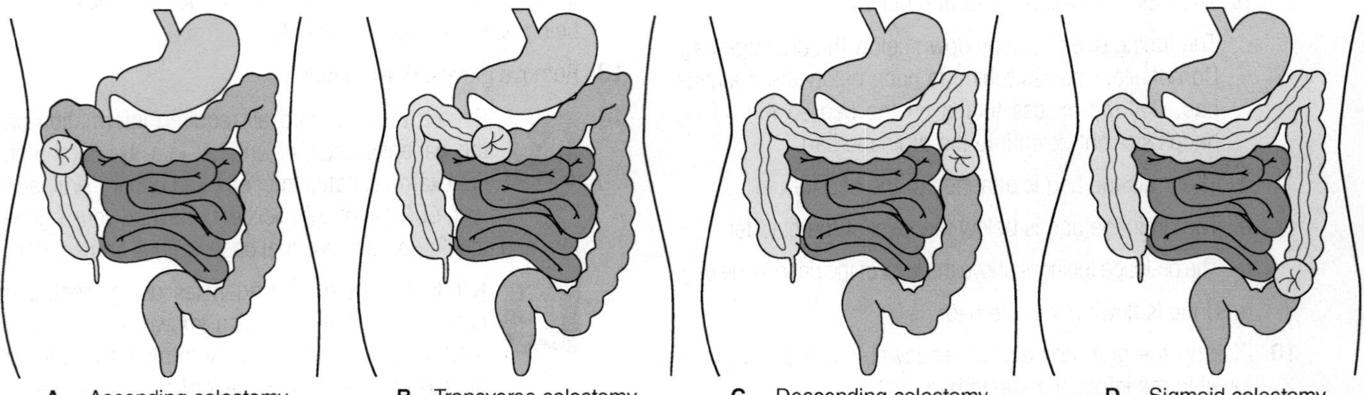

FIGURE 22–66 The type of colostomy depends on which part of the intestine is removed. Areas of intestine that remain after each type of colostomy are shown in blue.

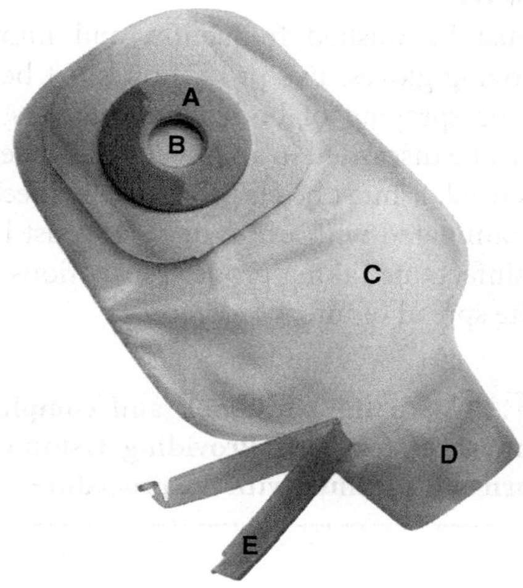

FIGURE 22–67 Most patients with ostomies wear a bag or pouch over the stoma, or opening, to collect the drainage.

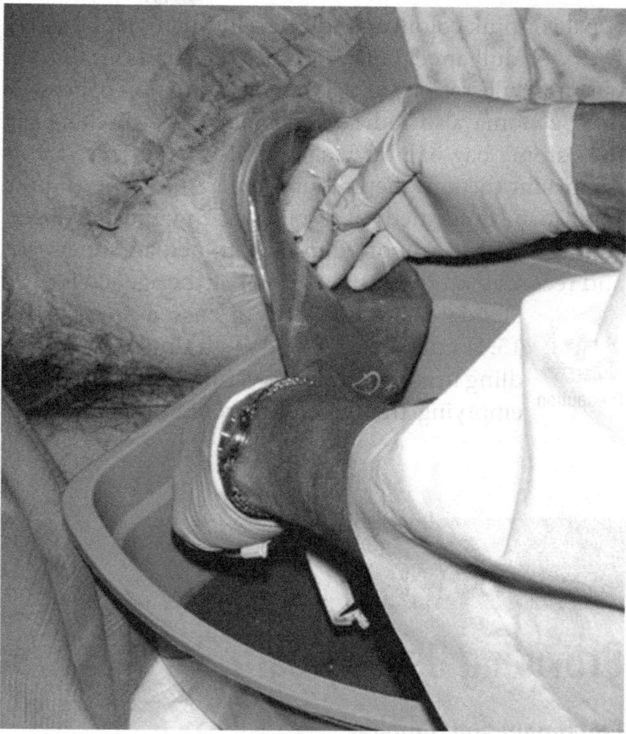

FIGURE 22–68 To empty the ostomy pouch, place the drainage end in a bedpan.

Good stoma and skin care is essential because of irritation caused by urine or stool drainage. Skin barriers such as wafers, pastes, powders, and liquid films frequently are applied to the skin around the stoma to prevent irritation from the removal of the pouch.

Legal

When an ostomy is first performed, care is provided by a registered nurse or wound care/ostomy nurse. For "older" ostomies, other trained and qualified health care workers may provide routine stoma care. It is essential to check the policy of your facility and to know your legal responsibilities before providing ostomy care. Eventually, most patients are taught to care for their own ostomies, if they are capable.

Patients with ostomies may experience psychological reactions. They may feel loss of personal worth and dignity because they are unable to eliminate body wastes in a routine manner. Even though clothing conceals the ostomy and pouch, the patient feels different. Some individuals have difficulty maintaining normal sexual relationships. Others may feel anger, anxiety, depression, fear, or hopelessness. If the ostomy is done because of a malignant tumor (cancer), fear and anxiety can be more severe. It is essential to allow the patient to express feelings and verbalize fears. Understanding and support from all health care providers is important during the initial adjustment period. Eventually, patients realize that thousands of people with ostomies live normal lives. Through ostomy support groups, made up of people with ostomies, and help from health care providers, most individuals learn to cope and live with their ostomies.

Comm

Careful observation is essential when providing care to the patient with an ostomy. The stoma is mucous membrane with no nerve endings. It is bright to dark red and looks wet because of the exposed mucosa (Figure 22–69). Rubbing or pressure can cause the stoma to bleed. Any abnormalities in appearance should be reported immediately. A blue-to-black color indicates interference with the blood supply.

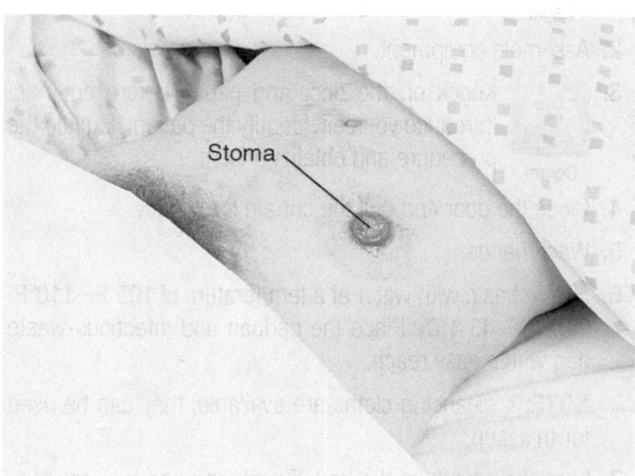

FIGURE 22–69 A stoma should be bright to dark red and look wet because of the exposed mucous membrane.

A pale or pink color can indicate a low hemoglobin level. A dry or dull appearance signifies dehydration. Profuse bleeding, ulcerations or cuts, or the formation of crystals on the stoma also indicate problems. The discharge in the ostomy bag or pouch should also be observed. It is important to note the amount, color, and type (liquid, semi-formed, formed) of discharge. Any unusual observations should be reported to your immediate supervisor and recorded on the patient's chart or the agency form.

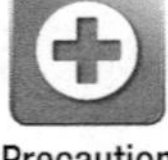
Precaution

Standard precautions (discussed in Chapter 15:4) must be observed at all times when handling urine or stool. Gloves must be worn when emptying the pouch or providing stoma care. Hands must be washed frequently, and immediately after removing gloves. Eye protection must be worn if splashing or spraying of body fluids is possible. The pouch must be discarded in an infectious-waste bag. If a bedpan is used, it must be cleaned and disinfected. Any areas contaminated with urine or stool must be wiped with a disinfectant. Taking proper precautions can help prevent the spread of infection.

STUDENT: **Go to the workbook and complete the assignment sheet for 22:9, Providing Ostomy Care. Then return and continue with the procedure.**

PROCEDURE 22:9

Providing Ostomy Care

Equipment and Supplies

Washcloth, towel, soap, basin, bed protector or underpad, bath blanket, ostomy pouch or bag, ostomy belt, adhesive (if needed), skin barrier or wafer (as ordered), toilet tissue, bedpan, disposable gloves, infectious-waste bag, paper and pen or computer

NOTE: If cleansing cloths are available, they can be used in place of the basin, soap, and washcloth.

Procedure

1. Check physician's orders or obtain authorization from your immediate supervisor.

   Legal

   CAUTION: Know your legal responsibilities before providing ostomy care.

2. Assemble equipment.

3.  Comm

   Knock on the door and pause before entering. Introduce yourself. Identify the patient. Explain the procedure and obtain consent.

4. Close the door and pull the curtain for privacy.

5. Wash hands.

6. Fill the basin with water at a temperature of 105°F–110°F (40.6°C–43.3°C). Place the bedpan and infectious-waste bag within easy reach.

   NOTE: If cleansing cloths are available, they can be used for this step.

7. Lock the wheels of the bed. Elevate the bed to a comfortable working height. If siderails are present and elevated, lower the siderail on the side where you are working.

8. Cover the patient with a bath blanket. Without exposing the patient, fanfold the top bed linen to the foot of the bed.

9. Place a bed protector or underpad under the patient's hips on the side of the stoma.

10. Put on disposable gloves.

    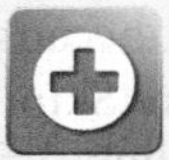
    Precaution

    CAUTION: Observe standard precautions at all times when handling urine or feces.

11. Open the belt, if used, and carefully remove the ostomy bag. Be gentle when peeling the bag away from the stoma. Note the amount, color, and type of drainage in the bag. Place the bag in the bedpan or infectious-waste bag. Follow agency policy.

    NOTE: Most ostomy bags are disposable, but some are reusable. To reuse a bag, drain the fecal material (or urine from a ureterostomy) by placing the clamp end of the bag over a bedpan. Then release the clamp and allow the fecal material to empty into the bedpan. Wash the inside of the bag with soap and water and allow it to dry before reapplying the bag. Most people use a second bag while the first bag is drying.

12. Use toilet tissue to gently wipe around the stoma to remove feces or drainage. Put the tissue in the bedpan or infectious-waste bag.

    NOTE: If the patient has a ureterostomy, wipe urine from the stoma area to prevent the urine from contacting the skin.

13. Carefully examine the stoma and surrounding skin. Check for irritated areas, bleeding, edema (or swelling), or discharge. Make sure you report any unusual observations to your immediate supervisor at the end of the procedure.

PROCEDURE 22:9 (CONT.)

14. Wash the ostomy area gently with soap and water. Use a circular motion, working from the stoma outward.
15. Rinse the entire area well to remove any soapy residue. Dry the area gently with a towel.

    NOTE: Make sure soap is removed. It has a drying effect and may irritate the skin.
16. Use a measuring chart to check the size of the stoma and determine the correct size barrier or wafer (Figure 22–70A). If the wafer is not self-adhesive, apply adhesive stoma paste to the skin around the stoma. Some pastes must dry a few minutes; follow the manufacturer's instructions. Peel the paper backing from the wafer. Position the wafer, adhesive side down, over the adhesive paste (Figure 22–70B).

    NOTE: The wafer serves as a barrier between the ostomy pouch or bag and the skin. It is not changed every time the pouch is changed. A new pouch can be snapped onto the existing wafer.

    NOTE: Some types of ostomy pouches and bags do not use wafers. Instead, barriers in the forms of pastes, liquids, or powders are applied to the skin to protect it. Follow the manufacturer's instructions.
17. If used, position the belt around the patient. If necessary, apply a clean belt.
18. Gently press to snap a clean ostomy bag in place over the wafer (Figure 22–70C). Seal the bag tightly to the wafer to prevent leakage.
19. If the pouch has a drainage area, make sure the clip or clamp sealing the drainage site is secure.
20. Remove the underpad or bed protector. If any linen on the bed is soiled, change the linen.
21. Remove gloves and discard in an infectious-waste bag.
22. Replace the top bed linen and remove the bath blanket. Make sure the patient is comfortable and positioned in correct body alignment.
23. Observe all checkpoints before leaving the patient: elevate the siderails (if indicated); lower the bed to its lowest level; and place the call signal, water, tissues, and other supplies within easy reach of the patient.
24. Wash hands thoroughly and put on gloves.
25. 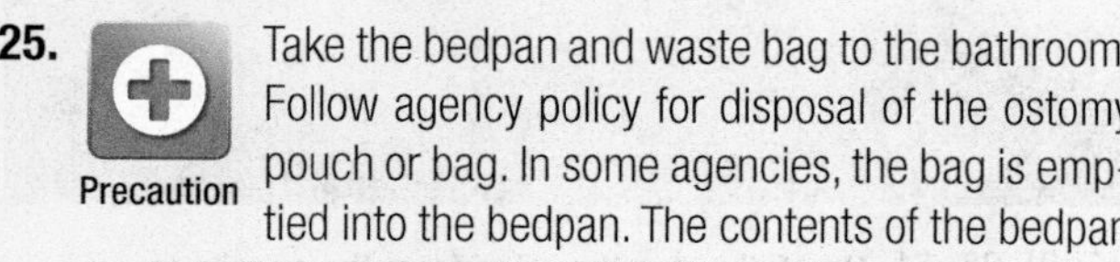

    Take the bedpan and waste bag to the bathroom. Follow agency policy for disposal of the ostomy pouch or bag. In some agencies, the bag is emptied into the bedpan. The contents of the bedpan are then flushed down the toilet. The ostomy pouch or bag

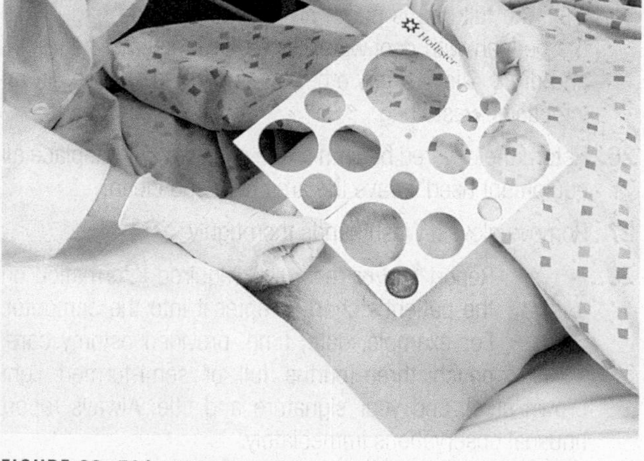

FIGURE 22–70A Check the size of the stoma to determine the correct size for the barrier or wafer.

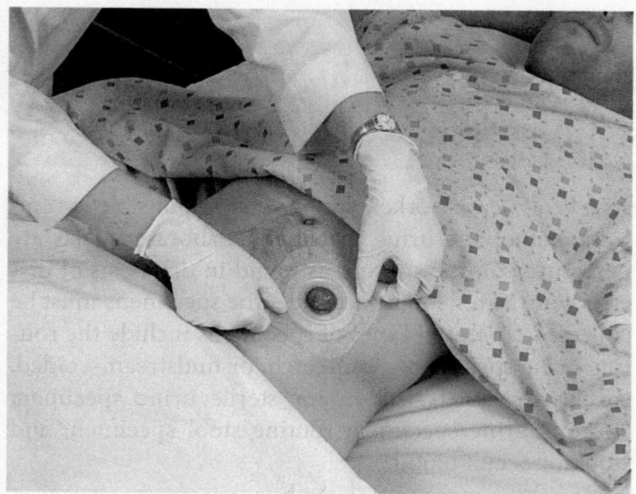

FIGURE 22–70B Position the wafer, adhesive side down, around the stoma.

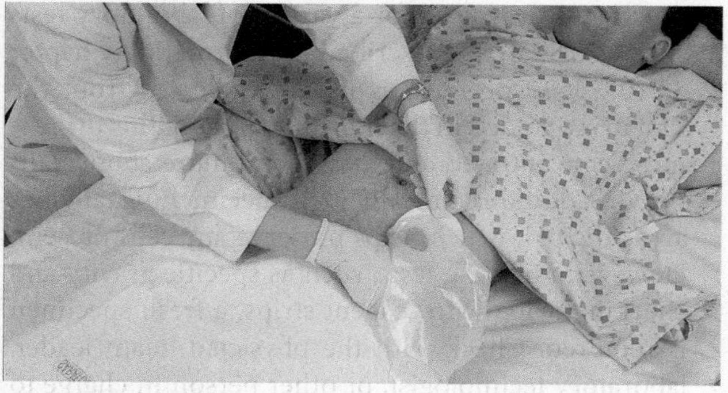

FIGURE 22–70C Gently press to snap the ostomy bag in place over the wafer.

(continues)

PROCEDURE 22:9 (CONT.)

is then placed in an infectious-waste bag. In other agencies, the full bag is put in an infectious-waste bag. Rinse the bedpan with cool water and a disinfectant. Then rinse and dry it. Discard any other contaminated supplies in an infectious-waste bag.

26. Return the covered bedpan to the patient's unit. Replace all equipment used. Leave the area neat and clean.
27. Remove gloves. Wash hands thoroughly.
28. 
Comm
Report and/or record all required information on the patient's chart or enter it into the computer. For example, date, time, provided ostomy care, pouch three-fourths full of semi-formed light brown stool, and your signature and title. Always report unusual observations immediately.

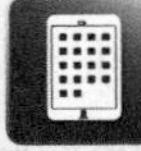
EHR
NOTE: In health care agencies using electronic health records (EHRs), also known as electronic medical records (EMRs), the information is entered directly into the patient's record on a computer.

PRACTICE: **Go to the workbook and use the evaluation sheet for 22:9, Providing Ostomy Care, to practice this procedure. When you believe you have mastered this skill, sign the sheet and give it to your instructor for further action.**

Check
FINAL CHECKPOINT: Using the criteria listed on the evaluation sheet, your instructor will grade your performance.

22:10 Collecting Stool/Urine Specimens

As a health care worker, you may be responsible for collecting stool and urine specimens. Laboratory tests are performed on the specimens to aid in diagnosis of disease. For the tests to be accurate, the specimens must be collected correctly. Types of specimens include the routine urine specimen; clean-catch, or midstream-voided, specimen; catheterization for sterile urine specimen; 24-hour urine specimen; routine stool specimen; and stool for occult blood.

Routine Urine Specimen

- A routine **urine specimen** is one of the most common specimens. It is used for a variety of laboratory tests such as urinalysis (described in information Chapter 20:10). The specimen is usually collected from the first urine voided in the morning because this urine is more concentrated and may reveal more abnormalities. In addition, a first-voided specimen usually has an acidic pH, which helps preserve any cells present. However, for some tests, such as specific gravity and checking urine with reagent strips, a fresh specimen is required. Check with the physician, team leader, laboratory technologist, or other person in charge to find out when the specimen should be collected.
- The specimen can be collected in a bedpan, urinal, or special specimen collector positioned on a toilet under the seat. The collected urine is then poured into the specimen container (Figure 22–71). It may also be collected by instructing the patient to void directly into the specimen container.
- Usually, 120 milliliters (mL) of urine is sufficient for this test. If the patient is unable to void this amount, obtain what is available and send this amount to the laboratory.
- The specimen should be sent to the laboratory immediately. If this is not possible, refrigerate the specimen until it can be sent to the laboratory.

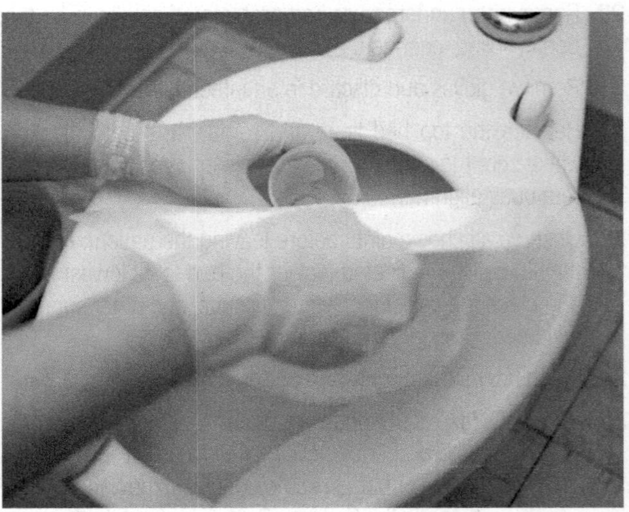
FIGURE 22–71 **Carefully pour the urine from the specimen collector into a specimen container.**

- If a specimen container is not available, any clean container can be used. Wash the container thoroughly with soap and water, then rinse and dry it. Patients should be cautioned against using containers that previously held medications, however, because using such containers can alter the results of the test.

Clean-Catch, or Midstream-Voided, Specimen

- A **midstream (clean-catch) specimen** is a urine specimen that is free from contamination. Because microorganisms are present on the genital area and on the specimen containers, special precautions are used to obtain a specimen.
- A sterile urine-specimen container, free from all microorganisms, is used to collect a midstream specimen.
- The genital area is cleansed thoroughly. This can be done by the health care worker, or the patient can be given careful instructions on how to do this procedure. Prepared wipes or clean cotton sponges or gauze squares and a mild antiseptic solution may be used.
- On a female patient, the genital area includes the perineum and the vulva. The vulva consists of two prominent folds, called the labia majora, and the structures within them: the labia minora, the urinary opening, the clitoris, and the vagina. Wipes are used to clean the external lips of the vulva. They are wiped from front to back. After each area is cleaned the wipe is discarded. The internal lips are then cleaned. Finally, the center area is cleaned from front to back. The center area contains the urinary opening (meatus).
- On a male patient, a circular motion is used. Starting at the urinary meatus (opening) at the tip of the penis, the end is cleaned thoroughly in a circular downward motion. Each wipe is discarded after each area is cleaned.

  NOTE: On uncircumcised male patients, the foreskin should be pushed back before cleaning. After the end of the penis is clean, gently push the foreskin back into its normal position.
- After the area has been cleaned, the patient is told to urinate, or void. A few drops of urine are allowed to flow into the bedpan or toilet bowl. The sterile container is then used to catch the urine that follows. The last few drops of urine should be discarded. In this way, the first and last part of the specimen are discarded, and only the middle, or midstream, urine is collected.
- The sterile lid of the container should be placed on this specimen immediately to prevent contamination. The specimen should immediately be sent to the laboratory or refrigerated.

Catheterization for Sterile Urine Specimen

- It is sometimes necessary to obtain a sterile urine specimen from a patient. In order to do this, the patient is catheterized. A narrow, hollow, sterile tube is inserted directly into the bladder. Urine from the tube is then placed in a sterile urine-specimen container.
- Specimen collection catheters are also available for obtaining a sterile urine specimen (Figure 22–72). These units contain a very small catheter attached to a collection test tube. The catheter is inserted into the bladder and urine drains directly into the tube. When the tube is full, the catheter is withdrawn. The catheter is then separated from the tube and discarded in a sharps container. The tube is sealed by pressing on the spout.
- Legal: Only a trained person should insert the catheter. However, if a catheter is already in place, you may collect a urine specimen in the sterile container (refer to Figures 22–63A and 22–63B). It is important that you work under supervision and use sterile technique to prevent contamination of the catheter when obtaining the specimen.

24-Hour Urine Specimens

- Special tests require a **24-hour urine specimen**. This means that all of the urine produced by the patient during a 24-hour period must be saved. This urine is used to check kidney function and components such as protein, creatinine, urobilinogen, hormones, and calcium.

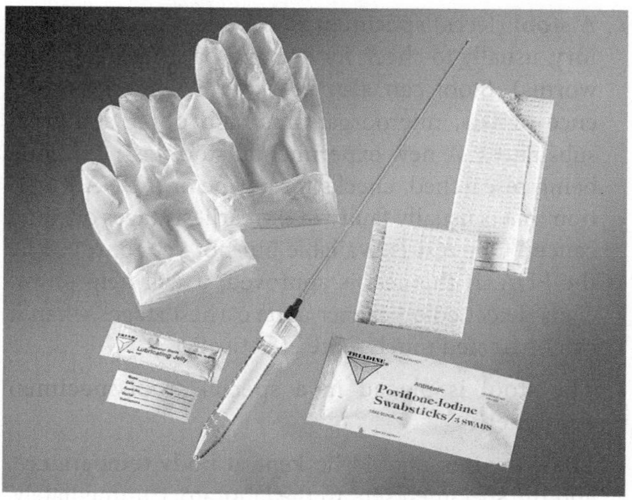

FIGURE 22–72 This Speci-Cath kit is designed to obtain a sterile urine specimen from a male patient. Courtesy of Medline Industries Inc., 1-860-MEDLINE

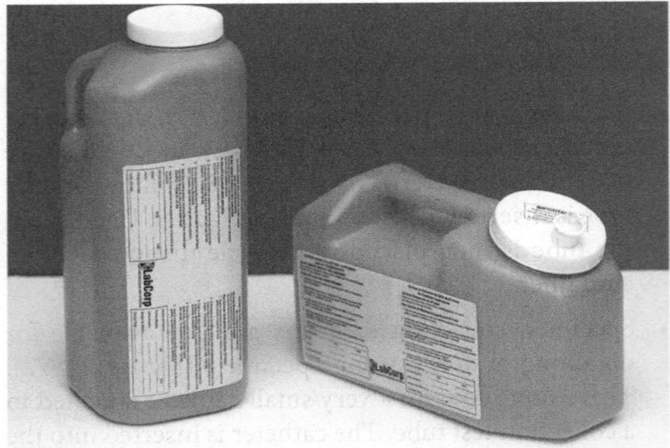

FIGURE 22–73 Different types of specimen collectors for collecting 24-hour urine specimens.

- The urine is preserved by chemicals or cold storage. The laboratory sends the correct container and instructions for preserving the specimen (Figure 22–73).
- To start, the patient voids to empty the bladder. This urine is discarded because it was produced before the start of the 24-hour period. The time of voiding is noted as the start of the 24-hour period. All urine voided in the next 24 hours is saved in the special container. At the end of the 24-hour period, the patient voids again for the final collection of urine.
- If any specimen is accidentally discarded during the 24-hour period, the test must be discontinued and restarted. In addition, toilet tissue cannot be discarded in any specimen. The tissue must be discarded in a plastic waste bag or toilet.

Routine Stool Specimen

- A **stool** (feces) **specimen** is examined by the laboratory, usually to check for ova and parasites (eggs and worms). Stool can also be examined for the presence of fats, microorganisms, and other abnormal substances. A new experimental stool test, currently being researched, checks for a gene or a DNA mutation that is usually faulty in the earliest stages of colon cancer. One test is available but not yet approved by the FDA. If this test is approved, it will help physicians detect colon cancer at its earliest stages when it can be treated much more effectively.
- The stool is placed in a special stool-specimen container.
- The container should be kept at body temperature, and the specimen sent to the laboratory immediately. For the most accurate results, it should be examined within 30 minutes.

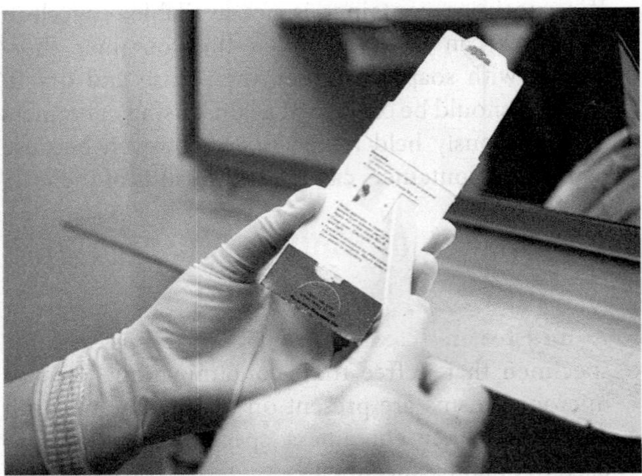

FIGURE 22–74 A small specimen of stool is placed on the Hemoccult card to test for occult blood.

Stool for Occult Blood

- Sometimes **occult blood** (blood from areas of the intestinal tract) can be found in the stool. Testing for occult blood requires only a small amount of stool.
- A special card is usually used for this test. The small specimen of stool is placed on a designated section(s) of the card (Figure 22–74).
- The card is sent to the laboratory or checked immediately by an authorized individual in some health care facilities. A few drops of a special developing solution, such as Hemoccult, is added to the area. A color change indicates a positive result.
- A positive test means that blood is present in the stool.
- The test for occult blood does not require that the stool be kept warm or that it be examined immediately. However, it should be sent to the laboratory as soon as possible so that the specimen is not misplaced.

Summary

All specimens must be labeled correctly, including the kind of specimen (urine or stool), the test ordered, the patient's name, room number or identification (ID) number, the date and time, and the physician's name. It is best to label the specimen container instead of the lid because errors could occur if the lid is misplaced. All required information must also be printed on the correct lab requisition form. A lab requisition must be sent with the labeled specimen. Health care agencies with electronic health records (EHRs), also called electronic medical records (EMRs), use computer-generated labels for the specimen container and lab requisition form.

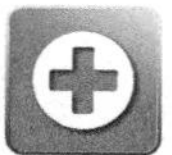
Precaution

Standard precautions (discussed in Chapter 15:4) must be observed when obtaining and handling urine or stool specimens. Gloves must be worn. Hands must be washed frequently and are always washed immediately after removing gloves. Eye protection must be worn if splashing or spraying of body fluids is possible. Any areas contaminated with urine or stool must be wiped with a disinfectant. To avoid contamination from spills, all urine or stool specimens are placed in special biohazard bags before being transported to the laboratory for testing. Taking proper precautions can help prevent the spread of infection.

STUDENT: Go to the workbook and complete the assignment sheet for 22:10, Collecting Stool/Urine Specimens. Then return and continue with the procedures.

PROCEDURE 22:10A

Collecting a Routine Urine Specimen

Equipment and Supplies

Bedpan with cover/urinal or specimen collector, urine-specimen container and label, toilet tissue, graduate or measuring pitcher, disposable gloves, infectious-waste bag, biohazard bag, paper and pen or computer

Procedure

1. Check physician's orders or obtain authorization from your immediate supervisor to be sure you are collecting the right type of specimen.

   NOTE: In most cases, the first-voided specimen of the day is collected.

2. Assemble equipment.

3. 
   Comm

   Knock on the door and pause before entering. Close the door and pull the curtain for privacy. Introduce yourself. Identify the patient. Explain the procedure and obtain consent.

4. Wash hands. Put on gloves.

   Precaution

   CAUTION: Observe standard precautions when obtaining and handling urine specimens.

5. If the patient is ambulatory, assist the patient to the bathroom.

   a. Place a specimen collector on the toilet and then reposition the toilet seat.

   b. Instruct the patient to discard the toilet tissue into the toilet and not into the specimen collector. An infectious waste bag can also be provided for the discarded tissue.

   c. Provide privacy while the patient voids. Make sure the call signal and toilet tissue are within reach.

   d. After the specimen has been collected, assist the patient back to a chair or bed.

6. If the patient is not ambulatory, offer the bedpan or urinal as previously instructed in Procedure 22:7A or 22:7B.

   a. Advise the patient not to put toilet tissue in the bedpan or urinal. Provide an infectious-waste bag for disposal of soiled toilet tissue.

   b. After the patient has voided, remove the bedpan or urinal. Place it on top of an underpad or bed protector that has been placed on the chair.

7. Remove gloves and wash hands thoroughly.

8. When the specimen has been obtained, allow the patient to wash his or her hands.

9. Observe all checkpoints before leaving the patient: position the patient comfortably and in correct body alignment, elevate the siderails (if indicated), place the call signal and supplies within easy reach of the patient, lower the bed to its lowest level, and leave the area neat and clean.

10. Put on clean gloves.

11. Take the bedpan or urinal to the patient's bathroom or remove the specimen collector from the toilet. Pour the urine into a measuring pitcher or graduate.

    NOTE: Record the amount if an intake and output (I&O) record is being kept for the patient (Figure 22–75).

12. Pour approximately 120 mL into the urine-specimen container.

13. Wash the outside of the container to remove any spilled urine. Remove gloves. Wash hands.

(continues)

PROCEDURE 22:10A (CONT.)

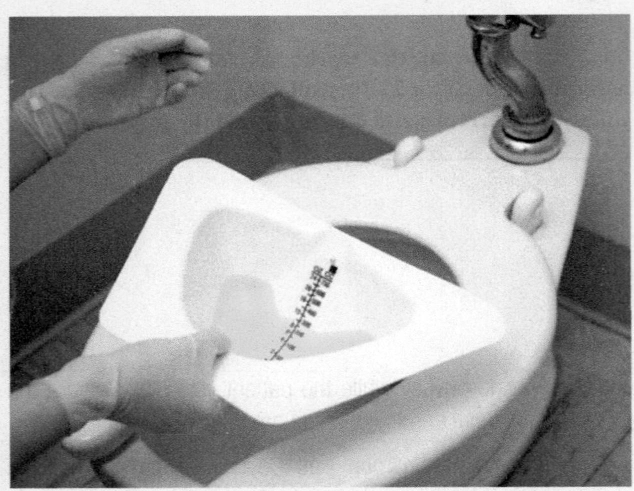

FIGURE 22–75 **If an I&O record is being kept for the patient, measure the amount of urine in the specimen collector.**

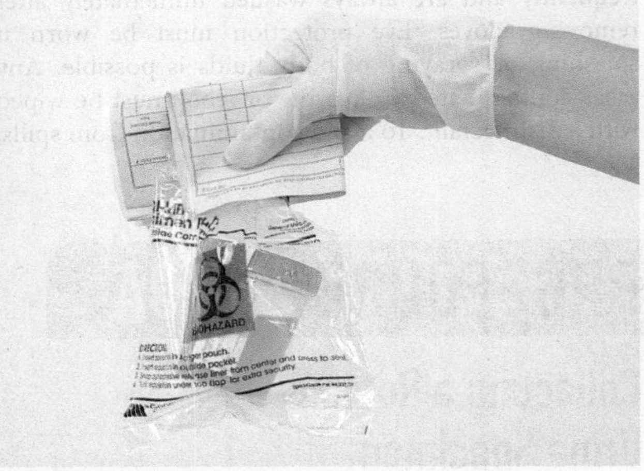

FIGURE 22–76 **All specimens must be placed in protective biohazard bags before being transported to the laboratory.**

Safety

CAUTION: Do not allow water to enter the container. Water will dilute the urine specimen and affect the accuracy of the test results.

14. Place the cover on the container.

15. 
Comm

Label the container or attach the computer-generated label. Include the date, time, patient's name, room or ID number, specimen type, test required, and physician's name. Print required information on the correct lab requisition; obtain the requisition from your immediate supervisor or use the computer-generated requisition. A lab requisition must be sent with the labeled specimen.

16. Clean and replace all equipment.

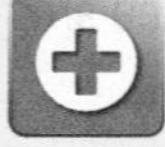
Precaution

CAUTION: Remember to wear gloves and observe standard precautions when cleaning any equipment or area contaminated with urine.

17. Precaution

Put the specimen in a protective biohazard bag for transport (Figure 22–76). Take or send the specimen to the laboratory immediately. Report the arrival of the specimen to laboratory personnel. If this is not possible, refrigerate the specimen until it can be sent to the laboratory.

18. Wash hands thoroughly.

19. 
Comm

Report and/or record all required information on patient's chart or enter it into the computer. For example, date, time, routine urine specimen collected and sent to lab, and your signature and title.

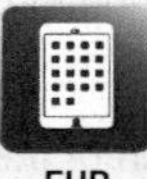
EHR

NOTE: In health care agencies using electronic health records (EHRs), also known as electronic medical records (EMRs), the information is entered directly into the patient's record on a computer.

PRACTICE: Go to the workbook and use the evaluation sheet for 22:10A, Collecting a Routine Urine Specimen, to practice this procedure. When you believe you have mastered this skill, sign the sheet and give it to your instructor for further action.

Check

FINAL CHECKPOINT: Using the criteria listed on the evaluation sheet, your instructor will grade your performance.

PROCEDURE 22:10B

Collecting a Midstream Urine Specimen

Equipment and Supplies

Sterile urine-specimen bottle and label, prepared wipes or gauze or cotton squares with antiseptic solution, small basin, infectious-waste bag, biohazard bag, disposable gloves, underpad or bed protector (if needed), paper and pen or computer

Procedure

1. Check physician's orders or obtain authorization from your immediate supervisor to be sure you are collecting the correct type of specimen.
2. Assemble equipment.
3. Comm Knock on the door and pause before entering. Introduce yourself. Identify the patient. Explain the procedure and obtain consent.
4. Wash hands.
5. Close the door and pull the curtain to provide privacy for the patient. Elevate the bed to a comfortable working height. If siderails are present and elevated, lower the siderail on the side where you are working. If the patient is ambulatory, the specimen can be collected in the bathroom. If the patient is not ambulatory, provide a bedpan or urinal as instructed in Procedure 22:7A or 22:7B.
6. Provide the patient with prepared wipes. If the wipes are not available, a gauze or cotton square and antiseptic solution can be used. In many agencies, a special kit is available for collecting midstream specimens. Follow the instructions that come with the kit, if one is used.
7. Put on disposable gloves.

   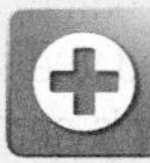
   Precaution

   CAUTION: Wear gloves and observe standard precautions when obtaining urine specimens.
8. Wash the genital area correctly or instruct the patient on how to do so.
   a. For a female patient, use the prepared wipes to clean the outer folds from front to back. Use a clean wipe for each area cleaned. Discard each wipe in the infectious-waste bag after one use. Clean the inner folds (lips) from front to back, using a clean wipe for each area cleaned. Discard each wipe after use. Finally, clean the innermost (middle) area from front to back. Discard soiled wipe.
   b. For a male patient, use a circular motion to clean from the urinary meatus outward and downward. Discard each wipe after one area is cleaned in the infectious-waste bag. Repeat at least two times or until the entire area is clean.

   NOTE: On uncircumcised male patients, the foreskin should be pushed back before cleaning. After cleaning, gently push the foreskin back to its normal position.
9. Instruct the patient to void. Allow the first part of the stream to escape. Catch the middle of the stream in the sterile specimen container. Allow the last part of the stream to escape.

   NOTE: If the amount must be measured because an intake and output (I&O) record is being kept for the patient, catch the first and last urine in a bedpan or urinal or in a specimen collector if the patient is on the toilet.
10. Place the sterile cap on the container immediately to prevent contamination of the specimen (Figure 22–77).

    Safety

    CAUTION: Do not touch the inside of the specimen container or the inside of the lid because this will contaminate the specimen.

    NOTE: Some midstream-specimen containers have a funnel that aids in the collection of the specimen. This is removed and discarded in the infectious-waste bag before the sterile cap is placed on the container.
11. Allow the patient to wash his or her hands.
12. Observe all checkpoints before leaving the patient: position the patient in correct body alignment, elevate the siderails (if indicated), lower the bed to its lowest level, place the call signal and supplies within easy reach of the patient, and leave the area neat and clean.

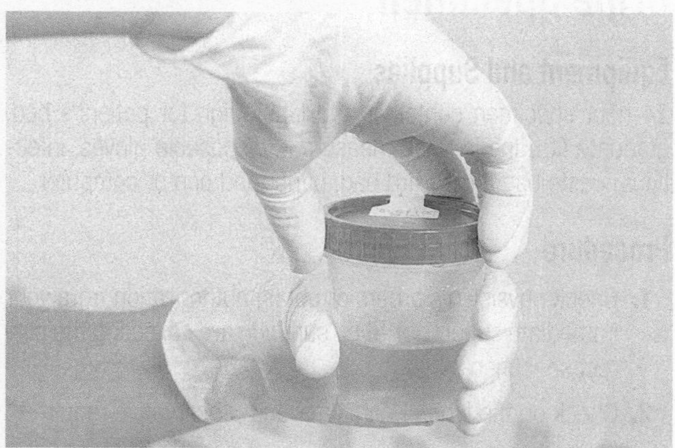

FIGURE 22–77 Place the sterile cap on the container immediately after collecting the urine specimen.

(continues)

PROCEDURE 22:10B (CONT.)

NOTE: Use a paper towel with a gloved hand or a one-glove method to avoid contaminating the environment.

13. Wash the outside of the container. Remove gloves and wash hands.
14. Comm Label the container as a "Midstream" or "Clean-Catch" specimen or attach a computer-generated label. Print the name of the ordered test, the patient's name, room number or ID number, the date and time, and physician's name on the label. Print required information on the correct lab requisition. Obtain the requisition from your immediate supervisor or use a computer-generated requisition. A lab requisition must be sent with the labeled specimen.
15. Clean and replace all equipment.

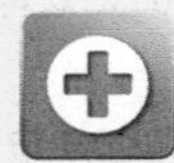
Precaution **CAUTION:** Remember to wear gloves and observe standard precautions when cleaning any equipment or area contaminated with urine.

16. Precaution Put the specimen in a protective biohazard bag for transport. Take or send the specimen to the laboratory immediately. Report the arrival of the specimen to laboratory personnel. If this is not possible, refrigerate the specimen until it can be sent to the laboratory.

NOTE: For the most accurate results, the specimen should be examined as soon as possible.

17. Wash hands thoroughly.
18.  Comm Report and/or record all required information on the patient's chart or enter it into the computer. For example, date, time, midstream urine specimen collected and sent to laboratory, and your signature and title.

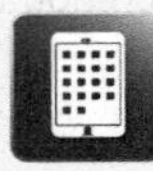
EHR **NOTE:** In health care agencies using electronic health records (EHRs), also known as electronic medical records (EMRs), the information is entered directly into the patient's record on a computer.

PRACTICE: **Go to the workbook and use the evaluation sheet for 22:10B, Collecting a Midstream Urine Specimen, to practice this procedure. When you believe you have mastered this skill, sign the sheet and give it to your instructor for further action.**

Check **FINAL CHECKPOINT:** Using the criteria listed on the evaluation sheet, your instructor will grade your performance.

PROCEDURE 22:10C

Collecting a 24-Hour Urine Specimen

Equipment and Supplies

24-hour specimen container and label, sign for patient's bed, graduate (if urine is to be measured), disposable gloves, infectious-waste bag, biohazard bag, paper and pen or computer

Procedure

1. Check physician's orders or obtain authorization from your immediate supervisor to be sure you are collecting the correct specimen.
2. Check on the type of container and preservative required.

   NOTE: Some containers for certain tests contain chemical preservatives. Others must be kept on ice or refrigerated during the 24 hours. The laboratory will supply information about the correct method for preserving the specimen.
3. Assemble equipment.
4. Comm Label the container with the patient's name, room number or ID number, the test ordered, the specimen type, the date, and the physician's name, or attach a computer-generated label.
5. Comm Knock on the door and pause before entering. Close the door and pull the curtain for privacy. Introduce yourself. Identify the patient. Explain the procedure and obtain consent. Tell the patient not to discard toilet tissue in the urine specimen. Provide a plastic waste bag for disposal of toilet tissue.

   NOTE: Make sure the patient understands the entire procedure. Stress the importance of saving all urine.
6. Wash hands. Put on disposable gloves.

PROCEDURE 22:10C (CONT.)

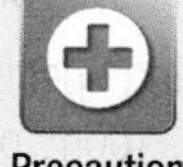
Precaution

CAUTION: Remember to wear gloves and observe standard precautions when obtaining urine and placing it in a 24-hour specimen container.

7. Allow the patient to void. Assist with the bedpan or urinal, if necessary. Measure the amount if an intake and output (I&O) record is being kept for the patient. Discard this specimen. Note the time of voiding as the start of the 24-hour period.

   NOTE: Urine voided at this time has been produced before the 24-hour time period. The patient must begin the 24-hour period with an empty bladder.

   NOTE: For female patients allowed to use the bathroom, a specimen collector can be placed under the seat in the toilet (refer to Figure 22–71). The patient must be told not to discard toilet tissue or defecate in the specimen collector.

8. Remove gloves. Wash hands thoroughly.
9. Place a sign on the patient's bed and/or in the bathroom to alert others that a 24–hour specimen is being collected. The sign usually states, "Save all urine—24-hour specimen."
10. During the 24-hour period, use the specimen container to collect all urine voided (Figure 22–78).

    NOTE: If any urine is discarded, the procedure must be stopped and started again.

11. At the end of the 24-hour period, ask the patient to void. Add this urine to the specimen container. It is the final voiding of the procedure.
12. Remove the sign from the patient's bed.
13.  Comm — Check the specimen label to make sure it is accurate and contains all the required information. Print the required information on the correct lab requisition. Obtain the requisition from your immediate supervisor or use a computer-generated requisition. A lab requisition must be sent with the labeled specimen.
14. Precaution — Put the specimen in a protective biohazard bag for transport. Take or send the specimen to the laboratory immediately. Notify laboratory personnel of the specimen's arrival.

    NOTE: For the most accurate results, urine should go to the laboratory as soon as possible.

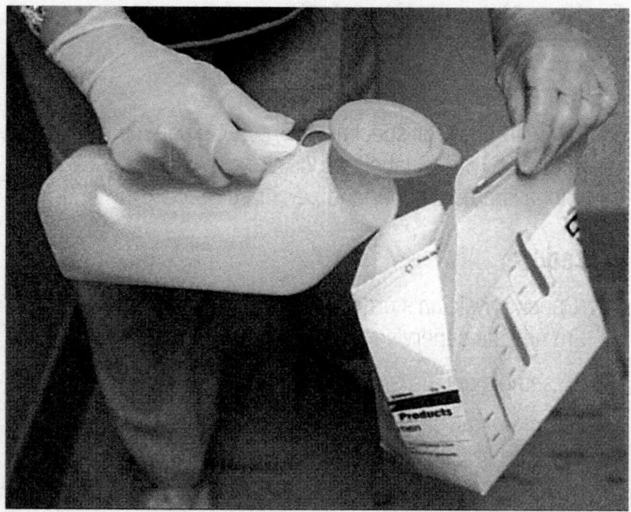

FIGURE 22–78 **All urine voided during the 24-hour period must be placed in the specimen container.**

15. Replace all equipment used.
16. Remove gloves. Wash hands thoroughly.
17.  Comm — Report and/or record all required information on the patient's chart or enter it into the computer. For example, date, time, 24-hour urine specimen completed and sent to laboratory, and your signature and title.

    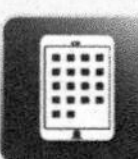 EHR

    NOTE: In health care agencies using electronic health records (EHRs), also known as electronic medical records (EMRs), the information is entered directly into the patient's record on a computer.

PRACTICE: Go to the workbook and use the evaluation sheet for 22:10C, Collecting a 24-Hour Urine Specimen, to practice this procedure. When you believe you have mastered this skill, sign the sheet and give it to your instructor for further action.

Check

FINAL CHECKPOINT: Using the criteria listed on the evaluation sheet, your instructor will grade your performance.

PROCEDURE 22:10D

Collecting a Stool Specimen

Equipment and Supplies

Bedpan with cover or specimen collector, stool-specimen container, tongue blades, label, disposable gloves, infectious-waste bag, biohazard bag, paper and pen or computer

Procedure

1. Check physician's orders or obtain authorization from your immediate supervisor; verify the type of specimen needed.
2. Assemble equipment.
3. 
Comm
Knock on the door and pause before entering. Close the door and pull the curtain for privacy. Introduce yourself. Identify the patient. Explain the procedure and obtain consent. Ask the patient to use the bedpan for his or her next bowel movement because a specimen is needed. Ask the patient not to void or place toilet tissue in the bedpan. Provide an infectious-waste bag for soiled toilet tissue.

   NOTE: In some agencies, specimen collectors that fit directly under the toilet seat are used.
4. Wash hands. Put on disposable gloves.

   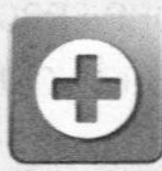
   Precaution
   CAUTION: Wear gloves and observe standard precautions when obtaining stool specimens.
5. Obtain the specimen in the bedpan. Allow the patient to wash his or her hands.

   NOTE: Assist with the bedpan, as necessary.
6. Take the bedpan to the bathroom.
7. Use two tongue blades to remove the stool from the bedpan. Place the stool in the specimen container. Discard the tongue blades in the infectious-waste bag.
8. Remove gloves and wash hands thoroughly.

   Safety
   CAUTION: Avoid contaminating the outside of the container.
9. Place the lid on the container. Make sure it is tightly in place.
10. 
Comm
Label the container correctly, including specimen type, test ordered, patient's name, room or ID number, date and time, and physician's name, or attach a computer-generated label. Print the required information on the correct lab requisition. Obtain the requisition from your immediate supervisor or use a computer-generated requisition. A lab requisition must be sent with the labeled specimen.
11. Put on gloves to clean the bedpan. Rinse the bedpan with cool water. Clean with a disinfectant, and rinse and dry. Replace all equipment used. Leave the area neat and clean.
12. Remove gloves and wash hands.
13. 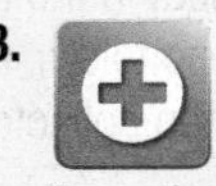
Precaution
Keep the specimen warm. Put the specimen in a protective biohazard bag for transport. Take or send it to the laboratory immediately. Report the arrival of the specimen to laboratory personnel.

    NOTE: The specimen should be examined within 30 minutes for most accurate results.
14. Wash hands.
15. 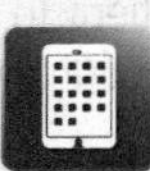
Comm
Report and/or record all required information on the patient's chart or enter it into the computer. For example, date, time, stool specimen collected and sent to laboratory, and your signature and title.

    EHR
    NOTE: In health care agencies using electronic health records (EHRs), also known as electronic medical records (EMRs), the information is entered directly into the patient's record on a computer.

PRACTICE: **Go to the workbook and use the evaluation sheet for 22:10D, Collecting a Stool Specimen, to practice this procedure. When you believe you have mastered this skill, sign the sheet and give it to your instructor for further action.**

Check
FINAL CHECKPOINT: Using the criteria listed on the evaluation sheet, your instructor will grade your performance.

PROCEDURE 22:10E

Preparing and Testing a Hemoccult Slide

Legal

NOTE: Legal requirements regarding who can perform this procedure vary from state to state. Check your legal responsibilities before performing this procedure.

Equipment and Supplies

Bedpan with cover/specimen collector, Hemoccult slide packet, Hemoccult developer, tongue blade, paper towel, disposable gloves, infectious-waste bag, biohazard bag, paper and pen or computer

Procedure

1. Obtain proper authorization to be sure of the type of specimen needed.
2. Assemble equipment. Read the manufacturer's instructions for the use of the Hemoccult slide packet and developer.
3.  Comm — Knock on the door and pause before entering. Close the door and pull the curtain for privacy. Introduce yourself. Identify the patient. Explain the procedure and obtain consent. Ask the patient to use the bedpan for his or her next bowel movement because a specimen is needed. Tell the patient not to void or place toilet tissue in the specimen in the bedpan. If necessary, provide an infectious-waste bag for disposal of soiled toilet tissue.

   NOTE: In some agencies, specimen collectors that fit directly under the toilet seat are used.
4. Wash hands. Put on gloves.

   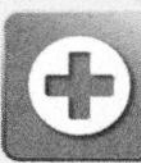 Precaution

   CAUTION: Wear gloves and observe standard precautions when obtaining stool specimens.
5. Obtain the specimen in the bedpan. Assist the patient, as necessary. Allow the patient to wash his or her hands.
6. Take the bedpan and specimen to the bathroom.
7. Place a paper towel on the counter. Put the Hemoccult slide packet on top of the towel.
8. Open the front cover or flap of the Hemoccult packet.
9. Use the tongue blade to smear a small amount of the stool specimen on the correct areas of the slide (refer to Figure 22–74). Use different parts of the stool specimen to obtain sample smears for each of the two areas.

   NOTE: Read the instructions. One or two small areas of exposed guaiac paper are present under the cover. Stool is placed on these areas.

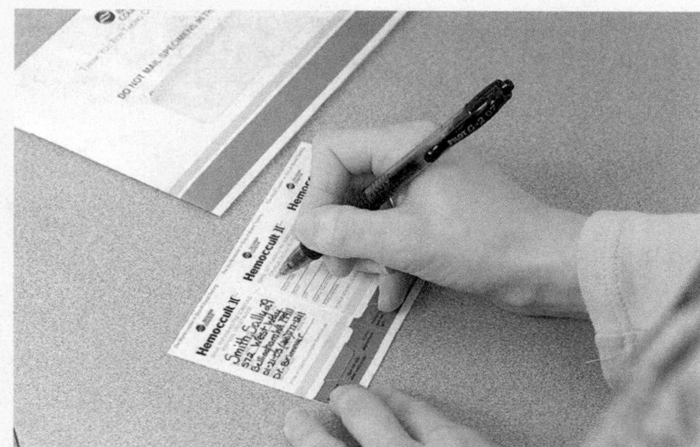

FIGURE 22–79A **Label the Hemoccult packet with all required information.**

10. Discard the tongue blade in an infectious-waste bag.
11. Remove gloves and wash hands.
12. Close the cover or flap of the Hemoccult packet.
13. Comm — Label the outside of the Hemoccult packet with all the required information, usually the date and time, patient's name, room or ID number, and physician's name (Figure 22–79A), or attach a computer-generated label. Print the required information on the correct lab requisition. Obtain the requisition from your immediate supervisor or use a computer-generated requisition. A lab requisition must be sent with the labeled specimen.
14. 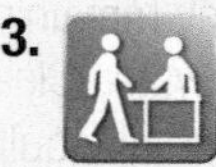 Precaution — Send the Hemoccult packet to the laboratory for developing. Put the specimen in a protective biohazard bag for transport. In some agencies, you may be required to complete the test. To develop the test, proceed as follows:
    a. Wash hands and put on gloves.
    b. Open the back tab of the Hemoccult packet to expose the back of the guaiac paper.
    c. Place the required number of drops (usually one to two) of Hemoccult developer on the exposed guaiac paper (Figure 22–79B). Some packets also have test areas to which developer is applied.

       NOTE: Read and follow manufacturer's instructions.
    d. Wait the correct amount of time, usually 30–60 seconds.
    e. Check the areas for color change. A positive test usually causes a blue or purple discoloration of the smear (Figure 22–79C).

(continues)

PROCEDURE 22:10E (CONT.)

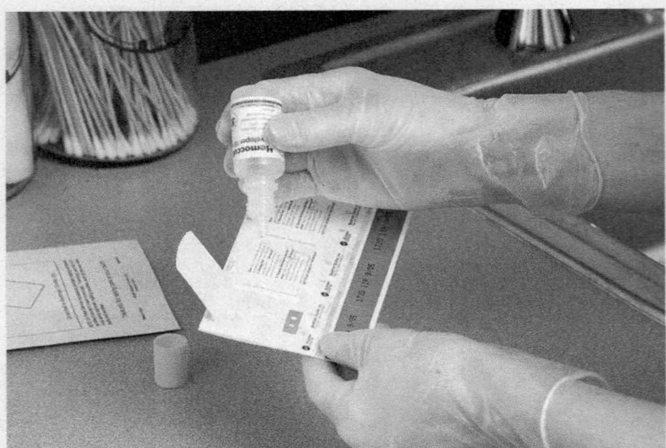

FIGURE 22–79B **Place the required number of drops of Hemoccult developing solution on the exposed guaiac paper.**

READING AND INTERPRETING THE HEMOCCULT® TEST

Negative Smears

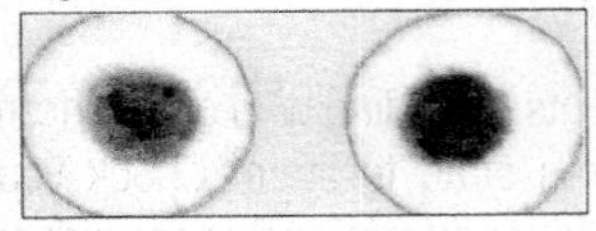

Sample report: negative
No detectable blue on or at the edge of the smears indicates the test is negative for occult blood.

Negative and Positive Smears

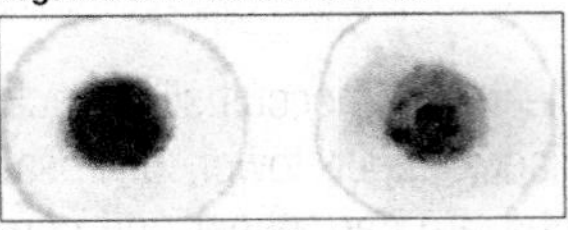

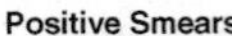

Positive Smears

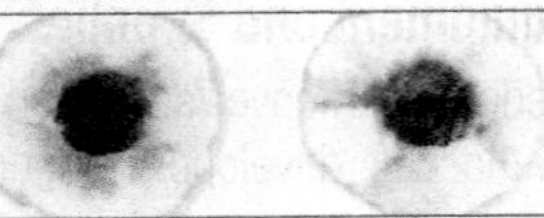

Sample report: positive
Any trace of blue on or at the edge of one or more of the smears indicates the test is positive for occult blood.

FIGURE 22–79C **A change in color indicates that blood is present in the stool.**

NOTE: A positive test indicates the presence of blood in the stool.

f. Remove gloves and wash hands.

15. Put on gloves to clean the bedpan. Discard any remaining stool in the toilet. Rinse the bedpan with cool water. Clean with a disinfectant, then rinse and dry. Replace all equipment used. Leave the area neat and clean.

16. Remove gloves and wash hands.

17. 

Report and/or record all required information on the patient's chart or enter it into the computer. For example, date, time, Hemoccult stool specimen obtained and sent to laboratory, and your signature and title.

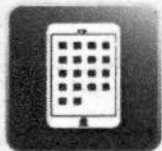

NOTE: In health care agencies using electronic health records (EHRs), also known as electronic medical records (EMRs), the information is entered directly into the patient's record on a computer.

PRACTICE: **Go to the workbook and use the evaluation sheet for 22:10E, Preparing and Testing a Hemoccult Slide, to practice this procedure. When you believe you have mastered this skill, sign the sheet and give it to your instructor for further action.**

FINAL CHECKPOINT: Using the criteria listed on the evaluation sheet, your instructor will grade your performance.

22:11 Enemas and Rectal Treatments

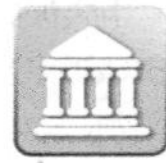

NOTE: Responsibility for performing these procedures varies from agency to agency. Check your agency's policy.

As a health care worker, you may be required to perform a number of rectal treatments. Equipment and solutions will vary from agency to agency, but the same basic principles are followed.

An **enema** is an injection of fluid into the large intestine through the rectum. The main purpose of an enema is to remove feces and flatus (gas) from the colon and rectum. In addition, enemas can be used to relieve intestinal congestion and give medication. Before some surgeries and imaging procedures, enemas may be ordered to clear the bowel of fecal material. The order may state, "enemas until clear." This means that enemas are given until the return solution is the same as that injected, and no fecal material is present. Check with your immediate supervisor to determine how many enemas can be given. Overuse of enemas can be dangerous. There is a risk of depleting minerals and electrolyte levels. No more than the maximum prescribed dose should be given.

Legal

A physician's order is required. The order usually states the type of enema and the amount of solution; it may also give other information such as time, purpose, or special instructions.

Enemas are frequently classified as retention or nonretention enemas:

- *Retention enemas* are small amounts of solution that are retained, or kept, in the intestine for a specified period after they are given. They are used to instill medications, soften stool, aid in elimination of intestinal parasites, lubricate the rectum, or expel flatus.
- *Nonretention enemas* are usually expelled in 5–10 minutes. Larger quantities of solution are usually given, and the enemas are generally used to clean the bowel of feces and flatus (gas).

Types of enemas frequently used are cleansing enemas, disposable enemas, and oil-retention enemas.

- *Cleansing enema*: This is usually a soap-solution, tap-water, or normal saline solution enema. Soap-solution enemas irritate the intestine and may kill beneficial bacteria (gut flora), so they are no longer used as frequently as tap-water or normal saline enemas. Normal saline is usually the preferred solution because it is an isotonic solution. It is the same concentration as body fluids and, therefore, does not cause fluid imbalances. A large amount of the solution, 750–1,000 milliliters (mL), is usually given. The main purpose is to remove stool and flatus.
- *Disposable enema*: This is also a cleansing enema, in most cases. However, these enemas come in prepared, disposable containers, each containing 4–6 ounces (120–180 mL) of solution. The solution tends to be hypertonic, meaning that it draws fluid from the body to stimulate peristalsis and elimination of stool and flatus.
- *Oil-retention enema*: Mineral or olive oil may be used. Commercially prepared enemas containing oil are also available. They usually contain 4–6 ounces of oil. These enemas are retained for at least 30–60 minutes. The main purpose is to soften fecal material so that it can be expelled. An oil-retention enema is sometimes followed with a cleansing enema.

The patient receiving an enema is usually placed in the Sims' (left lateral) position. This encourages the solution to flow from the rectum to the sigmoid portion of the colon. The patient should be encouraged to breathe deeply during enema administration. Deep breathing encourages relaxation and increases retention of the solution for more effective results.

Comm

Results must be observed after an enema is given. Amount, type, and color of stool, and the amount of flatus expelled should be recorded.

An **impaction** is a large, hard mass of fecal material lodged in the intestine or rectum. Oil-retention enemas are frequently ordered to soften the impaction so it can be expelled. If it cannot be removed by an enema, it is sometimes necessary to insert a lubricated, gloved finger into the rectum to break up the fecal material. The licensed supervisor or advanced care provider usually performs this procedure.

Gas (flatus) accumulation in the intestine is a frequent problem for surgical patients. A **rectal tube** may be inserted to aid in the expulsion of flatus. The tube is usually left in place for 20–30 minutes. Because fecal material may drain out of the tube, it is wise to place the open end of the tube in a basin or container. This procedure also is ordered by the physician.

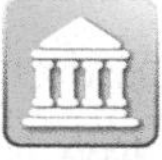
Legal

A **suppository** is a cone-shaped object that usually has a base material of cocoa butter or glycerin. It is inserted into the rectum and melts as a result of body heat. Suppositories are used to stimulate peristalsis and aid in expelling feces. Medicated suppositories have medication added to the base material. They can be used to relieve pain, decrease body temperature (aspirin suppositories), stop vomiting (antiemetics), and treat other conditions, depending on the medication given. A health care worker who is *not* authorized to administer medications is not allowed to insert medicated suppositories.

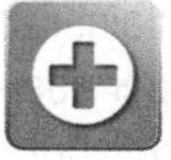
Precaution

Feces is contaminated with many microorganisms, so standard precautions (discussed in Chapter 15:4) must be observed when giving enemas and rectal treatments. Gloves must be worn. Hands must be washed frequently and are always washed immediately when gloves are removed. Eye protection must be worn if spraying or splashing of body fluids is possible. Any areas or equipment contaminated with fecal material must be cleaned with a disinfectant or sterilized. Most agencies use disposable enema kits and rectal tubes. These are discarded in an infectious-waste bag after use. Precautions must be taken at all times to prevent the spread of infection.

STUDENT: **Go to the workbook and complete the assignment sheet for 22:11, Enemas and Rectal Treatments. Then return and continue with the procedures.**

PROCEDURE 22:11A

Giving a Tap-Water, Normal Saline, or Soap-Solution Enema

Equipment and Supplies

Disposable enema kit (or irrigation container or bag with tubing, rectal tube, and liquid soap for a soap-solution enema), graduate or measuring pitcher, bath thermometer, paper towels, lubricating jelly, tray, two towels, toilet tissue, bedpan with cover, bath blanket, underpad or bed protector, disposable gloves, basin, washcloth, soap, infectious-waste bag, paper and pen or computer

NOTE: If cleansing cloths are available, they can be used in place of the basin, soap, and washcloth.

Procedure

1. Check physician's orders authorization from your supervisor.

   NOTE: The physician's order usually states the type of enema and amount to be given.

2. Assemble equipment.
3. Wash hands. Put on gloves.

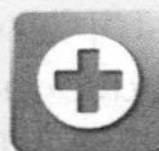

Precaution

CAUTION: Wear gloves and observe standard precautions when giving an enema.

4. Prepare the tray in the utility room or bathroom.
5. If necessary, attach the tubing to the irrigation container or bag (Figure 22–80A). Adjust the clamp to the proper position on the tubing (Figure 22–80B). Snap the clamp shut.

   NOTE: If the tubing does not have a rectal tube tip, attach a rectal tube.

6. Fill the irrigation container with tap water (or normal saline if ordered) to the 1,000-milliliter (mL) line or to the level ordered by the physician (Figure 22–80C). Use a bath thermometer to check the temperature of the water; it should measure 105°F (41°C) (Figure 22–80D).

Safety

CAUTION: Be sure the temperature is accurate. If the solution is too hot, it will burn the mucous membrane of the patient. If it is too cold, it could cause cramps and discomfort.

   NOTE: If the irrigation container does not have measurement markings, use a graduate or measuring pitcher to measure the amount needed. Then pour the solution into the irrigation container or bag.

   NOTE: Water is used for a tap-water or soap-solution enema. Prepared normal saline (NS) solution is used for an NS enema.

7. Put the packet of liquid soap into the water if a soap-solution enema is ordered (Figure 22–80E). Stir gently to prevent suds formation.

   NOTE: If a packet of soap is not provided, usually 20–30 mL of castile soap are added to the water. Soap is not added to the solution for a tap-water or NS enema.

8. Run the solution through the tubing to remove air from the tubing (Figure 22–80F). Clamp the tubing closed (Figure 22–80G).

   NOTE: This step can also be done immediately before insertion of the enema.

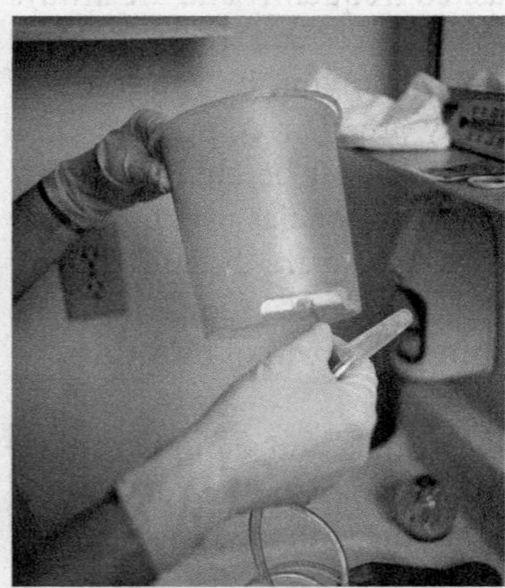

FIGURE 22–80A Attach the tubing to the enema container.

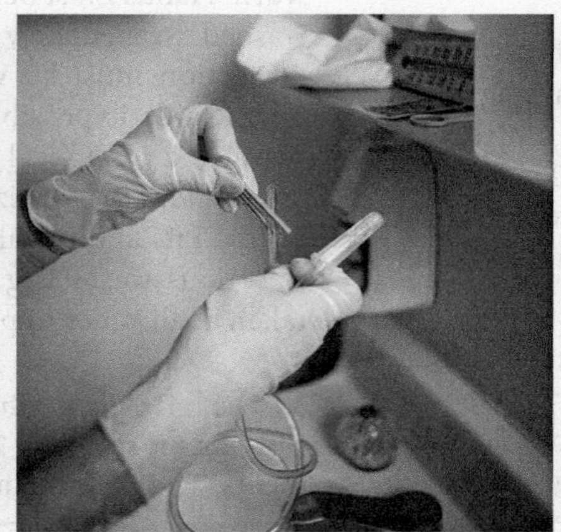

FIGURE 22–80B Slip the clamp into position on the tubing, and snap the clamp shut.

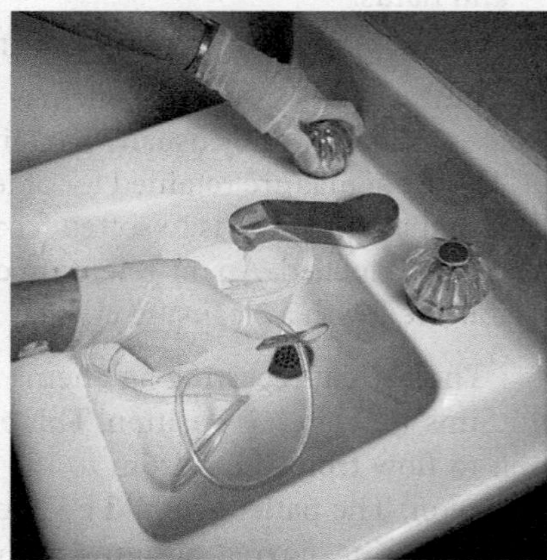

FIGURE 22–80C Fill the container with water to the 1,000-milliliter (mL) line or the level ordered by the physician.

PROCEDURE 22:11A (CONT.)

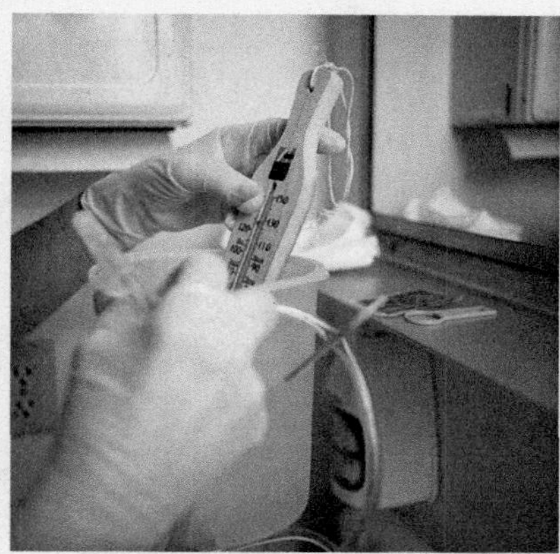

FIGURE 22–80D **Use a bath thermometer to check the temperature of the water; it must measure 105°F.**

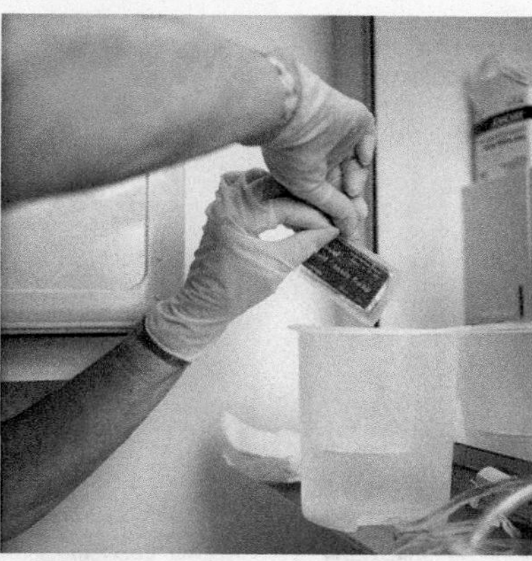

FIGURE 22–80E **Add the packet of soap to the container if a soap-solution enema is ordered.**

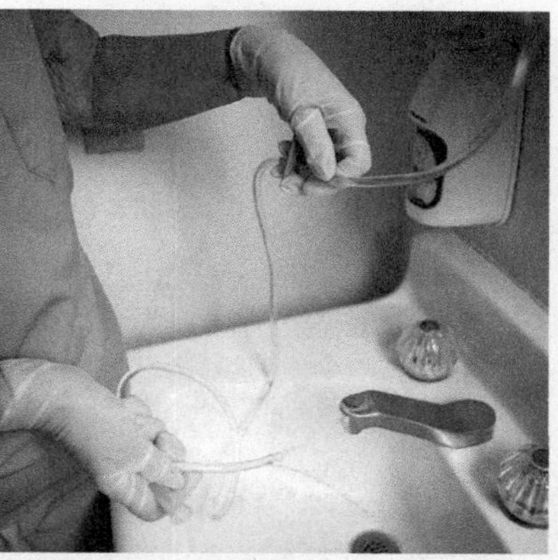

FIGURE 22–80F **Run the solution through the tubing to remove air from the tubing.**

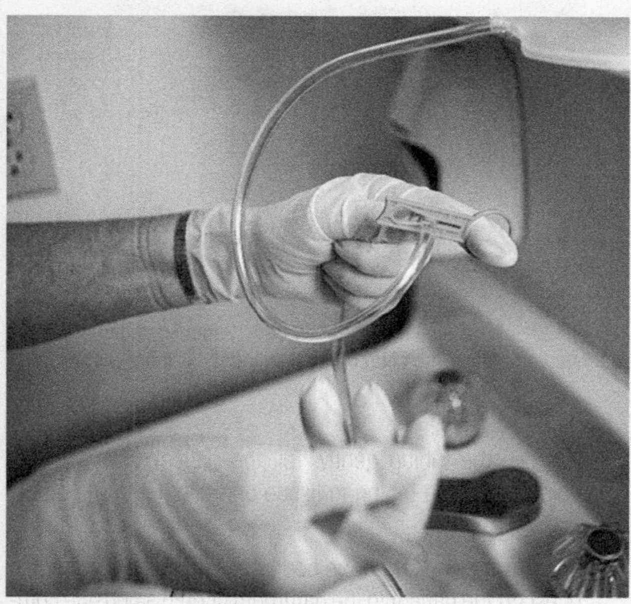

FIGURE 22–80G **Clamp the tubing.**

9. Place a small amount of lubricant on a paper towel. Place the tip of the tubing into the towel.

   NOTE: Even prelubricated tips usually require additional lubrication.

10. Place all equipment on the tray. Check to be sure all equipment is there. Cover the tray with a towel. Remove gloves and wash hands.
11. Take the tray to the patient's unit.
12. 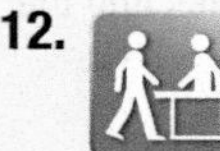 Comm Knock on the door and pause before entering. Introduce yourself. Identify the patient. Explain the procedure and obtain consent. Close the door and pull the curtain to provide privacy.
13. Wash hands. Put on gloves.

    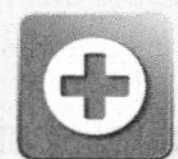 Precaution **CAUTION:** Observe standard precautions when giving an enema.

14. Place a chair by the bed and cover it with an underpad or bed protector. Then place the bedpan on it. Position all equipment conveniently.
15. Elevate the bed to a comfortable working height. If siderails are present and elevated, lower the siderail on the side where you are working.
16. Cover the patient with a bath blanket. Fanfold the top bed linens to the foot of the bed.
17. Place an underpad or bed protector under the patient's buttocks.

     Safety **CAUTION:** Use correct body mechanics. Bend at the hips and maintain a wide base of support.

18. Place the patient in the Sims' (left lateral) position. Fold the bath blanket back at an angle to expose the buttocks.

    NOTE: For patients who have difficulty retaining the enema, it is permissible to position them on the bedpan and in the dorsal recumbent position. Check with your immediate supervisor if you do not know which position to use.

(continues)

PROCEDURE 22:11A (CONT.)

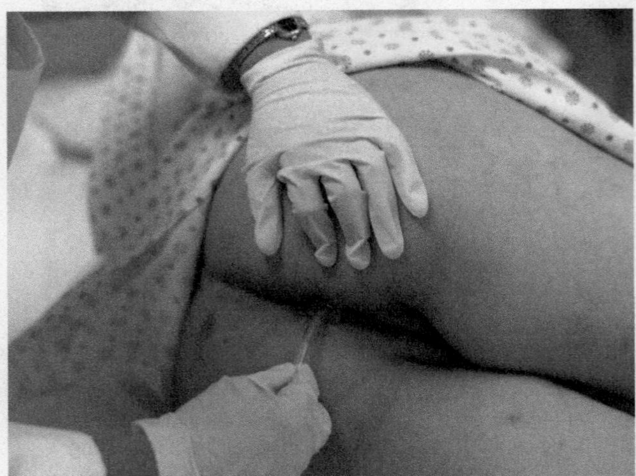

FIGURE 22–81A **Use one hand to raise the upper buttock and the other hand to gently insert the tip of the tubing 2–4 inches into the rectum.**

19. Check to be sure the tip is lubricated. Loosen the clamp and let some solution flow through the tubing and into the bedpan. Clamp the tubing off but make sure the solution is at the end of the tubing.

20. Comm Use one hand to carefully raise the upper buttock and expose the anus (the opening to the rectum). With your other hand, gently insert the tip 2–4 inches (5–10 centimeters) into the rectum (Figure 22–81A). Tell the patient you are inserting the tube. Encourage deep breathing and relaxation.

NOTE: If unable to insert the tube, pull back slightly and attempt to reinsert. If still unable to insert, discontinue the procedure and check with your immediate supervisor. A fecal impaction may be present.

21. Open the clamp. Raise the irrigation container or bag 12 inches (30 centimeters) above the level of the anus (Figure 22–81B). Make sure the solution flows in slowly. Encourage the patient to breathe deeply.

NOTE: If the patient complains of cramping or discomfort, clamp the tube to stop the flow and wait until the cramping stops.

NOTE: Regulate the rate of flow by raising (for a faster flow) or lowering (for a slower flow) the container or bag. The container may also be placed on an adjustable IV pole or stand.

22. When all of the solution has been drained, clamp the tubing before air enters the rectum.

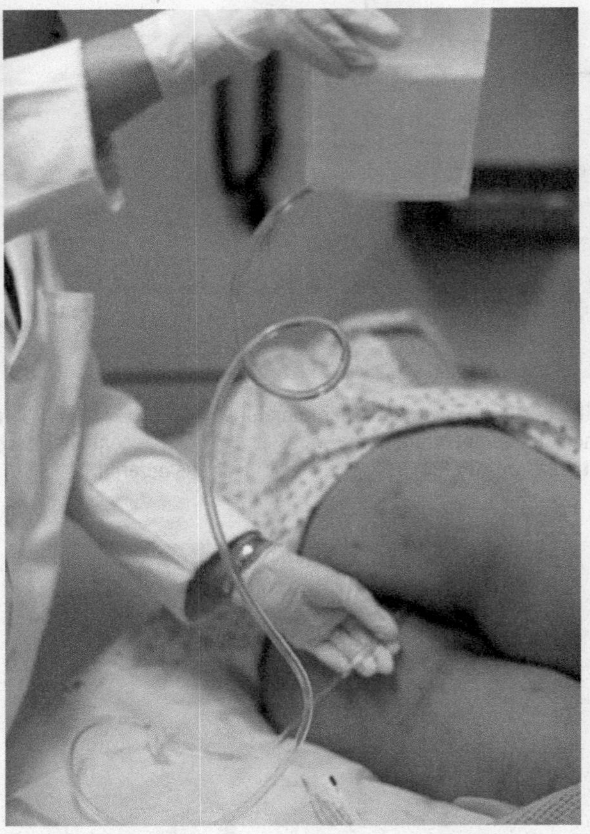

FIGURE 22–81B **Raise the irrigation bag 12 inches above the level of the anus to allow the solution to slowly flow into the rectum.**

23. Remove the tubing gently. Tell the patient what you are doing. Wrap the tubing in tissue and place it in the empty irrigation container.

24. Position the patient on the bedpan as previously instructed or escort the patient to the bathroom or onto a bedside commode, if the patient is ambulatory. Encourage the patient to retain the enema as long as possible. If the patient is ambulatory and will use the toilet, caution the patient not to flush the toilet until results are noted.

NOTE: Retention yields more effective results.

25. If the patient is on a bedpan, raise the patient's head to a comfortable position. Leave the call signal and toilet tissue within easy reach of the patient.

26. If the patient can be left alone, take the equipment to the bathroom for cleaning; if not, remain with the patient. Observe for signs of distress, weakness, excessive perspiration, paleness, or discomfort.

PROCEDURE 22:11A (CONT.)

27. Remove gloves and wash hands.
28. Answer the call signal immediately. Put on gloves. Remove the bedpan. Assist with cleaning the rectal area, if necessary. Assist with perineal care as needed.
29. Remove gloves. Provide washcloth or cleansing cloth so that the patient can wash his or her hands.
30. Reposition bed linens. Remove the bath blanket and underpad or bed protector.
31. Observe all checkpoints before leaving the patient: position the patient comfortably and in correct body alignment, elevate the siderails (if indicated), lower the bed to its lowest level, place the call signal and supplies within easy reach of the patient, and leave the area neat and clean.
32. Put on gloves. Take the bedpan to the bathroom. Observe contents before emptying the bedpan. Note the amount, type, and color of stool expelled, and the effectiveness of the enema.

Comm

NOTE: Words such as *good, poor, small,* or *no results* are used to describe the effectiveness of an enema.

33. Empty the bedpan. Rinse it with cold water. Clean it with a disinfectant. Rinse, dry, and return the bedpan to the patient's unit.
34. Clean and replace all other equipment used. If the irrigation container is disposable, place it in an infectious-waste bag.
35. Remove gloves and wash hands thoroughly.
36. 
Comm
Report and/or record all required information on the patient's chart or enter it into the computer. For example, date, time, 1,000 mL tap-water enema given with good results, retained 10 minutes, expelled four large dark-brown formed stools, tolerated procedure well, and your signature and title. Report any unusual observations immediately.

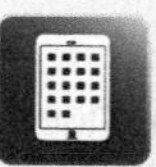
EHR

NOTE: In health care agencies using electronic health records (EHRs), also known as electronic medical records (EMRs), the information is entered directly into the patient's record on a computer.

PRACTICE: Go to the workbook and use the evaluation sheet for 22:11A, Giving a Tap-Water, Normal Saline, or Soap-Solution Enema, to practice this procedure. When you believe you have mastered this skill, sign the sheet and give it to your instructor for further action.

Check

FINAL CHECKPOINT: Using the criteria listed on the evaluation sheet, your instructor will grade your performance.

PROCEDURE 22:11B

Giving a Disposable Enema

NOTE: Approximately 4–6 ounces (120–180 mL) of hypertonic solution is usually contained in a plastic bottle with a prelubricated tip (for example, a Fleet enema).

Equipment and Supplies

Disposable enema unit, lubricating jelly, paper towels, tray with cover, bath blanket, underpad or bed protector, bedpan with cover, toilet tissue, disposable gloves, basin, towel, washcloth, soap, infectious-waste bag, paper and pen or computer

NOTE: If cleansing cloths are available, they can be used in place of the basin, soap, and washcloth.

Procedure

1. Check physician's orders or obtain authorization from your immediate supervisor. Verify the type of enema.
2. Assemble equipment.
3. Remove the enema from its package. Remove the cover from the tip. Add additional lubrication as needed by placing the tip in a paper towel with lubricating jelly.

   NOTE: Even prelubricated tips often need additional lubrication.

   NOTE: If the enema is to be warmed, place it in a basin of water at a temperature of 105°F (41°C). Disposable enemas are usually given at room temperature.

(continues)

PROCEDURE 22:11B (CONT.)

4. Place all equipment on the tray and cover with a towel. Go to the patient's unit.
5. Comm Knock on the door and pause before entering. Introduce yourself. Identify the patient. Explain the procedure and obtain consent.
6. Close the door and pull the curtain to provide privacy.
7. Wash hands. Put on gloves.

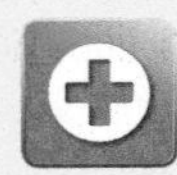
Precaution

CAUTION: Wear gloves and observe standard precautions when giving an enema.

8. Place a chair by the bed and cover it with an underpad or bed protector. Then place the bedpan on the chair. Position all equipment conveniently.
9. Elevate the bed to a comfortable working height. If siderails are elevated, lower the siderail on the side of the bed where you are working.
10. Cover the patient with a bath blanket. Fanfold the top bed linens to the foot of the bed. Place an underpad or bed protector under the patient's buttocks.
11. Place the patient in the Sims' position. Fold the bath blanket at an angle to expose the buttocks.
12. Squeeze the container slightly to get the solution to the top of the tip and eliminate air in the container (Figure 22–82).
13. Comm Use one hand to carefully raise the upper buttock and expose the anus (the opening to the rectum). With your other hand, gently insert the tip approximately 2 inches (5 centimeters). Explain each step to the patient to reduce anxiety and apprehension. Ask the patient to breathe deeply while the tip is being inserted.

    NOTE: If unable to insert the tip, pull it back slightly and try again. Sometimes, releasing a small amount of solution eases insertion. If still unable to insert, discontinue the procedure and check with your immediate supervisor.
14. To expel the solution, gently squeeze the container, starting from the bottom and progressing toward the tip in a spiral manner. Hold the container at a slight upward angle to prevent air bubbles. Encourage the patient to breathe deeply and to retain the enema solution.
15. When the solution has been injected and the container is empty, gently remove the tip from the rectum. Inform the patient as you do this. Place the container in an infectious-waste bag.

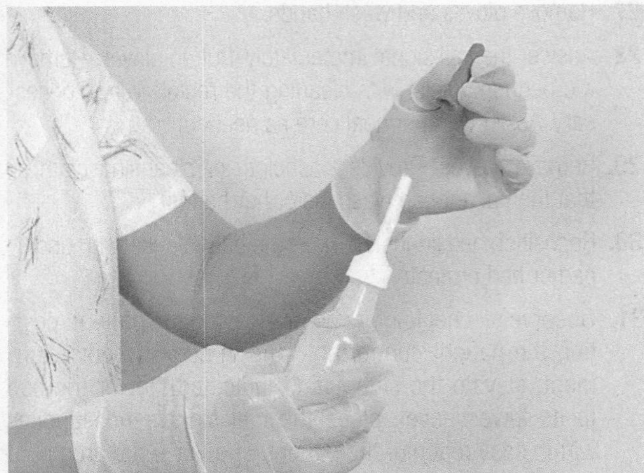

FIGURE 22–82 **Squeeze the container slightly to get the solution to the top of the tip of a disposable enema.**

16. Place the bedpan under the patient or assist the patient to the bathroom or onto a bedside commode. Encourage 5–10 minutes of retention.
17. If the patient is on a bedpan, position the patient comfortably. Elevate the head of the bed. Leave the call signal and toilet tissue within easy reach of the patient. Wash hands and remove gloves before leaving the room.

    NOTE: Remain with the patient, if necessary.
18. Answer the call signal immediately. Wash hands and put on gloves. Remove the bedpan. Assist the patient in cleaning the anal area, as needed. Assist with perineal care as needed.
19. Remove gloves and wash hands. Provide a washcloth or cleansing cloth. Allow the patient to wash his or her hands.
20. Replace the top bed linens. Remove the bed protector and bath blanket. Position the patient comfortably and in correct body alignment.
21. Observe all checkpoints before leaving the patient: elevate the siderails (if indicated), lower the bed to its lowest level, place the call signal and supplies within easy reach of the patient, and leave the area neat and clean.
22. Put on gloves. Take the bedpan to the bathroom. Observe the contents of the bedpan before emptying. Note amount, color, type, and any abnormalities. Record the results or effectiveness of the enema.
23. Empty the bedpan and rinse it with cold water. Clean it with a disinfectant. Rinse, dry, and return the bedpan to the patient's unit.
24. Clean and replace other equipment used.

PROCEDURE 22:11B (CONT.)

25. Remove gloves. Wash hands.

26.  Comm Report and/or record all required information on the patient's chart or enter it into the computer. For example, date, time, Fleet enema given with poor results, expelled one small formed dark-brown stool, patient complaining of "gas pains," and your signature and title. Report any unusual observations immediately.

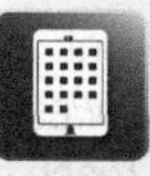 EHR **NOTE:** In health care agencies using electronic health records (EHRs), also known as electronic medical records (EMRs), the information is entered directly into the patient's record on a computer.

PRACTICE: Go to the workbook and use the evaluation sheet for 22:11B, Giving a Disposable Enema, to practice this procedure. When you believe you have mastered this skill, sign the sheet and give it to your instructor for further action.

 Check **FINAL CHECKPOINT:** Using the criteria listed on the evaluation sheet, your instructor will grade your performance.

PROCEDURE 22:11C

Giving an Oil-Retention Enema

Equipment and Supplies

Commercially prepared oil-retention enema (or 4–6 ounces mineral oil, olive oil, or other oil specified by physician and irrigation container with tubing, rectal tube, and clamp), lubricating jelly, paper towels, disposable gloves, tray with cover, bath blanket, underpad(s) or bed protector(s), toilet tissue, bedpan with cover, basin, soap, towel, washcloth, infectious-waste bag, paper and pen or computer

NOTE: If cleansing cloths are available, they can be used in place of the basin, soap, and washcloth.

Procedure

1. Check physician's orders or obtain authorization from your immediate supervisor. Verify the type and amount of enema.
2. Assemble equipment.
3. If a commercial enema unit is used, remove the enema from the outer package. Remove the protective cap from the tip and add lubrication as needed by rolling the tip in a paper towel with lubricating jelly.

   NOTE: If a commercial unit is not used, use 4–6 ounces of mineral oil, olive oil, or other oil specified in the order. Warm the oil by placing the container in a pan of warm water. Measure the correct amount of oil and place it in the irrigation container. Make sure the tubing is free of air and the clamp is shut. Lubricate the tip of the rectal tube.
4. Place all equipment on a tray. Cover and take to the patient's unit.
5.  Comm Knock on the door and pause before entering. Introduce yourself. Identify the patient. Explain the procedure and obtain consent.
6. Close the door and pull the curtain to provide privacy.
7. Wash hands. Put on gloves.

   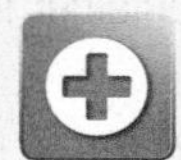 Precaution **CAUTION:** Wear gloves and observe standard precautions when giving an enema.
8. Place a chair by the bed and cover it with an underpad or bed protector. Then place the bedpan on the chair. Position all equipment conveniently.
9. Elevate the bed to a comfortable working height. If siderails are present and elevated, lower the siderail on the side where you are working.
10. Cover the patient with a bath blanket. Fanfold the top bed linens to the foot of the bed. Place an underpad or bed protector under the patient's buttocks.
11. Place the patient in the Sims' position (Figure 22–83). Fold the bath blanket at an angle to expose the buttocks.
12. Squeeze the container slightly to bring the oil to the tip and remove air.

    NOTE: If an irrigation container and tubing are used, open the clamp to allow oil to fill the tubing.
13.  Comm Use one hand to carefully raise the upper buttock and expose the anus (the opening to the rectum). With your other hand, gently insert the tip 2 inches into the rectum. Tell the patient what you are doing.

(continues)

PROCEDURE 22:11C (CONT.)

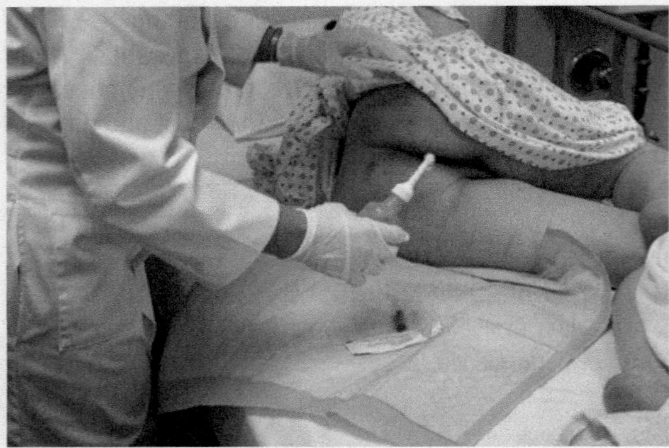

FIGURE 22–83 **Position the patient in a Sims' (left lateral) position with the right leg sharply flexed.**

14. Squeeze the container in a spiral fashion to expel the solution. Instill the solution slowly and gently. Encourage the patient to breathe deeply and to retain the enema solution.

NOTE: If a container and tubing are used, raise the container 12 inches to control the flow rate.

15. When the container is empty, gently remove the tip. Tell the patient what you are doing. Place the container in an infectious-waste bag.

16. Encourage the patient to retain the solution for at least 30–60 minutes. Leave the call signal within easy reach. Remove gloves and wash hands thoroughly.

NOTE: If the oil seeps, an additional underpad may be necessary.

17. Answer the call signal immediately. Wash hands and put on gloves. Position the patient on the bedpan or assist him or her to the bathroom or onto a bedside commode. Make sure toilet tissue and the call signal are within easy reach.

NOTE: Remain with the patient, if necessary.

18. Answer the call signal immediately. Remove the bedpan. Assist the patient in cleaning the anal area, as needed. Assist with perineal care as needed.

NOTE: A tap-water or soap-solution enema is sometimes ordered to follow an oil-retention enema, if the results are poor or the patient cannot expel the oil-retention enema.

19. Remove gloves and wash hands. Provide a washcloth or cleansing cloth for the patient to wash his or her hands.

20. Position the patient comfortably and in correct body alignment. Replace top bed linens. Remove underpad and bath blanket. If necessary, put a clean underpad under the patient's buttocks.

NOTE: Because some oil may continue to seep from the rectum after cleaning, it is usually wise to place a clean underpad under the patient's buttocks.

21. Observe all checkpoints before leaving the patient: elevate the siderails (if indicated), lower the bed to its lowest level, place the call signal and supplies within easy reach of the patient, and leave the area neat and clean.

22. Put on gloves. Take the bedpan to the bathroom. Note amount, color, and type of stool before emptying.

23. Empty the bedpan and rinse it with cold water. Clean with a disinfectant. Rinse, dry, and return the bedpan to the patient's unit.

24. Clean and replace all other equipment used.

25. Remove gloves. Wash hands.

26. 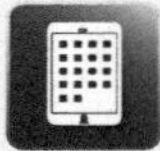
Comm

Report and/or record all required information on the patient's chart or enter it into the computer. For example, date, time, oil-retention enema given with good results, retained 30 minutes, expelled large amount of light brown semi-formed stool and flatus, patient stated, "I feel much better," and your signature and title. Report any abnormal observations immediately.

EHR

NOTE: In health care agencies using electronic health records (EHRs), also known as electronic medical records (EMRs), the information is entered directly into the patient's record on a computer.

PRACTICE: **Go to the workbook and use the evaluation sheet for 22:11C, Giving an Oil-Retention Enema, to practice this procedure. When you believe you have mastered this skill, sign the sheet and give it to your instructor for further action.**

Check

FINAL CHECKPOINT: Using the criteria listed on the evaluation sheet, your instructor will grade your performance.

PROCEDURE 22:11D

Inserting a Rectal Tube

Equipment and Supplies

Rectal tube and flatus bag, lubricating jelly, paper towel, tissue, underpad or protective bed cover, basin or specimen bottle (if needed), disposable gloves, tape, infectious-waste bag, paper and pen or computer

Procedure

1. Check physician's orders or obtain authorization from your immediate supervisor. Note time ordered.

   NOTE: This procedure may be ordered for a specific time, for example, a half hour after administration of a medication.

2. Assemble equipment. Place the tip of the rectal tube in lubricating jelly on a paper towel. Connect the opposite (open) end to the flatus bag (Figure 22–84).

   NOTE: Instead of connecting it to a flatus bag, the open end may be placed in a disposable glove and taped or in a basin or specimen bottle. Follow agency policy.

   NOTE: Many agencies now use disposable rectal tubes with flatus bags attached. The tip of the tube must still be lubricated. The tube and bag are discarded in an infectious-waste bag after one use.

3.  Comm Knock on the door and pause before entering. Introduce yourself. Identify the patient. Explain the procedure and obtain consent.

4. Close the door and pull the curtain for privacy.

5. Wash hands. Put on gloves.

   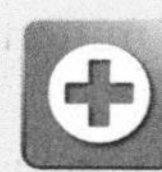 Precaution **CAUTION:** Wear gloves and observe standard precautions when inserting a rectal tube.

6. Elevate the bed to a comfortable working height. If siderails are elevated, lower the siderail on the side where you are working.

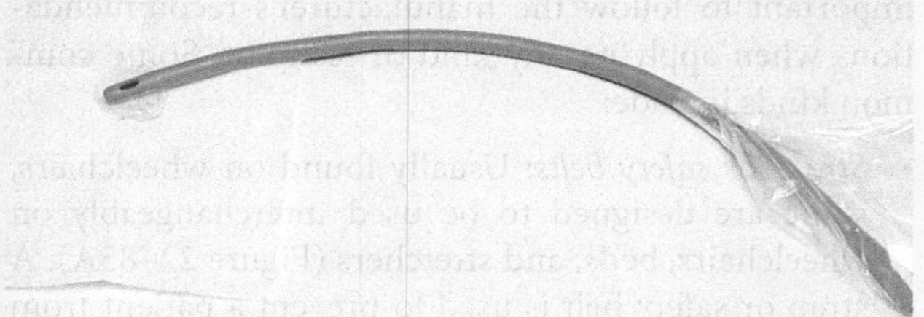

FIGURE 22–84 Place the tip of the rectal tube in lubricating jelly on a paper towel. Connect the opposite end to the flatus bag.

7. Place the patient in the Sims' position. Place an underpad under the patient's buttocks. Fold the bed linen at an angle to expose the buttocks.

8.  Comm Use one hand to carefully raise the upper buttock and expose the anus (the opening to the rectum). With your other hand, gently insert the rectal tube 2–4 inches into the rectum. Tell the patient what you are doing.

9. Tape the tube to the patient's buttocks to hold the tube in place.

10. If a flatus bag is not in use, place the free end of the tube in a basin, bedpan, or specimen bottle.

    NOTE: Fecal material may seep from tube.

11. Make sure the patient is as comfortable as possible before leaving. Elevate siderails, if indicated. Leave the call signal within easy reach of the patient.

12. Remove gloves and wash hands thoroughly.

13. Return at intervals to check the patient and rectal tube.

     Safety **CAUTION:** Do not leave if the patient is unconscious or not alert to surroundings.

14. Wash hands and put on gloves. Remove the tube promptly at the end of the ordered time, usually 20–30 minutes. Tell the patient what you are doing. Remove the tube gently.

     Safety **CAUTION:** The tube can irritate sensitive tissue if left in place too long.

15. 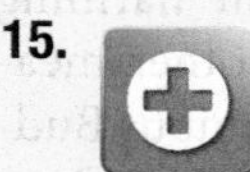 Precaution Place the rectal tube and bag in the infectious-waste bag. Clean the patient, as needed. Remove the underpad and replace the bed linens.

16. 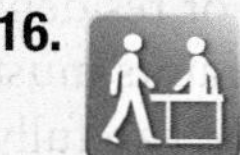 Comm Ask the patient how much flatus (gas) was expelled or if the patient feels better.

    NOTE: Licensed personnel may listen to bowel sounds immediately after the rectal tube is removed. Inform the correct person that you have removed the rectal tube.

17. Observe all checkpoints before leaving the patient: position the patient in correct body alignment, elevate the siderails (if indicated), lower the bed to its lowest level, place the call signal and supplies within easy reach of the patient, and leave the area neat and clean.

18. Note any result, including collection of air (flatus) in the bag, drainage, and the patient's comments following the procedure.

(continues)

PROCEDURE 22:11D (CONT.)

19. Clean and replace all equipment.
20. Remove gloves. Wash hands.
21. 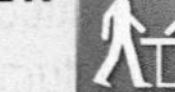

Report and/or record all required information on the patient's chart or enter it into the computer. For example, date, time, rectal tube inserted for 20 minutes, expelled large amount of flatus, no drainage noted, patient stated, "I feel much better," and your signature and title. Report any unusual observations immediately.

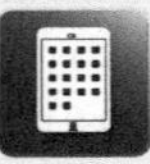

NOTE: In health care agencies using electronic health records (EHRs), also known as electronic medical records (EMRs), the information is entered directly into the patient's record on a computer.

PRACTICE: Go to the workbook and use the evaluation sheet for 22:11D, Inserting a Rectal Tube, to practice this procedure. When you believe you have mastered this skill, sign the sheet and give it to your instructor for further action.

FINAL CHECKPOINT: Using the criteria listed on the evaluation sheet, your instructor will grade your performance.

22:12 Applying Restraints

Although sick people are usually quiet and need encouragement to move, there are times when it is necessary to limit the movement of overactive patients. **Restraints** are used to limit movement. There are two kinds of restraints: chemical and physical. *Chemical restraints* are medications that affect the patient's behavior. Examples include tranquilizers, sedatives, and mood-altering medications. Licensed personnel are responsible for administering any chemical restraints.

Physical restraints are protective devices that limit a patient's movements. They should be used only to protect patients from harming themselves or others and when all other measures to correct the situation have failed. Omnibus Budget Reconciliation Act (OBRA) legislation clearly defines the limitations of using restraints. All patient or resident behavior that may necessitate the use of restraints must be documented. Alternatives must be tried and carefully documented. If alternate solutions are not successful, a physician must write the order for the restraint, and the order must state the type of restraint, the reason for its use, the length of time it can be used, and where or when it can be used. The least restrictive device must always be used first. A restraint applied unnecessarily can be considered false imprisonment. A health care worker should never apply a restraint without proper authorization.

Circumstances and conditions that may necessitate the use of restraints include:

- *Severe behavioral or cognitive issues*: Patients with a psychiatric diagnosis or in adverse mental health may demonstrate violent tendencies toward staff, self, or others. Restraints may have to be applied for their own safety and/or the safety of others.
- *Irrational or confused patients*: Patients can become irrational or confused because of anesthesia, medications, senility, sleep deprivation, and other factors. They may attempt to climb out of bed or over siderails, or they may wander about. Because they could fall and injure themselves, restraints must sometimes be applied to limit their movements.
- *Danger to self*: A patient may require restraints if he or she is unable to comprehend the need for treatment and is interfering with medical care or devices or attempting to pull out vital lines or tubes.
- *Skin conditions*: Patients, especially small children, with itchy skin conditions must sometimes have their hands restrained or encased in protective mittens to prevent scratching.
- *Paralysis or limited muscular coordination*: Patients under anesthesia or who are paralyzed by strokes are often unable to coordinate or control their muscular movements. They may require restraints.

There are different kinds of physical restraints. It is important to follow the manufacturer's recommendations when applying any kind of restraint. Some common kinds include:

- *Straps or safety belts*: Usually found on wheelchairs, some are designed to be used interchangeably on wheelchairs, beds, and stretchers (Figure 22–85A). A strap or safety belt is used to prevent a patient from falling out of the device. The strap or belt should not be applied too tightly because it can restrict breathing and interfere with circulation. Self-release belt restraints are also available for use. They are

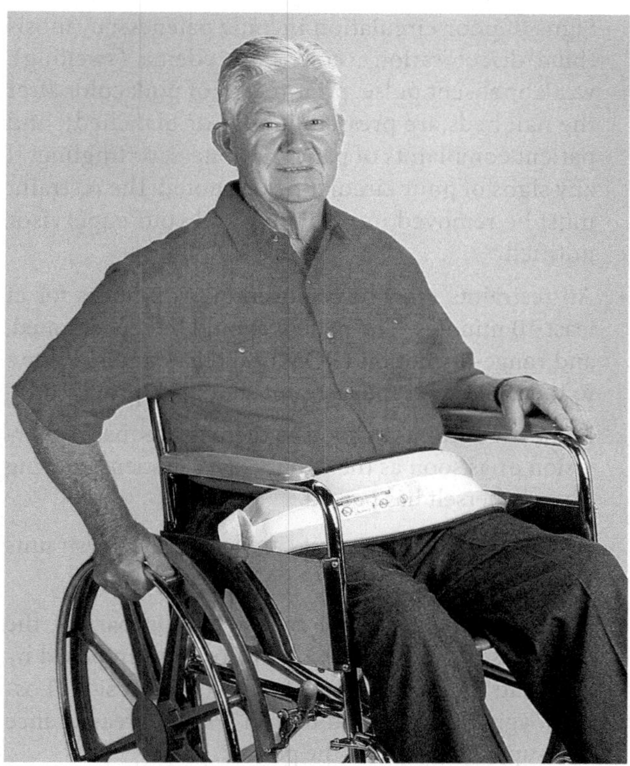

FIGURE 22–85A A belt restraint can be used to support a patient sitting in a wheelchair. Courtesy of J. T. Posey Company

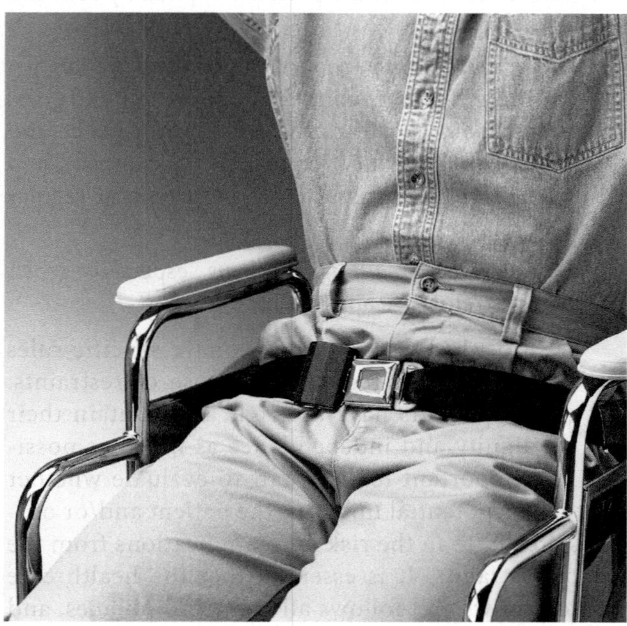

FIGURE 22–85B An alternative self-release belt sounds an alarm when the patient begins to open it. Courtesy of J. T. Posey Company

considered to be less restrictive because the patient can release the belt. However, when the patient does start to release the belt, an alarm sounds that alerts the staff (Figure 22–85B).

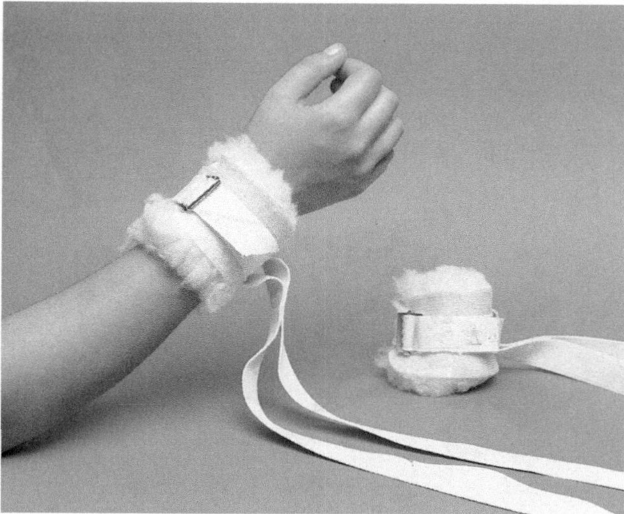

FIGURE 22–86 Place the soft edge of the limb restraint against the patient's skin. Courtesy of J. T. Posey Company

- *Limb restraints*: Usually, soft, padded restraints that are wrapped around the arm or leg to limit movement of the limb (Figure 22–86). The restraint straps are then attached to the movable part of the bed frame or stretcher to secure the limb into position. At least two fingers should be slipped between the restraint and the patient's skin to make sure the restraint is not too tight.
- *Restraint jackets*: These devices are used to prevent a patient from sitting up, rolling, getting out of bed, or falling out of a wheelchair. Jacket restraints are available in different sizes. It is important to follow manufacturer's directions and measure the patient carefully to make sure the correct size jacket restraint is used. Jacket restraints must also be applied so that they do not interfere with breathing or circulation.
- *Geriatric chair*: These are used for patients who may sit up in a chair but are at risk for falling because they are unsteady and confused. Most chairs contain a tabletop tray that locks into place to prevent patients from getting up unassisted (Figure 22–87).
- *Hand mitts*: These devices are similar to mittens that are applied to the hands to prevent the patient from scratching or injuring the skin (Figure 22–88). They can also be used to prevent patients from pulling on lines and tubes.

There are some important points to remember when using restraints:

- Use only when all other means of obtaining the patient's cooperation have failed.
- Restraints should be as unnoticeable to the patient as possible.

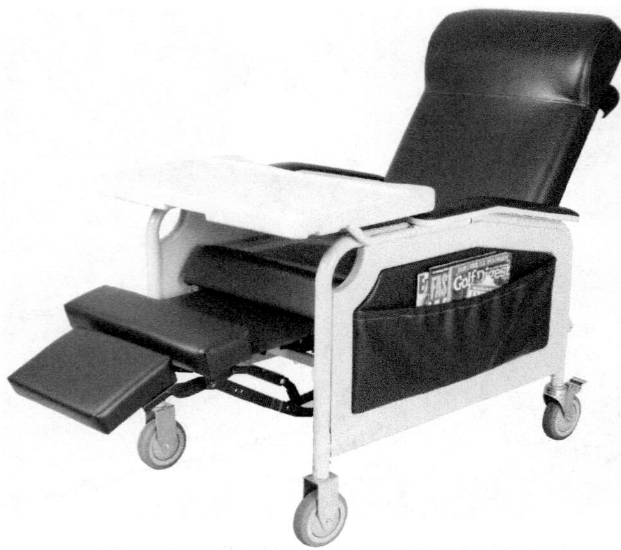

FIGURE 22–87 A geriatric chair can be used to position a patient comfortably in an upright or reclining position. When the tabletop is locked into position across the patient's lap, the patient is not able to get out of the chair. Courtesy, Winco

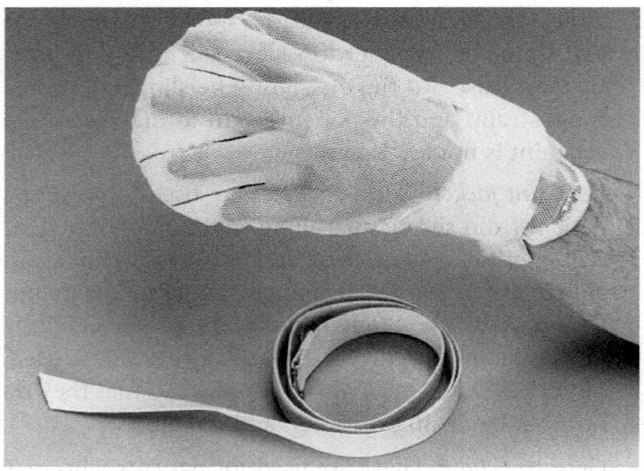

FIGURE 22–88 Hand mitts can be applied to prevent the patient from scratching or injuring the skin. Courtesy of J. T. Posey Company

- Patients should be allowed to move as much as possible without danger of self-injury.
- The patient should always be told why his or her movements are being restricted, even when the patient is irrational or confused.
- The restrained patient feels both physical and mental frustration. Therefore, it is important to reassure the patient frequently.
- Restraints should be checked frequently after they have been applied. Circulation below a limb restraint should be checked every 15–30 minutes. Signs of poor circulation include paleness; cyanosis (blue discoloration); cold skin; edema (swelling); weak or absent pulse; poor return of pink color after the nail beds are pressed lightly (or blanched); and patient complaints of pain, numbness, or tingling. If any signs of poor circulation are noted, the restraint must be removed immediately and your supervisor notified.
- All restraints *must* be removed every 2 hours for at least 10 minutes. The patient should be repositioned, and range-of-motion (ROM) exercises and skin care to the skin under the restraint should be provided.
- Remove restraints as soon as there is adequate supervision or as soon as the danger of the patient injuring him- or herself has passed.

Some complications that can occur when restraints are applied include:

- *Physical and mental frustration* on the part of the patient is common. The loss of freedom imposed by restraints can cause disorientation, depression, hostility, agitation, and withdrawal. Provide reassurance and supportive care to the patient.
- *Impaired circulation* can result. Check skin color and skin temperature frequently.
- *Pressure ulcers* from the pressure applied by restraint can develop.
- *Loss of muscle tone, joint stiffness, and discomfort* from immobility are common. The inability to go to the bathroom at will can lead to incontinence and constipation. Provide frequent ROM exercises and offer to take the patient to the bathroom at regular intervals.
- *Respiratory or breathing problems*, especially when jacket restraints are applied, may develop.

Legal

Most health care facilities have specific rules and policies regarding the use of restraints. All patients have the right to maintain their dignity and independence as much as possible. It is important for the staff to evaluate whether the risk for potential injury to the patient and/or others is greater than the risk for complications from the use of restraints. It is essential that the health care worker knows and follows all rules and policies, and is aware of legal responsibilities regarding the use of restraints.

STUDENT: **Go to the workbook and complete the assignment sheet for 22:12, Applying Restraints. Then return and continue with the procedures.**

PROCEDURE 22:12A

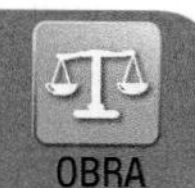
OBRA

Applying Limb Restraints

Equipment and Supplies

Adjustable limb restraint(s), paper and pen or computer

Procedure

1. Check physician's orders or obtain authorization from your immediate supervisor.

Legal

CAUTION: A restraint cannot be applied without a physician's order.

NOTE: The order must state the type of restraint and reason for its use. The least restrictive device must be used first.

2. Assemble equipment.
3. Comm — Knock on the door and pause before entering. Introduce yourself. Identify the patient. Explain the procedure even if the patient is irrational or confused, and obtain consent if possible.
4. Wash hands.
5. Close the door and pull the curtain to provide privacy. If the patient is in a bed, elevate the bed to a comfortable working height. If siderails are present and elevated, lower the siderail on the side where you are working. If the patient is in a wheelchair, lock the wheels of the chair. Position the patient in a comfortable position and in good body alignment.
6. Place the soft edge of the restraint against the patient's skin. Wrap the restraint smoothly around the limb (Figure 22–89A). Make sure there are no wrinkles.
7. Pull the ends of the straps through the tabs or rings on the restraint. Then pull the restraint securely, but not too tightly, against the patient's skin.

Safety

CAUTION: If applied too tightly, the restraint could stop circulation or cause a pressure sore.

8. Test for fit and comfort by inserting fingers between the restraint and the patient's skin (Figure 22–89B).
9. Position the arm or leg in a comfortable position. Limit movement only as much as is necessary.
10. Use a quick-release tie to secure the straps to the nonmovable part of the bed frame, stretcher frame, or other frame (Figure 22–89C). To make the quick-release tie, bring the end of the strap around the frame. Then bring the loose end up behind and around the back of the strap to create a hole. Fold the loose end of the strap into a loop and tuck the loop into the hole formed. Pull up on the descending part of the strap to tighten the loop in the hole. To release the tie, simply pull on the loose, exposed end of the strap.

NOTE: Many restraints have snap closures that make them easy to attach to the bed.

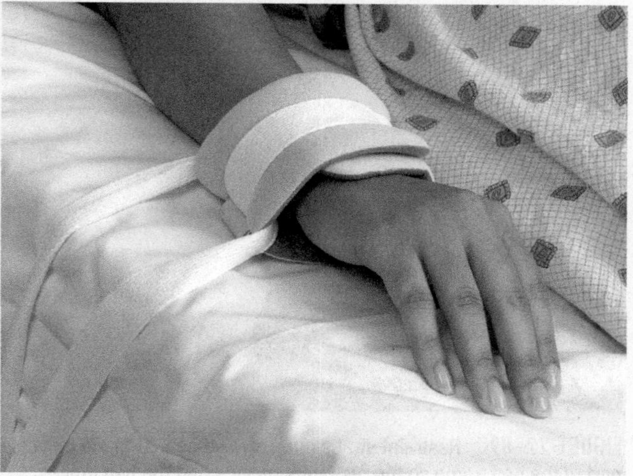

FIGURE 22–89A Wrap the restraint smoothly around the limb, making sure there are no wrinkles.

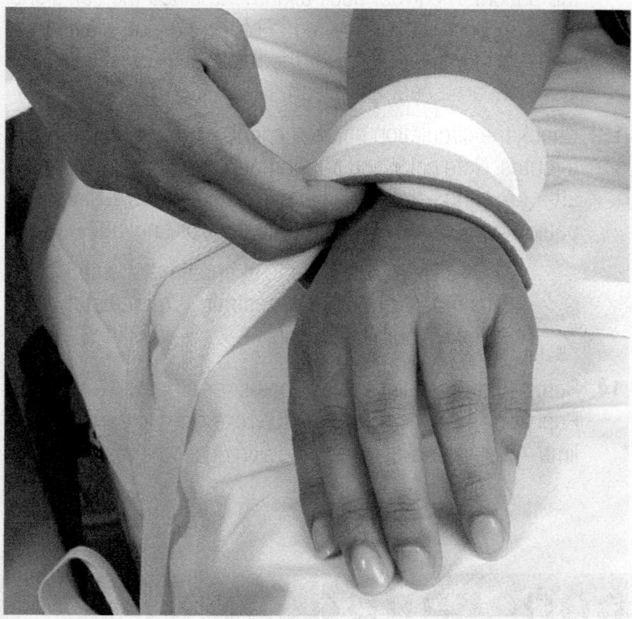

FIGURE 22–89B Insert two fingers between the restraint and the patient's skin to make sure the restraint is not too tight.

11. Recheck the patient before leaving.

Safety

CAUTION: Make sure the restraint is secure but not too tight.

(continues)

PROCEDURE 22:12A (CONT.)

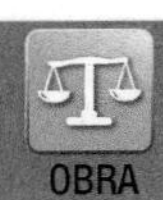

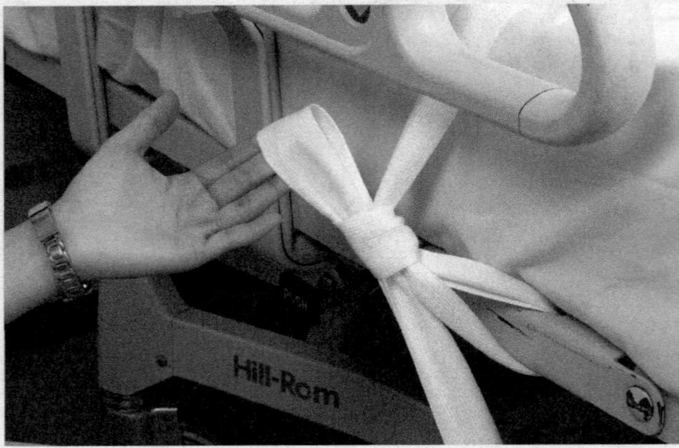

FIGURE 22–89C **Restraint straps must always be tied to the movable part of the bed frame so the restraints move when the bed moves.**

12. Observe all checkpoints before leaving the patient: position the patient in correct body alignment, place the call signal and supplies within easy reach of the patient, elevate the siderails (if indicated), lower the bed to its lowest level, and leave the area neat and clean.
13. Check the circulation below the limb restraint every 15–30 minutes. Note color and temperature of skin; return of color after pressing lightly on nail beds; edema (or swelling); and patient complaints of pain, numbness, or tingling.

CAUTION: If any signs of impaired circulation are noted, remove the restraint immediately and notify your supervisor.

14. Remove the restraint every 2 hours for at least 10 minutes. Reposition the patient. Provide ROM exercises to the restrained limb. Administer skin care to the skin under the restraint.
15. Remove the restraint when authorized to do so by your supervisor or the physician.

NOTE: Restraints are removed when the physician or supervisor feels that the danger of self-injury to the patient has passed. Restraints must always be removed as soon as is possible.

16. Replace all equipment.
17. Wash hands.
18. Report and/or record all required information on the patient's chart or enter it into the computer. For example, date, time, limb restraints applied to both arms while patient positioned in wheelchair, P 82 strong and regular at both wrists, patient appears to be resting quietly, and your signature and title. Report any unusual observations immediately.

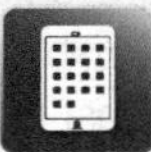

NOTE: In health care agencies using electronic health records (EHRs), also known as electronic medical records (EMRs), the information is entered directly into the patient's record on a computer.

PRACTICE: **Go to the workbook and use the evaluation sheet for 22:12A, Applying Limb Restraints, to practice this procedure. When you believe you have mastered this skill, sign the sheet and give it to your instructor for further action.**

FINAL CHECKPOINT: Using the criteria listed on the evaluation sheet, your instructor will grade your performance.

PROCEDURE 22:12B

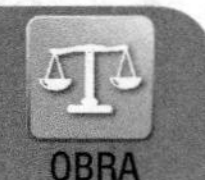

Applying a Jacket Restraint

Equipment and Supplies

Sleeveless jacket restraint, paper and pen or computer

Procedure

1. Check physician's orders or obtain authorization from your supervisor.

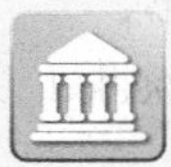

CAUTION: A restraint *cannot* be applied without a physician's order.

NOTE: The order must state the type of restraint and reason for its use. The least restrictive device must be used first.

2. Assemble equipment. Obtain the correct size restraint for the patient.

PROCEDURE 22:12B (CONT.)

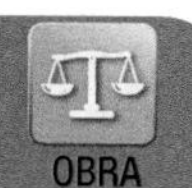
OBRA

Safety

CAUTION: Follow the manufacturer's instructions and carefully measure the patient to make sure the correct size jacket/vest restraint is used. If an incorrect size is used, the restraint will not provide proper support and could injure the patient.

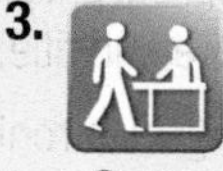
Comm

3. Knock on the door and pause before entering. Introduce yourself. Identify the patient. Explain the procedure even if the patient is irrational or confused, and obtain consent if possible.
4. Wash hands.
5. Close the door and pull the curtain to provide privacy. If the patient is in a bed, elevate the bed to a comfortable working height. If siderails are present and elevated, lower the siderail on the side where you are working. If the patient is in a wheelchair, lock the wheels of the chair. Place the patient in a comfortable position and in good body alignment.
6. Slip the sleeves of the jacket restraint onto the patient's arms. The solid part of the jacket restraint goes on the back, and the open or V-neck part of the restraint goes on the front (Figure 22–90A). It is essential to follow the manufacturer's instructions.

Safety

CAUTION: A restraint applied incorrectly may cause suffocation or injury.

7. Crisscross the straps in the back. Check all of the material to make sure it is free from wrinkles.
8. Bring the loose ends of the straps through the hole in the jacket. The jacket should now completely encircle the patient.
9. Check the restraint to be sure it is not too tight against the patient.

Safety

CAUTION: Excessive tightness could interfere with breathing.

10. Place the patient in a comfortable position. Allow as much movement as possible without risk of injury.
11. On each side of a bed or stretcher, use a quick-release tie to bring the straps down and secure them to the nonmovable part of the frame.
12. Straps should be brought down between the wheelchair and side plate. In a wheelchair, the straps can be attached to the kick bars at the rear of the wheelchair. Note that the kick bars' plastic end-caps must be in place to ensure that the ties will not slip off (Figure 22–90B).

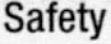
Safety

CAUTION: Never attach the straps to any parts of the wheels.

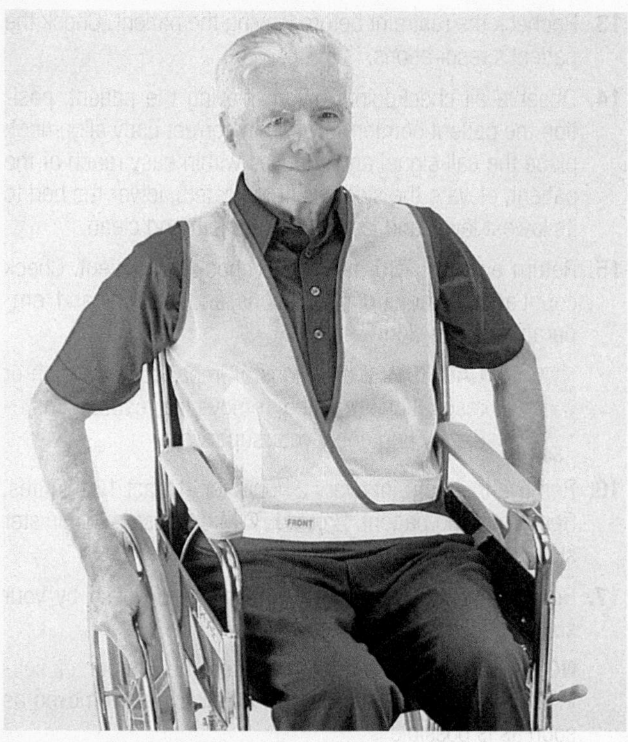

FIGURE 22–90A **Follow the manufacturer's instructions to measure a patient to make sure the jacket or vest is the correct size. Position the jacket restraint with the open or V-neck part of the restraint on the front.** Courtesy of J. T. Posey Company

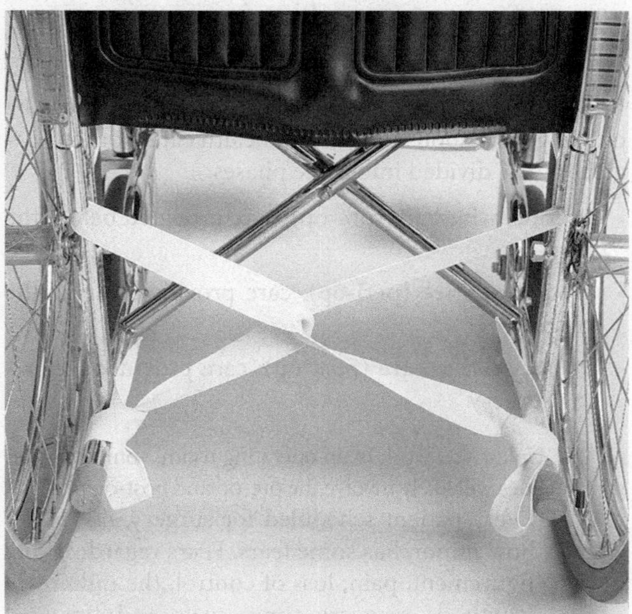

FIGURE 22–90B **Use a quick-release tie to secure the straps to the back frame of a wheelchair.** Courtesy of J. T. Posey Company

(continues)

PROCEDURE 22:12B (CONT.)

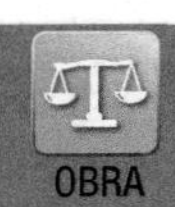

13. Recheck the restraint before leaving the patient. Check the patient's respirations.
14. Observe all checkpoints before leaving the patient: position the patient comfortably and in correct body alignment, place the call signal and supplies within easy reach of the patient, elevate the siderails (if indicated), lower the bed to its lowest level, and leave the area neat and clean.
15. Return every 15–30 minutes to check the patient. Check count and character of respirations, and the color and temperature of the skin.

CAUTION: If any signs of impaired circulation or respiration are noted, remove the restraint immediately and notify your supervisor.

16. Remove the restraint every 2 hours for at least 10 minutes. Reposition the patient. Provide ROM exercises. Administer skin care to the skin under the restraint.
17. Remove the restraint when authorized to do so by your supervisor or the physician.

NOTE: A restraint is removed when the danger of self-injury has passed. Restraints must always be removed as soon as is possible.

18. Replace all equipment.
19. Wash hands.
20.  Report and/or record all required information on the patient's chart or enter it into the computer. For example, date, time, jacket restraint applied, patient seated in wheelchair, and your signature and title.

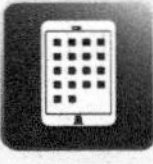

NOTE: In health care agencies using electronic health records (EHRs), also known as electronic medical records (EMRs), the information is entered directly into the patient's record on a computer.

PRACTICE: **Go to the workbook and use the evaluation sheet for 22:12B, Applying a Jacket Restraint, to practice this procedure. When you believe you have mastered this skill, sign the sheet and give it to your instructor for further action.**

FINAL CHECKPOINT: Using the criteria listed on the evaluation sheet, your instructor will grade your performance.

22:13 Administering Preoperative and Postoperative Care

Providing care to patients scheduled for surgery may be one of your responsibilities as a health care worker. Surgical care is divided into three phases:

- **Preoperative care** (pre-op): care provided before the surgery
- **Operative care** (peri-op): care provided during the surgery
- **Postoperative care** (post-op): care provided following surgery

NOTE: Unless you work in an operating room, your major responsibilities will likely involve the pre-op and post-op phases.

Every patient scheduled for surgery, no matter how minor, has some fears. Fears regarding disfigurement, pain, loss of control, the unknown, length of recovery time, costs and financial problems, a poor diagnosis after surgery, and even death create concerns for many patients. It is important to provide emotional support in addition to physical care. Answer all questions you can to the best of your ability. However, specific questions about the surgery, outcome, or anesthesia should be referred to the physician or your supervisor. Be sure to report these questions and the patient's fears to your immediate supervisor.

Preoperative Care

Preoperative care involves many aspects of care. Most of the preparation is ordered by the physician, depending on the type of operation. Possible aspects of preparation are:

-  *Operative permit*: This is a form signed by the patient to give permission for the anesthesia and surgery. If the patient is unable to sign due to a severe illness or confusion, the next of kin or an individual with a power of attorney (POA) can sign for them. Signatures must be witnessed by a legally authorized individual.
- *Laboratory tests*: These tests may include blood tests, urine tests, chest or other radiographs, electrocardiogram (ECG), and special tests ordered by the physician.
- *Enemas or vaginal irrigations*: These are ordered by the physician in preparation for certain types of surgery.

- *Baths*: Baths may be given both the night before surgery and the morning of surgery. The purpose is to remove as many microorganisms as possible in an effort to prevent infections. Some surgeries require a Hibiclens bath the night before and the morning of the surgery. Hibiclens is a cleanser that removes bacteria from the skin to prevent it from entering the surgical incision. Baths also give the patient a chance to talk and relieve some anxiety.
- *Vital signs*: These are taken and recorded. They are used as a standard to check vital signs during and after the surgery.
- *NPO*: The patient is allowed nothing by mouth for 8–12 hours before the surgery. The order usually starts at 12:00 AM (midnight). A sign is usually placed on the patient's bed. Water is removed from the area at the appointed time.
- *Valuables*: All the patient's valuables, including money and jewelry, should be placed in a hospital safe or with security to prevent loss. A patient is sometimes allowed to wear a wedding ring. However, it must be taped or tied to the finger to prevent loss.
- *Remove prosthetics*: All artificial parts are removed. This includes dentures, contact lenses or glasses, artificial arms or legs, and hearing aids.
- *Remove cosmetics*: Nail polish, makeup, hair pins, and wigs are all removed before surgery. The presence of cosmetics can mask skin or nail bed color changes.
- **Surgical shave** or *skin preparation*: This includes shaving and cleaning of the operative site. This may or may not be done. Some physicians feel that shaving the skin can cause superficial cuts that lead to infection, a concern supported by the Centers for Disease Control and Prevention (CDC). If a surgical shave is done, it can be done by a special skin-prep team, by the surgical staff immediately before the surgery, or, sometimes, by the nurse assistant before the patient is transferred to the operating room. Skin preparation sites for some specific surgeries are shown in Figure 22–91. Each agency has its own policy regarding what area is to be prepared. Sometimes, the physician specifies the area. The skin is shaved to prevent infection in and around the surgical site, and to remove longer hair that would interfere with surgery.
- *Clothing*: Usually, the patient must remove all clothing, including undergarments. A hospital gown is placed on the patient. Most agencies also place a surgical cap on the patient to cover the hair.
- Comm *Name band*: Before surgery, the patient's name band or identification band should be checked for accurate information. Because the patient frequently is unconscious during surgery, the name band is the only method of identifying the patient.
- *Voiding*: To make sure the bladder is empty during surgery, the patient should void immediately before being brought to the operating room. For some surgeries, a catheter is inserted in the bladder to constantly drain all urine. Only a qualified person should insert the catheter.
- *Surgical checklist*: Most agencies use surgical checklists to track most of the previously noted preparation items. As these items are completed, they are checked off the checklist. This provides a method for determining that the patient has been properly prepared for surgery. The checklist is usually attached to the patient's chart or entered into the computerized record.

Frequently, patients are not admitted to the hospital or surgical clinic until the morning of the surgery. In this case, many of the tests such as blood work, radiographs, and ECG are performed on an outpatient basis before the day of surgery.

Anesthesia

Anesthesia is prevention of pain by way of loss of sensation. Medication is administered by an anesthesiologist, anesthetist, or physician. The type of anesthetic used and the method of administration depends on the type of surgery, the length of time needed, and the physical condition of the patient. Three main kinds are:

- *General anesthesia*: Medication is given intravenously or is inhaled through a mask. This causes unconsciousness, which continues throughout the surgery. A common postoperative problem is nausea or vomiting.
- *Local anesthesia*: Medication is injected into the area around the operative site to stop the sensation of pain. The patient is awake when local anesthesia is used.
- *Spinal anesthesia*: Medication is injected into the spinal canal and causes loss of sensation (feeling) in all areas below the injection. This is often used for abdominal surgery because it produces good muscle relaxation. Patients must be told that they will not have any feeling or movement in the legs for a period of time. Patients sometimes complain of headaches after this type of anesthesia. This symptom should be reported.

Postoperative Care

While the patient is in surgery, the postoperative room or bed unit is prepared in such a way that all necessary equipment will be available when the patient returns from surgery. A recovery bed is made, an intravenous (IV) pole or stand and equipment for taking vital signs is put in place,

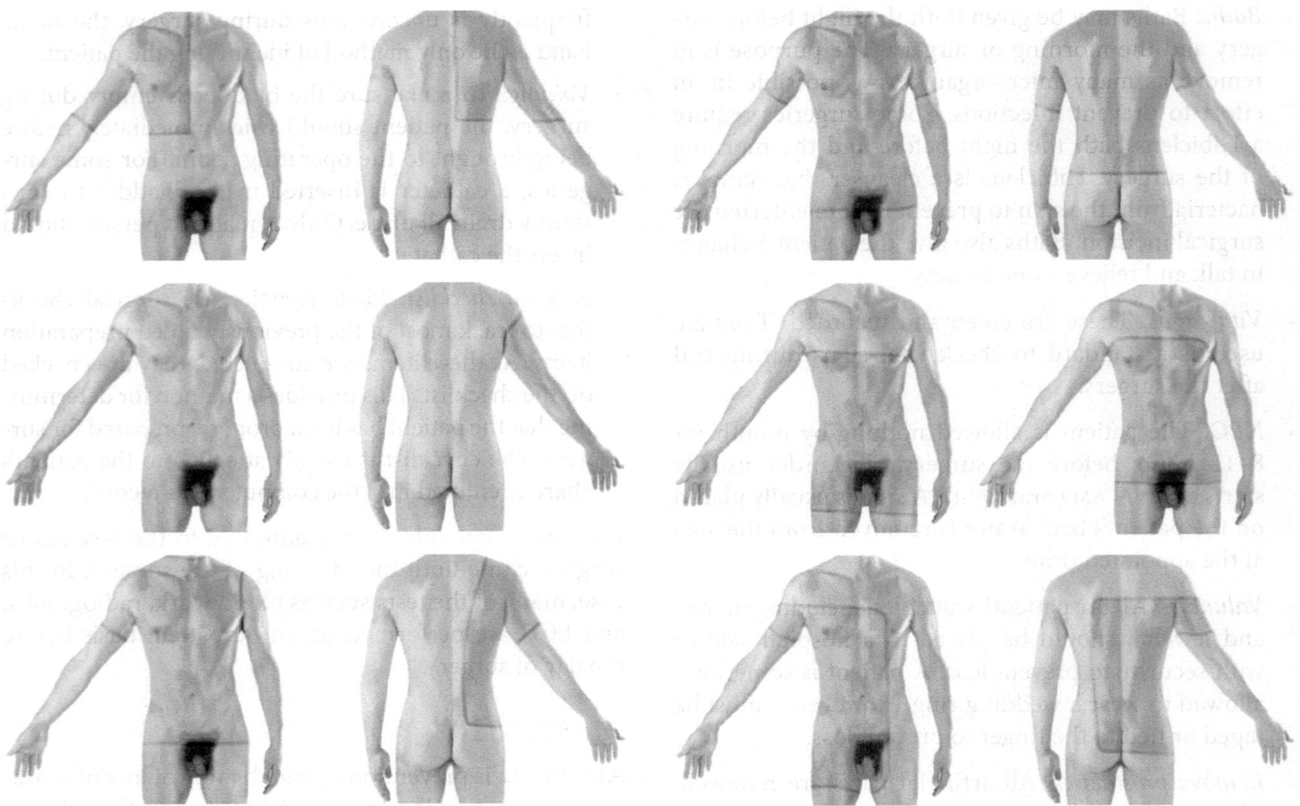
FIGURE 22–91 Shaded areas represent skin-preparation sites for some specific surgeries.

and an emesis basin and tissues are placed at the bedside. Necessary special equipment, such as a suction machine for drainage tubes or equipment for administering oxygen, is also placed in the unit. All unnecessary supplies or equipment are removed from the area. For example, the water pitcher and cup are removed until postoperative orders state that the patient can have fluids.

Postoperative care is an important aspect of surgical care. Some of the factors to be considered in immediate postoperative care are:

- *Vital signs*: These must be checked frequently and as ordered. They are sometimes taken every 15 minutes until the patient is stable. A sudden drop in blood pressure or change in pulse rate or character are often the first signs of hemorrhage or shock, so any changes or abnormal readings must be reported immediately.
- *Dressings*: These must be checked frequently (Figure 22–92). The color, amount, and type of drainage must be noted. Any unusual observations should be reported immediately.
- *IV*: The flow rate and injection site must be checked only by an authorized individual.
- *Level of pain*: An assessment must be made of the amount of pain a patient is experiencing. Frequently patients are asked to describe pain on a scale of 1 to 10, with 1 being mild pain and 10 being extreme pain. *Patient-controlled analgesics (PCAs)* are often used to control pain. An analgesic pump is attached to an IV line. The patient is taught to push a button when pain is felt. The pump delivers a specific dose of pain medication directly into the bloodstream to provide immediate relief. The patient cannot overdose on

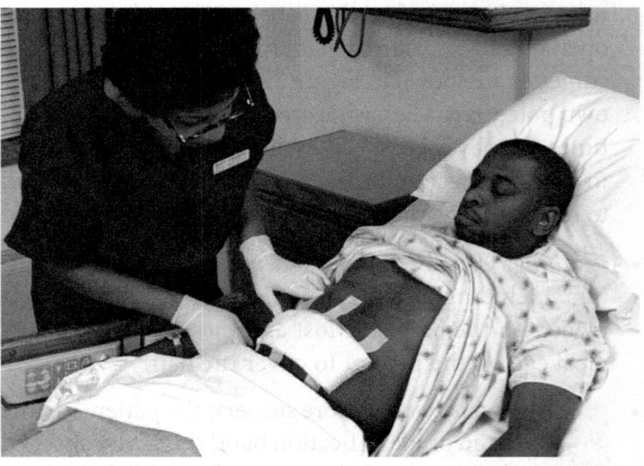
FIGURE 22–92 Dressings must be checked frequently after surgery.

the medication because the pump locks out delivery of medication for a set period. A change in position, if allowed, can also help alleviate pain. If patients do not seem to be able to get pain relief, this should be reported immediately.

- *Observations*: Restlessness, color and temperature of skin, nausea or vomiting, and similar observations should be noted and reported.
- *Position*: The patient's position must be changed when possible. Be sure you are aware of all movement restrictions. Some operations limit movement and positioning. Turn or move patients only after obtaining correct authorization.
- *Cough and deep breathe*: Most patients need to be encouraged to cough and deep breathe after general anesthesia (Figure 22–93). This exercise helps remove mucus from the lungs and respiratory tract and helps prevent pneumonia and other lung disorders.
- Comm *Tubes*: Surgical patients frequently have drainage tubes in place. The tubes are connected to drainage bottles or special drainage collectors. If the tubes are not draining, if they are clamped, if the drainage solution changes or seems unusual, if a tube is not connected to a drainage source, or if any unusual observations are noted, they should be reported immediately. Care must also be taken when turning or moving the patient to make sure that the tubes are not disconnected, twisted, or pulled out.

Binders are special devices that are ordered to hold dressings in place or provide support. (See Chapter 22:14 for information about binders.)

Surgical (elastic) hose, also called support or compression hose, may be ordered to support the veins of the legs and increase circulation. These hose help prevent formation of blood clots in the legs. The hose must be applied correctly. If they are applied too tightly, they can interfere with circulation.

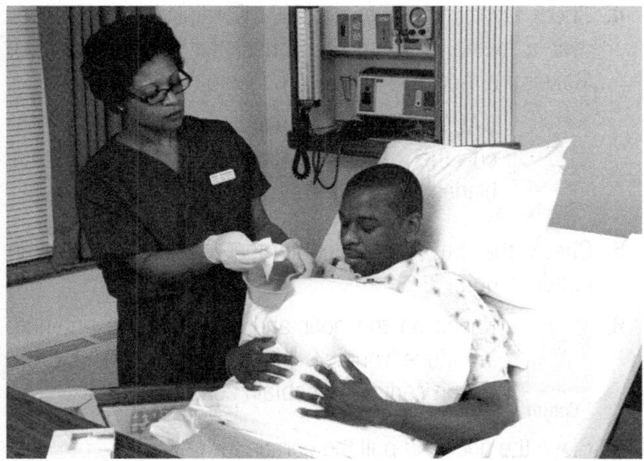

FIGURE 22–93 A pillow across the abdomen provides support when the patient is coughing and deep breathing.

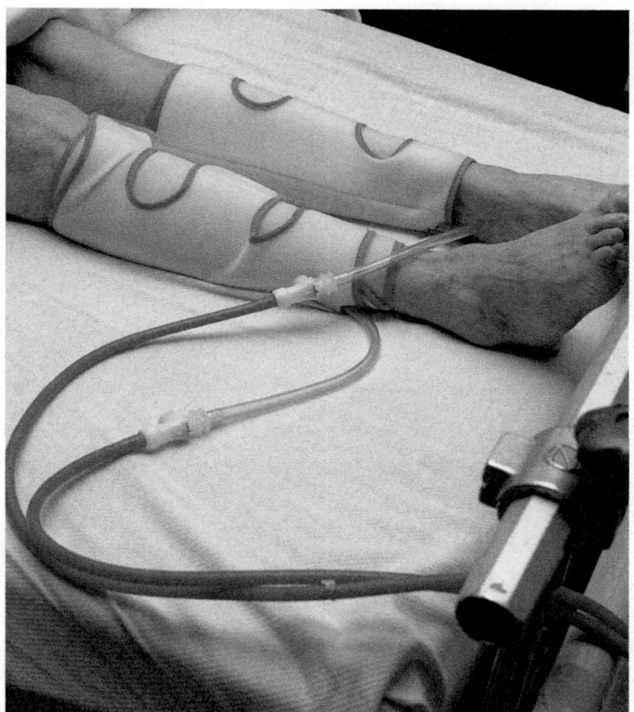

FIGURE 22–94 Compression stockings continually inflate and deflate to stimulate circulation in the legs.

Compression stockings, also called **sequential compression devices (SCDs)**, are attached to a pump that continually inflates and deflates the hose. They are frequently used to stimulate circulation in the legs by mimicking the action of the leg muscles on blood vessels (Figure 22–94). They increase the venous blood flow and prevent the formation of blood clots, or venous thromboembolism (VTE).

Montgomery straps are special adhesive strips that are applied when dressings must be changed frequently at the surgical site (Figure 22–95). The skin around the surgical site is cleaned thoroughly. A skin barrier, such as a liquid or paste, is applied to the skin to protect it from being irritated by the tape. The Montgomery straps are then applied on either side of the surgical site. The centers of the straps are nonadhesive and tied together. To change dressings, the straps are untied, the dressings are changed, and the straps are then tied in place on top of the dressings. This eliminates the need to remove and reapply adhesive tape during each dressing change.

Wound VACs provide negative-pressure wound therapy that can be used for recently closed surgical incisions or ones that were left open due to excessive

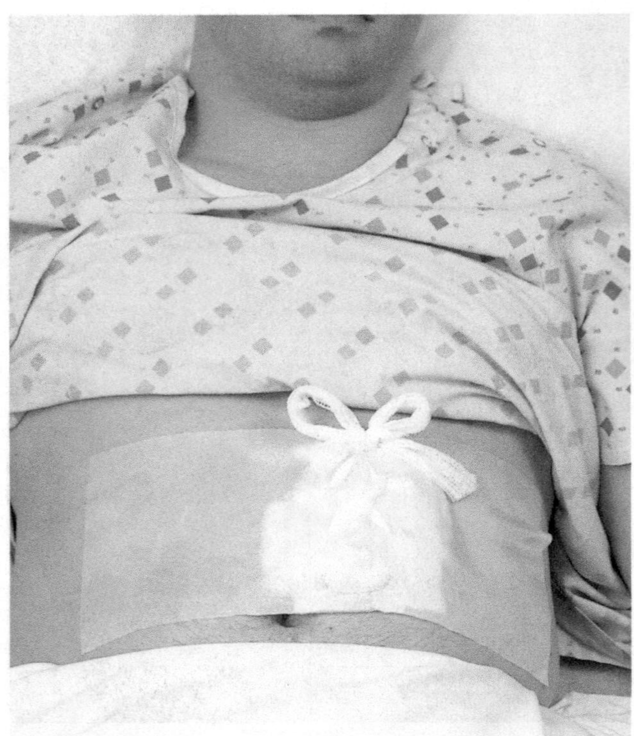

FIGURE 22–95 Montgomery straps are special adhesive strips that are applied when dressings must be changed frequently at the surgical site.

edema or drainage. They can also be used for incisions that were reopened for exploration or drainage (refer to Figure 22–7). This technique removes exudate and infectious material, and it reduces edema. It draws the wound edges together, promotes healing, and fights infection. It cannot be used if there are exposed vital organs or major vessels.

Summary

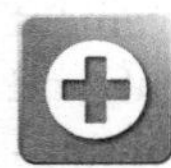

Precaution

It is essential that the nurse assistant follow all standard precautions whenever contact with blood or body fluids is possible. This helps prevent the spread of infection, including infection in the surgical patient after surgery.

It is essential for the nurse assistant to know and understand all aspects of care that have been ordered to properly care for the surgical patient. Good operative care can mean a faster recovery with fewer complications for the patient.

STUDENT: **Go to the workbook and complete the assignment sheet for 22:13, Administering Preoperative and Postoperative Care. Then return and continue with the procedures.**

PROCEDURE 22:13A

Shaving the Operative Area

NOTE: Disposable kits contain a bowl, razor, and most of the other supplies.

Equipment and Supplies

Skin-preparation kit, two bowls (if a kit is not used), razor and blades, ordered cleansing soap, gauze sponges, paper towels, applicator sticks, bath blanket, underpads or bed protectors, washcloth, towel, tray with cover, disposable gloves, gooseneck light or good light source, puncture-resistant sharps container, plastic waste bag, paper and pen or computer

Procedure

1. Check physician's orders or obtain authorization from your immediate supervisor. Clarify any questions about the area to be shaved.

Legal

NOTE: Sometimes, the physician's orders specify the area to be shaved; other times agency policy is followed.

2. Assemble equipment.
3. Prepare equipment in the utility room or bathroom. Fill both bowls (or sections of the skin-preparation kit) with water at 105°F (41°C). Add liquid cleansing soap to one bowl. Place the bowls on the tray.

   NOTE: Some kits contain sponges saturated with soap. Soap does not have to be added when using these kits.

4. Check razor and blades carefully. Carefully rub the blades over a folded gauze pad to check for damaged edges. Make sure there are no rough edges on the blades.

Safety

CAUTION: Rough or damaged blades can nick or cut the patient's skin. Discard any defective blades.

5. Check the tray for all equipment and take it to the patient's unit.
6. Knock on the door and pause before entering. Introduce yourself. Identify the patient. Explain the procedure and obtain consent.

Comm

7. Close the door and pull the curtain for privacy.
8. Wash hands.

PROCEDURE 22:13A (CONT.)

NOTE: Gloves may be put on at this point or immediately before shaving the patient.

9. Elevate the bed to a comfortable working height. If siderails are present and elevated, lower the siderail on the side where you are working. Cover the patient with a bath blanket. Fanfold the top bed linens to the foot of the bed. Place an underpad near the area to be shaved.
10. Position the gooseneck light or other light source so that the skin area is clearly illuminated. Make sure there are no glares or shadows.
11. Put on disposable gloves.

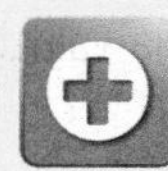
Precaution

CAUTION: If you nick the skin, observe standard precautions while controlling bleeding.

12. Start at the top of the area to be shaved. Apply soapy lather to a small area of skin.
13. Hold the skin taut. Shave in the direction of hair growth. If the hair is long, as may be the case with pubic, axillary, or chest hair, it may be clipped with scissors first. Take care to avoid cutting the patient's skin with the scissors.

NOTE: When scalp hair must be cut before brain or skull surgery, it is usually done in the operating room because it can be very traumatic for the patient.

Safety

CAUTION: Watch out for areas with moles or warts. Shave carefully around these areas.

14. Rinse the razor in the bowl of clean water. Remove excess hairs by rubbing the razor edge against a gauze square.
15. Repeat steps 12 to 14 on small areas until the entire operative site has been shaved. Work from top to bottom, side to side.
16. If the abdominal area is shaved, clean the umbilicus (navel) with cotton-tipped applicators. Shave with a circular motion, if necessary.
17. Carefully check the shaved area for any remaining hairs. Hold a light at an angle to the skin to see reflections of any remaining hairs. Remove all remaining hairs.
18. Wash the area with warm soapy water. Rinse thoroughly and dry.
19. Replace the top bed linens and remove the bath blanket and underpad.
20. Observe all checkpoints before leaving the patient: position the patient in correct body alignment, elevate the siderails (if indicated), lower the bed to its lowest level, place the call signal and supplies within easy reach of the patient, and leave the area neat and clean.
21. Clean and replace all equipment. Put the used blades or disposable razor(s) in a puncture-resistant sharps container.
22. Remove gloves. Wash hands.
23. 
Comm

Report and/or record all required information on the patient's chart or enter it into the computer. For example, date, time, abdominal skin prep completed, patient resting quietly, and your signature and title. Report any cuts, nicks, or unusual observations immediately.

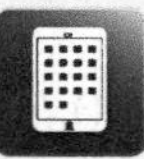
EHR

NOTE: In health care agencies using electronic health records (EHRs), also known as electronic medical records (EMRs), the information is entered directly into the patient's record on a computer.

PRACTICE: Go to the workbook and use the evaluation sheet for 22:13A, Shaving the Operative Area, to practice this procedure. When you believe you have mastered this skill, sign the sheet and give it to your instructor for further action.

Check

FINAL CHECKPOINT: Using the criteria listed on the evaluation sheet, your instructor will grade your performance.

PROCEDURE 22:13B

Administering Preoperative Care

Equipment and Supplies

Thermometer, stethoscope, sphygmomanometer, surgical gown and cap, nail polish remover, valuables envelope, tape or gauze (if needed), disposable gloves, paper and pen or computer

Procedure

1. Check physician's orders or obtain authorization from your immediate supervisor. Check the time of surgery.

   NOTE: Care should be completed 1 hour before surgery.

2. Assemble equipment.

(continues)

PROCEDURE 22:13B (CONT.)

3. 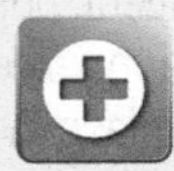 Comm — Knock on the door and pause before entering. Introduce yourself. Identify the patient. Explain the procedure and obtain consent. Make sure the operative permit has been signed (Figure 22–96A).

   NOTE: The patient may be frightened; reassure as needed.

4. Close the door and pull the curtain for privacy.
5. Wash hands. Puts on gloves.

   Precaution — **CAUTION:** Wear gloves and observe standard precautions. Contact with body fluids, secretions, or excretions is possible.

6. Elevate the bed to a comfortable working height. If siderails are present and elevated, lower the siderail on the side where you are working.
7.  Comm — Check the patient's identification band. Make sure it is secure. Verify name, room number, and other facts.
8. Assist with or instruct the patient to complete oral hygiene and bath.

   NOTE: Normally the bed is not made before surgery unless a Hibiclens bath is given. Then the bed is changed when the bath is complete.

   Safety — **CAUTION:** Because the patient is NPO (nothing by mouth), do not allow the patient to swallow any water when performing oral hygiene.

9. Put a surgical gown on the patient. No other clothing is permitted. Make sure the patient's underwear is removed.
10. Remove all hairpins, wigs, and other hair ornaments. Put a cap on the patient. Make sure all hair is inside the cap.
11. Remove nail polish. Check to be sure the patient is not wearing any makeup.
12. Remove all of the patient's jewelry and place it in a valuables envelope. Also place money and other valuables in the envelope. Follow hospital procedure for securing valuables.

    NOTE: Wedding rings may be tied or taped in place. Follow hospital procedure.

    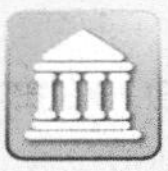 Legal — **CAUTION:** In some agencies, only certain health care workers are permitted to handle valuables. Follow agency policy.

13. Remove full or partial dentures. Place these in a denture cup labeled with the patient's name and room number. Place the cup in a drawer or safe area to prevent breakage.
14. Have the patient remove contact lenses, glasses, hearing aids, and all other prostheses (artificial parts). Place in a safe area.
15. Offer a bedpan or assist the patient to the bathroom. Encourage the patient to void. If a catheter and urinary-drainage unit is in place, empty the urinary-drainage unit and record the measurement.
16. Take vital signs and record correctly (Figure 22–96B).

     Safety — **CAUTION:** The vital signs must be accurate and correct. If in doubt about the results, ask your supervisor to check them.

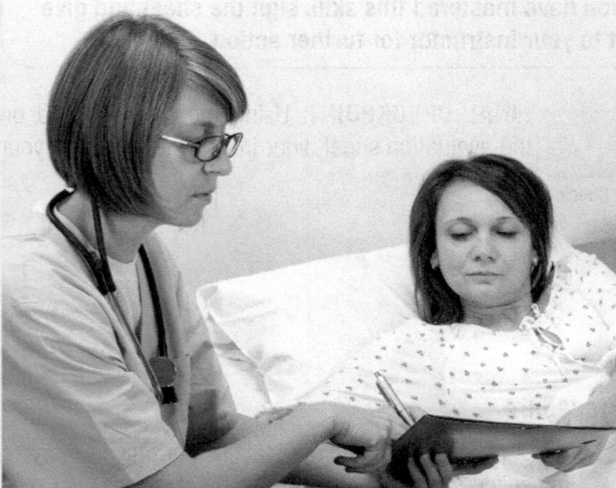

FIGURE 22–96A **Explain the procedure and make sure that the operative permit is signed. Remember that only authorized individuals can witness the signature.** ©iStock.com/Daniel Yordanov

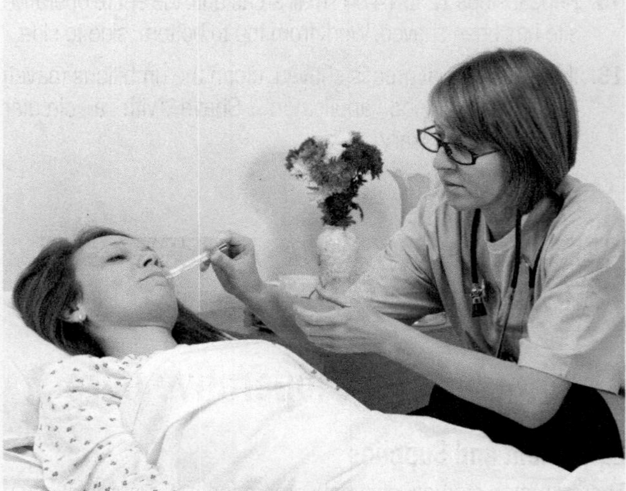

FIGURE 22–96B **Vital signs must be taken and recorded as part of preoperative care.** ©iStock.com/Daniel Yordanov

PROCEDURE 22:13B (CONT.)

17. Elevate the siderails immediately after preoperative medication has been given by an authorized person.

    NOTE: Preoperative medication is usually given 1 hour before surgery. It helps the patient relax, and it often contains medication to dry up nose and mouth secretions. Because the patient could become drowsy and fall out of bed, the siderails must be elevated immediately.

18. Place the patient in a comfortable position. Encourage the patient to rest.
19. Observe all checkpoints before leaving the patient: make sure the water pitcher has been removed from the unit, lower the bed to its lowest level, place the call signal within easy reach of the patient, and leave the area neat and clean.

    NOTE: Many hospitals use pre-op checklists, which are placed on patients' charts. If this is hospital policy, complete the checklist.

20. Clean and replace all equipment.
21. Remove gloves and wash hands.
22. 
Comm
Report and/or record all required information on the patient's chart or enter it into the computer. For example, date, time, pre-op care complete and noted on checklist, siderails elevated, patient resting quietly, and your signature and title. Report any unusual observations immediately.

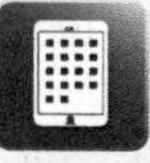
EHR
NOTE: In health care agencies using electronic health records (EHRs), also known as electronic medical records (EMRs), the information is entered directly into the patient's record on a computer.

PRACTICE: **Go to the workbook and use the evaluation sheet for 22:13B, Administering Preoperative Care, to practice this procedure. When you believe you have mastered this skill, sign the sheet and give it to your instructor for further action.**

Check
FINAL CHECKPOINT: Using the criteria listed on the evaluation sheet, your instructor will grade your performance.

PROCEDURE 22:13C

Preparing a Postoperative Unit

Equipment and Supplies

Bed linen for an unoccupied bed; extra draw sheet; underpads or protective covers; emesis basin; tissues; plastic bag and tape; gauze bandage; intravenous (IV) pole or stand; vital signs equipment (thermometer, blood pressure apparatus, watch with second hand); linen bag, hamper, or cart; gloves; paper and pen or computer

Procedure

1. Assemble equipment.

   NOTE: The post-op unit is prepared immediately after the patient leaves the area for the operating room.

2. Wash hands. Put on gloves.

   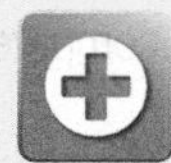
   Precaution
   CAUTION: Wear gloves. The linen may be contaminated with blood, body fluids, secretions, or excretions. Remove the gloves and wash hands thoroughly after removing the dirty linen and before applying the clean linen.

3. Remove any used linen from the bed and place in the linen bag, hamper, or cart. Remove gloves and wash hands.
4. Make the foundation (bottom sheet and draw sheet) of the bed as previously instructed for an unoccupied bed.
5. Place a cotton draw sheet over the head of the bed. Tuck in at the head of the bed as was done for bottom sheet. Make mitered corners and tuck in at the sides.

   NOTE: This protects the bed should the patient vomit.

   NOTE: Some agencies use underpads instead of draw sheets.

6. Place a top sheet and a spread on the bed. Let them fall loose.
7. Go to the foot of the bed and fold the top linen back. Make a cuff so that the top linen is even with the end of the mattress.

   NOTE: The top linen is not tucked in.

8. Go to the head of the bed. Make a cuff with the top linen.
9. Fanfold the top linen to the side of the bed opposite from where the patient will be brought in on the stretcher.

(continues)

PROCEDURE 22:13C (CONT.)

NOTE: In some agencies, the sheets are folded to the foot of the bed. Follow agency policy.

10. Cover the pillow with a pillowcase. Place the pillow in an upright position at the head of the bed.

    NOTE: This protects the patient's head against injury during the transfer to the bed.

11. Estimate the height of the stretcher and elevate the bed to this height.
12. Put a cuff on the plastic bag. Tape it to the side of the bed or bedside table.
13. Place underpads on the bed near where the operated body part will be resting.
14. Remove all unnecessary articles from the bedside stand. Place the emesis basin, tissues, and equipment for taking vital signs on the stand.

    NOTE: Make sure the water pitcher and cup are not on the bedside stand. Patients may be NPO (nothing by mouth) postoperatively.

15. Position the overbed table, chair, and other furniture so it will not be in the way of the stretcher.
16. Place the IV stand or pump in the most convenient location. It should be ready for the IV when the patient is transferred to the bed.
17. Check the area before leaving. Make sure that all equipment and supplies are ready for the patient's return from surgery (Figure 22–97).
18. Replace all equipment used.
19. Wash hands.
20. 

Report and/or record all required information on the patient's chart or enter it into the computer. For example, date, time, post-op unit prepared, and your signature and title.

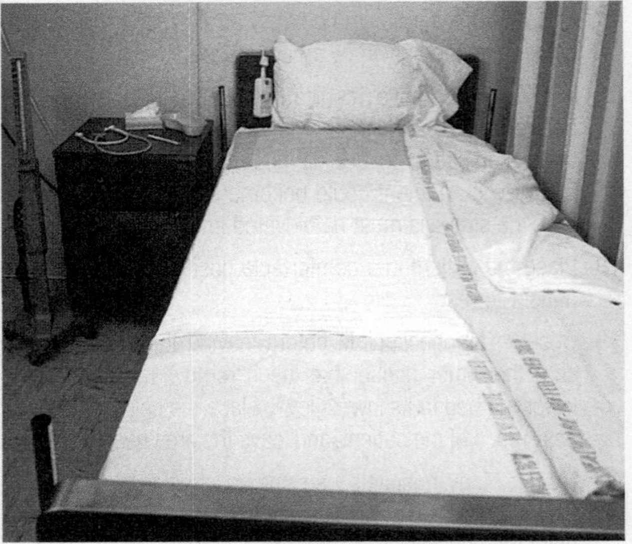

FIGURE 22–97 **Before leaving the post-op unit, check to make sure that all equipment and supplies are ready for the patient's return from surgery.**

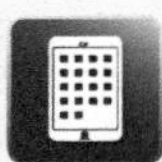

NOTE: In health care agencies using electronic health records (EHRs), also known as electronic medical records (EMRs), the information is entered directly into the patient's record on a computer.

PRACTICE: **Go to the workbook and use the evaluation sheet for 22:13C, Preparing a Postoperative Unit, to practice this procedure. When you believe you have mastered this skill, sign the sheet and give it to your instructor for further action.**

FINAL CHECKPOINT: Using the criteria listed on the evaluation sheet, your instructor will grade your performance.

PROCEDURE 22:13D

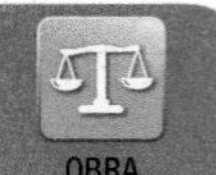

Applying Surgical Hose and Compression Stockings

NOTE: Surgical hose and compression stockings come in various sizes and lengths. This procedure deals with the application of knee-length surgical stockings and compression hose.

Equipment and Supplies

Correct size surgical hose and compression stockings, compression pump, measuring tape, paper and pen or computer

Procedure

1. Check physician's orders or obtain authorization from your immediate supervisor.

PROCEDURE 22:13D (CONT.)

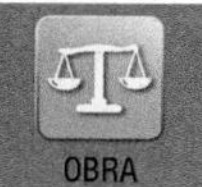

OBRA

2. Assemble equipment.
3.  Comm Knock on the door and pause before entering. Introduce yourself. Identify the patient. Explain the procedure and obtain consent.
4. Wash hands.
5. Check the hose and stockings to be sure they are clean and the correct size.

   NOTE: Hose and stockings from different companies are sized differently. Use the measuring tape and follow the instructions that came with the hose to determine the correct size for the patient.
6. Close the door and pull the curtain for privacy. Elevate the bed to a comfortable working height. If siderails are present and elevated, lower the side rail on the side where you are working. Expose the patient's legs.
7. Start with the surgical hose. Insert your hand into the top of the hose. Turn the hose so that the smooth side is on the outside.

   NOTE: This makes application easier and leaves the rough edge on the outside of the foot.
8. Grasp the heel area of the hose. Smoothly tuck the foot portion back into the stocking.
9. Stretch the hose open at the heel. Support the patient's leg and slide the foot and pocket of the heel into position on the patient's foot (Figure 22–98A).

    Safety **CAUTION:** Use correct body mechanics when applying hose. Stand with your feet apart and one leg ahead of the other, bending at the hips rather than the waist.
10. Make sure the heel of the stocking is secure over the patient's heel.
11. Grasp the top of the stocking. Pull it over the foot. Gather the material at the ankle. Use two hands and gentle pressure.

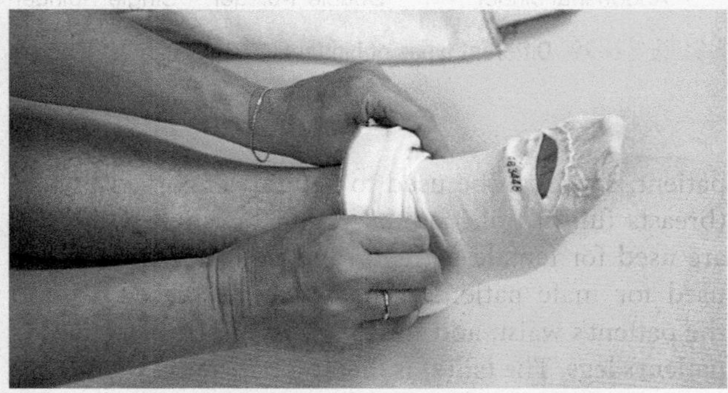

FIGURE 22–98A Slide the foot of the hose into position.

12. Begin gently pulling the hose up the leg to the area below the knee (Figure 22–98B). Work slowly to prevent wrinkles. Use both hands to smooth the hose into place.

     Safety **CAUTION:** Do not pull and stretch the hose. This will make it too tight and interfere with circulation.
13. Check the position of the hose. The top should be just below the knee. Smooth any excess material with your hands.
14. Pull the toe forward slightly to provide "toe room" (Figure 22–98C).
15. Repeat steps 7 to 14 for the opposite leg.
16. Once the surgical hose are in place, put the compression stockings, also called sleeves, on top of them.

    NOTE: Surgical hose and compression stockings/sleeves can be ordered together, or just one or the other may be ordered.

    a. Place the side of the compression sleeve with the printed instructions against the patient's leg.

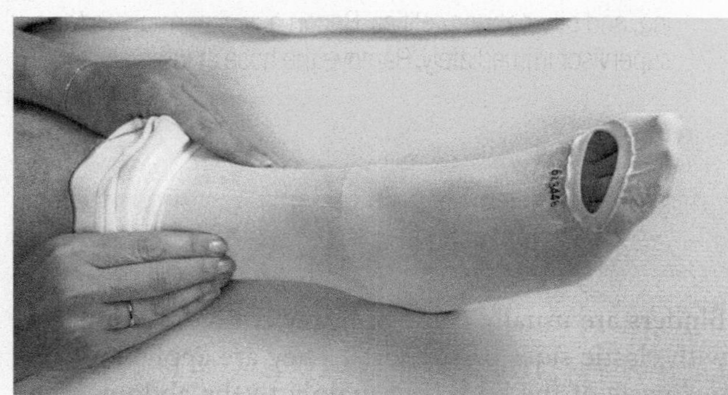

FIGURE 22–98B Draw the hose gently up the leg to the area below the knee.

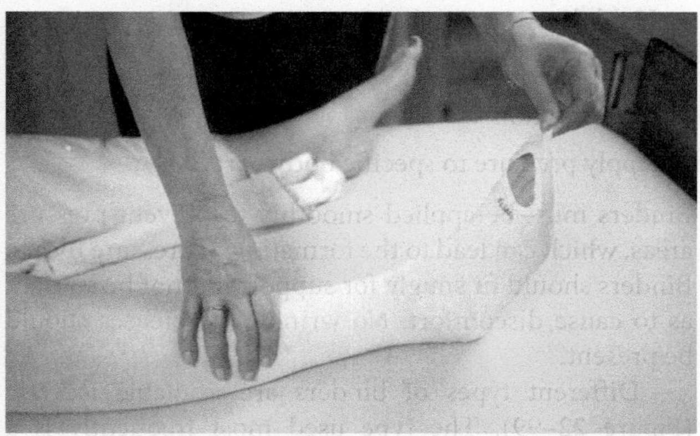

FIGURE 22–98C Pull the toe forward slightly to provide "toe room."

(continues)

PROCEDURE 22:13D (CONT.)

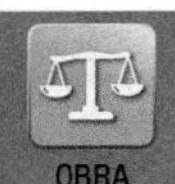

OBRA

b. Position the compression sleeve so it is centered behind the calf.

c. Wrap the sleeve securely around the calf, ensuring that two fingers can fit between the calf and the sleeve.

d. Secure the sleeve using the Velcro closures.

e. Repeat the process for the other leg (refer to Figure 22–94).

f. Attach the compression pump to the sleeves by snapping the connectors together.

g. Plug in the pump and turn it on.

h. Instruct the patient that he or she will feel the stockings inflating and deflating.

17. Observe all checkpoints before leaving the patient: position the patient in correct body alignment, elevate the siderails (if indicated), lower the bed to its lowest level, place the call signal and supplies within easy reach of the patient, and leave the area neat and clean.

18. Check the hose at intervals. Look for signs of impaired circulation, including abnormal skin color or temperature, swelling, and other abnormalities. Report any abnormalities to your supervisor immediately. Remove the hose at intervals, at least once every 8 hours. Administer skin care to the skin under the hose. If the hose become soiled, they can be washed.

19. Wash hands.

20. 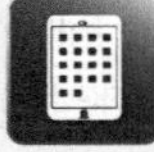

Comm

Report and/or record all required information on the patient's chart or enter it into the computer. For example, date, time, surgical hose applied to both legs, and your signature and title. Report any unusual observations immediately.

EHR

NOTE: In health care agencies using electronic health records (EHRs), also known as electronic medical records (EMRs), the information is entered directly into the patient's record on a computer.

PRACTICE: **Go to the workbook and use the evaluation sheet for 22:13D, Applying Surgical Hose, to practice this procedure. When you believe you have mastered this skill, sign the sheet and give it to your instructor for further action.**

Check

FINAL CHECKPOINT: Using the criteria listed on the evaluation sheet, your instructor will grade your performance.

22:14 Applying Binders

Binders are usually made of heavy cotton or flannelette with elastic sides or supports. They are applied to various parts of the body, but mainly to the abdomen and breasts. Functions of binders include the following:

- Provide support and relief from pain following surgery
- Hold dressings in place
- Provide support for engorged breasts
- Limit motion
- Apply pressure to specific body parts

Binders must be applied smoothly to prevent pressure areas, which can lead to the formation of pressure ulcers. Binders should fit snugly for support but not be so tight as to cause discomfort. No wrinkles or creases should be present.

Different types of binders are available for use (Figure 22–99). The type used most frequently is a straight binder. It can be applied to the abdomen, back, or rib cage. Straight binders are secured using Velcro tabs. Breast binders are used to support the breasts of a female patient. They can be used to support engorged breasts (breasts full of milk) after childbirth. Single T-binders are used for female patients, and double T-binders are used for male patients. The binder is placed around the patient's waist, and the tail(s) is passed between the patient's legs. The tail(s) is then pinned at the waist. This type of binder is used to hold perineal dressings in place or provide support. In most instances, T-binders have

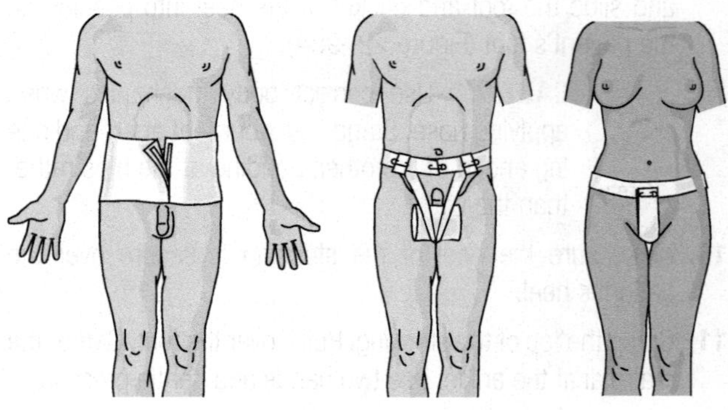

FIGURE 22–99 **Different types of binders.**

been replaced by scrotal supports for men and self-adhesive sanitary napkins for women.

Binders are applied from bottom to top for optimal support. In this way, organs can be supported correctly. Circulation and breathing should always be checked after binders are applied. A binder that is too tight can cause severe complications. In addition, binders should be removed at intervals, and skin care should be provided to the skin under the binder.

STUDENT: **Go to the workbook and complete the assignment sheet for 22:14, Applying Binders. Then return and continue with the procedure.**

PROCEDURE 22:14

Applying a Straight Binder

Equipment and Supplies

Straight binder, paper and pen or computer

Procedure

1. Check physician's orders or obtain authorization from your immediate supervisor.
2. Assemble supplies.
3.  Comm — Knock on the door and pause before entering. Introduce yourself. Identify the patient. Explain the procedure and obtain consent.
4. Wash hands.
5. Close the door and pull the curtain for privacy. Elevate the bed to a comfortable working height. If siderails are present and elevated, lower the siderail on the side where you are working.
6. Fanfold the top bed linen down to the patient's pubic area. Arrange the bedclothes so that the abdomen is exposed.
7. Assist the patient to move to the near side of the bed.

   Safety — **CAUTION:** Use correct body mechanics when applying binders.
8. With the inside facing out, fold the binder in half to determine where the center is.
9.  Comm — Ask the patient to flex the knees, place his or her weight on the heels, and raise the hips.

   NOTE: The patient can also turn on his or her side, if this is easier.
10. Unfold the binder and slide it under the patient (Figure 22–100A). Keep your thumbs at the edge of the center fold. Position the binder by putting the center fold at the center of the patient's spine. The bottom edge should be at the base of the spine but not so low as to interfere with the use of a bedpan.

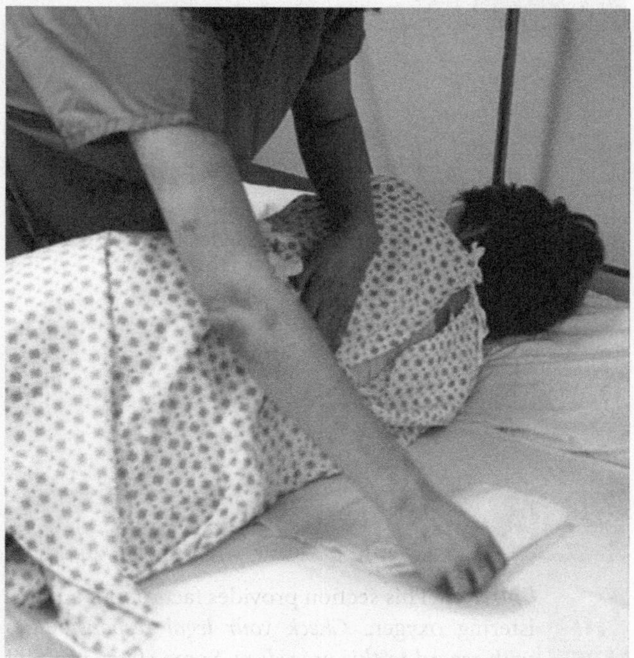

FIGURE 22–100A **Position the binder under the patient with the center fold at the patient's spine and the bottom edge at the base of the spine.**

11. Open the binder completely. Check placement. Make sure the binder is smooth and even, with no wrinkles.
12. Fasten the binder from the bottom to the top. Pull the sides together firmly. Start at the bottom edge and seal in an upward direction (Figure 22–100B).
13. Check the entire binder. Make sure it is snug but not too tight. Make sure it is smooth and positioned correctly. Check to be sure that it is not restricting breathing or circulation.
14. Replace all bed linens.
15. Observe all checkpoints before leaving the patient: position the patient in correct body alignment, elevate the siderails (if indicated), lower the bed to its lowest level, place the call signal and supplies within easy reach of the patient, and leave the area neat and clean.

(continues)

PROCEDURE 22:14 (CONT.)

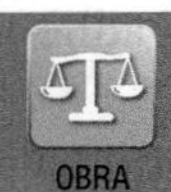
OBRA

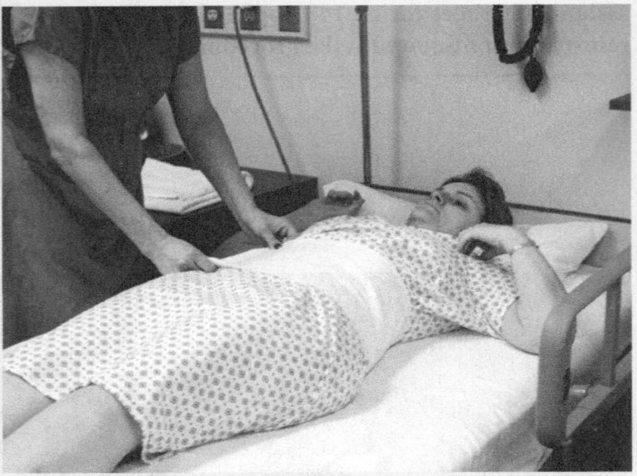

FIGURE 22–100B Secure the Velcro tabs of the binder by starting at the bottom edge and working in an upward direction.

16. Replace equipment.

17. Wash hands.

18. 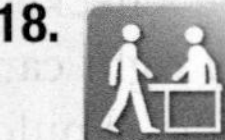 Comm Report and/or record all required information on the patient's chart or enter it into the computer. For example, date, time, straight binder applied to abdomen, and your signature and title.

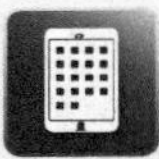 EHR **NOTE:** In health care agencies using electronic health records (EHRs), also known as electronic medical records (EMRs), the information is entered directly into the patient's record on a computer.

PRACTICE: **Go to the workbook and use the evaluation sheet for 22:14, Applying a Straight Binder, to practice this procedure. When you believe you have mastered this skill, sign the sheet and give it to your instructor for further action.**

 Check **FINAL CHECKPOINT:** Using the criteria listed on the evaluation sheet, your instructor will grade your performance.

22:15 Administering Oxygen

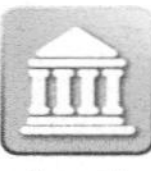 Legal **CAUTION:** This section provides facts about administering oxygen. *Check your legal responsibilities with regard to this procedure.* Some states prohibit administration of oxygen by a health care assistant.

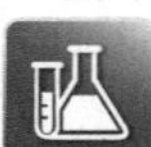 Science The blood must have oxygen. The blood's supply of oxygen is normally obtained from the air, which is approximately 23 percent oxygen. As a result of accident, injury, or respiratory disease, however, the body may be unable to take in enough oxygen or to use oxygen effectively. In such cases, oxygen can be given to the patient by various means.

The signs of an oxygen shortage are rapid and shallow respirations, rapid pulse, restlessness, anxiety, and cyanosis. A deficiency of oxygen is called hypoxia. Lack of oxygen can cause brain damage in 4–6 minutes.

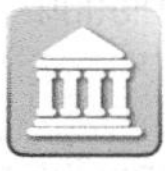 Legal A physician's order is usually required for the administration of oxygen. The order will include the method of administration and the concentration to be given. In cases of extreme emergency, oxygen can be started with standard concentrations, and the physician notified as soon as possible. Most rescue teams, ambulance personnel, and others involved in emergency work follow specific orders regarding oxygen administration.

Methods of Oxygen Administration

Oxygen is usually administered by one of the following methods:

- *Mask* (Figure 22–101A): The mask should cover the mouth and the nose. It should fit snugly to prevent loss of oxygen, but it should not be so tight as to cause discomfort to the patient. Oxygen by mask is the method of administration used most frequently by rescue personnel. It provides the highest concentration of oxygen. However, some patients are frightened by the mask. A careful explanation of its purpose along with constant reassurance are necessary. The rate of flow by mask is usually 6–10 liters per minute. Masks should never be used with flow rates less than 5 liters per minute because the patient will rebreathe carbon dioxide and feel smothered.
- *Cannula* (Figure 22–101B): The cannula consists of two small, curved, plastic tubes, which are placed one in each nostril. The other end of the cannula is attached to an oxygen tank or unit. The patient must be instructed to breathe through the nose. If the patient opens the mouth to breathe, the concentration of oxygen is reduced. The rate of flow by cannula is usually 2–6 liters per minute.

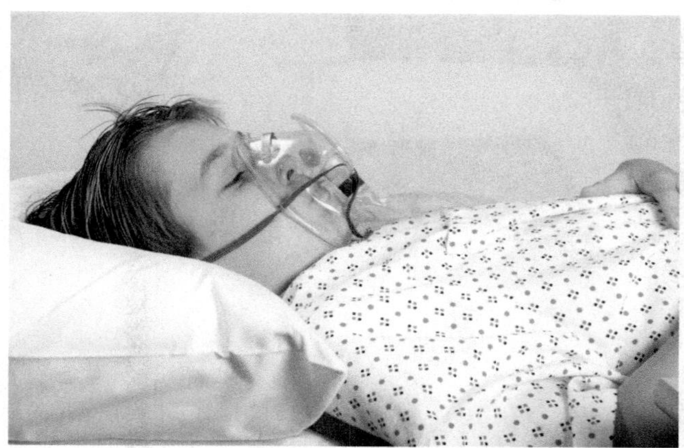
FIGURE 22–101A The oxygen mask covers the nose and mouth and provides a high concentration of oxygen. © Leah-Anne Thompson/Shutterstock.com

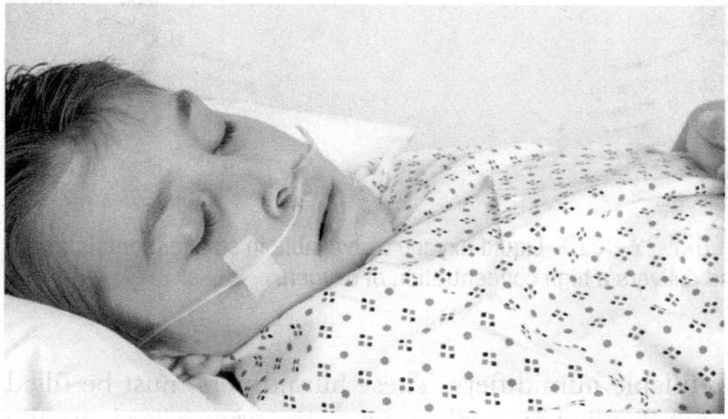
FIGURE 22–101B When a nasal cannula is used to provide oxygen, the patient must breathe through the nose. © Leah-Anne Thompson/Shutterstock.com

- *Tent*: The tent surrounds the patient with a high concentration of oxygen. It is often used for small children or restless patients who are not able to cooperate well with other methods. Oxygen and humidity are provided. A common example is a croupette used with infants and small children. The flow rate is usually 10–12 liters per minute.

Oxygen Delivery Systems

Different systems can be used to provide oxygen. Most hospitals pipe in oxygen through the wall. A flow meter for the oxygen is plugged into an adaptor in the wall (Figure 22–102A). When the flow meter is turned on, oxygen is delivered. Oxygen is color coded with a green label in the United States. The wall adaptor usually has a green label with the word oxygen or the symbol O_2. Portable oxygen cylinders are used while transporting patients, in emergencies, in some long-term care facilities, and in home situations (Figure 22–102B). Other health care facilities, such as some long-term care facilities, medical offices, or dental offices, may pipe in oxygen. However, in most cases, they use oxygen cylinders

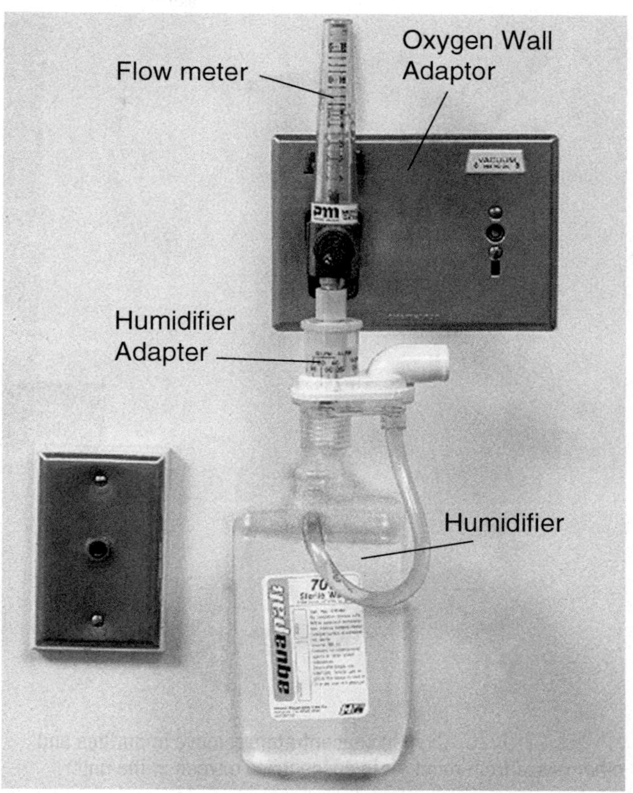

FIGURE 22–102A When oxygen is piped through a wall, the flow meter is plugged into a wall adaptor. A humidifier is used to moisturize the oxygen.

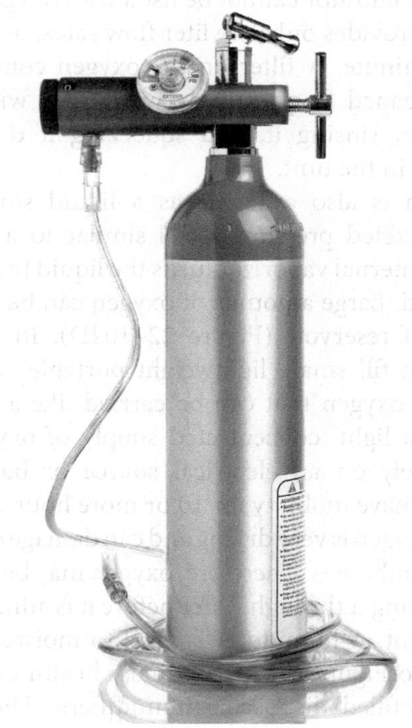
FIGURE 22–102B Portable oxygen cylinders can be used to provide oxygen in health care facilities, emergency care units, and homes. ©iStock.com/Thomas Acop

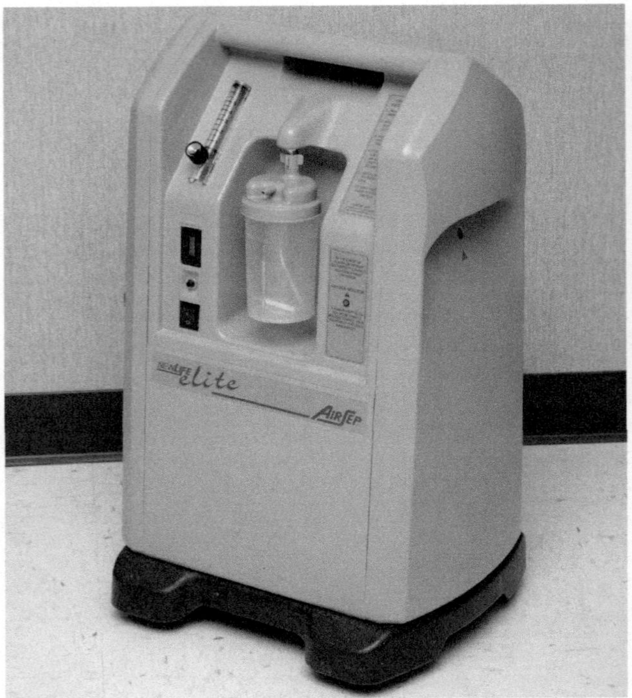

FIGURE 22–102C Oxygen concentrators remove impurities and other gases from room air to concentrate oxygen in the unit.

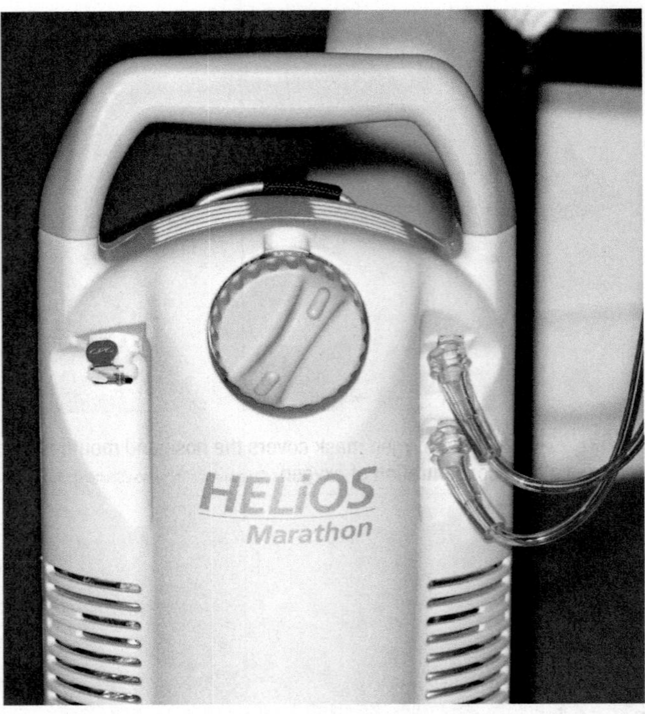

FIGURE 22–102D Liquid oxygen is available in smaller containers and delivers a high concentration of oxygen. Dr. P. Marazzi/Science Source

or oxygen concentrators. An oxygen concentrator removes impurities and other gases from room air to concentrate oxygen in the unit (Figure 22–102C). The oxygen concentrator cannot be used with oxygen masks because it provides only low liter flow rates, usually 2–4 liters per minute. A filter on the oxygen concentrator must be cleaned frequently by washing it with warm soapy water, rinsing it, and squeezing it dry before replacing it in the unit.

Oxygen is also available as a liquid stored in a vacuum-jacketed pressure vessel similar to a thermos bottle. An internal vaporizer turns the liquid to gas when it is released. Large amounts of oxygen can be stored in this type of reservoir (Figure 22–102D). In addition, patients can fill small, lightweight portable containers with liquid oxygen that can be carried like a shoulder bag. With a light, concentrated supply of oxygen that does not rely on an electrical source or batteries, a patient can have mobility for 10 or more hours.

Pure oxygen is very drying and can damage or irritate mucous membranes. Therefore, oxygen may be moisturized by passing it through water before it is administered to the patient. A humidifier is used to moisturize oxygen (refer to Figure 22–102A). Many health care facilities use prefilled disposable humidifiers. These units are changed and discarded when they are empty. They must be changed at least once each week or according to the manufacturer's instructions. Some facilities use refillable humidifiers. These humidifiers must be filled with distilled or sterile water to the proper level, usually one-half to two-thirds of the container; most humidifiers are marked for the proper level. Distilled or sterile water is usually used to prevent mineral deposits on the equipment. Refillable humidifiers must be washed and sterilized every 24 hours to prevent infection. A label is usually placed on the humidifier to indicate the date and time it was changed. Additional water should never be added to a partially filled humidifier.

Safety Precautions

Safety precautions must be observed when oxygen is in use. Although oxygen does not explode, burning is more rapid and intense in the presence of oxygen. Flammable materials (those that burn) will burn much more rapidly in the presence of oxygen. The following precautions should be taken whenever oxygen is in use:

- Smoking, lighting cigarettes or matches, burning candles, and the use of open flames are prohibited when oxygen is in use. In patient-care areas, where smoking is not already prohibited, a warning sign reading, for example, "No Smoking—Oxygen" is placed on the door to the patient's room, on the bed, or on the wall nearby. Warning labels are also sometimes placed on tanks used by emergency rescue personnel.

- 
Comm
The sign is not enough. The patient must be cautioned against smoking. Observers at the scene of an accident or emergency situation and visitors in a patient-care area must also be told to avoid smoking.
- The use of electrically operated equipment, which could cause sparks, should be avoided.
- Flammable liquids such as nail polish remover or adhesive tape remover should never be used while oxygen is in use. Alcohol-based aftershave lotions, hairspray, perfumes, and non-approved lip balms should not be used for patient care.
- Cotton blankets should be used in place of wool or nylon. In addition, all bed linen, bedspreads, and gowns or pajamas should be cotton instead of synthetic materials. Cotton is static-free, and its use decreases the danger of static electricity.
- Frequent inspections must be made of any area where oxygen is in use. Sources of sparks or static electricity should be removed.

Pulse Oximeters

Pulse oximeters may be used to monitor the patient who is receiving oxygen (Figure 22–103). An oximeter measures the level of oxygen in arterial blood. A photodetector probe is clipped on the patient's finger, toe, or earlobe. The percentage of oxygen in the arterial blood is displayed on the monitor screen of the oximeter. If the oxygen level falls below the minimum percentage programmed into the oximeter, an alarm will sound. Licensed personnel are responsible for programming and monitoring the oximeter. The health care assistant should make sure the probe is not disturbed and notify a supervisor if the alarm sounds.

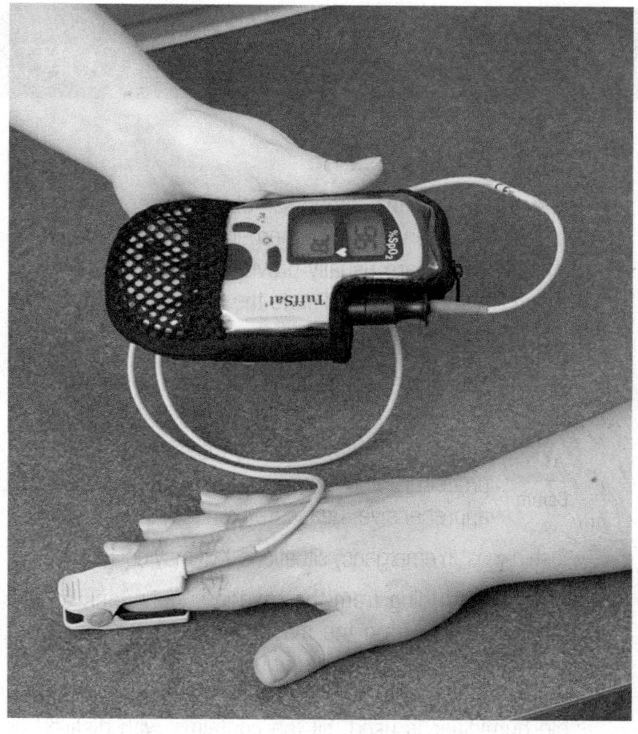

FIGURE 22–103 Pulse oximeters may be used to measure the level of oxygen in arterial blood.

Summary

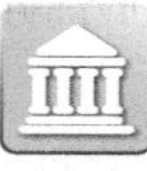
Legal

A patient who is receiving oxygen must be checked frequently. Quality of respirations should be noted. Mouth and nose care must be provided if a mask or cannula is used. The oxygen flow rate should be checked. Watch to make sure that the patient and visitors do not change the liter flow. If a humidifier is used, the water level must be checked and the humidifier replaced as indicated. Safety precautions must be checked frequently. In many facilities, oxygen administration is the responsibility of the respiratory therapy department. However, the health care worker, who is with the patient more frequently, should always be aware of safety precautions and check patients carefully. Any abnormal observations should be reported immediately.

STUDENT: **Go to the workbook and complete the assignment sheet for 22:15, Administering Oxygen. Then return and continue with the procedure.**

PROCEDURE 22:15

Administering Oxygen

Equipment and Supplies

Oxygen mask, cannula, or tent; tubing and gauge; oxygen tank or supply; distilled or sterile water (if refillable humidifier is used); paper and pen or computer

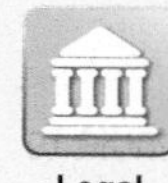
Legal

CAUTION: Some states prohibit the administration of oxygen by a health care assistant. Check your legal responsibilities in regard to this procedure.

(continues)

PROCEDURE 22:15 (CONT.)

Procedure

1. Read the physician's orders or obtain orders from your immediate supervisor. In emergency rescue situations, standard orders are usually provided for victims requiring oxygen. The orders should state the method of administration and liter flow per minute.
2. Assemble equipment.
3. 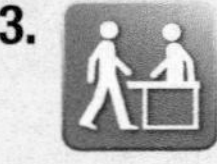 Comm Knock on the door and pause before entering. Introduce yourself. Identify the patient. Explain the procedure and obtain consent. Patients are often apprehensive. Reassure as needed.
4. Wash hands. In emergency situations, this may not be possible.
5. Connect the tubing from the oxygen supply (tank or wall unit) to the tubing on the mask or cannula. If a prefilled humidifier is used, follow manufacturer's instructions to release the seal and attach it to the flow meter. If a refillable humidifier is used, fill the container with distilled or sterile water. Distilled water prevents mineral deposits from forming inside the humidifier. Replace the lid and connect it to the flow meter or oxygen outlet.

   NOTE: If you are using oxygen from a wall unit, ensure that you are using the green flow meter marked oxygen. In many facilities, similar flow meters are used for air. They are yellow and marked as such.
6. Turn on the oxygen supply.

    Safety **CAUTION:** Do not insert the nasal cannula or apply the mask at this time. Regulate the gauge to the correct liter flow rate per minute first (Figure 22–104).

    Safety **CAUTION:** Make sure to follow specific manufacturer's instructions or agency policy for connecting and turning on the oxygen supply. Do not operate any oxygen equipment until you have been specifically instructed on how to use it.
7. Check to be sure that oxygen is passing through the tubing. Place your hand by the outlet on the mask or cannula.
8. Put on disposable gloves.

   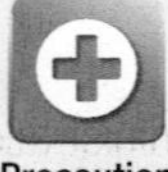 Precaution **CAUTION:** Observe all standard precautions. Contact with the patient's oral or nasal secretions is possible.
9. With the oxygen still flowing, apply the mask or cannula to the patient.
   a. If a mask is used, position it over the patient's nose and mouth. Adjust the strap so that it fits snugly but does not apply pressure to the face.

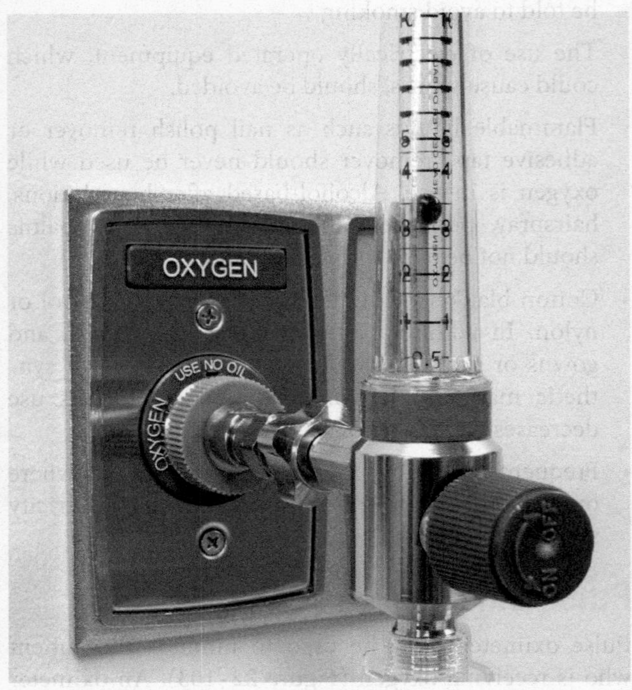

FIGURE 22–104 **Regulate the gauge to provide the correct liter flow rate for oxygen.** © Scott Milless/Shutterstock.com

   b. If a cannula is used, place the two tips in the patient's nostrils and loop the tubing around each ear. Adjust the straps at the neck so that the tips remain in position. Instruct the patient to breathe through the nose.
10. If a tent is used, it is first filled with oxygen. Then the prescribed liter flow is set. The humidifier is filled to the marked level with distilled or sterile water. Next, the tent is placed over the bed or crib, and the edges are tucked in on all sides to prevent oxygen loss. A cotton blanket, bath blanket, or sheet can be used to provide a cuff around the loose end covering the patient.
11. Check the surrounding area to make sure all safety precautions are being observed. Eliminate any sources of sparks or flames. In facilities where smoking is not already prohibited, caution any visitors and the patient against smoking while the oxygen is in use. In a patient-care area, make sure a sign is posted on the door or in the immediate area.
12. Check the patient at frequent intervals. Note respirations, color, restlessness, or discomfort. Provide skin care to the face and/or nose if a mask or cannula is used. Check the skin behind the ears and provide skin care if a nasal cannula is used. At times, it may be necessary to use a towel or cloth to dry the inside of the mask, because moisture will accumulate in the mask. If a nasal cannula is used, check

PROCEDURE 22:15 (CONT.)

the tips to make sure they are open and not plugged by mucus. Provide oral hygiene frequently. Check the water level, if a humidifier is used, and replace the humidifier as needed. Check the gauge and make sure the liter flow rate is correct. Report any abnormal conditions immediately.

13. When the oxygen is discontinued, make sure that the oxygen supply is turned off. Follow the specific manufacturer's instructions or agency policy. Clean and replace all equipment. Most masks and cannulas are disposable and discarded after use. If the items are not disposable, they should be cleaned and disinfected according to established agency policy.
14. Remove gloves. Wash hands.
15. Comm Report and/or record all required information on the patient's chart or enter it into the computer. For example, date, time, oxygen per mask at 6 L/min, R 16 deep and even, and your signature and title. Report any unusual observations immediately.

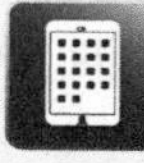
EHR

NOTE: In health care agencies using electronic medical records (EMRs), also known as electronic health records (EHRs), the information is entered directly into the patient's record on a computer.

PRACTICE: Go to the workbook and use the evaluation sheet for 22:15, Administering Oxygen, to practice this procedure. When you believe you have mastered this skill, sign the sheet and give it to your instructor for further action.

Check

FINAL CHECKPOINT: Using the criteria listed on the evaluation sheet, your instructor will grade your performance.

22:16 Giving Postmortem Care

OBRA

Providing care after death is a difficult but essential part of patient care. As a health care worker, you may perform or assist with this care.

Postmortem care is care given to the body immediately after death. It begins when a physician has pronounced the patient dead.

Dealing with death and dying is a difficult part of providing care. If a health care worker has cared for a patient for a time, it is natural for the worker to feel grief and a sense of loss on the patient's death. Crying is a natural expression of grief, and you should not feel embarrassed if you cry. However, it is also important for health care workers to try to control emotions because family members and other patients will need their support.

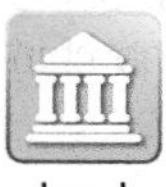
Legal

The patient's rights continue to apply after death. The body should be treated with dignity and respect. Privacy should be provided at all times.

If family members are not present when death occurs and want to view the body before it is taken to the morgue or funeral home, the body should be prepared for viewing. The patient should be positioned naturally, with the limbs straight. Elevate the head of the bed 30 degrees to prevent discoloration of the head and neck. Follow agency policy regarding dentures and glasses. Some facilities state dentures and glasses should be placed on the patient for family viewing. After the viewing, they are removed, packed safely, and sent to the funeral home with the body. Other facilities state that the dentures and glasses must be packed immediately and not placed on the body because the items could fall off and break. The bed linen should be neat and clean, and extra equipment should be removed from the unit. Provide privacy while the family views the body unless they request that you remain with them.

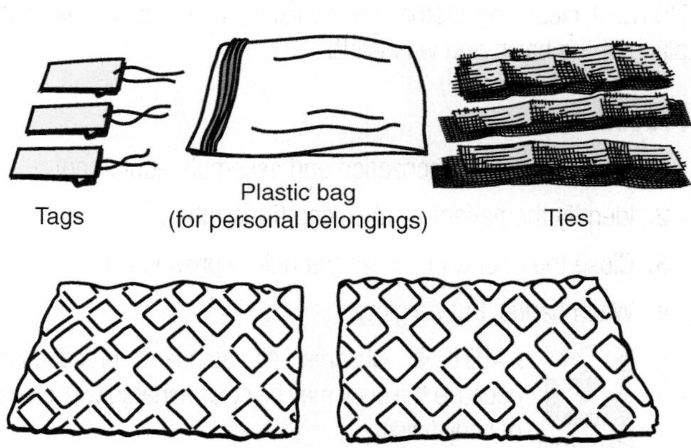

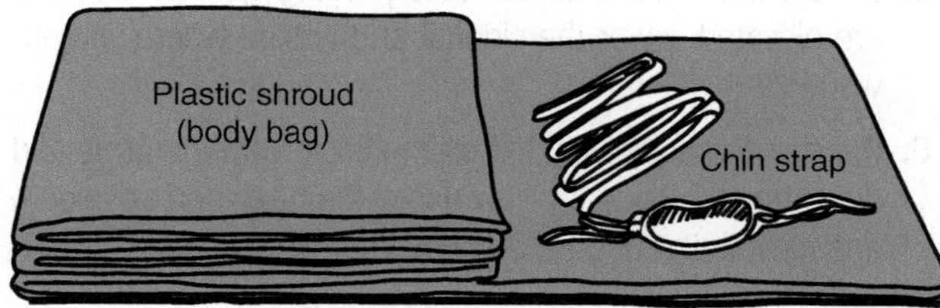

FIGURE 22–105 Supplies needed for postmortem care.

After the family has viewed the body, postmortem care is completed. The procedure for this care varies in different facilities. In some facilities, morgue personnel prepare the body and remove it to the morgue. In other facilities, the body is prepared and remains in the unit until the funeral home personnel arrive. In yet other facilities, funeral home personnel remove the body and provide postmortem care. Know and follow the procedure established by your facility.

Morgue kits often are used for postmortem care (Figure 22–105). Each kit usually contains a shroud or body bag, a gown, chin strap, pads, gauze squares, ties, two or three tags to identify the body, and safety pins. Procedure 22:16 describes one method of using these supplies to provide postmortem care.

Care of the patient's valuables and belongings is an important part of postmortem care. Each facility has a policy that should be followed. The personal inventory and valuables lists prepared on admission are often used to make sure that all items are present. These items are checked according to facility policy. Valuables in the safe or with security usually remain there until a family member signs for them. Jewelry is usually removed from the body, listed, and placed in the safe or with security until received by a family member. A wedding ring is frequently left on the body, but it should be taped in place and noted on the chart.

Legal

Frequently, two people work together to complete postmortem care. Some aspects of care, such as removal of tubes or IVs, may be the responsibility of the nurse or another authorized person. Follow your agency's policy and know your legal responsibilities with regard to giving or assisting with postmortem care.

STUDENT: **Go to the workbook and complete the assignment sheet for 22:16, Giving Postmortem Care. Then return and continue with the procedure.**

PROCEDURE 22:16

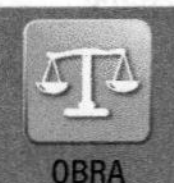
OBRA

Giving Postmortem Care

Equipment and Supplies

Postmortem kit (shroud or clean sheet, gown, tags, gauze squares, cotton balls, safety pins), underpads or bed protectors, basin, towels, washcloth, personal inventory and valuables lists, disposable gloves, plastic waste bag, paper and pen or computer

NOTE: If cleansing cloths are available, they can be used in place of the basin and washcloth.

Procedure

1. Obtain proper authorization and assemble equipment.
2. Identify the patient by checking the armband.
3. Close the door and screen the unit to provide privacy.
4. Wash hands. Put on gloves.

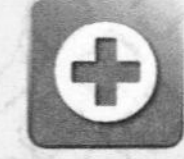
Precaution

CAUTION: Observe all standard precautions because the body may be contaminated with blood or body fluids.

5. Elevate the bed to a comfortable working height. If siderails are elevated, lower the siderail on the side where you are working.
6. Position the body lying flat on the back, with the arms and legs straight. Place a pillow under the head and shoulders and elevate the bed 30 degrees.

NOTE: The head is elevated to prevent the bluish purple discoloration of the head and neck that occurs when gravity causes blood to accumulate in the lowest areas of the body after death.

NOTE: Handle the body gently and with respect.

7. If the eyes are open, close them by gently pulling the eyelids over the eyes (Figure 22–106). Put a moist cotton ball on each eye if the eyes do not remain shut.
8. Follow agency policy regarding the use of dentures and chin straps. Some agencies state that dentures should be replaced in the mouth for family viewing. Others state that they should be packed securely in a denture cup because they could fall out of the mouth and break. Some agencies use a chin strap to hold the jaw shut. Other agencies feel that the chin strap can bruise or discolor the skin and that it should not be used. Some agencies use a rolled towel or padding under the chin to keep the mouth closed.
9. Remove soiled dressings and replace with clean ones, as necessary. If tubes, IVs, catheters, or drainage bags are in place, follow agency policy for removal. This is often the responsibility of the nurse. If an autopsy is to be performed, some tubes may have to be left in place.
10. Use warm water or cleansing cloths to bathe any soiled body areas. Dry all areas thoroughly. Comb the hair, if needed.

PROCEDURE 22:16 (CONT.)

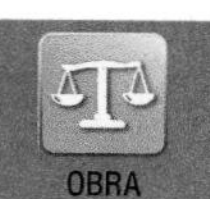

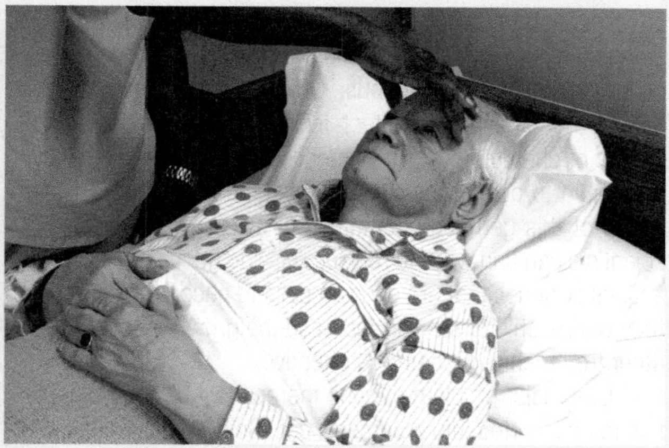

FIGURE 22–106 If the eyes are open after death, close them by gently pulling the eyelids over the eyes.

11. Place an underpad or padding under the buttocks at the anal area.

    NOTE: The bowels and bladder may empty after death.

12. Put a clean gown on the body.
13. Remove gloves and wash hands.
14. If jewelry is present, follow agency policy. Jewelry is usually removed, listed on a valuables list, and stored in a safe or with security until signed for by a family member. A wedding ring frequently is left on the body, but it should be taped in place and noted on the chart or postmortem form.
15. If the family is to view the body, use a sheet to cover the body to the shoulders. Make sure the room is neat and clean. Provide privacy for the family unless they request that you remain with them.
16. After the family visit, remove dentures and eyeglasses (if they were placed on the patient). Pack them securely, label them with the patient's name, and send them to the funeral home.
17. Comm Fill out the identification card or tag. One tag is usually placed on the patient's right ankle or right big toe.
18. Place the body in the shroud or body bag. Use safety pins or tape to hold the shroud in place. If a shroud is not available, use a sheet to cover the body.

    NOTE: Many facilities have plastic body bags with zippers.

    CAUTION: Handle the body carefully. Pressure from your hands can leave marks on the body.

    NOTE: Sometimes, padding is placed between the ankles and knees, and the legs are tied together lightly before the body is placed in the shroud.

19. If required, attach a second identification card or tag to the outside of the shroud or body bag.
20. Collect all belongings and make a list. This list frequently is checked against the admission personal inventory and valuables list to make sure that all items are present. Put the items in a bag or container and attach an identification card or tag. Follow agency policy for care of belongings until they are signed for by a family member.
21. Obtain assistance and transfer the body to a stretcher. Make sure doors to other patient's rooms are closed and the corridor is empty before transporting the body to the morgue.

    NOTE: In some facilities, morgue personnel or orderlies transport the body to the morgue. In other facilities, the body remains in the unit until funeral home personnel arrive.

22. Return to the unit. Wash hands and put on gloves. Strip the linen from the bed. Follow agency policy for cleaning the unit and equipment. Leave the area neat and clean.
23. Remove gloves. Wash hands.
24. 

    Report and/or record all required information on the patient's chart or enter it into the computer. For example, date, time, postmortem care given, body transported to morgue, belongings placed in locked closet by nurses' station, and your signature and title.

    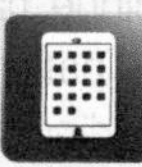

    NOTE: In health care agencies using electronic health records (EHRs), also known as electronic medical records (EMRs), the information is entered directly into the patient's record on a computer.

PRACTICE: Go to the workbook and use the evaluation sheet for 22:16, Giving Postmortem Care, to practice this procedure. When you believe you have mastered this skill, sign the sheet and give it to your instructor for further action.

FINAL CHECKPOINT: Using the criteria listed on the evaluation sheet, your instructor will grade your performance.

TODAY'S RESEARCH TOMORROW'S HEALTH CARE

Gene Therapy That Cures Cancer?

Liver cancer kills. The American Cancer Society estimates that more than 35,660 new cases of liver cancer are diagnosed each year in the United States with more than 700,000 cases worldwide. About 24,550 people die of liver cancer every year in the United States, and 600,000 die worldwide. How can these lives be saved?

Researchers are experimenting with many different treatments for liver cancer. One treatment involves the use of gene therapy. Every human has between 50,000 and 100,000 different genes. These genes determine what a person inherits, such as hair and eye color. Genes also carry instructions that tell cells to perform certain functions, such as when to reproduce and grow. Initially, scientists researching the spread of liver cancer to the colon and rectum identified a gene called p53. This gene is present in normal cells and regulates cell growth. In many types of cancer, it is missing or changed, allowing uncontrolled growth of the cancer cells. Another group of researchers in Japan studied hepatitis C (HVC) carriers and discovered that the presence of a gene identified as DEPDC5 SNP roughly doubles the chances that a hepatitis C carrier will develop liver cancer. Scientists at Cold Spring Harbor Laboratory in New York identified a gene called FGF-19 that becomes active in about 15 percent of liver cancer patients, causing healthy cells to become cancerous. However, these scientists also found that when an experimental antibody was applied, the gene's activity stopped, preventing the development of cancerous cells. Other scientists in Columbus, Ohio, found a gene called STAT3 that seems to protect liver cancer cells from the effects of chemotherapy (treatment with cancer drugs). They were able to design a synthetic substance that blocked the action of this gene so chemotherapy was more effective. If scientists can find ways to replace missing genes or block the actions of genes that are causing cells to become malignant, they will be able to stop or decrease the growth of cancer so other treatments will be more effective.

One major problem of gene therapy is the way the gene has to be inserted into a person's cell. Scientists cannot simply inject genes into cells. They must be transported into the cell by using a carrier called a vector. The most common vectors used are retroviruses. Scientists inactivate the retroviruses to keep them from causing disease and then use them to carry the gene into cells. The problems that occur with this method are that the genes might alter or change other normal cells, or that the new gene might be inserted into the wrong location, causing additional damage to the body. For these reasons, scientists must identify easier and better ways to deliver genes to body cells. Scientists throughout the world are trying to solve these problems. If they are successful, many people with cancer may be cured.

CHAPTER 22 SUMMARY

Many nurse assistant skills are directed toward providing quality personal care for the patient. Examples include bathing, caring for hair and nails, gowning or dressing the patient, giving backrubs, providing oral hygiene, shaving, feeding, assisting with bedpans or urinals, and bedmaking. It is essential that the nurse assistant learn and follow correct procedures to provide for the safety, comfort, and privacy of the patient.

Other nurse assistant skills include positioning, turning, moving, and transferring patients. During any move or transfer, the use of correct body mechanics is essential.

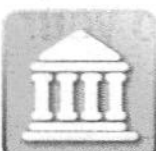
Legal

Nurse assistant skills are required for other special procedures, such as measuring intake and output (I&O), collecting stool and urine specimens, giving enemas, assisting the surgical patient, administering oxygen, applying restraints, providing catheter care, applying binders or surgical hose, and giving postmortem care. It is important to determine legal responsibility before performing some of these special procedures because some states or agencies do not allow all nurse assistants to perform the procedures.

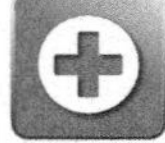
Precaution

While performing any nurse assistant skill, it is essential to use approved procedures and make every effort to provide quality care to the patient. In addition, standard precautions must be observed at all times. Contact with blood, body fluids, secretions, or excretions is possible. Finally, it is important to make careful observations of the patient while providing care, and to record or report these observations correctly. In this way, you will use nurse assistant skills to become an important member of the health care team.

INTERNET SEARCHES

Use the search engines suggested in Chapter 12:9 in this text to search the Internet for additional information about the following topics:

1. **Organizations:** Research nurse assisting careers, educational requirements, and duties at organizational sites such as the American Health Care Association, American Hospital Association, American Nurses Association, Association of Surgical Technologists, Foundation for Hospice and Homecare, National Association for Practical Nurse Education and Service, National League for Nursing, and the National Federation of Licensed Practical Nurses.
2. **Patient care:** Research patients' rights, hospice care, home health care, oncology care, surgical care, and postmortem care.
3. **Suppliers:** Find suppliers of hospital and medical equipment to compare the different products available.

REVIEW QUESTIONS

1. List six (6) specific tasks that must be performed while admitting a patient to a hospital or long-term care facility.
2. Describe four (4) ways to prevent pressure sores and contractures from developing.
3. Name three (3) main ways to make beds and explain when each type is made.
4. Identify all the areas of care that may provide personal hygiene to a patient.
5. Why is it important to constantly observe a patient while providing personal care? Identify six (6) observations that might be indicative of a medical problem.
6. What is a urinary catheter? Why is it used?
7. Differentiate between a routine, midstream (clean-catch), sterile, and 24-hour urine specimen.
8. Why is stool tested for occult blood?
9. Define each of the following words:
   a. ostomy
   b. suppository
   c. fecal impaction
   d. enema
   e. flatus
10. Differentiate between a retention and a nonretention enema. Give an example of each type.
11. List four (4) specific rules that OBRA legislation has placed on the use of restraints.
12. Identify five (5) specific aspects of care for both pre-op and post-op patients.
13. Name three (3) methods for administering oxygen. Describe the use for each method.
14. Explain five (5) standard precautions that must be observed while performing any nurse assisting procedure.

For additional information about nursing careers, contact the following associations:

- American Health Care Association
  1201 L Street NW
  Washington, DC 20005
  Internet address: *www.ahcancal.org*
- American Nurses Association
  8515 Georgia Avenue, Suite 400
  Silver Springs, MD 20910
  Internet address: *www.nursingworld.org*
- National Association for Practical Nurse Education and Service
  1940 Duke Street, Suite 200
  Alexandria, VA 22314
  Internet address: *www.napnes.org*
- National Association of Health Care Assistants
  501 East 15th Street
  Joplin, MO 64804
  Internet address: *www.nahcacares.org*
- National Federation of Licensed Practical Nurses
  3801 Lake Boone Trail, Suite 190
  Raleigh, NC 27607
  Internet address: *www.nflpn.org*
- National League for Nursing
  2600 Virginia Avenue, NW
  Washington, DC 20037
  Internet address: *www.nln.org*
- National Network of Career Nursing Assistants
  3577 Easton Road
  Norton, OH 44203
  Internet address: *www.cna-network.org*
- State nurses' associations

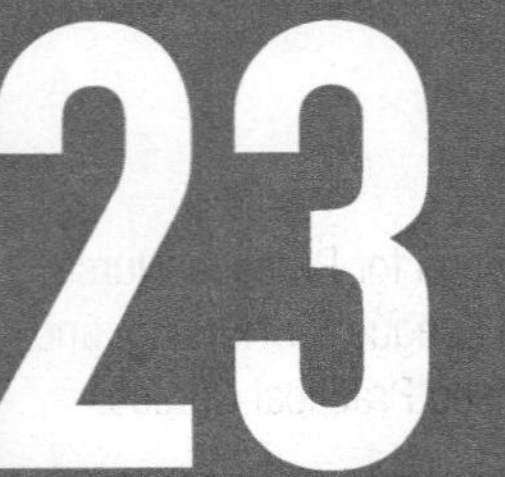

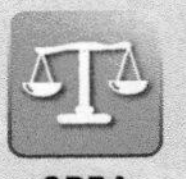

23 Physical Therapy Skills

CHAPTER OBJECTIVES

After completing this chapter, you should be able to:

- Perform range-of-motion (ROM) exercises on all body joints, observing all safety precautions.
- Ambulate a patient using a transfer (gait) belt.
- Check the correct measurements of patients for canes, crutches, and walkers.
- Ambulate a patient using the following crutch gaits: four point, three point, two point, swing to, and swing through.
- Ambulate a patient using a cane.
- Ambulate a patient using a walker.
- Apply an ice bag or ice collar, observing all safety precautions.
- Apply a warm-water bag, observing all safety precautions.
- Apply an aquamatic pad, observing all safety precautions.
- Apply a moist compress, observing all safety precautions.
- Administer a sitz bath.
- Define, pronounce, and spell all key terms.

KEY TERMS

aquathermia pads *(ak"-wah-thur'-me-ah)*
cane
compresses *(cahm'-press-ez)*
contracture *(kun-track'-shure)*
crutches
cryotherapy
dry cold
dry heat
hydrocollator packs
hypothermia blanket *(high"-poh-thur'-me-ah)*
ice bags
ice collars
moist cold
moist heat
paraffin wax treatment
range of motion (ROM)
sitz baths
thermal blankets
thermotherapy
transfer (gait) belt
vasoconstriction *(vay"-zow"-kon-strik'-shun)*
vasodilation *(vay'-zow"-di-lay'-shun)*
walker
warm-water bags

career highlights

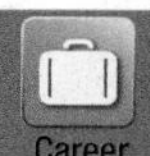

Physical therapist assistants (PTAs) provide treatment to improve mobility and prevent or limit permanent disability of patients with disabling injuries or disease. They are important members of the health care team. They work under the supervision of a physical therapist who has a master's degree from an accredited program and is licensed (required in all states). Most physical therapist assistants have an associate's degree from an accredited program and an internship. Licensure is required in most states.

The duties of physical therapist assistants vary but usually include performing exercises; providing ultrasound or electrical stimulation treatments; administering heat, cold, or moist applications; ambulating patients with assistive devices; and informing the physical therapist of the patient's response and progress. In addition to the knowledge and skills presented in this chapter, physical therapist assistants must also learn and master skills such as:

- Presenting a professional appearance and attitude
- Obtaining knowledge regarding health care delivery systems, organizational structure, and teamwork
- Meeting all legal responsibilities
- Communicating effectively
- Being sensitive to and respecting cultural diversity
- Learning medical terminology
- Comprehending anatomy, physiology, and pathophysiology with an emphasis on the skeletal, muscular, nervous, and circulatory systems
- Observing all safety precautions
- Practicing all principles of infection control
- Administering first aid and cardiopulmonary resuscitation
- Promoting good nutrition and a healthy lifestyle to maintain health
- Using computer and technology skills
- Cleaning and maintaining equipment
- Ordering and maintaining supplies and materials
- Performing administrative duties such as answering the telephone, scheduling appointments, completing insurance forms, and maintaining patient records

LEGAL ALERT

Before performing any procedures in this chapter, know and follow the standards and regulations established by the scope of practice; federal laws and agencies; state laws; state or national licensing, registration, or certification boards; professional organizations; professional standards; and agency policies.

It is your responsibility to learn exactly what you are legally permitted to do and to perform only procedures for which you have been trained.

23:1 Performing Range-of-Motion (ROM) Exercises

Activity and exercise are important for all individuals. When patients have limited ability to move, range-of-motion exercises help keep muscles and joints functioning.

Range-of-motion (ROM) exercises are done to maintain the health of the musculoskeletal system. Each joint and muscle in the body is moved through its full range of motion. Range-of-motion exercises are frequently ordered by physicians for patients with limited ability to move. These exercises are administered by a physical therapist, nurse, health care assistant, or other authorized person. Range-of-motion exercises can be done during the daily bath or at other times during the day.

Range-of-motion exercises are done to prevent the problems caused by lack of movement and by inactivity (Figure 23–1). Some of these problems include:

- **Contracture**: A contracture is a tightening and shortening of a muscle, resulting in a permanent flexing of a joint. Foot drop is a common contracture, but contractures can also affect the knees, hips, elbows, and hands (refer to Figure 22–8).
- *Muscle and joint function*: Muscles atrophy (shrink) and become weak. Joints become stiff and difficult to move.
- *Circulatory impairment*: The circulation of blood is affected, and blood clots and pressure ulcers (pressure sores) can develop.

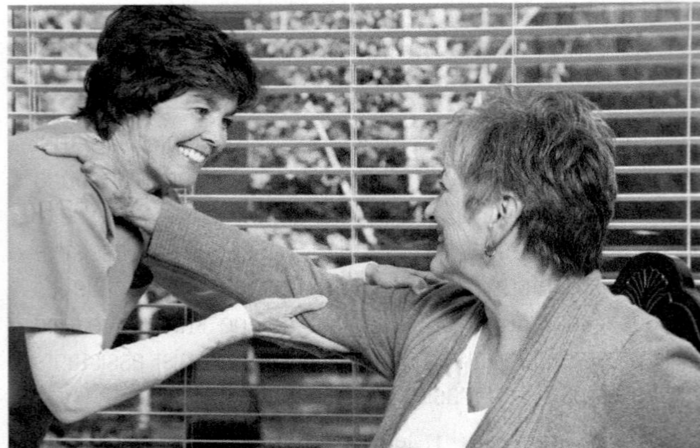

FIGURE 23–1 Range-of-motion (ROM) exercises are done to prevent problems caused by lack of movement and by inactivity.
© iStock.com/Pamela Moore

- *Mineral loss:* Inactivity causes mineral loss, especially of calcium from the bones. The bones become brittle, and fractures occur. As the blood calcium level increases, renal calculi (kidney stones) are more likely to form.
- *Other problems:* Lack of exercise can also cause poor appetite, constipation, urinary infections, respiratory problems, and hypostatic pneumonia.

There are four main types of ROM exercises:

- *Active ROM exercises:* These are performed by patients who are able to move each joint without assistance (Figure 23–2). This type of ROM exercise strengthens muscles, maintains joint function and movement, and helps prevent deformities.
- *Active assistive ROM exercises:* The patient actively moves the joints but receives assistance to complete the entire ROM. This type of ROM strengthens muscles, maintains joint function and movement, and helps prevent deformities. At times, equipment, such as a pulley, is used to complete the ROM.
- *Passive ROM exercises:* Another person moves each joint for a patient who is not able to exercise. This type of ROM maintains joint function and movement, and helps to prevent deformities. However, it does not strengthen muscles.
- *Resistive ROM exercises:* Administered by a therapist, these exercises are performed against resistance provided by the therapist. This type of ROM helps the patient develop increased strength and endurance.

Legal

The health care worker should find out what type of ROM exercises are to be performed and determine whether any limitations to the exercises exist before administering or assisting the patient with the exercises. In some states and health care facilities, only physical therapists or registered nurses may perform ROM exercises to the head and neck, especially if stretching is involved. After hip or knee replacement surgeries, some ROM exercises may be restricted or limited. Patients with osteoporosis, a condition in which the bones become porous and are prone to fracture, may have limitations on ROMs. It is your responsibility to check legal requirements regarding ROM exercises.

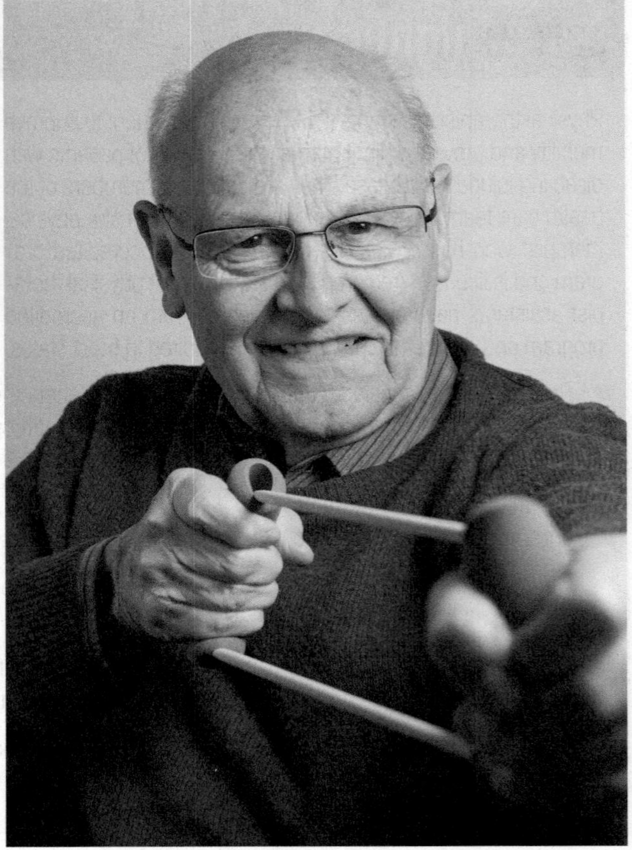

FIGURE 23–2 Patients who are able to move each joint without assistance perform active range-of-motion (ROM) exercises.
© Carme Balcells/Shutterstock.com

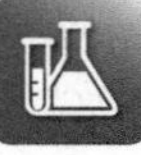
Science

Various movements are used when performing ROM exercises. The health care worker must be aware of the terms used for movements of each joint. The main movements are shown in Figure 23–3 and include:

- *Abduction:* moving a part away from the midline of the body
- *Adduction:* moving a part toward the midline of the body
- *Flexion:* bending a body part
- *Extension:* straightening a body part
- *Hyperextension:* excessive straightening of a body part
- *Rotation:* moving a body part around its own axis, for example, turning the head from side to side

- *Circumduction:* moving in a circle at a joint, or moving one end of a body part in a circle while the other end remains stationary, such as swinging the arm in a circle; involves all the movements of flexion, extension, abduction, adduction, and rotation

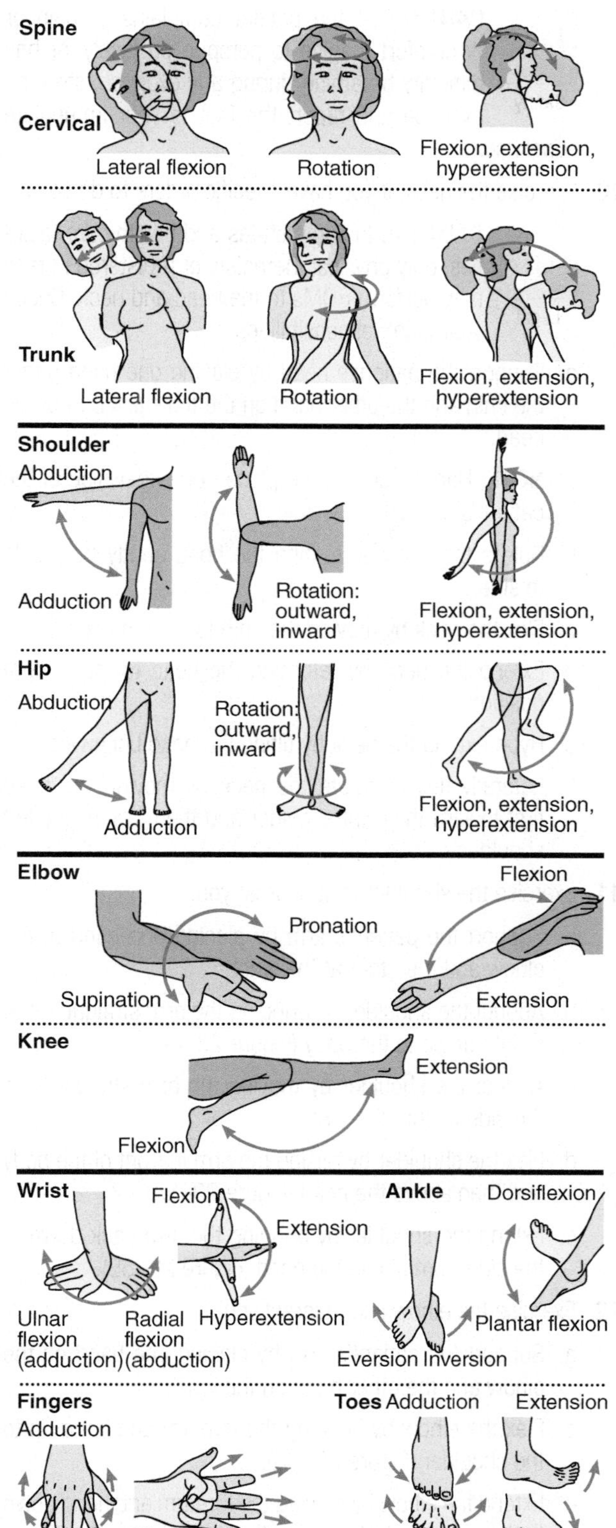

FIGURE 23–3 Range-of-motion (ROM) exercises for specific joints.

- *Pronation:* turning a body part downward (turning palm down)
- *Supination:* turning a body part upward (turning palm up)
- *Opposition:* touching each of the fingers with the tip of the thumb
- *Inversion:* turning a body part inward
- *Eversion:* turning a body part outward
- *Dorsiflexion:* bending backward (bending the foot toward the knee)
- *Plantar flexion:* bending forward (straightening the foot away from the knee)
- *Radial deviation:* moving toward the thumb side of the hand
- *Ulnar deviation:* moving toward the little finger side of the hand

Certain principles must be observed at all times when performing ROM exercises:

- Movements should be slow, smooth, and gentle to prevent injury.
- Support should be provided to the parts above and below the joint being exercised.
- A joint should never be forced beyond its ROM or exercised to the point of pain, resistance, or extreme fatigue.
- If a patient complains of pain, stop the exercise and report this fact to your immediate supervisor.
- Watch the patient closely. If you notice the patient is in pain, has shortness of breath, is perspiring profusely (diaphoresis), or is pale, stop the exercise and notify your supervisor.
- Each movement should be performed three to five times or as ordered.
- The patient should be encouraged to assist as much as possible.
- Prevent unnecessary exposure of the patient. Only the body part being exercised should be exposed.
- The door should be closed and/or the curtain pulled shut to provide privacy.
- Use correct body mechanics at all times to prevent injury.

STUDENT: **Go to the workbook and complete the assignment sheet for 23:1, Performing Range-of-Motion (ROM) Exercises. Then return and continue with the procedure.**

PROCEDURE 23:1

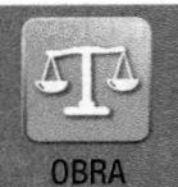

OBRA

Performing Range-of-Motion (ROM) Exercises

Equipment and Supplies

Bath blanket, paper and pen and/or computer

Procedure

1. Obtain proper authorization. Determine the type of ROM exercises and any limitations to movement.

Legal

CAUTION: Remember, it is your responsibility to check legal requirements regarding ROMs.

2. Assemble supplies.
3. 

Comm

Knock on the door and pause before entering. Introduce yourself. Identify the patient. Explain the procedure and obtain consent.

4. Close the door and pull the curtain for privacy. Lock the wheels of the bed to prevent movement.
5. Wash hands.
6. Elevate the bed to a comfortable working height. If siderails are present and elevated, lower the siderail on the side where you are working.
7. Position the patient in the supine position (on the back) and in good body alignment.

NOTE: Some ROM exercises can be done while the patient is sitting in a chair.

8. Use the bath blanket to drape the patient. Fanfold the top bed linens to the foot of the bed.
9. Administer the exercises in an organized manner. Start at the head and move to the feet. Complete one side of the body first and then work on the opposite side of the body. Perform each movement three to five times or as ordered. Provide support for the body parts above and below the joint being exercised. *Never* force any joint beyond its ROM or cause pain while exercising a joint.

Safety

CAUTION: Use proper body mechanics when administering ROM exercises. Get close to the patient by bending at your hips and knees and keeping your back straight. Stand with your feet apart and one foot slightly forward to provide a good base of support.

Safety

CAUTION: If the patient complains of pain or discomfort, begins to perspire profusely, or has difficulty breathing during any exercise, stop the exercise and report the fact to your immediate supervisor.

10. Exercise the neck, if you have specific orders to do so:

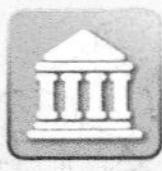

Legal

CAUTION: In some states and health care facilities, only physical therapists or registered nurses may perform ROMs to the head and neck. Check your legal responsibilities.

   a. Support the patient's head by placing one hand under the chin and the other hand on the top-back part of the head.

   NOTE: Hands can also be placed on either side of the patient's head.

   b. Rotate the neck by turning the head gently from side to side.
   c. Flex the neck by moving the chin toward the chest.
   d. Extend the neck by returning the head to the upright position.
   e. Hyperextend the neck by tilting the head backward.
   f. Laterally flex or rotate the neck by moving the head first toward the right shoulder and then toward the left shoulder.

11. Exercise the shoulder joint nearest you:
   a. Support the patient's arm by placing one hand at the elbow and the other at the wrist.
   b. Abduct the shoulder by bringing the arm straight out at a right angle to the body (Figure 23–4A).
   c. Adduct the shoulder by moving the arm straight in to the side (Figure 23–4B).
   d. Flex the shoulder by raising the arm in front of the body and then above the head (Figure 23–5A).
   e. Extend the shoulder by bringing the arm back down to the side from above the head (Figure 23–5B).
12. Exercise the elbow joint nearest you:
   a. Support the patient's arm by placing one hand on the elbow and the other hand on the wrist.
   b. Flex the elbow by bending the forearm and hand up to the shoulder (Figure 23–6A).
   c. Extend the elbow by moving the forearm and hand down to the side, or straightening the arm (Figure 23–6B).

PROCEDURE 23:1 (CONT.)

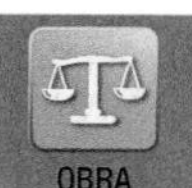

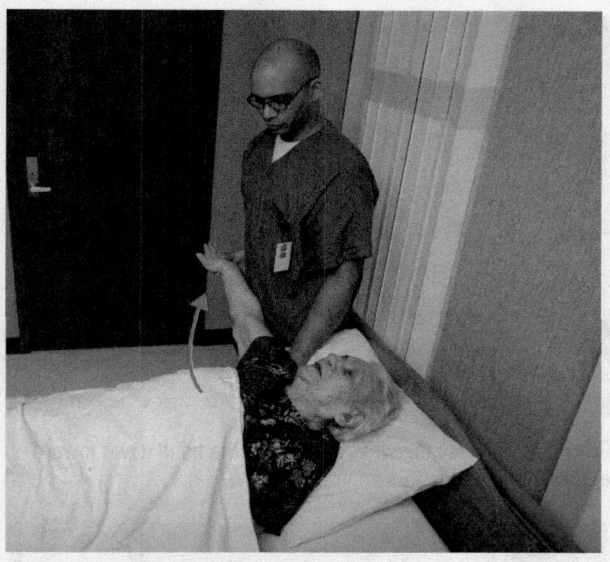

FIGURE 23–4A Abduct the shoulder by bringing the arm straight out at a right angle to the body.

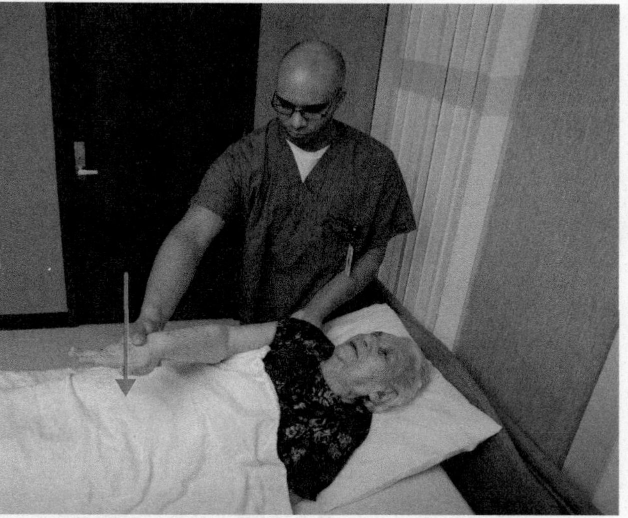

FIGURE 23–4B Adduct the shoulder by moving the arm straight in to the body.

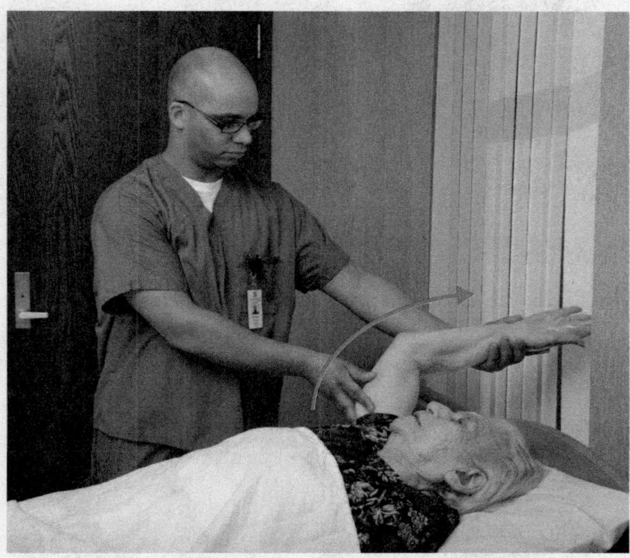

FIGURE 23–5A Flex the shoulder by raising the arm in front of the body and then above the head.

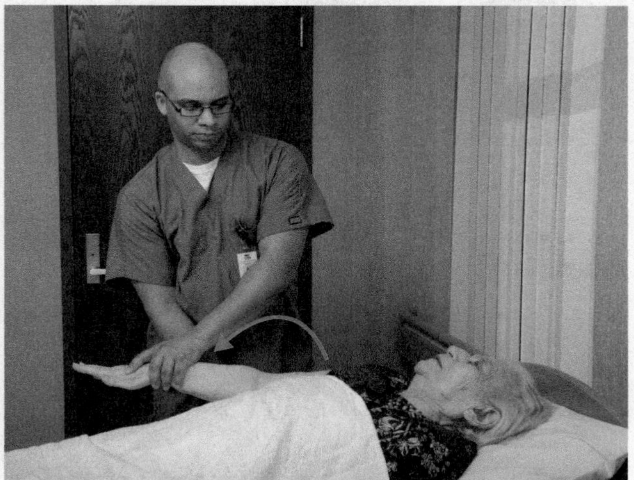

FIGURE 23–5B Extend the shoulder by bringing the arm back down to the side from above the head.

d. Pronate by turning the forearm and hand so that the palm of the hand is down.

e. Supinate by turning the forearm and hand so that the palm of the hand is up.

13. Exercise the wrist nearest you:

a. Support the patient's wrist by placing one hand above it and the other hand below it.

b. Flex the wrist by bending the hand down toward the forearm (Figure 23–7A).

c. Extend the wrist by straightening the hand (Figure 23–7B).

d. Hyperextend the wrist by bending the top of the hand back toward the forearm (Figure 23–7C).

e. Deviate the wrist in an ulnar direction by moving the hand toward the little finger side (Figure 23–8A).

f. Deviate the wrist in a radial direction by moving the hand toward the thumb side (Figure 23–8B).

(continues)

PROCEDURE 23:1 (CONT.)

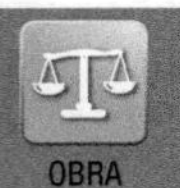

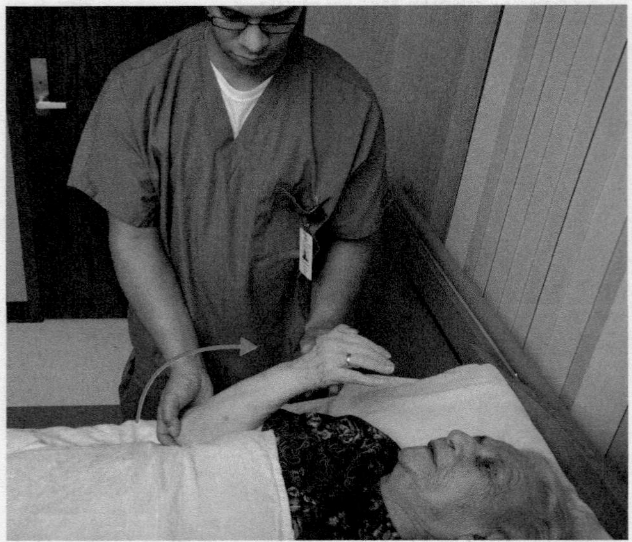

FIGURE 23–6A **Flex the elbow by bending the forearm and hand up to the shoulder.**

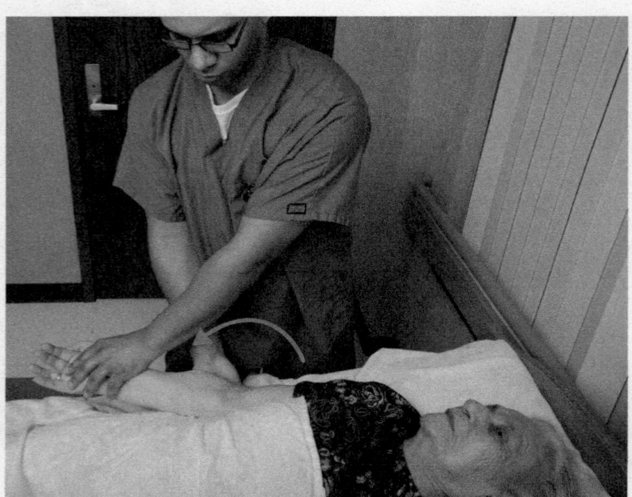

FIGURE 23–6B **Extend the elbow by moving the forearm and hand down to the side.**

14. Exercise the fingers and thumb on the hand nearest you:

a. Support the patient's hand by placing one hand at the wrist.

b. Flex the thumb and fingers by bending them toward the palm (Figure 23–9A).

c. Extend the thumb and fingers by straightening them (Figure 23–9B).

d. Abduct the thumb and fingers by spreading them apart (Figure 23–10A).

e. Adduct the thumb and fingers by moving them together (Figure 23–10B).

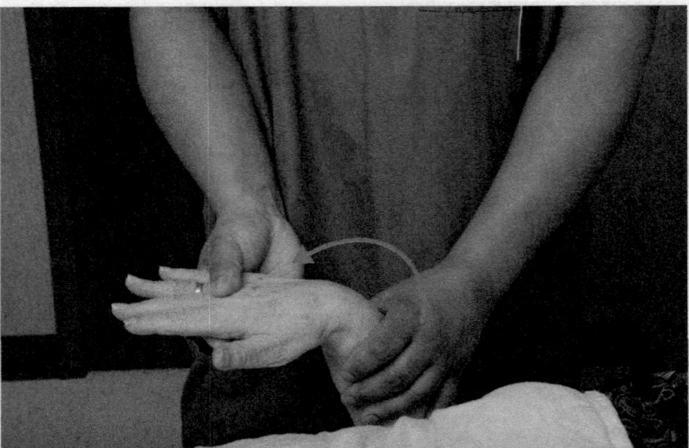

FIGURE 23–7A **Flex the wrist by bending the hand down toward the forearm.**

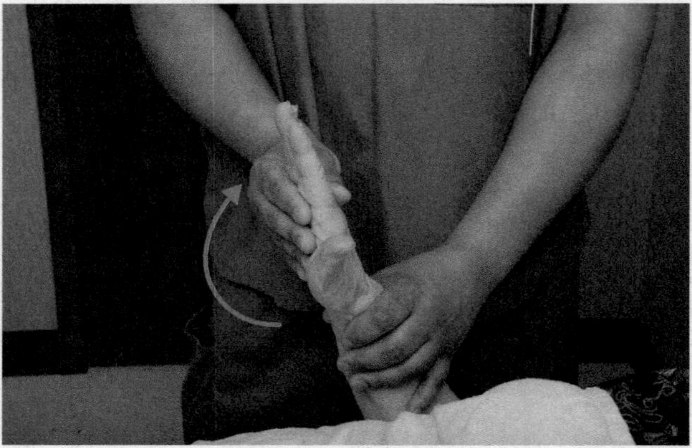

FIGURE 23–7B **Extend the wrist by straightening the hand.**

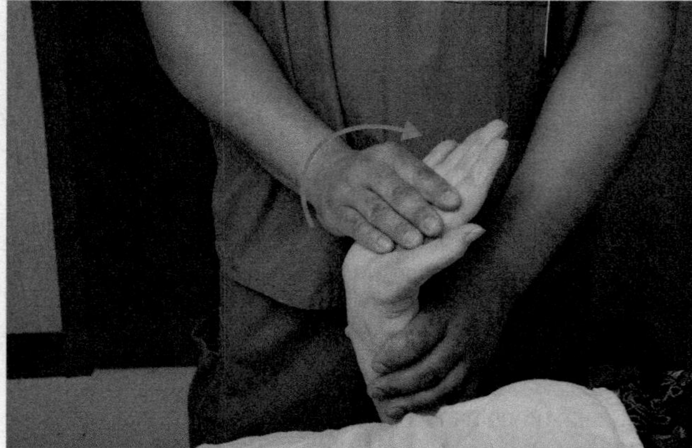

FIGURE 23–7C **Hyperextend the wrist by bending the top of the hand back toward the forearm.**

f. Perform opposition by touching the thumb to the tip of each finger.

g. Circumduct the thumb by moving it in a circular motion.

PROCEDURE 23:1 (CONT.)

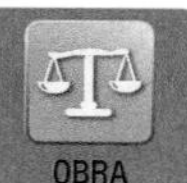

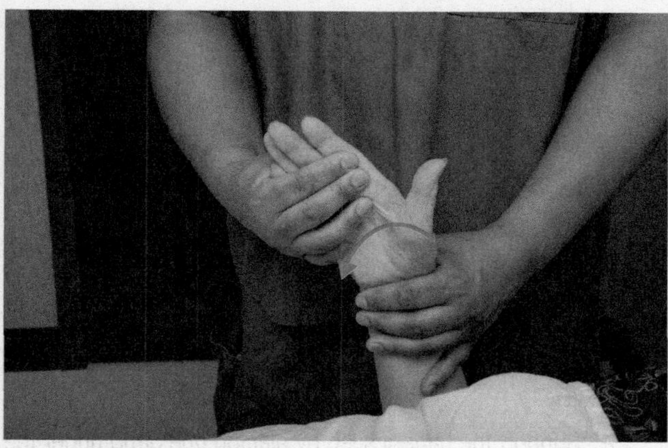

FIGURE 23–8A Deviate the wrist in an ulnar direction by moving the hand toward the little finger side.

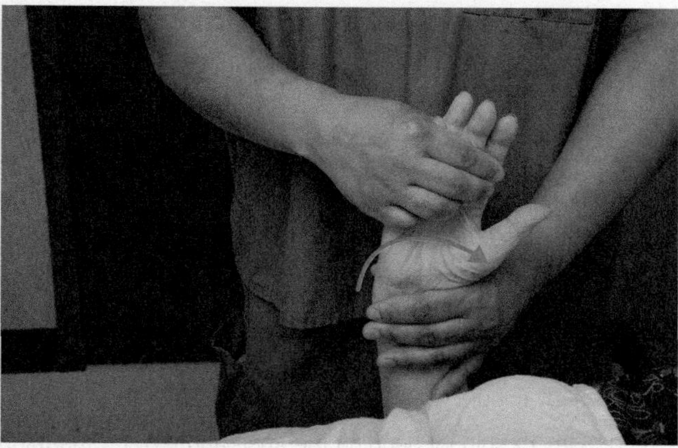

FIGURE 23–8B Deviate the wrist in a radial direction by moving the hand toward the thumb side.

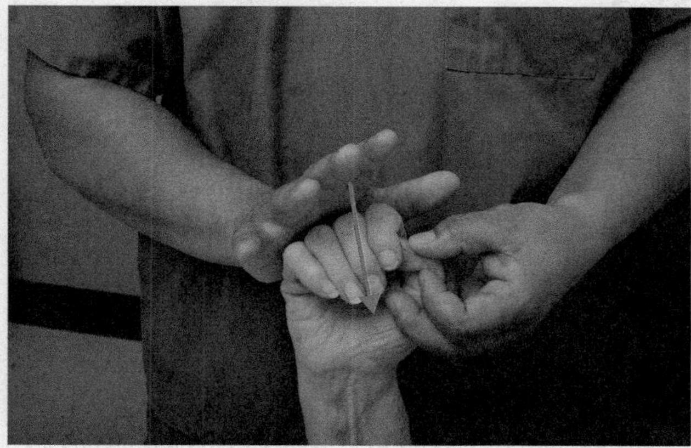

FIGURE 23–9A Flex the thumb and fingers by bending them toward the palm.

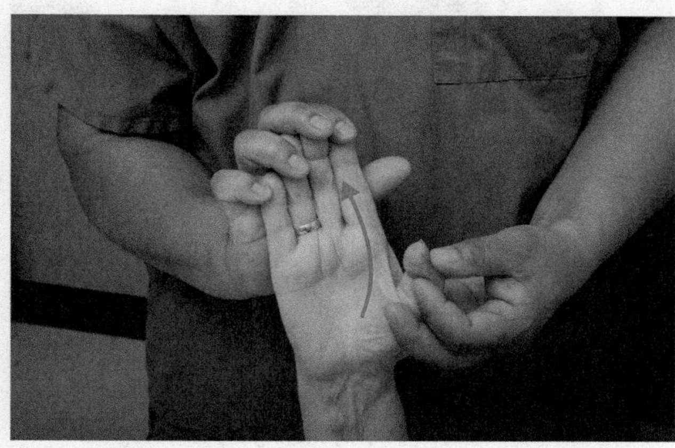

FIGURE 23–9B Extend the thumb and fingers by straightening them.

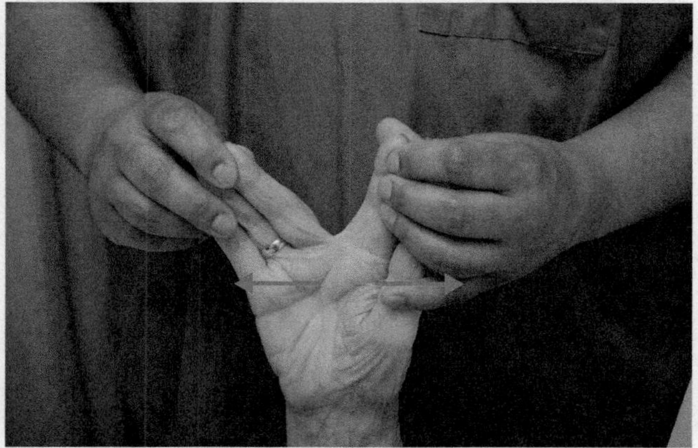

FIGURE 23–10A Abduct the thumb and fingers by spreading them apart.

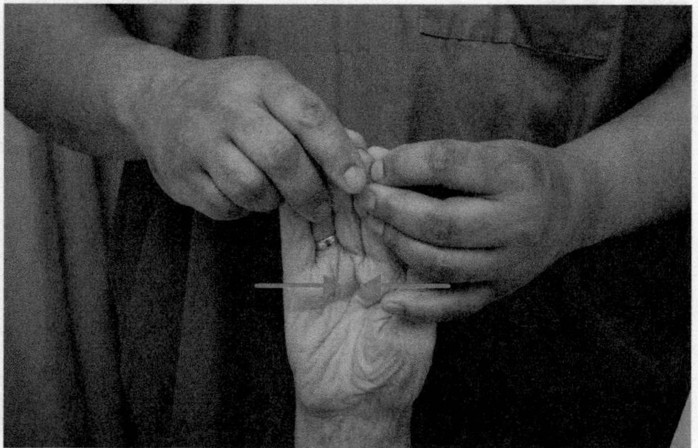

FIGURE 23–10B Adduct the thumb and fingers by moving them together.

(continues)

PROCEDURE 23:1 (CONT.)

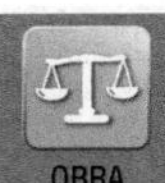

15. Uncover the leg nearest you and exercise the hip:

CAUTION: If the patient had hip or knee replacement surgery, check first for any limitations or restrictions to ROMs.

a. Support the patient's leg by placing one hand under the knee and the other hand under the ankle.

b. Abduct the hip by moving the entire leg out to the side (Figure 23–11A).

c. Adduct the hip by moving the entire leg back toward the body (Figure 23–11B).

d. Flex the hip by bending the knee and moving the thigh up toward the abdomen (Figure 23–12A).

e. Extend the hip by straightening the knee and moving the leg away from the abdomen (Figure 23–12B).

f. Medially rotate the hip by bending the knee and turning the leg in toward the midline.

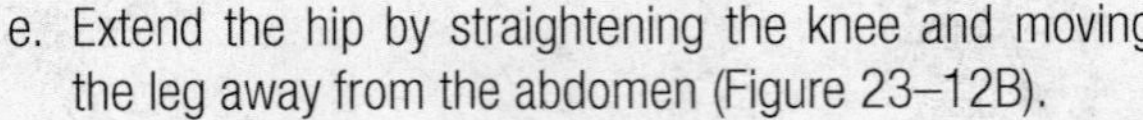

g. Laterally rotate the hip by bending the knee and turning the leg out away from the midline.

16. Exercise the knee nearest you:

CAUTION: If the patient had hip or knee replacement surgery, check first for any limitations or restrictions to ROM exercises.

a. Support the patient's leg by placing one hand under the knee and the other hand under the ankle.

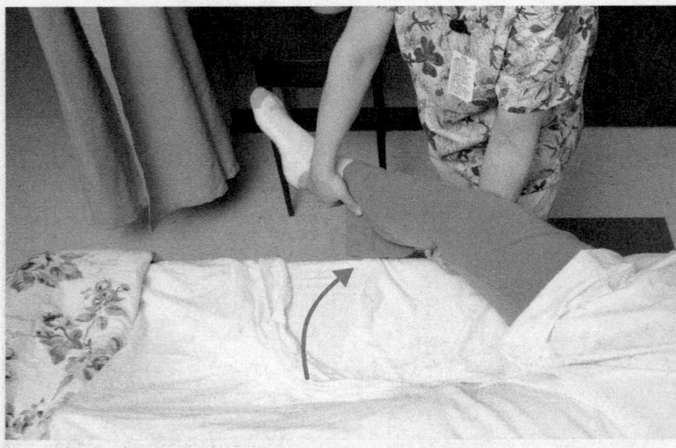

FIGURE 23–11A **Abduct the hip by moving the entire leg out to the side.**

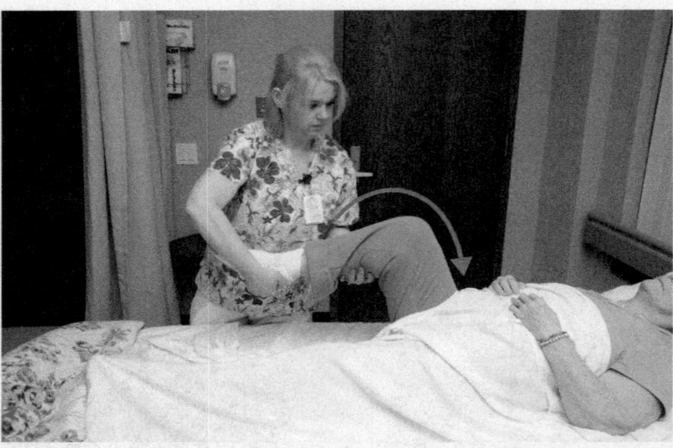

FIGURE 23–12A **Flex the hip by bending the knee and moving the thigh up toward the abdomen.**

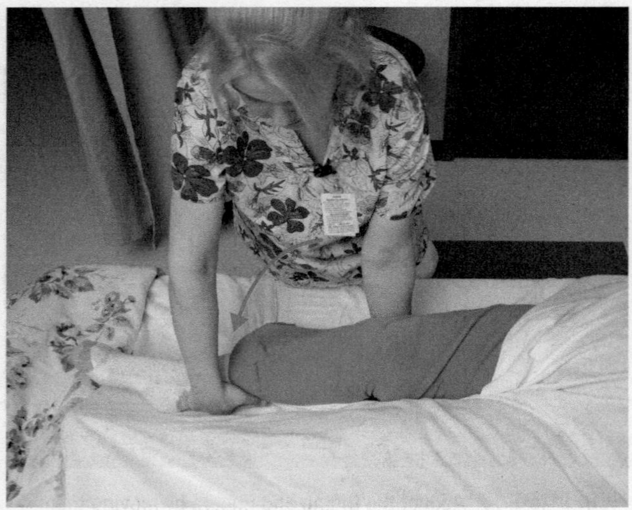

FIGURE 23–11B **Adduct the hip by moving the entire leg back toward the body.**

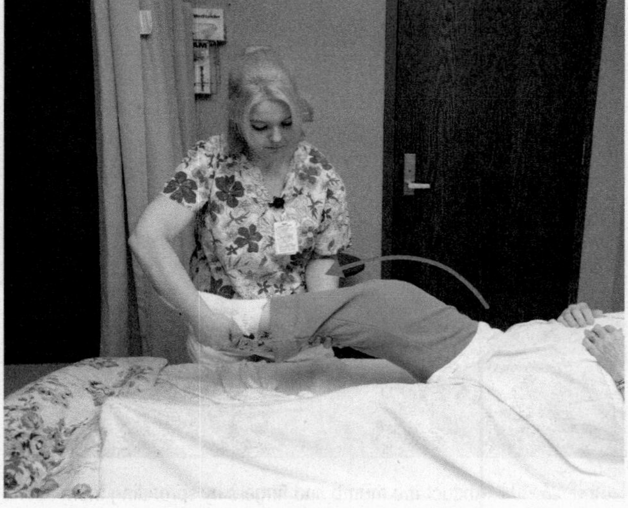

FIGURE 23–12B **Extend the hip by straightening the knee and moving the leg away from the abdomen.**

PROCEDURE 23:1 (CONT.)

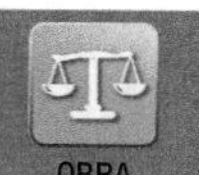

b. Flex the knee by bending the lower leg back toward the thigh.

c. Extend the knee by straightening the leg.

17. Exercise the ankle nearest you:

a. Support the patient's foot by placing one hand under the foot and the other hand behind the ankle.

b. Dorsiflex the ankle by moving the toes and foot up toward the knee (Figure 23–13A).

c. Plantar flex the ankle by moving the toes and foot down away from the knee (Figure 23–13B).

d. Invert the foot by gently turning it inward (Figure 23–14A).

e. Evert the foot by gently turning it outward (Figure 23–14B).

18. Exercise the toes on the foot nearest you:

a. Rest the patient's leg and foot on the bed for support.

b. Abduct the toes by separating them, or moving them away from each other.

c. Adduct the toes by moving them together.

d. Flex the toes by bending them down toward the bottom of the foot.

e. Extend the toes by straightening them.

19. Use the bath blanket to cover the patient. Raise the siderail, if indicated, and move to the opposite side of the bed. Lower the siderail if it is elevated.

20. Repeat steps 11–18 on the opposite side of the body.

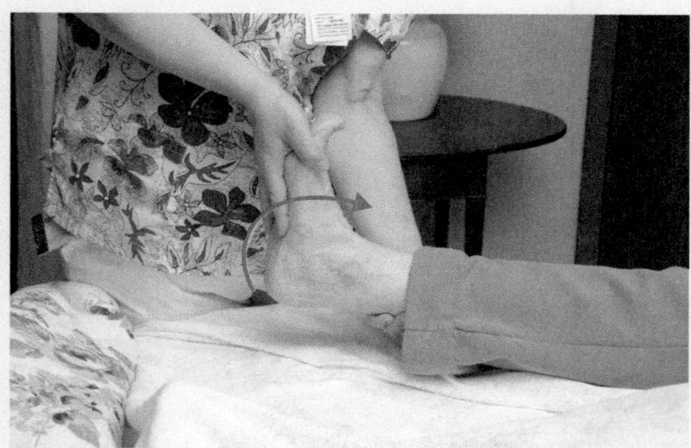

FIGURE 23–13A Dorsiflex the ankle by moving the toes and foot up toward the knee.

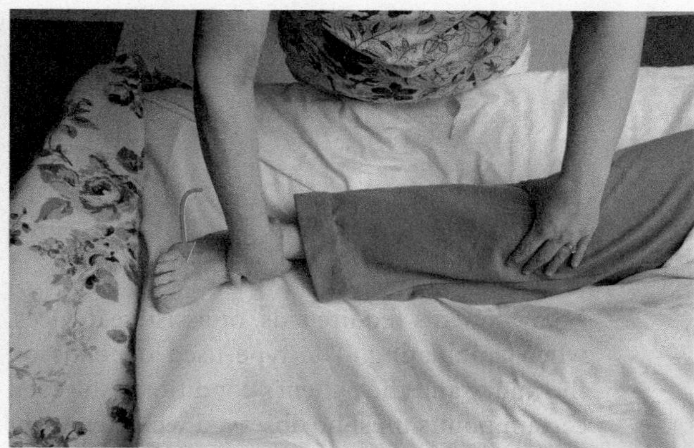

FIGURE 23–14A Invert the foot by gently turning it inward.

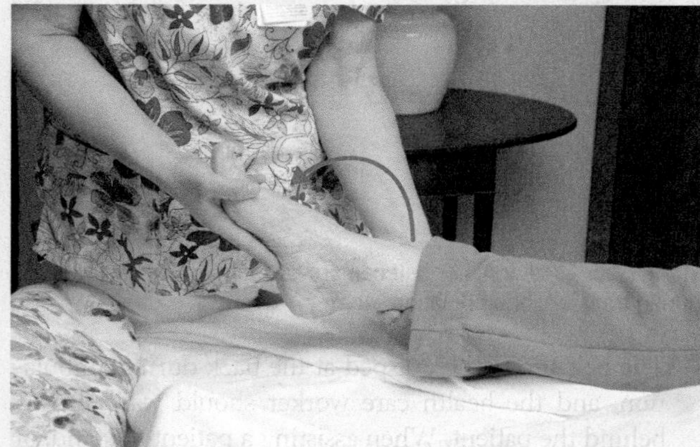

FIGURE 23–13B Plantar flex the ankle by moving the toes and foot down away from the knee.

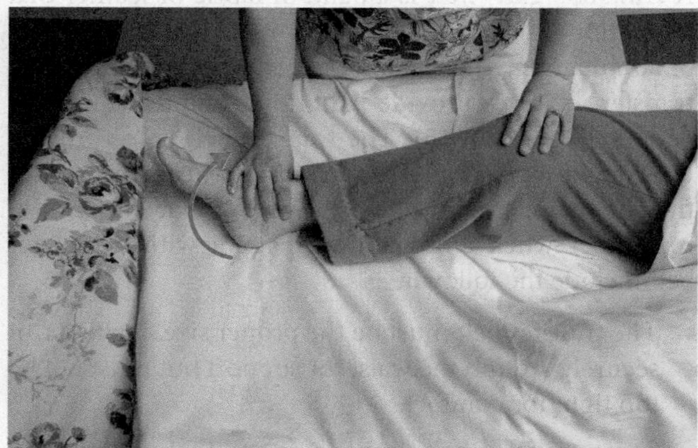

FIGURE 23–14B Evert the foot by gently turning it outward.

(continues)

PROCEDURE 23:1 (CONT.)

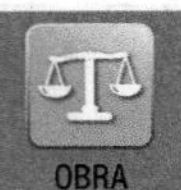

21. When ROM exercises are complete, comfortably position the patient in good body alignment. Replace the top bed linens and remove the bath blanket.
22. Observe all checkpoints before leaving the patient: elevate the siderails (if indicated), lower the bed to its lowest level, place the call signal and supplies within easy reach of the patient, and leave the area neat and clean.
23. Wash hands.
24.  Report and/or record all required information on the patient's chart or enter it into the computer. For example: date, time, ROM exercises performed on all joints, patient assisted with movements of arms and hands, and your signature and title. Report any unusual observations immediately.

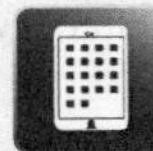

NOTE: In health care agencies using electronic health records (EHRs), also known as electronic medical records (EMRs), the information is entered directly into the patient's record on a computer.

PRACTICE: **Go to the workbook and use the evaluation sheet for 23:1, Performing Range-of-Motion (ROM) Exercises, to practice this procedure. When you believe you have mastered this skill, sign the sheet and give it to your instructor for further action.**

FINAL CHECKPOINT: Using the criteria listed on the evaluation sheet, your instructor will grade your performance.

23:2 Ambulating Patients Who Use Transfer (Gait) Belts, Crutches, Canes, or Walkers

Many patients require aids, or assistive devices, when ambulating. The type used depends on the injury and the patient's condition. However, certain points must be observed when a patient uses crutches, canes, or a walker.

Transfer (Gait) Belt

A **transfer (gait) belt** is a band of fabric or leather that is positioned around the patient's waist. During transfers or ambulation, the health care worker can grasp the transfer belt to provide additional support for the patient (Figure 23–15). The transfer belt helps provide the patient with a sense of security and helps to stabilize the patient's center of balance. Some important facts to remember when ambulating a patient with a transfer belt include the following:

- The transfer belt must be the proper size. It should fit securely around the waist for support but must not be too tight for comfort.
- Some transfer belts contain loops that are grasped when ambulating the patient. If loops are not present, an underhand grasp should be used to hold on to the belt during ambulation. The underhand grasp is more secure than grasping the belt from the top, because the hands are less likely to slip off the belt.

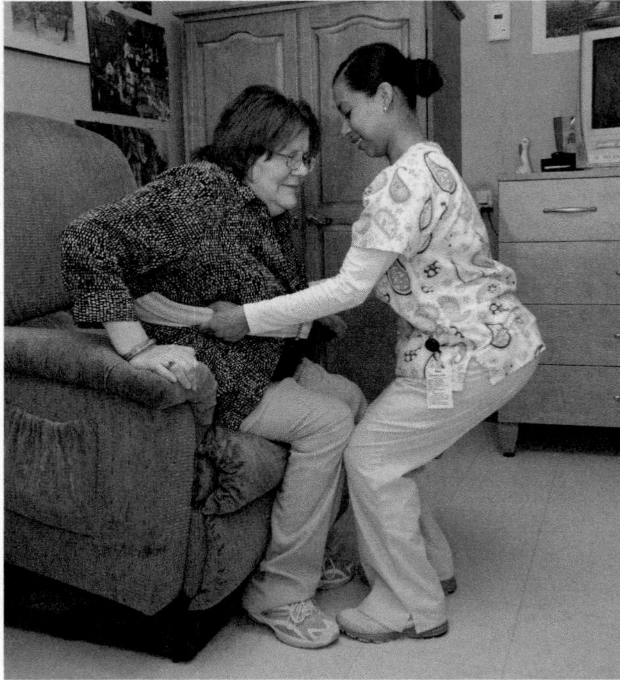

FIGURE 23–15 A transfer belt can provide support for the patient during transfers or ambulation.

- The belt should be grasped at the back during ambulation, and the health care worker should walk slightly behind the patient. When assisting a patient to stand, or during transfers such as transferring a patient to a wheelchair, grasp the belt on both sides while facing the patient.
- The transfer belt is applied over the patient's clothing. It should not be applied over bare skin because it can irritate the skin.

The use of a transfer belt is contraindicated in patients who have an ostomy, gastrostomy tube, abdominal pacemaker, severe cardiac or respiratory disease, fractured ribs, or recent surgery on the lower chest or abdominal area. It is also contraindicated for pregnant women.

Crutches

Crutches are artificial supports that assist a patient who needs help walking. Crutches are usually prescribed by a physician. A therapist or other authorized individual fits the crutches to the patient and teaches the appropriate gait. In addition, exercises to strengthen the muscles of the shoulders, arms, and hands are frequently prescribed by the physician or therapist. Health care workers should be aware of the criteria for fitting crutches and of the gaits so that they can properly ambulate patients.

There are three main types of crutches:

- *Axillary crutches* (Figure 23–16A): These crutches are made of wood or aluminum and are used for patients who need crutches for a short period of time. The patient must be taught to bear weight on the hand bars instead of the axillary supports. If pressure is applied on the axillary bar, it can injure axillary blood vessels and nerves. They are *not* recommended for weak or elderly patients since axillary crutches require good upper body and arm strength, and a good sense of balance and coordination.
- *Forearm or Lofstrand crutches* (Figure 23–16B): These crutches attach to forearms, are used for patients with weakness or paralysis in both legs, are recommended for patients who need crutches permanently or for a long period of time, and require upper arm strength and good coordination.
- *Platform crutches* (Figure 23–16C): These crutches are used for patients who cannot grip handles of other

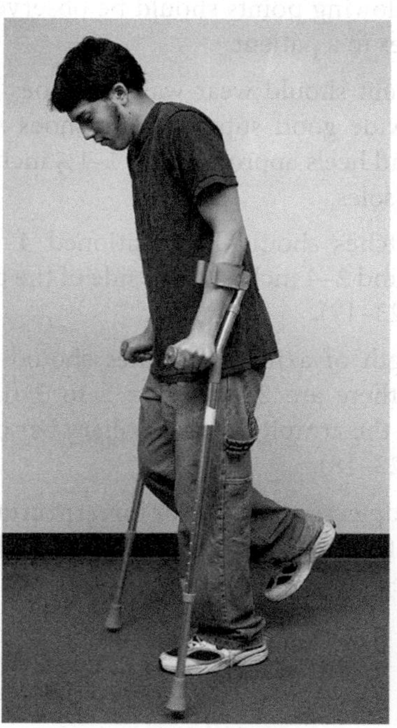

FIGURE 23–16B Forearm or Lofstrand crutches are recommended for patients who need crutches permanently or for a long period of time.

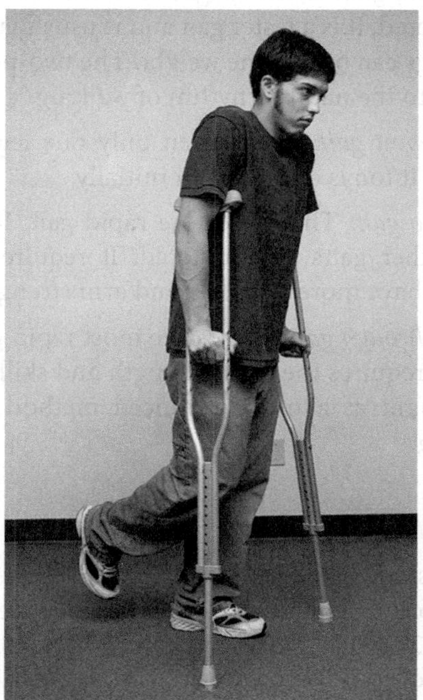

FIGURE 23–16A A patient using an axillary crutch must be taught to bear weight on the hand bars instead of on the axillary supports.

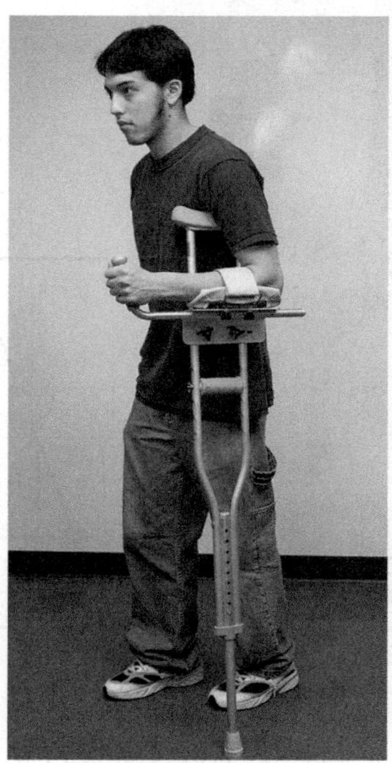

FIGURE 23–16C Platform crutches are used by patients who cannot grip the handles of other crutches or bear weight on the wrists and hands.

crutches or bear weight on their wrists and hands. They do not require as much upper body strength, but do require a good sense of balance and coordination. They require that elbows be flexed at a 90-degree or right angle so the patient can bear weight on the forearm.

The following points should be observed when fitting crutches to a patient.

- The patient should wear walking shoes that fit well and provide good support. The shoes should have low, broad heels approximately 1–1½ inches high and nonskid soles.
- The crutches should be positioned 4–6 inches in front of and 2–4 inches to the side of the patient's foot (Figure 23–17).
- The length of axillary crutches should be adjusted so that there are 2 inches or 2 to 3 finger widths between the armpit and the axillary bar of the crutch (Figure 23–18).
- The handpieces of axillary or forearm crutches should be adjusted so that each elbow is flexed at a 25- to 30-degree angle.

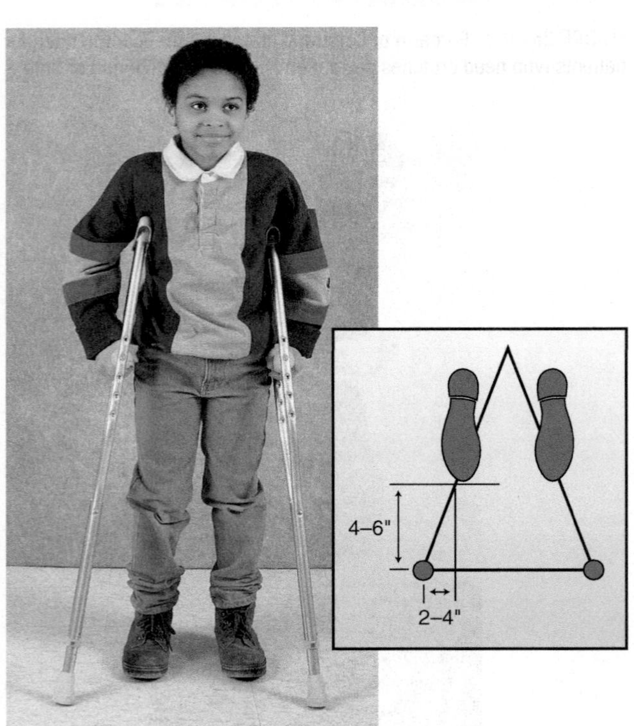

FIGURE 23–17 Crutches should be positioned 4–6 inches in front of and 2–4 inches to the side of the patient's foot.

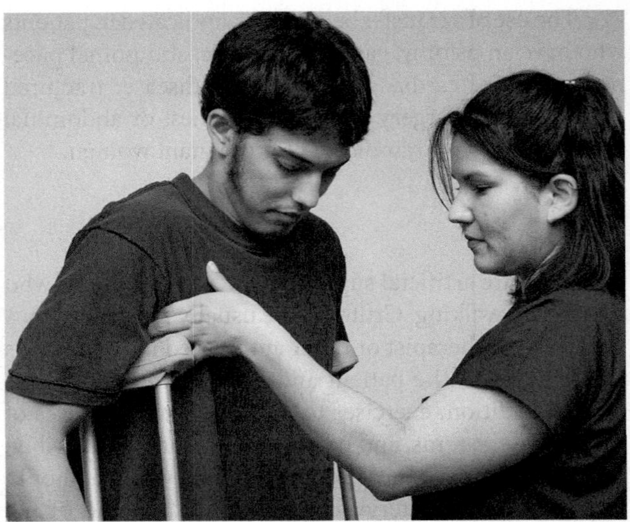
FIGURE 23–18 The length of axillary crutches should be adjusted so that there are 2 inches or 2 to 3 finger widths between the axillary area and the top of the crutches.

Some of the more common crutch-walking gaits are described. The gait taught by the therapist or authorized person depends on the injury and the patient's condition.

- *Four-point gait:* Used when both legs can bear some weight. It is a slow gait. Patients often are taught the four-point gait as the first gait and are then taught faster gaits when this one is mastered.
- *Two-point gait:* Often taught after the four-point gait is mastered. It is a faster gait and is usually used when both legs can bear some weight. The two-point gait is closest to the natural rhythm of walking.
- *Three-point gait:* Used when only one leg can bear weight. It too is a gait taught initially.
- *Swing-to gait:* This is a more rapid gait. It is taught after other gaits are mastered. It requires that the patient have more shoulder and arm strength.
- *Swing-through gait:* This is the most rapid gait. However, it requires the most strength and skill. It is usually taught as a more advanced method of crutch walking.

Cane

A **cane** is an assistive device that provides balance and support. There are several different types of canes (Figure 23–19A). *Standard* canes are single-tipped canes. They can have curved handles, T-handles, or J-handles with a handgrip. *Tripod* canes with three tips

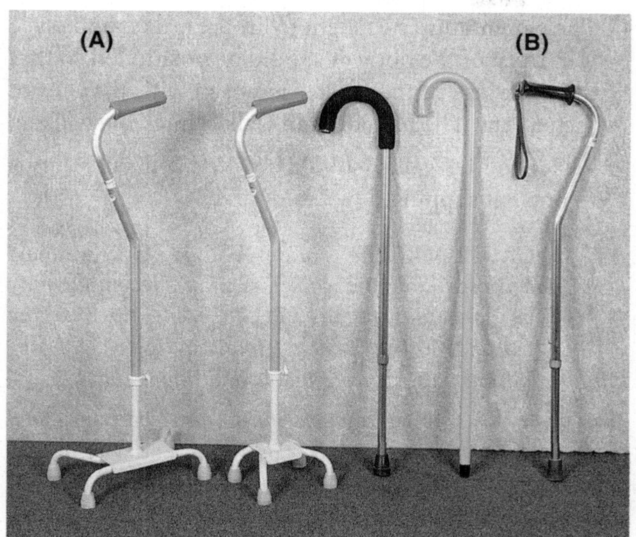

FIGURE 23–19A Different types of canes: (A) quad canes; (B) single-tipped canes.

and *quad* canes with four tips provide a wider base of support and more stability for the patient. A *walkcane*, also called a *Hemiwalker*, has four legs and a handlebar that the patient can grip (Figure 23–19B). It is used with patients who have *hemiplegia*, or paralysis on one side of the body. The bottom tip(s) of all canes should be fitted with a 1-inch rubber-suction tip to provide traction and prevent slipping. Basic principles for using canes include:

- A cane is used on the unaffected (good) side (Figure 23–19C). In this way, a wider base of support is provided to increase stability. This prevents the patient from leaning toward the cane and falling because of the weak or injured leg. In addition, in normal walking, the leg and opposite arm move together, so the cane and leg will follow the same pattern.
- Canes must be correctly fitted. The bottom tip of the cane should be positioned approximately 6–8 inches from the side of the unaffected foot. The cane handle should be level with the top of the femur at the hip joint. The patient's elbow should be flexed at a 25- to 30-degree angle.
- Several gaits for cane walking can be taught. In a two-point gait, the patient is taught to move the cane and affected leg together, and then move the unaffected leg. In a three-point gait, the patient is taught to move the cane, then the affected or involved leg, and finally the unaffected leg. The therapist or other authorized person determines the correct gait.

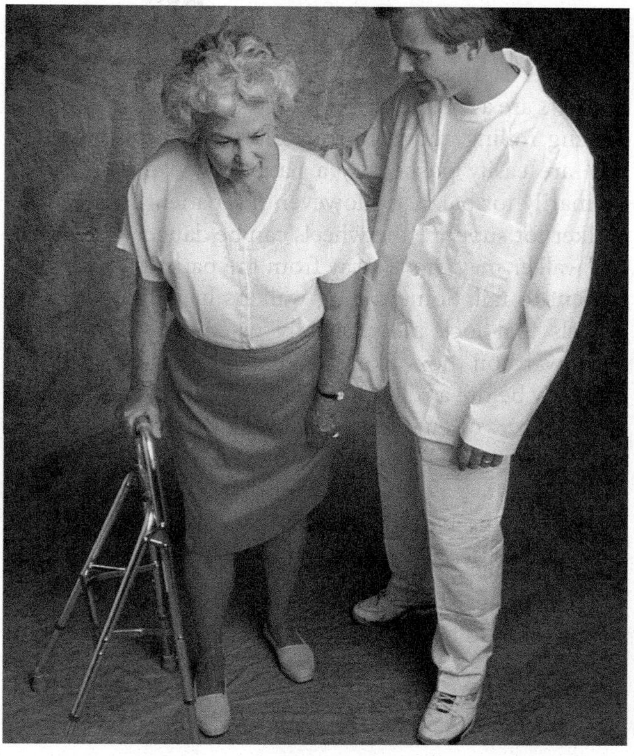

FIGURE 23–19B A walkcane has four legs and a handlebar that the patient can grip. Courtesy of Sunrise Medical

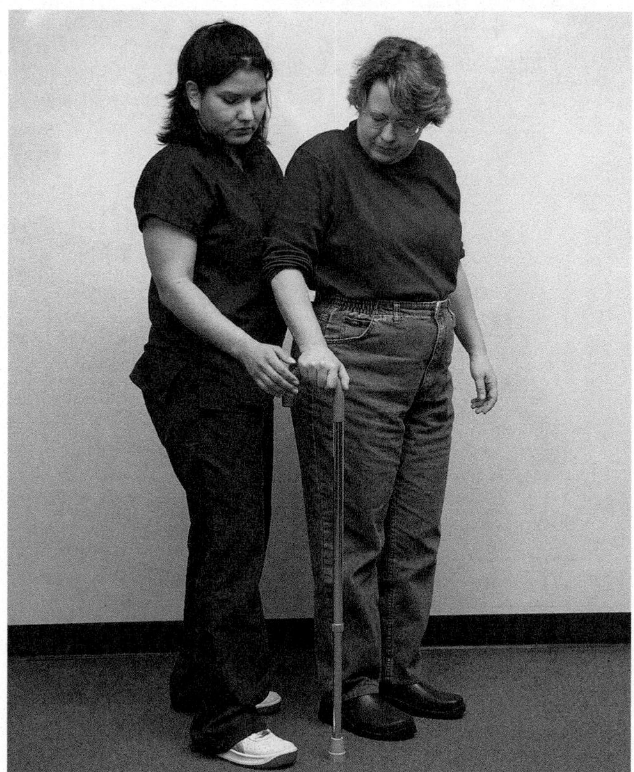

FIGURE 23–19C A cane is used on the unaffected (good) side to provide a wider base of support.

Walker

A **walker** is a four-legged device that provides support. Walkers are available in several styles, including standard, folding, rolling, and platform. Rolling walkers have wheels and are easily pushed by a patient who uses a walker primarily for balance. However, if a patient leans on the walker for support, the wheels can be dangerous because the walker may move away from the patient, causing the patient to fall. Some rolling walkers have brakes on the wheels that lock automatically when weight is placed downward on the walker. The patient must be evaluated carefully before a rolling walker is used (Figure 23–20).

Walkers often are used for weak patients who have a poor sense of balance even though no leg injuries may be present. To use a walker, patients must be strong enough to hold themselves upright while leaning on the walker. Basic principles for using a walker include:

- The walker should be fitted to the patient. The handles should be level with the top of the femurs at the hip joints. Each elbow should be flexed at a 25- to 30-degree angle.
- The patient must be taught to lift the walker and place it in front of the body. It should be positioned so that the back legs of the walker are even with the toes of the patient. The patient then walks "into" the walker.
- All legs of the walker should be fitted with rubber tips to prevent slipping.

FIGURE 23–20 Some walkers have wheels and a seat, but a patient must be evaluated carefully before this type of walker is used.

Safety

CAUTION: *The patient should be cautioned against sliding the walker. A sliding technique may be dangerous because it can easily tip over the walker. Most walkers are made of lightweight aluminum, so most patients are capable of lifting them.*

Safety

CAUTION: *Patients must also be cautioned against using the walker as a transfer device. If they try to hold on to the walker while getting out of bed or up from a chair, the walker can tip forward, causing the patient to fall. Patients should be taught how to use their arms to push against the bed or arms of a chair to rise to a standing position.*

Ambulation Precautions

Safety

It is essential that the health care worker remain alert at all times when ambulating a patient. Always walk on the patient's weak side and slightly behind the patient, and be alert for signs that the patient may fall. If the patient starts to fall, do *not* try to hold the patient in an upright position. Use your body to brace the patient, if at all possible. Keep your back straight, bend from the hips and knees, maintain a broad base of support, and try to grasp the patient under the axillary (armpit) areas. If the patient is wearing a transfer belt, keep a firm hold on the belt. The patient should be eased to the floor as slowly as possible (Figure 23–21). The patient's head and neck should be

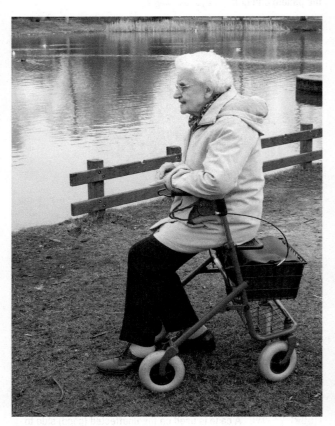

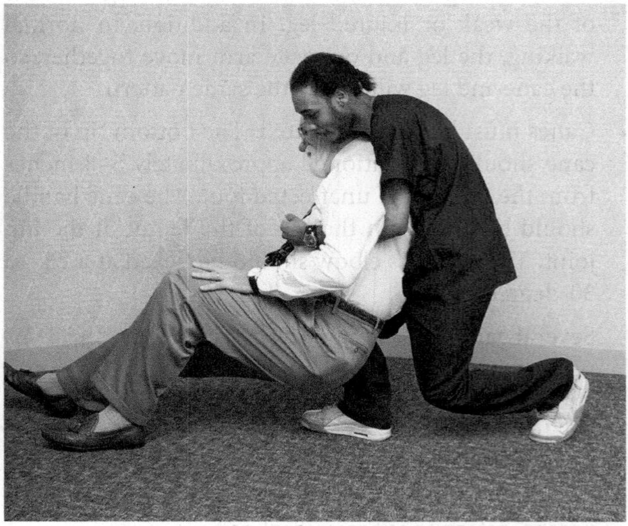

FIGURE 23–21 Ease a falling patient to the floor as slowly as possible. Try to protect the patient's head and neck.

protected, and the head should be prevented from striking the floor. Stay with the patient and call for help. Patients should not be moved until they have been examined for injuries. After a fall has occurred, most agencies require a written incident report. Follow agency policy for correct documentation of the incident.

STUDENT: Go to the workbook and complete the assignment sheet for 23:2, Ambulating Patients Who Use Transfer (Gait) Belts, Crutches, Canes, or Walkers. Then return and continue with the procedures.

PROCEDURE 23:2A

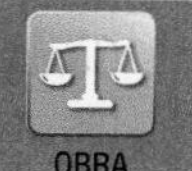

Ambulating a Patient with a Transfer (Gait) Belt

Equipment and Supplies

Transfer or gait belt, paper and pen and/or computer

Procedure

1. Check orders or obtain authorization from your immediate supervisor for ambulating the patient.
2. Assemble supplies.
3. Comm Knock on the door and pause before entering. Introduce yourself. Identify the patient, explain the procedure, and obtain consent.
4. Close the door and pull the curtain to provide privacy.
5. Wash hands.
6. Lock the wheels on the bed to prevent movement. If siderails are present and elevated, lower the siderail on the side where you are working.
7. Assist the patient into a sitting position. If the patient is wearing bedclothes, put a robe on the patient.
8. Check to be sure the transfer belt is the correct size. Position the belt around the patient's waist and on top of the clothing (Figure 23–22A). Position the buckle or clasp so that it is slightly off center in the front. Make sure the belt is smooth and free of wrinkles.
9. Tighten the belt so that it fits snugly; secure the clasp or buckle. Place three to four fingers under the belt to make sure it is not too tight (Figure 23–22B). Make sure the belt is comfortable and does not interfere with breathing. On a female patient, make sure the breasts are not under the belt.
10. Put shoes or slippers on the patient. For the most security, shoes should be worn. The shoes should have low, broad heels approximately 1–1½ inches high and nonskid soles. Make sure the patient's feet are on the floor. If the patient's feet are not on the floor, move the patient closer to the side of the bed or edge of a chair.

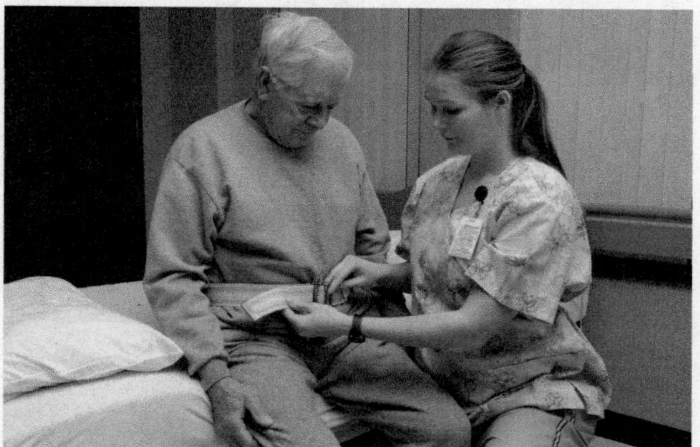

FIGURE 23–22A Position the transfer belt around the patient's waist and on top of the clothing.

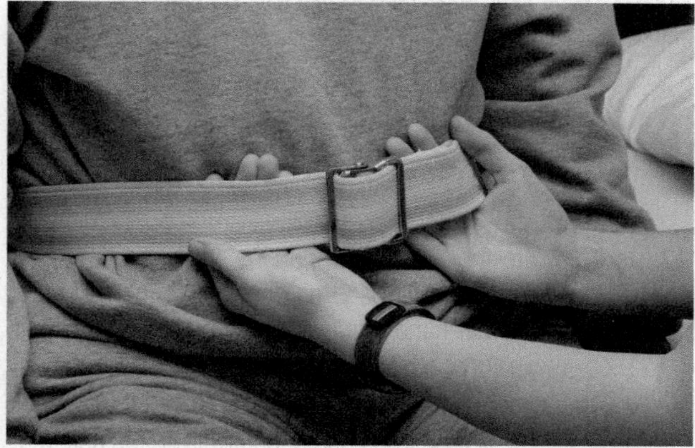

FIGURE 23–22B Check the transfer belt to make sure it is not too tight.

11. 

Assist the patient to a standing position. Face the patient and get a broad base of support. Grasp the loops on the side of the belt or place your hands under the sides of the belt. Ask the patient to assist by pushing against the bed with his/her hands at a given signal, such as "one, two, three, stand." Bend at your knees and give the signal for the patient to stand. Keep your back straight and straighten your knees as the patient stands (Figure 23–22C).

(continues)

PROCEDURE 23:2A (CONT.)

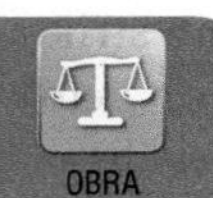
OBRA

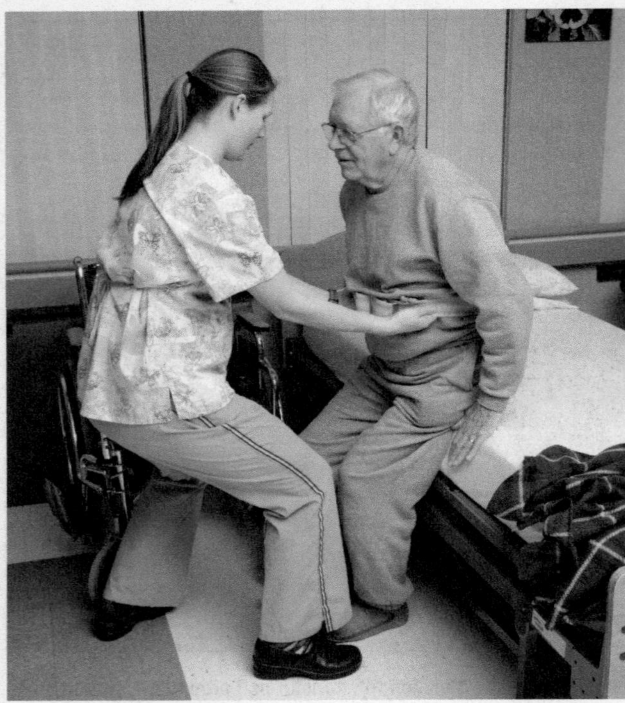

FIGURE 23–22C Place your hands under the sides of the belt and use proper body mechanics as you help the patient to a standing position.

Safety

CAUTION: Use correct body mechanics at all times.

12. To ambulate the patient, support the patient in a standing position. Keep one hand on one side of the belt while moving the other hand to the loops or the back of the belt. Then, move the second hand from the side to the loops or the back of the belt while you move behind the patient.

Safety

CAUTION: Keep one hand firmly on the belt at all times when changing position.

13. Ambulate the patient. Encourage the patient to walk slowly and use handrails, if available. Walk slightly behind the patient at all times and keep a firm, underhand grip on the belt or keep your hands firmly in the loops.

NOTE: If the patient has a weak side, position yourself on the patient's weak side.

14. If the patient starts to fall, keep a firm grip on the belt. Use your body to brace the patient. Keep your back straight. Gently ease the patient to the floor, taking care to protect his or her head. Stay with the patient and call for help. Do not try to stand the patient up until help arrives and the patient has been examined for injuries.
15. When ambulation is complete, assist the patient in returning to bed. Remove the transfer belt.
16. Observe all checkpoints before leaving the patient. Make sure the patient is comfortable and in good body alignment. Elevate the siderails (if indicated), lower the bed to its lowest level, place the call signal and supplies within easy reach of the patient, and leave the area neat and clean.
17. Replace all equipment.
18. Wash hands.
19. 
Comm
Report and/or record all required information on the patient's chart or enter it into the computer. For example: date, time, ambulated with a transfer belt, walked down to lounge and back, and your signature and title. Report any problems immediately.

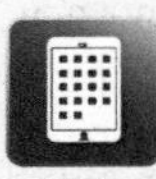
EHR

NOTE: In health care agencies using electronic health records (EHRs), also known as electronic medical records (EMRs), the information is entered directly into the patient's record on a computer.

PRACTICE: **Go to the workbook and use the evaluation sheet for 23:2A, Ambulating a Patient with a Transfer (Gait) Belt, to practice this procedure. When you believe you have mastered this skill, sign the sheet and give it to your instructor for further action.**

Check

FINAL CHECKPOINT: Using the criteria listed on the evaluation sheet, your instructor will grade your performance.

PROCEDURE 23:2B

Ambulating a Patient Who Uses Crutches

Equipment and Supplies

Adjustable crutches, paper and pen and/or computer

Procedure

1. Check orders or obtain authorization from your immediate supervisor. Ascertain which gait the therapist taught the patient.
2. Assemble equipment.
3. Check the crutches. Make sure there are rubber-suction tips on the bottom ends and that the tips are not worn down or torn. Check to be sure the axillary bars and hand rests are covered with padding.

   NOTE: Foam-rubber pads are usually placed on crutches.
4. Comm — Knock on the door and pause before entering. Introduce yourself. Identify the patient. Explain the procedure and obtain consent.
5. Wash hands.
6. Help the patient put on good walking shoes. The shoes should have low, broad heels approximately 1–1½ inches high and nonskid soles.
7. Place a transfer (gait) belt on the patient. Use an underhand grasp on the belt and assist the patient to a standing position. Advise the patient to bear his or her weight on the unaffected leg. Position the crutches correctly.
8. Check the fit of the crutches.
   a. Position the crutches 4–6 inches in front of the patient's feet.
   b. Move the crutches 2–4 inches to the sides of the feet.
   c. Make sure there is a 2-inch or 2 to 3 finger widths gap between the axilla (armpit) and the axillary bar or rest. If the length must be adjusted, check with your immediate supervisor.
   d. Each elbow must be flexed at a 25- to 30-degree angle. If the hand rests must be adjusted to achieve this angle, check with your immediate supervisor.

   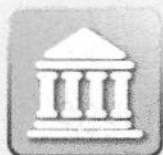
   Legal

   NOTE: In some agencies, the trained health care worker is permitted to adjust the crutches as necessary. The adjustments are then checked by the therapist or other authorized person. Follow your agency policy.
9. Assist the patient with the required gait. The gait used depends on the patient's injury and condition, and is determined by the therapist or other authorized person.

   Safety

   CAUTION: Remain alert at all times. Be ready to catch the patient if there are any signs of falling.
10. Four-point gait (Figure 23–23):
    a. The patient can bear weight on both legs. Start the patient in a standing position, with crutches at the sides.
    b. Move the right crutch forward.
    c. Move the left foot forward.
    d. Move the left crutch forward.
    e. Move the right foot forward.

    NOTE: This is a slow gait taught initially when both legs can bear weight.
11. Three-point gait (Figure 23–24):
    a. The patient can bear weight on one leg only. Start the patient in a standing position, with crutches at the sides.
    b. Advance both crutches and the weak or affected foot.
    c. Transfer the patient's body weight forward to the crutches.
    d. Advance the unaffected, or good, foot forward.

    NOTE: This is a slow gait taught initially when only one leg can bear weight.

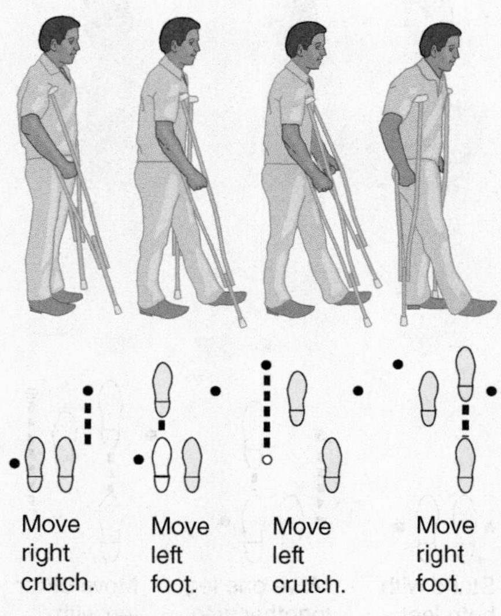
Move right crutch.
Move left foot.
Move left crutch.
Move right foot.

FIGURE 23–23 **Four-point gait for crutches.**

(continues)

PROCEDURE 23:2B (CONT.)

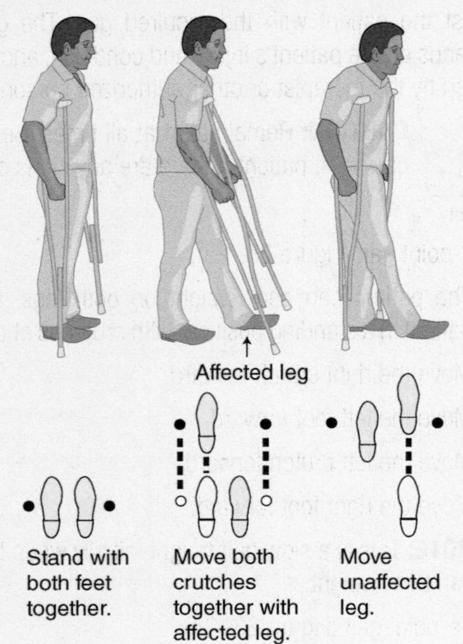

FIGURE 23–24 **Three-point gait for crutches.**

12. Two-point gait (Figure 23–25):

a. The patient can bear weight on both legs. Start with the crutches at the sides.

b. Move the right foot and left crutch forward at the same time.

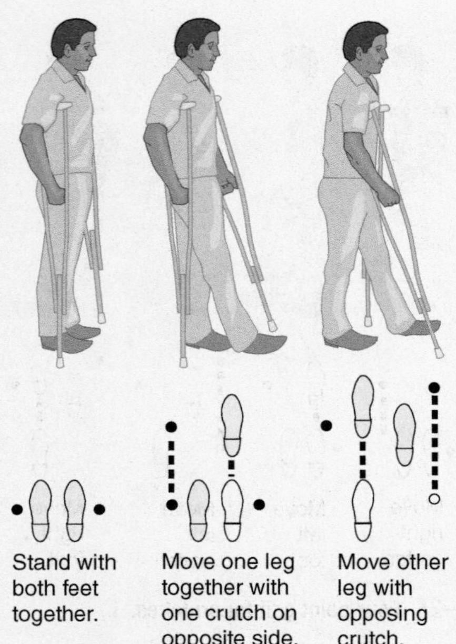

FIGURE 23–25 **Two-point gait for crutches.**

c. Move the left foot and right crutch forward at the same time.

NOTE: This is a more advanced and a more rapid gait used when the four-point gait has been mastered.

NOTE: The two-point gait is closest to the natural rhythm of walking.

13. Swing-to gait:

a. One or both of the patient's legs can bear weight. Start with the crutches at the sides.

b. Balance weight on foot or feet. Move both crutches forward.

c. Transfer weight forward.

d. Use shoulder and arm strength to swing feet up to crutches.

NOTE: This is a more rapid gait and requires more shoulder and arm strength and a good sense of balance and coordination.

14. Swing-through gait (Figure 23–26):

a. One or both of the patient's legs can bear weight. Start with the crutches at the sides. Balance weight on foot or feet.

b. Advance both crutches forward at the same time.

c. Transfer weight forward.

d. Use shoulder and arm strength to swing up to and through the crutches, stopping slightly in front of the crutches.

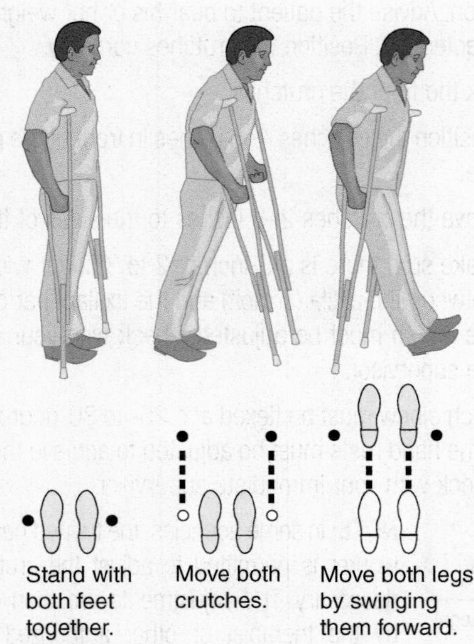

FIGURE 23–26 **Swing-through gait for crutches.**

PROCEDURE 23:2B (CONT.)

NOTE: This is the most rapid and advanced gait. It requires a great deal of shoulder and arm strength. It also requires an excellent sense of balance because at one point only the crutches are in contact with the ground.

15. When using crutches, the patient must *not* rest his or her body weight on the axillary rests. Shoulder and arm strength should provide movement on the crutches.

Safety

CAUTION: Warn the patient that nerve damage can occur if weight is supported constantly on the axillary rest.

16. Check to make sure that the patient is not moving too far forward at one time. Distances should be limited. If the patient attempts to move the crutches too far forward, he or she can very easily lose balance and fall forward.
17. Comm — Check the patient's progress. Report the progress to the therapist or your immediate supervisor. The therapist will determine when to teach the patient more advanced gaits.
18. When the patient is finished using the crutches, replace all equipment.
19. Assist the patient back to bed or position the patient in a chair. Remove the transfer belt. Observe all checkpoints before leaving the patient. Make sure the patient is comfortable and in good body alignment. If the patient is in bed, elevate the siderails (if indicated), lower the bed to its lowest level, place the call signal and other supplies within easy reach of the patient, and leave the area neat and clean.
20. Wash hands.
21.  Comm — Report and/or record all required information on the patient's chart or enter it into the computer. For example: date, time, ambulated with crutches, walked down the hall two times using two-point gait, no problems noted, and your signature and title. Report any problems immediately.

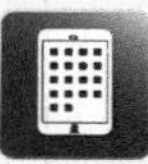
EHR

In health care agencies using electronic health records (EHRs), also known as electronic medical records (EMRs), the information is entered directly into the patient's record on a computer.

PRACTICE: Go to the workbook and use the evaluation sheet for 23:2B, Ambulating a Patient Who Uses Crutches, to practice this procedure. When you believe you have mastered this skill, sign the sheet and give it to your instructor for further action.

Check

FINAL CHECKPOINT: Using the criteria listed on the evaluation sheet, your instructor will grade your performance.

PROCEDURE 23:2C

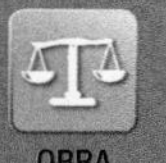
OBRA

Ambulating a Patient Who Uses a Cane

Equipment and Supplies

Adjustable cane, paper and pen and/or computer

Procedure

1. Check orders or obtain authorization from your immediate supervisor. Ascertain which gait the therapist taught the patient.
2. Assemble equipment.
3. Check the cane. Make sure the bottom has a rubber-suction tip. If the patient needs extra stability, use a tripod (three-legged) or quad (four-legged) cane.
4. Comm — Knock on the door and pause before entering. Introduce yourself. Identify the patient. Explain the procedure and obtain consent.
5. Wash hands.
6. Help the patient put on good walking shoes. The shoes should have low, broad heels approximately 1–1½ inches high and nonskid soles.
7. Place a transfer (gait) belt on the patient. Use an underhand grasp on the belt and assist the patient to a standing position. Advise the patient to bear his or her weight on the unaffected leg.
8. Check the height of the cane:
   a. Position the cane on the unaffected (good) side and approximately 6–8 inches from the side of the foot.

(continues)

PROCEDURE 23:2C (CONT.)

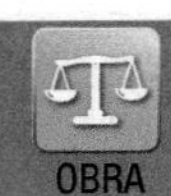

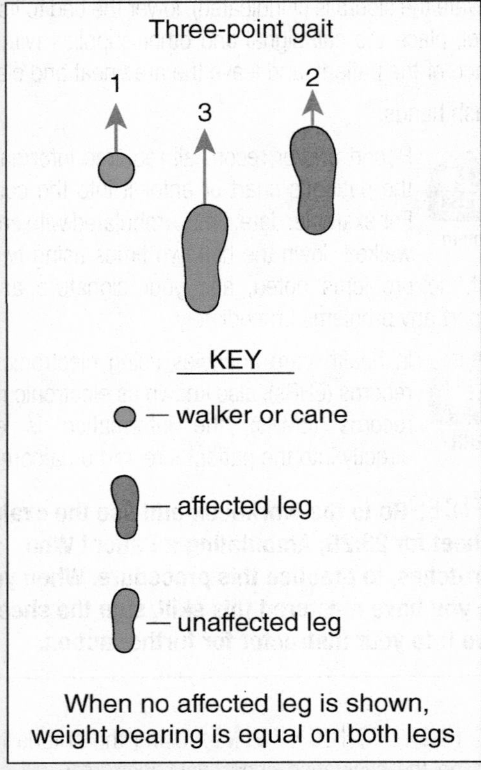

FIGURE 23–27A **Three-point gait for canes.**

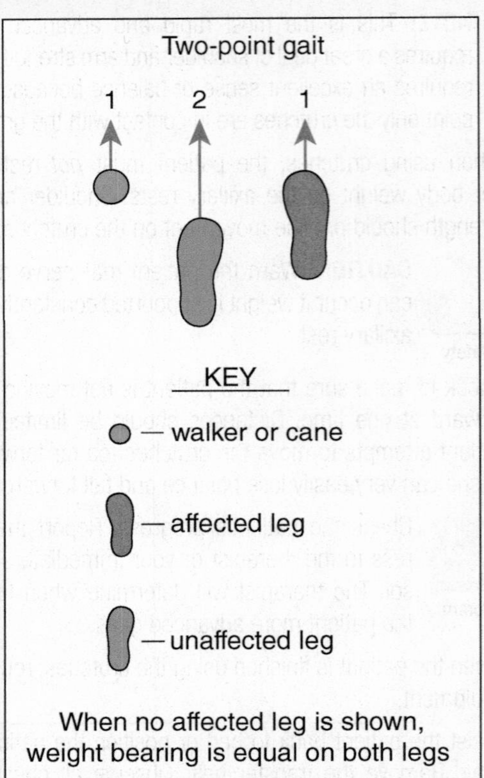

FIGURE 23–27B **Two-point gait for canes.**

b. The top of the cane should be level with the top of the femur at the hip joint.

c. The patient's elbow should be flexed at a 25- to 30-degree angle.

NOTE: If the height of the cane needs adjustment, follow agency policy. In some agencies, only the therapist adjusts canes. In other agencies, the trained health care worker can adjust canes.

9. Instruct the patient to use the cane on the good, or unaffected, side.

NOTE: This prevents leaning toward the weak or affected side and provides a broader base of support.

10. Assist the patient with the gait ordered. For a three-point gait (Figure 23–27A):

a. Balance the body weight on the strong or unaffected foot. Move the cane forward approximately 12–18 inches.

b. Move the weak or affected foot forward.

c. Transfer the weight to the affected foot and cane. Bring the unaffected foot forward.

For a two-point gait (Figure 23–27B):

a. Balance the weight on the strong or unaffected foot.

b. Move the cane and the weak or affected foot forward. Keep the cane fairly close to the body to prevent leaning.

c. Transfer body weight forward to the cane.

d. Move the good, or unaffected, foot forward.

CAUTION: Remain alert at all times. Be ready to catch the patient if there are any signs of falling.

NOTE: Maintain an underhand grasp on the transfer belt if the patient is not steady.

11. A common sequence to follow when assisting the patient up and down stairs is that of always starting with the good (unaffected) leg:

a. Step up with the unaffected leg.

b. Bring the cane and weak or affected leg up.

c. To go down steps, reverse this procedure. Step down on the good leg and follow with the cane and affected or weak foot.

NOTE: Remember this sequence by saying, "Good Guys Go First."

PROCEDURE 23:2C (CONT.)

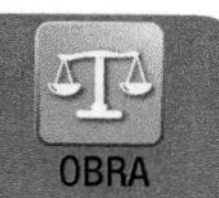

12. When walking with a cane, the patient should take small steps. Smaller steps are recommended to prevent leaning and/or loss of balance.
13. 

Note the patient's progress. Pay particular attention to any problems the patient experiences during ambulation. Report this information to your immediate supervisor or the therapist.
14. Assist the patient back to bed or position the patient in a chair. Remove the transfer belt.
15. Observe all checkpoints before leaving the patient. Make sure the patient is comfortable and in good body alignment. If the patient is in bed, elevate the siderails (if indicated), lower the bed to its lowest level, place the call signal and other supplies within easy reach of the patient, and leave the area neat and clean.
16. Replace all equipment.
17. Wash hands.
18. 

Report and/or record all required information on the patient's chart or enter it into the computer. For example: date, time, ambulated with tripod cane, walked to visitor's lounge and back to room, no problems noted, and your signature and title. Report any problems immediately.

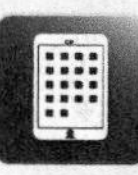

In health care agencies using electronic health records (EHRs), also known as electronic medical records (EMRs), the information is entered directly into the patient's record on a computer.

PRACTICE: **Go to the workbook and use the evaluation sheet for 23:2C, Ambulating a Patient Who Uses a Cane, to practice this procedure. When you believe you have mastered this skill, sign the sheet and give it to your instructor for further action.**

FINAL CHECKPOINT: Using the criteria listed on the evaluation sheet, your instructor will grade your performance.

PROCEDURE 23:2D

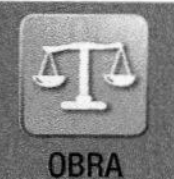

Ambulating a Patient Who Uses a Walker

Equipment and Supplies

Adjustable walker, paper and pen and/or computer

Procedure

1. Check orders or obtain authorization from your immediate supervisor for ambulating the patient.
2. Assemble equipment.
3. Check the walker. Make sure rubber-suction tips are secure on all of the legs. Check for rough or damaged edges on the hand rests.
4. Knock on the door and pause before entering. Introduce yourself. Identify the patient. Explain the procedure and obtain consent.
5. Wash hands.
6. Help the patient put on good walking shoes. The shoes should have low, broad heels approximately 1–1½ inches high and nonskid soles.
7. Place a transfer (gait) belt on the patient. Use an underhand grasp on the belt and assist the patient to a standing position. Position the walker correctly and ask the patient to grasp the hand rests securely.
8. Check the height of the walker to see whether the following requirements are met (Figure 23–28A):
   a. The hand rests are level with the tops of the femurs at the hip joints.
   b. The elbows are flexed at 25- to 30-degree angles.

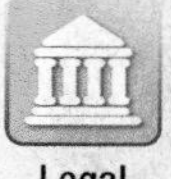

NOTE: If the height of the walker needs adjustment, follow agency policy. In some agencies, only the therapist makes such adjustments. In other agencies, a trained health care worker may adjust walkers.

(continues)

PROCEDURE 23:2D (CONT.)

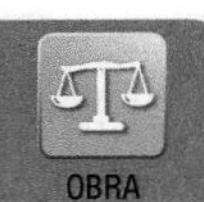
OBRA

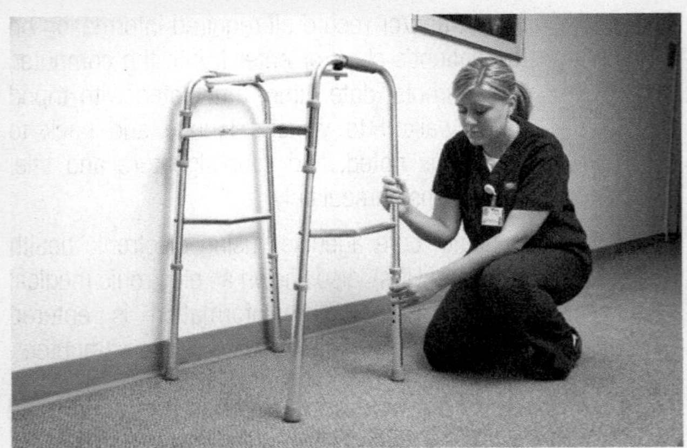

FIGURE 23–28A **Check the adjustment of the walker to make sure it is the correct height for the patient.**

9. Start with the walker in position. The patient should be standing "inside" the walker.

10.  Comm Tell the patient to lift the walker and place it forward so that the back legs of the walker are even with the patient's toes.

    Safety **CAUTION:** Tell the patient to avoid sliding the walker. The walker could fall forward and cause the patient to fall.

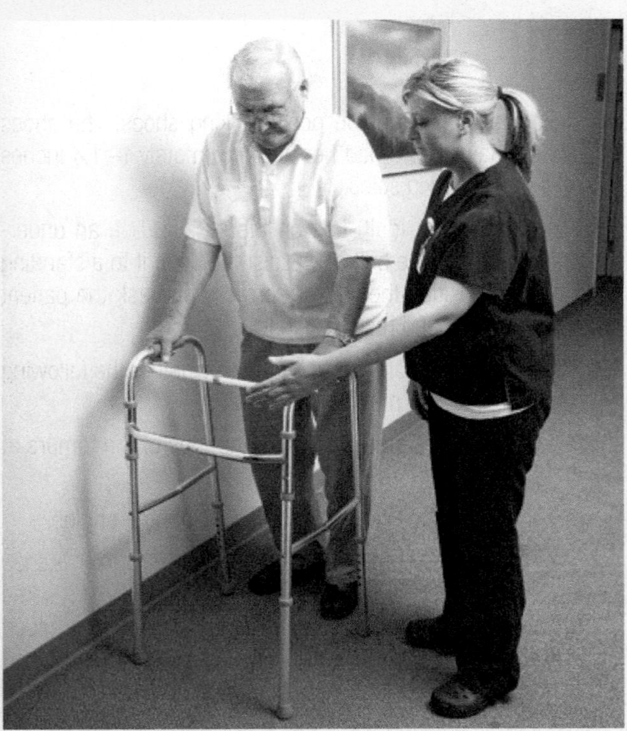

FIGURE 23–28B **Instruct the patient to use the walker for support while walking "into" the walker.**

11. Instruct the patient to transfer his or her weight forward slightly to the walker.

12. Instruct the patient to use the walker for support and to walk "into" the walker (Figure 23–28B). Do *not* allow the patient to "shuffle" his or her feet.

13. Repeat steps 10–12. While the patient is using the walker, walk to the side and slightly behind the patient. Be alert at all times. Be ready to catch the patient if there are any signs of falling.

    NOTE: If the patient has a weak side, position yourself on the patient's weak side.

14. Check constantly to make sure the patient is lifting the walker to move it forward. Also make sure the patient is placing the walker forward just to his or her toes and not attempting too large a step.

15. 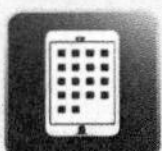 Comm Note the patient's progress. Pay particular attention to any problems the patient experiences during ambulation. Report this information to your immediate supervisor or the therapist.

16. Assist the patient back to bed or position the patient in a chair. Remove the transfer belt.

17. Observe all checkpoints before leaving the patient. Make sure the patient is comfortable and in good body alignment. If the patient is in bed, elevate the siderails (if indicated), lower the bed to its lowest level, place the call signal and other supplies within easy reach of the patient, and leave the area neat and clean.

18. Replace all equipment.

19. Wash hands.

20. Comm Report and/or record all required information on the patient's chart or enter it into the computer. For example: date, time, ambulated with walker, walked down the hall and back two times, needs encouragement to pick up walker and not slide it, and your signature and title. Report any problems immediately.

    EHR In health care agencies using electronic health records (EHRs), also known as electronic medical records (EMRs), the information is entered directly into the patient's record on a computer.

PRACTICE: **Go to the workbook and use the evaluation sheet for 23:2D, Ambulating a Patient Who Uses a Walker, to practice this procedure. When you believe you have mastered this skill, sign the sheet and give it to your instructor for further action.**

Check

FINAL CHECKPOINT: Using the criteria listed on the evaluation sheet, your instructor will grade your performance.

23:3 Administering Heat/Cold Applications

As a health care worker, you may be responsible for administering a variety of heat and cold applications. Some of the main principles involved are described in this section.

Cryotherapy is the use of cold for treatment. Cold applications are administered to relieve pain, reduce swelling, reduce body temperature, and control bleeding.

- **Moist cold** applications are cold and moist or wet against the skin. Examples are cold **compresses**, packs, and soaks. These applications are more penetrating than are dry cold applications.
- **Dry cold** applications are cold and dry against the skin. Examples are ice bags, ice collars, hypothermia blankets, and similar devices.
- **Ice bags** or **collars** are special containers filled with ice. Most health care facilities use disposable bags to prevent the spread of infection (Figure 23–29).

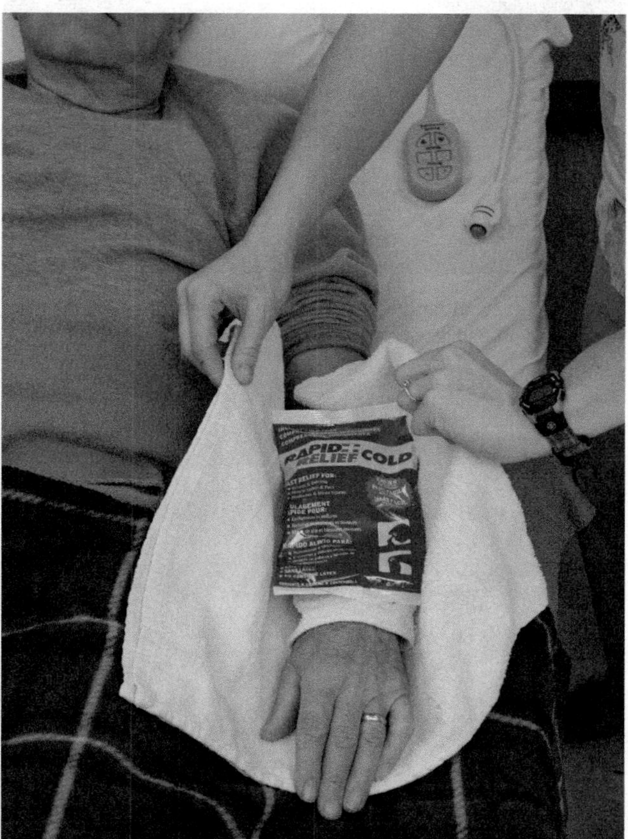

FIGURE 23–29 Most health care facilities use disposable ice bags to prevent the spread of infection. A towel or cover must be used because the bags should not be placed directly on the skin.

- **Hypothermia blankets**, also called *thermal blankets*, contain coils that are filled with cool fluid. They are used to reduce high body temperatures. A rectal probe is usually used to monitor the patient's temperature. When the patient's temperature reaches a preset level, the blanket decreases the circulation of the cooling fluid.

Thermotherapy is the use of heat for treatment. Heat applications are administered to relieve pain, increase drainage from an infected area, stimulate healing, increase circulation to an area, combat infection, and relieve muscle spasms or increase muscle mobility before exercise.

- **Moist heat** applications are warm and wet against the skin. These applications are more penetrating and more effective in relieving pain in deeper tissues than are dry heat applications. Examples are the sitz bath, hot soaks, compresses, hydrocollator packs, and paraffin wax treatments.
- **Sitz baths** provide warm moist heat to the perineal and rectal area. They are used postpartum (after birth) and after rectal surgery to provide comfort and promote healing.
- **Hydrocollator packs** are gel-filled packs that are warmed in a water bath at a temperature of 150°F–170°F, or 65.6°C–76.7°C. The gel maintains the warmth for approximately 30–40 minutes, and the pack can be contoured to fit smoothly over any area of the body (Figure 23–30). The pack must be covered with a thick terry cloth or flannel cover before being applied to the skin. Hydrocollator packs are frequently used prior to ROM exercises.
- **Paraffin wax treatments** are often used for chronic joint disease, such as arthritis, or prior to ROM exercises. A mixture of paraffin and a small amount of mineral oil are heated to the melting point. The physical therapist or authorized individual dips the patient's hand(s) or other body part into the warm paraffin three or four times to create a "glove" of wax (Figure 23–31A). The wax is left in place for 20–30 minutes before being peeled off (Figure 23–31B).
- **Dry heat** applications are warm and dry against the skin. Examples are warm-water bags, heating pads, thermal blankets, aquamatic pads or aquathermia pads, and heat lamps.
- **Warm-water bags** are special containers filled with warm water to provide heat to body parts. Most health care agencies use disposable bags to prevent the spread of infection.
- **Thermal blankets** contain coils that can be filled with air or fluid to warm or cool a patient (Figure 23–32). Usually, a rectal probe is used to monitor the patient's temperature. The unit automatically circulates warm or cool fluid or air to maintain a preset temperature.

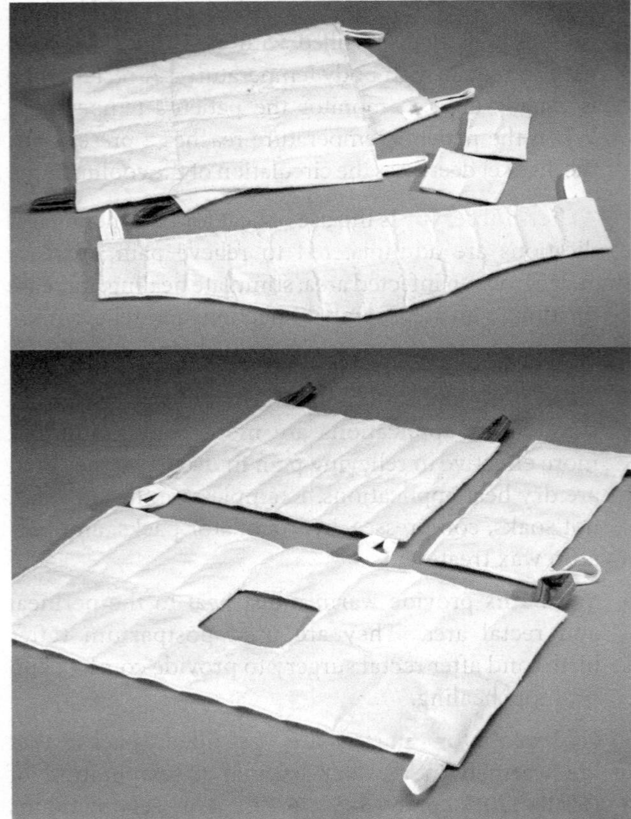

FIGURE 23–30 **Hydrocollator packs are gel-filled packs that are warmed in a water bath.** Courtesy of Briggs Corporation, Des Moines, IA

- **Aquathermia pads**, also called *aquamatic units*, are smaller pads that contain coils that fill with warm water. A control unit maintains a constant preset temperature of the water.

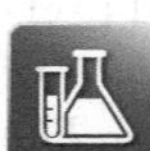

Science

Heat and cold applications are effective because of the reactions they cause in the blood vessels.

- Heat applications cause **vasodilation**. The blood vessels in the area become larger (dilated). More blood comes to the area. Therefore, more oxygen and nutrients are available to stimulate healing. Heat applications ease pain by allowing the blood to carry away fluids that cause inflammation and pain.
- Cold applications cause **vasoconstriction**. The blood vessels become smaller (constricted). Less blood comes to the area. Swelling decreases because fewer fluids are present. The cold also has a numbing effect, which decreases local pain.

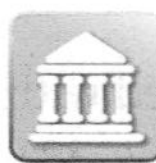

Legal

A physician's order is required for a heat or cold application. The order should state the type of application, duration of treatment, temperature (if not standard), and area of application. In some states and agencies, health care assistants are not

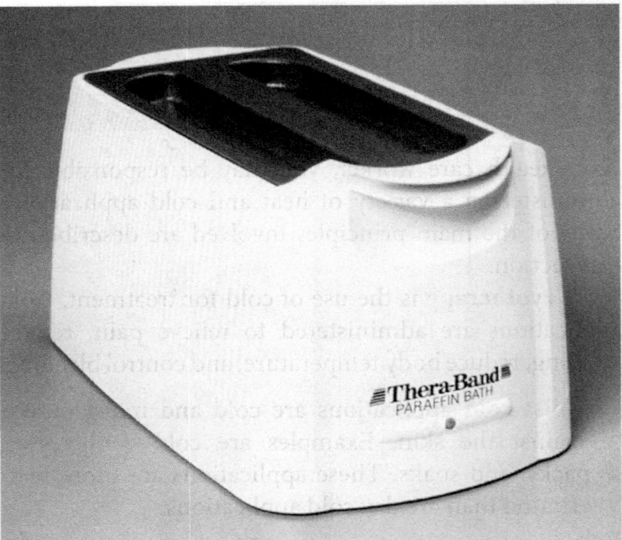

FIGURE 23–31A **A body part is dipped into the paraffin bath three or four times to create a layer of warm wax on the skin.** Courtesy of Briggs Corporation, Des Moines, IA

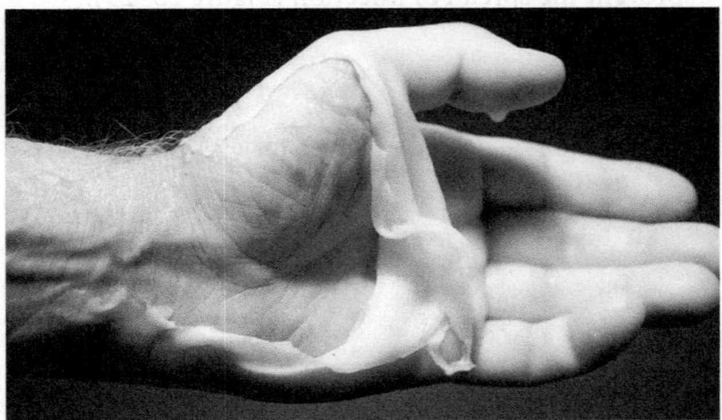

FIGURE 23–31B **After the wax has been in place for 20–30 minutes, it is peeled off and discarded.**

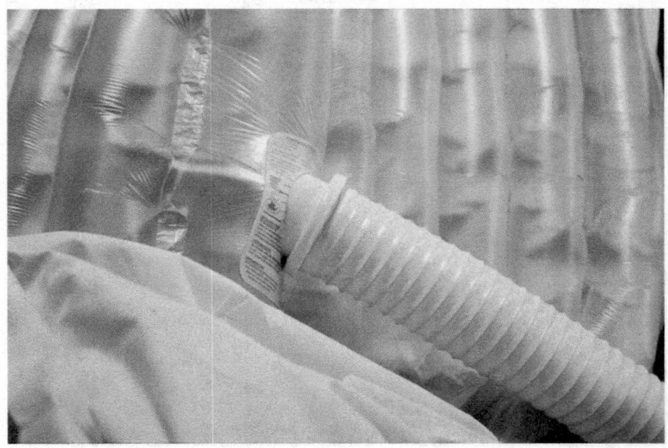

FIGURE 23–32 **A thermal blanket contains coils that are filled with water or air to warm or cool the body.**

allowed to administer heat or cold applications. It is important to check your agency's policy and be aware of your legal responsibilities.

Safety

CAUTION: The patient must be checked frequently when an application is in place. Color and temperature of the skin, amount of pain and bleeding, effect on circulation, and other signs and symptoms must be noted. Special attention must be given to infants, young children, and elderly patients, because the skin of these patients is less resistant and burns or injuries can occur rapidly. Metal objects, such as rings, bracelets, necklaces, watches, and zippers, readily conduct heat or cold. Patients should be asked to remove all metal objects in the treated area before a heat or cold application is administered. When administering heat or cold applications, the rubber or plastic should never come in contact with the skin. All rubber or plastic applications should be covered with a towel or special cloth cover. If any abnormal symptoms are noted, the application should be discontinued and the immediate supervisor notified. The health care worker must be alert at all times and observe all safety precautions when administering heat and cold applications.

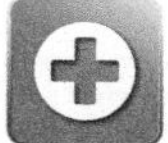
Precaution

Standard precautions (discussed in Chapter 15:4) must be observed if any contact with blood, body fluids, secretions, or excretions is possible. An example is a moist heat application placed on a draining wound. Gloves must be worn. Hands must be washed frequently and are always washed immediately after removing gloves. A mask and eye protection must be worn if splashing or spraying of body fluids is possible. A health care worker must always use proper precautions to prevent the spread of infection.

STUDENT: **Go to the workbook and complete the assignment sheet for 23:3, Administering Heat/Cold Applications. Then return and continue with the procedures.**

PROCEDURE 23:3A

Applying an Ice Bag or Ice Collar

Equipment and Supplies

Ice collar or ice bag and cap, cover or towel, tape, ice in basin, scoop or paper cup, paper and pen and/or computer.

Procedure

1. Check physician's orders or obtain authorization from your immediate supervisor for the application.
2. Assemble equipment.
3. Wash hands.
4. Fill the ice bag or collar with water. Check for leaks. Empty if no leaks are present.

   NOTE: Ice bags come in various sizes for different parts of the body. An ice collar is narrow and is used on the throat.
5. Use the scoop to fill the ice bag or collar half full (Figure 23–33A). To assist in filling, a paper cup with the bottom cut out can be placed in the neck of the bag and used as a funnel. Ice can then be scooped into the bag.

   NOTE: If ice cubes are used, rinse them with water to remove sharp edges.

   NOTE: In most agencies, disposable cold packs are used. To activate the chemicals in the cold pack, squeeze the pack or strike it against a solid surface. It does not need to be filled with ice. A cover must still be placed on the disposable cold pack because the plastic and cold can injure the skin.

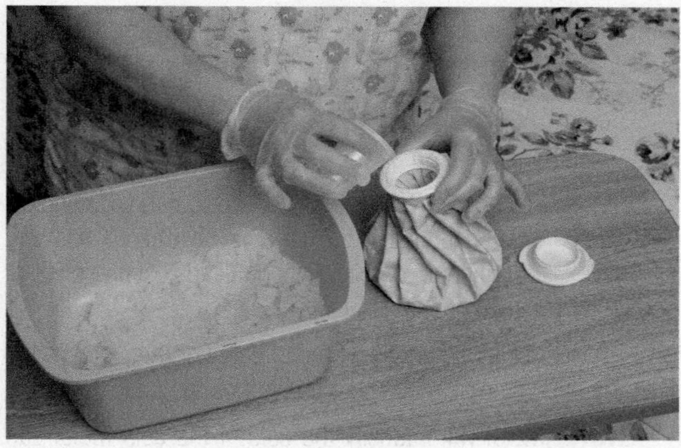

FIGURE 23–33A **Fill the ice bag half full.**

Safety

CAUTION: Chemical ice packs are *not* recommended for use on the face or head because of the danger of leaking chemicals.

6. Place the bag on a table or flat surface. Push gently on the bag to expel all air (Figure 23–33B). Tighten the cap.

   NOTE: If a rubber ring is present on the cap, make sure the ring is secure; it prevents leakage.
7. Wipe the outside of the bag dry.
8. Place a cover on the bag. If an ice bag or ice collar cover is not available, use a towel. Tape the towel in place.

(continues)

PROCEDURE 23:3A (CONT.)

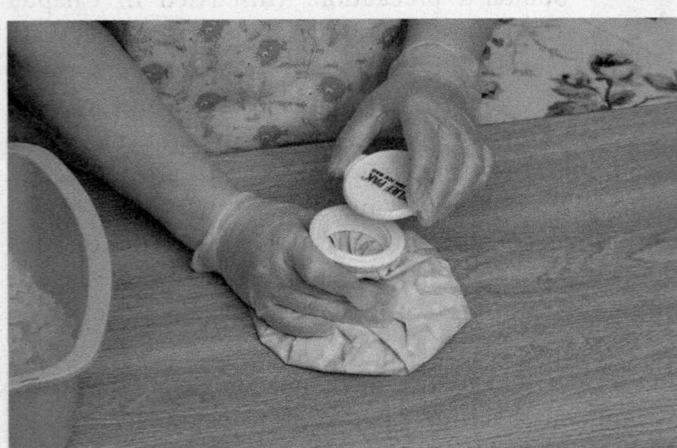

FIGURE 23–33B **Push gently on the bag to expel all air before tightening the cap.**

Safety

CAUTION: The bag *must* be covered. The rubber or plastic and the extreme cold can injure the skin.

9.  Comm

Knock on the door and pause before entering. Introduce yourself. Identify the patient. Explain the procedure and obtain consent.

10. Wash hands. Put on gloves if necessary.

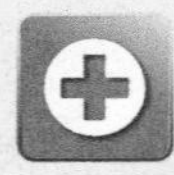
Precaution

CAUTION: Wear gloves and observe standard precautions if the area to be treated has any drainage of blood, body fluids, secretions, or excretions.

11. Place the ice bag gently on the affected area as ordered. If the cap is metal, make sure it is not on the patient's skin.

NOTE: Metal will intensify the cold. If the cold metal cap rests on the patient's skin, an injury can occur.

12. Make sure the patient is comfortable and the ice application is positioned correctly before leaving. Place the call signal within easy reach of the patient. Remove gloves, if worn, and wash hands before leaving the room.

13. Recheck the patient at least every 10 minutes. Make sure the bag is cold and refill it as needed. Check the condition of the skin. Check for pale or white skin, cyanosis (bluish color), or a mottled appearance. Ask the patient about numbness and pain.

Safety

CAUTION: If the skin is mottled or very discolored, or the patient complains of pain, remove the bag immediately and inform your immediate supervisor.

14. Leave the ice application in place for the length of time ordered. In some cases, continuous application is ordered; in others, a specific time period, such as 20 minutes, is ordered. Remove the bag when the designated time has elapsed.

15.  Comm

Carefully check the condition of the patient's skin. Note any comments the patient makes about the treatment. Report these to your supervisor.

16. Observe all checkpoints before leaving the patient: position the patient in correct body alignment, elevate the siderails (if indicated), lower the bed to its lowest level, place the call signal and supplies within easy reach of the patient, and leave the area neat and clean.

17. If the ice bag is disposable, discard it. If the ice bag is not disposable, empty it and clean it thoroughly. Wipe it with a disinfectant, rinse, and dry. Inflate it with air before storing. This prevents the sides from sticking. Replace all equipment.

18. Remove gloves, if worn. Wash hands.

19. Comm

Report and/or record all required information on the patient's chart or enter it into the computer. For example: date, time, ice bag applied to right forearm for 20 minutes, patient states arm feels better, and your signature and title. Report any unusual observations immediately.

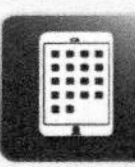
EHR

NOTE: In health care agencies using electronic health records (EHRs), also known as electronic medical records (EMRs), the information is entered directly into the patient's record on a computer.

PRACTICE: **Go to the workbook and use the evaluation sheet for 23:3A, Applying an Ice Bag or Ice Collar, to practice this procedure. When you believe you have mastered this skill, sign the sheet and give it to your instructor for further action.**

Check

FINAL CHECKPOINT: Using the criteria listed on the evaluation sheet, your instructor will grade your performance.

PROCEDURE 23:3B

Applying a Warm-Water Bag

Equipment and Supplies

Warm-water bag, cover or towel for bag, tape, measuring graduate or pitcher, bath thermometer, paper and pen and/or computer.

Procedure

1. Check physician's orders or obtain authorization from your immediate supervisor for the application.
2. Assemble equipment.
3. Wash hands.
4. Check for leaks by filling the warm-water bag with tap water or air. Expel the water or air if no leaks are present.
5. Fill the pitcher with water at a temperature of 110°F – 120°F, or 43°C – 49°C. Use the bath thermometer to check the temperature (Figure 23–34A).

Safety

CAUTION: The temperature should *not* exceed 120°F, or 49°C.

NOTE: Temperatures may vary. Follow agency policy.

NOTE: In most agencies, disposable heat packs are used. To activate the chemicals in the heat pack, squeeze the pack or strike it against a solid surface. It does not need to be filled with hot water. A cover must still be placed on the disposable heat pack because the plastic and heat can injure the skin.

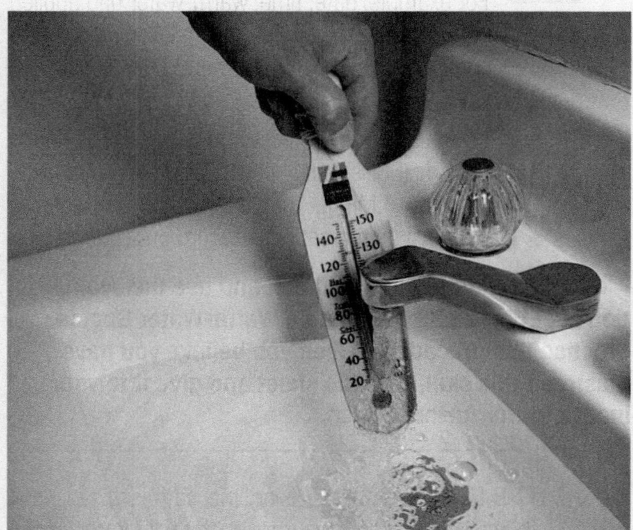

FIGURE 23–34A Use a bath thermometer to verify that the temperature of the water is 110°F – 120°F.

Safety

CAUTION: Chemical heat packs are *not* recommended for use on the face or head because of the danger of leaking chemicals.

6. Pour the measured hot water into the warm-water bag. Fill the bag one-third to one-half full (Figure 23–34B).
7. Expel remaining air by placing the warm-water bag on a flat surface, lifting and holding the neck portion of the bag upright, and pushing gently on the bag until the water reaches the neck (Figure 23–34C). Apply the screw cap or fold over the end.

   NOTE: If the bag has a fold end, note the letters *A*, *B*, and *C*. Fold *A* to *B*, *B* to *C*, and *C* to seal.

8. Wipe the outside of the bag dry. Check again for any signs of leaks.

Safety

CAUTION: Never use a warm-water bag or cap that leaks. The patient can be scalded.

9. Place a cover on the warm-water bag (Figure 23–34D). Use a standard cover, if available. If not, use a towel and tape the towel in place. The towel should be smooth and should completely cover the warm-water bag.

Safety

CAUTION: The warm-water bag *must* be covered to prevent injury to the skin.

10. Comm — Knock on the door and pause before entering. Introduce yourself. Identify the patient. Explain the procedure and obtain consent.

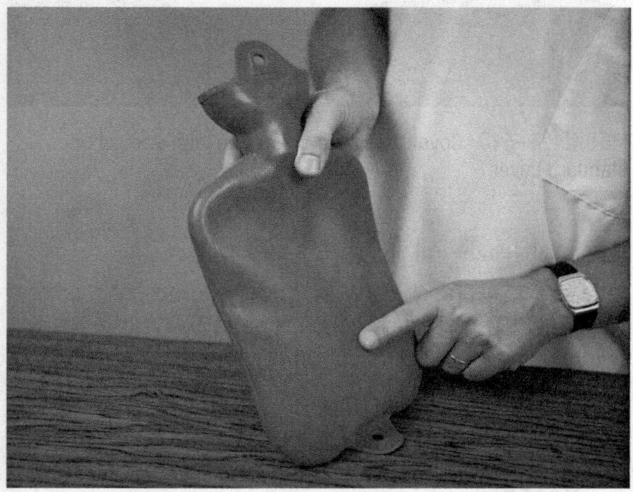

FIGURE 23–34B Fill the warm-water bag one-third to one-half full.

(continues)

PROCEDURE 23:3B (CONT.)

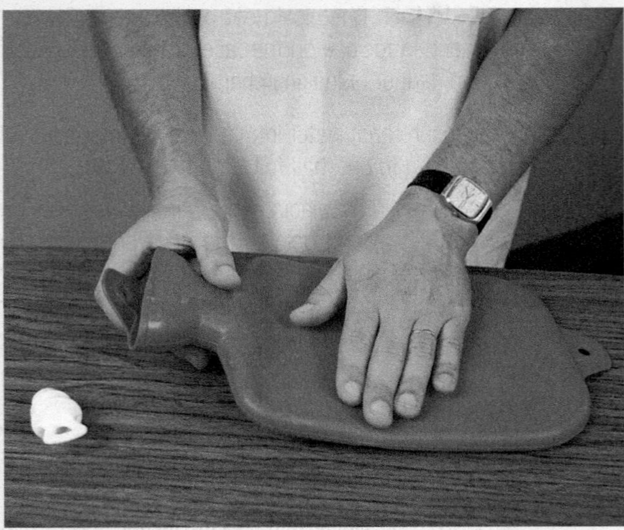

FIGURE 23–34C **Expel air from the warm-water bag by placing it on a flat surface and gently pressing it until the water reaches the neck of the bag.**

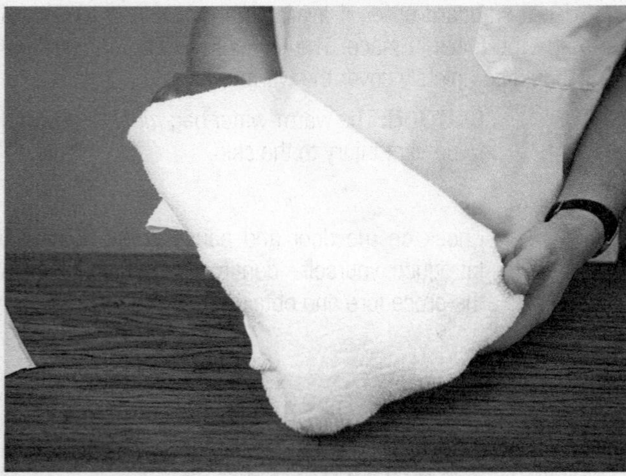

FIGURE 23–34D **Cover the warm-water bag with a towel or standard cover.**

11. Wash hands. Put on gloves if necessary.

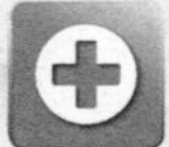

Precaution

CAUTION: Wear gloves and observe standard precautions if the area to be treated has any drainage of blood, body fluids, secretions, or excretions.

12. Apply the bag gently to the affected area as ordered. Make sure it is placed on top of the area. Never place heat under the body.

Safety

CAUTION: Do *not* allow any part of the patient's body to lie on top of the warm-water bag. The weight of the body part could intensify the heat.

13. Before leaving, check to be sure the patient is comfortable and the bag is properly positioned. Place the call signal within easy reach of the patient. Remove gloves, if worn, and wash hands before leaving the room.
14. Recheck the patient at least every 10 minutes. Refill the bag as needed to maintain warm temperature. Note any pain, extreme redness, or other conditions.

Safety

CAUTION: If signs of a burn are noted, remove the application immediately and report it to your immediate supervisor.

15. Remove the heat application when the time ordered has elapsed. Closely check the patient's skin.
16. Observe all checkpoints before leaving the patient: position the patient in correct body alignment, elevate the siderails (if indicated), lower the bed to its lowest level, place the call signal and supplies within easy reach of the patient, and leave the area neat and clean.
17. Discard a disposable heat pack. If the warm-water bag is not disposable, empty the warm-water bag and clean thoroughly. Wipe it with a disinfectant, rinse, and dry. Fill it with air before storing. This keeps the sides from sticking together. Replace all equipment.
18. Remove gloves, if worn. Wash hands.
19. Report and/or record all required information on the patient's chart or enter it into the computer. For example: date, time, warm-water bag applied to right knee for 20 minutes, patient stated pain relieved in knee, and your signature and title. Report any unusual observations immediately.

Comm

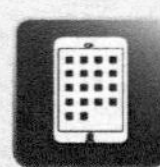

EHR

In health care agencies using electronic health records (EHRs), also known as electronic medical records (EMRs), the information is entered directly into the patient's record on a computer.

PRACTICE: **Go to the workbook and use the evaluation sheet for 23:3B, Applying a Warm-Water Bag, to practice this procedure. When you believe you have mastered this skill, sign the sheet and give it to your instructor for further action.**

Check

FINAL CHECKPOINT: Using the criteria listed on the evaluation sheet, your instructor will grade your performance.

PROCEDURE 23:3C

Applying an Aquathermia Pad

NOTE: Aquathermia or aquamatic pads can vary. Read the manufacturer's instructions before using.

Equipment and Supplies

Aquathermia unit and pad, cover, distilled water, paper and pen and/or computer

Procedure

1. Check physician's orders or obtain authorization from your immediate supervisor for the application.
2. Assemble equipment.
3.  Comm — Knock on the door and pause before entering. Introduce yourself. Identify the patient. Explain the procedure and obtain consent.
4. Wash hands. Put on gloves if necessary.

   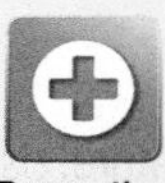 Precaution — **CAUTION:** Wear gloves and observe standard precautions if the area to be treated has any drainage of blood, body fluids, secretions, or excretions.

   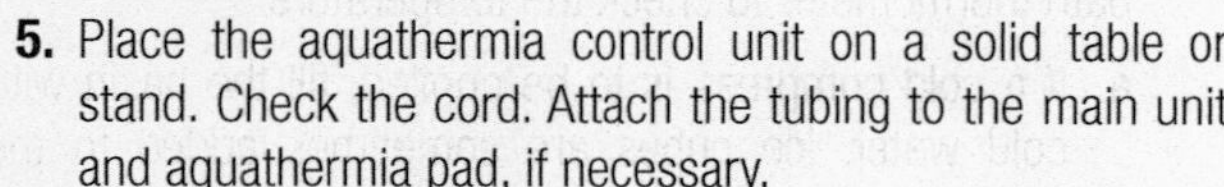
5. Place the aquathermia control unit on a solid table or stand. Check the cord. Attach the tubing to the main unit and aquathermia pad, if necessary.

   NOTE: Follow specific manufacturer's instructions. Some agencies use disposable pads. Tubing must be attached to these pads.
6. Unscrew the reservoir cap on the top of the unit. Use distilled water to fill the unit to the *fill* line.

   NOTE: Distilled water prevents formation of mineral deposits.
7. Screw the cap in place and then loosen it one-quarter turn. This allows for overflow of water and escape of steam.
8. Plug in the cord. Set the desired temperature by inserting the special key into the center of the dial or follow manufacturer's instructions. Temperature is usually set at 95°F – 105°F, or 35°C – 41°C. Turn the unit on.

   NOTE: Set the temperature according to physician's orders or agency policy.

    Safety — **CAUTION:** After setting the temperature, remove the key and store it in a safe area. Do not leave the key in position on the unit. Others could change or alter the temperature.
9. Check the pad for leaks. Also check that the unit is getting warm. Make sure the tubing is not bent or kinked. Recheck the level of water in the reservoir. A large amount of water is used when the pad is filled with water.

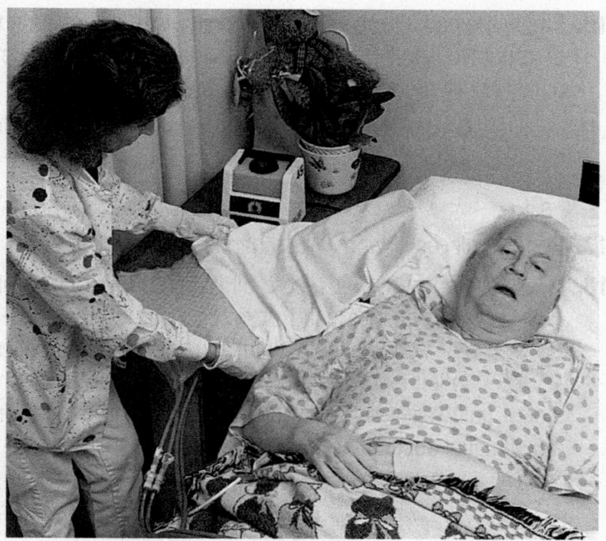

FIGURE 23–35 Cover the aquathermia pad before applying it to the patient.

10. Cover the pad (Figure 23–35). If a custom cover is not available, a pillowcase or towel can be used. Use tape to hold the cover in place.

     Safety — **CAUTION:** The pad must *never* be placed directly on the patient's skin. It can cause burns.
11. Place the pad on the correct area as ordered. Coil the tubing on the bed to facilitate the flow of water through the tubing. Do not allow the tubing to hang below the level of the bed. Check that the patient is comfortable. Place the call signal within easy reach of the patient. Remove gloves, if worn, and wash hands before leaving the room.
12. Recheck the patient at least every 10 minutes. Note the condition of the skin. If the skin is red or shows evidence of burns, or if the patient complains of pain, remove the pad and inform your immediate supervisor.
13. Refill the water unit with distilled water as necessary.
14.  Comm — When the ordered time has elapsed, remove the pad from the patient. Note the condition of the skin. Note the patient's comments to determine whether the application was effective.

    NOTE: The physician's orders may prescribe continuous application of the pad. If so, check the patient periodically.
15. Observe all checkpoints before leaving the patient: position the patient in correct body alignment, elevate the siderails (if indicated), lower the bed to its lowest level, place the call signal and supplies within easy reach of the patient, and leave the area neat and clean.

(continues)

PROCEDURE 23:3C (CONT.)

16. Empty the pad. Empty the control unit. Clean all equipment thoroughly. Disinfect the pad and unit according to agency policy or discard if disposable. Replace all equipment.

Safety

CAUTION: Do *not* put the electric control unit in water.

17. Remove gloves, if worn. Wash hands.

18. 
Comm

Report and/or record all required information on the patient's chart or enter it into the computer. For example: date, time, aquathermia pad applied to left elbow and forearm for 20 minutes, patient stated pain relieved, and your signature and title. Report any unusual observations immediately.

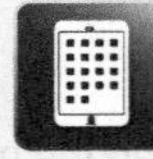
EHR

In health care agencies using electronic health records (EHRs), also known as electronic medical records (EMRs), the information is entered directly into the patient's record on a computer.

PRACTICE: **Go to the workbook and use the evaluation sheet for 23:3C, Applying an Aquathermia Pad, to practice this procedure. When you believe you have mastered this skill, sign the sheet and give it to your instructor for further action.**

Check

FINAL CHECKPOINT: Using the criteria listed on the evaluation sheet, your instructor will grade your performance.

PROCEDURE 23:3D

Applying a Moist Compress

Equipment and Supplies

Basin; bath thermometer; underpads or bed protectors; washcloth, towel, or gauze pads (for compress); bath towel; plastic sheet; paper and pen or and/or computer

Procedure

1. Check physician's orders or obtain authorization from your immediate supervisor for the application.
2. Assemble equipment.
3. 
Comm

Knock on the door and pause before entering. Introduce yourself. Identify the patient. Explain the procedure and obtain consent.

4. Wash hands. Put on gloves.

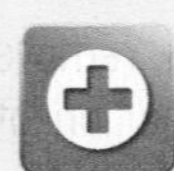
Precaution

CAUTION: Observe standard precautions if any contact with blood or body fluids is likely, such as when a compress is applied to a draining wound.

5. Close the door and/or pull the curtain closed for privacy. Elevate the bed to a comfortable working height. Fold the sheets back to expose the area to be treated.

   NOTE: A bath blanket can be used to drape the patient during the procedure.

6. Position an underpad or bed protector near the area to be treated. This will keep the patient's bedclothes and bed linens dry.
7. Fill the basin with water at the correct temperature. Use the bath thermometer to check the temperature.
   a. If a cold compress is to be applied, fill the basin with cold water. Ice cubes are sometimes added to the water. Do not add ice cubes unless you are told to do so.
   b. If a hot compress is to be applied, fill the basin with water at a temperature of 100°F – 105°F, or 37.8°C – 41°C.

   NOTE: Temperatures may vary. Follow physician's orders or agency policy.

8. Put the compress (washcloth, towel, or gauze pad) in the water. Wring out the compress to remove excess liquid (Figure 23–36A).
9. Apply the compress to the correct area (Figure 23–36B). Use a plastic sheet to cover the area. Then wrap a bath towel around the treated area.

   NOTE: The plastic sheet helps keep the compress moist and hot or cold.

   NOTE: An underpad or bed protector is sometimes used instead of a plastic sheet.

10. An ice bag or aquamatic pad is sometimes placed over the compress to help maintain the temperature. Follow agency policy or physician's orders.
11. Check the compress at frequent intervals. Change the compress and remoisten it as necessary. Check the condition of the skin under the compress. If the skin is discolored or the patient complains of pain, remove the compress immediately and inform your immediate supervisor.

PROCEDURE 23:3D (CONT.)

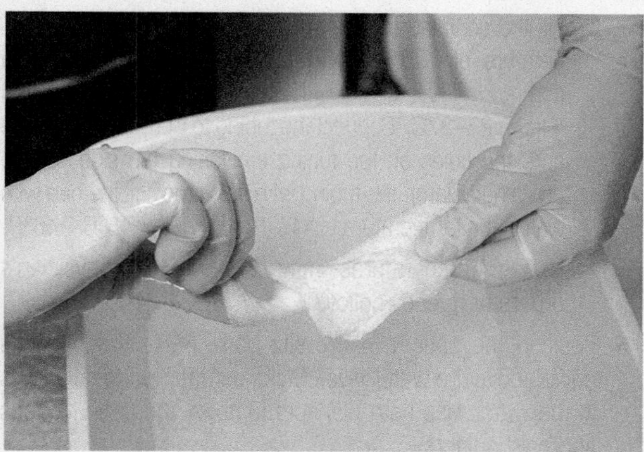

FIGURE 23–36A **After putting the compress in the water, wring it out to remove excess liquid.**

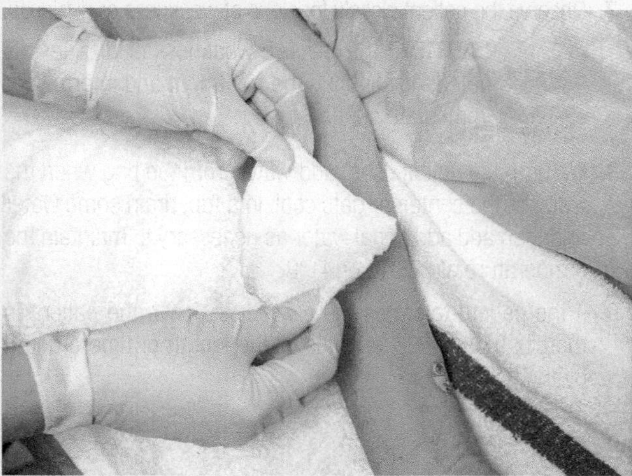

FIGURE 23–36B **Apply the compress to the correct area.**

12. Continue the treatment for the required period of time as ordered by the physician or per agency policy. Most compresses are left in place for 15–20 minutes.

13. When the ordered time has elapsed, remove the compress from the patient. Note the condition of the skin. Note the patient's comments to determine whether the application was effective.

14. Observe all checkpoints before leaving the patient: position the patient in correct body alignment, elevate the siderails (if indicated), lower the bed to its lowest level, place the call signal and supplies within easy reach of the patient, and leave the area neat and clean.

15. Clean and replace all equipment used. Discard gauze pads used as compresses. Place linen in a hamper or the laundry area.

16. Remove gloves. Wash hands.

17. 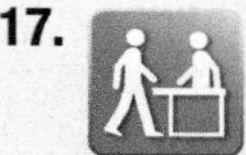
Comm
Report and/or record all required information on the patient's chart or enter it into the computer. For example: date, time, cold moist compresses applied to right knee for 20 minutes, no change in skin color noted, patient states knee still hurts, and your signature and title. Report any unusual observations immediately.

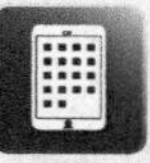
EHR
In health care agencies using electronic health records (EHRs), also known as electronic medical records (EMRs), the information is entered directly into the patient's record on a computer.

PRACTICE: **Go to the workbook and use the evaluation sheet for 23:3D, Applying a Moist Compress, to practice this procedure. When you believe you have mastered this skill, sign the sheet and give it to your instructor for further action.**

Check
FINAL CHECKPOINT: Using the criteria listed on the evaluation sheet, your instructor will grade your performance.

PROCEDURE 23:3E

Administering a Sitz Bath

Equipment and Supplies

Sitz-bath chair, disposable unit, or tub; one to two bath blankets; towels; gown; robe; slippers; bath thermometer; paper and pen and/or computer

Procedure

1. Check physician's orders or obtain authorization from your immediate supervisor for the treatment.
2. Assemble equipment.

(continues)

PROCEDURE 23:3E (CONT.)

3. Comm Knock on the door and pause before entering. Introduce yourself. Identify the patient. Explain the procedure and obtain consent. Ask the patient to put on a hospital gown. Assist as necessary.
4. Wash hands.
5. Prepare the sitz-bath unit:
   a. A *sitz chair* has an automatic temperature control, set the temperature at 105°F, or 41°C (Figure 23–37A). Fill the chair with water. Plug in the cord. Drape the bottom with a towel or bath blanket.
   b. Fill a *tub* or *sitz tub* to the correct level with water at a temperature of 105°F, or 41°C (Figure 23–37B). Place a towel or bath blanket in the bottom of the tub.

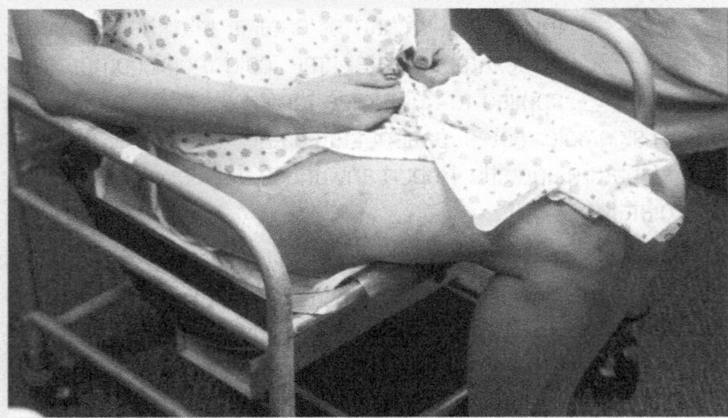

FIGURE 23–37A **The sitz chair has an automatic control to maintain the correct temperature while the patient is seated in the chair.**

   c. Fill the container on a *portable unit* with water at a temperature of 105°F, or 41°C. Place the container on a commode chair or toilet (lift the seat before positioning) (Figure 23–37C). Connect the tubing to the container. Make sure the holes on the tubing are facing the sides of the container. Clamp the tubing with its clamp. Fill the bag with water at a temperature of 110°F – 115°F, or 43°C – 46°C.

   NOTE: Temperatures may vary. Follow physician's orders or agency policy.
6. Position the patient in the sitz bath. Raise the patient's gown above the water level. Make sure the perineal area is in the water. Use bath blankets to cover the patient's legs and/or shoulders.

   NOTE: The gown can be removed if the patient is in a tub. Drape the patient with a bath blanket to prevent exposure.
7. Observe the patient closely for signs of weakness or dizziness.

   Safety
   CAUTION: If excessive weakness or dizziness is noted, discontinue the treatment and inform your immediate supervisor.
8. If a portable unit is used, add water from the bag when the water in the container gets cool. In a tub, drain some water and then add additional water as necessary to maintain the temperature at 105°F, or 41°C.
9. If the patient tolerates the procedure, leave the patient in the sitz bath for 20 minutes or the length of time ordered by the physician.

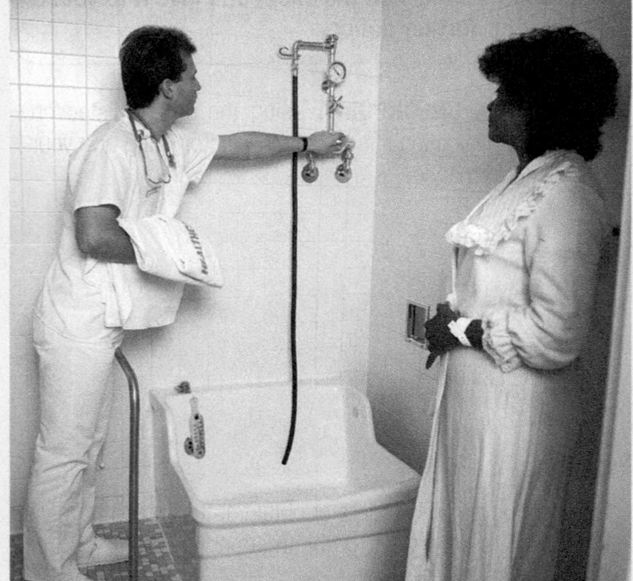

FIGURE 23–37B **Stationary sitz-bath tubs are available in many health care facilities.**

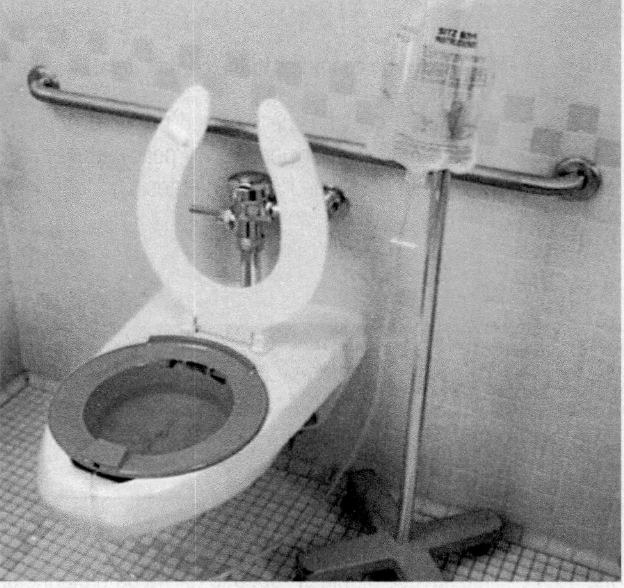

FIGURE 23–37C **A portable sitz-bath unit is positioned on the base of the toilet after the seat is elevated.**

PROCEDURE 23:3E (CONT.)

10. When the treatment is complete, assist the patient out of the chair, tub, or unit. Dry the patient with a towel. Put clean, dry clothing on the patient.
11. Assist the patient in returning to bed.
12. Observe all checkpoints before leaving the patient: position the patient in correct body alignment, elevate the siderails (if indicated), lower the bed to its lowest level, position the call signal and supplies within easy reach of the patient, and leave the area neat and clean.
13. Clean and replace all equipment used. Wear gloves to disinfect the tub, sitz tub, or sitz chair according to agency policy. Portable units are usually charged to the patient and kept in the patient's unit.
14. Remove gloves. Wash hands.
15. Comm Report and/or record all required information on the patient's chart or enter it into the computer. For example: date, time, sitz bath taken in sitz tub for 20 minutes, patient states she feels much better, and your signature and title. Report any unusual observations immediately.

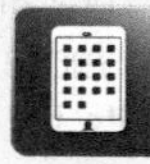

In health care agencies using electronic health records (EHRs), also known as electronic medical records (EMRs), the information is entered directly into the patient's record on a computer.

PRACTICE: Go to the workbook and use the evaluation sheet for 23:3E, Administering a Sitz Bath, to practice this procedure. When you believe you have mastered this skill, sign the sheet and give it to your instructor for further action.

FINAL CHECKPOINT: Using the criteria listed on the evaluation sheet, your instructor will grade your performance.

TODAY'S RESEARCH TOMORROW'S HEALTH CARE

Rewire the Brain to Treat Tinnitus?

According to the American Tinnitus Association, tinnitus—a condition that causes people to hear a constant ringing or buzzing sound in the ear—affects nearly 50 million people in the United States. Tinnitus can range from a dull buzzing in the ear, like static on a telephone, to a loud ringing that keeps people from thinking clearly and even from sleeping. Estimates are that approximately 2 million people are severely disabled by tinnitus. The most common cause is hearing loss, especially from long exposure to loud noises. Most of the available treatments are not very effective.

Researchers know that tinnitus is a problem in the brain, not just the ear. An initial theory is that after a hearing loss, the brain remaps itself so that nerve cells that responded to a specific frequency start to respond to other frequencies. However, the nerve cells do not respond correctly to the new frequencies, so odd sounds are created. Recently, scientists at the University of California at Berkeley conducted research that they believe shows the exact opposite. Their experiments with rats showed that the brain does not remap itself, and that the affected nerve cells do not receive any sensory input. In a person with normal hearing, the sensory input controls how the nerve cells send signals to communicate with each other. When the damaged nerve cells do not receive any input, the nerve cells send signals constantly, creating the sounds associated with tinnitus. This concept is similar to "phantom limb" pain, in which an amputee feels pain or itching in the body part that is no longer there. Phantom limb syndrome is also caused by nerve cells that are sending signals even though a body part is missing. The Berkeley team feels that if scientists can find a way to rewire the brain so the damaged cells receive sensory input, or if scientists could create a medication that turns off the nerve cell signals, tinnitus could be treated more effectively. Researchers at the University of Texas are examining areas of the hippocampus in the brain, a region not usually considered a part of the brain involved with hearing. In studies with rats exposed to loud noises for 30 minutes, they have found nerve cells in this region fire off signals that last for almost a day. They plan to test a substance called D-cycloserine to see if it decreases or eliminates the signals sent by these nerve cells. A research project at the University of Michigan plans to develop an implantable electrode that will be tested in a guinea pig to determine whether it can alter abnormal electrical signals causing tinnitus.

Many other researchers are currently conducting studies to determine which parts of the brain are causing tinnitus, how nerve cells communicate to create the sounds, and methods that can be used to stop the abnormal electrical nerve cell signals. If the research is successful, the ringing or buzzing sounds of tinnitus may finally be turned off.

CHAPTER 23 SUMMARY

Physical therapy techniques are utilized by a wide variety of health care workers. Physical therapy involves using physical means to treat the patient.

Range-of-motion (ROM) exercises are done to maintain the health of the muscles and skeletal system. They are frequently ordered for patients with limited ability to move. Each joint and muscle in the body is moved through its full ROM. By following the correct procedures and using proper body mechanics, the health care worker can help the patient maintain as much mobility as possible.

Proper techniques must also be used when ambulating patients using transfer (gait) belts, crutches, canes, or walkers. By understanding the different gaits, proper ways of fitting the devices to patients, and safety precautions, the health care worker can provide support and guidance for patients relying on these aids.

Heat and cold applications are administered for a wide variety of conditions. Careful observation of temperature and condition of the skin is essential to prevent injury to the patient. Again, correct techniques must be used at all times when these applications are administered.

Physical therapy is frequently an important part of the patient's treatment. By learning and understanding basic principles, the health care worker can help provide this part of the patient's care.

INTERNET SEARCHES

Use the search engines suggested in Chapter 12:9 in this text to search the Internet for additional information about the following topics:

1. **Organizations:** Research physical therapy careers, educational requirements, and duties at sites such as the American Athletic Trainer's Association, the American Physical Therapy Association, and the American Massage Therapy Association.
2. **Physical therapy:** Research range-of-motion exercises, massage therapy, ultrasound therapy, cryotherapy, thermotherapy, and physical therapy.
3. **Suppliers:** Find suppliers of physical therapy equipment to compare the different types of equipment available.

REVIEW QUESTIONS

1. What are the four (4) main types of range-of-motion (ROM) exercises? How is each type performed?
2. List eight (8) different types of joint movements and briefly describe each movement.
3. What are the basic rules that must be followed while measuring a patient for crutches?
4. You are ambulating a patient with a transfer belt. The patient starts to fall. What do you do?
5. Differentiate between a three-point and a two-point gait for canes.
6. What is the difference between moist heat and dry heat? Give two (2) examples for each type of application.
7. Define each of the following:
   a. vasodilation
   b. vasoconstriction
8. Identify five (5) safety measures or checkpoints that must be observed whenever a heat or cold application is applied to a patient.

For additional information on physical therapy careers, contact the following:

- American Physical Therapy Association
  1111 North Fairfax Street
  Alexandria, VA 22314
  Internet address: *www.apta.org*

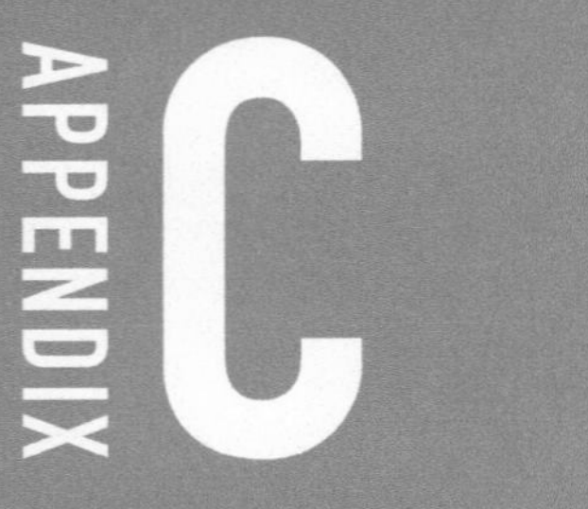

Metric Conversion Charts

The metric system, frequently called the International System of Units, or simply SI, is used in many health care fields. The following information and charts will assist you in converting measurements between the metric system and the U.S. customary system, commonly called the English or household system of measurement.

1. *Temperature measurements:*
   - To convert Fahrenheit (F) temperatures to Celsius (centigrade) (C) temperatures, subtract 32 from the Fahrenheit temperature and then multiply the result by 5/9, or 0.5556. Use one of the following formulas:

     $C = (F - 32) \times 5/9$ or $C = (F - 32) \times 0.5556$
   - To convert Celsius (C) temperatures to Fahrenheit (F) temperatures, multiply the Celsius temperature by 9/5, or 1.8, and then add 32 to the total. Use one of the following formulas:

     $F = (9/5 \times C) + 32$ or $F = (1.8 \times C) + 32$
   - The chart on the following page provides some major temperature equivalents.
2. *Linear measurements:*
   - To convert inches to centimeters, multiply the number of inches by 2.54 (1 inch = 2.54 centimeters).
   - To convert feet to centimeters, multiply the number of feet by 30.48 centimeters (1 foot = 30.48 centimeters).
   - To convert centimeters to inches, divide the number of centimeters by 2.54.
   - To convert centimeters to feet, divide the number of centimeters by 30.48.
   - The chart on the following page provides additional linear metric equivalents.
3. *Weight measurements:*
   - To convert pounds to kilograms, divide the number of pounds by 2.2 (1 kilogram = 2.2 pounds).
   - To convert kilograms to pounds, multiply the number of kilograms by 2.2.
4. *Liquid measurements:*
   - Note that 1 cubic centimeter (cc) is equal to 1 milliliter (mL).
   - To convert household measurements (for example, cups, ounces, quarts, or pints) to metric measurements, multiply the household measurement by the equivalent number of milliliters (mL). For example, 1 teaspoon equals 5 mL. Therefore, 3 teaspoons converted to metric would be 3×5, or 15 mL.
   - To convert metric measurements to household measurements, divide the metric measurement by the number of metric units in one of the household units. For example, there are 30 mL in 1 ounce. Therefore, 180 mL converted to ounces would be $180 \div 30$, or 6 ounces.
5. The chart on the following page provides additional liquid metric equivalents.

Fahrenheit–Celsius (Centigrade) Equivalents

F°	C°	F°	C°	F°	C°
32	0	102	38.9	116	46.7
70	21.1	103	39.4	117	47.2
75	23.9	104	40	118	47.8
80	26.7	105	40.6	119	48.3
85	29.4	106	41.1	120	48.9
90	32.2	107	41.7	125	51.7
95	35	108	42.2	130	54.4
96	35.6	109	42.8	135	57.2
97	36.1	110	43.3	140	60
98	36.7	111	43.9	150	65.6
98.6	37	112	44.4	212	100
99	37.2	113	45		
100	37.8	114	45.6		
101	38.3	115	46.1		

Linear English–Metric Equivalents

1 inch (in) = 0.0254 meters (m) = 2.54 centimeters (cm)
12 inches = 1 foot (ft) = 0.3048 meters (m) = 30.48 centimeters (cm)
3 feet = 1 yard (yd) = 0.914 meters (m) = 91.4 centimeters (cm)
5,280 feet = 1 mile = 1,609.344 meters (m)
39.372 inches = 3.281 feet = 1 meter (m)
1.094 yards = 1 meter (m)
0.621 miles = 1 kilometer (km)

Liquid English–Metric Equivalents

1 drop (gtt) = 0.0667 milliliter (mL)
15 drops (gtts) = 1.0 milliliter (mL)
1 teaspoon (tsp) = 5.0 milliliters (mL)
3 teaspoons = 1 tablespoon (tbsp) = 15.0 milliliters (mL)
1 ounce (oz) = 30.0 milliliters (mL)
8 ounces (oz) = 1 cup (cp) = 240.0 milliliters (mL)
2 cups (cp) = 1 pint (pt) = 500.0 milliliters (mL)
2 pints (pt) = 1 quart (qt) = 1,000.0 milliliters (mL)

Glossary

A

abbreviation—A shortened form of a word, usually just letters.

abdominal—Pertaining to the cavity or area in the front of the body and containing the stomach, the small intestine, part of the large intestine, the liver, the gallbladder, the pancreas, and the spleen.

abduction—Movement away from the midline.

abrasion—Injury caused by rubbing or scraping the skin.

absorption—Act or process of sucking up or in; taking in of nutrients.

abuse—Any care that results in physical harm or pain, or mental anguish.

accelerator—A chemical substance that increases the rate of a chemical reaction; a catalyst.

acceptance—The process of receiving or taking; approval; belief.

accreditation—Process where an educational program is recognized and/or approved for meeting and maintaining standards that qualify its graduates for professional practice.

acculturation—Process of learning the beliefs and behaviors of a dominant culture and assuming some of the characteristics.

acidosis—A pathological condition resulting from a disturbance in the acid-base balance in the blood and body tissues.

acquired immune deficiency syndrome (AIDS)—A disease caused by the human immunodeficiency virus (HIV) which attacks the immune system destroying the body's ability to fight infections.

activities of daily living (ADL)—Daily activities necessary to meet basic human needs, for example, feeding, dressing, and elimination.

acupuncture—Puncturing the skin at specific points with thin needles to relieve pain and/or treat disease.

acute—Lasting a short period of time but relatively severe (for example, an acute illness).

addiction—State of being controlled by a habit, as can happen with alcohol and drugs.

adduction—Movement toward the midline.

adenitis—Inflammation of a gland or lymph node.

adipose—Fatty tissue; fat.

adolescence—Period of development from 12 to 18 years of age; teenage years.

adrenal—One of two endocrine glands located one above each kidney.

advance directive—A legal document designed to indicate a person's wishes regarding care in case of a terminal illness or during the dying process.

aerobic—Requiring oxygen to live and grow.

afebrile—Without a fever.

affection—A warm or tender feeling toward another; fondness.

agar plate—Special laboratory dish containing agar, a gelatinous colloidal extract of a red alga, which is used to provide nourishment for growth of organisms.

agent—Someone who has the power or authority to act as the representative of another.

agglutination—Clumping together, as in the clumping together of red blood cells.

agnostic—Person who believes that the existence of God cannot be proved or disproved.

AIDS—*See* **acquired immune deficiency syndrome**.

air compressor—Machine that provides air under pressure; used in dental areas to provide air pressure to operate handpieces and air syringe.

airborne precautions—Methods of infection control that must be used for patients known or suspected to be infected with pathogens transmitted by airborne droplet nuclei.

albino—Absence of all color pigments.

alginate—Irreversible, hydrocolloid, dental impression material.

alignment—Positioning and supporting the body so that all body parts are in correct anatomical position.

alimentary canal—The digestive tract from the esophagus to the rectum.

alopecia—Baldness.
alternative therapy—Method of treatment used in place of biomedical therapies.
alveolar process—Bone tissue of the maxilla and mandible that contains alveoli (sockets) for the roots of the teeth.
alveoli—Microscopic air sacs in the lungs.
Alzheimer's disease—Progressive, irreversible disease involving memory loss, disorientation, deterioration of intellectual function, and speech and gait disturbances.
amalgam—Alloy (mixture) of various metals and mercury; restorative or filling material used primarily on posterior teeth.
ambulate—To walk.
amino acid—The basic component of proteins.
amputation—The cutting off or separation of a body part from the body.
anaerobic—Not requiring oxygen to live and grow; able to thrive in the absence of oxygen.
analgesia—The state of inability to feel pain yet still being conscious.
anaphylactic shock—An extreme, sometimes fatal, allergic reaction or sensitivity to a specific antigen such as a medication, insect sting, or specific food.
anatomy—The study of the structure of an organism.
anemia—Disease caused by lack of blood or an insufficient number of red blood cells.
anesthesia—The state of inability to feel sensation, especially the sensation of pain.
anesthetic carpules (cartridges)—Glass cylinders containing premeasured amounts of anesthetic solutions.
anger—Feeling of displeasure or hostility; mad.
angles—Measurements in degrees of the distance between a reference plane and a line drawn from a point on the plane.
anorexia—Loss of appetite.
anorexia nervosa—Psychological disorder involving loss of appetite and excessive weight loss not caused by a physical disease.
anoxia—Without oxygen; synonymous with suffocation.
antecubital—The space located on the inner part of the arm and near the elbow.
anterior—Before or in front of.
anterior teeth—Teeth located toward the front of the mouth; includes incisor and cuspids.
antibody—Substance, usually a protein, formed by the body to produce an immunity to an antigen or pathogen.
antibody screen—Test that checks for antibodies in the blood prior to a transfusion.
anticoagulant—Substance that prevents clotting of the blood.
antigen—Substance that causes the body to produce antibodies; may be introduced into the body or formed within the body.
antioxidants—Enzymes or organic molecules; help protect the body from harmful chemicals called *free radicals*.
antisepsis—Aseptic control that inhibits, retards growth of, or kills pathogenic organisms; not effective against spores and viruses.
anuria—Without urine; producing no urine.
anus—External opening of the anal canal, or rectum.
aorta—Largest artery in the body; carries blood away from the heart.
aortic valve—Flap or cusp located between the left ventricle of the heart and the aorta.
apathy—Indifference; lack of emotion.
apex—The pointed extremity of a conelike structure; the rounded, lower end of the heart, below the ventricles; the bottom tip of a tooth.
aphasia—Language impairment; loss of ability to comprehend or speak normally.
apical foramen—The opening in the apex of a tooth; allows nerves and blood vessels to enter tooth.
apical pulse—Pulse taken with a stethoscope and near the apex of the heart.
apnea—Absence of respirations; temporary cessation of respirations.
apoplexy—A stroke; *see* **cerebrovascular accident**.
apothecary system—A system used for weighing drugs and solutions, brought to the United States from England during the colonial period.
appendicular skeleton—The bones that form the limbs or extremities of the body.
application form—A form or record completed when applying for a job.
appointment—A schedule to do something on a particular day and time.
aquathermia pad—Temperature-controlled unit that circulates warm liquid through a pad to provide dry heat.
aqueous humor—Watery liquid that circulates in the anterior chamber of the eye.
aromatherapy—Use of natural scents and smells to promote health and well-being.
arrhythmia—Irregular or abnormal rhythm, usually referring to the heart rhythm.
arterial—Pertaining to an artery.
arteriole—Smallest branch of an artery; vessel that connects arteries to capillaries.
arteriosclerosis—Hardening and/or narrowing of the walls of arteries.
artery—Blood vessel that carries blood away from the heart.
arthritis—Inflammation of a joint.
asepsis—Being free from infection.
aspirate—To remove by suction.
aspirating syringe—Special dental anesthetic syringe designed to hold carpules or cartridges of medication.
aspiration—Process of inhaling food, fluid, or a foreign substance into the respiratory tract.
assault—Physical or verbal attack on another person; treatment or care given to a person without obtaining proper consent.
assistant—Level of occupational proficiency where an individual can work in an occupation after a period of education or on-the-job training.
associate's degree—Degree awarded by a vocational-technical school or community college after successful completion of a two-year course of study or its equivalent.

astigmatism—Defect or blurring of vision caused by irregularity of the cornea of the eye.
atheist—Person who does not believe in any deity.
atherosclerosis—Form of arteriosclerosis characterized by accumulation of fats or mineral deposits on the inner walls of the arteries.
athletic trainers—Individuals who prevent and treat athletic injuries and provide rehabilitative services to athletes.
atrium—Also called an *auricle*; an upper chamber of the heart.
atrophy—Wasting away of tissue; decrease in size.
audiologist—Individual specializing in diagnosis and treatment of hearing disorders.
audiometer—Instrument used to test hearing and determine hearing defects.
auditory acuity—Ability to perceive and comprehend sound waves; hearing.
aural temperature—Measurement of body temperature at the tympanic membrane in the ear.
auricle—Also called the *pinna*; external part of the ear.
auscultation—Process of listening for sounds in the body.
autoclave—Piece of equipment used to sterilize articles by way of steam under pressure and/or dry heat.
automated external defibrillator (AED)—Machine used to assess the heart rhythm and provide an electric shock to restore normal heart rhythm.
autonomic nervous system—That division of the nervous system concerned with reflex, or involuntary, activities of the body.
autopsy—Examination of the body after death to determine the cause of death.
avulsion—A wound that occurs when tissue is separated from the body.
axial skeleton—The bones of the skull, rib cage, and spinal column; the bones that form the trunk of the body.
axilla—Armpit; that area of the body under the arm.
Ayer blade—Wooden or plastic blade used to scrape cells from the cervix of the uterus; used for Pap tests.

B

bachelor's degree—Degree awarded by a college or university after a person has completed a four-year course of study or its equivalent.
backup—Copying or saving data in a secure location to prevent loss in the event of computer failure or a disaster.
bacteria—One-celled microorganisms, some of which are beneficial and some of which cause disease.
bandage—Material used to hold dressings in place, secure splints, and support and protect body parts.
bandage scissors—Special scissors with a blunt lower end used to remove dressings and bandages.
bargaining—Process of negotiating an agreement, sale, or exchange.
Bartholin's glands—Two small mucous glands near the vaginal opening.
basal metabolic rate (BMR)—The rate at which the body uses energy to maintain life when the subject is at complete rest.
base—Protective (dental) material placed over the pulpal area of a tooth to reduce irritation and thermal shock.
base of support—Standing with feet 8–10 inches apart to provide better balance.
battery—Unlawfully touching another person without that person's consent.
bed cradle—A device placed on a bed to keep the top bed linens from contacting the legs and feet.
benign—Not malignant or cancerous.
bias—A preference that inhibits impartial judgment.
bicuspids—Also called *premolars;* the teeth that pulverize or grind food and are located between cuspids and molars.
bifurcated—Having two roots (as in teeth).
bile—Liver secretion that is concentrated and stored in the gallbladder; aids in the emulsification of fats during digestion.
binders—Devices applied to hold dressings in place, provide support, apply pressure, or limit motion.
bioethics—Branch of medicine concerned with moral issues resulting from technological advances and medical research.
biohazardous—Contaminated with blood or body fluids and having the potential to transmit disease.
biological (medical) scientists—Individuals who study living organisms and assist in the development of vaccines, medicines, and treatments for diseases; evaluate the relationship between organisms and the environment; and administer the programs for testing food and drugs.
biological technicians—Individuals who work under the supervision of biological scientists to assist in the study of living organisms.
biomedical (clinical) engineers—Individuals who combine the knowledge of engineering with the knowledge of biology and biomechanical principles to assist in the operation of health care facilities.
biomedical equipment technicians (BETs)—Individuals who work with the many different machines used to diagnose, treat, and monitor patients.
biopsy—Excision of a small piece of tissue for microscopic examination.
biotechnological engineers (bioengineers)—Individuals who use engineering knowledge to develop solutions to complex medical problems.
biotechnology—The use of the genetic and biochemical processes of living systems and organisms to develop or modify useful products.
bioterrorism—The use of biological agents, such as pathogens, for terrorist purposes.
bite-wing—Also called a *cavity-detecting X-ray;* a dental radiograph that shows only the crowns of the teeth.
bladder—Membranous sac or storage area for a secretion (gallbladder); also, the vesicle that acts as the reservoir for urine.
bland diet—Diet containing only mild-flavored foods with soft textures.
block style—Letter format in which all parts of the letter start at the left margin.
blood—Fluid that circulates through the vessels in the body to carry substances to all body parts.
blood pressure—Measurement of the force exerted by the heart against the arterial walls when the heart contracts (beats) and relaxes.

blood smear—A drop of blood spread thinly on a slide for microscopic examination.
bloodborne—An infectious disease or pathogenic organism that is transmitted through blood.
body—Main content, or message part, of a letter.
body mass index (BMI)—A calculation that measures weight in relation to height and correlates this with body fat; used to determine if an individual is underweight, has ideal weight, or is overweight.
body mechanics—The way in which the body moves and maintains balance; proper body mechanics involves the most efficient use of all body parts.
bolus—Food that has been chewed and mixed with saliva.
bowel—The intestines.
Bowman's capsule—Part of the renal corpuscle in the kidney; picks up substances filtered from the blood by the glomerulus.
brachial—Pertaining to the brachial artery in the arm, which is used to measure blood pressure.
bradycardia—Slow heart rate, usually below 60 beats per minute.
bradypnea—Slow respiratory rate, usually below 10 respirations per minute.
brain—Soft mass of nerve tissue inside the cranium.
brand name—Company or product name given to a medication or product.
breast—Mammary, or milk, gland located on the upper part of the front surface of the body.
bronchi—Two main branches of the trachea; air tubes to and from the lungs.
bronchioles—Small branches of the bronchi; carry air in the lungs.
bronchitis—Acute or chronic inflammation of the bronchial tubes, or air tubes in the lungs.
buccal surface—Outside surface of the posterior teeth; surface facing the cheek; facial surface of bicuspids and molars.
budget—An itemized list of income and expected expenditures for a period of time.
buffer period—Period of time kept open on an appointment schedule to allow for emergencies, telephone calls, and other unplanned situations.
bulimarexia—Psychological condition in which a person eats excessively and then uses laxatives or vomits to get rid of the food.
bulimia—Psychological condition in which a person alternately eats excessively and then fasts or refuses to eat.
burn—Injury to body tissue caused by heat, caustics, radiation, and/or electricity.
burs—Small, rotating instruments of various types; used in dental handpieces to prepare cavities for filling with restorative materials.

C

calcaneus—Large tarsal bone that forms the heel.
calculus—Also called *tartar;* hard, calcium-like deposit that forms on the teeth; a stone that forms in various parts of the body from a variety of different substances.
calorie—Unit of measurement of the fuel value of food.
cancer—A group of diseases caused by abnormal cell division and/or growth.
cane—A rod used as an aid in walking.
capillary—Tiny blood vessel that connects arterioles and venules and allows for exchange of nutrients and gases between the blood and the body cells.
carbohydrate-controlled diet—Diet in which the number and types of carbohydrates are restricted or limited.
carbohydrates—Group of chemical substances including sugars, cellulose, and starches; nutrients that provide the greatest amount of energy in the average diet.
carcinogen—Any cancer-causing substance.
carcinoma—Malignant (cancerous) tumor of connective tissue.
cardiac—Pertaining to the heart.
cardiac arrest—Sudden and unexpected stoppage of heart action.
cardiopulmonary—Pertaining to the heart and lungs.
cardiopulmonary resuscitation (CPR)—Procedure of providing oxygen and chest compressions to a victim whose heart has stopped beating.
cardiovascular—Pertaining to the heart and blood vessels.
cardiovascular technologist—An individual who assists with cardiac catheterization and angioplasty procedures, monitors patients during open-heart surgery, and performs tests to check circulation in blood vessels.
caries—Tooth decay, an infectious disease that destroys tooth tissue.
carious lesion—An occurrence of tooth decay.
carpal—Bone of the wrist.
carpule—A glass cartridge that contains a premeasured amount of anesthetic solution; used for dental anesthesia.
catalyst—A chemical substance that increases the rate of a chemical reaction; an accelerator.
cataract—Condition of the eye where the lens becomes cloudy or opaque, leading to blindness.
catheter—A rubber, metal, or other type of tube that is passed into a body cavity and used for injecting or removing fluids.
caudal—Pertaining to any tail or tail-like structure.
cavitation—The cleaning process employed in an ultrasonic unit; bubbles explode to drive cleaning solution onto article being cleaned.
cavity—A hollow space, such as a body cavity (which contains organs) or a hole in a tooth.
cell—Mass of protoplasm; the basic unit of structure of all animals and plants.
cell membrane—Outer, protective, semipermeable covering of a cell.
cellulose—Fibrous form of carbohydrate.
Celsius—A scale of temperature on which water freezes at 0 degrees and boils at 100 degrees under standard conditions.
cement—Dental material used to seal inlays, crowns, bridges, and orthodontic appliances in place.
cementum—Hard, bonelike tissue that covers the outside of the root of a tooth.
centigrade—A scale of temperature on which water freezes at 0 degrees and boils at 100 degrees under standard conditions.

central nervous system (CNS)—The division of the nervous system consisting of the brain and spinal cord.
centrifuge—A machine that uses centrifugal (driving away from the center) force to separate heavier materials from lighter ones.
centrosome—That area of cell cytoplasm that contains two centrioles; important in reproduction of the cell.
cerebellum—The section of the brain that is dorsal to the pons and medulla oblongata; maintains balance and equilibrium.
cerebrospinal fluid—Watery, clear fluid that surrounds the brain and spinal cord.
cerebrovascular accident (CVA)—Also called a *stroke* or *apoplexy*; an interrupted supply of blood to the brain, caused by formation of a clot, blockage of an artery, or rupture of a blood vessel.
cerebrum—Largest section of brain; involved in sensory interpretation and voluntary muscle activity.
certification—The issuing of a statement or certificate by a professional organization to a person who has met the requirements of education and/or experience and who meets the standards set by the organization.
cervical—Pertaining to the neck portion of the spinal column or to the lower part of the uterus.
cervix—Anatomical part of a tooth where the crown joins with the root; entrance to or lower part of the uterus.
chain of infection—Factors that lead to the transmission or spread of disease.
character—The quality of respirations (for example, deep, shallow, or labored).
charge slip—A record on which charges or costs for services are listed.
check—A written order for payment of money through a bank.
chemical—The method of aseptic control in which substances or solutions are used to disinfect articles; does not always kill spores and viruses.
chemical abuse—Use of chemical substances without regard for accepted practice; dependence on alcohol or drugs.
chemotherapy—Treatment of a disease by way of chemical agents.
Cheyne-Stokes respirations—Periods of difficult breathing (dyspnea) followed by periods of no respirations (apnea).
chiropractic—System of treatment based on manipulation of the spinal column and other body structures.
cholelithiasis—Condition of stones in the gallbladder.
cholesterol—Fatlike substance synthesized in the liver and found in body cells and animal fats.
choroid—Middle or vascular layer of the eye, between the sclera and retina.
chromatin network—That structure in the nucleus of a cell that contains chromosomes with genes, which carry inherited characteristics.
chronic—Lasting a long period of time; reoccurring.
cilia—Hairlike projections.
circumduction—Moving in a circle at a joint, or moving one end of a body part in a circle while the other end remains stationary.
citizenship—Status of being a citizen (including associated duties, rights, and privileges).
civil law—Laws that focus on the legal relationships between people and the protection of a person's rights.
clavicle—Collarbone.
clean—Free from organisms causing disease.
clear-liquid diet—Diet containing only water-based liquids; nutritionally inadequate.
client—Person receiving service or care; a patient in health care.
clinic—Institution that provides care for outpatients; a group of specialists working in cooperation.
closed bed—Bed that is made following the discharge of a patient.
coccyx—The tailbone; lowest bones of the vertebral column.
cochlea—Snail-shaped section of the inner ear; contains the organ of Corti for hearing.
cognitive—Relating to intellectual activity such as solving problems, making judgments, and dealing with situations.
collection—To receive; a letter requesting payment on an account.
colon—The large intestine.
colostomy—An artificial opening into the colon; allows for the evacuation of feces.
communicable disease—Disease that is transmitted from one individual to another.
communication—Process of transmission; exchange of thoughts or information.
compensation—Something given or received as an equivalent for a loss, service, or debt; defense mechanism involving substitution of one goal for another goal to achieve success.
competent—Able, capable.
complementary therapy—Method of treatment used in conjunction with biomedical therapies.
complete bed bath—A bath in which all parts of a patient's body are bathed while the patient is confined to bed.
complimentary close—Courtesy closing of a letter (for example, *Sincerely*).
composite—The dental restorative or filling material used most frequently on anterior teeth.
compress—A folded wet or dry cloth applied firmly to a body part.
computer literacy—A basic understanding of how a computer works that allows an individual to feel comfortable using a computer.
computer-aided design (CAD)—Software that is used to create precision drawings, technical illustrations, or two- or three-dimensional models.
computer-assisted instruction (CAI)—Teaching method in which a computer and computer programs are used to control the learning process and deliver the instructional material to the learner.
computerized tomography (CT)—A scanning and detection system that uses a minicomputer and display screen to visualize an internal portion of the human body; formerly known as *CAT (computerized axial tomography)*.
concave—Curved inward; depressed.
concierge medicine—A type of personalized health care where an enhanced level of care is provided by a primary care physician for a monthly or annual fee.

confidential—Not to be shared or told; to be held in confidence, or kept to oneself.
congenital—Acquired during development of the infant in the uterus and present at birth.
conjunctiva—Mucous membrane that lines the eyelids and covers the anterior part of the sclera of the eye.
connective tissue—Body tissue that connects, supports, or binds body organs.
constipation—Difficulty in emptying the bowel; infrequent bowel movements.
constrict—To contract or narrow; to make smaller.
consultation—Process of seeking information or advice from another person.
Consumer Bill of Rights and Responsibilities—A list of patient's rights, implemented by the Department of Health and Human Services, that must be recognized and honored by health care providers.
contact precautions—Methods of infection control that must be used for patients known or suspected to be infected with epidemiological microorganisms that can be transmitted by either direct or indirect contact.
contagious—Easily spread; communicable.
contaminated—Containing infection or infectious organisms or germs.
contra angle—Attachment used on dental handpieces to cut and polish.
contract—To shorten, decrease in size, or draw together; an agreement between two or more persons.
contracture—Tightening or shortening of a muscle.
contusion—An injury that results in a hemorrhage (bleeding) beneath intact skin; a bruise.
conventional-speed handpiece—Low-speed handpiece in dental units; used to remove caries and for fine-finishing work.
convex—Curved outward; projected.
convulsion—Also called a *seizure*; a violent, involuntary contraction of muscles.
cornea—The transparent section of the sclera; allows light rays to enter the eye.
cortex—The outer layer of an organ or structure.
cost containment—Procedures used to control costs or expenses.
Cowper's glands—The pair of small mucous glands near the male urethra.
cranial—Pertaining to the skull or cranium.
cranium—Part of the skull; the eight bones of the head that enclose the brain.
criminal law—Law that focuses on behavior known as crime; deals with the wrongs against a person, property, or society.
criticism—Judgment regarding worth; censure, disapproval; evaluation.
cross-index/reference—A paper or card used in filing systems to prevent misplacement or loss of records.
cross-match—A blood test that checks the compatibility of the donor's blood and the recipient's blood before a transfusion.
crown—The anatomical portion of a tooth that is exposed in the oral cavity, above the gingiva, or gums.
crust—A scab; outer covering or coat.
crutches—Artificial supports that assist a patient in walking.
cryotherapy—Use of cold applications for treatment.
cultural assimilation—Absorption of a culturally distinct group into a dominant or prevailing culture.
cultural diversity—Differences among individuals based on cultural, ethnic, and racial factors.
culture—Values, beliefs, ideas, customs, and characteristics passed from one generation to the next.
culture specimen—A sample of microorganisms or tissue cells taken from an area of the body for examination.
cuspid—Also called a *canine* or *eyetooth*; the type of tooth located at angle of lips and used to tear food.
cuspidor—A bowl or cup that can be used to allow a patient to expectorate (spit out) particles and water during a dental procedure.
custom tray—Dental impression tray specially made to fit a particular patient's mouth.
cyanosis—Bluish color of the skin, nail beds, and/or lips due to an insufficient amount of oxygen in the blood.
cyst—A closed sac with a distinct membrane that develops abnormally in a body structure; usually filled with a semisolid liquid.
cystitis—Inflammation of the urinary bladder.
cystoscope—Instrument for examining the inside of the urinary bladder.
cytoplasm—The fluid inside a cell; contains water, proteins, lipids, carbohydrates, minerals, and salts.

D

dangling—Positioning the patient in a sitting position with his or her feet and legs over the side of the bed prior to ambulation.
database—An organized collection of information stored in a computer.
day sheet—A daily record listing all financial transactions and/or patients seen.
daydreaming—Defense mechanism of escape; dream-like musing while awake.
deciduous teeth—Also called *primary teeth*; the first set of 20 teeth.
decimals—One way of expressing parts of numbers or anything else that has been divided into parts, with the parts being expressed in units of 10.
decubitus ulcer—*See* **pressure (decubitus) ulcer.**
deduction—Something subtracted or taken out (for example, monies taken out of a paycheck for various purposes).
defamation—Slander or libel; a false statement that causes ridicule or damage to a reputation.
defecate—To evacuate fecal material from the bowel; to have a bowel movement.
defense mechanism—Physical or psychological reaction of an organism used in self-defense or to protect self-image.
defibrillate—Use of an electric shock to restore normal heart rhythm.

degenerative disease—A disease caused by the deterioration of the function or structure of body tissues and organs, either by normal aging or lifestyle choices.
degrees—A unit of measurement.
dehydration—Insufficient amounts of fluid in the tissues.
delirium—Acute, reversible mental confusion caused by illness, medical problems, and/or medications.
delusion—A false belief.
dementia—Loss of mental ability characterized by decrease in intellectual ability, loss of memory, impaired judgment, and disorientation.
denial—Declaring untrue; refusing to believe.
dental assistants (DAs)—Individuals who work under the supervision of dentists to prepare a patient for dental procedures and assist with the procedures.
dental chair—Special chair designed to position a patient comfortably while providing easy access to the patient's oral cavity.
dental hygienist (DH)—A licensed individual who works with a dentist to provide care and treatment for the teeth and gums.
dental laboratory technicians (DLTs)—Individuals who make and repair a variety of dental prostheses such as dentures, crowns, bridges, and orthodontic appliances.
dental light—Light used in dental units to illuminate the oral cavity.
dentin—Tissue that makes up the main bulk of a tooth.
dentists (DMDs or DDSs)—Doctors who specialize in diagnosis, prevention, and treatment of diseases of the teeth and gums.
dentition—The number, type, and arrangement of teeth in the mouth.
denture—An entire set of teeth; usually refers to artificial teeth designed to replace natural teeth.
dependable—Capable of being relied on; trustworthy.
deposit slip—A bank record listing all cash and checks that are to be placed in an account, either checking or savings.
depression—Psychological condition of sadness, melancholy, gloom, or despair.
dermis—The skin.
Designation of Health Care Surrogate—A legal document that permits an individual (principal) to appoint another person to make any decisions regarding health care if the principal becomes unable to make decisions.
development—Changes in the intellectual, mental, emotional, social, and functional skills that occur over time.
diabetes mellitus—Metabolic disease caused by an insufficient secretion or utilization of insulin and leading to an increased amount of glucose (sugar) in the blood and urine.
diabetic coma—An unconscious condition caused by an increased level of glucose (sugar) and ketones in the bloodstream of a person with diabetes mellitus.
diagnosis—Determination of the nature of a person's disease.
diagnostic related groups (DRGs)—Method of classifying diagnoses into specific payment or reimbursement categories.
dialysis—Removal of urine substances from the blood by way of passing solutes through a membrane.
dialysis technicians—Individuals who operate the kidney hemodialysis machines used to treat patients with limited or no kidney function.
diaphoresis—Profuse or excessive perspiration, or sweating.
diaphysis—The shaft, or middle section, of a long bone.
diarrhea—Frequent bowel movements with watery stool.
diastole—Period of relaxation of the heart.
diastolic pressure—Measurement of blood pressure taken when the heart is at rest; measurement of the constant pressure in arteries.
diathermy—Treatment with heat.
diencephalon—The section of the brain between the cerebrum and midbrain; contains the thalamus and hypothalamus.
dietetic technicians (DTs)—Individuals who work under the supervision of dietitians to plan menus, order foods, test recipes, assist with food preparation, and provide information on dietary instructions and proper nutrition.
dietitian (RD)—An individual who specializes in the science of diet and nutrition.
differential count—Blood test that determines the percentage of each kind of leukocyte (white blood cell).
digestion—Physical and chemical breakdown of food by the body in preparation for absorption.
digital—Pertaining to fingers or toes; examination with the fingers.
dilate—Enlarge or expand; to make bigger.
direct smear—A culture specimen placed on a slide for microscopic examination.
disability—A physical or mental handicap that interferes with normal function; incapacitated, incapable.
discretion—Ability to use good judgment and self-restraint in speech or behavior.
disease—Any condition that interferes with the normal function of the body.
disinfection—Aseptic-control method that destroys pathogens but does not usually kill spores and viruses.
dislocation—Displacement of a bone at a joint.
disorientation—Confusion with regard to the identity of time, place, or person.
displacement—Defense mechanism in which feelings about one person are transferred to someone else.
distal—Most distant or farthest from the trunk, center, or midline.
distal surface—Side surface of teeth that is toward the back of the mouth, or away from the midline of the mouth.
diuretics—Drugs that increase urinary output; "water pills."
doctorate/doctoral degree—Degree awarded by a college or university after completion of a prescribed course of study beyond a bachelor's or master's degree.
dorsal—Pertaining to the back; in back of.
dorsal recumbent position—The patient lies on the back with the knees flexed and separated; used for vaginal and pelvic examinations.
dorsiflexion—Bending backward or bending the foot toward the knee.
dressing—Covering placed over a wound or injured part.
droplet precautions—Methods of infection control that must be used for patients known or suspected to be

infected with pathogens transmitted by large particle droplets expelled during coughing, sneezing, talking, or laughing.
dry cold—Application that provides cold temperature but is dry against the skin.
dry heat—Application that provides warm temperature but is dry against the skin.
duodenum—First part of the small intestine; connects the pylorus of the stomach and the jejunum.
Durable Power of Attorney—A legal document that permits an individual (principal) to appoint another person to make any decisions regarding health care if the principal becomes unable to make decisions.
dyspepsia—Difficulty in digesting food; indigestion.
dysphagia—Difficulty in swallowing.
dyspnea—Difficult or labored breathing.
dysrhythmia—An abnormal rhythm in the electrical activity of the brain or heart.
dystrophy—Progressive weakening (atrophy) of a body part, such as a muscle.
dysuria—Difficult or painful urination.

E

early adulthood—Period of development from 19 to 40 years of age.
early childhood—Period of development from 1 to 6 years of age.
Ebola—A filovirus that causes hemorrhagic fever disease.
echocardiograph—A diagnostic test that uses ultra-high-frequency sound waves to evaluate the structure and function of the heart.
edema—Swelling; excess amount of fluid in the tissues.
ejaculation—Expulsion of seminal fluid from the male urethra.
ejaculatory duct—In the male, duct or tube from the seminal vesicle to the urethra.
electrocardiogram (ECG)—Graphic tracing of the electrical activity of the heart.
electroencephalogram (EEG)—Graphic recording of the brain waves or electrical activity in the brain.
electroneurodiagnostic (END) technologist—An individual who performs nerve conduction tests, measures responses to stimuli, measures brain responses, and operates monitoring devices to assist with diagnosing disorders and diseases of the brain and nervous system.
electronic health record (EHR)—Also called an *electronic medical record (EMR)*; a computerized version of all of a patient's medical information.
electronic mail—Also called *e-mail*; a form of communication that is sent, received, and forwarded online from one computer to another by means of an Internet connection.
embalmers—Individuals who prepare the body of a deceased person for interment or burial.
emblem—A symbol; identifying badge, design, or device.
embolus—A blood clot or mass of material circulating in the blood vessels.
embryo—Unborn infant during the first 3 months of development.
emergency medical technician (EMT)—An individual who provides emergency prehospital care to victims of accidents, injuries, or sudden illness.
emesis—Vomiting; expulsion of the contents of the stomach and/or intestine through the mouth and/or nose.
emotional—Pertaining to feelings or psychological states.
empathy—Identifying with another's feelings but being unable to change or solve the situation.
emphysema—A chronic respiratory condition that occurs when the walls of the alveoli deteriorate and lose their elasticity resulting in poor exchanges of gases in the lungs.
enamel—Hardest tissue in the body; covers the outside of the crown of a tooth.
endocardium—Serous membrane lining of the heart.
endocrine—Ductless gland that produces an internal secretion discharged into the blood or lymph.
endodontics—Branch of dentistry involving treatment of the pulp chamber and root canals of the teeth; root canal treatment.
endogenous—Infection or disease originating within the body.
endometrium—Mucous membrane lining of the inner surface of the uterus.
endoplasmic reticulum—Fine network of tubular structures in the cytoplasm of a cell; allows for the transport of materials in and out of the nucleus and aids in the synthesis and storage of protein.
endorsement—A written signature on the back of a check; required in order to receive payment.
endoscope—A lighted instrument used to examine the inside of the body.
endosteum—Membrane lining the medullary canal of a bone.
enema—An injection of fluid into the large intestine through the rectum.
enthusiasm—Intense interest or excitement.
entrepreneur—Individual who organizes, manages, and assumes the risk of a business.
enunciate—To speak clearly, using correct pronunciation.
enuresis—Bedwetting; loss of bladder control while sleeping.
enzyme—A chemical substance that causes or increases the rate of a chemical reaction.
epidemic—An infectious disease that affects a large number of people within a population, community, or region at the same time.
epidemiologists—Individuals who identify and tract diseases as they occur in a group of people.
epidemiology—The study of the history, cause, and spread of an infectious disease.
epidermis—The outer layer of the skin.
epididymis—Tightly coiled tube in the scrotal sac; connects the testes with the vas or ductus deferens.
epigastric—Pertaining to the area of the abdomen above the stomach.
epiglottis—Leaf-shaped structure that closes over the larynx during swallowing.
epilepsy—A chronic disease of the nervous system characterized by motor and sensory dysfunction, sometimes accompanied by convulsions and unconsciousness.
epiphysis—The end or head at the extremity of a long bone.

epistaxis—Nosebleed.
epithelial tissue—Tissue that forms the skin and parts of the secreting glands, and that lines the body cavities.
eponyms—Terms used in medicine that are named after people, places, or things.
ergonomics—An applied science used to promote the safety and well-being of a person by adapting the environment and using techniques to prevent injuries.
erythema—Redness of the skin.
erythrocyte—Red blood cell (RBC).
erythrocyte count—Blood test that counts the number of red blood cells (normally 4.5–6 million per cubic millimeter of blood).
erythrocyte sedimentation rate (ESR)—Blood test that determines the rate at which red blood cells settle out of the blood.
esophagus—Tube that extends from the pharynx to the stomach.
essential nutrients—Those elements in food required by the body for proper function.
esteem—Place a high value on; respect.
estimating—Calculating the approximate answer.
ethics—Principles of right or good conduct.
ethnicity—Classification of people based on national origin and/or culture.
ethnocentric—Belief in the superiority of one's own ethnic group.
etiology—The study of the cause of a disease.
eupnea—Normal breathing pattern.
eustachian tube—Tube that connects the middle ear and the pharynx, or throat.
eversion—Turning a body part outward.
exacerbation—Period of time during which the signs and symptoms of a chronic disease become more severe.
excretion—Process of eliminating waste products from the body.
exocrine—Gland with a duct that produces a secretion.
exogenous—Infection or disease originating outside of or external to the body.
expectorate—To spit; to expel mucus, phlegm, or sputum from the throat or respiratory passages.
expiration—The expulsion of air from the lungs; breathing out air.
expressed contracts—A contract or an agreement that is stated in distinct and clear language, either orally or in writing.
extended family—A family group that includes the nuclear family plus grandparents, aunts, uncles, and cousins.
extension—Increasing the angle between two parts; straightening a limb.
external auditory canal—Passageway or tube extending from the auricle of the ear to the tympanic membrane.
externship—Learning opportunities offered by educational institutions to give students short, practical experiences in their field of study.

F

facial surface—The tooth surface nearest the lips or cheek; includes the labial and buccal surfaces.
facsimile—Machine that utilizes telephone lines to send messages and/or documents from one location to another location; a fax.
fainting—Partial or complete loss of consciousness caused by a temporary reduction in the supply of blood to the brain.
Fahrenheit—A scale of temperature on which water freezes at 32° and boils at 212° under standard conditions.
Fallopian tubes—Oviducts; in the female, passageway for the ova (egg) from the ovary to uterus.
false imprisonment—Restraining an individual or restricting an individual's freedom.
fanfolding—Folding in accordion pleats; done with bed linens.
fascia—Fibrous membrane covering, supporting, and separating muscles.
fasting blood sugar (FBS)—Blood test that measures blood serum levels of glucose (sugar) after a person has had nothing by mouth for a period of time.
fat—Overweight.
fat-restricted diets—Diets with limited amounts of fats, or lipids.
fats—Also called *lipids*; nutrients that provide the most concentrated form of energy; highest-calorie energy nutrients.
fax—*See* **facsimile**.
febrile—Pertaining to a fever, or elevated body temperature.
feces—Also called *stool*; waste material discharged from the bowel.
Federation Dentaire International (FDI) System—Abbreviated means of identifying the teeth that uses a two-digit code to identify the quadrant and tooth.
feedback—A method used to determine if communication was successful which occurs when the receiver of a message responds to the message.
fee-for-service compensation—A health payment plan in which doctors or providers are paid for each service they render.
femur—Thigh bone of the leg; the longest and strongest bone in the body.
fertilization—Conception; impregnation of the ovum by the sperm.
fetus—Unborn infant from the end of the third month of pregnancy until birth.
fever—Elevated body temperature, usually above 101°F, or 38.3°C, rectally.
fibula—Outer and smaller bone of the lower leg.
fields—Specific data categories within a computer database, for example, the entry of an address in a patient information database.
file—A group of related records that have been combined together.
filing—Arranging in order.
fire extinguisher—A device that can be used to put out fires.
firewalls—Software programs or hardware devices designed to prevent unauthorized access to a computer system.
first aid—Immediate care given to a victim of an injury or illness to minimize the effects of the injury or illness.
first responder—The first person to arrive at the scene of an illness, injury, or accident.
fixed expenses—Those items in a budget that are set and usually do not change (for example, rent and car payments).
flatus—Air or gas in the intestines.

flexion—Decreasing the angle between two parts; bending a limb.
fomite—Any substance or object that adheres to and transmits infectious material.
fontanel—Area between the cranial bones where the bones have not fused together; "soft spots" in the skull of an infant.
Food and Drug Administration (FDA)—A federal agency responsible for regulating food and drug products sold to the public.
foramina—A passage or opening; a hole in a bone through which blood vessels or nerves pass.
forensic science technicians—Individuals who investigate crimes by collecting and analyzing physical evidence.
Fowler's position—The patient lies on the back with the head elevated at one of several different angles.
fractions—A way of expressing numbers that represent parts of a whole.
fracture—A break (usually, a break in a bone or tooth).
frontal (coronal) plane—Imaginary line that separates the body into a front section and a back section.
frostbite—Actual freezing of tissue fluid resulting in damage to the skin and underlying tissue.
full liquid diet—Diet consisting of liquids and foods that are liquid at body temperature.
funeral directors—Individuals who manage and operate a funeral home; also called *morticians or undertakers*.
fungi—Group of simple, plantlike animals that live on dead organic matter (for example, yeast and molds).

G

gait—Method or manner of walking.
gait belt—A belt placed around a patient's waist to assist with transfer and/or ambulation.
gallbladder—Small sac near the liver; concentrates and stores bile.
gastric—Pertaining to the stomach.
gastrostomy—Surgical opening through the abdominal wall into the stomach; used for inserting a feeding tube.
generic name—Chemical name of a drug; name not protected by a trademark.
genes—The structures on chromosomes that carry inherited characteristics.
genetic counselors—Individuals who provide information to patients and/or their families on genetic diseases or inherited conditions.
genital—Pertaining to the organs of reproduction.
genome—The total mass of genetic instruction humans inherit from their parents.
genomic (genetic) testing—The use of specific tests to check for the presence of inherited genes known to cause disease.
genomics—The study of all the genes in the human genome, or the complete set of DNA within a single cell of an organism.
geriatrics, gerontology—The study of the aged or old age and treatment of related diseases and conditions.
gingiva—The gums (tissues surrounding the teeth).
glaucoma—Eye disease characterized by increased intraocular pressure.
glomerulus—Microscopic cluster of capillaries in Bowman's capsule of the nephron in the kidney.
glucose—The most common type of sugar in the body.
glucose meter—Instrument used to measure blood-glucose (blood-sugar) level.
glucose tolerance test—A diagnostic test that evaluates how well a person metabolizes a calculated amount of glucose.
glycohemoglobin test—A blood test that measures the amount of glucose that attaches to hemoglobin on red blood cells to determine the average blood-sugar levels for the previous 2 to 3 months; commonly called HbA1C or A1C test.
glycosuria—Presence of sugar in the urine.
goal—Desired result or purpose toward which one is working.
Golgi apparatus—That structure in the cytoplasm of a cell that produces, stores, and packages secretions for discharge from the cell.
gonads—Sex glands, ovaries in the female and testes in the male.
goniometer—An instrument that measures the angle of a joint's range of motion (ROM).
Gram's stain—Technique of staining organisms to identify specific types of bacteria present.
graphic chart—Record used to record vital signs (for example, temperature, pulse, and respirations) and other information.
groin—Area between the abdomen and upper inner thigh.
gross income—Amount of pay earned before deductions are taken out.
growth—Measurable physical changes that occur throughout a person's life.
gynecology—The study of diseases of women, especially those affecting the reproductive organs.

H

halitosis—Bad breath.
hantavirus—A virus spread by contact with rodents (rats and mice) or their excretions.
hard copy—Computer term for a printed copy of information.
hard palate—Bony structure that forms the roof of the mouth.
hardware—Machine or physical components of a computer system (usually, the parts of the computer and the peripherals).
heading—That section of a letter containing the address of the person sending the letter and the date of writing.
health care administrators—Individuals who plan, direct, coordinate, and supervise the delivery of health care in a health care facility.
health information exchange (HIE)—A federally established system that allows all health care agencies to readily transfer patient electronic health records (EHRs) between agencies in a national network.
health information (medical records) technicians (HITs)—Individuals who organize and code medical records, gather statistical information, and monitor records to ensure confidentiality.

Health Insurance Portability and Accountability Act (HIPAA)—Set of federal regulations adopted to protect the confidentiality of patient information and the ability to retain health insurance coverage.
health maintenance organizations (HMOs)—A type of health insurance that provides a health care delivery system which administers health care directed toward preventive care.
heart attack—*See* **myocardial infarction.**
heat cramp—Muscle pain and spasm resulting from exposure to heat and inadequate fluid and salt intake.
heat exhaustion—Condition resulting from exposure to heat and excessive loss of fluid through sweating.
heat stroke—Medical emergency caused by prolonged exposure to heat, resulting in high body temperature and failure of sweat glands.
helminths—A parasitic worm (for example, a tapeworm or leech).
hematemesis—Vomiting of blood.
hematocrit—Blood test that measures the percentage of red blood cells per a given unit of blood.
hematology—The study of blood and blood diseases.
hematoma—A localized mass of blood.
hematopoiesis—Formation of blood cells.
hematuria—Blood in the urine.
hemiplegia—Paralysis on one side of the body.
hemodialysis—Mechanical method of circulating blood through semipermeable membranes to remove body wastes; procedure used for kidney failure.
hemoglobin—The iron-containing protein of the red blood cells; serves to carry oxygen from the lungs to the tissues.
hemolysis—Disintegration of red blood cells, causing cells to dissolve or go into solution.
hemoptysis—Spitting up blood; blood-stained sputum.
hemorrhage—Excessive loss of blood; bleeding.
hemorrhoids—Varicose veins of the anal canal or anus.
hemostat—Instrument used to compress (clamp) blood vessels to stop bleeding.
heparin—A substance formed in the liver to prevent the clotting of blood; an anticoagulant.
hepatitis—Inflammation of the liver.
high-fiber diet—Diet containing large amounts of fiber, or indigestible food.
high-protein diet—Diet containing large amounts of protein-rich foods.
high-speed handpiece—A piece of dental equipment that is held in the hand and used to do most of the cutting and preparation of the tooth during dental procedures.
high-velocity oral evacuator—Dental handpiece used to remove particles and large amounts of liquid from the oral cavity.
HIPAA—*See* **Health Insurance Portability and Accountability Act.**
histology—Study of tissue.
holistic health care—Care that promotes physical, emotional, social, intellectual, and spiritual well-being.
home health care—Any type of health care provided in a patient's home environment.
homeostasis—A constant state of natural balance within the body.
honesty—Truthfulness; integrity.
horizontal recumbent position—*See* **supine position.**
hormone—Chemical substance secreted by an organ or gland.
HOSA—A national organization for students enrolled in health science programs.
hospice—Program designed to provide care for the terminally ill while allowing them to die with dignity.
hospital—Institution that provides medical or surgical care and treatment for the sick or injured.
household system—A system of units developed so patients could measure out dosages at home using ordinary containers found in the kitchen.
humerus—Long bone of the upper arm.
hydrocollator packs—Gel-filled packs that are warmed in a water bath to provide a moist heat application.
hygiene—Principles for health preservation and disease prevention.
hyperglycemia—Presence of sugar in the blood; high blood sugar.
hyperopia—Farsightedness; defect in near vision.
hyperpnea—An increased respiratory rate.
hypertension—High blood pressure.
hyperthermia—Condition that occurs when body temperature exceeds 104°F, or 40°C, rectally.
hypoglycemia—Low blood sugar.
hypotension—Low blood pressure.
hypothalamus—That structure in the diencephalon of the brain that regulates and controls many body functions.
hypothermia—Condition in which body temperature is below normal, usually below 95°F (35°C) and often in the range of 78°F–95°F (26°C–35°C).
hypothermia blanket—Special blanket containing coils filled with a cooling solution; used to reduce high body temperature.
hypoxia—Without oxygen; a deficiency of oxygen.

I

ice bag/collar—Plastic or rubber device filled with ice to provide dry-cold application.
idiopathic—Without recognizable cause; condition that is self-originating.
ileostomy—A surgical opening connecting the ileum (small intestine) and the abdominal wall.
ileum—Final section of small intestine; connects the jejunum and large intestine.
image-guided surgery (IGS)—A surgical procedure in which a surgeon uses preoperative and intraoperative images to guide or direct the surgery.
immunity—Condition of being protected against a particular disease.
impaction—A large, hard mass of fecal material lodged in the intestine or rectum; a tooth that does not erupt into the mouth.
implied contracts—A contract or agreement that creates obligations without verbally expressed terms.

impression—Negative reproduction of a tooth or dental arch.
improper fractions—Fractions that have numerators that are larger than the denominators.
incisal surface—The cutting or biting surface of anterior teeth.
incision—Cut or wound of body tissue caused by a sharp object; a surgical cut.
incisors—Teeth located in the front and center of the mouth; used to cut food.
income—Total amount of money received in a given period (usually a year); salary is usually the main source.
incontinent—Unable to voluntarily control urination or defecation.
index—To put names in proper order for filing purposes.
infancy—Period of development from birth to 1 year of age.
infarction—Area of tissue that is necrotic (dead) after the cessation of a blood supply; death of tissue.
infection—Invasion by organisms; contamination by disease-producing organisms, or pathogens.
inferior—Below; under.
inflammation—Tissue reaction to injury characterized by heat, redness, swelling, and pain.
informed consent—Permission granted voluntarily by a person who is of sound mind and aware of all factors involved.
ingestion—Taking food, fluids, or medications into the body through the mouth.
inguinal—Pertaining to the region of the body where the thighs join the trunk; the groin.
inhalation—Breathing in.
inherited disease—A disease transmitted from parents to child genetically.
initiative—Ability to begin or follow through with a plan or task; determination.
inquiry—Search for information.
insertion—End or area of a muscle that moves when the muscle contracts.
inside address—That section of a letter that contains the name and address of the person or firm to whom the letter is being sent.
inspiration—Breathing in; taking air into the lungs.
insulin—A hormone secreted by the islets of Langerhans in the pancreas; essential for the metabolism of glucose.
insulin shock—Condition that occurs in individuals with diabetes when there is an excess amount of insulin and a low level of glucose (sugar) in the blood.
insurance form—A form used to apply for payment by an insurance company.
intake and output (I&O)—A record that notes all fluids taken in or eliminated by a person in a given period of time.
integrative (integrated) health care—A form of health care that uses both mainstream medical treatments and complementary and alternative therapies to treat a patient.
integumentary—Pertaining to the skin or a covering.
intercostal—Pertaining to the space between the ribs (costae).
Internet—Worldwide computer network.
internship—A system of on-the-job training that provides students with an opportunity to gain experience in their field of study.
interproximal space—The area between two adjoining teeth.
intestine—That portion of the alimentary canal from the stomach to the rectum and anus.
intradermal—Inserted or put into the skin.
intramuscular (IM)—Injected or put into a muscle.
intravenous (IV)—Injected or put into a vein.
intubate—To insert a tube.
invasion of privacy—Revealing personal information about an individual without his or her consent.
invasive—Pertains to a test or procedure that involves penetrating or entering the body.
inversion—Turning a body part inward.
involuntary—Independent action not controlled by choice or desire.
iris—Colored portion of the eye; composed of muscular, or contractile, tissue that regulates the size of the pupil.
ischemia—Inadequate blood flow to the body tissues caused by an obstruction in circulation.
isolation—Method or technique of caring for persons who have communicable diseases.

J

jackknife (proctologic) position—The patient lies on the abdomen with both the head and legs inclined downward and the rectal area elevated.
jaundice—Yellow discoloration of the skin and eyes, frequently caused by liver or gallbladder disease.
jejunum—The middle section of the small intestine; connects the duodenum and ileum.
job interview—A face-to-face meeting or conversation between an employer and an applicant for a job.
joint—An articulation, or area where two bones meet or join.

K

kcal-controlled diet—Diet containing low-calorie foods; frequently prescribed for weight loss.
ketone—Chemical compound produced during an increased metabolism of fat.
ketonuria—Presence of ketones in the urine.
kidney—Bean-shaped organ that excretes urine; located high and in back of the abdominal cavity.
knee-chest position—The patient rests his or her body weight on the knees and chest; used for sigmoidoscopic and rectal examinations.

L

labia majora—Two large folds of adipose tissue lying on each side of the vulva in the female; hairy outer lips.
labia minora—Two folds of membrane lying inside the labia majora; hairless inner lips.
labial surface—Crown surface of the anterior teeth that lies next to the lips; facial surface of the anterior teeth.
laboratory—A room or building where scientific tests, research, experiments, or learning takes place.
laceration—Wound or injury with jagged, irregular edges.
lacrimal—Pertaining to tears; glands that secrete and expel tears.
lactation—Process of secreting milk.

lacteal—Specialized lymphatic capillary that picks up digested fats or lipids in the small intestine and transports them to the thoracic duct.
lancet—Sharp, pointed instrument used to pierce the skin to obtain blood.
larynx—Voice box, located between the pharynx and trachea.
lasers—Light beams that can be focused precisely.
late adulthood—Period of development beginning at 65 years of age and ending at death.
late childhood—Period of development from 6 to 12 years of age.
lateral—Pertaining to the side.
lead—An angle or view of the heart that is recorded in an electrocardiogram.
leadership—Ability to lead, guide, and direct others.
ledger card—A card or record that shows a financial account of money charged, received, or paid out.
left lateral position—*See* **Sims' position.**
legal—Authorized or based on law.
legal disability—A condition in which a person does not have legal capacity and is therefore unable to enter into a legal agreement (for example, as is the case with a minor).
lens—Crystalline structure suspended behind the pupil of the eye; refracts or bends light rays onto the retina; also, the magnifying glass in a microscope.
lethargy—Abnormal drowsiness or sluggishness; state of indifference or stupor.
letterhead—Preprinted heading at the top of paper used for written correspondence.
leukocyte—White blood cell (WBC).
leukocyte count—Blood test that counts the total number of white blood cells (normally 4,500 to 11,000 cells per cubic millimeter of blood).
liability—A legal or financial responsibility.
libel—False written statement that causes a person ridicule or contempt or causes damage to the person's reputation.
licensed practical/vocational nurses (LPNs/LVNs)—Individuals who work under the supervision of physicians or registered nurses and provide patient care requiring basic technical knowledge.
licensure—Process by which a government agency authorizes individuals to work in a given occupation.
life stages—Stages of growth and development experienced by an individual from birth to death.
ligament—Fibrous tissue that connects bone to bone.
light diet—Also called a *convalescent diet*; diet that contains easy-to-digest foods.
line angle—Area on crown surfaces of a tooth formed by a line drawn between two surfaces.
liner—Dental material that covers or lines exposed tooth tissue, usually in the form of a varnish.
lingual surface—The crown surface of teeth that is next to the tongue.
lipids—Organic compounds commonly called fats and oils; provide the most concentrated form of energy for the body.
listen—To pay attention, make an effort to hear.
lithotomy position—The patient lies on the back with the feet in stirrups and knees flexed and separated.
liver—Largest gland in the body; located in the upper right quadrant of the abdomen; two of its main functions are excreting bile and storing glycogen.
living will—A legal document stating a person's desires on what measures should or should not be taken to prolong life when his or her condition is terminal.
low-cholesterol diet—Diet that restricts foods high in saturated fat.
low-protein diet—Diet that limits foods high in protein.
low-residue diet—Diet that limits foods containing large amounts of residue, or indigestibles.
low-speed handpiece—Slower handpiece in dental units; used to remove caries and for fine finishing work.
lung—Organ of respiration located in the thoracic cavity.
lymph—Fluid formed in body tissues and circulated in the lymphatic vessels.
lymph node—A round body of lymph tissue that filters lymph.
lymphatic duct—Short tube that drains purified lymph from the right sides of the head and neck and the right arm.
lymphatic vessels—Thin-walled vessels that carry lymph from tissues.
lysosomes—Those structures in the cytoplasm of a cell that contain digestive enzymes to digest and destroy old cells, bacteria, and foreign matter.

M

macule—A discolored but neither raised nor depressed spot or area on the skin.
magnetic resonance imaging (MRI)—Process that uses a computer and magnetic forces, instead of X-rays, to visualize internal organs.
mainframe computer—Largest type of computer; many users can access this computer at the same time.
malignant—Harmful or dangerous; likely to spread and cause destruction and death (for example, cancer).
malnutrition—Poor nutrition; without adequate food and nutrients.
malpractice—Providing improper or unprofessional treatment or care that results in injury to another person.
mammogram—Radiographic (X-ray) examination of the breasts.
managed care—A health care delivery system designed to reduce the cost of health care while providing access to care through designated providers.
mandible—Horseshoe-shaped bone that forms the lower jaw; only movable bone of the skull.
massage therapists—Individuals who use massage, bodywork, and therapeutic touch to provide pain relief, improve circulation, and relieve stress and tension.
master's degree—Degree awarded by a college or university after completion of one or more years of prescribed study beyond a bachelor's degree.
mastication—The process of chewing with the teeth.
matriarchal—Social organization in which the mother or oldest woman is the authority figure.
maxilla—Upper jawbone; two bones fused or joined together.
meatus—External opening of a tube (for example, the urinary meatus).

mechanical lifts—Special devices used to move or transfer a patient.
medial—Pertaining to the middle or midline.
Medicaid—Government program that provides medical care for people whose incomes are below a certain level.
medical assistants (MAs)—Individuals who work under the supervision of physicians and perform tasks to assist physicians with patient care.
medical history—A record that shows all diseases, illness, and surgeries that a patient has had.
medical record—Also called a *patient chart*; written record of a patient's diagnosis, care, treatment, test results, and prognosis.
Medicare—Government program that provides medical care for elderly and/or disabled individuals.
medication—Drug used to treat a disease or condition.
Medigap policy—An insurance plan that serves as supplemental insurance to Medicare; usually pays deductible for Medicare and co-payments of care.
medulla—Inner, or central, portion of an organ.
medulla oblongata—The lower part of the brainstem; controls vital processes such as respiration and heartbeat.
medullary canal—Inner, or central, portion of a long bone.
meiosis—The process of cell division that occurs in gametes, or sex cells (ovum and spermatozoa).
melanin—Brownish black pigment found in the skin, hair, and eyes.
memorandum—A short, written statement or message.
meninges—Membranes that cover the brain and spinal cord.
menopause—Permanent cessation of menstruation.
mental—Pertaining to the mind.
mesial surface—The side surface of teeth that is toward the midline of the mouth.
metabolism—The use of food nutrients by the body to produce energy.
metacarpal—Bone of the hand between the wrist and each finger.
metastasis—The spread of tumor or cancer cells from the site of origin.
metatarsal—Bone of the foot between the instep and each toe.
metric system—A decimal measuring system based on the meter, liter, and gram as units of length, capacity, and weight or mass.
microbiology—Branch of biology dealing with the study of microscopic organisms.
microcomputer—Desktop or personal computer found in the home or office.
microorganism—Small, living plant or animal not visible to the naked eye; a microbe.
microscope—Instrument used to magnify or enlarge objects for viewing.
micturate—Another word for *urinate*; to expel urine.
midbrain—That portion of the brain that connects the pons and cerebellum; relay center for impulses.
middle adulthood—Period of development from 40–65 years of age.
midsagittal—An imaginary line drawn down the midline of the body to divide the body into a right side and a left side.
midstream (clean-catch) specimen—Urine specimen in which urination is begun before catching the specimen in the specimen cup.
military time—A convention of time keeping in which the day runs from midnight to midnight and is divided into 24 hours.
minerals—Inorganic substances essential to life.
mitered corner—Special folding technique used to secure linen on a bed.
mitochondria—Those structures in a cell that provide energy and are involved in the metabolism of the cell.
mitosis—Process of asexual reproduction by which cells divide into two identical cells.
mitral valve—Flap or cusp between the left atrium and left ventricle in the heart.
model—Also called a *cast*; a positive reproduction of the dental arches or teeth in plaster or similar materials.
modified block—Letter-writing format in which all parts of the letter start at the left margin except the heading, complimentary close, signature, and title, which start at the center line.
moist cold—An application that provides cold temperature and is wet against the skin.
moist heat—An application that provides warm temperature and is wet against the skin.
molars—Teeth in the back of the mouth; largest and strongest teeth; used to grind food.
monotheists—Individuals who believe in the existence of one God.
Montgomery straps—Special adhesive strips that are applied when dressings must be changed frequently at a surgical site.
motivated—Stimulated into action; incentive to act.
mouth—Oral cavity; opening to the digestive tract, or alimentary canal.
mucus—Thick, sticky fluid secreted by mucous membranes.
muscle tissue—Body tissue composed of fibers that produce movement.
muscle tone—State of partial muscle contraction providing a state of readiness to act.
myocardial infarction—Heart attack; a reduction in the supply of blood to the heart resulting in damage to the muscle of the heart.
myocardium—Muscle layer of the heart.
myopia—Nearsightedness; defect in distant vision.
myth—A false belief; an established belief with no basis.

N

nanotechnology—The manipulation of atoms and molecules at the nanometer scale (a very small particle) to create new materials and devices.
nasal cavity—Space between the cranium and the roof of the mouth.
nasal septum—Bony and cartilaginous partition that separates the nasal cavity into two sections.
nasogastric tube—A tube that is inserted through the nose and goes down the esophagus and into the stomach.

National Institutes of Health (NIH)—A federal agency that is involved in research on disease.
nausea—A feeling of discomfort in the region of the stomach accompanied by the tendency to vomit.
necrosis—Death of tissue.
need—Lack of something required or desired; urgent want or desire.
needle holder—Instrument used to hold or support a needle while sutures (stitches) are being inserted.
negligence—Failure to give care that is normally expected, resulting in injury to another person.
neonate—Newborn infant.
neoplasm—New growth or tumor.
nephritis—Inflammation of the kidney.
nephron—Structural and functional unit of the kidney.
nerve—Group of nerve tissues that conducts impulses.
nerve tissue—Body tissue that conducts or transmits impulses throughout the body.
net income—Amount of pay received for hours worked after all deductions have been taken out; take-home pay.
network—Connection of two or more computers to share data and hardware.
neurology—The study of the nervous system.
neuron—Nerve cell.
nocturia—Excessive urination at night.
nomenclature—A method of naming.
noninvasive—Pertaining to a test or procedure that does not require penetration or entrance into the body.
nonpathogens—Microorganisms that are not capable of causing disease.
nonverbal—Without words or speech.
nonverbal communication—The use of facial expressions, body language, gestures, eye contact, and touch to convey messages or ideas; communication that is not spoken.
nose—The projection in the center of the face; the organ for smelling and breathing.
nosocomial—Pertaining to or originating in a health care facility such as a hospital.
nuclear family—A family group that usually consists of a mother, father, and children, but can consist of a single parent and children.
nucleolus—The spherical body in the nucleus of a cell that is important in reproduction of the cell.
nucleus—The structure in a cell that controls cell activities such as growth, metabolism, and reproduction.
nurse assistants—Individuals who work under the supervision of registered or licensed practical nurses to provide basic patient care.
nutrition—All body processes related to food; the body's use of food for growth, development, and health.
nutritional status—The state of one's nutrition.

O

obesity—Excessive body weight 20 percent or more above the recommended weight, or a BMI equal to or greater than 30.
objective observation—An observation about a patient that is visible, palpable, or measurable; commonly called a *sign*.
observation—To look at, watch, perceive, or notice.
obstetrics—The branch of medicine dealing with pregnancy and childbirth.
occlusal surface—The chewing or biting surface of posterior teeth.
occult—Hidden, concealed, not visible (for example, an internal [occult] hemorrhage).
occult blood—Blood that is hidden; also, a test done on stool to check for the presence of blood.
Occupational Safety and Health Administration (OSHA)—A federal agency that establishes and enforces standards that protect workers from job-related injuries and illnesses.
occupational therapy—Treatment directed at preparing a person requiring rehabilitation for a trade or for return to the activities of daily living.
occupied bed—A bed that is made while the patient is in bed.
odontology—Study of the anatomy, growth, and diseases of the teeth.
olfactory—Pertaining to the sense of smell.
oliguria—Decreased or less-than-normal amounts of urine secretion.
ombudsman—Specially trained individual who acts as an advocate for others to improve care or conditions.
Omnibus Budget Reconciliation Act (OBRA) of 1987—Federal law that regulates the education and testing of nursing assistants.
oncology—The branch of medicine dealing with tumors or abnormal growths (for example, cancer).
open bed—A bed with the top sheets fanfolded to the bottom.
operative care—Care that is provided before, during, and after a surgical procedure.
ophthalmologist—A medical doctor who specializes in diseases of the eye.
ophthalmology—The study of the eye and diseases and disorders affecting the eye.
ophthalmoscope—An instrument used to examine the eye.
opportunistic infection—An infection that occurs when the body's immune system cannot defend itself from pathogens normally found in the environment.
optician—An individual who makes or sells lenses, eyeglasses, and other optical supplies.
optometrist (OD)—A licensed, nonmedical practitioner who specializes in the diagnosis and treatment of vision defects.
oral—Pertaining to the mouth.
oral cavity—The mouth.
oral hygiene—Care of the mouth and teeth.
oral surgery—Surgery on the teeth, mouth, and/or jaw and facial bones; also called *maxillofacial surgery*.
oral-evacuation system—Special machine that uses water to form a suction or vacuum system to remove liquids and particles from the oral cavity.
organ—Body part made of tissues that have joined together to perform a special function.
organ of Corti—Structure in the cochlea of the ear; organ of hearing.
organelles—Structures in the cytoplasm of a cell, including the nucleus, mitochondria, ribosomes, lysosomes, and Golgi apparatus.

organizational structure—A line of authority or chain of command that indicates areas of responsibility and leads to the efficient operation of a facility.
origin—End or area of a muscle that remains stationary when the muscle contracts.
originator—The person who writes a check to issue payment.
orthodontics—The branch of dentistry dealing with prevention and correction of irregularities of the alignment of teeth.
orthopedics—The branch of medicine/surgery dealing with the treatment of diseases and deformities of the bones, muscles, and joints.
orthopnea—Severe dyspnea in which breathing is very difficult in any position other than sitting erect or standing.
orthotist—An individual skilled in straightening or correcting deformities by the use of orthopedic appliances (for example, braces or special splints).
os coxae—The hip bone; formed by the union of the ilium, ischium, and pubis.
ossicles—Small bones, especially the three bones of the middle ear that amplify and transmit sound waves.
osteopathy—A field of medicine and treatment based on manipulation, especially of the bones, to treat disease.
osteoporosis—Condition in which bones become porous and brittle because of lack or loss of calcium, phosphorus, and other minerals.
ostomy—A surgically created opening into a body part.
otoscope—An instrument used to examine the ear.
ovary—Endocrine gland or gonad that produces hormones and the female sex cell, or ovum.
overweight—A body weight that is 10–20 percent greater than the average recommended weight for a person's height, or a BMI from 25 to 29.9.

P

pain—An unpleasant sensation that is perceived in the nervous system when illness or injury occurs.
palate—Structure that separates the oral and nasal cavities; roof of the mouth.
palliative—Measures taken to treat symptoms and/or pain even though it will not cure a disease; comfort measures.
pallor—Paleness; lack of color.
palpation—The act of using the hands to feel body parts during an examination.
pancreas—Gland that is dorsal to the stomach; secretes insulin and digestive juices.
pandemic—An infectious disease that affects many people over a wide geographic area; a worldwide epidemic.
panoramic—Dental radiograph that shows the entire dental arch, or all of the teeth and related structures, on one film.
Papanicolaou test—Also called a *Pap test*; a test to classify abnormal cells obtained from the vagina or cervix.
papule—Solid, elevated spot or area on the skin.
paraffin wax treatment—Heated mixture of paraffin and mineral oil; used to provide a moist heat application.
paralysis—Loss or impairment of the ability to feel or move parts of the body.
paramedic (EMT-P)—An individual who can perform all of the basic emergency medical technician duties in addition to in-depth patient assessment and care; the highest level of an emergency medical technician.
paraplegia—Paralysis of the lower half of the body.
parasite—Organism that lives on or within another living organism.
parasympathetic—A division of the autonomic nervous system.
parathyroid—One of four small glands located on the thyroid gland; regulates calcium and phosphorus metabolism.
parenteral—Other than by mouth.
paresis—Weakness and/or paralysis of an extremity.
parliamentary procedure—A set of rules or guidelines that determine the conduct and order that is followed during a meeting.
partial bath—Bath in which only certain body parts are bathed or in which the health care provider bathes those parts of the body that the patient is unable to bathe.
patella—The kneecap.
pathogens—Disease-producing organisms.
pathology—The study of the cause or nature of a disease.
pathophysiology—Study of how disease occurs and the responses of living organisms to disease processes.
patience—Ability to wait, persevere; capacity for calm endurance.
Patient Protection and Affordable Care Act (PPACA)—A federal statute signed into law and designed to expand access to affordable health coverage in the United States.
Patient Self-Determination Act (PSDA)—A federal law that mandates that every individual has the right to make decisions regarding medical care, including the right to refuse treatment and the right-to-die.
patients' rights—Factors of care that all patients can expect to receive.
patriarchal—Social organization in which the father or oldest male is the authority figure.
patriotism—Love and devotion to one's country.
payee—Person receiving payment.
pediatrics—The branch of medicine dealing with care and treatment of diseases and disorders of children.
pedodontics—The branch of dentistry dealing with treatment of teeth and oral conditions of children.
pegboard system—Method of maintaining financial accounts and records in an office.
pelvic—Pertaining to the pelvis area below the abdominal region and near the sacrum and hip bones.
penis—External sex organ of the male.
percentages—Numbers used to express either a whole or part of a whole.
percussion—Process of tapping various body parts during an examination.
percussion (reflex) hammer—Instrument used to check reflexes.
perfusionists—Individuals who are members of the open-heart surgical team and operate the heart-lung machines used in coronary bypass surgery.
periapical—Around the apex of a root of a tooth; dental X-ray that shows the entire tooth and surrounding area.

pericardium—Membrane sac that covers the outside of the heart.

perineum—Region between the vagina and anus in the female and between the scrotum and anus in the male.

periodontal ligament—Dense fibers of connective tissue that attach to the cementum of a tooth and the alveolus to support or suspend the tooth in its socket.

periodontics—The branch of dentistry dealing with the treatment of the gingiva (gum) and periodontium (supporting tissues) surrounding the teeth.

periodontium—Structures that surround and support the teeth.

periosteum—Fibrous membrane that covers the bones except at joint areas.

peripheral—That part of the nervous system apart from the brain and spinal cord; also, a device connected to a computer.

peristalsis—Rhythmic, wavelike motion of involuntary muscles.

peritoneal—Pertaining to the body cavity containing the liver, stomach, intestines, urinary bladder, and internal reproductive organs.

permanent (succedaneous) teeth—The 32 teeth that make up the second, or permanent, set of teeth.

personal hygiene—Care of the body including bathing, hair and nail care, shaving, and oral hygiene.

personal protective equipment (PPE)—Protective barriers such as a mask, gown, gloves, and protective eyewear that help protect a person from contact with infectious material.

personal space—The distance people require to feel comfortable while interacting with others; also called *territorial* space.

perspiration—The secretion of sweat.

pH—A scale of 0–14 used to measure the degree of acidity or alkalinity of a substance, with 7 being neutral.

phalanges—Bones of the fingers and toes.

pharmacists (PharmDs)—Individuals who dispense medications per written orders from physicians, dentists, and other health care professionals authorized to prescribe medications.

pharmacogenomics—Using a person's genetic makeup, or genome, to choose the drugs and drug doses that are likely to work best for that individual.

pharmacology—The study of drugs.

pharmacy technicians—Individuals who work under the supervision of pharmacists to help prepare medication for dispensing and perform other duties as directed by pharmacists.

pharynx—The throat.

phlebitis—Inflammation of a vein.

phlebotomist—Also called a *venipuncture technician*; individual who collects blood and prepares it for tests.

physiatrist—Medical doctor specializing in rehabilitation.

physical—Of or pertaining to the body.

physical therapy—Treatment by physical means, such as heat, cold, water, massage, or electricity.

physicians—Doctors who examine patients, obtain medical histories, order tests, make diagnoses, perform surgery, treat diseases/disorders, and teach preventive health.

physician assistants (PAs)—Individuals who work under the supervision of physicians and take medical histories, perform routine physical examinations and basic diagnostic tests, make preliminary diagnoses, treat minor injuries, and prescribe and administer treatments.

Physicians' Desk Reference (PDR)—Reference book that contains essential information on medications.

physiological needs—Basic physical or biological needs required by every human being to sustain life.

physiology—The study of the processes or functions of living organisms.

pineal—Glandlike structure in the brain.

pinna—Also called the *auricle*; external portion of the ear.

pituitary—Small, rounded endocrine gland at the base of the brain; regulates function of other endocrine glands and body processes.

placenta—Temporary endocrine gland created during pregnancy to provide nourishment for the fetus; the afterbirth.

plane—Flat or relatively smooth surface; an imaginary line drawn through the body at various parts to separate the body into sections.

plantar flexion—Bending forward or bending the foot away from the knee.

plaque—Thin, tenacious, filmlike deposit that adheres (sticks) to the teeth and can lead to decay; made of protein and microorganisms.

plasma—Liquid portion of the blood.

plaster—A gypsum material used to form dental models.

platelet—*See* **thrombocyte**.

pleura—A serous membrane that covers the lungs and lines the thoracic cavity.

podiatrist—An individual who specializes in the diagnosis and treatment of diseases and disorders of the feet.

point angle—Area on the crown surface of a tooth that is formed when three surfaces meet.

poisoning—Condition that occurs when contact is made with any chemical substance that causes injury, illness, or death.

polycythemia—Excess number of red blood cells.

polydipsia—Excessive thirst.

polyphagia—Excessive ingestion of food.

polytheists—Individuals who worship and believe in many Gods.

polyuria—Increased production and discharge of urine; excessive urination.

pons—That portion of the brainstem that connects the medulla oblongata and cerebellum to the upper portions of the brain.

positron emission tomography (PET)—Computerized body scanning technique in which the computer detects a radioactive substance injected into a patient.

posterior—Toward the back; behind.

posterior teeth—Teeth toward the back of the oral cavity, including the bicuspids and molars.

postmortem care—Care given to the body immediately after death.

postoperative—After surgery.

postpartum—Following delivery of a baby.
Power of Attorney (POA)—A legal document authorizing a person to act as another person's legal representative or agent.
PPACA—*See* **Patient Protection and Affordable Care Act.**
preferred provider organization (PPO)—A type of managed care health insurance plan usually provided by large industries or companies to their employees.
prefix—An affix attached to the beginning of a word.
prejudice—Strong feeling or belief about a person or subject that is formed without reviewing facts or information.
prenatal—Before birth.
preoperative—Before surgery.
pressure (decubitus) ulcer—A pressure sore; a bedsore.
primary (deciduous) teeth—Also called *deciduous teeth*; the first set of 20 teeth.
privileged communications—All personal information given to health personnel by a patient; must be kept confidential.
process technicians—Individuals who operate and monitor the machinery that is used to produce biotechnology products.
proctoscope—Instrument used to examine the rectum.
professionalism—A blending of many different personal qualities such as good judgment, proper behavior, courtesy, good communication skills, honesty, politeness, responsibility, integrity, competence, and a proper appearance to meet the standards expected in a health care career.
prognosis—Prediction regarding the probable outcome of a disease.
projection—Defense mechanism in which an individual places the blame for his or her actions on someone else or circumstances.
pronation—Turning a body part downward; turning "palm down."
prone position—The patient lies on the abdomen, with the legs together and the face turned to the side.
prophylactic—Preventive; agent that prevents disease.
prophylaxis angle—Dental handpiece attachment that holds polishing cups, disks, and brushes used to clean the teeth or polish restorations.
proportion—A statement of equality between two ratios, or the relationship of one part to another part.
prostate gland—In the male, gland near the urethra; contracts during ejaculation to prevent urine from leaving the bladder.
prosthesis—An artificial part that replaces a natural part (for example, dentures or a limb).
prosthodontics—The branch of dentistry dealing with the construction of artificial appliances for the mouth.
protective isolation—*See* **reverse isolation.**
proteins—Basic components of all body cells; one of six essential nutrients needed for growth and repair of tissues.
proteomics—Scientific study of the structure and function of proteins.
protoplasm—Thick, viscous substance that is the physical basis of all living things.
protozoa—Microscopic, one-celled animals often found in decayed materials and contaminated water.
proximal—Closest to the point of attachment or area of reference.
pruritus—Itching.
psychiatrists—Physicians who specialize in diagnosing and treating mental illness.
psychiatry—The branch of medicine dealing with the diagnosis, treatment, and prevention of mental illness.
psychologists—Individuals who study human behavior and use this knowledge to help patients deal with the problems of everyday living.
psychology—The study of mental processes and their effects on behavior.
psychosomatic—Pertaining to the relationship between the mind or emotions and the body.
puberty—Period of growth and development during which secondary sexual characteristics begin to develop.
pulmonary—Pertaining to the lungs.
pulmonary valve—Flap or cusp between the right ventricle of the heart and the pulmonary artery.
pulp—Soft tissue in the innermost area of a tooth and made of nerves and blood vessels held in place by connective tissue.
pulse—Pressure of the blood felt against the wall of an artery as the heart contracts or beats.
pulse deficit—The difference between the rate of an apical pulse and the rate of a radial pulse.
pulse oximeter—A device that measures the oxygen level in arterial blood.
pulse pressure—The difference between systolic and diastolic blood pressure.
puncture wound—Injury caused by a pointed object such as a needle or nail.
pupil—Opening or hole in the center of the iris of the eye; allows light to enter the eye.
pustule—Small, elevated, pus- or lymph-filled area of the skin.
pyrexia—Fever.
pyuria—Pus in the urine.

Q

quadrant—One-fourth of a specific area.
quadriplegia—Paralysis below the neck; paralysis of arms and legs.

R

race—Classification of people based on physical or biological characteristics.
radial deviation—Moving toward the thumb side of the hand.
radiation therapy—The use of high-energy particles to decrease the size of tumors and treat cancer.
radiograph—X-ray; an image produced by radiation.
radiologic technologists (RTs)—Individuals who use X-rays, radiation, nuclear medicine, ultrasound, and magnetic resonance to diagnose and treat disease.
radiology—The branch of medicine dealing with X-rays and radioactive substances.
radiolucent—Transparent to X-rays; permitting the passage of X-rays or other forms of radiation.

radiopaque—Not transparent to X-rays; not permitting the passage of X-rays or other forms of radiation.
radius—Long bone of the forearm, between the wrist and elbow.
rale—Bubbling or noisy sound caused by fluid or mucus in the air passages.
range of motion (ROM)—The full range of movement of a muscle or joint; exercises designed to move each joint and muscle through its full range of movement.
rate—Number per minute, as with pulse and respiration counts.
rationalization—Defense mechanism involving the use of a reasonable or acceptable excuse as explanation for behavior.
ratios—Comparison used to show relationships between numbers or like values; for example, how many of one number or value is present as compared with the other.
reagent strip—Special test strip containing chemical substances that react to the presence of certain substances in the urine or blood.
reality orientation (RO)—Activities to help promote awareness of time, place, and person.
recall—To call back; letter or notice that reminds a patient to return for periodic treatment or examination.
receipt—Written record that money or goods has been received.
reciprocal—The multiplicative inverse of a number or fraction; a fraction that has been inverted or turned upside down so the denominator becomes the numerator.
record—A collection of related information in a database; a document that contains all of a patient's information.
rectal, rectum—Pertaining to or the lower part of the large intestine, the temporary storage area for indigestibles.
rectal tube—Tube inserted into the rectum to aid in the expulsion of flatus (gas).
red blood cell—*See* **erythrocyte.**
red marrow—Soft tissue in the epiphyses of long bones.
reference initials—Initials placed at the bottom of a letter to indicate the writer and/or preparer.
reference plane—A real or imaginary flat surface from which an angle is measured.
refractometer—An instrument used to measure the specific gravity of urine.
registered nurses (RNs)—Licensed individuals who work under the direction of physicians to provide total care to patients.
registration—Process whereby a regulatory body in a given health care area administers examinations and/or maintains a list of qualified personnel.
regression—A defense mechanism that involves retreating to a previous developmental level that provided more safety and security than the current level the individual is experiencing.
rehabilitation—The restoration to useful life through therapy and education.
religion—Spiritual beliefs and practices of an individual.
remission—Period of time during which the signs and symptoms of a chronic disease are less severe or not present.
repression—Defense mechanism involving the transfer of painful or unacceptable ideas, feelings, or thoughts into the subconscious.
resident—An individual who lives in a long-term care facility.
resistant—Able to oppose; organisms that remain unaffected by harmful substances in the environment.
respiration—The process of taking in oxygen (inspiration) and expelling carbon dioxide (expiration) by way of the lungs and air passages.
responsibility—Being held accountable for actions or behaviors; willing to meet obligations.
restoration—Process of replacing a diseased portion of a tooth or a lost tooth by artificial means, including filling materials, crowns, bridges, or dentures.
restraints—Protective devices that limit or restrict movement.
résumé—A summary of a person's work history and experience, submitted when applying for a job.
retina—The sensory membrane that lines the eye and is the immediate instrument of vision.
retractor—Instrument used to hold or draw back the lips or sides of a wound or incision.
reverse isolation—Technique used to provide care to patients requiring protection from organisms in the environment.
rheostat—Foot control in dental units; used to operate handpieces.
rhythm—Referring to regularity; regular or irregular.
ribs—Also called *costae*; 12 pairs of narrow, curved bones that surround the thoracic cavity.
rickettsiae—Parasitic microorganisms that live on other living organisms.
right to die—A legal right under the Patient Self-Determination Act that allows an individual to determine whether or not to accept medical care to continue life.
robotic surgery—Performing surgery with a mechanical device that is computer controlled.
Roman numerals—Symbols in the old Roman notation that represent numbers.
root—The anatomic portion of a tooth that is below the gingiva (gums); helps hold the tooth in the mouth.
rotation—Movement around a central axis; a turning.
rounding numbers—Changing numbers to the nearest ten, hundred, thousand, and so on.
rubber base—Dental impression material that is elastic and rubbery in nature.

S

Safety Data Sheet (SDS)—Information sheet that must be provided by the manufacturer for all hazardous products.
safety standards—Set of rules designed to protect both the patient and the health care worker.
saliva ejector—Handpiece in dental units that provides a constant, low-volume suction to remove saliva and fluids from the mouth.
salivary glands—Glands of the mouth that produce saliva, a digestive secretion.

salutation—A greeting; the greeting in a letter (for example, "Dear").
sarcoma—Tumor of connective tissue; frequently malignant.
satisfaction—Fulfillment or gratification of a desire or need.
scalpel—Instrument with a knife blade used to incise (cut) skin and tissue.
scapula—Shoulder blade or bone.
sclera—White outer coat of the eye.
scope of practice—The procedures, processes and actions that health care providers are legally permitted to perform in keeping with the terms of their professional license.
screen—To evaluate; to determine the purpose of telephone calls so they can be referred to the correct person.
scrotum—Double pouch containing the testes and epididymis in the male individual.
search engine—Computer program designed to locate specific information on the Internet.
sebaceous gland—Oil-secreting gland of the skin.
secretion—Substance produced and expelled by a gland or other body part.
seizure—A convulsion; involuntary contraction of muscles.
self-actualization—Achieving one's full potential.
self-esteem—Satisfaction with oneself.
self-motivation—Ability to begin or to follow through with a task without the assistance of others.
semicircular canals—Structures of the inner ear that are involved in maintaining balance and equilibrium.
seminal vesicle—One of two saclike structures behind the bladder and connected to the vas deferens in the male individual; secretes thick, viscous fluid for semen.
senile lentigines—Dark-yellow or brown spots that develop on the skin as aging occurs.
senility—Feebleness of body or mind caused by aging.
sensitive—Susceptible to a substance; organisms that are affected by an antibiotic in a culture and sensitivity study.
sensitivity—Ability to recognize and appreciate the personal characteristics of others.
sepsis—Presence of pus-forming pathogens and their toxins in the blood.
septum—Membranous wall that divides two cavities.
sequential compression device (SCD)—A device that continually inflates and deflates compression hose on the legs to stimulate circulation in the legs.
serrated—Notched; toothed.
sexuality—Sexual life and experience; people's feelings concerning their masculine/feminine natures, their ability to give and receive love and affection, and their roles in reproduction of the species.
sharps container—A puncture-resistant container for disposal of needles, syringes, and other sharp objects contaminated with blood or body fluids.
shock—Clinical condition characterized by various symptoms and resulting in an inadequate supply of blood and oxygen to body organs, especially the brain and heart.
sigmoidoscope—Instrument used to examine the sigmoid, or S-shaped, section of the large intestine.
sign—Objective evidence of disease; something that is seen.
signature—A person's name written by that person.
silicone—An impression material, usually polysiloxane or polyvinylsiloxane, used to take impressions of the teeth and or dental arches.
Sims' position—The patient lies on his or her left side with the right leg bent up near the abdomen.
sinus—Cavity or air space in a bone.
sitz bath—Special bath given to apply moist heat to the genital or rectal area.
skeleton—The bony structure of the body.
skill—Expertness, dexterity; an art, trade, or technique.
skin puncture—A small puncture made in the skin to obtain capillary blood.
slander—Spoken comment that causes a person ridicule or contempt or damages the person's reputation.
small intestine—That section of the intestine that is between the stomach and large intestine; site of most absorption of nutrients.
smear—Material spread thinly on a slide for microscopic examination.
Snellen charts—Special charts that use letters or symbols in calibrated heights to check visual acuity.
social—Pertaining to relationships with others.
social workers (SWs)—Individuals who assist patients who have difficulty coping with various problems by helping them make adjustments in their lives and/or referring them to community resources for assistance.
sodium hypochlorite—Household bleach.
sodium-restricted diets—Special diets containing low or limited amounts of sodium (salt).
soft diet—Special diet containing only foods that are soft in texture.
soft palate—Tissue at the back of the roof of the mouth; separates the mouth from the nasopharynx.
software—Programs or instructions that allow computer hardware to function intelligently.
specific gravity—Weight or mass of a substance compared with an equal amount of another substance that is used as a standard.
speculum—Instrument used to dilate, or enlarge, an opening or passage in the body for examination purposes.
sphygmomanometer—Instrument calibrated for measuring blood pressure in millimeters of mercury (mm Hg).
spinal—Pertaining to the vertebral column or spinal cord.
spinal cord—A column of nervous tissue extending from the medulla oblongata of the brain to the second lumbar vertebra in the vertebral column.
spirituality—Individualized and personal set of beliefs and practices that evolve and change throughout an individual's life.
spleen—Ductless gland below the diaphragm and in the upper-left quadrant of the abdomen; serves to form, store, and filter blood.
splinter forceps—Instruments with sharp points used to remove splinters and foreign objects from the skin and/or tissues.
sprain—Injury to a joint accompanied by stretching or tearing of the ligaments.
spreadsheet—A computer document created by special software that is used to access a computer's ability to perform high-speed math functions.

sputum—Substance coughed up from the bronchi; contains saliva and mucus.
standard precautions—Recommendations that must be followed to prevent transmission of pathogenic organisms by way of blood and body fluids.
statement-receipt—Financial form that shows charges, amounts paid, and balance due.
statistical data—Record containing basic facts about a patient, such as address, place of employment, insurance, and similar items.
stem cells—Cells that are capable of becoming any of the specialized cells in the body; two main types include embryonic stem cells from a developing fetus and somatic or adult stem cells.
stereotyping—Process of assuming that everyone in a particular group is the same.
sterile—Free of all organisms, including spores and viruses.
sterile field—An area that is set up for certain procedures and is free from all organisms.
sterilization—Process that results in total destruction of all microorganisms; also, surgical procedure that prevents conception of a child.
sternum—Breastbone.
stethoscope—Instrument used for listening to internal body sounds.
stoma—The opening of an ostomy on the abdominal wall.
stomach—Enlarged section of the alimentary canal, between the esophagus and the small intestine; serves as an organ of digestion.
stone—A gypsum material used to form dental models.
stool—Material evacuated from the bowels; feces.
strain—Injury caused by excessive stretching, overuse, or misuse of a muscle.
stress—Body's reaction to any stimulus that requires a person to adjust to a changing environment.
stress test—An electrocardiogram (ECG) that is obtained while the patient is exercising or after the patient has been given medication to create a heart response similar to active exercise.
stroke—*See* **cerebrovascular accident.**
subcutaneous—Beneath the skin.
subcutaneous fascia (hypodermis)—Layer of tissue that is under the skin and connects the skin to muscles and underlying tissues.
subjective observation—An observation about a patient that is felt by the patient but cannot be seen, palpated, or measured; commonly called a *symptom*.
sublingual—Under the tongue.
succedaneous teeth—The 32 teeth that make up the second set of teeth; also called *permanent* or *secondary teeth*.
sudoriferous gland—Sweat-secreting gland of the skin.
suffix—An affix attached to the end of a word.
suicide—Killing oneself.
superior—Above, on top of, or higher than.
supination—Turning a body part upward; turning "palm up."
supine position—The patient lies flat on the back, face upward.
suppository—Solid medication that has a base of cocoa butter or glycerin and is designed to melt after insertion into a body cavity (for example, the rectum or vagina).
suppression—Defense mechanism used by an individual who is aware of unacceptable feelings or thoughts but refuses to deal with them.
surgery—The branch of medicine dealing with operative procedures to correct deformities, repair injuries, or treat disease.
surgical (elastic) hose—Elastic or support hose used to support leg veins and increase circulation.
surgical scissors—Special scissors used to cut tissue.
surgical shave—Removal of hair and cleansing of skin prior to an operation.
suture—Surgical stitch used to join the edges of an incision or wound; also, an area where bones join or fuse together.
suture-removal set—Set of instruments, including suture scissors and thumb forceps, used to remove stitches (sutures).
sympathetic—That division of the autonomic nervous system that allows the body to respond to emergencies and stress; also, to understand and attempt to solve the problems of another.
symptom—A subjective indication of disease that is felt by the patient.
syncope—Fainting; temporary period of unconsciousness.
system—A group of organs and other parts that work together to perform a certain function.
systemic—Pertaining to the whole body.
systole—Period of work, or contraction, of the heart.
systolic pressure—Measurement of blood pressure taken when the heart is contracting and forcing blood into the arteries.

T

tachycardia—Fast, or rapid, heartbeat (usually more than 100 beats per minute in an adult).
tachypnea—Respiratory rate above 25 respirations per minute.
tactful—Able to do or say the correct thing; thoughtful.
tarsal—One of seven bones that forms the instep of the foot.
tartar—*See* **calculus.**
teamwork—Cooperative effort by the members of a group to achieve a common goal.
technician—A level of proficiency usually requiring a 2-year associate's degree or 3 to 4 years of on-the-job training.
technologist—A class of expertise in a health career field, usually requiring at least 3 to 4 years of college plus work experience.
teeth—Structures in the mouth that physically break down food by chewing and grinding.
telemedicine—The use of video, audio, and computer systems to provide medical and/or health care services.
telepharmacies—The use of video, audio, and computer systems to manage and dispense medications.
temperature—The measurement of the balance between heat lost and heat produced by the body.
temporal temperature—Measurement of body temperature at the temporal artery on the forehead.
temporary—Dental material used for restorative purposes for a short period of time until permanent restoration can be done.

tendon—Fibrous connective tissue that connects muscles to bones.
tension—Uncomfortable inner sensation, discomfort, strain, or stress that affects the mind.
terminal illness—An illness that will result in death.
testes—Gonads or endocrine glands that are located in the scrotum of the male and that produce sperm and male hormones.
thalamus—That structure in the diencephalon of the brain that acts as a relay center to direct sensory impulses to the cerebrum.
therapeutic diets—Diets used in the treatment of disease.
therapy—Remedial treatment of a disease or disorder.
thermal blankets—Special blankets which contain coils that can be filled with air or fluid to warm or cool a patient's body.
thermometer—Instrument used to measure temperature.
thermotherapy—Use of heat applications for treatment.
thoracic—Pertaining to the chest or thorax.
thoracic duct—Main lymph duct of the body; drains lymph from the lymphatic vessels into the left subclavian vein.
thrombocyte—Also called a *platelet*; blood cell required for clotting of the blood.
thrombus—A blood clot.
thymus—Organ in the upper part of the chest, lymphatic tissue and endocrine gland that atrophies at puberty.
thyroid—Endocrine gland that is located in the neck and regulates body metabolism.
tibia—Inner and larger bone of the lower leg, between the knee and ankle.
time management—System of practical skills that allows an individual to use time in the most effective and productive way.
tissue—A group of similar cells that join together to perform a particular function.
tissue forceps—An instrument with one or more fine points (teeth) at the tips of blades; used to grasp tissue.
tongue—Muscular organ of the mouth; aids in speech, swallowing, and taste.
tongue blade/depressor—A wood or plastic stick used to depress the tongue so the throat can be examined.
tonsil—Mass of lymphatic tissue found in the pharynx (throat) and mouth.
tort—A wrongful or illegal act of civil law not involving a contract.
tourniquet—Device used to compress the blood vessels.
towel clamps—Instruments with pointed ends that lock together; used to attach surgical drapes to each other and/or clamp dissected tissue.
trachea—Windpipe; air tube from the larynx to the bronchi.
tracheostomy—Creation of an opening into the trachea to facilitate breathing.
transcultural health care—Health care based on the cultural beliefs, emotional needs, spiritual feelings, and physical needs of a person.
transdermal—Through the skin.
transfer (gait) belt—Band of fabric or leather that is placed around a patient's waist; grasped by the health care worker during transfer or ambulation to provide additional support for the patient.
transfusion—Transfer of blood from one person to another person; injection of blood or plasma.
transient ischemic attacks—A brief episode that disrupts the blood flow to the brain and causes the same symptoms as a cerebrovascular accident or stroke; frequently called a *ministroke*.
transmission-based precautions—Methods or techniques of caring for patients who have communicable diseases.
transverse plane—Imaginary line drawn through the body to separate the body into a top half and a bottom half.
Trendelenburg position—The patient lies on the back with the head lower than the feet, or with both the head and feet inclined downward.
triage—A method of prioritizing treatment.
TRICARE—The U.S. government health insurance plan for all military personnel.
tricuspid valve—Flap or cusp between the right atrium and right ventricle in the heart.
tri-flow (air-water) syringe—Handpiece in dental units that provides air, water, or a combination of air and water for various dental procedures.
trifurcated—Having three roots (as do some teeth).
tuning fork—An instrument that has two prongs and is used to test hearing acuity.
24-hour urine specimen—Special urine test in which all urine produced in a 24-hour period is collected in a special container.
tympanic membrane—The eardrum.
typing and crossmatch—A determination of blood types and antigens prior to a blood transfusion.

U

ulcer—An open lesion on the skin or mucous membrane.
ulna—Long bone in the forearm, between the wrist and elbow.
ulnar deviation—Moving toward the little finger side of the hand.
ultrasonic units—Pieces of equipment that clean using sound waves.
ultrasonography—Noninvasive, computerized scanning technique that uses high-frequency sound waves to create pictures of body parts.
ultra-speed handpiece—High-speed handpiece used in dental units to cut and prepare a tooth during a dental procedure.
umbilicus—Navel; in slang, "belly button."
underweight—A body weight that is 10–15 percent less than the desired weight, or a BMI less than 18.5.
uninterrupted power supply (UPS)—A device that provides battery backup when the electrical power fails or drops to an unacceptable voltage level.
Universal/National Numbering System—Abbreviated means of identifying the teeth.
uremia—Excessive amounts of urea (a waste product) in the blood.
ureter—Tube that carries urine from the kidney to the urinary bladder.
ureterostomy—Formation of an opening on the abdominal wall for drainage of urine from a ureter.

urethra—Tube that carries urine from the urinary bladder to outside the body.
urinalysis—Examination of urine by way of physical, chemical, or microscopic testing.
urinary-drainage unit—Special device used to collect urine and consisting of tubing and a collection container usually connected to a urinary catheter.
urinary meatus—External opening of the urethra.
urinary sediments—Solid materials suspended in urine.
urinate—To expel urine from the bladder.
urine—The fluid excreted by the kidney.
urinometer—Calibrated device used to measure the specific gravity of urine.
urology—The branch of medicine dealing with urine and diseases of the urinary tract.
urticaria—Hives.
uterus—Muscular, hollow organ that serves as the organ of menstruation and the area for development of the fetus in the female body.

V

vaccine—Substance given to an individual to produce immunity to a disease.
vagina—Tube from the uterus to outside the body in a female individual.
value-based compensation—A health payment plan in which doctors and providers are paid a certain amount for each diagnosis or disease regardless of the number of services provided.
variable expense—In a budget, an expense that can change or be adjusted (for example, expenses for clothing and entertainment).
varicose—Pertaining to distended, swollen veins.
vas deferens—Also called the *ductus deferens*; the tube that carries sperm and semen from the epididymis to the ejaculatory duct in the male body.
vascular—Pertaining to blood vessels.
vasoconstriction—Constriction (decrease in diameter) of the blood vessels.
vasodilation—Dilation (increase in diameter) of the blood vessels.
vector—A carrier of disease; an insect, rodent, or small animal that transmits disease.
vein—Blood vessel that carries blood back to the heart.
venipuncture—Surgical puncture of a vein; inserting a needle into a vein.
venous—Pertaining to the veins.
ventilation—Process of breathing.
ventral—Pertaining to the front, or anterior, part of the body; in front of.
ventricle—One of two lower chambers of the heart; also, a cavity in the brain.
venule—The smallest type of vein; connects capillaries and veins.
vertebrae—Bones of the spinal column.
vertigo—Sensation of dizziness.
vesicle—Blister; a sac full of water or tissue fluid.
vestibule—Small space or cavity at the beginning of a canal.
veterinary—Pertaining to the medical treatment of animals.
villi—Tiny projections from a surface; in the small intestine, projections that aid in the absorption of nutrients.
virus—One of a large group of very small microorganisms, many of which cause disease.
viruses—Programs that contain instructions to alter the operation of computer programs, erase or scramble data on the computer, and/or allow access to information on the computer.
visceral—Pertaining to organs.
visual acuity—Ability to perceive and comprehend light rays; seeing.
vital signs—Determinations that provide information about body conditions; include temperature, pulse, respirations, and blood pressure.
vitamins—Organic substances necessary for body processes and life.
vitreous humor—Jelly-like mass that fills the cavity of the eyeball, behind the lens.
void—To empty the bladder; urinate.
volume—The degree of strength of a pulse (for example, strong or weak).
voluntary—Under one's control; done by one's choice or desire.
vomit—To expel material from the stomach and/or intestine through the mouth and/or nose.
vulva—External female genitalia; includes the labia majora, labia minora, and clitoris.

W

walker—A device that has a metal framework and aids in walking.
warm-water bag—Rubber or plastic device designed to hold warm water for dry-heat application.
wellness—State of being in good health; well.
wheezing—Difficult breathing with a high-pitched whistling or sighing sound during expiration.
white blood cell—*See* **leukocyte**.
whole numbers—Numbers that are traditionally used to count (1, 2, 3, …); they do not contain fractions.
withdrawal—Defense mechanism in which an individual either ceases to communicate or physically removes self from a situation.
word root—Main word or part of word to which prefixes and suffixes can be added.
Workers' compensation—Payment and care provided to an individual who is injured on the job.
World Health Organization (WHO)—An international agency sponsored by the United Nations and concerned with compiling statistics and information on disease and addressing serious health problems throughout the world.
wound—An injury to tissues.
wound VAC—A medical device that applies negative pressure to a wound to promote healing and prevent infections.

X

xiphoid process—The small, bony projection at the lower end of the sternum (breastbone).

Y

yellow marrow—Soft tissue in the diaphysis of long bones.

References

Acello, B. (2002). *The OBRA guidelines for quality improvement* (4th ed.). Clifton Park, NY: Cengage Learning.

Acello, B. (2002). *The OSHA handbook: Guidelines for compliance in health care facilities* (3rd ed.). Clifton Park, NY: Cengage Learning.

Acello, B. (2007). *Advanced skills for health care providers* (2nd ed.). Clifton Park, NY: Cengage Learning.

Aehlert, B. (2016). *ECGs made easy* (5th ed.). St. Louis, MO: Mosby.

Agency for Instructional Technology. (2002). *Communicating with your team* (2nd ed.). Cincinnati, OH: South-Western.

Agency for Instructional Technology. (2002). *Communication and diversity* (2nd ed.). Cincinnati, OH: South-Western.

Agency for Instructional Technology. (2002). *Communication 2000: Resolving problems and conflicts* (2nd ed.). Cincinnati, OH: South-Western.

Aiken, T. D. (2008). *Legal and ethical issues in health occupations* (2nd ed.). Philadelphia: W. B. Saunders.

Allen, E., & Marotz, L. (2013). *Developmental profiles: Pre-birth to eight* (7th ed.). Clifton Park, NY: Cengage Learning.

Alternative Link Systems Inc. (2001). *The state legal guide to complementary and alternative medicine and nursing*. Clifton Park, NY: Cengage Learning.

Altman, G. (2010). *Fundamental and advanced nursing skills* (3rd ed.). Clifton Park, NY: Cengage Learning.

American Heart Association. (2004). *Recommendations for blood pressure measurements in humans*. Dallas, TX: American Heart Association.

American Heart Association. (2010). *2010 Handbook of emergency cardiovascular care for healthcare providers*. Dallas, TX: American Heart Association.

American Heart Association. (2011). *BLS for healthcare providers*. Dallas, TX: American Heart Association or check online courses at *www.heart.org*.

American Heart Association. (2013). *Heart diseases and stroke statistics*. Dallas, TX: American Heart Association.

American Hospital Association. (2016). *ICD-10-CM and ICD-10-PCS coding handbook 2016*. Chicago: American Hospital Association.

American Medical Association. (2012). *Health care careers directory, 2012–2013*. Chicago: American Medical Association.

American Medical Association. (2014). *Current Procedural Terminology (CPT)*. Chicago: American Medical Association.

Andrews, M., & Boyle, J. (2011). *Transcultural concepts in nursing care* (6th ed.). Philadelphia: Lippincott Williams & Wilkins.

Anspaugh, D., Hamrick, M., & Rosato, F. (2010). *Wellness: Concepts and applications* (8th ed.). New York: McGraw-Hill.

Association of Surgical Technologists. (2014). *Surgical technology for the surgical technologist: A positive care approach* (4th ed.). Clifton Park, NY: Cengage Learning.

Atkinson, P., & Timme, D. (2011). *Medical office practice* (8th ed.). Clifton Park, NY: Cengage Learning.

Bailey, L. (2013). *Working* (5th ed.). Clifton Park, NY: Cengage Learning.

Beck, M. (2011). *Theory and practice of therapeutic massage* (5th ed.). Clifton Park, NY: Cengage Learning.

Beebe, R., & Funk, D. (2010). *Fundamentals of emergency care* (3rd ed.). Clifton Park, NY: Cengage Learning.

Beers, M., & Jones, T. V. (2005). *The Merck manual of geriatrics* (3rd ed.). Whitehouse Station, NJ: Merck and Company.

Beers, M., & Jones, T. V. (2005). *The Merck manual of health and aging*. Whitehouse Station, NJ: Merck and Company.

Bird, D., & Robinson, D. S. (2011). *Torres and Ehrlich modern dental assisting* (10th ed.). Philadelphia: W. B. Saunders.

Blesi, M., Wise, B.A., & Kelley-Arney, C. (2012). *Medical assisting administrative and clinical competencies* (7th ed.). Clifton Park, NY: Cengage Learning.

Bonewit-West, K., Fulcher, E., & Burton, B. (2015). *Clinical procedures for medical assistants* (9th ed.). Philadelphia: W. B. Saunders.

Bowie, M. J., & Schaffer, R. M. (2012). *Understanding ICD-9-CM coding* (3rd ed.). Clifton Park, NY: Cengage Learning.

Bowie, M. J., & Schaffer, R. M. (2014). *Understanding ICD-10-CM and ICD-10-PCS: A worktext* (2nd ed.). Clifton Park, NY: Cengage Learning.

Bowie, M. J., & Smith, G. (2014). *2013 ICD-10-CM and ICD-10-PCS workbook*. Clifton Park, NY: Cengage Learning.

Bowman, M., & Lawlis, G. F. (2003). *Complementary and alternative medicine management*. Clifton Park, NY: Cengage Learning.

Boyd, L. B. (2015). *Dental instruments* (5th ed.). Philadelphia: W. B. Saunders.

Brunzel, N. A. (2012). *Fundamentals of urine and body fluid analysis* (3rd ed.). Philadelphia: W. B. Saunders.

Buck, G. (2002). *Preparing for biological terrorism: An emergency services guide*. Clifton Park, NY: Cengage Learning.

Buck, G., Buck, L., & McGill, B. (2003). *Preparing for terrorism: The public safety communicator's guide*. Clifton Park, NY: Cengage Learning.

Buckley, W., & Okrent, K. (2015). *Torts and personal injury law* (5th ed.). Clifton Park, NY: Cengage Learning.

Burke, L., & Weill, B. (2013). *Information technology for the health profession* (4th ed.). Upper Saddle River, NJ: Prentice Hall.

Burkhardt, M., & Nathaniel, A. (2014). *Ethics and issues in contemporary nursing* (4th ed.). Clifton Park, NY: Cengage Learning.

Burkhardt, M. A., & Naqai-Jacobson, M. G. (2002). *Spirituality: Living our connectedness*. Clifton Park, NY: Cengage Learning.

Burton, G. R., & Engelkirk, P G. (2015). *Microbiology for the health sciences* (10th ed.). Philadelphia: Lippincott Williams & Wilkins.

Campbell, M. (2016). *Certification exam review for dental assisting: Prepare, practice, and pass*. Clifton Park, NY: Cengage Learning.

Capellini, S. (2006). *Massage therapy career guide for hands-on success* (2nd ed.). Clifton Park, NY: Cengage Learning.

Carlton, R. R., & McKenna Adler, A. (2013). *Principles of radiographic imaging* (5th ed.). Clifton Park, NY: Cengage Learning.

Charlesworth, R. (2013). *Understanding child development* (9th ed.). Clifton Park, NY: Cengage Learning.

Chernega, J. (2013). *Emergency guide for dental auxiliaries* (4th ed.). Clifton Park, NY: Cengage Learning.

Cohen, B. (2012). *Memmler's structure and function of the human body* (10th ed.). Philadelphia: Lippincott Williams & Wilkins.

Cohen, B. (2012). *Memmler's the human body in health and disease* (12th ed.). Philadelphia: Lippincott Williams & Wilkins.

Colbert, B. J. (2006). *Workplace readiness for health occupations*. (2nd ed.). Clifton Park, NY: Cengage Learning.

Colbert, B. J., Ankney, J., Wilson, J., & Havrilla, J. (2012). *An integrated approach to health sciences: Anatomy and physiology, math, chemistry, and medical microbiology* (2nd ed.). Clifton Park, NY: Cengage Learning.

Colwell Systems. (n. d.). *Appointment control system*. Roselle, IL: Colwell Systems.

Conklin, W. A., White, G., Cothren, C., Williams, D., & Davis, R. (2011). *Principles of computer security* (3rd ed.). New York: McGraw-Hill.

Correa, C. (2010). *Getting started in the computerized medical office: Fundamentals and practice* (2nd ed.). Clifton Park, NY: Cengage Learning.

Covell, A. (2015). *Coding workbook for the physician's office*. Clifton Park, NY: Cengage Learning.

Cowan, M., & Park Talaro, K. (2015). *Microbiology: A systems approach*. (4th ed.). New York: McGraw-Hill.

Craig, R., Powers, J., & Wataha, J. (2012). *Dental materials: Properties and manipulation* (10th ed.). St. Louis, MO: Mosby.

Cronin, A., & Mandich, M. B. (2015). *Human development and performance throughout the lifespan* (2nd ed.). Clifton Park, NY: Cengage Learning.

Cumming, A., Simpson, K., & Brown, D. (2007). *Complementary and alternative medicine*. New York: Churchill Livingstone.

Dalton, M., Hoyle, D. G., & Watts, M. W. (2010). *Human relations* (4th ed.). Cincinnati, OH: South-Western.

Damjanov, I. (2011). *Pathology for the health professions* (4th ed.). Philadelphia: W. B. Saunders.

Daniels, R. (2015). *Delmar's guide to laboratory and diagnostic tests* (3rd ed.). Clifton Park, NY: Cengage Learning.

Daniels, R., & Nicoll, L. (2012). *Contemporary medical-surgical nursings* (2nd ed.). Clifton Park, NY: Cengage Learning.

D'Avanzo, C. (2008,). *Mosby's Pocket guide to cultural health assessment* (4th ed.). St. Louis, MO: Mosby.

Davies, J. (2008). *Essentials of medical terminology* (3rd ed.). Clifton Park, NY: Cengage Learning.

Davies, J. J. (2016). *Illustrated guide to medical terminology* (2nd ed.). Clifton Park, NY: Cengage Learning.

Davis, B. K. (2011). *Phlebotomy: From student to professional* (3rd ed.). Clifton Park, NY: Cengage Learning.

DeLaune, S. C., & Ladner, P. K. (2011). *Fundamentals of nursing, standards and practice* (4th ed.). Clifton Park, NY: Cengage Learning.

Delmar, Cengage Learning. (2002). *Flash! medical terminology flashcard software* (2nd ed.). Clifton Park, NY: Cengage Learning.

Dennerll, J. T. (2007). *Medical terminology made easy* (4th ed.). Clifton Park, NY: Cengage Learning.

Dennerll, J. T., & Davis, P. (2010). *Medical terminology: A programmed systems approach* (10th ed.). Clifton Park, NY: Cengage Learning.

DesJardins, T. (2013). *Cardiopulmonary anatomy and physiology: Essentials of respiratory care* (6th ed.). Clifton Park, NY: Cengage Learning.

Deter, L. L. (2011). *Medication administration*. Clifton Park, NY: Cengage Learning.

Deutsch, J. E., & Anderson, E. S. (2008). *Complementary therapies for physical therapy*. Philadelphia: W. B. Saunders.

Diamond, M. (2012). *Understanding hospital coding and billing* (2nd ed.). Clifton Park, NY: Cengage Learning.

Dietz-Bourguignon, E. (2002). *Safety standards and infection control for dental assistants*. Clifton Park, NY: Cengage Learning.

Dietz-Bourguignon, E. (2006). *Materials and procedures for today's dental assistants*. Clifton Park, NY: Cengage Learning.

Dikel, M., & Roehm, F. (2007). *Guide to Internet job searching*. Indianapolis, IN: Jist Works.

Diller, J. (2015). *Cultural diversity: A primer for the human services* (5th ed.). Clifton Park, NY: Cengage Learning.

Dofka, C. (2013). *Dental terminology* (3rd ed.). Clifton Park, NY: Cengage Learning.

Dorland's illustrated medical dictionary (32nd ed.). (2011). Philadelphia: W. B. Saunders.

Doscher, M. (2005). *HIPAA: A short- and long-term perspective for health care*. Chicago: American Medical Association.

Edge, R., & Groves, J. (2006). *Ethics of health care: A guide for clinical practice* (3rd ed.). Clifton Park, NY: Cengage Learning.

Ehrlich, A., & Schroeder, C. L. (2015). *Introduction to Medical Terminology* (3rd ed.). Clifton Park, NY: Cengage Learning.

Ehrlich, A., & Schroeder, C. L. (2013). *Medical terminology for health professions* (7th ed.). Clifton Park, NY: Cengage Learning.

Elahi, A. (2006). *Data, network, and Internet communications technology*. Clifton Park, NY: Cengage Learning.

Engelkirk, P., & Burton, G. (2015). *Burton's microbiology for the health sciences* (10th ed.). Philadelphia: Lippincott Williams & Wilkins.

Estes, M. E. Z. (2014). *Health assessment* (5th ed.). Clifton Park, NY: Cengage Learning.

Estridge, B., Reynolds, A., & Walters, N. (2012). *Basic clinical laboratory techniques* (6th ed.). Clifton Park, NY: Cengage Learning.

Farr, M. (2006). *Job searching fast and easy*. Clifton Park, NY: Cengage Learning.

Feldstein, P. J. (2012). *Health care economics* (7th ed.). Clifton Park, NY: Cengage Learning.

Finkbeiner, B., & Finkbeiner, C. A. (2011). *Practice management for the dental team* (7th ed.). St. Louis, MO: Mosby.

Flight, M. R. (2011). *Law, liability, and ethics for the medical office professional* (5th ed.). Clifton Park, NY: Cengage Learning.

Fordney, M. (2014). *Insurance handbook for the medical office* (13th ed.). Philadelphia: W. B. Saunders.

Fosegan, J. S. (2003). *Alphabetic indexing rules: Application by computer* (4th ed.). Cincinnati, OH: South-Western.

Frazier, M. S., & Drzymkowski, J. (2012). *Essentials of human disease and conditions* (5th ed.). Philadelphia: W. B. Saunders.

Fremgen, B. F. (2011). *Medical law and ethics* (4th ed.). Upper Saddle River, NJ: Prentice Hall.

French, L. L., & Fordney, M. (2013). *Administrative medical assisting* (7th ed.). Clifton Park, NY: Cengage Learning.

Frey, K., & Price, P. (2006). *Surgical anatomy and physiology for surgical technologists*. Clifton Park, NY: Cengage Learning.

Frisch, B. (2007). *Correct coding for medicare, compliance, and reimbursement*. Clifton Park, NY: Cengage Learning.

Fry, R. (2013). *101 great answers to the toughest interview questions* (6th ed.). Clifton Park, NY: Cengage Learning.

Fry, R. (2013). *101 great resumes* (3rd ed.). Clifton Park, NY: Cengage Learning.

Fry, R. (2013). *101 smart questions to ask on your interview* (3rd ed.). Clifton Park, NY: Cengage Learning.

Fry, R. (2012). *Get organized* (4th ed.). Clifton Park, NY: Cengage Learning.

Fry, R. (2012). *How to study* (7th ed.). Clifton Park, NY: Cengage Learning.

Gerlach, M. J. (2014). *Assisting in long-term care* (6th ed.). Clifton Park, NY: Cengage Learning.

Giger, J. N. (2013). *Transcultural nursing: Assessment and intervention* (6th ed.). St. Louis, MO: Mosby.

Gould, B. (2010). *Pathophysiology for the health related professions* (4th ed.). Philadelphia: W. B. Saunders.

Green, M. (2014). *3-2-1 code* (4th ed.). Clifton Park, NY: Cengage Learning.

Green, M., & Bowie, M. J. (2011). *Essentials of health information management: Principles and practices* (2nd ed.). Clifton Park, NY: Cengage Learning.

Green, M., & Rowell, J. C. (2014). *Understanding health insurance: A guide to billing and reimbursement* (11th ed.). Clifton Park, NY: Cengage Learning.

Hanan, Z. I., & Durgin, J. M. (2015). *Pharmacy Practice for Technicians* (5th ed.). Clifton Park, NY: Cengage Learning.

Hansen, M. (2010). *Business math* (17th ed.). Cincinnati, OH: South-Western.

Haroun, L. (2011). *Career development for health professionals* (3rd ed.). Philadelphia: Saunders.

Hegner, B., & Acello, B. (2008). *On the job: The essentials of nursing assisting* (2nd ed.). Clifton Park, NY: Cengage Learning.

Hegner, B., Acello, B., & Caldwell, E. (2008). *Nursing assistant: A nursing process approach* (10th ed.). Clifton Park, NY: Cengage Learning.

Heller, M., & Krebs, C. (2013). *Cengage learning's clinical handbook for the medical office* (3rd ed.). Clifton Park, NY: Cengage Learning.

Heller, M., & Veach, L. (2009). *Clinical medical assisting.* Clifton Park, NY: Cengage Learning.

Henderson, D. A., O'Toole, T., & Inglesly, T. V. (Eds.) (2005). *Bioterrorism: Guidelines for medical and public health management.* Chicago: American Medical Association.

Hoeltke, L. (2013). *Complete textbook of phlebotomy* (4th ed.). Clifton Park, NY: Cengage Learning.

Hoeltke, L. (2013). *Phlebotomy, procedures and practice* (2nd ed.). Clifton Park, NY: Cengage Learning.

Hoffman, S. M. (2006). *Child care in action: Infants and toddlers.* Clifton Park, NY: Cengage Learning.

Hogan, M. (2012). *Four skills of cultural diversity competence.* (4th ed.). Pacific Grove, CA: Brooks/Cole.

Hover-Kramer, D. (2002). *Healing touch: A guide book for practitioners* (2nd ed.). Clifton Park, NY: Cengage Learning.

Jennings, D. (2013). *Emergency guide for dental auxiliaries* (4th ed.). Clifton Park, NY: Cengage Learning.

Johnson, S., & McHugh, C. (2013). *Understanding medical coding: A comprehensive guide* (3rd ed.). Clifton Park, NY: Cengage Learning.

Jones, B. D. (2011). *Comprehensive medical terminology* (4th ed.). Clifton Park, NY: Cengage Learning.

Kalanick, K. (2012). *Phlebotomy technician specialist* (2nd ed.). Clifton Park, NY: Cengage Learning.

Keegan, L. (2001). *Healing with complementary and alternative therapies.* Clifton Park, NY: Cengage Learning.

Keegan, L. (2002). *Healing nutrition* (2nd ed.). Clifton Park, NY: Cengage Learning.

Kelz, R. (1999). *Conversational Spanish for health professions.* Clifton Park, NY: Cengage Learning.

Kennamer, M. (2005). *Math for health care professionals.* Clifton Park, NY: Cengage Learning.

Klinoff, R. (2012). *Introduction to fire protection* (4th ed.). Clifton Park, NY: Cengage Learning.

Koprucki, V. (2007). *Client-centered care for clinical medical assisting.* Clifton Park, NY: Cengage Learning.

Krager, D., & Krager, C. (2005). *HIPAA for medical office personnel.* Clifton Park, NY: Cengage Learning.

Krantman, S. (2013). *The resume writer's workbook* (4th ed.). Clifton Park, NY: Cengage Learning.

Kubler-Ross, E. (1997). *Death: The final stage of growth.* Englewood Cliffs, NJ: Prentice-Hall.

Kuhns, D. J., Noonan Rice, P., & Winslow, L. L. (2006). *Health unit coordinator, 21st century professional.* Clifton Park, NY: Cengage Learning.

Lamkin, C. (2014). *Dental Office Management* (2nd ed.). Clifton Park, NY: Cengage Learning.

Leonard, P. C. (2014). *Quick and easy medical terminology* (7th ed.). Philadelphia: W. B. Saunders.

Lesmeister, M. B. (2007). *Writing basics for the health care professional* (2nd ed.). Upper Saddle River, NJ: Prentice Hall.

Lesmeister, M. B. (2014). *Math basics for health care professionals* (4th ed.). Upper Saddle River, NJ: Prentice Hall.

Lewis, K. (2010). *ECG practical applications pocket reference guide.* Clifton Park, NY: Cengage Learning.

Limmer, D., O'Keefe, M., Dickinson, E., Grant, H., Murray, B., & Bergeron, J. D. (2011). *Emergency care* (12th ed.). Upper Saddle River, NJ: Brady/Prentice Hall.

Lindh, W., Pooler, M., Tamparo, C., Dahl, B., & Morris, J. (2014). *Comprehensive medical assisting: Administrative and clinical competencies* (5th ed.). Clifton Park, NY: Cengage Learning.

Luckmann, J. (2000). *Transcultural Communication in Health Care.* Clifton Park, NY: Cengage Learning.

Maki, S. E., & Petterson, B. (2014). *Using the electronic health record in health care provider practice.* (2nd ed.). Clifton Park, NY: Cengage Learning.

Malarkey, L. M., & McMorrow, M. E. (2011). *Saunders nursing guide to laboratory and diagnostic tests* (2nd ed.). Philadelphia: W. B. Saunders.

Mandleco, B. (2004). *Growth and development handbook: Newborn through adolescent.* Clifton Park, NY: Cengage Learning.

Mappes, T., Ballard, J., & DeGrazia, D. (2010). *Biomedical ethics* (7th ed.). New York: McGraw-Hill.

Marotz, L., Cross, M. Z., & Rush, J. (2012). *Health, safety, and nutrition for the young child* (8th ed.). Clifton Park, NY: Cengage Learning.

Maville, J. (2013). *Health promotion in nursing.* Clifton Park, NY: Cengage Learning.

McArdle, W., Katch, F., & Katch, V. (2014). *Exercise physiology: Energy, nutrition, and human performance* (8th ed.). Philadelphia: Lippincott Williams & Wilkins.

McCutcheon, M., & Phillips, M. (2006). *Exploring health careers* (3rd ed.). Clifton Park, NY: Cengage Learning.

McElroy, O. H., & Grabb, L. L. (2010). *Spanish-English English-Spanish medical dictionary* (4th ed.). Philadelphia: Lippincott Williams & Wilkins.

McWay, D. (2010). *Legal aspects of health information management* (3rd ed.). Clifton Park, NY: Cengage Learning.

Means, T. (2009). *Business communications* (2nd ed.). Cincinnati, OH: South-Western.

The Merck manual of diagnosis and therapy (19th ed.). (2011). Porter, R. S., & Kaplan, J. L., Eds. Whitehouse Station, NJ: Merck and Company.

Miller, C. H., & Palenik, C. J. (2014). *Infection control and management of hazardous materials for the dental team* (5th ed.). St. Louis, MO: Mosby.

Milliken, M. E. (2011). *Understanding human behavior* (8th ed.). Clifton Park, NY: Cengage Learning.

Mitchell, J., & Haroun, L. (2012). *Introduction to health care* (3rd ed.). Clifton Park, NY: Cengage Learning.

Mitchell, M. (2011). *Dental instruments: A pocket guide to identification* (2nd ed.). Philadelphia: Lippincott Williams & Wilkins.

Mitchell, M. K. (2008). *Nutrition across the life span*. Philadelphia: W. B. Saunders.

Moisio, M. (2008). *Medical terminology: A student centered approach* (2nd ed.). Clifton Park, NY: Cengage Learning.

Moisio, M. (2014). *A guide to health insurance billing* (4th ed.). Clifton Park, NY: Cengage Learning.

Mosby's dictionary of medicine, nursing, and health professions (9th ed.). (2013). St. Louis, MO: Mosby.

Moule, J. (2012). *Cultural competence: A primer for educators* (2nd ed.). Clifton Park, NY: Cengage Learning.

Mullins, D. F. (2006). *501 human diseases*. Clifton Park, NY: Cengage Learning.

Mulvihill, M. L., Zelman, M., Holdaway, P, Tompary, E., & Raymond, J. (2009). *Human diseases: A systemic approach* (7th ed.). Upper Saddle River, NJ: Prentice Hall.

Munoz, C., & Luckmann, J. (2005). *Transcultural communication in nursing* (2nd ed.). Clifton Park, NY: Cengage Learning.

Nasso, J., & Celia, L. (2007). *Dementia care*. Clifton Park, NY: Cengage Learning.

National Health Council. (2002). *300 ways to put your talent to work in the health field*. New York: National Health Council.

National Health Council. (2008). *Guide to voluntary health agencies*. New York: National Health Council.

National Safety Council. (2012). *Advanced first aid, CPR, and AED* (2nd ed.). New York: McGraw-Hill.

Neighbors, M., & Tannehill-Jones, R. (2015). *Human diseases* (4th ed.). Clifton Park, NY: Cengage Learning.

Nettina, S. (2014). *Lippincott manual of nursing practice* (10th ed.). Philadelphia: Lippincott Williams & Wilkins.

Nix, S. (2012). *Williams' basic nutrition and diet therapy* (14th ed.). St. Louis, MO: Mosby.

Olson, M. (2002). *Healing the dying* (2nd ed.). Clifton Park, NY: Cengage Learning.

Papalia, D. E., & Duskin Feldman, R. (2014). *A child's world: Infancy through adolescence* (13th ed.). New York: McGraw-Hill.

Parry, J., & Ryan, A. (2003). *A cross-cultural look at death, dying, and religion*. New York: McGraw-Hill.

Payne, R. A. (2010). *Relaxation techniques: A practical handbook for the health care professional* (4th ed.). New York: Churchill Livingston.

Peden, A. (2012). *Comparative health information management* (3rd ed.). Clifton Park, NY: Cengage Learning.

Phinney, D., & Halstead, J. (2014). *Dental assisting instrument guide* (2nd ed.). Clifton Park, NY: Cengage Learning.

Phinney, D., & Halstead, J. (2009). *Delmar's dental materials guide*. Clifton Park, NY: Cengage Learning.

Phinney, D., & Halstead, J. (2013). *Dental assisting: A comprehensive approach* (4th ed.). Clifton Park, NY: Cengage Learning.

Physicians' desk reference. (2015). Montvale, NJ: Thomson Healthcare.

Potts, N., & Mandleco, B. (2012). *Pediatric nursing: Caring for children and their families* (3rd ed.). Clifton Park, NY: Cengage Learning.

Quill, T. (1993). *Death and dignity*. New York: W. W. Norton and Company.

Quill, T., & Battin, M. P. (2004). *Physician-assisted dying: The case for palliative care and patient choice*. Baltimore, MD: Johns Hopkins University Press.

Raffel, M. W., & Barsukiewicz, C. K. (2011). *The US health system origins and functions* (6th ed.). Clifton Park, NY: Cengage Learning.

Rice, J. (2011). *Principles of pharmacology for medical assisting* (5th ed.). Clifton Park, NY: Cengage Learning.

Rios, J., & Fernandez, J. (2010). *Spanish for health care providers* (2nd ed.). New York: McGraw-Hill.

Rizzo, D. (2010). *Fundamentals of anatomy and physiology* (3rd ed.). Clifton Park, NY: Cengage Learning.

Robertson, C. (2013). *Safety, health, and nutrition in early education* (5th ed.). Clifton Park, NY: Cengage Learning.

Robinson, J., & McCormick, D. J. (2011). *Concepts in health and wellness*. Clifton Park, NY: Cengage Learning.

Roth, R. A. (2014). *Nutrition and diet therapy* (11th ed.). Clifton Park, NY: Cengage Learning.

Ryan, J. S. (2009). *Managing your personal finances* (6th ed.). Cincinnati, OH: South-Western.

Saba, V., & McCormick, K. (2011). *Essentials of nursing informatics* (5th ed.). New York: McGraw-Hill.

Scott, A., & Fong, E. (2014). *Body structures and functions* (12th ed.). Clifton Park, NY: Cengage Learning.

Short, M. J. (2013). *Head, neck, and dental anatomy* (4th ed.). Clifton Park, NY: Cengage Learning.

Shortell, S., & Kaluzny, A. (2012). *Health care management, organization, design, and behavior* (6th ed.). Clifton Park, NY: Cengage Learning.

Simmers, L., Simmers-Nartker, K., & Simmers-Kobelak, S. (2013). *Practical problems in mathematics for health science careers* (3rd ed.). Clifton Park, NY: Cengage Learning.

Smeltzer, S., Bare, B., Hinkle, J., & Cheever, K. (2014). *Brunner and Suddarth's textbook of medical surgical nursing* (13th ed.). Philadelphia: Lippincott Williams & Wilkins.

Sormunen, C. (2010). *Terminology for allied health professionals* (6th ed.). Clifton Park, NY: Cengage Learning.

Sorrentino, S. (2014). *Mosby's essentials for nursing assistants* (5th ed.). St. Louis, MO: Mosby.

Spatz, A., & Balduzzi, S. (2005). *Homemaker/home health aide* (6th ed.). Clifton Park, NY: Cengage Learning.

Spratto, G., & Woods, A. (2013). *PDR: Nurse's drug handbook* (22nd ed.). Clifton Park, NY: Cengage Learning.

Stedman's alternative and complementary medicine words (2nd ed.). (2004). Philadelphia: Lippincott Williams & Wilkins.

Stedman's medical dictionary for the health professions and nursing (7th ed.). (2011). Philadelphia: Lippincott Williams & Wilkins.

Tamparo, C. D., & Lindh, W. (2008). *Therapeutic communications for health care* (3rd ed.). Clifton Park, NY: Cengage Learning.

Terryberry, K. (2005). *Writing for the health professions.* Clifton Park, NY: Cengage Learning.

Thibodeau, G., & Patton, K. (2013). *Anatomy and physiology* (8th ed.). St. Louis, MO: Mosby.

Thibodeau, G., & Patton, K. (2014). *Human body in health and disease* (6th ed.). St. Louis, MO: Mosby.

Thibodeau, G., & Patton, K. (2011). *Structure and function of the body* (14th ed.). St. Louis, MO: Mosby.

Thomson Cengage Learning. (2005). *Quick reference for health care providers.* Clifton Park, NY: Cengage Learning.

Thomson, L., & Trocquet, C. (2014). *Clinical Rotations* (2nd ed.). Clifton Park, NY: Cengage Learning.

Throop, R. K., & Castellucci, M. (2006). *Personal excellence.* Clifton Park, NY: Cengage Learning.

Tideiksaar, R. (2006). *Avoiding falls: A guideline for certified nursing assistants.* Clifton Park, NY: Cengage Learning.

U.S. Department of Agriculture. (2015). *2015 Dietary guidelines for Americans.* Washington, DC: U.S. Government Printing Office.

U.S. Department of Health and Human Services. (2007). *Guidelines for isolation precautions in hospitals.* Retrieved from *http://www.cdc.gov/incidod/dhqp/gl_isolation.html*

U.S. Department of Health and Human Services. (2012). *International classification of diseases.* Washington, DC: U.S. Government Printing Office.

U.S. Department of Labor. (2014). *Occupational outlook handbook.* Washington, DC: U.S. Government Printing Office.

Villemarie, L., & Villemarie, D. (2006). *Grammar and writing skills for the health care professional* (2nd ed.). Clifton Park, NY: Cengage Learning.

Wallace, H. R., & Masters, A. (2010). *Personal development for life and work* (10th ed.). Cincinnati, OH: South-Western.

Walz, B. J. (2011). *Foundations of EMS systems.* (2nd ed.). Clifton Park, NY: Cengage Learning.

Weiss, R. (2009). *Physical therapy aide: A worktext* (3rd ed.). Clifton Park, NY: Cengage Learning.

Wendleton, K. (2013). *Mastering the job interview and winning the money game.* Clifton Park, NY: Cengage Learning.

Wendleton, K. (2013). *Packaging yourself: The targeted resume.* Clifton Park, NY: Cengage Learning.

White, L. (2011). *Foundations of basic nursing* (3rd ed.). Clifton Park, NY: Cengage Learning.

White, L., & Duncan, G. (2013). *Medical-surgical nursing: An integrated approach* (3rd ed.). Clifton Park, NY: Cengage Learning.

Williams, S. J., & Torrens, P. (2008). *Introduction to health services* (7th ed.). Clifton Park, NY: Cengage Learning.

Williams, S., Schlenker, E., & Long, S. (2014). *Essentials of nutrition and diet therapy* (11th ed.). St. Louis, MO: Mosby.

Wischnitzer, S., & Wischnitzer, E. (2010). *Top 100 health-care careers.* Indianapolis, IN: Jist Works.

Woelfel, J., & Scheid, R. (2011). *Dental anatomy: Its relevance to dentistry* (8th ed.). Philadelphia: Lippincott Williams & Wilkins.

Wolfinger, A. (2009). *Best career and education Web sites* (6th ed.). Indianapolis, IN: Jist Works.

Woodrow, R. (2015). *Essentials of pharmacology for health occupations* (7th ed.). Clifton Park, NY: Cengage Learning.

Zalenski, R., & Stone, S. C. (2011). *Emergency palliative care.* St. Louis, MO: McGraw-Hill.

Zedlitz, R. H. (2013). *How to get a job in health care* (2nd ed.). Clifton Park, NY: Cengage Learning.

Index

A

D

E

I

J

K

L

M

N

Q

R

U

CHAPTER 2 Health Care Systems

ASSIGNMENT SHEET

Grade ______________________________ Name____________________________________

INTRODUCTION: An awareness of the many different kinds of health care systems is important for any health care worker. This assignment will help you review the main facts on health care systems.

INSTRUCTIONS: Read the information on Health Care Systems. Then follow the instructions in each section to complete this assignment.

A. Completion or Short Answer: In the space provided, print the word(s) that best completes the statement or answers the question.

1. Unscramble the following words to identify some health care facilities.

   a. RAALOTBYRO

   b. TLEHHA NNCIAMTNAEE

   c. OLGN ETMR AREC

   d. UNLTISIDAR ETHLAH

   e. MNCEGEREY AECR

   f. LNTEMA LHTEHA

   g. LNCCII

   h. EAIINRIABHTLTO

   i. POTSAHIL

2. Place the name of the type of health care facility next to the brief description of the facility.

   a. ____________________ provide assistance and care mainly for elderly patients

   b. ____________________ provide special care for accidents or sudden illness

   c. ____________________ deal with mental disorders and diseases

   d. ____________________ health centers located in large companies or industries

   e. ____________________ offices owned by one or more dentists

   f. ____________________ perform special diagnostic tests

   g. ____________________ provide care in a patient's home

   h. ____________________ provide physical, occupational, and other therapies

   i. ____________________ check for genetic abnormalities and birth defects

   j. ____________________ prepare and dispense medications

3. Hospitals are classified into four types depending on the sources of income received. List the four (4) main types.

4. Differentiate between residential care facilities, extended care facilities, and independent living facilities.

5. List three (3) services offered by medical offices.

6. Identify at least three (3) different types of clinics.

7. List three (3) examples of services that can be provided by home health care agencies.

8. What is palliative care?

9. What is the purpose or main goal of the care provided by rehabilitation facilities?

10. Identify three (3) services offered by school health services.

11. An international agency sponsored by the United Nations is the ____________________. A national agency that deals with health problems in America is the ____________________. Another national organization that is involved in the research of disease is the ____________________. A federal agency that establishes and enforces standards that protect workers from job-related injuries and illnesses is the ____________________. The federal agency that researches the quality of health care delivery and identifies the standards of treatment that should be provided is the ____________________.

12. List four (4) services that can be offered by state and local health departments.

13. Nonprofit or voluntary agencies provide many services.
    a. How do these agencies receive their funding?

    b. What was the purpose of creating the Joint Commission?

    c. List two (2) services provided by nonprofit agencies.

CHAPTER 5 LEGAL AND ETHICAL RESPONSIBILITIES

ASSIGNMENT SHEET

Grade ______________________ Name ______________________

INTRODUCTION: All health care workers must understand the legal and ethical responsibilities of their particular health care career. This assignment will help you review the basic facts on legal and ethical responsibilities.

INSTRUCTIONS: Read the information on Legal and Ethical Responsibilities. In the space provided, print the word(s) that best completes the statement or answers the question.

1. Use the Key Terms to fill in the blanks.

   a. C _ _ _ _ _ _ _ (agreement between two or more parties)

   b. _ O _ _ _ (wrongful acts that do not involve contracts)

   c. _ _ _ N _ _ _ (spoken defamation)

   d. _ _ F _ _ _ _ _ _ _ (a false statement)

   e. _ I _ _ _ (written defamation)

   f. _ _ _ _ _ D _ _ _ _ _ _ _ _ _ (without legal capacity)

   g. _ E _ _ _ (authorized or based on law)

   h. _ _ _ N _ (person working under principal's direction)

   i. _ T _ _ _ _ (principles morally right or wrong)

   j. _ _ _ _ _ I _ _ _ _ _ _ _ _ _ _ _ _ (restricting an individual's freedom)

   k. _ _ _ _ _ A _ _ _ _ _ (bad practice)

   l. _ _ _ _ _ L _ (threat or attempt to injure)

   m. _ _ _ _ I _ _ _ _ _ (failure to give expected care)

   n. _ _ _ _ _ _ T _ _ _ _ _ _ _ (factors of care patients can expect)

   Y

2. Differentiate between criminal law and civil law.

3. Describe a situation that provides an example that could lead to legal action for each of the following torts.

   a. malpractice:

   b. negligence:

   c. assault and battery:

   d. invasion of privacy:

   e. false imprisonment:

   f. abuse:

   g. defamation:

4. How are slander and libel the same? How are they different?

5. What are the three (3) parts of a contract?

6. What is the difference between an implied contract and an expressed contract?

7. List three (3) examples of individuals who have legal disabilities.

Name ______________________________

8. What legal mandate must be followed when a contract is explained to a non-English-speaking individual?

9. Who is responsible for the actions of an agent? Why is it important for a health care worker to be aware of his or her role as an agent?

10. What are privileged communications?

What is required before privileged communications can be shared with anyone else?

11. List three (3) examples of information that is exempt by law and not considered to be privileged communications.

12. Who has ownership of health care records?

What rights do patients have in regard to their health care records?

13. What should you do if you make an error while recording information on health care records?

14. List three (3) ways health care facilities create safeguards to maintain computer confidentiality.

15. List three (3) advantages associated with a health information exchange (HIE).

16. What standards provide federal protection for privacy of health care records?

17. What information must be on the authorization form for the release of patient information?

18. The procedures, processes, and actions that health care providers are legally permitted to perform in keeping with the terms of their professional license or registration is called the ____________________. Some regulations are mandated by ____________________ such as HIPAA, PSDA, and the PPACA. Other standards and regulations are issued by ____________________ such as the CDC, OSHA, and the FDA. Professional organizations in all of the health care careers assist in the establishment of ____________________ requirements, ____________________ standards, and a code of ____________________ that must be followed. Health care agencies also have standards and regulations that are found in the ____________________ for the facility. It is your responsibility to learn exactly what you are ____________________ permitted to do.

19. What are ethics?

20. What should you do in the following situations to maintain your legal/ethical responsibilities?

   a. A patient with a *Do Not Resuscitate (DNR)* order tells you he has saved a supply of sleeping pills and intends to commit suicide.

   b. You work in a nursing home and see a coworker shove a patient into a chair and then slap the patient in the face.

   c. You work as a dental assistant and a patient asks you, "Will the doctor be able to save this tooth or will it have to be pulled?"

   d. A patient has just been admitted to an assisted care facility. As you are helping the patient undress and get ready for bed, you notice numerous bruises and scratches on both arms.

21. What are patient's rights?

Name ______________________________

22. Identify five (5) rights provided by the Consumer Bill of Rights and Responsibilites.

23. What is the name of the act that guarantees certain rights to residents in long-term care facilities?

24. Choose three (3) rights provided to consumers under the Patient Protection and Affordable Care Act (PPACA). State why you think they are important.

25. What is the purpose for each of the following advance directives for health care?

   a. Living will:

   b. Durable Power of Attorney (POA):

26. What is the purpose of the Patient Self-Determination Act (PSDA)?

27. Describe three (3) ways you can identify a patient.

28. What should you do in the following situations to maintain professional standards?

   a. The doctor you work for asks you to give a patient an allergy shot, but you are not qualified to give injections.

   b. An elderly patient, who is frequently confused and disoriented, refuses to let you take his temperature.

   c. You work in a medical laboratory. A patient's wife asks you if her husband's blood test was positive for an infectious disease.

29. What is a *DNR* order? What does it mean?

CHAPTER 13 MEDICAL MATH

ASSIGNMENT SHEET

Grade ______________________ Name Jaren Lighthart

INTRODUCTION: Working in health care requires the use of math skills for many different aspects of patient care. This assignment will help you review math concerns and concepts that are essential to working in health care.

INSTRUCTIONS: Read the information on Medical Math. In the space provided, print the word(s) that best completes the statement or answers the question.

1. Identify four (4) applications of math skills in health care.

2. Numbers are what we traditionally use to count; they do not contain fractions or decimals. decimals are one way of expressing parts of numbers and are expressed in units of ten. Fractions have a numerator and a denominator. It is easier to calculate Fractions if you first convert them to decimals. denominator show relationships between numbers or like values or how many of one number or value is present as compared to the other. Rounding a number means changing it to the nearest ten, hundred, thousand, and so on.

3. List four (4) guidelines to make estimating useful.

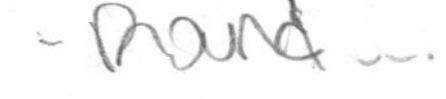

4. Perform the calculations indicated for whole numbers.

   a. 742 + 1,259 = 2001

   b. 1,138 + 1,423 + 2,557 + 924 = 6042

   c. 238,031 − 152,987 = 85044

   d. 18,654 − 8,986 = 9668

   e. 22 × 156 = 3432

   f. 1,057 × 324 = 342,468

   g. 555 ÷ 15 = 37

   h. 171,450 ÷ 9,525 = 18

5. Perform the calculations indicated for decimals.

a. 5.893 + 87.32 + 0.5 = 93.713

b. 54.5 + 0.05455 + 5,450 + 5.00456 = 5509.55911

c. 78.3 − 49.538 = 28.762

d. 485.782 − 396.99 = 88.792

e. 28.561 × 5.39 = 153.94379

f. 0.614 × 0.00568 = .00348752

g. 125.49 ÷ 2.35 = 53.4

h. 1,027.08 ÷ 6.34 = 162

6. Perform the calculations indicated for fractions.

a. $\frac{1}{8} + \frac{3}{4} + \frac{1}{2} =$ 1.375

b. $3\frac{5}{8} + 20\frac{3}{5} =$ 24.225

c. $\frac{15}{16} - \frac{3}{8} =$ .5625

d. $46\frac{3}{4} - 37\frac{1}{3} =$ $10.08\overline{3}$

e. $\frac{7}{12} \times \frac{8}{21} =$ $.\overline{2}$

f. $12\frac{2}{5} \times 5\frac{5}{8} =$ 14.625

g. $\frac{7}{8} \div \frac{5}{6} =$ $.0291\overline{6}$

h. $27\frac{1}{2} \div 5\frac{1}{2} =$ 27.6

7. Perform the calculations indicated for percentages.

a. 38% + 53.5% = 91.5%

b. 54.3% − 11.4% = 42.9%

c. 230 × 5% = 46%

d. 563 ÷ 2% = 281.5%

Name ______________________

8. Round the following numbers to the place indicated.

   a. 9,837 to the nearest ten

   b. 652 to the nearest hundred

   c. 1,479 to the nearest thousand

9. Use proportions to calculate the following problems.

   a. How many 250 milligram (mg) tablets must be given for a total dosage of 750 mg?

   b. How many 5-grain aspirins must be given for a total dosage of 7.5 grains?

   c. How many milligrams of medication should you give an 80-pound person if dosage requires 20 mg for every 10 pounds of weight?

   d. If 45 milliliters (mL) of water are required to mix 100 grams (g) of plaster, how many mL would you need for 250 g of plaster?

10. Convert the following numbers to Roman numerals.

    a. 55

    b. 109

    c. 595

    d. 788

    e. 2,367

11. Interpret the following Roman numerals.

    a. XII

    b. CCXIX

    c. XLIV

    d. DCXCII

    e. MMMDXXXIII

12. Give three (3) examples of how angles are used in health care.

13. What are the six (6) steps used for performing conversions between systems of measurement?

14. Convert the following as indicated. Use the approximate equivalents shown in the textbook to calculate your answers.

a. 5 teaspoons = ______________________ milliliters

b. 1,250 milliliters = ______________________ quarts

c. 33 kilograms = ______________________ pounds

d. 6 ounces = ______________________ milliliters

e. 121 pounds = ______________________ kilograms

f. 2 feet = ______________________ centimeters

15. Convert the following temperatures from Fahrenheit to Celsius and round off the answers to the nearest one-tenth of a degree.

a. 35°F

b. 72°F

c. 99.6°F

d. 103°F

16. Convert the following temperatures from Celsius to Fahrenheit and round off the answers to the nearest one-tenth of a degree.

a. 30°C

b. 62°C

c. 15°C

d. 25.6°C

17. Define *military time.*

Name ______________________________

18. Convert the following to military time.

    a. 1:00 PM

    b. 2:00 AM

    c. 12:00 NOON

    d. 3:00 AM

    e. 8:35 PM

    f. 5:05 AM

    g. 11:48 PM

    h. 12:00 MIDNIGHT

19. A dental laboratory technician (DLT) earns $14 per hour when she works days and $18 per hour when she works nights. One month she works six 4-hour days, three 8-hour days, three 10-hour days, five 6-hour nights, and four 8-hour nights. What is her total pay for the month?

20. A pharmacy technician is preparing a prescription for a patient. The physician ordered a dosage of 1 capsule before meals and 2 capsules at bedtime every day. How many capsules should the technician dispense for a 14-day supply of medication?

21. A staining solution bottle in a medical laboratory contains 30 ounces (oz). A blood staining test requires 3/4 oz of solution. A tissue staining test requires 1/2 oz of solution. If four blood tests and five tissue tests are performed, how many ounces of solution are left in the bottle?

22. A child with asthma is given aminophylline. The recommended dosage is 0.6 milligrams (mg) per kilogram (kg) of body weight. If the child weighs 54 pounds (lb), what dosage should the child receive? Round off to tenths. (*Hint:* 1 kg = 2.2 pounds)

23. A pharmacy technician must prepare 120 ounces (oz) of infant formula for the neonatal intensive care unit. The mixture is 1/4 formula and 3/4 water. How much formula should she use? How much water?

24. A study shows that an influenza (flu) vaccine is 71.4% effective in preventing a particular type of influenza. If 15,422 people receive the vaccine, how many would not be protected and would be likely to get influenza? Round off to the nearest whole number.

25. A pharmacist orders medications for a total of $6,439.65. A 6 ¼% discount is given if payment is made within 15 days, and a 2.5% discount is given if payment is made within 30 days. How much money can be saved by paying in 15 days instead of 30 days?

26. A hospital emergency room treated 36 people in one day. If 24 of the people were children, what was the ratio of children to adults that day?

27. A hemoglobin (Hgb) test measures 14.5 grams (g) of Hgb per 100 milliliters (mL) of blood. If the patient has 5.5 quarts (qt) of blood in her body, how many grams of Hgb are present? (*Hint:* 1 qt = 1,000 mL)

28. A pharmacy technician reviews a prescription that orders Sumycin suspension 250 milligrams (mg) by mouth every 6 hours. Sumycin suspension is available as 125 mg/5 mL. How many milliliters should the technician dispense for a 6-day supply?

29. The cornerstone of a hospital shows the date when the hospital was built as MCMXLVII. When was the hospital built?

30. The normal range for body temperature is 97°F–100°F. What is the normal range for body temperature in °C?

31. A patient has surgery for a knee replacement. Operating room charges are $3,286.00, anesthesia is $1,554.80, the charge for a hospital room for 3 days is $1,952.42 per day, medications total $1,297.59, and miscellaneous charges are $739.15. The insurance company pays $10,187.84.

    a. What is the balance the patient must pay?

    b. What percent of the bill was paid by the insurance company?

32. A physician orders 525 milligrams (mg) of Cefaclor suspension for a patient with pharyngitis. Cefaclor is available as 375 mg/5 mL of solution. How many milliliters should be given?

33. A pharmacy technician must prepare 350 milliliters (mL) of a 3% boric acid solution. How many grams (g) of boric acid crystals will he use?

34. A physician orders 1 milligram (mg) of atropine intravenous (IV) for a patient in cardiac arrest. Atropine is available as 0.5 mg/5 mL. The nurse administers the medication at 8:30 PM and charts the time given as 1830.

    a. How many milliliters of solution should be given to the patient?

    b. Did the nurse note the time correctly? If not, how should the time be expressed in military time?

CHAPTER 14:1 Using Body Mechanics

ASSIGNMENT SHEET

Grade ______________ Name Jason Lightfoot

INTRODUCTION: The correct use of body mechanics is essential to protect both the worker and the patient. This assignment will allow you to review the main facts.

INSTRUCTIONS: Read the information on Using Body Mechanics. In the space provided, print the word(s) that best completes the statement or answers the question.

1. Define body mechanics.

   The way body moves & maintains balance.

2. List four (4) reasons for using correct body mechanics.

   - Muscles work better
   - Makes pulling, lifting, & pushing easier
   - saves energy
   - prevents self injury

3. Identify four (4) principles of good posture.

   - shoulder back - chin up
   - chest up - feet flat

4. In the following diagrams, certain rules for correct body mechanics are not being observed. At least three rules are being broken in each diagram. In the space provided for each diagram, list three rules not being observed.

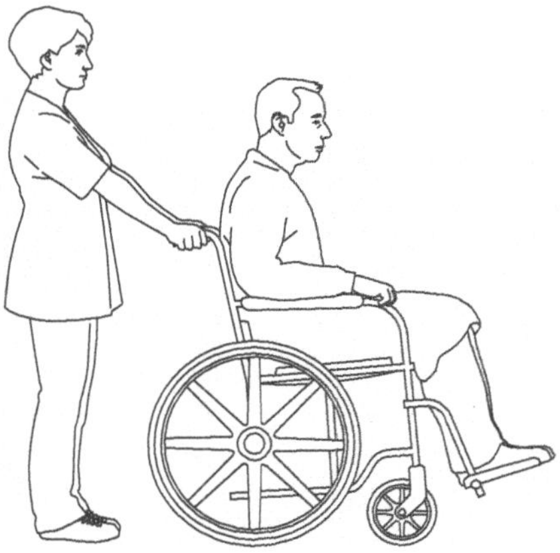

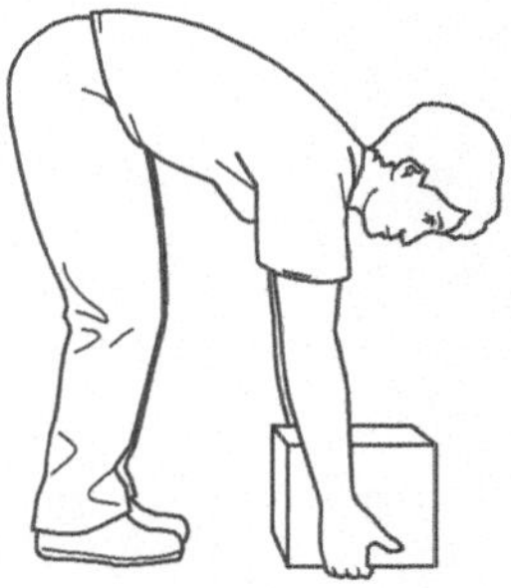

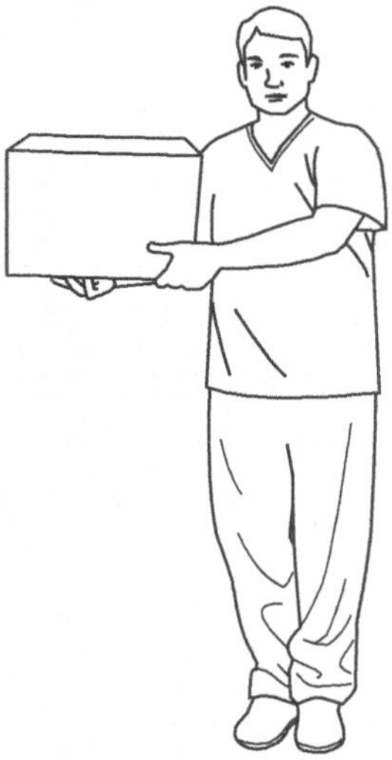

Diagram 1:
(1) Feet too close
(2) shoulder not back
(3) elbows locked

Diagram 2:
(1) feet too close
(2) weigh shifted.
(3) holding box weird

Diagram 3:
(1) feet to close
(2) lifting with back
(3) leg not bent

CHAPTER 14:3 OBSERVING FIRE SAFETY

ASSIGNMENT SHEET

Grade ______________________ Name Jason Lightfoot

INTRODUCTION: Knowing how to respond to a fire can save your life. This assignment will help you review the main facts of fire safety.

INSTRUCTIONS: Read the text information about Observing Fire Safety. In the space provided, print the word(s) that best completes the statement or answers the question.

1. Fires need three (3) things to start. What are they?

   Heat, fuel, oxygen

2. List four (4) causes of fires.

   Smoking, matches, electricity, heating systems

3. List three (3) rules for preventing fires.

   - Dont light matches
   - Dont through cigs on ground
   - Keep electrical stuff safe

4. Where is the nearest fire alarm box located?

   Nearest Exit

5. a. What is the location of the nearest fire extinguisher?

   Probably at the nearest falicity

   b. What class of fire extinguisher is it? What kind of fire will it extinguish?

   - Probably class C.
   - electrical fires

6. Fill in the following chart about fire extinguishers.

Class	Used on what type of fires?
A	paper, cloth, wood
B	flamable liquids
C	Applhereess
D	metals

7. Identify the class of fires on which each of the following types of fire extinguishers can be used:
   a. water: A
   b. halon: C
   c. dry chemical: ABC
   d. carbon dioxide: BC

8. Which types of fire extinguishers leave a dangerous residue?

   Class C

9. For what does the acronym *RACE* stand?
   R: Rescue
   A: Activate Alarm
   C: Contain fire
   E: Extinguish

10. List three (3) special precautions that must be observed when a patient is receiving oxygen.

    - No fires around - No firerisk
    - No sparky things

11. Identify three (3) basic principles that must be followed when any type of disaster occurs.

    - Extinguish - Rescue - Alarm

12. Health care workers are legally responsible for familiarizing themselves with disaster policies so appropriate action can be taken when a disaster strikes.

CHAPTER 15:1 UNDERSTANDING THE PRINCIPLES OF INFECTION CONTROL

ASSIGNMENT SHEET

Grade ______________________ Name ______________________

INTRODUCTION: This assignment will allow you to gain a basic knowledge of how disease is transmitted and the main ways to prevent it.

INSTRUCTIONS: Read the information on Understanding the Principles of Infection Control. In the space provided, print the word(s) that best completes the statement or answers the question.

1. Use the Key Terms to complete the crossword puzzle.

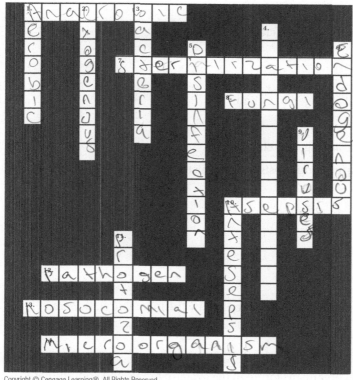

ACROSS

1. Organisms that live and reproduce in the absence of oxygen Anaerobic
7. Process that destroys all microorganisms, including spores and viruses Sterilization
8. Plant-like organisms that live on dead organic matter 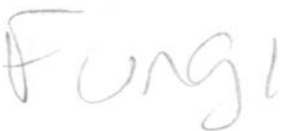

10. Absence of pathogens Asepis

12. Germ- or disease-producing microorganism pathogens

13. Infections acquired in a health care facility nosocomial

14. Small living plant or animal organism not visible to naked eye micro organism

DOWN

1. Organisms that require oxygen to live Aerobic
2. Disease that originates outside the body Exogenous
3. One-celled plant-like organisms that multiply rapidly bacteria
4. Factors that must be present for disease to occur [illegible]
5. Process that destroys or kills pathogens Disinfection
6. Disease that originates within the body Endogenous
9. Smallest microorganisms Viruses
10. Process that inhibits or prevents the growth of pathogenic organisms Antisepsis
11. One-celled animal organisms found in decayed materials and contaminated water Protozoa

---

2. How do nonpathogens differ from pathogens?

   Pathogens cause infection

3. Identify the following shapes of bacteria.
   a. rod shaped: streptococci
   b. comma shaped: Flagellated
   c. round or spherical arranged in a chain: Bacilli
   d. spiral or corkscrew: Spirochetes
   e. round or spherical arranged in clusters: staphylococci

4. Identify the following antibiotic-resistant organisms.
   a. MRSA: Methicillin-resistant staphylococcus aureus
   b. VRE: Vancomycin-resistant enterococcus
   c. MRAB: Multidrug-resistant acinetobacter baumannii
   d. CRE: Carbapenem-resistant enterobacteriaceae
   e. ESBL: Extended spectrum beta lactamese

5. Identify the class of microorganisms described by the following statements.
   a. smallest microorganisms: viruses
   b. parasitic microorganisms: Rickettsiae
   c. one-celled animal organisms found in decayed materials and contaminated water: Protozoa or ~~Bacteria~~
   d. plant-like organisms that live on dead organic matter: Fungi
   e. microorganisms that live on fleas, lice, ticks, and mites: Rickettsiae
   f. cause diseases such as gonorrhea and syphilis: Diplococci
   g. cause diseases such as measles and mumps: Viruses
   h. cause diseases such as ringworm and athlete's foot: Fungi

Name ______________________________

6. Identify the following viruses.
   a. mosquito-borne flavivirus: Ebola
   b. virus that causes avian or bird flu: H5N1
   c. variant of the coronavirus that can lead to respiratory failure and death: SARS
   d. virus affecting monkeys, other primates, and rodents: Monkeypox
   e. viruses that cause hemorrhagic fever: Filoviruses
   f. virus that causes AIDS: HIV
   g. virus that affects the liver and can lead to destruction and scarring of liver cells: Filoviruses
   h. virus that causes swine flu: H1N1
7. What does federal law require of employers in regard to the hepatitis B vaccine?
   Free shot
8. List three (3) things needed for microorganisms to grow and reproduce.
   host, darkness, wetness
9. Identify two (2) ways pathogenic organisms can cause infection and disease.
   Produce toxins, attach cells
10. What is the difference between an endogenous disease and an exogenous disease?
    endo - starts in body exo - outside body
11. Name three (3) common examples of nosocomial infections.
    Staphylococcus, pseudomonas, & enterococci
12. What do health care facilities do to prevent and deal with nosocomial infections?
    Give Antibiotics, keep things clean
13. Identify the part(s) of the chain of infection that has been eliminated by the following actions.
    a. thorough washing of the hands: infectious agent
    b. intact, unbroken skin: Reservoir
    c. healthy, well-rested individual: portal of exit
    d. cleaning and sterilizing a blood-covered instrument: Mode of transmission
    e. spraying to destroy mosquitoes: Portal of entry
    f. rapid, accurate identification of organisms: susceptible host
14. List four (4) common aseptic techniques.
    handwashing, good personal hygiene, gloves, clean instruments
15. Define the following.
    a. antisepsis: Prevent growth of pathogenic, not spores or viruses
    b. disinfection: kills pathogenic organisms
    c. sterilization: destroys all microorganisms

CHAPTER 15:3 WASHING HANDS

ASSIGNMENT SHEET

Grade ______________ Name Javen Lightfoot

INTRODUCTION: Handwashing is the most important method used to practice aseptic technique. This assignment will help you review the main facts.

INSTRUCTIONS: Read the information on Washing Hands. In the space provided, print the word(s) that best completes the statement or answers the question.

1. What is an aseptic technique?

   Washing hands

2. List two (2) reasons for washing the hands.

   kill germs ; keep from spreading harmful Bacteria

3. List six (6) times when the hands should be washed.

   - Before handling food - If your hands become contaminated
   - After using toilet - After touching a patient
   - After blowing nose - before TOUCHING a SICK PERSON.

4. Why is soap used as a cleansing agent?

   Because it kills 99.9% of germs

5. How should the fingertips be pointed while washing hands?

   Down

   Why?

   So germs dont drip down to your arm

6. What temperature water should be used?

   Warm

   Why?

   Hot hurts the skin.

7. Why are paper towels used while turning on and off the faucet?

   There could be germs on the faucet

8. List three (3) surfaces on the hands that must be cleaned.

   finger nails, Between fingers, forearm

Name ______________________________

9. Name two (2) items that can be used to clean the nails.

Orange stick, hand brush

10. Why are long or artificial fingernails prohibited in most health care facilities?

cant wear gloves

11. What type of handwashing is recommended by the Centers for Disease Control and Prevention (CDC) for each of the following situations?

   a. hands are not visibly dirty or are not soiled with blood or body fluids:

   b. caring for a patient on specific organism transmission-based precautions:

   c. routine cleansing when the hands are visibly dirty or soiled with blood or other body fluids:

   d. prior to invasive procedures:

Wash your hands for all these situations

12. What do most waterless hand cleaners contain?

Ultroucolet black lights

13. How long should the hands be rubbed with a waterless hand cleaner?

Awhile

14. How many times can you use a waterless hand cleaner before you need to use soap and water?

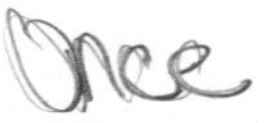

CHAPTER 15:4 OBSERVING STANDARD PRECAUTIONS

ASSIGNMENT SHEET

Grade ______________ Name Jaren Lightfoot

INTRODUCTION: Observing standard precautions is one way the chain of infection can be broken. This assignment will allow you to review the main principles of standard precautions.

INSTRUCTIONS: Read the information on Observing Standard Precautions. In the space provided, print the word(s) that best completes the statement or answers the question.

1. Name three (3) pathogens spread by blood and body fluids that are a major concern to health care workers.

   - HBV, HCV, HIV

2. What federal agency established standards for contamination with blood or body fluids that must be followed by all health care facilities?

   OSHA

3. Name four (4) types of personal protective equipment (PPE) that an employer must provide.

   Written control plan, free HBV vac-, handwashing facilities, provide PPE equipment

4. Can a health care worker drink coffee in a laboratory where blood tests are performed? Why or why not?

   No, not safe

5. What responsibilities does an employer have if an employee is splashed with blood when a tube containing blood breaks?

   To clean themselves

6. List the four (4) main requirements that employers must meet as a result of the Needlestick Safety and Prevention Act.

   - Use effective medical devices.
   - Incorporate changes to updates of control plan
   - Solicit input from nonmangerial employees
   - Sharps injury log

7. When must standard precautions be used?

   ~~Everyday~~
   At all times.

8. Describe four (4) situations when gloves must be worn.

contacting: Blood, body fluids, secretions, excretions

9. When must gowns be worn?

splashing or spraying of Blood

10. Describe three (3) examples of situations when masks, protective eyewear, or face shields must be worn.

Spray of blood, body fluids, secretions

11. When must masks be changed?

Every 30 min.

12. How must needles and syringes be handled after use?

bent or broken after use

13. During a blood test, some blood splashes on the laboratory counter. How must it be removed?

gloves on; disposable cleaning suplies

14. What is the purpose of mouthpieces or resuscitation devices?

to avoid mouth-to-mouth resuscitation

15. Where must you discard a dressing contaminated with blood and pus?

immediatly

16. What must you do if you stick yourself with a contaminated needle?

reported immediately

CHAPTER 15:8 USING STERILE TECHNIQUES

ASSIGNMENT SHEET

Grade ______________________ Name Jaren Lightfoot ______________________

INTRODUCTION: Following correct sterile technique is essential in many different procedures. This assignment will help stress the main facts.

INSTRUCTIONS: Read the information on Using Sterile Techniques. In the space provided, print the word(s) that best completes the statement or answers the question.

1. Define *sterile*.

   Clean

   Define *contaminated*.

   not clean

2. How can you avoid allowing sterile articles to touch the skin or clothing?

   by being careful

3. What part of a sterile field or tray is considered to be contaminated?

   if its been touched by an organism

4. List three (3) methods for removing sterile articles from wraps and placing them on a sterile field or tray. Briefly describe each method.

   assemble all equipment, wash hands, check date of sterility

5. Why must a sterile field be kept dry?

   water carrys bacteria

6. What should you do if you spill solution on a sterile field?

   Clean it

7. What part of sterile gloves is considered contaminated?

   None if its sterile

8. Before applying the sterile gloves, what must you make sure has been done in relation to the sterile tray?

   Washed hands

9. Once gloves have been applied, where should you hold your hands to avoid contamination?

   above waist

10. What should you do if you suspect an article is contaminated?

    Dont use it ; clean it

CHAPTER 16:1 MEASURING AND RECORDING VITAL SIGNS

ASSIGNMENT SHEET

Grade ______________________ Name Jasen Lightfoot

INTRODUCTION: Vital signs are important indicators of health states of the body. This assignment will help you review the main facts about vital signs.

INSTRUCTIONS: Read the information on Measuring and Recording Vital Signs. In the space provided, print the word(s) that best completes the statements or answers the questions.

1. Use the Key Terms to complete the crossword puzzle.

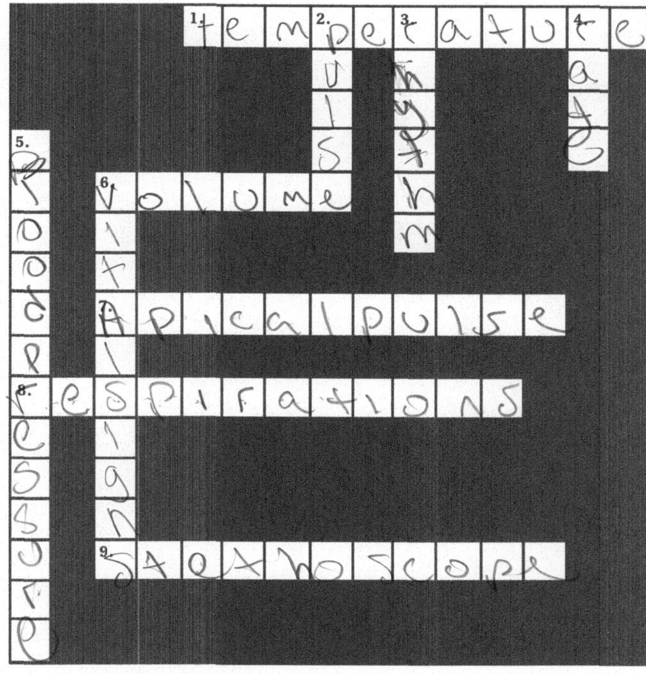

ACROSS

1. Measurement of the balance between heat lost and heat produced
6. Strength of the pulse
7. Pulse taken at the apex of the heart with a stethoscope
8. Measurement of breaths taken by a patient
9. Instrument used to take apical pulse

DOWN

2. Pressure of the blood felt against the wall of an artery
3. Regularity of the pulse or respirations Rythym
4. Number of beats per minute

5. Measurement of the force exerted by the heart against arterial walls
6. Various determinations that provide information about body conditions

---

2. List the five (5) vital signs.

temp., pulse, resporations, BP, and Pain.

3. Why is it essential that vital signs are measured accurately?

First indication of Disease

4. Identify four (4) common sites in the body where temperature can be measured.

Mouth, rectum, ear, Arm pit

5. Define *pulse*.

Pressure of Blood felt against artery

List three (3) factors recorded about a pulse.

Rate, rhythm, Volume

6. What three (3) factors are noted about respirations?

Count, rhythm, Character

7. Identify the two (2) readings noted on a blood pressure.

systolic & Diastolic

8. What is pain?

unpleasant sensation

9. How can you assess a patient's pain level?

1-10 scale

10. How often should pain be assessed? Why?

2 hours

11. List three (3) times when you may have to take an apical pulse.

illness, hardening of arteries and weak pulse

12. What should you do if you note any abnormality or change in any vital sign?

report to supervisor

Name ______________________

13. What should you do if you cannot obtain a correct reading for a vital sign?

Get someone else to check the patient

14. Convert the following Fahrenheit (F) temperatures to Celsius (C) temperatures. Use the formula: C = (F–32) × 5/9 or 0.5556.

For example: Fahrenheit (F) temperature is equal to 120°. What is Celsius temperature?

Subtract 32 from F: 120 – 32 = 88

Multiply the answer by 5/9 or 0.5556: 88 × 0.5556 = 48.8928 or 48.9

Celsius temperature is 48.9°.

Note: Round off answers to nearest tenth or one decimal point.

a. 140°F 60°
b. 70°F 21.1
c. 50°F 10°
d. 38°F 3.3°
e. 86°F 30°
f. 105°F 40.5°
g. 138°F 58.8°
h. 204°F 95.5°
i. 99.6°F 37.5°
j. 25°F -3.8°

15. Convert the following Celsius (C) temperatures to Fahrenheit (F) temperatures. Use the formula:

F = (C × 9/5 or 1.8) + 32

For example: Celsius (C) temperature is equal to 22°. What is Fahrenheit (F) temperature?

Multiply C by 9/5 or 1.8: 22 × 1.8 = 39.6

Add 32 to the answer: 39.6 + 32 = 71.6

Fahrenheit temperature is 71.6°.

Note: Round off answers to nearest tenth or one decimal point.

a. 32°C 89.6°
b. 54°C 129.2
c. 8°C 46.4°
d. 91°C 195.8
e. 0°C 32°
f. 72°C 161.6
g. 26°C 78.8°
h. 81°C 177.8°
i. 99.8°C 211.64°
j. 46.1°C 114.98°

CHAPTER 16:3 MEASURING AND RECORDING PULSE

ASSIGNMENT SHEET

Grade ______________________ Name Jaren Lightfoot

INTRODUCTION: One of the vital signs you will be required to record is pulse. This assignment sheet will assist you in learning the sites for taking pulse and the important aspects about pulse.

INSTRUCTIONS: Read the information about Measuring and Recording Pulse. In the space provided, print the word(s) that best completes the statement or answers the question.

1. Define *pulse.* Pressure of Blood against the wall artery in the heart.

2. (a) Study the outlined figure. As you identify each pulse site, enter the name beside the corresponding letter on the following list.

   A. temporal

   B. carotid

   C. Brachial

   D. Radial

   E. Femorall

   F. Popliteal

   G. Dorsalis Pedis

   H. Posterior tibial

   (b) Circle the site (on the sketch) that is used most frequently for taking pulse.

A.
B.
C.
D.
E.
F.
G.
H.

Copyright © Cengage Learning®. All Rights Reserved.

3. List three (3) factors that must be noted about each and every pulse.

   rate, rythm, and volume

4. What is the normal pulse range for each of the following?

   a. Adults: 60-100

   b. Children over 7 years old: 70-100

   c. Children from 1–7 years old: 80-110

   d. Infants: 100-160

5. List three (3) factors that could cause an increase in a pulse rate.

   drugs, exitment, fever

6. List three (3) factors that could cause a decrease in a pulse rate.

   sleep, coma, heart desease

7. In an adult, a pulse rate under 60 beats per minute is called Bradycardia. A pulse rate above 100 beats per minute is called tachycardia. An irregular or abnormal rhythm is a/an arrhythmia.

CHAPTER 16:7 MEASURING AND RECORDING BLOOD PRESSURE

ASSIGNMENT SHEET #1

Grade ______________________ Name Jaren Lightfoot

INTRODUCTION: The following assignment will help you review the main facts regarding blood pressure.

INSTRUCTIONS: Read the information about Measuring and Recording Blood Pressure. Then answer the following questions in the spaces provided.

1. Define *blood pressure.* The pressure of your blood circulating through your body

2. Define *systolic.* pressure occurs in the walls of the arteries when the left ventricle

3. Define *diastolic.* Pressure is the constant pressure in the walls of arteries

4. The average reading for systolic pressure is <120 with a range of 100-120.
5. The average reading for diastolic pressure is <80 with a range of 60-80.
6. What is the pulse pressure if the blood pressure is 136/72?

   64

7. What is *prehypertension*? Why is it important for health care professionals to recognize this condition in a patient?

   It means high BP will develope
   Prehypertension could develope

8. Hypertension is indicated when pressures are greater than 140 systolic and 90 diastolic.
9. List three (3) causes of hypotension.

   anxiety, stress, obesity, high salt intake

10. What is orthostatic, or postural, hypotension? What causes it?

    Low Blood Presure
    heart failure, dehydration, depression

Name ______________________________

11. List three (3) factors that can increase blood pressure.

-anxiety - Exercise
-stress

12. List three (3) factors that can decrease or lower blood pressure.

- lying down - Dehydration
- Old age

13. Why does the Occupational Health and Safety Administration (OSHA) discourage the use of mercury sphygmomanometers?

Poisons our body by contact

14. a. Record the following blood pressure readings correctly.

Systolic	128	Diastolic	92	— 128/92
Diastolic	84	Systolic	188	— 188/84
Systolic	136	Diastolic	76	— 136/76
Diastolic	118	Systolic	210	— 118/210

b. List the above readings that fall within normal range.

128/92 136/76

c. List the above readings that do not fall within normal range.

188/84 118/210

15. Why is it important to use the correct size cuff?

To get a correct reading

CHAPTER 17:1 PROVIDING FIRST AID

ASSIGNMENT SHEET

Grade ______________________ Name Jaren Lightfoot

INTRODUCTION: The following assignment will help you review the main facts on general guidelines for providing first aid.

INSTRUCTIONS: Study the information on Providing First Aid. In the space provided, print the word(s) that best answers the question or completes the statement.

1. Define *first aid*. emmidiate care given to prevent further enjurey until experts can take over

2. Using the correct first aid methods can mean the difference between life and death, or recovery versus permant disability

3. The type of first aid treatment you provide will vary depending on several factors. List three (3) factors that may affect any action taken.
   - No breathing - Poisoning
   - Blood loss

4. Identify three (3) senses that can alert you to an emergency.
   Screaming, Screaching car tires, fire

5. What action should you take if you notice that it is not safe to approach the scene of an accident?
   Call 911

6. What is the first thing you should determine when you get to the victim?
   If theyre consious

7. Why is it important to avoid moving a victim whenever possible?
   spinal injuries

8. List five (5) kinds of information that should be reported when calling emergency medical services (EMS).
   situation, actions taken, exact locations, telephone #, and condition of victim

9. What should you do if a person refuses to give consent for care?

Dont Give Care ; call EMS

10. What is triage? Priortizing Treatment

11. Identify six (6) life-threatening emergencies that must be cared for first.

- No Breathing - Vomiting
- No pulse - Poisoning
- Present pain - Shock

12. List four (4) sources of information you can use to find out the details regarding an accident, injury, or illness.

Victim, persons present, examination of Items

13. How can you reassure the victim?

Act calm & confident

14. Why shouldn't you discuss the victim's condition with observers at the scene?

Victims confidentiality

15. While providing first aid to the victim, make every attempt to avoid further injury. Provide only the treatment you are able to provide.

CHAPTER 21:2 Positioning a Patient

ASSIGNMENT SHEET

Grade ____________________ Name Jaren Lightfoot

INTRODUCTION: To position patients correctly for various procedures, you must know the different positions and their uses. This assignment will help you review the facts.

INSTRUCTIONS: Review the information on Positioning a Patient. Place the letter of the position in Column B next to the numbered item in Column A that applies to the position. Letters may be used once, more than once, or not at all.

Column A

C B ____ 1. Used to examine the breasts and abdomen
H ____ 2. Used for enemas and rectal temperatures
E H ____ 3. Used for sigmoidoscopic examinations
H D ____ 4. Used for rectal surgery
B ____ 5. Used for breathing problems
B ____ 6. Head elevated at 25, 45, or 90-degree angles
G ____ 7. Patient lying flat on abdomen
H ____ 8. Patient lying on left side
A F ____ 9. Used for Pap tests and vaginal examinations
A F ____ 10. Used for pelvic surgery
I ____ 11. Used for circulatory shock
G ____ 12. Used to examine the back and spine
C ____ 13. Also called the supine position
C ____ 14. Patient lying flat on back
B ____ 15. Used to encourage drainage
A F ____ 16. Feet elevated in stirrups
H ____ 17. Also called the left lateral position
E ____ 18. Patient rests body weight on knees and chest
E H ____ 19. Used for rectal examinations and treatments
C ____ 20. Used to examine the chest

Column B

A. Dorsal recumbent
B. Fowler's
C. Horizontal recumbent
D. Jackknife
E. Knee-chest
F. Lithotomy
G. Prone
H. Sims'
I. Trendelenburg

21. How can you learn how to operate an examination table before positioning a patient?

Read manual

22. List two (2) ways to avoid exposing a patient during an examination or a procedure.

- Make sure they tie their gown
- Put them in the correct positions

CHAPTER 22:15 ADMINISTERING OXYGEN

ASSIGNMENT SHEET

Grade ______________________ Name Jasen Lightfoot

INTRODUCTION: The following assignment will help you learn the main points of oxygen administration.

DIRECTIONS: Review the information on Administering Oxygen. In the space provided, print the word(s) that best completes the statement or answers the question.

1. Why is it important to check your legal responsibilities before administering oxygen?

   because its just like administering medication

2. Define *hypoxia.* Oxygen deficiency

3. List three (3) signs of oxygen shortage. - rapid & shallow respirations
   - rapid pulse
   - restlessness

4. List the three (3) main methods of administering oxygen. Then list the usual flow rate for each method.

Method	*Flow Rate*
- Mask	- 5 L/m
- cannula	- 2-6 L/m
- tent	- 10-12 L/m

5. What is an oxygen concentrator? What does it do?

   A machine that removes impurities and other gases from room air to concentrate oxygen in the unit.

6. Why is oxygen usually passed through water before being administered to a patient?

   to moisten it

7. List four (4) safety rules that must be observed when oxygen is in use.

   - No burning, sparking, or smoking
   - Dont use electrical equipment
   - patients must be cautioned against smoking
   - flammable liquids

8. What does a pulse oximeter measure?

   Oxygen in Arterial blood

9. A patient who is receiving oxygen must be checked frequently. List three (3) special checkpoints that must be observed.

   humidifiers must be washed every 24hrs

10. Who is usually responsible for oxygen administration in health care facilities?

    Physicians

CHAPTER 23:1 Performing Range-of-Motion (ROM) Exercises

ASSIGNMENT SHEET

Grade ______________________ Name Jaren Lightfoot

INTRODUCTION: Range-of-motion (ROM) exercises help keep muscles and joints functioning. This assignment will help you review the information on ROMs.

INSTRUCTIONS: Read the information on Performing Range-of-Motion (ROM) Exercises. In the space provided, print the word(s) that best completes the statement or answers the question.

A: Short Answer

1. Why are range-of-motion (ROM) exercises done? to maintain healt and musculoskeletal system

2. Who performs ROM exercises? physical therapist, nurse, health care assistant

3. Identify six (6) problems caused by lack of movement and inactivity.

   - lack of appetite - respiratory problems
   - constipation - hypostatic pneumonia
   - urinary infections - mineral loss

4. Briefly describe each of the following types of range-of-motion exercises and identify who does each type.
   a. active: strengthens muscle; patient are able to move without assis
   b. active assistive: strengthens muscle, joint function; can move but is assis
   c. passive: joint function, Another person moves each joint
   d. resistive: increased strength + endurance; therapist

5. In some states or health care facilities, only PTs and RNs may perform range-of-motion exercises to the head and neck. Some exercises may be restricted, or limited, after knee or hip replacement surgery.

6. Where should support be provided when ROMs are being performed?
   At the joint being moved

7. How many times should each movement be performed?
   - 5-15 times
   - at least.

8. What should you do if a patient complains of pain during ROMs?

Stop; report to supervisor

9. Identify two (2) ways to provide privacy for the patient while providing ROMs.

Close door & shut curtains

B. Matching: Place the letter of the term in Column B next to the numbered item in Column A that defines the term. Letters may be used once, more than once, or not at all.

	Column A	Column B
___	1. Bending a body part	A. Abduction
___	2. Turning a body part downward	B. Adduction
___	3. Moving toward thumb side of hand	C. Circumduction
___	4. Turning a body part outward	D. Dorsiflexion
___	5. Moving a part toward the midline	E. Eversion
___	6. Swinging the arm in a circle	F. Extension
___	7. Excessive straightening of a body part	G. Flexion
___	8. Moving the lower arm away from upper arm	H. Hyperextension
___	9. Moving toward little finger side of hand	I. Inversion
___	10. Turning palm up	J. Opposition
___	11. Turning a body part inward	K. Plantar flexion
___	12. Straightening the foot away from the knee	L. Pronation
___	13. Moving the arm out to the side	M. Radial deviation
___	14. Turning the head from side to side	N. Rotation
___	15. Moving a part away from the midline	O. Supination
___	16. Bending the fingers to make a fist	P. Ulnar deviation
___	17. Straightening a body part	
___	18. Bending top of hand back toward the forearm	
___	19. Bending the foot toward the knee	
___	20. Touching each of the fingers with the tip of the thumb	

CHAPTER 23:2 AMBULATING PATIENTS WHO USE TRANSFER (GAIT) BELTS, CRUTCHES, CANES, OR WALKERS

ASSIGNMENT SHEET

Grade ______________________ Name Joren Lightfoot

INTRODUCTION: This assignment will help you review the main facts on ambulation aids.

INSTRUCTIONS: Review the information on Ambulating Patients Who Use Transfer (Gait) Belts, Crutches, Canes, or Walkers. In the space provided, print the word(s) that best completes the statement or answers the question.

1. What type of grasp should be used with a transfer belt? Why?

   fingers under belt

2. Identify the following types of crutches.

   a. crutches that are used for short periods of time and require that the patient bear weight on the hand bars instead of the axillary supports:

      Axillery

   b. crutches that require the patient to flex the elbows at a right angle so he or she can bear weight on the forearm:

      Forearm

   c. crutches for patients who cannot grip handles or bear weight on the wrist or hands:

      Platform

3. When a patient is being fitted for crutches, the following measurement points should be noted:
   Height of heels on shoes: wrists

   Position of crutches: 4-6" inches in front of, and 2-4" inches to the side of, the patient's foot.

   Distance between axilla and axillary bar: 2 in

   Degree angle for elbows: 25°-30°

4. If a patient can bear weight on both legs, the four point gait gait is usually taught first. When the patient has mastered this gait, the two point gait is taught next. After the patient gains strength in the arms and shoulders, faster gaits such as the swing through or ______ are taught.

5. If a patient can bear weight on only one leg, the first crutch gait taught is the three point. When the patient gains strength in the arms and shoulders, faster gaits such as the swing through and two point are taught.

Name ____________________

6. Why is it important to avoid putting pressure on the axillary area when fitting a patient for crutches?

to get the right measurment

7. Canes should generally be used on the good side.
8. The bottom tip of a cane should be positioned approximately 6 to 8 inches from the side of the unaffected foot. The cane handle should be level with femur. The elbow should be flexed at a/an 25-30 degree angle while cane is being used.
9. Why are walkers with wheels dangerous?

Could slip & fall

10. What major criteria is used to determine whether a patient should use a walker?

if both feet are okay

11. Handles on a walker should be level with the top femur. The elbows should be flexed at a/an 25-30 degree angle.
12. Why are the legs of the walker fitted with rubber tips?

No slip

13. Why is it important to caution a patient against sliding a walker?

to not slip

14. You are walking a patient with a transfer belt. The patient starts to fall forward. What should you do?

use your body to catch and cutien them to the ground. Call for help and report insident.

